Contents

List of Canadian Research Boxes

1.1 Gleason, M. (2002). Race, class, and health: School medical inspection and "healthy" children in British 'Columbia, 1890–1930. *Canadian Bulletin of Medical History/Bulletin Canadien d'histoire de la médecine, 19*(1), 95–112.

1.2 McPherson, K. (2003). Nursing and colonization: The work of Indian Health Service nurses in Manitoba, 1945–1970. In G. Feldberg, M. Ladd-Taylor, A. Li, & K. McPherson (Eds.), *Women, health, and nation: Canada and the United States since 1945* (pp. 222–246). Montreal & Kingston: McGill–Queen's University Press.

2.1 Underwood, J. M., et al. (2009b). Building community and public health nursing capacity: A synthesis report of the National Community Health Nursing Study. *Canadian Journal of Public Health, 100*(5), I1–I11.

2.2 Ganann, R., Underwood, J., Matthews, S., Goodyear, R., Stamler, L. L., Meagher-Stewart, D., & Munroe, V. (2010). Leadership attributes: A key to optimal utilization of the community health nursing workforce. *Canadian Journal of Nursing Leadership, 23*(2), 60–71.

3.1 Aston, M., Meagher-Stewart, D., Edwards, N., & Young, L. M. (2009). Public health nurses' primary health care practice: Strategies for fostering citizen participation. *Journal of Community Health Nursing, 26*(1), 24–34.

3.2 Underwood, J., Baumann, A., Akhtar-Danesh, N., MacDonald-Rencz, & Matthews, S. (2009, March). *National community health nursing study: Comparison of enablers and barriers for nurses working in the community.* (No. 14). Hamilton, ON: McMaster University School of Nursing and the Nursing Health Services Research Unit.

4.1 Cohen, B. E., & Gregory, D. (2009). Community health clinical education in Canada: Part II—Developing competencies to address social justice, equity, and the social determinants of health. *International Journal of Nursing Education Scholarship, 6*(1), 1–15.

4.2 Browne, A. J., Hartrick Doane, G., Reimer, J., MacLeod, M. L. P., & McLellan, E. (2010). Public health nursing practice with "high priority" families:

The significance of contextualizing risk. *Nursing Inquiry, 17*(1), 27–38.

5.1 Bottoroff, J. L., Johnson, J. L., Carey, J., Hutchinson, P., Sullivan, D., Mowatt, R., & Wardman, D. (2010). A family affair: Aboriginal women's efforts to limit second-hand smoke exposure at home. *Canadian Journal of Public Health, 101*, 32–35.

5.2 Reid, J. L., Hammond, D., & Driezen, P. (2010). Socio-economic status and smoking in Canada, 1999–2006: Has there been any progress on disparities in tobacco use? *Canadian Journal of Public Health, 101*, 73–78.

6.1 Veuglers, P., Sithole, F., Zhang, S., & Muhajarine, N. (2008). Neighborhood characteristics in relation to diet, physical activity and overweight of Canadian children. *International Journal of Pediatric Obesity, 3*, 152–159.

6.2 Bottorff, J., Carey, J., Mowatt, R., Varcoe, C., Johnson, J., Hutchinson, P., . . . Wardman, D. (2009). Bingo halls and smoking: Perspectives of First Nations women. *Health and Place.* doi:10.1016/j.health place.2009.04.005

7.1 Smith, D., Edwards, N., Martens, P. J., Varcoe, C., & Davies, B. (2008). The influence of governance on organizations' experiences of improving care for Aboriginal people: Decolonizing possibilities. *Pimatisiwin: A Journal of Aboriginal and Indigenous Community Health, 6*(1), 1–30.

7.2 Edwards, N., & Roelofs, S. *Strengthening nurses' capacity in HIV policy development in Sub-Saharan Africa and the Caribbean* (Year 3 Progress Report, February 1, 2009–January 31, 2010). Ottawa, ON: University of Ottawa.

8.1 Maddalena, V. J., Bernard, W. T., Etowa, J., Murdoch, S. D., Smith, D., & Jarvis, P. M. (2010). Cancer care experiences and use of complementary and alternative medicine at end of life in Nova Scotia's Black communities. *Journal of Transcultural Nursing, 21*(2), 114–122. doi:10.1177/1043659609357634

8.2 Koskinen, L., Campbell, B., Aarts, C., Chassé, F., Hemingway, A., Juhansoo, T., & Nordstrom, P. M. (2009). Enhancing cultural competence: Trans-Atlantic experiences of European and Canadian nursing students. *International Journal of Nursing*

Preface

We would like to begin by thanking both students and faculty who welcomed the first two editions and provided excellent and insightful feedback for this third edition. This book has been useful not only at multiple levels within a basic or post-RN curriculum, but also in preparation for the Canadian Nurses Association certification examination in community health. To know that the first editions were informative and easy to read and had challenged their thinking made developing this new edition even more meaningful.

In the preface to the first edition we posed the question, "Why should we choose to write a community health nursing book from a Canadian perspective?" The response to the first and second editions has solidified our beliefs. We believe that there are historical, political, legislative, cultural, and social influences that are unique to Canadians. They have shaped the evolution of Canada as a society, our definitions of health, and our expectations relative to healthcare delivery. Community health nurses are both a product of those influences and an influence themselves. Community health nursing has evolved differently in Canada than in other countries. We believe that new practitioners in community health nursing must understand these influences to continue to practise in and shape community health nursing.

OUR APPROACH

Over time there has been much discourse on community health nursing versus public health nursing versus community-based nursing. A cadre of authors have offered different definitions that attempt to discriminate among these terms. They base their conclusions on factors such as who is the client, what is the setting, what is the educational preparation of the nurse, and who is the employer. Historically, "community health nursing" was used to describe all nursing outside the hospital setting. In this book, community health nursing is defined as a specialty in nursing that encompasses a number of sub-specialties, such as public health nursing and home health nursing. The client may be an individual, group, community, or population, but care is rendered with an eye to the health of the population. The setting may be a home, institution, community, or agency serving the population. The common academic preparation is the basic education leading to the designation Registered Nurse; however, it is clear that additional educational preparation is frequently required, especially if the basic preparation is not a baccalaureate degree. The employer may be an individual, family, community, government, or non-governmental agency. Whether the chapter authors are addressing a specific health issue or a specific population or aggregate, all are speaking about a segment within the larger whole of community health nursing.

It is our belief that community health nursing functions within a multiplicity of theories and understandings. Some theories are common to all facets of the nursing profession, such as ethical treatment of clients, family assessment, or the meaning of health. In some cases, nursing drove the development of the theory; in others, we have used the work of theorists in other disciplines. This text reflects that multiplicity, and the authors have described how the theories relate to community health nursing.

Community Health Nursing: A Canadian Perspective, Third Edition, has been written with the undergraduate student in mind. We continue to hear that faculty and students are looking for a concise text that will provide an overview of community health nursing. We have made every effort to provide as broad and comprehensive an overview of this field as possible. Each topic is written with the understanding that this will be the student's first foray into the community nursing spectrum. We have chosen to incorporate individual, family, and community as client perspectives throughout the text.

NEW TO THE THIRD EDITION

The new edition brings many changes. As is appropriate to the pace of change in community health and community health nursing, you will notice that the chapters have been extensively updated, with new content, statistics, and Canadian research. Further, the focus is more on the health of the aggregate or population, rather than on the specific clients. We have added four new chapters to this edition:

- Chapter 15: Maternal and Child Health
- Chapter 18: Gender and Community Health
- Chapter 19: Older Adult Health
- Chapter 31: Global Health

Several other chapters have changed in terms of direction. These include Chapter 2: Financing, Policy, and Politics of Healthcare Delivery, where leadership has been added to the discourse on financing, policy, and politics. Chapter 24: Environmental and Occupational Health has been expanded to focus on occupational health in the context of environmental health. Chapter 30: Emergency Preparedness and Disaster Nursing has expanded the role of the Public Health Agency of Canada and included the new Ontario Public Health Standards (OPHS).

Canadian Research Boxes and Case Studies throughout the text have been thoroughly updated. We also have new contributors, who offer a fresh perspective and insights to various chapters.

We have continued to build on the features of the third edition, with the addition of multiple-choice Review Questions at the end of each chapter. These critical thinking and application questions intend to assist students to prepare for the Canadian Registered Nurse Examination (CRNE). Additional readings, websites, and videos are also listed to enrich the chapter contents. New to this addition, **MyNursingLab** gives students the opportunity to test themselves on key concepts and skills. Students can track their own progress through the course and use a personalized study plan to achieve success. Both teachers and students will find additional resources and background information related to the relevant chapters on MyNursingLab.

ABOUT THE CONTRIBUTORS

This third edition brings new and former authors to the book. As before, some hold academic positions, some are in management or policy positions, and others are front-line practitioners. All came with a commitment to contribute to a Canadian community health nursing text, and this further demonstrates the cyclical nature of theory and practice. Each brought expertise and knowledge to a particular chapter and topic. Each has presented the various historical, geographical, and theoretical perspectives that assist in explaining and describing community nursing practice. All have made a meaningful contribution to introducing nursing students to this specialty. You will find a list of the contributors, their affiliations, and the chapters they authored following the preface. To provide context on the varied experience and expertise of our contributors, we have also provided a short biographical sketch for each contributor immediately following the chapter(s) they wrote.

CHAPTER ORGANIZATION

The chapters in *Community Health Nursing: A Canadian Perspective* are organized into five parts:

- Part I: The Context of Community Health Nursing in Canada
- Part II: Foundations and Tools for Community Health Nursing Practice
- Part III: Nursing Care of Community Aggregates
- Part IV: Selected Community Problems
- Part V: Looking Ahead

Part I: The Context of Community Health Nursing in Canada introduces students to the general topic area. **Chapter 1: The History of Community Health Nursing in Canada** presents an historical perspective on Canadian community health nursing so that students may be enlightened by lessons from the past. **Chapter 2: Financing, Policy, and Politics of Healthcare Delivery** presents the administration of community health from legislative, cultural, and political perspectives. In this edition the importance of strong leadership to assist in meeting healthcare delivery challenges has been highlighted. This chapter is followed by an Appendix, which outlines healthcare delivery to Aboriginal populations. **Chapter 3: Nursing Roles, Functions, and Practice Settings** presents a discussion of the variety of settings, competencies, roles, and functions germane to community health nursing, such as public health nursing and home health nursing. The authors of **Chapter 4: Advocacy, Ethical, and Legal Considerations** have used the Canadian Community Health Nursing Standards of Practice (found in Appendix A) to frame a discussion on legal and ethical issues for CHNs. These chapters form the underpinning for the subsequent sections.

Part II: Foundations and Tools for Community Health Nursing Practice builds the base upon which the sub-specialties rest. It begins in **Chapter 5: Concepts of Health** with a discourse on health from a variety of perspectives. Health promotion is examined from a variety of theoretical frameworks in **Chapter 6: Population Health Promotion Models and Strategies**, demonstrating how the philosophy and framework can influence the decisions about interventions. **Chapter 7: Primary Health Care** provides an examination of the principles of primary health care and the CHN's role regarding social justice and its relationship to health inequities. **Chapter 8: Cultural Diversity** adds current critiques of transcultural nursing and includes Community Health Nurses Association of Canada's Public Health Nursing category of Diversity and Inclusiveness, as well as providing explicit discussion of cultural safety, cultural competencies, intersections, and diversity. **Chapter 9: Epidemiology** describes the science of epidemiology and how it can inform community health nurses' practice. Guided information on finding, using, and participating in community health nursing research is the focus of **Chapter 10: Research**. In **Chapter 11: Information Technology** you will find a discussion of information technology and how it contributes to community nursing practice. **Chapter 12: Communicable Diseases** describes concepts related to communicable disease and discusses the role of CHNs in communicable disease control and management in relation to the legislative mandate locally, provincially/territorially, and federally. **Chapter 13: Community Care** provides an overview of the community health nursing process, including community assessment, selected community health practice models, population health promotion, community development, and community participatory tools. It provides a new section on Population, Intervention, Setting, and Outcome (PISO) statement formulation to reinforce the need to formulate evidence-based questions in community assessment. This section continues with **Chapter 14: Community Health Planning, Monitoring, and Evaluation**, where the authors examine specifics around planning, monitoring, and evaluating community health programs, with additional information on the logic model and Gantt charts. We believe the topics in Parts I and II are essential for an understanding of community health nursing.

Parts III and IV, composed of focus chapters, examine groups and issues that make the picture of community health nursing more complete. In **Part III**, the spotlight is on **Nursing Care of Community Aggregates**, which has been deliberately focused on health rather than challenges. **Chapter 15: Maternal and Child Health** examines population health promotion approaches with socio-environmental perspectives on enhancing maternal and child health. **Chapter 16: Family Health** provides an overview of the social and cultural context of the family in family care. It has a new section on family visits related to the CCHN standard of Building Relationships and Facilitating Access and Equity. **Chapter 17: School Health** has updated information on the comprehensive school health programs and the common health concerns in school settings. **Chapter 18: Gender and Community Health** focuses on applying a gender lens to community health nursing practice. **Chapter 19: Older Adult Health** highlights the aging population in Canada and expands on factors related to the assessment, maintenance, and promotion of the health of older adults. **Chapter 20: Gay, Lesbian, Bisexual, and Transgender Clients** describes the factors in Canadian society that contribute to ill health in gay, lesbian, bisexual, and transgender individuals, and identifies strategies that community health nurses can use to mitigate these influences. **Chapter 21: Mental Health** discusses challenges facing persons with mental illness, available services, and strategies to promote mental health within Canadian society. It now has more emphasis on mental health in Aboriginal individuals. **Chapter 22: Aboriginal Health** examines the historical and current influences on the health of Aboriginal populations in Canada. First Nations healthcare, including cultural issues for CHNs in Aboriginal communities, are discussed. **Chapter 23: Rural Health** looks at the large portion of Canada's population that lives in rural settings. It examines the diversity of this aggregate, as well as the realities of CHN practice in rural communities. **Chapter 24: Environmental and Occupational Health** replaces the occupational health chapter. The discussion has been expanded to include the environmental burden of disease, as well as the nurse's role in assessment and prevention. **Chapter 25: Correctional Health** looks at nursing within a controlled environment. The divergent concepts of custody and caring are examined within the current Canadian context.

In contrast, **Part IV** focuses on **Selected Community Problems** that may apply to a variety of populations. Each chapter focuses on one of five specific issues. **Chapter 26: Violence in Societies** describes how theoretical frameworks help CHNs identify violence in individuals' lives, families, groups, communities, and societies; raise critical awareness of the health impacts of violence; and guide prevention, health promoting, and empowering strategies to eliminate violence in society. **Chapter 27: Poverty and Homelessness** examines these phenomena within Canadian society and uses the framework of Determinants of Health to illustrate how both poverty and homelessness contribute to difficulty in achieving and maintaining health. **Chapter 28: Substance Use** looks at licit as well as illicit drug use in Canada. Both the harmful consequences of substance use and health promotion activities are presented. **Chapter 29: Sexually Transmitted Infections and Blood Borne Pathogens** presents the variety of types of infections, as well as how public policy in Canada has been developed around these illnesses. Prevention campaigns are a highlight of this chapter. **Chapter 30: Emergency Preparedness and Disaster Nursing** provides an overview of the role of CHNs in community emergency preparedness planning and in disaster situations. It highlights different types of disasters and how the Incident Management System (IMS) functions as a comprehensive model to manage major incidents. In these chapters, the authors have explored the issue first and then identified the populations most affected.

The final section, **Part V: Looking Ahead**, contains another new chapter, **Chapter 31: Global Health**. This chapter provides an overview of global health and selected global health issues that impact communities as well as the nursing profession. The text concludes with a brief look at where the field of community health nursing is headed and the coming opportunities and challenges in **Chapter 32: Challenges and Future Directions**.

As you read through the book, you will notice that some concepts and items are mentioned in several of the chapters. This is because they are often seminal documents or definitions that may be viewed through the lenses of the various topics and authors. For instance, many of the chapters will talk about the Lalonde Report, the Epp Report, or the *Declaration of Alma Ata*. You will note that each author views the reports differently, depending on the chapter topic. For example, proponents of health promotion may view some of the reports from one perspective, while the author of the chapter on primary health care may discuss a slightly different perceived influence of the same report. Similarly, cross-cultural nursing is mentioned in the family health and the cultural diversity chapters but may also be mentioned in the Aboriginal health chapter and the violence in societies chapter. We anticipate that students and teachers will see this not as redundancy, but rather as an example of multiple perspectives and how and why a multiplicity of theory and practice exists in community health nursing.

A Note on Appendices

In this edition, the core competencies for public health are now found in MyNursingLab. These were developed with broad national consultation, and led to the creation of the discipline-specific competencies that are included in the text. As in previous editions, we include the Canadian Community Health Nursing Standards of Practice. Revised and re-released in 2008, this document explicitly reflects the current practice standards for Canadian community health nurses. In our appendix, we have included the Canadian Community Health Nursing Practice Model, along with a complete outline and description of the standards. In several chapters, contributors have made reference to the standards to enhance the discussion.

Appendices B and C are the discipline-specific competencies. Appendix B is the Public Health Nursing Discipline Specific Competencies published by the Community Health Nurses of Canada in 2009. They were developed using several source documents and a Delphi process to arrive at consensus. Appendix C includes the Home Health Nursing Competencies. They were developed by the Community Health Nurses of Canada (CHNC) in partnership with the CHNC Certification, Standards and Competencies Committee and Advisory Group.

Chapter Features

A special effort has been made with this book to incorporate features that will facilitate learning and enhance an understanding of community health nursing in Canada.

- **Chapter Objectives** outline the salient points of the chapter and clarify the skills and knowledge to be learned in that chapter.

- **Canadian Research Boxes** present specific studies from the literature or the authors' knowledge to illustrate or augment the material covered in the chapter. Either the researchers themselves are nurses, or we have chosen health research that community health nurses can use in their practice. Each Research Box is followed by a few Discussion Questions to assist students in using the results.

CANADIAN RESEARCH BOX

Can the Internet be used as a health promotion marketing tool?

Gosselin, P., & Poitras, P. (2008). Use of an Internet "viral" marketing software platform in health promotion. *Journal of Medical Internet Research, 10*, e47.

An online health promotion game named the "The Crazy Race" was promoted through the use of viral marketing with the aim of increasing traffic to a Canadian government health promotion website (Canadian Health Network). Viral marketing relies on person-to-person electronic communications about a topic, which are self-generating—an electronic version of "word-of-mouth"

- **Case Studies** illustrate a practice application of the information presented in the chapter, followed by Discussion Questions.

CASE STUDY: Testing Website Accessibility

Identify your favourite health information website or your current clinical placement agency website. Once you have located the website, highlight and copy the URL (Universal Resource Locator—a unique identifier that provides an address for an Internet site). Then proceed to an accessibility checker website. W3C has listed many website accessibility checkers (http://www.w3.org/WAI/

- **Key Terms** are boldfaced where they are introduced in the body of the text. For convenience, the key terms are listed at the end of each chapter in the order in which they appear.

- **Review Questions** test students' knowledge using a format similar to the Canadian Registered Nurse Examination that all basic students must pass to become a Registered Nurse in Canada. Using this format will help students to prepare for this examination. Answers to these questions are included at the end of the book.

- **Study Questions** test students' knowledge of the facts and concepts in the chapter. Answers to the study questions are included at the end of the book.

STUDY QUESTIONS

1. Identify different ways that the "digital divide" has been conceptualized since the term first appeared.
2. Describe three tools that can be used to enhance Internet accessibility for disabled populations.
3. What is HON code and what is its purpose?
4. Describe three online health promotion interventions that show promise.
5. Where can community health nurses get access to evidence-based information on the Web to guide their decision making in practice?

- **Individual** and **Group Critical Thinking Exercises** challenge students to reflect on the content of the chapter and apply it in different situations.

INDIVIDUAL CRITICAL THINKING EXERCISES

1. What criteria would you use to evaluate a health promotion intervention, such as a smoking-cessation website?
2. What would you need to consider when working as a community health nurse with a client who is visually impaired and wants to use the Internet?
3. Discuss the merits and drawbacks of the HON code. Review the editorial and the response to it found in the *Journal of Medical Internet Research* by Eysenbach (2000).

- **References** cited in the chapter are presented in APA format.
- **Additional Resources** direct students to further information on the chapter topic. These include references to books, journal articles, and websites. Students will also find references to specific government and nongovernmental agencies relevant to the chapter topics.

TEACHING SUPPORT

The following supplements are designed to aid instructors in presenting classes, fostering classroom discussion, and encouraging learning.

- **Instructor's Resource Manual** Each chapter begins with an overview, a list of learning objectives from the text, and an outline. This is followed by suggestions for classroom activities and discussion points for the Individual and Group Critical Thinking Exercises found at the end of each chapter, as well as the discussion questions found in the Case Studies and Canadian Research Boxes throughout the text. The lecture suggestions, classroom activities, and out-of-class assignments tied to each of the five parts in the text have been updated to reflect changes made to the third edition. The Instructor's Resource Manual with Solutions is available for download from Pearson Education Canada's online catalogue at **http://vig.pearsoned.ca** and on the Instructor's Resource CD-ROM that accompanies this textbook.

- **TestGen Testbank** This computerized testbank has been extensively revised for the new edition. This computerized testbank contains CRNE-style multiple-choice questions. Some of the questions are presented within cases, in which a brief description of a case is followed by a group of three to five questions. The remainder of the testbank consists of single, independent questions that are unrelated to a case or to other questions on the exam. Rationales for the correct and incorrect options for each multiple-choice item are provided. Each question has been checked for accuracy and is available in the latest version of TestGen software. This software package allows instructors to custom design, save, and generate classroom tests. The test program permits instructors to edit, add, or delete questions from the test bank; edit existing graphics and create new ones; analyze test results; and organize a database of tests and student results. This software allows for greater flexibility and ease of use. It provides many options for organizing and displaying tests, along with search and sort features. This TestGen testbank is available for download from Pearson Education Canada's online catalogue at **http://vig.pearsoned.ca** and on the Instructor's Resource CD-ROM that accompanies this textbook.

- The testbank is also available in **MyTest** format. **MyTest** from Pearson Education Canada is a powerful assessment generation program that helps instructors easily create and print quizzes, tests, and exams, as well as homework or practice handouts. Questions and tests can all be authored online, allowing instructors ultimate flexibility and the ability to efficiently manage assessments at any time, from anywhere. These questions are also available in Microsoft Word format on the Instructor's Resource CD-ROM.

- **PowerPoint® Presentations.** A variety of PowerPoint® slides accompany each chapter of the textbook.

- **Image Library (on IRCD only).** The Image Library provides access to many of the images, figures, and tables in the textbook.

- The Instructor's Resource Manual, the TestGen testbank, the Test Item File in Word format, the PowerPoint® Presentations, and the Image Library are provided in electronic format on the **Instructor's Resources CD-ROM** (ISBN: 978-0-13-262794-8).

- **CourseSmart** goes beyond traditional expectations, providing instant, online access to the textbooks and course materials you need at a lower cost for students. And even as students save money, you can save time and hassle with a digital eTextbook that allows you to search for the most relevant content at the very moment you need it. Whether it's evaluating textbooks or creating lecture notes to help students with difficult concepts, CourseSmart can make life a little easier. See how when you visit **www.coursesmart.com/instructors.**

- **Technology Specialists** Pearson's Technology Specialists work with faculty and campus course designers to ensure that Pearson technology products, assessment tools, and online course materials are tailored to meet your specific needs. This highly qualified team is dedicated to helping schools take full advantage of a wide range of educational resources, by assisting in the integration of a variety of instructional materials and media formats. Your local Pearson Education sales representative can provide you with more details on this service program.

NEW mynursinglab

Each MyNursingLab course matches the organization of the accompanying textbook. Preloaded content for every chapter of the accompanying textbook allows instructors to use MyNursingLab as is or to customize MyNursingLab with their own materials. Some features for instructors include:

- MyTest
- Instructor's Manual
- PowerPoints
- Image Library

FEATURES FOR STUDENTS

- **Pearson eText** gives students access to the text whenever and wherever they have access to the Internet. eText pages look exactly like the printed text, offering powerful new functionality for students and instructors. Users can create notes, highlight text in different colours, create bookmarks, zoom, click hyperlinked words and phrases to view definitions, and view in single-page or two-page view. Pearson eText allows for quick navigation to key parts of the eText using a table of contents and provides full-text search. The eText may also offer links to associated media files, enabling users to access videos, animations, or other activities as they read the text.

- **Customized Study Plan**—based upon the results of the Chapter Pre-Test, students receive a plan to help them remediate important concepts and applications where they need improvement. Some of the tools the study plan provides include:
  - **E-book pages from the student textbook**
  - **PowerPoint presentations of key concepts**
  - **Videos and Real-Life Stories**
  - **Glossary flashcards**
- **Assessment tools** including
  - Test Your Terminology
  - CRNE-style Review Questions
  - Case Studies
- **Additional resources** including
  - Clinical Guidelines
  - Real-Life Stories
  - Weblinks
  - MySearchLab
  - Multiple Pathways to Learning
  - StudyLife

ACKNOWLEDGEMENTS

In the creation of a book such as this, there are so many people to thank. First, we need to thank students and colleagues for encouraging us to start the project and then move on to a third edition. As the third edition began to take shape, we were thankful for the many authors who once again agreed to contribute to the book or suggested others who had the expertise we required. Many of our authors took time from other projects to add their knowledge to the book, making this book a priority. We would like to thank Dr. Bridey Stirling for all the work she did creating the new MyNursingLab that accompanies this book. Dr. Stirling has been a Registered Nurse for 14 years. Bridey is an Epidemiologist, focusing primarily on cancer and HIV prevention. She has practiced internationally in countries such as Kenya, Malawi and India. She has created a mathematical model to predict the cases of HIV averted and associated costs saved in Nairobi. She worked at the University of Toronto's Centre for Global Health Research prior to returning to British Columbia. Bridey is currently an Adjunct Professor of Medicine at the University of British Columbia.

We are grateful to the talented team at Pearson Education Canada. Mr. Maurice Esses, Mr. John Polanszky, and Ms. Michelle Sartor guided us through the whole process of development of this edition. Ms. Cheryl Jackson provided expertise, ideas, and support, which were invaluable in moving through production. The reviewers, who were nameless to us at the time, contributed significant time and effort in assisting us to make this text strong and representative of Canadian community health nursing. Their names are listed below. Each of us had particular friends and family members who were supportive as we moved through the process of completing a major text. We are grateful to all of you. Finally, as teachers, we thank our students, who were guiding forces in considering the project at all.

Many nurses across the country have contributed countless hours to portray community health nursing with passion and pride. We are very excited with this new edition. We hope teachers and learners will also be excited as they continue to learn, explore, and discuss community health nursing as a distinct specialty in Canadian nursing.

Lynnette Leeseberg Stamler and Lucia Yiu

REVIEWERS

Cheryl Armistead, McGill University
Carol Bassingthwaighte, University of British Columbia
Freida Chavez, University of Toronto
Sally Dampier, Confederation College
Susanna Edwards, Ryerson University
Judy Gleeson, Mount Royal College
Susan Hammond, Douglas College
Corinne Hart, Ryerson University
Beverley Jones, St. Clair College
Roberta Mercier, Douglas College
Donna M. Romyn, Athabasca University
Anne Sochan, University of Ottawa
Roxie Thompson Isherwood, University of Calgary
Sasha Wiens, University of Calgary

This edition is dedicated to Anne Marie Leeseberg,
and Cheryl Ann Davis, both nurses who inspired me.
It is also dedicated to my husband Allan, for his unwavering support,
and finally, all my students who continue to inspire me.
—L.S.

This book is dedicated to my daughters, Tamara, Camillia,
and Tiffany who love to learn; to the community health nurses
who devote themselves to promoting the health of their communities;
and to our students whose love for learning will help shape the future directions
for community health nursing.
—L.Y.

Contributors

Amy Bender, RN, PhD
Assistant Professor, Lawrence S. Bloomberg Faculty of Nursing, University of Toronto
Chapter 31—Global Health

Claire Betker, RN, MN, CCHN(C)
Director of Research, Early Child Development, National Collaborating Centre for Determinants of Health
Chapter 2—Financing, Policy, and Politics of Healthcare Delivery

Diane Bewick, RN, BScN, MScN, DPA, CCHN(C)
Director of Family Health Services and Chief Nursing Officer, Middlesex-London Health Unit
Chapter 2—Financing, Policy, and Politics of Healthcare Delivery

Helen Brown, RN, PhD
Assistant Professor, School of Nursing, University of British Columbia
Chapter 15—Maternal and Child Health

Irene Buckland, RN, BScN, MScN
Manager, Child Health Team, Family Health Services, Middle-London Health Unit
Chapter 17—School Health

Kathleen Carlin, RN, MSc, PhD
Instructor, Department of Philosophy, Ryerson University
Chapter 4—Advocacy, Ethical, and Legal Considerations

Freida S. Chavez, RN, MHSc, CHE
Senior Lecturer and Director, International Office, Lawrence S. Bloomberg Faculty of Nursing, University of Toronto
Chapter 31—Global Health

Donna Ciliska, RN, PhD
Professor, School of Nursing, McMaster University; Nursing Consultant, Hamilton Public Health and Community Services
Chapter 10—Research

Benita Cohen, RN, PhD
Associate Professor, Faculty of Nursing, University of Manitoba
Chapter 6—Population Health Promotion Models and Strategies

Kathryn Edmunds, RN, BN, MSN, PhD (C)
Doctoral student, School of Nursing, University of Western Ontario; Adjunct Assistant Professor, Faculty of Nursing, University of Windsor
Chapter 8—Cultural Diversity

Nancy C. Edwards, RN, PhD
Professor, School of Nursing and Department of Epidemiology and Community Medicine, University of Ottawa
Chapter 14—Community Health Planning, Monitoring, and Evaluation

Josephine Etowa, RN, PhD
Associate Professor School of Nursing, University of Ottawa
Chapter 14—Community Health Planning, Monitoring, and Evaluation

Linda Ferguson, RN, PhD
Professor, College of Nursing, University of Saskatchewan
Chapter 11—Information Technology

Aaron Gabriel, RN, BA, BSN
Master's student, College of Nursing, University of Saskatchewan
Chapter 27—Poverty and Homelessness

Rebecca Ganann, RN, MSc
Instructor, School of Nursing, McMaster University
Chapter 10—Research

Denise Gastaldo, PhD
Associate Professor, Lawrence S. Bloomberg Faculty of Nursing and Associate Director, Centre for Critical Qualitative Health Research, University of Toronto
Chapter 31—Global Health

Elizabeth Battle Haugh, RN, BA, MScN
Director of Health Promotion, Windsor-Essex County Health Unit;
Adjunct Associate Professor, Faculty of Nursing, University of Windsor
Chapter 3—Nursing Roles, Functions, and Practice Settings

Roberta Heale, RN (EC), BScN, MN
Assistant Professor, School of Nursing, Laurentian University
Chapter 3—Nursing Roles, Functions, and Practice Settings

Janet B. Hettler, RN, DipN, BScN, MN
Manager, Crisis Nursery, Calgary Children's Cottage Society
Chapter 29—Sexually Transmitted Infections and Blood Borne Pathogens

Joan Wharf Higgins, PhD
Professor, School of Exercise Science, Physical and Health Education, University of Victoria
Chapter 5—Concepts of Health

Joy L. Johnson, RN, PhD, FCAHS
Professor, School of Nursing, University of British Columbia;
Scientific Director, Canadian Institutes of Health Research,
Institute of Gender and Health
Chapter 18—Gender and Community Health

Anne Katz, RN, PhD
Adjunct Professor, University of Manitoba
Chapter 20—Gay, Lesbian, Bisexual, and Transgender Clients

Margaret Ann Kennedy, RN, PhD
Director of Standards, Standards Collaborative, Canada
Health Infoway; President-Elect, Canadian Nursing
Informatics Association
Chapter 14—Community Health Planning, Monitoring,
and Evaluation

Elizabeth Kinnaird Iler, RN, BScN, MSc
Manager, Healthy Babies Healthy Children Program,
Windsor-Essex County Health Unit
Chapter 8—Cultural Diversity

Shelley Kirychuk, BSN, MSc, MBA, PhD
Assistant Professor, University of Saskatchewan
Chapter 24—Environmental and Occupational Health

Niels Koehncke, MD, MSc, FRCPC
Assistant Professor, University of Saskatchewan; Director,
Occupational Medicine Clinic, Royal University Hospital
Chapter 24—Environmental and Occupational Health

Judith C. Kulig, RN, DNSc
Professor, Nursing Program, School of Health Sciences,
University of Lethbridge
Chapter 23—Rural Health

Yvette Laforêt-Fliesser, RN, BScN, MScN, CCHN (c)
Adjunct Associate Professor, University of Western Ontario;
Independent Consultant
Chapter 17—School Health

Wendi Lokanc-Diluzio, BN, MN
Sexual and Reproductive Health Specialist, Alberta
Health Services
Chapter 29—Sexually Transmitted Infections and Blood
Borne Pathogens

Carol MacDougall, RN, BSc, MA
Public Health Manager, School and Sexual Health, Perth
District Health Unit, Stratford, Ontario
Chapter 17—School Health

Martha L. P. MacLeod, RN, PhD
Professor and Chair, School of Nursing, University of
Northern British Columbia
Chapter 23—Rural Health

Margaret M. Malone, RN, PhD
Associate Professor, School of Nursing, Ryerson University
Chapter 26—Violence in Societies

Sheila Marchant-Short, RN, BScN, MScN
Regional Manager, Communicable Disease Control Programs,
Community Health Services and Public Health, Eastern
Health, St. John's, Newfoundland
Chapter 12—Communicable Diseases

Lori Schindel Martin, RN, BA, BScN, MScCHN, PhD
Associate Professor, School of Nursing, Faculty of Community
Health Services, Ryerson University
Chapter 19—Older Adult Health

Marion McKay, RN, PhD
Senior Instructor and Associate Dean, Undergraduate
Programs, Faculty of Nursing, University of Manitoba
Chapter 1—The History of Community Health Nursing
in Canada

Gladys McPherson, RN, PhD
Assistant Professor, School of Nursing, University of British
Columbia
Chapter 15—Maternal and Child Health

Elaine Mordoch, RN, PhD
Assistant Professor, Faculty of Nursing, University of
Manitoba
Chapter 21—Mental Health

Alison Nelson, BScN, MN
Manager of Health Promotion, Cancer Screening Programs,
Alberta Health Services
Chapter 29—Sexually Transmitted Infections and Blood
Borne Pathogens

John L. Oliffe, RN, MEd, PhD,
Associate Professor, School of Nursing, University of British
Columbia
Chapter 18—Gender and Community Health

Elizabeth Peter, RN, BScN, BA, MScN, PhD
Associate Professor and Associate Dean, Academic Programs,
Lawrence S. Bloomberg Faculty of Nursing, University of
Toronto
Chapter 4—Advocacy, Ethical, and Legal Considerations

Cindy Peternelj-Taylor, RN, MSc, DF-IAFN
Professor, College of Nursing, University of Saskatchewan;
Distinguished Fellow—International Association of Forensic
Nurses
Chapter 25—Correctional Health

Wendy E. Peterson, RN, PhD
Associate Professor, School of Nursing, University of Ottawa
Chapter 14—Community Health Planning, Monitoring, and Evaluation

Roger Pitblado, PhD
Professor Emeritus and Senior Research Fellow, Centre for Rural and Northern Health Research, Laurentian University
Chapter 23—Rural Health

Zaida Rahaman, BScN, MN
Doctoral Student in Nursing, University of Ottawa
Chapter 7—Primary Health Care

Rose Alene Roberts, RN, BScN, MSc, PhD
Assistant Professor, College of Nursing, University of Saskatchewan
Chapter 22—Aboriginal Health

Betty Schepens, RN, BScN, DPA
Public Health Nurse and Emergency Preparedness Coordinator, Chatham-Kent Public Health Unit, Chatham, Ontario
Chapter 30—Emergency Preparedness and Disaster Nursing

Patricia A. Sealy, RN, BA, BScN, MScN, PhD
Nurse Researcher Educator and Adjunct Assistant Professor, Labatt Family School of Nursing, University of Western Ontario
Chapter 16—Family Health

Dawn Smith, RN, BScN, MN, PhD
Assistant Professor, School of Nursing, University of Ottawa
Chapter 7—Primary Health Care

Julia O. Smith, RN, BSc, MSc(A), PhD (c)
Epidemiology and Biostatistics University of Western Ontario
Chapter 16—Family Health

Jane Sparkes, RN, BSN, MSc eHealth
Chapter 11—Information Technology

Lynnette Leeseberg Stamler, RN, BSN, MEd, PhD
Professor and Assistant Dean, College of Nursing, University of Saskatchewan
Chapter 9—Epidemiology
Chapter 27—Poverty and Homelessness
Chapter 32—Challenges and Future Directions

Norma J. Stewart, RN, PhD
Professor, College of Nursing, University of Saskatchewan
Chapter 23—Rural Health

Bridey Stirling, RN, BScN, PhD
Adjunct Professor of Medicine, University of British Columbia
MyNursingLab

Louise R. Sweatman, RN, BScN, LLB, MSc
Nurse Lawyer; Chief Operating Officer of Assessment Strategies, Inc.
Chapter 4—Advocacy, Ethical, and Legal Considerations

Ruta Valaitis, RN, PhD
Associate Professor, School of Nursing, McMaster University
Chapter 11—Information Technology

Kim Van Herk, BScN, MN
Community Health Nurse
Chapter 7—Primary Health Care

Claire Warren, RN, BScN, MN, CCHN (C)
Manager of Professional Practice and Development and Community Nurse Specialist, Sudbury & District Health Unit
Chapter 3—Nursing Roles, Functions, and Practice Settings

Janet L. Wayne, BScN, MN
Director of Accreditation for Southern Alberta, Alberta Health Services
Chapter 29—Sexually Transmitted Infections and Blood Borne Pathogens

Leeann Whitney, RN, BScN, MAEd
Nursing and Public Health Consultant
Chapter 12—Communicable Diseases

Hélène Philbin Wilkinson, RN, BScN, MN
Forensic Program Director, Northeast Mental Health Centre, North Bay, Ontario
Chapter 28—Substance Use

Phil Woods, RPN, PhD
Professor and Associate Dean Research, Innovation and Global Initiatives, College of Nursing, University of Saskatchewan
Chapter 25—Correctional Health

Lucia Yiu, RN, BScN, BA, BSc, MScN
Associate Professor, Faculty of Nursing, University of Windsor; Educational and Training Consultant
Chapter 13—Community Care
Chapter 30—Emergency Preparedness and Disaster Nursing
Chapter 32—Challenges and Future Directions

Lynne E. Young, RN, PhD
Associate Professor, School of Nursing, University of Victoria
Chapter 5—Concepts of Health

chapter

1

The History of Community Health Nursing in Canada

Marion McKay

OBJECTIVES

After studying this chapter, you should be able to:

1. Identify the social conditions and beliefs that were the impetus for the development of community health nursing in Canada.
2. Discuss the theoretical and practical distinctions between the practices of visiting nurses and public health nurses.
3. Describe how the emergence of the welfare state shaped the evolution of public health and visiting nursing programs.
4. Discuss the role that women played in the development of public health and visiting nursing programs.
5. Compare and contrast the work of community health nurses in urban, rural, and remote areas of Canada.

INTRODUCTION

Many nurses practise in the community. Over time, a variety of terms have been used to define and classify their practice. These terms vary from one country to the next, so it is important that educators, students, and practitioners consistently use the terminology as it is understood in the specific setting in which the practice is taking place. In Canada, the term community health nurse (CHN) is used to describe nurses who work in the community. Two types of CHNs are defined by the Community Health Nurses of Canada (Community Health Nurses Association of Canada, 2008). One is the public health nurse (PHN), whose practice focuses on promoting, protecting, and preserving the health of populations. These nurses work in a variety of community settings to meet the health needs of specific populations or the community as a whole. The second type of CHN is the home health nurse (HHN), whose practice focuses on prevention, health restoration, health maintenance, or palliative care. These nurses work in homes, schools, and workplaces to deliver nursing care to individuals and groups who live in the community.

In the United States, a different approach to the definition and description of the practices of nurses who work in the community is used. Community nursing is divided into two broad categories. The first, community-oriented nursing, is defined as nursing that focuses on the care of either the whole community or a population of individuals, families, and groups living in the community. Two specific types

of nursing practices fall within this definition: public health nursing and community health nursing. Public health nursing has as its primary focus the provision of healthcare to communities and populations with the goal of disease prevention and the preservation, promotion, and protection of the community's health. Community health nursing, on the other hand, aims to preserve, protect, promote, or maintain the health of individuals, families, and groups in the community. The second category of nursing practice in the community is community-based nursing. Community-based nurses focus on the provision of acute and long-term care to individuals and families living in the community (Stanhope & Lancaster, 2006).

The purpose of this chapter is to explore the history of community health nursing programs delivered by professionally educated nurses in Canada. From their origins in the late nineteenth century, community health nursing programs have been profoundly influenced by a variety of social, political, and economic forces. The public health movement, well established in Canada by the beginning of the twentieth century, put the health of Canadians on the public agenda. Maternal feminists, who believed that the unique nurturing capacity of women made them particularly suited to the development of programs to assist women and children (Ladd-Taylor, 1994), also played a major role in the creation of the Canadian welfare state. Their searching critiques of the prevailing social order sparked many of the social reform programs established in early twentieth-century

Canada, including the child welfare movement, services for childbearing women, and the establishment of mothers' allowances and other programs to assist families in need (Christie & Gauvreau, 1996). In addition, social beliefs about gender and appropriate roles for women shaped the social system in which community health nurses (CHNs) lived and practised. Finally, the tensions between professional medicine and nursing created both opportunities for and barriers to the development of nursing practice in the community.

It is impossible in the space of a single chapter to describe and analyze the development of community health nursing in each Canadian province and territory. Instead, this chapter will trace trends in the development of community health nursing using specific examples drawn from published sources and from research in progress. It will trace the evolution of community health nursing from its dual origins in philanthropic healthcare organizations and publicly funded municipal health departments, examining the role that the evolving concepts of charity and citizenship played in shaping current models of community health nursing. It will also examine the challenges that confronted nurses as they carved out a role in the community. In the final analysis, community health nursing was always both a response to and a product of its particular time and place.

THE ORIGINS OF COMMUNITY HEALTH NURSING IN CANADA

Community health nursing evolved in two streams. The earliest form was **district nursing** or **visiting nursing**, which evolved in late nineteenth-century Britain, the United States, and Canada. Charitable agencies, often organized and operated by maternal feminists, employed visiting nurses (VNs) to provide care to poor and destitute families. Working-class and lower-middle-class families also were recipients of visiting nursing services. These families could not afford to hire full-time private-duty nurses, and their homes were not large enough to provide accommodation for a nurse during the term of her employment. In Canada, visiting nursing services were organized at both the national and the local level. The best known of these, the Victorian Order of Nurses for Canada (VON), was founded in 1897 "to supply nurses, thoroughly trained in Hospital and District Nursing, and subject to one Central Authority, for the nursing of the sick who are otherwise unable to obtain trained nursing in their own homes, both in town and country districts" (Lady Aberdeen, cited in Gibbon, 1947, p. 8).

The public health nurse (PHN) was a civil servant employed by the local, provincial, or federal government. **Public health nursing** emerged in Canada in the early twentieth century when civic departments of health established health education and preventive programs to combat communicable disease, infant mortality, and morbidity in school-age children. Nurses were perceived as the ideal professionals to deliver these programs because of their medical knowledge

and their ability to interact with women and children in private homes and in the public school setting (Sears, 1995).

Although these definitions are theoretically distinct, in practice there was considerable blurring of the boundaries between the practices of VNs and PHNs. For example, in some Canadian cities the VON provided programs on behalf of the local health department. In other communities, the VON provided public health programs to supplement those provided by the local government. PHNs in rural and remote areas of the country, however, often provided bedside nursing care and obstetrical care because no VNs were available to undertake this work.

In her analysis of twentieth-century Canadian nursing, McPherson (1996) divides the profession into three sectors: hospital nurses, private-duty nurses, and public health (including visiting) nurses. During the late nineteenth and early twentieth centuries, when community health nursing emerged as a distinct specialty, the majority of all nurses were self-employed as private-duty nurses. Public health and visiting nurses were counted among the profession's elite. Employment in this specialty practice required additional clinical skills such as midwifery training and, particularly after World War I, post-diploma training at a university (Baldwin, 1997; Green, 1974; McPherson, 1996; Miller, 2000; Penney, 1996). Myra (Grimsley) Bennett, who worked for 50 years as a nurse along Newfoundland's northwestern coast, took two courses in midwifery prior to leaving England (Green, 1974).

As an occupational group, nurses came from a variety of social backgrounds, including middle-class, working-class, and agricultural families. The majority were female, white, and Canadian or British born. Nursing, one of the few respectable careers available to women, offered young women seeking autonomy from their family the prospect for both financial independence and social status (McPherson, 1996). Many women married and left the profession soon after completing their hospital training programs. Others, usually those who remained single or those whose marriages had ended, forged life-long careers in nursing.

Public health and visiting nurses were different from nurses employed in other sectors of the healthcare system in several ways. They tended to remain in their community practices longer than those employed in hospitals and private-duty nursing. They also enjoyed greater financial stability and higher salaries (McPherson, 1996). Published biographical material also indicates that these nurses actively sought opportunities that combined challenging work with travel and adventure. "I had always wanted to travel," wrote Margaret Giovannini, another Newfoundland outpost nurse, ". . . and when the opportunity arose to work as well as travel I liked it" (Giovannini, 1988, p. 1). Other pioneer CHNs wrote of their eagerness to find a place where they could fulfill their desire to use their hard-won knowledge and skills in a meaningful way (Colley, 1970; Miller, 2000). "When I first arrived at my little northern hospital in Granite Springs," wrote Mary E. Hope, "I felt that my search for the end of the rainbow was over. . . . With my shining new public health nursing diploma under my arm, I was a consecrated scientist about to enlighten this benighted wilderness village. . . . This was my kingdom"

(Hope, 1955, pp. 5–6). Still others sought a practice free (or at least more distant) from the hierarchy and constraints of supervisors and large institutions (Green, 1974). Bessie J. Banfill, who worked in rural Saskatchewan, found that her work among that province's settlers, many of whom were immigrants from Eastern Europe, fulfilled a deep personal need. "[I]mpulsive by nature, and restless and dissatisfied with hospital routine and nursing patients surrounded by luxury, I longed for more challenging adventure and freedom" (Banfill, 1967, p. 9). Many genuinely enjoyed interaction with people and embraced opportunities to learn about other cultures (Baldwin, 1997). Banfill (1967) wrote that her "Scottish blood boiled" in response to comments that foreigners were not welcome in Canada. Their sense of adventure, independence, courage, and humanitarianism led pioneering Canadian CHNs to offer their services in Canada's poorest urban districts and most isolated rural communities. These qualities also placed them at the forefront of efforts to place healthcare within reach of all Canadians.

HEALTH, THE INDIVIDUAL, AND THE STATE

The idea that healthcare was a right of citizenship, rather than a privilege based upon social rank and income, developed slowly during Canada's first century. The British North America Act (1867) made only limited provisions for the establishment and maintenance of a healthcare system. The Act specified that the federal government was responsible for quarantine and for the establishment of Marine Hospitals. All other responsibilities for the organization of healthcare, including public health services, devolved to the provinces. These responsibilities were not specified within the Act, nor did the provinces, in the early years after Confederation, make much effort to undertake them. Such organized healthcare as did exist was provided at the local (municipal) level through public welfare or, more frequently, charitable organizations. Many provinces passed enabling legislation in the late nineteenth century, which allowed for the establishment of local and provincial departments of health. However, even at the local level, there was considerable reluctance to provide public health services on an ongoing basis. Most early health departments were organized in response to specific local emergencies. When the emergency was over, they were dissolved (Bilson, 1980; Bliss, 1991). Similarly, medical officers of health (MOHs) were appointed on a part-time basis until the 1880s. Toronto, for example, appointed its first full-time MOH in 1883 (MacDougall, 1990). Nurses were an even later addition to the staff of local health departments.

These arrangements were consistent with the social attitudes of the time. The state neither undertook nor was expected to undertake any responsibility for the healthcare of individuals and families. Those who could afford to pay for their own healthcare did so. Those who did not have the financial means to make these arrangements either went without care or, if sufficiently desperate or destitute, turned to local governments or charitable organizations for assistance.

The poverty, poor health, and social unrest created by industrial capitalism, immigration, and urbanization demonstrated the inadequacy of nineteenth-century assumptions about individual and collective responsibility for the provision of healthcare. They also shaped the organization and financing of the public health system and the nature of community health nursing.

The Emergence of the Public Health Nurse

The Rise of Urban Health Departments The establishment of urban health departments was fraught with controversy. In an era when individuals were expected to provide for their own healthcare and governments were not permitted to intrude into the personal lives of individual citizens, health departments threatened to blur the boundaries between the private and public domains. Further, they did so at considerable expense to the public purse. A. J. Douglas, Winnipeg's first full-time MOH, summed up the challenges of his office as follows:

> [W]hen I first took office, the health officer, in my community at least, was looked upon by most people as a rather unnecessary appendage to the municipal pay-roll—not only unnecessary, but very often pernicious, for sometimes he had the temerity to interfere with citizens, particularly the so-called best citizens' inalienable right to do as they please. . . . It was considered that his proper sphere was to supervise the collection of city wastes, to keep the streets clean, to juggle with statistics (always with a view to emphasizing the salubrity of his own locality), and to occasionally show some activity during outbreaks of the more serious communicable diseases. . . . He was always to use discretion as to whose toes he trod upon; he was not to point out glaring sanitary defects in his community as this spoiled business and kept visitors away. (Douglas, 1912, p. 85)

At the end of the nineteenth century, Canada's major urban centres faced a health crisis which matched in substance, if not quite in magnitude, that of cities in the United States and Great Britain. Major Canadian cities such as Montreal, Toronto, and Winnipeg possessed inadequate or non-existent sanitary infrastructures at the time of their most rapid expansion (Artibise, 1975; Bliss, 1991). The problems were most acute in areas populated by new immigrants and the working poor. The unsanitary living conditions, overcrowding, and inadequate nutrition created by urban poverty were a recipe for disaster. Infant and maternal mortality rates climbed steadily (see Figure 1.1). Periodic outbreaks of communicable diseases such as smallpox, cholera, typhoid, and influenza killed thousands of Canadians. Tuberculosis (TB) emerged as the leading cause of death for urban dwellers who had survived early infancy (Humphreys, 1999).

The first cohort of Canadian public health officials focused their efforts on creating adequate systems of waste disposal and a safe water supply. In addition, drawing on the new science of bacteriology, efforts were directed toward

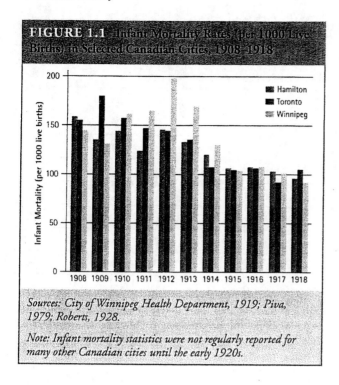

FIGURE 1.1 Infant Mortality Rates (per 1000 Live Births) in Selected Canadian Cities, 1908–1918

Sources: *City of Winnipeg Health Department, 1919; Piva, 1979; Roberts, 1928.*

Note: *Infant mortality statistics were not regularly reported for many other Canadian cities until the early 1920s.*

establishing a safe food supply. Particular attention was focused on the health hazards created by unpasteurized milk. Many Canadian cities enacted by-laws that required the inspection of meat, milk, and bread sold within the city limits, and hired inspectors to enforce these regulations.

In the early twentieth century, public health officials identified health education as another strategy to combat unnecessary disease and death. It was at this point that nurses were first employed as civil servants in local health departments. Although the exact chronology varies from one city to another, the first PHNs were responsible for TB control, child hygiene programs, or school inspection programs (see Table 1.1). Two important trends can be identified from these pioneering initiatives. First, the employment of nurses by civic authorities was often undertaken with considerable reluctance and only after voluntary programs had foundered in the face of overwhelming need and inadequate financial resources. Second, early PHNs were appointed to single, specific programs rather than to a generalist practice.

From Voluntary to Civic Public Health Programs In 1907 in Toronto, the first civic nurse was employed to provide health education and nursing care in the home to TB patients. However, this nurse and her predecessors had previously been employed by the Toronto General Hospital through a special fund donated by a concerned Toronto citizen. When this arrangement ended, Toronto's city council agreed to include the salary of the TB nurse in the health department's budget. Her work went on virtually unchanged, except that she was now required to report to the MOH twice a week (Royce, 1983). That same year in Montreal, the Tuberculosis League hired a nurse from the VON to provide instruction to those suffering from TB (Gibbon, 1947). In Winnipeg, TB nursing was established in 1909 by the Anti-Tuberculosis

Society, a voluntary association of physicians and interested citizens (City of Winnipeg Health Department, 1910). The health visiting and health education provided by the Society's TB nurse was carefully coordinated with the city's sanitation and health inspection programs. The Winnipeg Health Department took over the TB nursing program in 1914. A major reason for the change from voluntary to civic funding was to enable the TB nurses to "have the power to make people carry out our regulations where at present persuasion and argument are about the only weapons she can personally use" (City of Winnipeg Health Department, 1915, p. 7).

In other cities, the first PHNs participated in initiatives to preserve and promote the health of school-age children. As working-class children were removed from economic production and placed in the public school system, the significant health problems from which they suffered became fully visible (Peikoff & Brickey, 1991). In the opinion of public officials and social reformers, this situation was intolerable. Ill health detracted from the child's educational attainment, and, worse still, it was feared that the sickly child of the present was destined to become the poverty-stricken and dependent citizen of the future. Programs for the medical inspection of school children were established in major cities across Canada. School-based inspections were often augmented by home visits to educate the parents and to ensure that all recommendations were followed (Sutherland, 1981). In many cities, such as Montreal, Toronto, Winnipeg, and Vancouver, school health programs were initially established by the board of education. They were subsequently taken over by the health department as part of the process of consolidating all public health programs under one jurisdiction (City of Winnipeg Health Department, 1910; MacDougall, 1990).

Finally, many early PHNs were employed in programs to reduce infant mortality. Despite all efforts to improve urban sanitation and to regulate food and milk supplies, infant mortality rates in Canadian cities continued to climb until well into the second decade of the twentieth century. What made this state of affairs a national crisis rather than a family tragedy was a shift in beliefs about the role that children played in industrial society and in the process of nation building. Every child, even the Canadian-born child of an Eastern European immigrant, became a precious element in the patriotic process of nation building (Peikoff & Brickey, 1991). An equally powerful concern, which particularly preoccupied Canadian-born, Anglo-Celtic members of the elite and middle classes, was the fear that they would soon be overwhelmed as a social and political force by the waves of immigrants arriving from Southern and Eastern Europe (McLaren & McLaren, 1997). As the failure of sanitarian and bacteriological strategies to reduce infant mortality became evident, MOHs across North America and Western Europe re-examined their assumptions about its etiology and the role that public health might legitimately play in its reduction. Their experiences with poor and immigrant populations convinced them that other factors, particularly those embedded in family and cultural practices, also influenced infant mortality (Meigs, 1916).

TABLE 1.1 Evolution of Community Health Nursing Programs in Canada

1891–1900: Laying the Groundwork for Community Health Nursing

1897	Victorian Order of Nurses for Canada founded	Ottawa
1897	District nurse employed by general hospital outpatient department	Winnipeg
1898	First VON local branch established	Ottawa

1901–1910: Emergence of Specialized Community Health Nursing Programs

1901–10	Milk depots and child hygiene programs established by voluntary agencies	Toronto, Montreal, Winnipeg
1901	National anti-tuberculosis society founded	Ottawa
1904	Margaret Scott Nursing Mission founded	Winnipeg
1905	TB nurse employed by general hospital outpatient department	Toronto
1906	TB nurse employed by City Health Department	Ottawa
1907	Medical inspection of school children inaugurated by school board	Montreal
1909	Nurses employed by school board for school inspection program	Winnipeg
1909	Lethbridge Nursing Mission founded	Lethbridge, AB
1910	Civic funding provided to support child hygiene program and milk depot	Winnipeg

1911–1930: Elaboration and Consolidation of Community Health Nursing Programs

1914	Child Hygiene program transferred to City Health Department	Toronto, Winnipeg
1914	School Board nurses transferred to City Health Department	Toronto
1914	Public Health Nursing reorganized as a generalist program	Toronto
1916	First provincial public health nurses employed	Manitoba
1918–20	VD control programs established under federal-provincial program	Canada
1919	Provincial District Nursing Service established	Alberta
1919	Red Cross funding supports establishment of public health nursing programs at five Canadian universities	Canada
1920	Provincial school health program established with Red Cross funding	Prince Edward Island
1920	County nursing program established with Red Cross funding	Nova Scotia
1920	Provincial public health nurses employed to work in Northern Ontario	Ontario
1920	First full-time provincial health unit in Canada established	Saanich, BC
1921	Provincial child hygiene program established with Red Cross funding	New Brunswick

1931–1980: Community Health Nursing in the Evolving Welfare State

1941–42	Buck Commission recommends major reorganization of public health and visiting nursing programs	Manitoba
1943	Margaret Scott Nursing Mission closes	Winnipeg
1943	VON transfers prenatal, postnatal, and child health programs to provincial health department	Manitoba
1968–70	VON establishes home care demonstration projects	Ontario
1973	*Pickering Report* recommends VON be mandated to deliver home care programs in Canada	Canada
1974	VON included in first publicly funded provincial home care program	Manitoba

Note: Events identified are those found in current literature, and may not, in all instances, be the first such program established in Canada.

Canadian efforts to reduce infant mortality were initiated by elite and middle-class women. Their desire to alleviate the suffering of women and children was inspired by both the **social gospel movement** and maternal feminism. The social gospel movement, which placed priority on the quality of human life on earth, united clergy, politicians, and ordinary citizens in efforts to reform Canadian society (Merkley, 1987). The movement found important allies among maternal feminists, who were also advocating sweeping social reform, particularly to protect the interests of women, children, and families (Christie & Gauvreau, 1996).

Public health officials and maternal feminists also turned their attention to the care that infants received from their mothers (Meigs, 1916). They concluded that many parents, particularly the mothers, were "ignorant" and barely capable of providing a safe and healthy environment for the nation's future citizens. Because removing children from their parents was no longer a viable option, educating mothers about infant feeding and hygiene became the intervention of choice (Peikoff & Brickey, 1991). Infant/child welfare/hygiene programs were carried out at milk depots, well baby clinics, and in private homes (Locke, 1918; MacNutt, 1913). VNs staffed the clinics and visited the homes of newborn infants in the early postpartum period. They assessed the health of the infant and mother, the family's childcare practices, and the hygienic conditions in the home. A major focus was to promote the breastfeeding of newborn infants.

In Toronto, a variety of women's groups, settlement houses, and church missions established milk depots and well baby clinics for the city's poorest citizens (MacDougall, 1990; Royce, 1983). Twenty "gouttes de lait" (clinics where mothers unable to breastfeed learned how to properly use cow's milk) were established in Montreal by the Fédération nationale Saint-Jean-Baptiste between 1910 and 1912 (Baillargeon, 2002). In 1915, the VON undertook responsibility for child welfare work in Edmonton, and in 1922 a similar program was established in Ottawa (Gibbon, 1947). In Winnipeg, a child hygiene program was founded in 1910 by the Margaret Scott Nursing Mission (MSNM) with funding from the city's health department.

Although voluntary programs confirmed the overwhelming need for both milk depots and child hygiene programs, they could not be sustained. In Winnipeg, for example, the Margaret Scott Nursing Mission encountered such severe financial problems that the health department took over the program in 1914. A similar pattern of municipal takeover of voluntary programs occurred in other Canadian cities, with PHNs taking the place of VNs in the delivery of child hygiene and milk depot services.

From Specialist to Generalist Practice In the second decade of the twentieth century, urban PHNs began to deliver general rather than specialized services in the community. This change was pioneered in Toronto, where the community health system had gradually evolved into a confusing mix of programs under the auspices of a variety of private and civic organizations. School health nurses were employed by the board of education. VNs were employed by philanthropic

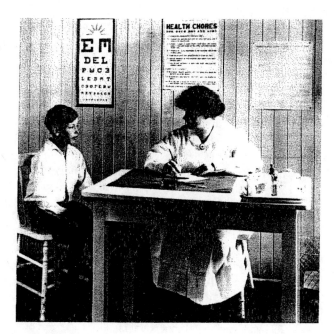

Photo 1.1

In Winnipeg, the first public health nurses were hired by the School Board to carry out medical inspections of school-age children. This 1923 photograph shows a provincial public health nurse conducting a health inspection of a school boy in Brooklands, a working-class suburb of Winnipeg.

Credit: Provincial Archives of Manitoba: Public Health Collection 63 (N13039)

organizations to staff milk depots and child hygiene programs. PHNs employed by the health department were assigned to several programs, including TB control, measles control, and child welfare. In 1914, Toronto's Child Hygiene and the Communicable Disease programs were amalgamated at the service delivery level and each PHN provided direct care in the home for both programs. The rationale for this reorganization was that the family, rather than the individual, was the basic unit of intervention in public health nursing. "We decided to specialize in homes rather than diseases," stated Eunice Dyke, superintendent of Toronto's PHNs, "and to safeguard the interests of the medical specialist by office organization rather than multiplication of health visitors" (cited in Royce, 1983, p. 49). In 1917, the board of education nurses were transferred to the City of Toronto Health Department, and their responsibilities were integrated into the role of the generalist PHN (Royce, 1983). Visiting nursing services continued to be provided by the VON and the St. Elizabeth Visiting Nursing Association. These were coordinated with the preventive and health education programs provided by the PHNs (MacDougall, 1990).

The Establishment of Rural Public Health Nursing Public health services in rural and small-town Canada were relatively unorganized until after World War I. A severe shortage of nurses occurred during and after the war (Riddell, 1991), and the majority of available nurses were unprepared for work in

CANADIAN RESEARCH BOX

How were healthy children in British Columbia assessed historically?

Gleason, M. (2002). Race, class, and health: School medical inspection and "healthy" children in British Columbia, 1890–1930. *Canadian Bulletin of Medical History/Bulletin Canadien d'histoire de la médecine, 19*(1), 95–112.

This historical analysis examines the efforts of social reformers and public health professionals to impose urban, Anglo-Celtic, middle-class values about health on school-age children and their parents. Interventions in the school setting included daily personal hygiene inspection of the children by teachers, a regular program of medical inspections, health education, communicable disease control, and home visits by school/public health nurses to ensure that families both understood and complied with health professionals' recommendations to improve identified medical and health problems. Rural families and those of Aboriginal, Asian, Eastern European, and East Indian origin were the primary targets of these programs because their health practices and beliefs were more likely to deviate from the standards set by the white urban middle class. The author concludes (1) that the standards for school health programs and medical inspection of school children could not be attained in rural and working-class school districts, (2) that these programs stigmatized children whose families were unwilling or unable to conform to white middle-class models of health, (3) that reform programs that targeted non–Anglo-Celtic families were powerful instruments to strengthen and legitimize the existing social and political system, and (4) that public health professionals contributed to this process, both deliberately and inadvertently, through their paternalistic and sometimes judgmental interactions with both children and parents.

Discussion Questions

1. How do these findings compare with other descriptions you have read about the impact of public health programs on school-age children and their families?

2. If you were asked to plan a school health program, how would you use the findings of this study?

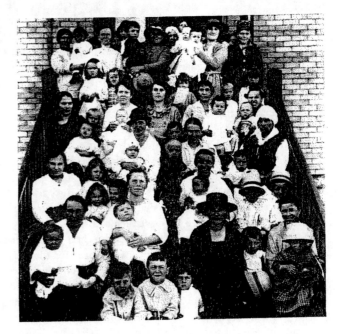

Photo 1.2

Child hygiene programs offered public health officials an opportunity to both monitor the health of young children and encourage their mothers to adopt Canadian child-rearing practices. This group, which includes 34 infants and children, gathered on the steps of All People's Mission, Winnipeg, in 1921 after having attended a child health clinic staffed by Dr. Ellen Douglas and several nurses.

Credit: Provincial Archives of Manitoba: L.B. Foote Collections 1452 (N2377)

CANADIAN RESEARCH BOX

What is the link between nursing and colonization in Manitoba?

McPherson, K. (2003). Nursing and colonization: The work of Indian Health Service nurses in Manitoba, 1945–1970. In G. Feldberg, M. Ladd-Taylor, A. Li, & K. McPherson (Eds.), *Women, health, and nation: Canada and the United States since 1945* (pp. 222–246). Montreal & Kingston: McGill–Queen's University Press.

This article analyzes the work of Indian Health Service (IHS) nurses working in Zone 6 of the IHS after 1945. It first reviews historical approaches to the "complex relationship of gender, professionalism, and colonization" (p. 223) and then discusses how these categories of analysis have been used to examine the experiences of nurses working with government-sponsored Aboriginal health programs in the United States and Canada. Drawing on this body of literature, McPherson argues that nurses working in Aboriginal communities have had an ambiguous impact on the health and cultural practices of the populations that they served. For example, because of their gender, nurses could forge closer relationships with Aboriginal women than could male physicians and Indian agents, and were thus more able to offer "medical" care and health teaching. As

public health nursing. Post-diploma programs to prepare nurses for public health work were unavailable in Canada. The VON had established training centres in several Canadian cities, including Ottawa, Toronto, and Winnipeg, to prepare registered nurses interested in joining the Order (Gibbon, 1947). However, the impact of the training centres was constrained by the Order's limited financial resources.

Fiscal constraints were another factor that delayed the development of rural public health services. Urban centres with a reasonably large tax base found it difficult enough to fund health departments. The challenge of raising sufficient funds in small towns and unorganized rural districts was nearly insurmountable. As well, power over the allocation of members of a profession often subordinated to medicine, nurses working in isolated Aboriginal communities often enjoyed considerable autonomy and had many opportunities to practise in expanded roles. Their role within the larger colonial project is more problematic. Given that medicine was a primary tool by which European settlers sought to undermine Aboriginal peoples' cultural beliefs and practices, IHS nurses were full participants in the process of imposing Western cultural practices upon Canada's indigenous populations. However, depending on their own attitudes and beliefs, nurses could also choose to support or at least tolerate the use of traditional healing practices in the communities in which they worked.

McPherson and others caution against an inappropriately benign interpretation of the impact of Westernized healthcare services in Aboriginal communities. All nurses, they argue, wielded professional, cultural, and racial power over Aboriginal people. Their interventions drew on middle-class standards of hygiene and child care, which often had little relevance to populations experiencing poverty, cultural disruption, the depletion of traditional sources of food, and environmental pollution. As well, Canadian IHS nurses worked within a bureaucracy that both defended and perpetuated a system of healthcare based on charity, not citizenship.

Using Zone 6 as a case study, McPherson draws additional examples and provides further analysis of how gender, professional status, and colonialism both helped and hindered the work of IHS nurses working in Manitoba and Northwestern Ontario. Further analysis, she argues, is needed to understand the extent to which individual nurses may have "managed to work around racism and colonialism" (p. 240) to forge gender-based bonds with Aboriginal women. In the final analysis, sweeping generalizations about the impact of IHS nurses contribute little to the debate. "Understanding women's relationships with the state and with medicine demands that we ask, which women in what historical circumstances and in what relations of power?" (p. 241).

Discussion Questions

1. To what extent do you think that today's health education and health promotion programs contain cultural, racial, and gender biases that limit their effectiveness and create barriers between community health nurses and the populations that they serve?

2. What forums would you use to lobby for reform of current community health programs?

scarce financial resources rested with far fewer individuals in non-urban settings. Both Stuart (1987) and Riddell (1991) contain first-person accounts by early rural PHNs about the impact that "penny pinching" local officials had on the development of local public health programs.

Popular conceptions about the relative healthiness of urban and rural settings also delayed the development of rural public health programs. Prior to the war, cities had been perceived as more unhealthy environments (Stuart, 1987). The visibility of urban squalor and the relative invisibility of its rural equivalent lulled many social reformers into believing that the pastoral nature of rural life was a healthy antidote to the evils of the city.

After World War I, the development of public health nursing was facilitated by a change in the mandate of the International Red Cross. To support more general efforts at rebuilding social structures in the post-war era, the International Red Cross prioritized the development of public health nursing (Hutchinson, 1996). The Canadian Red Cross possessed a substantial fund that had been originally earmarked to support the war effort (VON Minutes, Feb. 1920). In the immediate post-war period, it used these funds to establish cottage hospitals and public health nursing services in rural and isolated communities (Miller, 2000; Riddell, 1991; Stuart, 1987), to support visiting nursing services in urban centres (MSNM Minutes, Feb. 1920; VON Minutes, Feb. 1920), and to provide funding for post-diploma programs in public health nursing at several Canadian universities (Riddell, 1991; Stuart, 1987). In British Columbia, for example, successive classes of nurses graduating from the University of British Columbia's post-diploma and baccalaureate nursing programs accelerated the pace at which rural public health programs could be established (Green, 1984; Riddell, 1991; Zilm & Warbinek, 1995).

The poor health of many military personnel recruited from rural Canada and the horrific loss of life during World War I also redirected political and public attention to the establishment of rural public health programs (Stuart, 1987). The agrarian protest movement in Ontario and the Prairie Provinces also accelerated the development of rural public health services in the post-war era. In Ontario, for example, the election of an agrarian/labour coalition government in 1919 was rapidly followed by the implementation of rural public health programs (Stuart, 1987).

At the local level, rural women's groups such as the Women's Institute and the United Farm Women made community development and the development of healthcare services a priority. These women lobbied local officials, served tea at child welfare clinics, sewed layettes for destitute families, provided transportation, made referrals, raised funds, and in untold other ways tried to enable the PHNs to fulfill their professional obligations to the fullest extent possible (Miller, 2000; Riddell, 1991; Stuart, 1987).

Unlike their counterparts in urban settings, the first rural PHNs were generalists. Blurring the boundaries between visiting nursing and public health nursing, these nurses delivered programs in health education, school health, maternal/child health, communicable disease control, social welfare, dental health, and medical/surgical nursing (Riddell, 1991; Stuart, 1987). In addition, they delivered babies and provided emergency medical, dental, and even veterinary assistance during the frequent occasions when these professionals were not available (Giovannini, 1988; Miller, 2000; Riddell, 1991; Stuart, 1987).

To accomplish this work, rural PHNs faced formidable challenges created by distance and climate. Although their

Photo 1.3

Immunization of school-age children was an important part of a rural PHN's work. Small schools and long distances made this a challenging task. In 1932, public health nurse Ina Grenville and an unidentified physician were photographed immunizing a group of school children at Algoma School in Northern Ontario.

Credit: Archives of Ontario. Reference code: RG 10-30-2 (I0005225) Immunizing Children, Algoma, Ontario, 1932

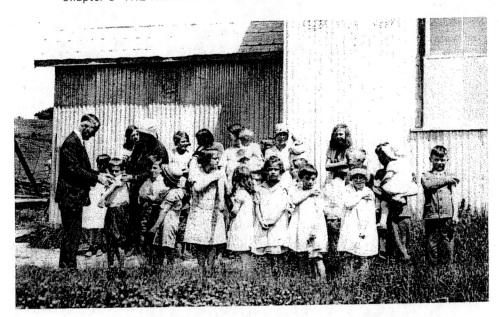

urban counterparts, particularly in the early years, often walked many miles to visit homes at considerable distances from streetcar routes, urban nursing districts were measured in mere city blocks. Rural districts were enormous. As Olive Matthews reported in *The Canadian Nurse* in 1920: "I have a car for my school inspection, given voluntarily by Argyle and Clear Lake districts. It is the only way of covering 925 miles twice a year and paying home visits" (Matthews, 1920, p. 16). The first-hand accounts of early rural PHNs contain vivid descriptions of the various modes of transportation used in the course of their work, and the dangerous road and weather conditions in which they travelled (Colley, 1970; Giovannini, 1988; Miller, 2000; Nevitt, 1978).

In the interwar years, the development of public health services was uneven and often unsuccessful. The time available to follow up on individuals and families needing health education or preventive services was limited, and the nurses' ability to provide long-term follow-up in complex situations was significantly constrained. The need for primary care in rural and isolated areas also limited the successful establishment of public health nursing programs. Many communities wanted VNs who provided bedside nursing care, rather than PHNs who focused on health education and prevention of illness (Matthews, 1920; Stuart, 1987).

On the other hand, local physicians sometimes did not support public health programs because they feared that the PHNs would provide primary care and thus compete with them for both patients and income. It took considerable effort on the part of the nurses to assuage these concerns. Stuart (1987), in her analysis of rural public health nursing in northern Ontario, found that PHNs often avoided giving advice to families about the prevention of communicable diseases even when they knew more about immunization programs than did the local physicians. One of the strategies employed to mute the protests of local physicians was to refer all individuals found to have "abnormal" conditions to the attending physician for further follow-up, even in cases

where the nurses could have provided this care themselves (Riddell, 1991).

However, tensions surrounding which level of government should finance the public health system likely had the most negative impact on the development of PHN services in rural areas in the interwar years. For example, the nurses sent out to establish a public health system in northern Ontario were not permanently stationed in a community. Instead, they were expected to provide a short-term "demonstration" of the benefits of public health programs, then move on to another location. Should the local authorities agree that these services were necessary, the financing to continue them was to be allocated at the local level. Local authorities were often very happy to accept the services of PHNs financed by the provincial government, but reluctant to employ them out of local funds (Stuart, 1987).

Visiting Nursing in Canada

As is evident from the preceding discussion, previously private health concerns, such as TB and infant hygiene, were redefined as public health concerns in the early part of the twentieth century. In some communities, public health programs replaced services pioneered by visiting nursing organizations. In others, visiting nursing organizations either entered into contractual arrangements with local health departments to provide these services or continued to provide them on their own initiative in the absence of government action. In addition to their occasional involvement in public health programs, visiting nursing organizations also continued to fulfill their original mandate to provide bedside nursing care in the home. This section will examine the experiences and challenges of Canadian visiting nursing organizations between 1897 and 1945.

Established in 1897, the VON is Canada's only national community health nursing organization. Its capacity to respond to local needs and opportunities stemmed from its organizational structure. Local branches were established in communities that had enough volunteers to sustain the organization. They reported to the central board, located in Ottawa, which set out guiding principles for the operation of local branches. It also encouraged local branches to seize opportunities to extend their work and to demonstrate the VON's capacity to deliver the whole range of community health nursing services. Visiting nursing services were the backbone of the local branches. In most communities, bedside nursing care was provided to a full range of destitute, working-class, and middle-class families who could not afford to hire private-duty nurses. Families paid what they could for these services. The difference between the actual cost of the service and what was paid in fees was underwritten by charitable donations, fundraising, and, in some cases, grants from city or provincial governments. In this way, the local branches fulfilled a dual mandate: charitable work among the poor and the provision of affordable nursing care to the working and middle classes. The history of the VON has been documented in two monographs, one written on the occasion of its 50th anniversary (Gibbon, 1947) and one to celebrate its 100th year of service in Canada (Penney, 1996). The experience of the Winnipeg Branch of the VON will be used as a case study to illustrate how the unique characteristics of specific communities shaped the services offered by the local branches.

In Winnipeg, charitable visiting nursing was pioneered by the Margaret Scott Nursing Mission, founded in 1904 to support the charitable work that Margaret Scott had been carrying out in the immigrant districts of Winnipeg since the 1890s (MSNM Minutes, May 1904). Scott was not a nurse, but in the course of her visits she encountered many people requiring medical and nursing assistance. The Mission performed an important role in preventing the admission of indigent patients to the charity wards of the Winnipeg General Hospital, thus reducing the cost of their care for local taxpayers. In keeping with the goals of the social gospel movement and maternal feminism, the majority of the Mission's patients in the early years were children and pregnant women. After hospital-based obstetrical care became the norm even for poor women, the majority of individuals receiving services from the MSNM were elderly or chronically ill.

The incursion of the Winnipeg branch of the VON into visiting nursing in 1905 forced the two organizations to coordinate their work so that they would not duplicate services. Ultimately, they agreed that the VON would provide services to those who ". . . did not wish to be classed as charity patients & who were willing to pay moderately for the services of a nurse," while the MSNM would continue to focus its attention on Winnipeg's poor and destitute populations (MSNM Minutes, May 1910). For the first few years, the Winnipeg Branch struggled to establish a non-charitable visiting nursing program in the city and the growth of the organization was relatively slow.

However, new life was injected into the Winnipeg Branch after WWI. In 1919, a new superintendent of nurses brought fresh ideas gleaned from her extensive experience in other communities. In 1920, the local Red Cross Society provided the funds to put some of these ideas into action.

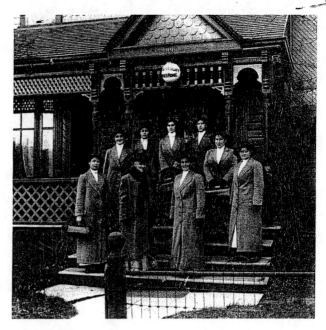

Photo 1.4

The Margaret Scott Nursing Mission provided charitable visiting nursing services to Winnipeg's poor and immigrant citizens from 1904–1943. It was located at 99 George St. on the south edge of Winnipeg's famous North End. This photograph, circa 1914, was taken just prior to the takeover of their child hygiene program by the City Health Department. Margaret Scott is front row centre.

Credit: Allan D. McKay (private collection)

Between 1919 and 1925, the Winnipeg Branch expanded its visiting nursing services into several suburbs adjacent to Winnipeg. It also established child welfare clinics, mothercraft classes, special clinics for immigrant women, and prenatal visiting in urban and suburban Winnipeg. It pioneered the use of mothers' helpers to assist mothers whose primary need was respite rather than nursing care. In addition, the Winnipeg Branch entered into agreements with two major Winnipeg employers to provide industrial (occupational health) nursing services to their employees and opened a dental clinic to provide dental care to working-class and indigent families. In 1923, they inaugurated an hourly nursing service for middle-class families who could afford to pay nurses on an hourly basis but not full-time (VON Minutes, May 1923). The enlarged scope of their programs was coordinated with other agencies such as the city and provincial PHNs, the outpatient departments of the Winnipeg General and Children's Hospitals, and the MSNM.

One very important function distinguished VNs employed by charitable organizations from publicly employed PHNs. This was the VNs' responsibility to ensure that the nursing care they provided did not **pauperize** their clients by diminishing their personal initiative and rendering them permanently dependent on the state. Because the provision of charitable health and welfare services was a responsibility of local governments and the wealthy elite (Taylor, 1987), the possibility that charitable assistance might be

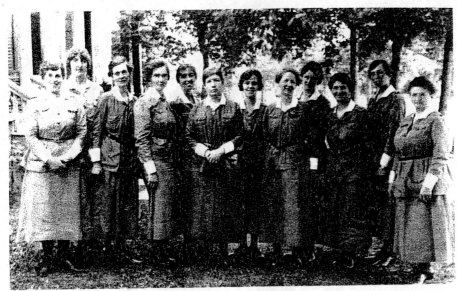

Photo 1.5

Annah L. Prichard, Distr___
Superintendent, with the nursing
the Winnipeg Branch VON. Prichard
served in this capacity between 1919 and
1925, during an era of rapid expansion of
the Winnipeg Branch.

*Credit: Victorian Order of Nurses,
Manitoba Branch Photographic
Collection*

given indiscriminately was a significant concern for its providers. Charity relieved the suffering of the poor, but it might also pauperize them. Because PHNs were paid out of public funds, they were, at least in theory, required to assist all who requested their services. Visiting nursing services, however, were at least partially funded by charitable donations. Part of their responsibility, therefore, was **investigation work**, which involved the financial assessment of the family and the determination of what portion of the cost of the nursing visit the family could afford. Paying at least part of the cost mitigated the humiliation of accepting charity and enabled families to avoid being classified as paupers. Thus, the VON's major role in their Winnipeg dental clinic was to visit the homes of the clinic patients and determine their ability to pay. In the same vein, the nurses of the Lethbridge Nursing Mission (LNM) could provide charitable assistance to destitute families in addition to providing bedside nursing care, because they had the necessary mandate and experience (Richardson, 1997). Even the MSNM encouraged its clients to pay anything, even a penny, for the services of its nurses.

By the beginning of World War II, the essential elements of community health nursing services had been put in place across the country. Provincial health departments had been organized and local health departments operated in the majority of Canadian cities. The scope of work in health education and prevention of illness had enlarged to include programs such as mental health, venereal disease control, pre-school health, and prenatal education. The VON continued to flourish by using its success in the provision of bedside nursing care in the home as a springboard to also provide public health programs in communities where local attitudes and gaps in services made this possible. The only irony was that, although it had been envisioned by its founders as a nursing service for those living in rural and isolated "country districts," the VON had attained its greatest success and stability in Canada's urban centres.

COMMUNITY HEALTH NURSING IN THE WELFARE STATE

The Political and Economic Context

Even prior to World War II, the provision of healthcare services had undergone significant change in Canada. The federal, provincial, and local governments now funded, albeit at times reluctantly, many services that had previously been the responsibility of the individual, the family, or a charitable organization. The provision of publicly funded health and social welfare programs by federal and provincial governments is known as the **welfare state.** The transition from laissez-faire government to the welfare state gained momentum during the 1930s. The Great Depression dramatically demonstrated the limited capacity of local and provincial governments to provide health and social welfare services during times of greatest need. However, the federal government's ability to intervene was limited under the provisions of the BNA Act. In 1937, the Royal Commission on Dominion-Provincial Relations was appointed to determine how federal and provincial powers might be modified to improve the social welfare of all Canadians. It tabled its report in 1940, recommending that the federal government assume responsibility for unemployment insurance and old age pensions and that the provincial governments retain responsibility for public health programs and hospital care (Owram, 1986). However, concerns about how the government could protect citizens from the economic consequences of prolonged illnesses persisted. Several private and provincial medical and hospital insurance programs evolved after World War II, but these did not provide all Canadians with equitable access to healthcare. In 1948, the federal government established health grants for a variety of health programs offered at the provincial level (Shillington, 1972). Universal insured medical and hospital services were established with the passage of the Hospital Insurance and Diagnostic Services Act in 1957 and the Medical Care Insurance Act in 1968.

However, community and public health agencies across Canada never benefited from federal legislation and funding in the same way as did the acute and long-term healthcare sector. Despite the recommendations of the 1943 Report of the Advisory Committee on Health Insurance (the Heagerty Report), the funding of the Canadian public health system remained the responsibility of local and provincial governments (Government of Canada, 1943). In many instances, provincial legislation concerning the establishment of local health units was enabling rather than mandatory. Funding to support these health units was usually obtained though cost-sharing arrangements between the local and provincial governments, with the latter providing anywhere from one-third to two-thirds of the necessary funding. In some instances, charitable organizations such as the Canadian Red Cross and the Rockefeller Foundation provided funding to establish local or provincial public health programs and/or health units (Archives of Manitoba, The Garson Papers, 1942; Baldwin, 1997; Canadian Public Health Association [CPHA], 1940; Miller, 2000). Thus, public health services were available only in communities that possessed both the interest to request them and the financial resources to fund them (CPHA, 1940; Government of Canada, 1943). Federal financial contributions to the public health system were confined to specific programs, often for specific periods of time. For example, the venereal disease campaign received federal funding between 1919 and 1932. More recently, the National Immunization Strategy, a five-year federal transfer program, was established in 2003. Despite the limited federal support for the community health sector, federal/provincial cost-sharing arrangements for the acute and long-term healthcare sector had a significant impact on the programs offered by both public health nursing and visiting nursing programs.

New Roles for Visiting Nurses: The Emergence of Home Care Programs

Publicly funded healthcare programs changed the organization and work of visiting nursing associations in several ways. First, philanthropic support of local VNAs such as the MSNM and the LNM waned. Most closed in the decade immediately following World War II, unable to sustain either their funding or the quality of their nursing programs (MSNM, 1943; Richardson, 1997).

Although the VON continued to grow during the postwar years, it was also forced to respond to the changing face of healthcare in Canada. Expanded local and provincial departments of health took over public health programs that previously had been provided by the VON (Penney, 1996). Hospital admission became the norm for most Canadians requiring obstetrical, medical, or surgical care. This development shifted the VON visiting nursing caseloads to the care of convalescent and chronically ill individuals. Further, the erosion of charitable donations, which had at least partially offset the cost of caring for the poor in the past, meant that VNs were more likely to be providing care to those who could afford to pay for these services either directly or through third-party insurance arrangements.

In the early 1970s, rising hospital costs created both an opportunity and a crisis for the VON. Patients were discharged from hospital earlier, and required longer and more complex follow-up care in the community. However, these individuals were often unable to obtain bedside nursing care in their homes during their convalescence. No publicly insured programs for home care services existed until 1974, when the first such program was established in Manitoba (Shapiro, 1997). The VON realized that participation in publicly insured home care programs was an opportunity to both consolidate and strengthen their organization. It commissioned a national report, which recommended that Canada's oldest and most experienced visiting nursing organization be given the mandate to deliver publicly insured home care programs (Pickering, 1976). However, individual provincial governments made a variety of decisions about the organization and funding of home care programs, and these did not always include the VON (Penney, 1996). Today, as it did in the past, the VON continues to function by offering a mix of services shaped by local circumstances, with a particular focus on creating programs to respond to unmet needs among specific segments of the population (Penney, 1996).

New Mandates for Public Health Nurses

Increased government responsibility for the healthcare of Canadians also had a significant impact on public health nursing. Between 1940 and 1970, health departments focused on the elaboration of existing programs. However, this process also included a general shift of emphasis from traditional programs such as child health, immunization, and communicable disease control to programs focusing on the reduction of morbidity and mortality from chronic illnesses and injuries. Early postpartum discharge programs, a modification of the traditional postpartum home visit, placed significant demands on the time and resources of PHNs. In some instances, staffing patterns in health units and community health centres were modified to provide seven-day-a-week early postpartum services to mothers and neonates.

The reduction in government spending during the 1980s and 1990s affected PHNs both directly and indirectly. Static or reduced nursing staffs decreased levels of service for many programs. Infrastructures for communicable disease control were particularly hard hit. The loss of capacity to monitor, identify, and follow up on communicable diseases has been identified as one of the major reasons for the resurgence of TB and the recent emergence of new diseases, such as AIDS, SARS, and H1N1 influenza (Garrett, 1994, 2000).

Challenges Old and New

Community health nurses have always been conscious of the impact that political, economic, and other macro systems have on individual, family, aggregate, and population health. Knowledge development in health promotion, healthy public policy, and the determinants of health enabled nurses to shape their practices in ways that sought to engage both healthcare professionals and community members in finding new and innovative ways to achieve health for all. More about these ideas and their application to the practices of community health nurses will be found in subsequent chapters of this book.

In a similar vein, working with individuals, families, and groups from diverse cultures, traditions, and languages has always been an integral part of the practices of both VNs and PHNs. Health-seeking behaviours are enmeshed in both cultural and scientific knowledge. Thus, avoiding the imposition of healthcare practices that simply reflect the beliefs and values of the dominant culture requires sensitivity, adaptability, and openness on the part of nurses who practise in their clients' homes and neighbourhoods. History provides us with many examples of well-meaning individuals and groups who failed to recognize and/or respond to the healthcare needs of specific populations in a culturally appropriate manner. Rather than creating a false sense of complacency about the progress of nursing knowledge and practices, these examples should remind today's nurses that embracing and nurturing the cultural diversity of contemporary Canadian society is both a privilege and an ongoing challenge.

SUMMARY

At the end of the twentieth century, many aspects of community health nursing had come full circle. Publicly funded home care programs have created a tremendous growth in the number of nurses working in community settings. However, the role of home care nurses, who provide bedside nursing care and health education to the sick and convalescent, is similar to that fulfilled by the VNs of the late nineteenth and early twentieth centuries. The number of PHNs, on the other hand, has remained relatively stable. Their mandate has continued to emphasize health promotion, communicable disease control, healthy child development, prevention of chronic illness, and the identification of other factors that create morbidity and mortality in the population. What has changed is their visibility. Although PHNs have worked in the community for nearly a century, their small numbers and the presence of many other community-based service providers have rendered them less visible and more likely to be overlooked by both the funders and the users of the healthcare system. The challenge for the community health nurses of the future is to regain the visibility of their predecessors and to continue to demonstrate the capacity of nurses to provide leadership in the community health systems of tomorrow.

KEY TERMS

community health nurse, p. 1
public health nurse, p. 1
home health nurse, p. 1
community-oriented nursing, p. 1
community-based nursing, p. 1
public health movement, p. 1
maternal feminist, p. 1
district nursing, p. 2
visiting nursing, p. 2
public health nursing, p. 2
social gospel movement, p. 6
pauperize, p. 10
investigation work, p. 11
welfare state, p. 11

REVIEW QUESTIONS

1. Which statement about the earliest Canadian visiting nurses is correct?
   a) They were employed by local health departments.
   b) They were employed by provincial health departments.
   c) They were employed by charitable organizations.
   d) They were self-employed.

2. In 1900, what was the leading cause of death for Canadian adults?
   a) cardiovascular disease
   b) tuberculosis
   c) typhoid fever
   d) cancer

3. What statement about early Canadian public health nurses working in urban settings is correct?
   a) They worked in specific programs such as child hygiene, TB control, or school inspection.
   b) They worked in generalist practices delivering a variety of programs to families living in a specific district of their community.
   c) They provided bedside nursing services to poor families living in the community.
   d) Their salaries were paid by charitable donations.

4. What statement about the Victorian Order of Nurses is correct?
   a) The VON was established to provide nursing care to poor people living in urban areas of Canada.
   b) The VON has never accepted charitable donations to support its programs.
   c) In many communities, the VON contracted with local and provincial governments to provide public health nursing services.
   d) The VON depended on hospital training schools to prepare their nurses for practice in the community.

5. A careful examination of the American and Canadian definitions of community nursing practice reveals both similarities and differences. Which American nurse working in the community appears to have the role the most similar to the Canadian home health nurse?
   a) public health nurse
   b) community health nurse
   c) community-oriented nurse
   d) community-based nurse

STUDY QUESTIONS

1. Describe the two forms of community health nursing that evolved in Canada in the early twentieth century.

2. What social movements supported the emergence of community health nursing?

3. Which segments of the population were the focus of early community nursing programs?

4. Briefly describe the three earliest public health programs in which nurses were involved and the reasons for their implementation.

5. How did the British North America Act (1867) and nineteenth-century beliefs about the role of government influence the development of community health services?

6. Describe the emergence of the Canadian welfare state.

7. Describe the role that non-governmental organizations, such as the VON, the Red Cross, and local philanthropic agencies, played in the development of community health nursing programs.

After working through these questions, go to the MyNursingLab at www.pearsoned.ca/mynursinglab to check your answers.

INDIVIDUAL CRITICAL THINKING EXERCISES

The sources listed at the end of each question are cited in full in either the References or the Additional Resources section of this chapter. Each source will provide additional insights into the controversies and debates surrounding the history of public health and visiting nursing.

1. Meryn Stuart (1989), in her analysis of the development of rural public health nursing in northern Ontario, states that "The Board's focus on health education, however delivered by the nurses, would not erase the effects of poverty. . . . Health education was a facile solution to the serious problem of the lack of permanent human and material resources" (p. 111). Analyze the apparent lack of congruency between the needs of the populations that public health programs served and the typical services that these programs offered. (Sources: Piva, 1979; Stuart, 1989)

2. Physicians and nurses assumed different roles in early community health organizations. What role did gender play in the assignment of these roles? (Sources: McPherson, 1996, Chapter 1; Stuart, 1992)

3. Community health nursing has frequently been described as more autonomous than nursing practice in institutional settings. However, Eunice Dyke, Toronto's first supervisor of public health nursing, once stated that ". . . public health nursing has in the medical profession its greatest friend and not infrequently its greatest stumbling block." How autonomous was the practice of early community health nurses? (Sources: Comacchio, 1993, Chapter 7; Stuart, 1992)

4. What role did middle-class ideas about class, ethnicity, and gender play in the development of public health programs to protect the health of infants and children? (Sources: Gleason, 2002; Comacchio, 1993, Chapter 3)

5. Reflect on the constraints/limits on the scope of practice of PHNs in the 1920s and '30s. Do you see any parallels in the practice of PHNs today? Are there recurring patterns, and, if so, what are they? (Sources: Stuart, 1989; 1992)

6. Examine the community-based nursing programs available in your community. What do they, as individual organizations, contribute to the practice of community health nursing? Taken as a whole, do all of these organizations cover the practice of community health nursing as discussed in this textbook?

GROUP CRITICAL THINKING EXERCISES

1. Social historians such as Alan Hunt (1999) argue that charity, philanthropy, and welfare programs are essentially efforts by the elite and middle classes to impose their behaviour, values, and culture upon others. Hunt describes these programs of moral or social regulation as being inspired by ". . . the passionate conviction that there is something inherently wrong or immoral about the conduct of others" (p. ix). Locate an issue of an early public health or nursing journal such as *The Public Health Journal* (now the *Canadian Journal of Public Health*) or *The Canadian Nurse* (particularly the section on public health). Conduct a brief content analysis of the issue, paying close attention to how the recipients of public health interventions are described. What conclusions can be drawn about the attitudes of healthcare professionals? What anxieties seem to underlie the interventions they describe and recommend to other healthcare practitioners?

2. Nurses were the intermediaries between the clients they served and the social and political elite who employed them to work in the community. However, their perspective on the objectives and effectiveness of community health programs is often absent from published histories of public health. To fill this gap in the historical record, do one of the following: 1) locate a biographical account written by an early visiting or public health nurse, 2) locate an oral history of an early visiting or public health nurse in an archive, or 3) interview a retired visiting or public health nurse. How does their account resemble and differ from the history of community health nursing presented in this chapter? How would you account for any differences you identify?

3. Based on what you have learned about the history of community health nursing in Canada, what do you believe are the greatest challenges facing nurses in this practice setting today and in the future?

PRIMARY SOURCES

Archives of Manitoba, The Garson Papers, P2357, Folder 11, Dr. Carl Buck. Notes on Meeting of Council dated January 21, 1942.

Margaret Scott Nursing Mission, Board of Management. (n.d.). *Minutes 1904–1943.* (Archives of Manitoba. MG10 B9 Box IV).

Victorian Order of Nurses for Canada, Winnipeg Branch. (n.d.). *Minutes of Board Meetings 1901–1927.*

REFERENCES

Artibise, A. F. (1975). *Winnipeg: A social history of urban growth, 1874–1914.* Montreal, QC: McGill–Queen's University Press.

Baillargeon, D. (2002). Entre la "Revanche" et la "Veillée" des berceaux: Les médecins québécois francophones, la mortalité infantile et la question nationale, 1910–40. *Canadian Bulletin of Medical History/Bulletin Canadien d'histoire de la médecine, 19*(1), 113–137.

Baldwin, D. O. (1997). *She answered every call: The life of public health nurse Mona Gordon Wilson (1894–1981).* Charlottetown, PE: Indigo Press.

Banfill, B. J. (1967). *Pioneer nurse.* Toronto, ON: Ryerson Press.

Bilson, G. (1980). *A darkened house: Cholera in nineteenth-century Canada.* Toronto, ON: University of Toronto Press.

Bliss, M. (1991). *Plague: A story of smallpox in Montreal.* Toronto, ON: HarperCollins.

Canadian Public Health Association. (1940). *The development of public health in Canada.* Toronto, ON: University of Toronto Press.

Christie, N., & Gauvreau, M. (1996). *A full-orbed Christianity: The Protestant churches and social welfare in Canada.* Toronto, ON: University of Toronto Press.

City of Winnipeg Health Department. (1910). *Annual report for the year ending December 1909.* Winnipeg, MB: City of Winnipeg.

City of Winnipeg Health Department. (1915). *Annual report for the year ending December 1914.* Winnipeg, MB: City of Winnipeg.

City of Winnipeg Health Department. (1919). *Annual report for the year ending December 1918.* Winnipeg, MB: City of Winnipeg.

Colley, K. B. (1970). *While rivers flow: Stories of early Alberta.* Saskatoon, SK: Prairie Books.

Community Health Nurses Association of Canada. (2008). *Canadian community health nursing standards of practice.* Toronto, ON: Author.

Douglas, A. J. (1912). Chairman's Address, Section of Municipal Health Officers, American Public Health Association. *American Journal of Public Health, 2*(2), 85–86.

Garrett, L. (1994). *The coming plague: Newly emerging diseases in a world out of balance.* New York, NY: Penguin Books.

Garrett, L. (2000). *Betrayal of trust: The collapse of global public health.* New York, NY: Hyperion Press.

Gibbon, J. M. (1947). *The Victorian Order of Nurses for Canada: 50th anniversary, 1897–1947.* Montreal, QC: Southam Press.

Giovannini, M. (1988). *Outport nurse.* St. John's, NL: Memorial University, Faculty of Medicine.

Government of Canada. (1943). *Report of the advisory committee on health insurance* [the Heagerty Report]. Ottawa, ON: Minister of Pensions and National Health.

Green, H. G. (1974). *Don't have your baby in the dory!: A biography of Myra Bennett.* Montreal, QC: Harvest House.

Green, M. (1984). *Through the years with public health nursing: A history of public health nursing in the provincial government jurisdiction British Columbia.* Ottawa, ON: Canadian Public Health Association.

Hope, M. E. (1955). *Lamp on the snow.* London, UK: Angus & Robertson.

Humphreys, M. (1999). Tuberculosis: The "consumption" and civilization. In K. F. Kiple (Ed.), *Plague, pox and pestilence: Disease in history* (pp. 136–141). London, UK: Phoenix Illustrated.

Hutchinson, J. F. (1996). *Champions of charity: War and the rise of the Red Cross.* Boulder, CO: Westview Press.

Kerr, J., & MacPhail, J. (1996). *An introduction to issues in community health nursing in Canada.* Toronto, ON: Mosby.

Ladd-Taylor, M. (1994). *Mother-work, women, child welfare and the state, 1890–1930.* Urbana, IL: University of Illinois Press.

Locke, H. L. F. (1918). The problem of our infant population with special reference to the opportunity of the welfare nurse. *American Journal of Nursing, 18*(7), 523–526.

MacDougall, H. (1990). *Activists and advocates: Toronto's Health Department, 1883–1983.* Toronto, ON: Dundurn Press.

MacNutt, J. S. (1913). The Board of Health nurse: What she can do for the public welfare in a small city. *American Journal of Public Health, 3*(4), 1913.

Matthews, O. (1920). Child welfare. *The Canadian Nurse, 16*(1), 15–16.

McLaren, A., & McLaren, A. T. (1997). *The bedroom and the state: The changing practices and politics of contraception and abortion in Canada, 1880–1997* (2nd ed.). Oxford, UK: Oxford University Press.

McPherson, K. (1996). *Bedside matters: The transformation of Canadian nursing, 1900–1990.* Toronto, ON: Oxford University Press.

Meigs, G. L. (1916, August). Other factors in infant mortality than the milk supply and their control. *American Journal of Public Health, 6,* 847–853.

Merkley, P. (1987). The vision of the good society in the social gospel: What, where and when is the kingdom of God? *Historical Papers: Canadian Historical Association,* pp. 138–145.

Miller, G. L. (2000). *Mustard plasters and handcars: Through the eyes of a Red Cross outpost nurse.* Toronto, ON: Natural Heritage/Natural History.

Nevitt, J. (1978). *White caps and black bands: Nursing in Newfoundland to 1934*. St. John's, NL: Jefferson Press.

Owram, D. (1986). *The government generation: Canadian intellectuals and the state, 1900–1945*. Toronto, ON: University of Toronto Press.

Peikoff, T., & Brickey, S. (1991). Creating precious children and glorified mothers: A theoretical assessment of the transformation of childhood. In R. Smandych, G. Dodds, & A. Esau (Eds.), *Dimensions of childhood: Essays on the history of children and youth in Canada* (pp. 29–61). Winnipeg, MB: Legal Research Institute of the University of Manitoba.

Penney, S. (1996). *A century of caring: The history of the Victorian Order of Nurses for Canada*. Ottawa, ON: Victorian Order of Nurses for Canada.

Pickering, E. A. (1976). *A case for the VON in home care*. Ottawa, ON: Victorian Order of Nurses for Canada.

Piva, M. J. (1979). *The condition of the working class in Toronto, 1900–1921*. Ottawa, ON: University of Ottawa Press.

Richardson, S. (1997). Women's enterprise: Establishing the Lethbridge Nursing Mission, 1909–1919. *Nursing History Review, 5*, 105–30.

Riddell, S. E. (1991). *Curing society's ills: Public health nurses and public health nursing in rural British Columbia, 1916–1946*. Unpublished master's thesis, Simon Fraser University, Vancouver, BC.

Roberts, J. (1928). Twenty-three years of public health. *The Public Health Journal, 19*, 554.

Royce, M. (1983). *Eunice Dyke: Health care pioneer: From pioneer public health nurse to advocate for the aged*. Toronto, ON: Dundurn Press.

Sears, A. (1995). Before the welfare state: Public health and social policy. *Canadian Review of Sociology and Anthropology/ Revue canadienne de sociologie et d'anthropologie, 32*(2), 169–188.

Shapiro, E. (1997). *The cost of privatization: A case study of home care in Manitoba*. Ottawa, ON: Canadian Centre for Policy Alternatives.

Shillington, C. H. (1972). *The road to medicare in Canada*. Toronto, ON: Del Graphics.

Stanhope, M., & Lancaster, J. (2006). *Foundations of nursing in the community: Community-oriented practice* (2nd ed.). St. Louis, MO: Mosby Elsevier.

Stuart, M. E. (1987). *"Let not the people perish for lack of knowledge": Public health nursing and the Ontario rural child welfare project, 1916–1930*. Unpublished doctoral dissertation, University of Pennsylvania, Philadelphia, PA.

Sutherland, N. (1981). "To create a strong and healthy race": School children in the public health movement, 1880–1914. In S. E. D. Shortt (Ed.), *Medicine in Canadian society: Historical perspectives* (pp. 361–393). Montreal, QC: McGill–Queen's University Press.

Taylor, M. G. (1987). *Health insurance and Canadian public policy*. Montreal, QC: McGill–Queen's University Press.

Zilm, G., & Warbinek, E. (1995). Early tuberculosis nursing in British Columbia. *The Canadian Journal of Nursing Research, 27*(3), 65–81.

ADDITIONAL READINGS

Monographs and Articles

Buhler-Wilkerson, K. (1989). *False dawn: The rise and decline of public health nursing, 1900–1930*. New York, NY: Garland.

Buhler-Wilkerson, K. (2001). *No place like home: A history of nursing and home care in the United States*. Baltimore, MD: Johns Hopkins University Press.

Comacchio, C. (1993). *Nations are built of babies: Saving Ontario's mothers and children 1900–1940*. Montreal, QC: McGill–Queen's University Press.

Copp, T. (1981). Public health in Montreal, 1870–1930. In S. E. D. Shortt (Ed.), *Medicine in Canadian society: Historical perspectives* (pp. 395–416). Montreal, QC: McGill–Queen's University Press.

Gleason, M. (2002). Race, class and health: School medical inspection and "healthy" children in British Columbia, 1890–1930. *Canadian Bulletin of Medical History/Bulletin Canadien d'histoire de la médecine, 19*(1), 95–112.

Hunt, A. (1999). *Governing morals: A social history of moral regulation*. Cambridge, UK: Cambridge University Press.

Stuart, M. (1989). Ideology and experience: Public health nursing and the Ontario Rural Child Welfare Project, 1920–25. *Canadian Bulletin of Medical History/Bulletin Canadien d'histoire de la médecine, 6*, 111–131.

Stuart, M. (1992). "Half a loaf is better than no bread": Public health nurses and physicians in Ontario, 1920–1925. *Nursing Research, 41*(1), 21–27.

FURTHER READING

A comprehensive synthesis of the history of community health nursing in Canada has never been written. This chapter does not fill that gap. It focuses almost exclusively on the work of "trained nurses" and their work in formal community health programs, both of which originated in the late nineteenth century. While facilitating a thematic approach to the subject, this approach also has limitations. It omits the significant contributions of lay and religious women who visited and cared for the sick in their homes from the time that the first European settlers arrived in Canada. The contributions of national and regional community nursing organizations such as the VON, the Saint Elizabeth Visiting Nurses' Association of Ontario, and the Lethbridge Nursing Mission receive limited attention. The chapter also does not discuss in any detail the experiences and practices of outpost nurses working with, for example, the Canadian Red Cross, the Grenfell Mission (Labrador), le service médical aux colons (Quebec), and Alberta's District Nursing Service. Although the influence of maternal feminist lay women is discussed in some detail in this chapter, the role of other non-governmental groups instrumental in the establishment of community and public health nursing is not discussed in any detail. For example, both the Red Cross and the Rockefeller Foundation funded demonstration projects in public health nursing in several

Canadian provinces. These programs were eventually integrated into provincial public health systems.

This chapter is also limited by the existing historiography. Most of the existing monographs and articles focus on the development of public health and community health nursing programs prior to 1970. This is not entirely unexpected. For many historians, more recent developments are not yet history. More recent developments in public health nursing await historical analysis. Finally, the historiography of community health nursing in Canada is unevenly developed. Some provinces and regions have been blessed with historians who have written extensively on the subject. Others have not. The following bibliography provides further resources for those interested in learning more about the history of community health nursing in Canada, particularly those aspects of the subject that are not adequately discussed in the chapter itself.

Canada

Allemang, M. (2000). Development of community health nursing in Canada. In M. Stewart (Ed.), *Community health nursing in Canada* (2nd ed.) (pp. 3-29). Toronto, ON: W. B. Saunders.

Arnup, M. K. (1991). *Education for motherhood: Women and the family in twentieth century English Canada.* Unpublished doctoral dissertation, University of Toronto.

Bates, C., Dodd, D., & Rousseau, N. (2005). *On all frontiers: Four centuries of Canadian nursing.* Ottawa, ON: University of Ottawa Press.

Buckley, S., & McGinnis, J. D. (1982). Venereal disease and public health reform in Canada. *Canadian Historical Review, 63*(3), 337–354.

Dodd, D. (1991). Advice to parents: The Blue Books, Helen MacMurchy, MD, and the Federal Department of Health, 1920–34. *Canadian Bulletin of Medical History, 8*(2), 203–230.

Duncan, S. M., Leipert, B. D., & Mill, J. E. (1999). Nurses as health evangelists?: The evolution of public health nursing in Canada, 1918–1939. *Advances in Nursing Science, 22*(1), 40–51.

Emory, F. H. M. (1953). *Public health nursing in Canada.* Toronto, ON: Macmillan.

Harrison, H. E. (2001). *"In the picture of health": Portraits of health, disease and citizenship in Canada's public health advice literature, 1920–1960.* Unpublished doctoral dissertation, Queen's University, Kingston, ON.

Lewis, J. (1986). The prevention of diphtheria in Canada and Britain 1914–1945. *Journal of Social History, 20*(1), 163–176.

McCuaig, K. (1999). *The weariness, the fever, and the fret: The campaign against tuberculosis in Canada, 1900–1950.* Montreal, QC: McGill–Queen's University Press.

McKay, M. (2009). Public health nursing in early 20th century Canada. *Canadian Journal of Public Health, 100*(4), 249–250.

Nesmith, T. (1985). The early years of public health: The Department of Agriculture, 1867–1918. *Archivist, 12*(5), 1–3.

Newfoundland

House, E. (1990). *The way out: The story of NONIA, 1920–1990.* St. John's, NL: Creative Publishers.

Neary, P. (1998). "And gave just as much as they got": A 1941 American perspective on public health in Newfoundland. *Newfoundland and Labrador Studies, 14*(1), 50–70.

Neary, P. (1998). Venereal disease and public health administration in Newfoundland in the 1930s and 1940s. *Canadian Bulletin of Medical History, 15*(1), 129–151.

Nova Scotia

Farley, J. (2002). The Halifax diphtheria epidemic (1940 to 1944): A disaster waiting to happen or a blessing in disguise? *Journal of the Royal Nova Scotia Historical Society, 5*, 44–63.

Gregor, F. (2004). Mapping the demise of the St John Ambulance Home Nursing Program in Nova Scotia, 1950–1975. *Canadian Bulletin of Medical History, 21*(2), 351–375.

Gregor, F. (2005). "Home nursing has continued to present problems": The St. John Ambulance Home Nursing Program in Nova Scotia. In J. Fingard & J. Guildford (Eds.), *Mothers of the municipality: Women, work, and social policy in post 1945 Halifax* (pp. 226–252). Toronto, ON: Toronto University Press.

Penney, S. (1990). *Inventing the cure: Tuberculosis in twentieth century Nova Scotia* (Unpublished doctoral dissertation). Dalhousie University, Halifax.

Twohig, P. (2001). Public health in industrial Cape Breton, 1900–1930s. *Journal of the Royal Nova Scotia Historical Society, 4*, 108–131.

Twohig, P. (2005). The Rockefellers, the Cape Breton Island Health Unit and public health in Nova Scotia. *Journal of the Royal Nova Scotia Historical Society, 5*, 122–133.

Prince Edward Island

Baldwin, D. (1990). The volunteers in action: The establishment of government health care on Prince Edward Island, 1900–1931. *Acadiensis, 19*(2), 121–147.

Baldwin, D. (1993). Amy MacMahon and the struggle for public health. *Island Magazine, 34*, 20–27.

Baldwin, D. (1995). Interconnecting the personal and public: The support networks of Public Health Nurse Mona Wilson. *Canadian Journal of Nursing Research, 27*(3), 19–37.

Beck, B., & Townshend, A. (1993). The Island's Florence Nightingale. *Island Magazine, 34*, 16.

Lanigan, H., & Beck, B. (2005). The great white plague: Tuberculosis on Prince Edward Island. *Island Magazine, 57*, 22–29.

Palmer, D. (2005). Public health nursing on Prince Edward Island in the 1930s. *Island Magazine 57*, 30–33.

Quebec

Baillargeon, D. (1993). Les infirmières de la Métropolitaine au service des Montréalaises. In Les bâtisseuses de la cité, Actes du colloque "Les bâtisseuses de la cité," Section d'études féministes, congrès de l'Acfas, Montréal, ACFAS, *Les cahiers scientifiques* no. 79, 1993, pp. 107–120.

Baillargeon, D. (1996). Fréquenter les gouttes de lait: L'expérience des mères Montréalaises, 1910–65. *Revue d'Histoire de l'Amérique Française, 50*(1), 29–68.

Baillargeon, D. (1998). Gouttes de lait et soif de pouvoir. Les dessous de la lutte contre la mortalité infantile à Montréal, 1910–1953. *Canadian Bulletin of Medical History, 15*(1), 27–57.

Baillargeon, D. (2002). Care of mothers and infants in Montreal between the wars: The visiting children's nurses of the Metropolitan Life, milk deposits and maternal assistance. In M. D. Behiels (Ed.), *Quebec since 1800: Selected reading* (pp. 93–209). Toronto, ON: Irwin.

Braithwaite, C., Keating, P., & Viger, S. (1996). The problem of diphtheria in the Province of Quebec: 1894–1909. *Histoire Sociale, 29*(57): 71–95.

Cohen, Y. (2004). Rapports de genre, de classe et d'ethnicité: l'Histoire des infirmières au Québec. *Canadian Bulletin of Medical History, 21*(2), 387–409.

Cohen, Y., & Gélinas, M. (1989). Les infirmières hygiénistes de la Ville de Montréal: Du service privé au service civique. *Histoire Sociale, 22*(44), 219–246.

Copp, T. (1981). Public health in Montreal, 1870–1930. In S. E. D. Shortt (Ed.), *Medicine in Canadian society: Historical perspectives* (pp. 395–416). Montreal, QC: McGill–Queen's University Press.

Daigle, J. (2007). The call of the north: Settlement nurses in the remote areas of Québec. In J. Elliott, M. Stuart, & C. Toman (Eds.), *Place and practice in Canadian nursing history* (pp. 111–136). Vancouver, BC: UBC Press.

Daigle, J., & Rousseau, N. (1998). Le service médical aux colons: Gestation et implantation d'un service infirmier au Québec (1932–1943). *Revue d'Histoire de l'Amérique Française, 52*(1), 47–72.

Desrosiers, G., Gaumer, B., & Keel, O. (1998). *La santé publique au Québec: Histoire des unités sanitaires de comté: 1926–1975.* Montreal, QC: University of Montreal Press.

Gagnon, F. (1994). *État, médecine et santé communautaire au Québec (1970–1988): La construction d'un discours* (Unpublished doctoral dissertation). University of Laval, Quebec City.

Gaumer, B., Desrosiers, G., & Keel, O. (2002). *Histoire du Service de Santé de la Ville de Montréal, 1865–1975.* Sainte-Foy, QC: University of Laval Press.

Goulet, D., Lemire, G., & Gauvreau, D. (1996). Des bureaux d'hygiène municipaux aux unités sanitaires le conseil d'hygiène de la province de Québec et la structuration d'un système de santé publique, 1886–1926. *Revue d'Histoire de l'Amérique Française, 49*(4), 491–520.

Guérard, F. (1996). L'hygiène publique au Québec de 1887 à 1939: Centralisation, normalisation et médicalisation. *Recherches Sociographiques, 37*(2), 203–227.

Guillaume, P. (1990). Épiscopat Québecois et santé publique dans la deuxième moitié du XIXe siècle. *Revue d'Histoire Moderne et Contemporaine, 37*(Apr–June), 324–336.

Merrick, E., Daigle, J., Rousseau, N., & Saillant, F. (1993). Des traces sur la neige: La contribution des infirmières au

développpment des régions isolées du Québec au XXe siècle. *Recherches feminists, 6*(1), 93–103.

Rousseau, N., & Daigle, J. (2000). Medical service to settlers: The gestation and establishment of a nursing service in Quebec, 1932–1943. *Nursing History Review, 8,* 95–116.

Ontario

Bator, P. (1979*). "Saving lives on the wholesale plan": Public health reform in the City of Toronto, 1900–1930* (Unpublished doctoral dissertation). University of Toronto, Toronto.

Comacchio, C. (1988). "The mothers of the land must suffer": Child and maternal welfare in rural and outpost Ontario, 1918–1940. *Ontario History, 80*(3), 183–205.

Comacchio, C. (1993). *Nations are built of babies: Saving Ontario's mothers and children 1900–1940.* Montreal, QC: McGill–Queen's University Press.

Dehli, K. (1990). Health scouts for the state? School and public health nurses in early twentieth-century Toronto. *Historical Studies in Education, 2*(2), 247–264.

Dodd, D. (2001). Helen MacMurchy, MD: Gender and professional conflict in the medical inspection of Toronto schools, 1910–1911. *Ontario History, 93*(2), 127–149.

Gagan, R. (1989). Mortality patterns and public health in Hamilton, Canada, 1900–14. *Urban History Review, 17*(3), 161–175.

Rafael, A. R. F. (1999). The politics of health promotion: Influences on public health in Ontario, Canada from Nightingale to the nineties. *Advances in Nursing Science, 22*(1), 23–39.

Risk, M. (1973). *The origins and development of public health nursing in Toronto, 1890–1973* (Master's thesis). University of Toronto, Toronto.

Stuart, M. (1989). Ideology and experience: Public health nursing and the Ontario Rural Child Welfare Project, 1920–25. *Canadian Bulletin of Medical History, 6*(2), 111–131.

Stuart, M. (1992). "Half a loaf is better than no bread": Public health nurses and physicians in Ontario, 1920–1925. *Nursing Research, 41*(1), 21–27.

Stuart, M. (1994). Shifting professional boundaries: Gender conflict in public health 1920–1925. In D. Dodd & D. Gorham (Eds.), *Caring and curing: Historical perspectives on women and healing in Canada* (pp. 49–70). Ottawa, ON: University of Ottawa Press.

The Prairies

Bramadat, I., & Saydak, M. (1993). Nursing on the Canadian Prairies, 1900–1930: Effects of Immigration. *Nursing History Review, 1,* 105–117.

Burnett, K. (2008). The healing work of Aboriginal women in indigenous and newcomer communities. In J. Elliott, M. Stuart, & C. Toman (Eds.), *Place and practice in Canadian nursing history* (pp. 40–52). Vancouver, BC: UBC Press.

Kozak, N. (2005). Advice ideals and rural prairie realities: National prairie scientific motherhood advice, 1920–1929. *Unsettled pasts: Reconceiving the West through women's history.* Calgary, MB: University of Calgary Press.

Manitoba

Jones, E. (2007). *Influenza 1918: Disease, death, and struggle in Winnipeg*. Toronto, ON: University of Toronto Press.

McKay, M. (2008). Region, faith, and health: The development of Winnipeg's visiting nursing agencies, 1897–1926. In J. Elliott, M. Stuart & C. Toman (Eds.), *Place and practice in Canadian nursing history* (pp. 70–90). Vancouver, BC: UBC Press.

McPherson, K. (2003). Nursing and colonization: The work of Indian Health Service Nurses in Manitoba, 1945–1970. In G. Fedlberg, M. Ladd-Taylor, A. Li, & K. McPherson (Eds.), *Women, health, and nation: Canada and the United States since 1945* (pp. 223–246). Montreal, QC: McGill–Queen's University Press.

Miller, T. (2009). "All our friends and patients know us": The Margaret Scott Nursing Mission. In E. Jones & G. Friesen (Eds.), *Prairie metropolis: New essays on Winnipeg social history* (pp. 82–100). Winnipeg, MB: University of Manitoba Press.

Saskatchewan

Drees, L. M., & McBain, L. (2001). Nursing and Native peoples in Northern Saskatchewan: 1930s–1950s. *Canadian Bulletin of Medical History, 18*(1), 43–65.

Lux, M. (1997). "The Bitter Flats": The 1918 influenza epidemic in Saskatchewan. *Saskatchewan History, 49*(1), 313.

Alberta

Gahagan, A. C. (1979). *Yes father: Pioneer nursing in Alberta*. Manchester, NH: Hammer Publications.

Richardson, S. (1998). Frontier health care: Alberta's District Nursing Service. *Alberta History, 46*(1), 2–9.

Richardson, S. (1998). Political women, professional nurses, and the creation of Alberta's District Nursing Service, 1919–1925. *Nursing History Review, 6*, 25–50.

Richardson, S. (2002). Alberta's provincial travelling clinic. *Canadian Bulletin of Medical History, 19*(1), 245–263.

Stewart, I. (1979). *These were our yesterdays: A history of district nursing in Alberta*. Altona, MB: D. W. Friesen and Sons.

British Columbia

Davies, M. (2005). Night soil, cesspools, and smelly hogs on the streets: Sanitation, race, and governance in early British Columbia. *Histoire Sociale, 38*(75), 135.

Gleason, M. (2002). Race, class, and health: School medical inspection and "healthy" children in British Columbia, 1890 to 1930. *Canadian Bulletin of Medical History, 19*(1), 95–112.

Hayes, M., & Foster, L. (2002). Too small to see, Too big to ignore: Child health and wellbeing in British Columbia. *Canadian Western Geographical Series*, no. 35. Victoria, BC: Western Geographical Press.

Territories/Yukon

Crnkovich, Mary (Ed.). (1990). *Gossip: A spoken history of women in the North*. Ottawa, ON: Canadian Arctic Resources Committee.

Goodwill, J. (1984). Nursing Canada's Indigenous People. *Canadian Nurse, 80*(1), 6.

Goodwill, J. (1988). Indian and Inuit Nurses of Canada. *Saskatchewan Indian Federated College Journal, 4*(1), 93–104.

Rutherdale, M. (2008). Cleaners, cautious caregivers, and optimistic adventurers: A proposed typology of Arctic Canadian nurses. In J. Elliott, M. Stuart, & C. Toman (Eds.), *Place and practice in Canadian nursing history* (pp. 53–69). Vancouver, BC: UBC Press.

Scott, J. K., with Kieser, J. E. (Ed.). (2002). *Northern nurses: True nursing adventures from Canada's North*. Oakville, ON: Kokum Publications.

Zelmanovits, J. (2003). "Midwife preferred": Maternity care in outpost nursing stations in Northern Canada, 1945–1988. In G. Fedlberg, M. Ladd-Taylor, A. Li, & K. McPherson (Eds.), *Women, health, and nation: Canada and the United States since 1945* (pp. 161–188). Montreal, QC: McGill–Queen's University Press.

VOLUNTARY ORGANIZATIONS

Canadian Red Cross

Elliott, J. (2004). Blurring the boundaries of space: Shaping nursing lives at the Red Cross outposts in Ontario, 1922–1945. *Canadian Bulletin of Medical History, 21*(2), 303–325.

Elliott, J. (2004). *"Keep the flag flying": Medical outposts and the Red Cross in Northern Ontario, 1922–1984* (Unpublished doctoral dissertation). Queen's University, Kingston.

Elliott, J. (2007). (Re)constructing the identity of a Red Cross outpost nurse: The letters of Louise de Kirline. In J. Elliott, M. Stuart, & C. Toman (Eds.), *Place and practice in Canadian nursing history* (pp. 136–152). Vancouver, BC: UBC Press.

Massie, M. (2004). Ruth Dulmage Shewchuk: A Saskatchewan Red Cross outpost nurse. *Saskatchewan History, 56*(2), 35–44.

Perry, A. A. (1930). Guarding settlers on outposts of North: How railway Red Cross hospitals and hospital car on Canadian National System watch over welfare of pioneer families. *Canadian National Railways Magazine, 16*(89), 33.

Quiney, L. (2007). "Suitable young women": Red Cross Nursing pioneers and the crusade for healthy living in Manitoba, 1920–1930. In J. Elliott, M. Stuart, & C. Toman (Eds.), *Place and practice in Canadian nursing history* (pp. 91–110). Vancouver, BC: UBC Press.

Sheehan, N. (1987). The Red Cross and relief in Alberta, 1920s–1930s. *Prairie Forum, 12*(2), 277–293.

Grenfell Mission

Bulgin, I. (2001). *Mapping the self in the utmost purple rim: Published Labrador memoirs of four Grenfell nurses* (Unpublished doctoral dissertation). Memorial University, St. John's.

Coombs, H. (2004). "I guess I should have been a suffragette!!!!": A profile of Lesley Diack, nurse with the Grenfell Mission, 1950–1988. *Newfoundland Quarterly, 97*(2), 28–32.

Diack, L. (1963). *Labrador nurse.* London, UK: Victor Gollancz.

Merrick, E. (1942). *Northern nurse.* New York, NY: Charles Scribner's Sons.

Perry, J. (1997). *Nursing for the Grenfell Mission: Maternal and moral reform in Northern Newfoundland and Labrador, 1894–1938* (Unpublished M.A. thesis). Memorial University, St. John's.

Victorian Order of Nurses for Canada

Bienvenue, L. (1998). Le Victorian Order of Nursing dans la croisade hygiéniste Montréalaise, 1897–1925. *Bulletin d'Histoire Politique, 6*(2), 64–73.

Boutilier, B. (1994). *Gender, organized women, and the politics of institution building: Founding the Victorian Order of Nurses for Canada, 1893–1900* (Unpublished doctoral dissertation). Carlton University, Ottawa.

MacDonald, C. (1997). From founding to frontier: The VON in the Klondike. *Beaver, 77*(5), 13–18.

Religious Groups

Duchaussois, P. (1919). *The Grey Nuns in the far North (1867–1919).* Toronto, ON: McClelland & Stewart.

Mitchell, E. (c.1987). *The Grey Nuns of Montréal at the Red River, 1844–1984.* Winnipeg[?], MB: Publisher unknown.

Paul, P. (1994). The contribution of the Grey Nuns to the development of nursing in Canada: Historiographical issues. *Canadian Bulletin of Medical History, 11*(1), 207–217.

WEBSITES

American Association for the History of Nursing
http://www.aahn.org

AMS Nursing History Research Unit
http://www.health.uottawa.ca/nursinghistory/

B.C. History of Nursing Group
http://www.bcnursinghistory.ca/cmss/

Canadian Association for the History of Nursing
http://www.cahn-achn.ca

College & Association of Registered Nurses of Alberta
http://www.nurses.ab.ca/museum/intro.html

Margaret M. Allemang Centre for the History of Nursing
http://www.allemang.on.ca

Nurses Association of New Brunswick
http://www.nanb.nb.ca

United Kingdom Centre for the History of Nursing
http://www.ukchnm.org

About the Author

Marion McKay, RN, PhD, holds a bachelor's and master's degree in nursing and an MA and PhD in history. She recently completed two SSHRC research projects, one exploring contemporary PHNs' experiences in working with families living in poverty, and the other exploring how nurses and their work contributed to changing notions of health, citizenship, and national belonging in Canada. Prior to joining the Faculty of Nursing at the University of Manitoba, she worked for several years as a public health nurse.

The author acknowledges with deep gratitude the assistance and advice of several valued colleagues and friends, including Meryn Stuart, Nicole Rousseau, Janet Beaton, Benita Cohen, and Sandra Gessler. Special thanks to Ulysses Lahaie, who translated several articles written in French and got hooked on nursing history in the process. Thank you also to the anonymous reviewers whose comments did much to improve previous drafts of this chapter. A SSHRC Doctoral Fellowship supported the research necessary for the preparation of this manuscript and is acknowledged with thanks.

Financing, Policy, and Politics of Healthcare Delivery

Claire Betker and Diane Bewick

OBJECTIVES

After studying this chapter, you should be able to:

1. Summarize milestones in the development of the Canadian healthcare system with a focus on community health.
2. Identify federal, provincial, regional, and municipal responsibilities for the delivery of healthcare in Canada.
3. Examine delivery models and funding mechanisms for healthcare in Canada, specifically those that apply to community healthcare.
4. Critique the leadership role individual nurses and organizations play in ensuring the quality of care provided in the community.
5. Examine the leadership role of the Community Health Nurse (CHN) within the current Canadian healthcare system.

INTRODUCTION

To many Canadians, the Canada Health Act provides for a healthcare system that contributes to how we define our country. The **Canada Health Act** is the legislation that is held up as symbolizing the values that represent Canada and articulating a social contract that defines healthcare as a basic right (Auditor General of Canada, 2002, p. 13). Evolving from the traditions of the religious orders that first provided healthcare in Canada, the Canadian healthcare system, or **Medicare**, reflects the values of social justice, equity, and community. A Community Health Nurse's (CHN's) professional practice occurs in a wide variety of settings within the healthcare system. In their professional practice, CHNs are "accountable to a variety of authorities and stakeholders; the public, the regulatory body, and the employer; and are governed by legislative and policy mandates from multiple sources both internal and external to their employment situation" (Meagher-Stewart et al., 2004, p. 3). The structure, process, and **leadership** within the organizations and agencies in which CHNs work affects their practice; enabling and constraining it through its funding, governance, values, policies, goals, and standards (Gannon et al., 2010; Meagher-Stewart et al., 2004; Underwood et al., 2009b).

Almost every day, reports in the media suggest that healthcare in Canada is in crisis, that spending is out of control, wait times are unreasonable, and that substantive changes are needed to ensure sustainability. At the same time, there has been a repetitive chorus regarding the significance of health promotion and prevention as well as the critical role of public and community health. It is important for CHNs to understand how Canada's healthcare system evolved and what factors influence healthcare reform. The impact of leadership at all levels has been identified as a particularly significant factor in the evolution of the healthcare system, and in supporting community health nursing practice across the country. Throughout this evolution, CHN practice has changed. The last section of this chapter will outline key concerns nationally for CHNs at this time in history.

BIRTH OF CANADIAN MEDICARE

Although the 1867 Constitution Act (also known as the British North America Act) did not explicitly assign responsibility for health policy to either the federal or provincial governments, both have been involved in ensuring the availability of and funding for health services. With only a few exceptions, such as the direct health services provided by the federal government to Aboriginal populations, veterans, and military personnel, provincial governments have assumed responsibility for the delivery of healthcare. However, funding for healthcare is another matter. The Canadian Constitution contains an equalization clause requiring provinces to provide "reasonably comparable levels of public service for reasonably comparable levels of taxation" (Sullivan & Baranek, 2002, p. 21). Because provincial and territorial wealth varies considerably, the federal government's involvement has been necessary to equalize services across provinces and territories. Since 1957, the federal government has done that in two ways: first by contributing money (in effect, transferring money from wealthier to poorer provinces and territories), and second by stipulating specific conditions the provinces and territories must meet in order to receive that money.

In 1919, access to medical care was of sufficient concern that the Liberal party included national health insurance as part of its platform (Rachlis & Kushner, 1994). Provincial objections to federal involvement in healthcare thwarted early attempts to implement national insurance for both hospital and physicians' services. As a result, the first universal health insurance program was actually implemented at a provincial level. In Saskatchewan, in 1947, Tommy Douglas and the Cooperative Commonwealth Federation (CCF) party introduced legislation to institute Medicare. Tommy Douglas is still referred to as the Father of Medicare. It was not until 10 years later, in 1957 that similar legislation, the Hospital Insurance and Diagnostic Services Act (HIDS), was passed by the federal government (Rachlis & Kushner, 1994).

The Hospital Insurance and Diagnostic Services Act (HIDS) provided financial incentives for the provinces to establish hospital insurance plans. The federal government would pay half the costs if the insurance plans met five key criteria. Those criteria, still the legal cornerstone of Medicare, include comprehensiveness, accessibility, universality of coverage, public administration, and portability of benefits. The incentive provided the needed motivation for the provinces to participate, resulting in rapid expansion of cost-shared institutional care. However, the development of programs that focused on health promotion, prevention, and home care support was neglected.

In 1962, Saskatchewan again led the country with legislation providing universal, **publicly funded** medical insurance. In 1966, the federal government followed suit with the passage of the National Medical Care Insurance Act (Medicare). This act, enshrining the right of Canadians to physicians' services, stipulated that the same five principles as required by the HIDS Act were necessary to ensure the federal government's payment of 50% of provincial healthcare costs. The act was passed in 1968, and by 1971 all provinces were fully participating (Rachlis & Kuschner, 1994).

The 50/50 cost-sharing relationship strained the federal budget (Rafael, 1997) and as a result, in 1977, the federal government passed the Established Programs Financing Act (EPF), which changed the federal share of health costs from a 50/50 cost-sharing to per capita block grants. This federal funding contribution decreased several times over the next 20 years (Begin, 1988). The changes also have represented decreased federal involvement in healthcare.

Soon after the passage of the Established Programs Financing Act, Monique Begin was appointed federal Minister of Health and Welfare (Begin, 2002). She quickly became aware that extra-billing by physicians and user fees by provincial institutions were rising dramatically. Begin believed the extra-billing and user-fee trends posed a serious threat to

Medicare and so on December 12, 1983, she introduced to parliament Bill C-3, the Canada Health Act.

Passage of the Canada Health Act (CHA) in April 1984 was a proud moment in Canadian nursing history. Mme Begin faced tough opposition to the Act from lobby groups, opposition parties, and even from members of the Liberal cabinet (Begin, 2002). Intense lobbying and support by the Canadian Nurses Association was instrumental in the bill being passed. In the words of Begin: "Nursing became a big player during the Canada Health Act. They made the difference; it's as simple as that" (Rafael, 1997). This invaluable support by Canadian nurses was acknowledged by the Honorable Monique Begin at the Canadian Public Health Association (CPHA) conference in Toronto in June 2010. She noted that not only were nurses instrumental in passing the Canada Health Act into law, but they were also successful in amending it. As it was introduced into Parliament in 1983, Bill C-3 identified only physicians as providers of insurable services. The Canadian Nurses Association amendment changed the language to include other healthcare workers as potential providers of insurable services (Mussallem, 1992). Under the Canada Health Act, federal funding for essential medical services would continue so long as the provinces' health insurance plans met the criteria of being **publicly administered** (administered by a public authority accountable to the provincial government); **comprehensive** (must cover necessary in-hospital, medical, and surgical–dental services); **universal** (100% of residents must be covered); **portable** (available after a maximum of three months of residency and no extra charge for care out of province); and **accessible** (no user fees and healthcare providers must be reimbursed adequately). The Canada Health Act is significant in ensuring that Canadians have access to healthcare regardless of their ability to pay or where they live. However, the Canada Health Act identified only essential medical and hospital services as those qualifying for federal cost-sharing. Health promotion, prevention of disease and injury, health protection, and home health were not emphasized. More than 25 years later, this focus remains. Tommy Douglas envisioned a second more ambitious phase to Medicare—one with a focus to keep people well—as he understood that illness prevention and improved health were essential to controlling healthcare costs (Campbell & Marchildon, 2007). This requires shifting focus from individual conditions and behaviour to the social and economic **determinants of health** such as poverty, hunger, and inadequate housing (McBane, 2004). In October 2006, CNA again spoke up with the then-president, Dr. Marlene Smadu, presenting *A Healthy Nation Is a Wealthy Nation* to the House of Commons Standing Committee on Finance. This paper outlined the position of nurses in Canada that health promotion, funding for the determinants of health, and support for control of drug costs were as important considerations as wait times and fears about financial sustainability (CNA, 2006).

The Established Programs Financing Act continued until 1996 to be the **financing** mechanism for transferring money from federal to provincial governments for healthcare. At that time, the EPF and the existing payment plan for welfare, the

TABLE 2.1 Comparisons of Health Outcomes by Country

	Infant Mortality Rate/1000			Life Expectancy at Birth in Years: Females			Life Expectancy at Birth in Years: Males		
	1970	2000	2008	1970	2000	2008	1970	2000	2008
Australia	17.9	5.1	4.1	74.2	82.0	83.7	67.4	76.6	79.2
Canada	18.8	5.3	5.1*	75.2	81.7	83.0	68.8	76.3	77.1
Germany	22.5	4.4	3.5	73.6	81.2	82.7	67.5	75.1	77.6
Japan	13.1	3.2	2.6	74.7	84.6	86.1	69.3	77.7	79.3
New Zealand	16.7	6.3	4.9	74.5	80.8	82.4	68.4	75.9	78.4
Sweden	11.0	3.4	2.5	77.1	82.0	83.2	72.2	77.4	79.1
United Kingdom	18.5	5.6	4.7	75.0	80.3	81.8	68.7	75.5	77.6
United States	20.0	6.9	6.7**	74.7	79.3	80.4	67.1	74.1	75.3

*2007 & **2006 figures; 2008 data not available.
Source: Data based on OECD (2010), OECD Health Data 2010: Statistics and Indicators, http://www.oecd.org/health/healthdata

Canada Assistance Plan (CAP), were replaced by the Canada Health and Social Transfer (CHST) block fund, which included federal transfer payments for health, post-secondary education, and welfare (Sullivan & Baranek, 2002). **Allocations** or transfers of funds to provinces and territories continued in the same proportion as the previous combined EPF and CAP entitlements. As a result of cuts in federal funding, fiscal constraints were imposed on healthcare spending, fuelling the debate regarding the quality, affordability, and sustainability of a publicly funded healthcare system (Burnett, 2008).

In assessing the degree to which the Canada Health Act was successful in ensuring that all Canadians have access to the healthcare they need, we need to look at the purpose of the Act and the extent to which other aspects of healthcare, addressed by the Act, have been implemented. In addition to its stated purpose, the Canada Health Act implicitly and explicitly suggests a broader purpose. For example, Section 3 of the Act endorses health promotion, stating the "primary objective of Canadian healthcare policy" is twofold: to facilitate reasonable access to health services and "to protect, promote, and restore the physical and mental well-being of residents of Canada" (Canada House of Commons, 1984, Section 3). Despite this, the focus on adequate funding of community health services has been limited. Because the Canada Health Act establishes that only medically necessary physician services and hospital services are publicly funded, services such as home care fall outside the legislation.

Protective, promotive, and preventive services were not required to meet the five criteria of Medicare and were not subject to the conditions of the Act. Thus these services, which were provided largely by provincial and territorial public health systems and which added a critical balance to the treatment-focused insured service delivery addressed by the Canada Health Act, were left unprotected by federal legislation. Each province, territory, and region thus determines the extended services that are covered and to what extent. The result is varied and fragmented community health service across the country (Tsasis, 2009).

The two aspects of the Canadian healthcare system that can be compared with other countries are the level of health Canadians enjoy and the relative cost of our healthcare system. The Organization for Economic Cooperation and Development (OECD) provides data that are helpful in making such international comparisons. Table 2.1 reports selected health outcomes by country for 1970, 2000, and 2008. Infant mortality rates per 100 live births and life expectancy in years at birth for males and females are accepted measures of the health of populations. They are data that can be compared internationally. Table 2.2 reports three different expenditure measures of the healthcare system. First, total healthcare expenditures per capita represent how much was spent on healthcare for every person in that country expressed in U.S. dollars. The second reports healthcare expenditures as a percentage of gross domestic product (GDP), which is the percentage of the total market value of all goods and services produced in a country in a given year. The third reports the percentage of total health expenditure that was public funding.

Canada's life expectancies for both women and men rank among the highest in the world. Although Canadian infant mortality rates have dropped since 1970, the 2007 rate of 5.1 deaths per 1000 live births is still higher than the same rate in a number of other developed countries. When comparing health outcomes to expenditures, one message is very clear: increased spending on healthcare does not result in better health. In 2000 and 2008, the United States spent more per capita on healthcare than any of the other 29 countries compared by the OECD. Health expenditures in the United States also represented the highest percentage of gross domestic product (GDP). Yet American health outcomes compare poorly with those of other countries. Japan, for example, spent less than half as much per capita on healthcare as the United States, yet ranks very high on all three measures of health outcome. Canada's per capita spending in 2008 was about 54% that of the United States, and healthcare spending amounted to 10.4% of the GDP, compared with 16% in the United States. However, on all three health outcomes, Canada

TABLE 2.2   Comparisons of Health Expenditure by Selected Country

	Total per Capita Expenditures in U.S.$			Total Expenditures as Percentage of GDP			Public Expenditure as a Percentage of Total Health Expenditure		
	1970	2000	2008	1970	2000	2008	1970	2000	2008
Australia	176	2266	3353	4.1	8.0	8.5*	57.0	67.0	67.5
Canada	294	2519	4079	6.9	8.8	10.4	70.0	70.0	70.2
Germany	268	2669	3737	6.0	10.3	10.5	73.0	80.0	88.0
Japan	151	1969	2729	4.6	7.7	8.1*	70.0	81.0	82.0*
New Zealand	214	1607	2683	5.2	7.7	9.8	80.0	78.0	80.0
Sweden	311	2286	3470	6.8	8.2	9.4	86.0	85.0	82.0
United Kingdom	159	1837	3129	4.5	7.0	8.7	87.0	79.0	83.0
United States	356	4703	7538	7.1	13.4	16.0	36.0	43.0	46.5

*2007 figures; 2008 data not available.

Source: Data based on OECD (2010), OECD Health Data 2010: Statistics and Indicators, http://www.oecd.org/health/healthdata.

fared substantially better than the United States. Perhaps this is related to the fact that the American healthcare industry relies to a larger extent on private funding (53.5%) than any of the other countries.

On March 23, 2010, President Barack Obama introduced one of the most significant pieces of social policy legislation in 50 years (Gruber, 2010). The Patient Protection and Affordable Care Act will dramatically increase health insurance coverage but concerns abound about the impact on healthcare expenditures (Gruber, 2010).

Data analyses suggest that Canada's universal health coverage is less costly and more effective than the privatized U.S. health system (Evans, 2008; Rachlis, 2008; Rachlis, Evans, Lewis, & Barer, 2001; Starfield, 2010); however, there is room for improvement, as noted by the Commissioner on the Future of Healthcare.

When we first started debating Medicare 40 years ago, "medically necessary" health care could be summed up in two words: hospitals and doctors. Today, hospital and physician services account for less than half of the total cost of the system. More money is spent on drugs than on physicians. There are more specialists and more care is delivered in homes, in communities, and through a wide array of healthcare providers. In short, the practice of health care has evolved. And despite efforts to keep pace, Medicare has not. (Romanow, 2002, p. 2)

Effective chronic disease prevention and management will require broad policy options including amending the Canada Health Act; promoting interdisciplinary teamwork; and supporting further integration between public health, home care, and other sectors of the healthcare system (Tsasis, 2009). Palliative care and community mental health services are also areas that need to be strengthened within the Canada Health Act (Marchildon, 2005). The review of the Act will require the involvement of professionals, citizens, and communities to provide insight and direction for delivery and funding of healthcare.

THE FEDERAL ROLE

As Mr. Romanow observed, when the legislative pillars of Canadian Medicare were enacted in 1957, 1966, and 1984, the biomedical model dominated public and political thinking about health. The clinical definition of health was the absence of disease and the term "health promotion" was often used interchangeably with "disease prevention." Labelling the illness-oriented, treatment-focused physician and hospital services that were insured under the Acts as "healthcare" contributed to this confusion. As challenges to the idea that health was related exclusively to a country's illness emerged, the federal government responded and provided leadership in the development of health promotion policies and resources.

An important acknowledgement of the limitations of the primacy of the funded medical treatment system in Canada was The Lalonde Report of 1974 (Lalonde, 1974). It presented a vision for health promotion services as a critical component of Canada's healthcare system. The proposed framework identified four determinants of health: environment, lifestyle, human biology, and the healthcare system. The Lalonde Report was considered revolutionary globally, and led to a reconceptualization of health promotion.

Four years later, in 1978, Canada and other countries around the world met at The International Conference on Primary Health Care in Alma Ata, USSR. They urged governments to take action to "protect and promote the health" of the people of the world by issuing the Declaration of Alma Ata (World Health Organization, 1978), to which Canada was a signatory.

In the years following Alma Ata, federal leadership in health promotion policy continued. In 1986, the federal Minister of Health, the Honourable Jake Epp, published the document Achieving Health for All: A Framework for Health Promotion (Epp, 1986). The Epp Framework expanded Lalonde's definition of health promotion; incorporated some of the tenets of primary health care; and emphasized the role

CASE STUDY: Healthcare Reform in Canada

Canada's healthcare system, while widely cherished and considered a hallmark of Canadian culture, clearly has some problems. Issues such as the skewed distribution of funding toward acute care and curative services, the dominance of a biomedical approach in insured services, and increasing inequities in uninsured services warrant substantial changes to create the equitable, accessible, integrated healthcare system that was envisioned when Medicare was initially conceived. Healthcare practices have changed: for example, patients are discharged "sicker and quicker" to their homes. Concerns that an aging population will place increasing demands on the healthcare system give rise to discussion and debate that the healthcare system will be inadequate or is unsustainable.

Difficulty recruiting and retaining healthcare personnel, economic recessions, and the election of governments with an agenda to slash taxes and decrease government involvement in health and social services have all contributed to a difficult situation. Media reports of unreasonable waiting lists and relocation practices that transport Canadians in need of medical interventions away from their homes to urban centres, other provinces, and the United States alarm Canadians and lead them to consider whether alternative models such as privatization could provide a better, sustainable healthcare system.

Discussion Questions

1. Consider your personal and your family's situation and experience with the healthcare system locally. How does your experience compare with what you read or hear in the media?

2. How do these issues impact the practice of CHNs?

3. Describe the "debate" that you hear or participate in regarding financing of the healthcare system in Canada.

of broad social, environmental, and political determinants of health. The document concluded with a denouncement of strategies that focus on individual responsibility for health, or "blaming the victim," while ignoring the social and economic conditions that contribute to disease and disability.

The Epp Framework formed the basis for the Ottawa Charter for Health Promotion that emerged from the First International Conference on Health Promotion, hosted by the federal government in Ottawa in November, 1986 (Epp, 1986). The Ottawa Charter, authored jointly by Health Canada, the CPHA, and the World Health Organization (WHO), identified prerequisites for health, strategies for promoting health, and outcomes of those strategies. The Ottawa Charter acknowledged that caring for one's self and others is conducive to health and identified caring, holism, and ecology as essential concepts in health promotion (WHO, 1986). Federal government support for health promotion through policy and development of resources has continued. Many of

the resources that have been developed, such as the *Population Health Template* (Health Canada, 2001) and the *Population Health Promotion Model* (Hamilton & Bhatti, 1996) have been used to guide the practice and education of CHNs.

More than 30 years after the declaration of Alma Ata, the seventh Global Conference on Health Promotion was held in Nairobi in October 2009. Organized by the WHO and the Kenyan Ministry of Public Health, the conference closed with the adoption and declaration of the *Nairobi Call to Action* developed using multiple participatory processes. The *Call to Action* identifies key strategies and commitments urgently required to close the implementation gap in health and development through health promotion (WHO, 2009).

Public Health Agency of Canada

The report of the Expert Panel on SARS and Infectious Disease Control (Walker, 2004), the National Advisory Committee on SARS and Public Health (Naylor, 2003), and the two interim SARS Commission Reports (Campbell, 2004, 2005) highlighted the central importance of public health in preventing the spread of disease. These reports posed questions about how the current system is funded, governed, and managed. The writing of these reports followed a series of communicable disease outbreaks and their focus was on the health system's ability to respond adequately.

In response to concerns raised, the Public Health Agency of Canada (PHAC) was established in September 2004 to strengthen public health in Canada. It was confirmed as a legal entity in December 2006 through the Public Health Agency of Canada Act. It is one of six departments that make up the federal government's health portfolio and reports to the Parliament of Canada through the Minister of Health. In 2010 there were over 2200 PHAC staff working in headquarters in Ottawa and in six regions across Canada. The Public Health Agency of Canada is led by the Chief Public Health Officer (CPHO) who is the lead federal public health professional tasked with communicating directly with Canadians and government on important public health matters. The mission of the Public Health Agency of Canada is to promote and protect the health of Canadians. The PHAC brings together scientists, researchers, policy makers, and public health professionals, including physicians, nurses, and epidemiologists. They are committed to the well-being of communities and the Canadian population as a whole.

The development of a public health agency has strengthened public health leadership in Canada, leadership required to address factors that contribute to illness and injury in times of crisis and emergency, as well as in other times. PHAC concentrates, within one agency, the required resources to focus efforts to advance public health nationally and internationally.

While the PHAC was a federal response, each province and territory also responded to the e. coli and SARS outbreaks, and took steps to review and strengthen the public health component of the health system within their jurisdiction. In Ontario, for example, the provincial government launched Operation Health Protection in 2003 (Ontario, 2004), a three-year plan to rebuild public health. The intent was to address the concerns of infectious disease control as well as concerns related to disease prevention and health promotion. Related activities included the establishment of two provincial committees to move forward public health renewal. The first committee, the Capacity Review Committee, was to assess and make recommendations as to the capacity and organizational framework for public health, and the second was to provide recommendations and a plan to establish a provincial arms-length agency that would focus on research and practise excellence in public health. The newly developed Ontario Agency for Health Protection and Promotion (OAHPP) provides provincial leadership on funding, policy, standards–setting, and accountability in public health programs. All these directly impact the practice of community health nursing in Ontario.

ORGANIZATION OF HEALTHCARE IN THE COMMUNITY

Many factors have influenced how community health services are organized and delivered across Canada. Over the last few decades many provinces have moved to regional health authority structures for all health service delivery. This approach strives to integrate most or all health services (including CHN services) into a single organization. The timing and organization of the regional health authorities has been unique to each province or territory. The size and population served varies across Canada. For example British Columbia's five Regional Health Authorities serve a population of 4.3 million people, while Saskatchewan's 12 Regional Health Authorities provide services for a population of approximately 1 million. Community health services are organized and delivered differently across Canada. However, each province and territory provides primary health care, public health, and home care services. These will be briefly discussed in the next section.

Primary Health Care and Primary Care

Primary health care in the *Declaration of Alma Ata* is defined as accessible, acceptable, affordable healthcare (WHO, 1978). Other specific tenets of primary health care include a basis in research; a continuum of services from promotive to rehabilitative; the identification of health education, proper nutrition, disease prevention and control, and maternal and child healthcare as minimum services; the recognition that intersectoral and interdisciplinary approaches are necessary for success; and an emphasis on community participation and empowerment. It encompasses the determinants of health and their influence on health and well-being (WHO, 1978). CHNs have participated in and are well prepared to play a leadership role in primary health care.

Primary care, on the other hand, refers to services commonly accessed at the first point of contact with the health system. Primary care, a core component of primary health care, is more narrowly focused. In many "developed" countries, primary care services focus on acute care and treatment of disease. While the largest group of primary care providers in Canada is physicians, other primary care providers include nurses, nurse practitioners, dentists, chiropractors, pharmacists, dietitians, midwives, optometrists, and public health nurses. Current funding mechanisms favour physicians and, as a result, most Canadians access primary care in the community physicians' office, commonly through a family or general practitioner, who is reimbursed on a fee-for-service basis.

Physicians' fees account for 13.6% of total healthcare costs (Evans, 2007). The most expensive form of remuneration for physicians' services is fee-for-service; the overwhelming majority of physicians earn almost all their income in this way. Hutchinson, Abelson, and Lavis (2001) noted that "for the 89% of Canadian family physicians/general practitioners who receive some fee-for-service income, fee-for-service payments account for an average of 88% of their total income" (p. 117). Increasing criticism for this traditional and costly model of primary care has led to some innovations over the past quarter century.

Primary care reform began at a national level and sought to move toward an integrated systems approach, which would more broadly provide the full spectrum of health services in communities or neighbourhoods. It was envisioned that health promotion and disease and injury prevention services would be enhanced as the focus shifted "up-stream" with the implementation of primary health care.

In the early 1970s, community health centres (CHCs) were recognized for more "fully reflecting the objectives, priorities, and relationships which society wishes to establish for healthcare in the future" (Canadian Council on Social Development, Research and Development Branch, 1972, p. ii). An inquiry was commissioned to examine the place of CHCs as part of a plan aimed at restructuring healthcare delivery and funding mechanisms.

Quebec introduced one of the first primary care reforms in the form of a model based on Centres Locaux de Service Communautaires (CLSCs). Philosophically, CLSCs are based on the ideal of a global, integrated system of care, delivering a broader, less costly range of services (Hutchinson, Abelson, & Lavis, 2001) to neighbourhoods across the province. In addition to providing primary care treatment, these local community service centres emphasize health promotion, disease prevention, and the provision of expanded services including social services and a mental health program (Shah, 2003). There are more than 145 CLSCs in Quebec, which employ approximately 1500 salaried physicians and more than 5000 full-time-equivalent nurses. CLSCs are required to provide services during regular and extended hours and on the weekend to increase access to community health services.

Community Health Centres (CHCs) in Ontario focus on the determinants of health providing interdisciplinary primary health care services, which include health promotion, illness prevention, health protection, chronic disease management, and individual and community capacity building. In November of 2009, there were 66 CHCs in Ontario, a number with satellite offices, each serving on average 5500 individuals. By the end of 2010, it is anticipated that this number will increase to 74 CHCs. Each centre is incorporated as a non-profit agency with a volunteer, community-elected board of directors (Ontario Ministry of Health and Long Term Care, 2009).

The most recent primary care reform initiative of the Ontario government has been to establish Family Health Teams (FHTs). Family health teams are composed of physicians, nurse practitioners, nurses, social workers, dietitians, and other professionals who work together to provide healthcare to a community. Each team is set up based on local health and community needs and focuses on chronic disease management, disease prevention, and health promotion as well as working with other organizations such as public health, home care, and hospitals. Since April of 2005, 170 teams have been created across the province and it is expected this will result in improved healthcare for 2.7 million Ontarians. Thirty more teams are planned (Ontario Ministry of Health and Long Term Care, 2009).

Nurse practitioners (NP) have the potential to significantly contribute to primary care reform and frequently practise in CHCs and Family Health Teams. NPs are registered nurses with advanced education who provide a full range of services, including assessing, diagnosing, and treating illnesses. NPs also focus on many health promotion and illness preventing issues. The Canada Health Act allows provinces to establish reimbursement mechanisms for healthcare professionals other than physicians and dentists. Although all provinces and territories have enacted legislation that defines an extended scope of practice for nurse practitioners, only some provinces established associated funding mechanisms for their reimbursement (Canada, House of Commons, 1984).

Public Health

Whereas hospital and physicians' services have been governed by federal legislation for the last half of the 20th century, public health was decentralized at the outset so the responsibility rested with the provinces and in some cases the municipalities. The same principles of comprehensiveness, universality, portability, public administration, and accessibility have been hallmarks of Canadian public health services. Public health augmented Medicare by ensuring that health promotion and protection services were among the affordable, acceptable, essential health services that were "universally accessible to individuals and families in the community" (WHO, 1978). Together, Canada's public health services and national healthcare system provided health services that were consistent with the tenets of primary health care.

Over the last several decades, the public health infrastructure in Canada has been severely eroded. In 1996, the Canadian Public Health Association (CPHA) warned of the erosion by noting that in some jurisdictions "Public Health units and specific categories of workers (e.g., Public Health Nurses) are disappearing" (CPHA, 1996, p. 1–12). In 2001, the CPHA identified "increasing complexity and decreased funding" as challenges facing public health (p. 7). Sullivan (2002) reported the key findings of a report of the Federal, Provincial, and Territorial Advisory Committee on Population Health that identified severe problems in public health in Canada, such as disparities among provinces and regions, severely inadequate

and decreasing funding, critical human resource issues, and the development of public health policies without consideration of relevant data. There was a consensus that the water contamination in Walkerton, Ontario, in 2000 was a "wake-up call" for Canadian public health, occurring because "institutions vital to the infrastructure of public health were neglected" (Schabas, 2002, p. 1282). Funding of public health services depends in large part on provincial governance and delivery structures. Funds are distributed to regions and municipalities through various funding formulas. CPHA (2010a) proposed the development of a National Public Health Infrastructure Fund as a transfer payment scheme dedicated to public health that demands a certain percentage of matching dollars from the provinces and territories to ensure a stable level of funding for the public health system across the country (p. 9).

Home Health

Health Canada defines home care as "a wide range of health services delivered at home and throughout the community to recovering, disabled, chronically, or terminally ill persons in need of medical, nursing, social, or therapeutic treatment and/or assistance with the essential activities of daily living" (Health Canada, 2010). "Home health nurses are committed to the provision of accessible, responsive, and timely care which allows people to stay in their homes with safety and dignity" (CHNC, 2010c, p. 4). The use of home care services has been steadily growing in Canada over the past 35 years, and government spending on home care reached $3.4 billion in 2003–2004 (Canadian Institute of Health Informatics, 2007).

The increase in use and funding has been attributed to several factors, most significantly the belief that services provided in the home are both less costly and a more desirable means of receiving necessary care. These claims, however, have yet to be proven. Another issue is that as the services shift to the home and community, they shift beyond the boundaries of public insurance (Deber, 2003). While all of the provinces offer a package of basic services, there are significant provincial variations in the degree to which services are publicly funded versus privately financed resulting in significant inequity in accessing publicly funded home care across different regions of the country. Although the actual figure is difficult to verify, Coyte and McKeever (2001) calculated that private payment (a combination of out-of-pocket and private insurance coverage) for home care services approximated almost 20% of total home care expenditures in 1997. Thus savings associated with the provision of services in the home versus in an acute care setting may not so much reflect an actual decrease in cost but rather a transfer of costs to patients and their families (Shah, 2003). Nursing care, pharmaceuticals, and physiotherapy services are among those services that are being debated (Deber, 2003).

Some provinces have legislation that addresses the financing and provision of home care services at provincial and regional levels (Public Health Agency of Canada, 2006). However, in the absence of common national standards, legitimate concerns exist in relation to equal access to type, amount, and quality of home care services (Sullivan & Baranek, 2002).

Home care is an expanding area of health spending in Canada. However, home care expenditures represent less than 5% of total health spending (Coyte & McKeever, 2001). In all 13 provinces and territories, the ministries or departments of health and/or social/community services maintain control over home care budgets and funding levels. As part of regionalization, most provinces have delegated responsibility for service delivery decisions to regional or local health authorities, while maintaining control over policy guidelines, standards for regional service delivery, reporting requirements, and monitoring outcomes. For example, in British Columbia, Alberta, Saskatchewan, Manitoba, Newfoundland and Labrador, Nunavut, and the Northwest Territories, the delivery of home care services has been completely devolved to local or regional authorities. In Quebec, the 146 Centre Local de Services Communautaires (CLSCs) deliver home care services. In New Brunswick, two programs under the department of health and community services administer home care, whereas in Nova Scotia, regional offices of the department of health administer and make delivery decisions about home care. In the Yukon, the social services branch of the department of health and social services administers home care.

In Ontario, home care is provided through 14 Community Care Access Centres (CCACs), which manage healthcare services to those at home or in school. In the early part of 2000, the 43 local Community Care Access Centres amalgamated to 14 in alignment with the restructuring of certain aspects of healthcare in Ontario into 14 Local Health Integration Networks. Funding for many components of the health system was transferred to the LHINs including funding for home care and CCACs. Each CCAC is staffed by professionals, including nurses, who will assess individual health needs, determine requirements for care, answer questions, and develop a customized health plan with the client. The range of professional services provided include nursing, physiotherapy, social work, dietetics, occupational therapy, speech therapy, personal support, and case management.

Across Canada, home care services are delivered using several funding frameworks. The models all provide some element of streamlining (intake, assessment, referral, case management), but vary in their approach to delivery of care, most significantly in the degree to which contracting out services to private agencies (both for-profit and not-for-profit) occurs.

Within their home care budget, each region must decide how much is allocated to home care versus acute care services versus public health and health promotion services. Public funding for home care is allocated to home care organizations which then coordinate and/or deliver home care services. While major budgetary decisions are made at the regional level, case managers are then required to make decisions at the individual or family level.

Denton et al. (2002) found that while there is increased demand for home care, there is a paucity of research on the impact of restructuring. The impact of the changing of the governance and organizational structures on the quality of care and on the workers (including nurses) requires investigation.

Service providers, a mix of for-profit agencies and not-for-profit agencies, compete for contracts to provide the required in-home services. This process allows private, for-profit agencies to profit from public funding earmarked for the delivery of health services. This new situation, sometimes referred to as passive privatization, has sparked significant debate and concern. A number of papers have been produced that challenge the competitive bidding process. While the expectation is that the competitive process will lead to efficiencies, it can result in downward pressure on wages, skill mix, and working conditions (Deber, 2003). The process by which service providers are obtained will have a significant impact on the quality of care individuals will receive.

CURRENT AND FUTURE CHALLENGES FOR COMMUNITY HEALTH NURSES

Over the past decade, there has been a slow growth in research and literature that describes the current situation for CHNs across Canada. This literature points to the current strengths CHNs bring to positively influence the health of individuals and communities. It also paints a picture of some of the challenges before them. Four of these challenges are outlined below.

Health System Challenges

Community health nursing practice occurs in a sociopolitical environment. Nurses' ability to shape this environment and thus take an active role in evolving healthcare, and thus the health of communities, is often met with multiple challenges and barriers. Despite numerous calls for a strengthening of primary health care (Romanow, 2002) and a shift to community health and preventive care, an emphasis on illness care remains the current paradigm. Inadequate funding and resources for prevention and health promotion remain an issue and what exists is under constant and real threat. The lack of stable, long-term funding is cited as a major barrier to effective practice and service delivery (Underwood et al., 2009b). CHNs themselves identify as a priority the need for advocacy to shape system change (CHNC, 2010a; Schofield et al., 2010).

CANADIAN RESEARCH BOX

What is the current capacity of community health nurses?

Underwood, J. M., et al. (2009b). Building community and public health nursing capacity: A synthesis report of the National Community Health Nursing Study. *Canadian Journal of Public Health*, 100(5), 11–111.

Information describing community health nursing (CHNsg) professionals in Canada and the contributions they made was difficult to find. Similarly, pertinent human resource considerations for CHNs were relatively absent from the literature. However, in the past five years, administrators and researchers have shown renewed interest in this area. A Canadian study, *Building Community and Public Health Nursing Capacity: A Synthesis Report of the National Community*

Health Nursing Study, begins to uncover important elements of this critical nursing issue. The study sought to describe the CHNsg workforce in Canada and to compare across jurisdictions and CHNsg sectors what helps and hinders CHNs to work effectively. The authors looked specifically at public health nurses to identify organizational attributes that support them to practise to the full scope of their competencies.

Mixed methods were used for this study, and data were obtained from three sources. An analysis of the Canadian Institute for Health Information nursing databases (1996–2007) was conducted, a survey of over 13 000 CHNs across Canada was completed, and, finally, 23 focus groups composed of policy makers and front-line public health nurses were conducted across Canada.

The demographic analysis identified that approximately 53 000 RNs and licensed practical nurses (LPNs) were working in community health in 2007. This represented 18% of all RNs and 10% of LPNs. The number of RNs working in community health centres increased over the past 10 years, from 39% to 60% of all RNs working in community settings. On average, RNs working in community health were older than the rest of the profession. In 2007, 28% of CHNs were over 55 years of age or older. This reflects an increase from 13% a decade earlier. Nurses working in the community who are under the age of 30 decreased significantly over the past 10 years (from 9% to 5%).

In 2007, more than 54% of RNs working in the community were employed full time, and they were more likely than RNs in other sectors to have a university degree. In terms of leadership positions in 2007, less than 15% of RNs in chief executive positions or in chief nursing officer roles were in community settings or organizations, the lowest proportion since 1996. However, the number of nursing consultants in the community increased (from 30% to 53%).

Sixty percent of RNs (6180) responded to the survey. The response rate varied across the country from 42.6% to 67%. The three work settings that were most frequently identified by respondents were public health (34%), home health agency (21%), and community health centres (19%). A series of questions were posed in order to identify enablers and barriers for CHNs to practise to their full competence. Survey results were divided into four main themes: professional confidence, team relationships, work environment, and community context. Most community nurses felt confident in their practice and relationships with other nurses and professionals, although less so with physicians. Most nurses would like more learning opportunities, policy and practice information, and chances to debrief on their work.

Focus group data were collected from the public health sector—12 groups of front-line public health nurses and 11 combined groups of policy makers and managers (n = 156). Participants came from all provinces/territories of Canada. Appreciative inquiry was used to uncover organizational attributes that promote optimal public health nursing practice. Nurses identified a number of organizational attributes, including

- government and system attributes,
- flexible and adequate funding structure,
- champions for public health,
- public health planning and co-ordination,
- organizational values and leadership characteristics,
- a shared vision for public health,
- effective leadership,
- culture of creativity and responsiveness,
- management practices,
- clear program planning,
- promoting and valuing public health nursing,
- supporting autonomous practice,
- commitment to learning and professional development,
- effective human resource practices and staffing,
- supporting partnership and community development,
- effective communication, and
- healthy workplace policies.

Focus group participants provided in-depth information regarding how organizations, as well as the broader systems, have a significant impact on the practice of public health nursing and thus the care public health is able to provide to families and communities. Adequate time, flexible funding, and management support enable CHNs to develop effective relationships with the communities and people they work with, as well as with other members of the interprofessional team.

Discussion Questions

1. The perspectives of about 7000 nurses are reflected in the research described above. How might these data assist nurse leaders in the community and employers to plan for and ensure that work in an environment that promotes continued professional development?

2. How might provincial and national policy makers, currently focused on healthy human resource and workforce planning, ensure that CHNs will be there and able to address the determinants of health, as well as meet the growing health needs of communities?

3. To what extent could the transformational leadership characteristics identified in Figure 2.1 act to strengthen the organizational attributes listed above?

Role Clarity Although coming from a long and rich history, community health nursing is in a vulnerable position today. The Community Health Nurses of Canada (CHNC) conducted a survey in 2008 to establish a vision for community health nursing in the year 2020 in Canada (CHNC, 2009). This visioning initiative included a national survey and several focus groups with CHNs in different regions across Canada. The resulting document, *Community Health Nursing Vision 2020: Shaping the Future* (CHNC, 2009) contains the following expressions of how community nurses experience their roles:

> I think public health nurses are undervalued by the community, by the consumer, by the nursing profession, by colleagues in different areas of nursing . . . people view it (community

health nursing) as not really nursing while it is really and truly the highest level of nursing that you're going to do. (p. 9)

This undervaluing mirrors the previous decades of diminished funding and resources. Others have identified the relative invisibility of CHNs. Two such examples can be found in post-SARS national and provincial reports. Campbell's report spoke generally of the public health system as "broken and need[ing] to be fixed . . . [T]he overall system is woefully inadequate . . . unprepared, fragmented, poorly led, uncoordinated, inadequately resourced, professionally impoverished and generally incapable of discharging its mandate" (Campbell, 2005, p.24). Naylor, in his report *Learning from SARS: Renewal of public health in Canada*, wrote: "the essential role of public health nurses throughout and following SARS received little attention" (Naylor, 2003, p. 131).

The need for greater role clarity for CHNs is consistently noted in the literature (Brookes, Davidson, Daly & Hancock, 2004; Kennedy et al., 2008) and provides the basis for articulating the value of community health nursing. Across Canada there are differences in how CHNs are identified on official registration forms and in organizational structures. It remains unknown how many nurses actually work in the various sectors of community health as well as any associated demographics. A 2010 synthesis paper reviewed eight recent community health nursing reports, examining the common issues associated with community health nursing (CHNC, 2010b). Of the eight reports reviewed, seven specifically identified role clarity as an issue. Role clarity includes components such as shared common language to describe the role, working to the full scope of practice within the role, and understanding of the role by others within the health system and the public. The ability to describe with confidence the CHN's role can contribute to a greater valuing of the role by other professionals, the community, and policy makers. As clear professional roles are foundational to both a strong healthcare system and an ability to work effectively on interprofessional teams, CHNs, the organizations within which they work, and the professional associations that support them must continue to address this challenge. In response to this issue, the CPHA and CHNC recently released an updated role document for Public Health Nursing in Canada (CPHA, 2010b). Produced in partnership with the Canadian Public Health Association, the document provides a common vision for the role and activities of Community Public Health Nursing in Canada.

Leadership A third issue expressed is the decline in visible community health nursing leadership. In 2005 Falk-Rafael and colleagues surveyed the changing roles of public health nurses in Ontario. Thirty-nine percent of public health nurses who responded to the survey did not know if their health unit had a designated chief nursing officer or designated Senior Nurse Leader. A further 25% answered "no" when asked if such a role existed in their agency. These results followed a provincial directive from the provincial Medical Officer of Health directing each Health Unit to appoint a senior nurse to a chief nursing officer role. In this same study, public health nurses saw themselves as 9th out of a list of 10 possible groups who could influence nursing practice in their organization. In

2005 an Ontario survey of all public health employees was conducted as part of a review to assess the capacity of Public Health in Ontario (Capacity Review, 2006). Keeping in mind that over 55% of the workforce is nurses, the following key issues were identified:

- need for stronger discipline specific communities of practice and more opportunities to meet with peers to discuss and solve professional issues,
- substantial level of concern regarding leadership within health units and management skills at the senior management level, and
- lack of career paths and opportunities for advancement.

The areas most cited as needing attention were organizational cultures, a sense of being valued and appreciated, the quality of leadership, the quality of supervision and management, and access to ongoing education and training (Capacity Review, 2005, p. 34).

A national study of community health nursing using an appreciative inquiry process found three important organizational attributes that support community and public health nursing practice (Meagher-Stewart et al., 2009; Underwood et al., 2009b):

- management practice;
- local organizational culture, which includes values and leadership characteristics; and
- government policy, including system attributes.

The results of surveys such as the ones identified above spurred dialogue about options for action on the issues. One proposal is the development of a national Centre of Excellence for Public Health Nursing. In support of this concept, the CHNC commissioned a document that synthesized key community health nursing reports and provided recommendations to improve the state of community health nursing in Canada (CHNC, 2010b). Development and support of strong and effective leadership was an important recommendation.

Interprofessional Relationships The relationships nurses have with each other and with other professionals that enable them to achieve a common vision to deliver care, and to strengthen the health system and those who are impacted by it, are referred to as interprofessional relationships. Developing and strengthening these relationships, including intersectoral partnerships, is critical to achieving effective health outcomes. The future success of CHNs and nursing in leading the health system—from individual client and family care to broad population health interventions—requires a focus on the significance of professional and client and community collaboration and partnership.

Nurses regard interprofessional and intersectoral partnerships as important; however, recent studies also indicate they have identified learning needs in this area (CHNC, 2010a; Schofield et al., 2008). Foundational to effective partnerships is the need to understand the roles of healthcare partners and the contribution that each can make. Contributions include the ability to make or influence care and service decisions,

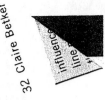

implement organizational change, empower policy and administrative decisions, or develop educational curricula. Establishing positive and effective partnerships and processes for working together requires time, leadership, and mutual understanding.

ROLE OF LEADERSHIP IN RESPONDING TO CHALLENGES FOR CHNS

As described in the preceding sections, Community Health Nursing in the current healthcare system faces significant challenges. Although there are many necessary elements to ensure sustaining effective community health nursing care, leadership development is essential. Leadership is about influence that moves individuals, groups, communities, and systems toward achieving goals that will result in better health. While senior leaders often occupy formal leadership positions, all CHNs have the opportunity within their practice to function as leaders with various levels of influence. Leadership is proposed as a strategy for all CHNs to embrace in order to effectively meet the challenges outlined above.

While the key attributes of leaders have been articulated (Ganann et al., 2010), awareness of oneself is of key importance. Insight into one's beliefs, strengths, weaknesses, and style of relating is fundamental to effective leadership. Similarly, understanding the impact of one's behaviour on others and being able to moderate and modify that behaviour or style is essential to effectively steering organizations toward a vision. Creating and articulating a clear purpose and vision is critical and to do that effectively, nurses must be able to see the long view, incorporating multiple aspects of the broader environment, political environment, and the larger system.

Strategic thinking and action must be evident in the vision as well as evidence of hearing the perspectives or voices of others including staff and the community. Multiple perspectives must be taken into account. The ability to lead others involves the ability to engage their hearts, minds, and feet through expertise in building and sometimes mending relationships. Strong problem solving, conflict management, and interpersonal skills promote emotional engagement and foster motivation. Leaders understand their role in developing an organizational culture and do so in a deliberate, intentional fashion grounded in clear, strong values and principles, which encompass honesty and integrity.

An effective leader not only copes with change, but understands change and the change process. Effective leaders bring energy, enthusiasm, action, and humour to the process as well as the tasks at hand, while keeping a focus on the desired results (Cummings et al., 2010). The literature does not identify any single discipline as having superior leadership skills but rather each brings a unique set of perspectives, experiences, knowledge, and skills that can be channelled into effective leadership.

The outcomes of effective leadership have been described extensively. One such document is the Registered Nurses Association of Ontario's *Best Practice Guideline: Developing and Sustaining Nursing Leadership*, discusses the significant impact of leadership and community. For example, primary health service organizations with strong strate increased organizational commit organizational effectiveness, greater sen organizational goals, and increased abil. workforce.

Personal resources for nurse leaders in a community health setting that contribute to effective leadership practices include the personal characteristics one brings to a leadership role as well as personal supports, learned behaviours, and expertise that has been honed over time. Personal growth is dependent on individual self-awareness and understanding of how one's behaviour influences those around you, as well as events in an organization and in the broader community. As community health work is so interconnected to organizations and political bodies, self-awareness and self-concept are critical to effectively influence or lead within these systems (Cummings et al., 2010).

Research completed through the development of the *Best Practice Guidelines on Nursing Leadership* (RNAO, 2006) found that the following attributes of nurse leaders contribute to effectiveness:

- communication and listening;
- resilience, persistence, and hardiness;
- comfort with ambiguity, uncertainty, and complexity;
- willingness to take risks;
- working from a moral framework;
- confidence in own values and beliefs;
- self-confidence, self-awareness, social awareness;
- knowledgeable; and
- cultivation of professional and personal supports.

CANADIAN RESEARCH BOX

What leadership attributes contribute to CHN practice?

Ganann, R., Underwood, J., Matthews, S., Goodyear, R., Stamler, L. L., Meagher-Stewart, D., & Munroe, V. (2010). Leadership attributes: A key to optimal utilization of the community health nursing workforce. *Canadian Journal of Nursing Leadership, 23*(2), 60–71.

The purpose of this research was to examine the leadership attributes that support the optimal use and practice of Community Health Nurses. This study included an analysis of the Canadian Institute for Health Information nursing database, a survey of over 13 000 CHNs across Canada, and 23 focus groups composed of policy makers and front-line public health nurses. Leadership was identified as an essential attribute of organizations that influences their utilization and support of CHNs, which in turn affects the quality of care and impacts on health outcomes.

The study found that the percentage of nursing leaders working in community settings was the lowest in 10 years. However, leadership attributes emerged as the strongest health nu ... on the CHNs' ability to practise effectively. Front-... anagers were reported to have the greatest impact on ...ne nurses' ability to practise to the full scope of their competencies. Leadership was identified as important at various levels. At the governmental or larger systems level, the study found that having "champions" or advocates for community health services was important. These leaders were seen as able to advocate for systems change, adequate funding, and co-ordinated planning for community health services. At a local organization or agency level, supportive leadership included valuing community health roles and contributions, and showing trust and respect for CHNs. Taking risks, being innovative, and supporting healthy workplaces were considered important activities of leaders.

Leadership development was found to be important within organizations, both for those in leadership positions and as part of succession planning.

Discussion Questions

1. The perspectives of about 7000 nurses are reflected in the research described above. How might these data assist nurse leaders in the community and employers to plan for and ensure nurses work in an environment that promotes continued leadership development?

2. How might provincial and national policy makers, currently focused on health human resource and workforce planning, provide the leadership required so that CHNs will be there and able to address the determinants of health, as well as meet the growing health needs of communities?

3. To what extent could the transformational leadership characteristics identified in Figure 2.1 support the practice of CHNs?

Figure 2.1 is a conceptual model outlining individual and system components that contribute to effective nursing leadership (RNAO, 2006). This model (Figure 2.1) identifies contextual and personal factors that impact a nurse's approach to transformational leadership. For example, a nurse leader who strongly values professional nursing supports will approach relationship building in a way that is more likely to result in healthy and effective outcomes than a nurse leader who values individual successes and works alone in a chaotic environment where budgets are unstable. Leadership growth builds on organizational supports, personal resources, and past outcome experiences.

Organizational Supports

An organizational assessment tool is contained in Table 2.3. The tool builds on the leadership conceptual model, particularly the components of organizational support, and provides a series of activities leaders may champion that are essential to ensuring effective and healthy work environments. These strategies (left column) support employees to focus on developing personal resources as well as assisting managers and leaders (right column) to develop system-wide infrastructure. The individual strategies focus on the community health professional as an individual who is growing within their discipline. They focus on formalized communication networks, broader community partnerships, and meaningful involvement of staff in organization and agency decision making. As leaders of organizations, it is important to be continually assessing the current strategies to ensure effective individual and organizational systems are in place to ensure excellence in practice and outcomes. This tool can be used to assess organizational supports to leadership and invite reflection and dialogue on local and larger systems (PHAC, 2006).

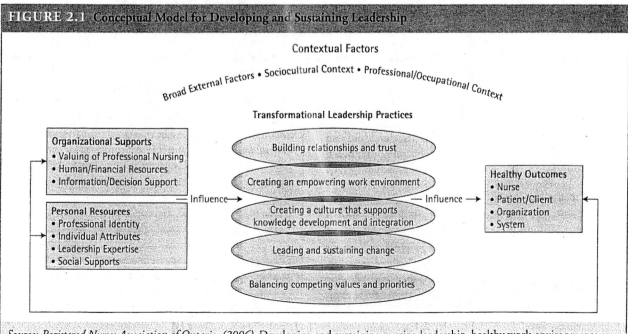

FIGURE 2.1 Conceptual Model for Developing and Sustaining Leadership

Contextual Factors

Broad External Factors • Sociocultural Context • Professional/Occupational Context

Transformational Leadership Practices

Organizational Supports
• Valuing of Professional Nursing
• Human/Financial Resources
• Information/Decision Support

Personal Resources
• Professional Identity
• Individual Attributes
• Leadership Expertise
• Social Supports

Building relationships and trust

Creating an empowering work environment

Creating a culture that supports knowledge development and integration

Leading and sustaining change

Balancing competing values and priorities

— Influence →   — Influence →

Healthy Outcomes
• Nurse
• Patient/Client
• Organization
• System

Source: Registered Nurses Association of Ontario. (2006). Developing and sustaining nursing leadership, healthy work environments, best practice guidelines. *Toronto, Canada: Registered Nurses' Association of Ontario.*

TABLE 2.3   Organizational Supports

A. Employee Development/Enrichment	Yes	No	B. Community Health Organization	Yes	No
1. Employee retention plan	___	___	1. Clear connection between agency vision, mission and mandate, and service delivery. Articulated vision to drive mandate	___	___
2. Recruitment and succession plan	___	___			
3. Orientation and mentoring program for all new staff	___	___	2. Articulated cultural vision and implementation plan to support workplace environment	___	___
4. Regular performance feedback mechanisms that include a variety of inputs such as manager, peer, client, colleague, community partner	___	___	3. Committee/planning structures, which include all levels of staff in a meaningful way	___	___
			4. Stable and predictable funding resources dedicated to a systematic organizational review (e.g., accreditation)	___	___
5. Personal learning plans/professional development plans	___	___	5. Clear boundaries/program mandates with flexibility to address realities of individual community	___	___
6. Employee satisfaction feedback systems and a process for addressing outcomes	___	___	6. Opportunities to nurture discussions on relevant research, practice changes	___	___
7. Continuing education policies	___	___	7. Encouragement to engage with communities and form joint ventures and partnerships	___	___
8. Staff education and training opportunities that include development of affective domain (i.e., values, assumptions, feelings)	___	___	8. Opportunities for disciplines to work together based on collaborative practice principles	___	___
9. Formalized career development opportunities	___	___	9. Formalized student preceptor programs	___	___
10. Leadership development plan	___	___	10. Formalized agreements with the academic community, which include cross appointments, joint research, and student clinical experiences	___	___
11. Opportunities for communities of practice to meeting together regularly	___	___			
12. Appreciation/acknowledgement events where achievements are recognized (department, team, individual)	___	___	11. Infrastructure support—technical, informational, safety	___	___
			12. Mechanisms for regular meetings with unions and other associations	___	___
13. Development and role modelling aimed at mid-career nurses and late-career nurses	___	___	13. Quality Practice Council(s)	___	___
			14. Formalized communication mechanisms such as all-staff meetings, newsletter, intranet, bulletin board, department updates	___	___
			15. Well-established networks within the organization and with key community organizations	___	___

Within the context of community health nursing practice, important organizational supports that positively influence practice include a work culture that

- values the unique and combined contribution of staff,
- deliberately establishes leadership and mentoring plans,
- has a clear vision engendering commitment, and
- has stable funding and access to necessary resources to accomplish work.

Collaborative leadership at a national level will be strengthened by developing intersectoral relationships, promoting community health solutions across sectors, and addressing the wider determinants of health (PHAC, 2006).

SUMMARY

To varying degrees, federal, provincial, regional, and municipal levels of government are involved in Canadian healthcare. Medicare is one of the great achievements of Canada, and is more than a public insurance program (Campbell & Marchildon, 2007). A universally accessible, publicly funded, not-for-profit-delivered healthcare system is steeped in Canadian values and embraced by the Canadian public. Efforts to enshrine those values in federal legislation began as early as 1919. The present legislation, the Canada Health Act, is limited in that its principles of public administration, portability, accessibility, universality, and public administration apply only to essential medical and hospital services. Nevertheless, the publicly funded and largely privately delivered healthcare system has served Canadians well with respect to both health outcomes and cost-effectiveness (Starfield, 2010).

Pressures to reform Medicare come not only because of its narrow focus but also because some favour augmenting the public system with services provided by the for-profit sector. Numerous reports at provincial and federal levels have recommended reforms to the healthcare system. The most comprehensive of those, the *Romanow Commission Report*, made 47 recommendations for both the immediate future and for the next 20 years (Romanow, 2002).

The federal government has played a leadership role, not only in Canada but also in the world, in health promotion policy. However, a co-ordinated approach to implementing health promotion policy at the community and population levels has been hampered by the lack of a national public health plan.

Prior to SARS in 2004, there had been a steady and declining emphasis on the role of community health in the Canadian health system, in large part to its exclusion from the Canada Health Act. Restructuring of provincial health systems to regional models that include community health has played a role in the declining emphasis on community health. Community health issues compete with more pressing acute care concerns. Demands on limited home/health and primary health care nursing services have challenged the community health system. Serious erosions to public health in Canada have led to the withdrawal and reduction of many public health nursing services.

Community health nurses practise at the intersection of public policy and private lives and can include political advocacy and efforts to influence healthy public policy in their practice (Falk Rafael, 2005). A strong call for a revitalized public health and community health system is being made. Strong leadership and action at all levels and situations is required to answer the call. Falk Rafael (2005) states that CHNs are well positioned and morally obligated to act and provide leadership.

KEY TERMS

Canada Health Act, p. 21
Medicare, p. 21
leadership, p. 21
publicly funded, p. 22
publicly administered, p. 22
comprehensive, p. 22
universal, p. 22
portable, p. 22
accessible, p. 22
determinants of health, p. 22
financing, p. 22
allocations, p. 23
public health, p. 23
delivery, p. 23
primary health care, p. 26
primary care, p. 26
home care, p. 27

REVIEW QUESTIONS

1. The organizational attributes that community health nurses identified as promoting optimal nursing practice included
   a) non-governmental organizations' characteristics.
   b) having strong and narrow mandates.
   c) a culture of creativity and responsiveness.
   d) many individual visions.
2. Primary care reform has resulted in
   a) closing community health centres.
   b) privatizing nursing services.
   c) establishing Family Health Teams.
   d) closing many physician private practices.
3. CHNs across Canada describe a number of challenges to them making strong health impacts. These challenges include
   a) a decrease in opportunities for formal education.
   b) an emphasis on acute care which impacts funding for health promotion and prevention.
   c) an increased ability to clearly articulate the contributions of CHNs.
   d) visible community health nurse leaders.
4. Transformational leadership practices, which lead to quality nursing practice and professional development, are based on a number of contextual factors that determine effective implementation. Contextual factors include
   a) community members making demands for more nurses.
   b) lifelong learning being promoted and supported.
   c) relationships within nursing organizations being developed when time permits.
   d) ensuring employment for nurses is guaranteed.
5. One of the key limitations of the Canada Health Act is
   a) it is not portable from province to province.
   b) it allows for user fees if certain procedures cost more money.
   c) the focus is on essential hospital and medical services.
   d) it is not publicly funded.

STUDY QUESTIONS

1. Identify the origins of Medicare in Canada and summarize the laws that created the present Canadian healthcare system. What is considered to be phase 2 of the implementation of Medicare?
2. Discuss the events that led up to and necessitated passage of the Canada Health Act.
3. What role did organized nursing play in the passage of the Canada Health Act?
4. Discuss the federal and provincial responsibilities for health according to the Canadian Constitution Act.
5. Contrast the funding mechanisms for public health and home health nursing services with the rest of the system.
6. Describe how the Canada Health Act was or was not successful in achieving the intended goals. Are there issues with it?

*After working through these questions, go to the MyNursingLab at **www.pearsoned.ca/mynursinglab** to check your answers.*

INDIVIDUAL CRITICAL THINKING EXERCISES

1. List your core values for healthcare in Canada. How do your values compare with the values reflected in the five key funding criteria described in the Canada Health Act (1984)?

2. How would your life be different if healthcare in this country were provided based on ability to pay, rather than need?

3. This chapter has shown that health policy decisions leave a legacy for generations. Describe briefly one policy revision you would make in the areas of primary care/primary health care, public health, and home care.

4. What examples can you describe of nurses' work to bring about healthcare systems change?

5. What opportunities have you encountered to promote the second phase of Medicare development?

6. Leadership development is an ongoing process. What ideas do you have to develop your leadership skills and knowledge?

GROUP CRITICAL THINKING EXERCISES

1. What are the values on which the healthcare system is founded? How do your own values fit with the societal values that are reflected in the five funding criteria described in the Canada Health Act (1984)?

2. What are some of the solutions that you and your group can generate to address the real issues in Canada's healthcare system. What role can community health nurses play?

3. In an ideal world, create a healthcare system designed to provide the best care, to the most people, in the most cost-effective manner. Describe mechanisms for financing, allocation, and delivery. Compare and contrast this system with the current Canadian system.

REFERENCES

Auditor General of Canada. (2002). *1999 report of the Auditor General of Canada to the House of Commons* (chapter 29). Retrieved from http://www.oag-bvg.gc.ca/internet/English/parl_oag_199911_29_e_10158.html

Begin, M. (1988). *Medicare: Canada's right to health.* Translated by David Homel and Lucille Nelson. Montreal, QC: Optimum.

Begin, M. (2002). *Revisiting the Canada Health Act (1984): What are the impediments to change?* Address to the Institute for Research on Public Policy, 30th Anniversary Conference, Ottawa, ON. Retrieved from http://www.irpp.org/events/archive/020218e.pdf

Brookes, K., Davidson, P., Daly, J., & Hancock, K. (2004). Community health nursing in Australia: A critical literature review and implications for professional nursing. *Contemporary Nursing, 16*(3), 195–207.

Burnett, S. (2008). Financing the health care system: Is long term sustainability possible? *Canadian Centre for Policy Alternatives.* Retrieved from http://www.policyalternatives.ca/publications/reports/financing-health-care-system

Campbell, A. (2004). *SARS Commission. Interim report: SARS and public health in Ontario.* Toronto, ON: Ministry of Health and Long Term Care. Retrieved from http://www.health.gov.on.ca/english/public/pub/ministry_reports/campbell04/campbell04.html

Campbell, A., 2005. *SARS Commission. Second interim report: SARS and public health legislation.* Toronto, ON: Ministry of Health and Long-Term Care. Retrieved from http://www.health.gov.on.ca/english/public/pub/ministry_reports/campbell05/campbell05.pdf

Campbell, B., & Marchildon, G. (2007). Completing Tommy's vision. *Canadian Centre for Policy Alternatives.* Retrieved from http://www.policyalternatives.ca/publications/commentary/completing-tommys-vision

Canada, House of Commons. (1984). An Act Relating to Cash Contributions by Canada in Respect of Insured Health Services Provided Under Provincial Health Care Insurance Plans and Amounts Payable by Canada in Respect of Extended Health Care Services and to Amend and Repeal Certain Acts in Consequence Thereof. (The Canada Health Act). Ottawa, ON: Government of Canada.

Canadian Council on Social Development, Research and Development Branch. (1972). *Case studies in social planning: Planning under voluntary councils and public auspices.* Ottawa, ON: Author.

Canadian Institute for Health Information. (2007). *Government home care spending reaches $3.4 billion in 2003–2004.* Retrieved from http://secure.cihi.ca/cihiweb/dispPage.jsp?cw_page=media_22mar2007_e

Canadian Nurses Association. (2006). *A healthy nation is a wealthy nation.* Retrieved from http://www.cna-aiic.ca/CNA/documents/pdf/publications/Standing_Committee_Submission-2006_e.pdf

Canadian Public Health Association. (1996). *Focus on health: Public health in health services restructuring.* Ottawa, ON: Author.

Canadian Public Health Association. (2001). *Creating conditions for health: Recommendations to the Commission.* Ottawa, ON: Author.

Canadian Public Health Association. (2010a). *Enhancing the public health human resource infrastructure in Canada.* A presentation by CPHA to the House of Commons Standing Committee on Health. Ottawa, ON: Author. Retrieved from http://www.cpha.ca/uploads/policy/enhance_ph_e.pdf

Canadian Public Health Association (2010b). *Public health - Community health nursing practice in Canada: Roles and Activities* (4th ed.). Ottawa: ON. Author. Retrieved from http://www.cpha.ca/uploads/pubs/3-1bk04214.pdf

Capacity Review Committee. (2005). *Interim report. Revitalizing Ontario's public health capacity: A discussion of issues and options.* Toronto, ON: Author. Retrieved from http://www.health.gov.on.ca/english/public/pub/ministry_reports/capacity_review05/capacity_review05.pdf

Capacity Review Committee. (2006). *Final report: Revitalizing Ontario's public health capacity.* Toronto, ON: Author. Retrieved from http://www.health.gov.on.ca/english/public/pub/ministry_reports/capacity_review06/capacity_review06.pdf

Community Health Nurses of Canada. (2009). *Vision statement and definition of community health nursing practice in Canada.* Toronto, ON: Author. Retrieved from http://www.chnc.ca/documents/2009EnglishCHNDefinition_VisionStatement.pdf

Community Health Nurses of Canada. (2010a). *Community health nurses speak out! Key Findings from an environmental scan about the future of community health nursing in Canada.* Retrieved from http://www.chnc.ca/documents/Environmentalscan-CHNsspeakout.pdf

Community Health Nurses of Canada (2010b). *A synthesis of Canadian community health nursing reports.* Retrieved from http://www.chnc.ca/documents/ CommunityHealthNursingkeyreportssynthesis2010.doc

Community Health Nurses of Canada (2010c). *Home health nursing competencies: Version 1.0.* Toronto, ON: Author. Retrieved from http://chnc.ca/documents/ HomeHealthNursingCompetenciesVersion1.0March2010.pdf

Coyte, P., & McKeever, P. (2001). Home care in Canada: Passing the buck. *Canadian Journal of Nursing Research, 33*(2), 11–25.

Cummings, G., MacGregor, T., Davey, M., Lee, H., Wong, C., Lo, E., Muise, M., & Stafford, E., (2010). Leadership styles and outcome patterns for the nursing workforce and work environment: A systematic review. *International Journal of Nursing Studies, 4,* 363–385.

Deber, R. (2003). Health care reform: Lessons from Canada. *American Journal of Public Health, 93*(1), 20–24.

Denton, M., Zeytinoglu, I. U., Davies, S., & Lian, J. (2002). Job stress and job dissatisfaction of home care workers in the context of health care restructuring. *International Journal of Health Services, 32*(2), 327–357.

Epp, J. (1986). *Achieving health for all: A framework for health promotion.* Ottawa, ON: Health and Welfare Canada.

Evans, R. (2007). *Economic myths and political realities: The inequality agenda and the sustainability of Medicare.* Retrieved from http://www.chspr.ubc.ca/files/publications/ 2007/chspr07-13W.pdf

Evans, R. (2008). Reform, re-form, and reaction in the Canadian health care system. *Health Law Journal. Special Edition,* 265–286.

Falk-Rafael, A. (2005). Speaking truth to power: Nursing's legacy and moral imperative. *Advances in Nursing Science, 28*(3), 212–223.

Falk-Rafael, A., Fox, J., & Bewick, D. (2005). Report of a 1999 survey of public health nurses: Is public health restructuring in Ontario Canada moving toward primary health care? *Primary Health Care Research & Development, 6*(2), 172–183.

Gannon, R., Underwood, J., Matthews, S., Goodyear, R., Stamler, L. L., Meagher-Stewart, D., & Munroe, V. (2010). Leadership attributes: A key to optimal utilization of the community health nursing workforce. *Canadian Journal of Nursing Leadership, 23*(2), 60–71.

Gruber, J. (2010). The cost implications of health care reform. *The New England Journal of Medicine, 29*(5), 1050–1051.

Hamilton, N., & Bhatti, T. (1996). *Population health promotion.* Ottawa, ON: Health Canada, Health Promotion and Development Division. Retrieved from http://www.phac-aspc.gc.ca/ph-sp/php-psp/index-eng.php

Health Canada. (2001). *The population health template: Key elements and actions that define a population health approach.* Retrieved from http://www.phac-aspc.gc.ca/ph-sp/pdf/ discussion-eng.pdf

Health Canada. (2010). *Home and continuing care.* Retrieved from http://www.hc-sc.gc.ca/hcs-sss/homedomicile/ index-eng.php

Hutchison, B., Abelson, J., & Lavis, J. (2001). Primary care in Canada: So much innovation, so little change. *Health Affairs, 20*(3), 116–131.

Kennedy, C., Christie, J., Harbison, J., Maxton, F., Rutherford, I., & Moss, D. (2008). Establishing the contribution of nursing in the community to the health of the people of Scotland: Integrative literature review. *Journal of Advanced Nursing, 64*(50), 416–439.

Lalonde, M. (1974). *A new perspective on the health of Canadians: A working paper.* Ottawa, ON: Health and Welfare Canada.

Marchildon, G. (2005). *Health systems in transition: Canada.* Edited by S. Allin and E. Mossialos. Toronto, ON: University of Toronto Press.

McBane, M. (2004). December 2004: Medicare still on life-support. *Canadian Centre for Policy Alternatives.* Retrieved from www.policyalternatives.ca

Meagher-Stewart, D., Aston, M., Edwards, N., Smith, D., Young, L., & Woodford, E. (2004). *Fostering citizen participation and collaborative practice: Tapping the wisdom and voices of public health nurses in Nova Scotia. The study of public health nurses primary health care practice.* Retrieved from http://preventionresearch.dal.ca/pdf/ PHN_study_nov25.pdf

Meagher-Stewart, D., Underwood, J., Schoenfeld, B., Lavoie-Tremblay, M., Blythe, J., MacDonald, M., . . . Munroe, V. (2009). *Building Canadian public health nursing capacity: Implications for action.* Hamilton, ON: McMaster University, Nursing Health Services Research Unit (Health human resources series No. 15).

Mussallem, H. K. (1992). Professional nurses' associations. In A. J. Baumgart & J. Larsen (Eds.), *Canadian nursing faces the future* (2nd ed., pp. 495–518). Toronto, ON: Mosby.

Naylor, D. (2003). *Learning from SARS: Renewal of public health in Canada: A report of the National Advisory Committee on SARS and Public Health.* Ottawa, ON: Health Canada.

Ontario Ministry of Health and Long Term Care. (2004). *Operation health protection: An action plan to prevent threats to our health and to promote a healthy Ontario.* Retrieved from http://www.health.gov.on.ca/english/public/pub/ ministry_reports/consumer_04/oper_ healthprotection04 .pdf

Ontario Ministry of Health and Long Term Care. (2009). *McGuinty government expanding Community Health Centres.* Retrieved from http://ogov.newswire.ca/ ontario/GPOE/2005/11/10/c3426.html?lmatch= &lang=_e.html

Organization for Economic Co-operation and Development. (2010). *OECD health data 2010: Statistics and indicators for 30 countries.* Retrieved from http://www.ecosante.org/ index2.php?base=OCDE&langs=ENG&langh=ENG

Public Health Agency of Canada (2006). *Health is everyone's business.* Retrieved from http://www.phac.health.govt.nz/ moh.nsf/pagescm/761/$File/health-everyones-business .pdf

Rachlis, M. (2008). *Operationalizing health equity: How Ontario's health services can contribute to reducing health disparities.* Wellesley Institute. Retrieved from http://wellesleyinstitute. com/files/OperationalizingHealthEquity.pdf

Rachlis, M., & Kushner, C. (1994). *Strong medicine: How to save Canada's health care system.* Toronto, ON: Harper Perennial.

Rachlis, M., Evans, R. G., Lewis, P., & Barer, M. L. (2001). *Revitalizing medicare: Shared problems, public solutions.* Tommy Douglas Research Institute. Retrieved from http://www.chspr.ubc.ca/files/publications/2001/hpru01-02D_tommydouglaspaper.pdf

Rafael, A. (1997). *Every day has different music: An oral history of public health nursing in Southern Ontario, 1980–1996* (Unpublished doctoral dissertation). University of Colorado, Denver, CO.

Registered Nurses Association of Ontario. (2006). *Healthy work environments best practice guidelines: Developing and sustaining nursing leadership.* Toronto, ON: Author. Retrieved from http://www.rnao.org/Storage/16/1067_BPG_Sustain_Leadership.pdf

Romanow, R. (2002). *Shape the future of health care: Interim report.* Retrieved from http://dsp-psd.pwgsc.gc.ca/Collection/CP32-76-2002E.pdf

Schabas, R. (2002). Public health: What is to be done? *Canadian Medical Association Journal, 166*(10), 1282–1283.

Schofield, R., Ganann, R., Brooks, S., McGugan, J., Dalla Bona, K., Betker, C., . . . Whitford, J. (2008). *Community health nursing vision 2020: Wait or shape? Fact sheet.* Toronto, ON: CHNC. Retrieved from http://www.chnc.ca/documents/CHNVision2020FactSheetAug2008.pdf

Schofield, R., Ganann, R., Brooks, S., McGugan, J., Dalla Bona, K., Betker, C., Dilworth, K., Parton, L. et al. (2010, in press). Community health nursing vision for 2020: Shaping the future. *Western Journal of Nursing Research XX*(X), 1–22.

Shah, C.P. (2003). *Public health and preventive medicine in Canada* (5th ed.). Toronto, ON: Elsevier Press.

Starfield, B. (2010). Reinventing primary care: Lessons from Canada for the United States. *Health Affairs, 29*(5), 1030–1036.

Sullivan, P. (2002). Canada's public health system beset by problems: Report. *Canadian Medical Association Journal, 166*(10), 1319.

Sullivan, T., & Baranek, P. (2002). *First do no harm: Making sense of Canadian health reform.* Toronto, ON: Malcolm Lester & Associates.

Tsasis, P., (2009). Chronic disease management and the home-care alternative in Ontario, Canada. *Health Services Management Research, 22,* 136–139.

Underwood, J., Deber, R., Baumann, A., Dragan, A., Laporte, A., Alameddine, M., & Wall, R. (2009a). *Demographic profile of community health nurses in Canada 1996–2007.* Hamilton, ON: McMaster University, Nursing Health Services Research Unit (Health human resources series No. 13).

Underwood, J. M., Mowat, D. L., Meagher-Stewart, D. M., Deber, R. B., Baumann, A. O., MacDonald, M. B., . . . Munroe, V. J. (2009b). Building community and public health nursing capacity: A synthesis report of the National Community Health Nursing Study. *Canadian Journal of Public Health, 100*(5), I–1–I–13.

Walker D. (2004). *For the public's health: A plan for action. Final report of the Ontario Expert Panel on SARS and Infectious Disease Control.* Toronto, ON: Ministry of Health and Long-Term Care. Retrieved from http://www.health.gov.on.ca/english/public/pub/ministry_reports/walker04/walker04_mn.html

World Health Organization. (1978). *Declaration of Alma Ata.* Retrieved from http://www.who.int/hpr/NPH/docs/declaration_almaata.pdf

World Health Organization. (1986). *Ottawa Charter for Health Promotion.* Ottawa: WHO. Retrieved from http://www.who.int/hpr/NPH/docs/ottawa_charter_hp.pdf

World Health Organization. (2009). *Promoting health and development: Closing the implementation gap, The 7th Global Conference on Health Promotion.* Retrieved from http://www.who.int/mediacentre/events/meetings/7gchp/en/index.html

ADDITIONAL RESOURCES

Canada's Health Infrastructure: History 1994–2004
http://www.hc-sc.gc.ca/hcs-sss/ehealth-esante/infostructure/hist-eng.php

Canadian Broadcasting Corporation – a variety of audio and video clips related to the history of Medicare
http://archives.cbc.ca/health/health_care_system/
http://archives.radio-canada.ca/sante/sante_publique/

Canadian Council on Social Development – A profile of Health in Canada
http://www.ccsd.ca/factsheets/health/index.htm

Canadian Health Services Research Foundation (CHSRF) –Discussion papers submitted to the Romanow Commission and papers on key issues in the commission's final report
http://www.chsrf.ca/other_documents/romanow/index_e.php

Canadian Healthcare Association, (2006) – A Strong Publicly-Funded Health System: Keeping Canadians Healthy and Securing Our Place in a Competitive World. A Brief submitted to the House of Commons Standing Committee on Finance
http://www.cha.ca/documents/pa/FINAL_Pre-budget_brief_September_26_2006.pdf

Canadian Museum of Civilization Making Medicare: The history of health care in Canada, 1914–2007
http://www.civilisations.ca/cmc/exhibitions/hist/medicare/medic00e.shtml

Canadian Nurses Association (2006) – A healthy nation is a wealthy nation
http://www.cna-aiic.ca/CNA/documents/pdf/publications/Standing_Committee_Submission-2006_e.pdf

Canadian Women's Health network – A Women's Guide to Health Care Debates
http://www.cwhn.ca/network-reseau/5-3/5-3pg4.html

Health Canada – Canada's Health Care System (Medicare)
http://www.hc-sc.gc.ca/hcs-sss/medi-assur/index_e.html

Medicare: A People's Issue – a virtual exhibition produced by the Saskatchewan Council of Archives and Archivists, 2004
http://scaa.usask.ca/gallery/medicare/

The Council of Canadians: Health care
http://www.canadians.org/healthcare/index.html

Tommy Douglas Research Institute
http://www.tommydouglas.ca/

About the Authors

Claire Betker, RN, MN, CCHN(C), has worked in community health for more than 30 years at a local, regional, provincial, and national level in Mental Health, Home Health, Primary Health Care, and Public Health. She is currently the Director of Research, Early Child Development with the National Collaborating Centre for Determinants of Health.

Claire was recently (2010) awarded the Canadian Public Health Association and the Public Health Agency of Canada's Human Resources Individual Award for her contribution to Public Health workforce development in Canada. As a volunteer, Claire has been involved with the Community Health Nurses of Canada in Manitoba and nationally, most recently as the Past President. She is newly elected to the Board of Directors of the Canadian Nurses Association. She is currently a PhD student at the University of Saskatchewan where her interest is in theory and its contribution to public health nursing practice and leadership development.

Diane Bewick, RN, BScN, MScN, DPA, CCHN(C), has extensive experience working in community health. She is currently the Director of Family Health Services and the Chief Nursing Officer with the Middlesex-London Health Unit in Ontario. Diane has been an active member of numerous boards and commissions such as the RNAO expert panel developing the Leadership Best Practice Guideline, the Canadian Nurse Practitioner Initiative Advisory Panel, the Ontario Public Health Association (OPHA), and the Ontario Public Health Nursing Management Association (ANDSOOHA).

She is an Assistant Professor in the Faculty of Health Sciences at University of Western Ontario and is the recipient of the Sigma Theta Thau Leadership Award (Nursing Honour Society). She is currently working with others to strengthen community health nursing leadership nationally, including developing a Centre for Public Health Nursing Excellence.

Appendix 2A
Funding for Health Services for First Nations and Inuit in Canada   ROSE ALENE ROBERTS

First Nations, Inuit, and Aboriginal Health (FNIAH) is a branch within Health Canada (HC) that is responsible for the delivery of health services in First Nations and Inuit communities. Services are federally funded and regionally managed. FNIAH is divided into seven regions (Atlantic, Quebec, Ontario, Manitoba, Saskatchewan, Alberta, and British Columbia) that roughly correspond to the provincial boundaries. Atlantic Region includes all four Atlantic provinces. The Yukon, Northwest Territories, and Nunavut are overseen by the Northern Secretariat.

FNIAH regions are separate, parallel structures to the HC regional offices that exist in each region. Regional authority is decentralized and each region has its own unique organizational structure and relationship to its First Nations (FN) constituents. Most of the First Nations and Inuit (FN/I) communities in Atlantic, Quebec, and British Columbia regions manage their own healthcare services in whole or in part. In the remainder, the non-transferred community-based health services are managed by the regional office.

First Nations people are Canadian citizens, and as such, have access to provincially and territorially funded health services that fall under the Canada Health Act, 1984. Aboriginal people, who include the Métis and Inuit, are included in the per capita allocations of federal funding that are transferred to the provinces for "medically necessary" health services. However, First Nations communities (legally known as reserves)

below the 60th parallel are federal or crown land. For this reason, the federal government has historically funded public health and primary health care services on reserves. "North of 60" Aboriginal people comprise most of the population of the Canadian territories; reserves are largely absent; and health services for Aboriginal people are completely integrated into the health and social services systems.

Indian Health Policy, 1979

The Federal Indian Health policy is one of the cornerstones of current policy regarding First Nations people and the Canadian Government. The Indian Health Policy of 1979 stated that it was based on the special relationship of the First Nations people to the federal government and to the Crown (Health Canada, 2007a). This relationship is committed to addressing access issues and health disparities that exist for this specific population.

Policy for federal programs for First Nations people (of which the health policy is an aspect), flows from constitutional and statutory provisions, treaties, and customary practice. It also flows from the commitment of First Nations people to preserve and enhance their culture and traditions. It recognizes the intolerable conditions of poverty and community decline, which affect many communities, and seeks a framework in which communities can remedy these conditions. The federal government recognizes its legal and traditional responsibilities to Aboriginal populations, and seeks to promote the ability of Aboriginal communities to pursue their aspirations within the framework of Canadian institutions (Health Canada 2007a)

Many First Nations communities exhibit conditions that are comparable to the level of poverty and community decline present in many rural and remote parts of Canada. Combined with this economic disadvantage are cultural isolation and the effects of a colonial past. For this reason, addressing the determinants of health is a key feature of federal policy for FN communities. Thus the Indian Health Policy of 1979 noted that improving the level of health in First Nations communities is founded on three pillars

- community development (socioeconomic, cultural, and spiritual) to remove the conditions of poverty and powerlessness that prevent the members of the community from achieving a state of physical, mental, and social well-being;
- the traditional relationship of the First Nations people to the federal government, in which the federal government promotes the capacity of First Nations communities to manage their own local health services; and
- the Canadian health system, consisting of specialized and interrelated services funded by federal, provincial, or municipal governments, First Nations bands, or the private sector.

The federal role lies in public health activities on reserves, health promotion, and the detection and mitigation of hazards to health in the environment. The most significant provincial and private roles are in the diagnosis and treatment of acute and chronic disease and rehabilitation services (Health Canada–FNIAH, 2007a).

In 1989, the "Treasury Board approved authorities and resources to support the transfer of Indian health services from Medical Services, Health and Welfare Canada (now Health Canada) to First Nations and Inuit wishing to assume responsibility" (Health Canada–FNIAH, 2005a). This "transfer process" (also called the "transfer initiative")

- permits health program control to be assumed at a pace determined by the community; that is, the community can assume control gradually over a number of years through a phased transfer;
- enables communities to design health programs to meet their needs;
- requires that certain mandatory public health and treatment programs be provided; and
- strengthens the accountability of Chiefs and Councils to community members.

Further, the transfer process

- gives communities the financial flexibility to allocate funds according to community health priorities and to retain unspent balances,

- gives communities the responsibility for eliminating deficits and for annual financial audits and evaluations at specific intervals,
- permits multi-year (three- to five-year) agreements,
- does not prejudice treaty or Aboriginal rights,
- operates within current legislation, and
- is optional and open to all First Nations communities south of the 60th parallel (Health Canada–FNIAH, 2005a).

Financial Highlights

First Nations Inuit Health Branch (FNIHB) is responsible for funding the delivery of community-based health services to 606 Aboriginal communities and about 805 750 persons, most south of the 60th parallel (Health Canada–FNIAH, 2009). FNIHB directly manages health services in about half those communities and administers integrated agreements and transfer agreements for the rest, who manage their own health services in whole or in part following the process outlined above.

The total budget for FNIHB in 2008–2009 was estimated at $2 billion (Health Canada–FNIAH, 2009). Incorporated into the budgetary programming are the following: management and support, 3%; facilities, 2%; NIHB service delivery, 2%; NIHB benefits, 43%; territorial grants, 1%; hospitals, 1%; and community programs, 48%. (Health Canada–FNIAH, 2009) The Non-Insured Health Benefits program (NIHB) and community programs take up the greatest percentage of the budget (43% and 48%, respectively). The NIHB is a payer of last resort for health services that are not covered under the Canada Health Act for all status Indians in Canada, both on and off reserve. This includes, for example, drugs, dental care, eyeglasses, other assistive devices, short-term crisis intervention, mental health services, and medical transportation (Health Canada–FNIAH, 2005b). Community programs include primary care nursing, communicable diseases, addictions, community health services, environmental health, and chronic diseases (Health Canada–FNIAH, 2009).

Demographic Highlights: South of the 60th Parallel

There are 606 FN/I communities that receive services through the First Nations and Inuit Health Branch in the provincial regions. Delivery of health services is administered in First Nations and Inuit communities in various ways. Those communities interested in having more control of their health services can decide from a menu of approaches: health services transfer, integrated community-based health services, and self-government, based on their eligibility, interests, needs, and capacity.

Since 1989, when the transfer process was initiated, 83% of eligible First Nations communities are now involved in the First Nations Control Process; 46% have signed Community-Based Transfer Agreements, 33% have signed Integrated

3

Nursing Roles, Functions, and Practice Settings

Claire Warren, Roberta Heale, Elizabeth Battle Haugh, and Lucia Yiu

OBJECTIVES

After studying this chapter, you should be able to:

1. Discuss the standards of practice for community health nurses in Canada.
2. Examine the public health nursing discipline specific core competencies and home health nursing competencies in Canada.
3. Contrast the roles of the public health nurse and home health nurse.
4. Explain the diversity of roles and practice settings within community health nursing.
5. Describe the roles and scope of practice for nurses working as nurse practitioners, as entrepreneurs, and in faith community nursing, forensic nursing, and military nursing.
6. Identify the emerging trends for community health nurses.

INTRODUCTION

Community health nurses (CHNs) are registered nurses who work in a variety of roles within the community. They partner with individuals, families, communities, and populations in various settings, such as homes, schools, workplaces, streets, shelters, churches, community health centres, outpost nursing stations, etc. The goal of community health nursing (CHNsg) is to promote the clients' health. In doing so, it is assumed that such determinants of health as socioeconomic and physical environments as well as education are strong predictors and play a large role in supporting the health of the individuals in the community (Community Health Nurses Association of Canada [CHNAC], 2008). CHNsg interventions must also take other determinants of health, such as culture, biological endowment, etc., into consideration when they attempt to achieve the goal of healthier communities. This long-term goal is achieved through a comprehensive variety of health promoting strategies. The complex interplay of individual-, group-, community-, and population-level interventions in promoting, protecting, and/or restoring health and preventing illness, makes CHNsg unique and challenging. CHNs may undertake many roles and implement a range of interventions within the broad goal of promoting health.

Community nursing provides a continuum of care from health promotion and protection and prevention of illness, to treatment, restorative and palliative care (CHNAC, 2008). This chapter describes the goals and practice competencies of

CHNs across a broad range of community nursing roles and settings, with an emphasis on home health and public health, which compose the majority of CHNsg positions. The roles of nurse entrepreneur, nurse practitioner, faith/parish nurse, forensic nurse, and military nurse will be described, while some of the other specialized community nursing roles are elaborated upon in other chapters. Also included in this chapter are the standards of practice for CHNs, core competency expectations for Public Health Nurses (PHNs) and Home Health Nurses (HHNs), and the evolving trends affecting CHN practice.

STANDARDS OF COMMUNITY HEALTH NURSING PRACTICE

According to the Canadian Nurses Association (CNA) (2008a), in 2006, CHNs composed more than 13.6% (36 928) of nurses in Canada. CHNs embrace their specialty nursing practice within a diversity of roles, functions, and practice settings. Combining their foundational nursing education with specialized knowledge of community nursing concepts and competencies, they use a multiplicity of frameworks and theories in their practice that span the complete continuum from **primary prevention** (reducing risks for a potential problem) to **secondary prevention** (providing screening and early detection and treatment) and **tertiary prevention** (maintaining health).

Standards of practice set the minimum level of expected performance for each professional nurse. They provide standardized guidelines for practice, education, and research, as well as criteria for evaluation. In the 1980s, we saw early initiatives to develop standards for CHN practice. An example is the *Standards of Nursing Practice for Community Health Nurses in Ontario*, which were jointly developed by nursing groups representing public health and home health, and by the College of Nurses, Ontario Nurses' Association, the Registered Nurses' Association of Ontario, and the Canadian Association of University Schools of Nursing (Craig, 1985). Today, national standards are set to unify the community health nursing profession. The *Canadian Community Health Nursing* (CCHN) *Standards of Practice* were released in 2003 and later updated in 2008. They were developed by the Community Health Nurses Association of Canada (CHNAC) [now called the Community Health Nurses of Canada (CHNC)], an associate member of the Canadian Nurses Association (CNA). These standards (see Appendix A) were developed to facilitate CHN professional practice in any domain—including education, administration, and research—and reflect the values of Canadian CHNs. They denote the generic nursing practice expectations and identify the principles specific to CHNsg practice (CHNAC, 2008).

In November 2009, the CHNC further developed a vision statement and a common definition of CHN practice in Canada (CHNCa, 2009). All CHNs are expected to know and apply these Standards to their practice, while expert CHNs would practise beyond these standards (CHNAC, 2008). The five main standards are necessarily broad to account for the breadth and scope of practices in community health nursing. They are

1. promoting health,
   a. health promotion
   b. prevention and health protection
   c. health maintenance, restoration and palliation
2. building individual and community capacity,
3. building relationships,
4. facilitating access and equity, and
5. demonstrating professional responsibility and accountability.

CHNAC recognizes that the standards need to be made meaningful to CHNs and that employers require support to ensure that the standards are integrated directly into nursing practices. Hence, a *Canadian Community Health Nursing Standards of Practice Toolkit* was developed to provide a framework for integrating the standards into basic human resource management processes (CHNAC & PHAC, 2006). The standards include continuing education and reflective practice, hiring practices, job descriptions and interview tools, orientation and mentoring programs for new nursing staff, and performance appraisals. The *Toolkit* gives concrete and prescriptive guidance to organizations in implementing the standards into policy and practice. It also provides a basis for integration into undergraduate baccalaureate curriculum in the classroom and clinical setting for nursing students.

In 2006, the first CNA Community Health Nursing Certification Examination was offered. It is now one of 19 recognized specialty nursing areas in Canada (CNA, 2009). In 2008, 338 RNs wrote the Community Health Nursing Specialty Exam (CNA, 2009). This is a voluntary national nursing credential based on national standards released by CNA in 2003 and competencies developed by CHNAC in 2005 (CNA, 2005a). National certification is valid for five years.

Public Health, Public Health Nursing, and Home Health Nursing Competencies

Over the years, various initiatives have occurred to define the areas of practice for community health nursing. Within the context of strengthening the public health system in Canada, the Public Health Agency of Canada (PHAC) developed and released a set of core competencies (version 1.0) for all public health sector workers in Canada in September 2007. These represent cross-cutting knowledge, skills, and attitudes required to practise in the public health field in Canada (PHAC, 2007) (see MyNursingLab). There are 36 public health competencies grouped into seven domains:

1. public health sciences
2. assessment and analysis
3. policy and program planning, implementation and evaluation
4. partnership, collaboration, and advocacy
5. diversity and inclusiveness
6. communication
7. leadership

These domains and competencies are a generic foundation to the practice of public health by its multidisciplinary workers. There are many disciplines working within public health that are developing discipline-specific competencies to complement and build on the generic ones (e.g., nursing, dietetics, epidemiology, dental practitioners, etc.).

A set of public health nursing discipline-specific competencies (version 1.0) was released in May 2009. With the commitment of CHNC's Certification, Standards, Competency Standing Committee and an expert group, and funding from PHAC, the development of these discipline-specific competencies was made possible. There are a total of 66 public health nursing competencies grouped into eight domains. The first seven domains are basically identical to PHAC's with the addition of an eighth domain: professional responsibility and accountability (CHNC, 2009b) (see Appendix B).

The relationship between core competencies and standards likely requires some clarification. **Standards** define the scope of practice or professional expectations (CHNAC, 2008), while **competencies** encompass the knowledge, skills, and attitudes required for practice (PHAC, 2007).

Key characteristics of CHNs are reflected in the standards and core competencies and include a high level of independence, autonomy, resourcefulness, collaboration with the client/family/community, strong community and individual health assessment skills, critical thinking and problem solving, and an understanding of the community and its resources and the overall healthcare system. All CHNs work within an array of legislations (written and approved laws), Acts (e.g., Nursing Act 1991; Regulated Health Professions Act; Canada Health Act; Health Insurance Act; Protection of Privacy Act; in Ontario the Health Protection and Promotion Act, the Community Care Access Corporations Act, etc.), mandates (e.g., Ontario Public Health Standards) and standards (professional standards set by each provincial College of Nurses), but the concepts of health promotion and primary health care are the foundation of their practice.

Health promotion is most commonly defined in global terms by the World Health Organization (WHO, 1984) as "the process of enabling people to increase control over and to improve their health." It is a broad definition and includes the spectrum of health enhancement, health protection, disease prevention, health restoration/recovery, and care and support.

Primary health care (PHC) was defined at the 1978 Alma Ata conference as healthcare that is scientifically sound, socially acceptable, universally accessible to individuals and families, through their full participation, and at a cost the community and country can afford within the spirit of self-reliance and self-determination (WHO, 1978). This definition has evolved to include all broad health determinants and the services that can influence health, such as income, housing, education, and social and physical environments (Health Canada, 2006; Raphael, 2008). All CHNs have a mandate to integrate the principles of PHC into their care of individuals, groups, communities, and populations (see Chapter 7). CHNsg competencies common to all include

- knowledge of community resources beyond health in order to link the client to appropriate ongoing resources to support their health goals (e.g., social services, housing, and employment services);
- understanding and utilization of ethics and culture care principles;
- knowledge of advocacy, health policy development and the overall health system; and
- client teaching strategies.

The CHNAC describes in its standards two distinct groups of CHNs: home health nurses (HHNs) and public health nurses (PHNs). The differences between the roles of an HHN and a PHN are best articulated in the CCHN's Standards of Practice document:

> The HHN begins with a close-up lens zooming in and focusing on the individual client and family, then shifting to a wide-angle lens to encompass groups and the supports in the community. The move from wide-angle to close-up lens is useful for the PHNs shifting their focus between systems, population health and intersectoral partnerships and the health of individual clients and families. (CHNAC, 2003, p. 3)

There may be provincial differences in roles and functions of the CHNs. For example, in Quebec, there is a blended community health nursing model where a nurse may function within both domains. Figure 3.1 depicts the various types of hospital and community nursing.

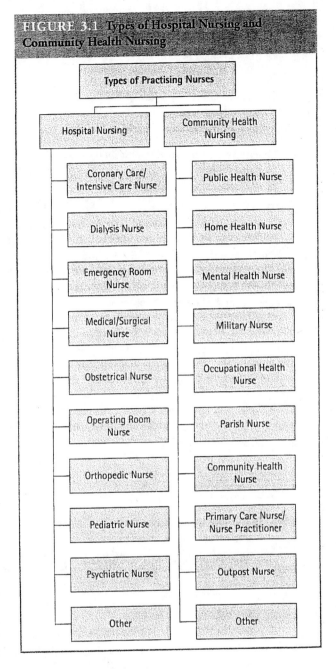

FIGURE 3.1 Types of Hospital Nursing and Community Health Nursing

Home health nursing consists of a broad spectrum of services that aim at "providing accessible, responsive, and timely care which allows people to stay in their homes with safety and dignity" (Community Health Nurses of Canada [CHNC], 2010, p. 7). Home health nursing "encompasses disease prevention, rehabilitation, restoration of health, health protection, and health promotion with the goal of managing existing problems and preventing potential problems" (p. 7).

In 2010, the CHNC developed a framework for home health nursing competencies (see Appendix C). The framework consists of the following nursing activities:

A. Elements of home health nursing practice
    a. Assessment, monitoring and clinical decision making
    b. Care planning and care coordination
    c. Health maintenance, restoration, and palliation

d. Teaching and education
e. Communication
f. Relationships
g. Access and equity-building capacity

B. Foundations of home health nursing
a. Health promotion
b. Illness prevention and health protection

C. Quality and professional responsibility
a. Quality care
b. Professional responsibility (p. 8)

To carry out the expected nursing practice competencies, CHNs must carry out a variety of roles and activities depending on their practice settings (see Table 3.1, p. 49). The Canadian Public Health Association (2010) addressed that CHNs play key roles in health promotion, disease and injury prevention, health protection, health surveillance, population health assessment, and emergency preparedness and response. Depending on the settings they work in, CHNs engage in the following activities: advocacy; building capacity; building coalition and networks; care/counselling; case management; communication; community development; consultation; facilitation; health education; health threat response; leadership; outreach; policy development and implementation; referral and follow-up; research; resource management; program planning, coordination, and evaluation; screening; surveillance; and team building and collaboration.

Public Health Nursing

Public health nursing touches everyone's life throughout the life span through activities such as prenatal classes, newborn home visiting, routine immunization, school and workplace health, infectious disease control, healthy lifestyle promotion, substance abuse prevention, injury prevention including infant and child injury, safe driving, preventing falls in the elderly, and environmental health.

A **public health nurse** (PHN) utilizes knowledge from public health, nursing, social and environmental sciences, and research, and integrates the concepts of primary health care, social determinants of health, and health inequities, in order to promote, protect, and maintain the health of populations (CHNAC, 2008). The *goal of public health nursing,* as with public health, is to increase the health of the community (i.e., reduce mortality and morbidity rates) by preventing disease and promoting healthy behaviours and environments. PHNs work under the mandate of provincial public health legislation in official public health agencies (i.e., a health unit or health department within municipal, regional, or provincial government/authorities) and their clients range from individuals, families, and groups, to populations in schools, workplaces, and the entire community.

PHNs work on interdisciplinary teams that may include public health professionals, such as public health inspectors and dietitians, epidemiologists, health promotion and program evaluation specialists, communication specialists, graphic designers, dental professionals, family support personnel, social workers, and physicians. Volunteers are also an important part of the team. In smaller agencies and rural and remote communities, PHNs often assume a generalist role in providing a variety of services to a geographic community as opposed to the specialist role in larger agencies.

Individual as Client The most common practice settings for individuals as recipients of public health nursing services are clinics and occasionally homes; however, telephone counselling reaches clients wherever they may be and is one strategy that is used uniquely for providing individualized client health teaching. Most public health agencies have PHN staff telephone help lines that triage all client calls for health information. The PHN (or nurse-on-call) provides callers with information, referral, and consultation services on topics such as newborns and childcare, breastfeeding and nutrition, healthy lifestyle advice, sexual health issues, smoking cessation, immunization, and communicable diseases (see Photo 3.1).

A variety of clinical services are also offered in public health. These range from communicable disease control and follow-up (e.g., HIV; TB; hepatitis A, B and C; sexually transmitted infections [STIs]), to birth control and safer sexual practices, travel health, immunization, breastfeeding, and well baby and child health clinics, where developmental screening, child health, and anticipatory counselling are provided. The level and specificity of service can differ from one jurisdiction to the next. The majority of nursing interventions within the clinic setting involve client assessment and counselling. Some sexual health clinics have certification training for nurses to perform Pap tests and urethral swabs or to treat genital warts with liquid nitrogen or sexually transmitted infections under medical directives. However, providing immunization, TB screening, and taking swabs or drawing blood for lab samples are the limits of potential hands-on intervention for most PHNs.

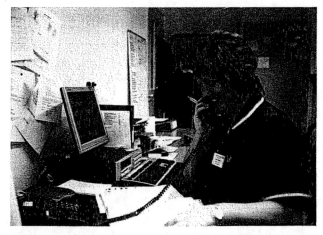

Photo 3.1

Public health nurse working on the telephone information line.

Credit: John Cole / Photo Researchers, Inc.

Family as Client An inclusive concept of the term "family" is always assumed in community health nursing. This includes any significant others for any given person, whether they are living together or related by blood or marriage. Family-centred nursing is a substantive part of public health nursing practice in the multitude of practice settings in which a PHN may work. The nurse's interventions can include all family members in the reinforcement of health teaching and as part of the entire assessment. Visiting in the client's home provides the nurse with an opportunity for a very holistic assessment. Socioeconomic, cultural, environmental, and psychological issues are more obvious in the home setting and therefore the nursing intervention can be more individualized to meet the specific needs of each unique family (see Chapter 16).

The birth of a new baby is always a stressful time for families. The addition of another family member can often cause intergenerational family patterns and roles to change while family members try to adapt to new roles as parents, grandparents, and siblings. A shift in family dynamics is inevitable. PHNs have a long tradition of being pivotal in the support to families as they adapt to the complexities of these role changes and caring for a new infant (see Photo 3.2).

Working with families requires the recognition of cultural sensitivities, which may be different among other generational family members. The composite of the family value system, including religious beliefs and family dynamics, is a major part of the PHN's holistic assessment (Alligood & Tomey, 2006). As nurses establish a relationship with the family, they are able to assess priorities and capitalize on the strengths of some family members to support and empower others (see Chapters 8, 15, and 16).

Group as Client Many public health nursing services are provided in a small-group setting, such as in schools, the workplace, or various community organizations. PHNs apply adult learning theory to engage the group in the health promotion issue. Adult learning or education theory identifies the adult learner as having unique needs (Barstable, 2008). Adult teaching strategies are routinely incorporated into the PHN practice, but in the group setting they assist the nurse to meet the common learning needs of a group of individuals who are potentially very diverse demographically. Prenatal classes are a prime example of education about a health issue that is relevant only to a small subset of the population in the reproductive stage. The group may have very different cultural and socioeconomic status, but the learning objectives are similar. The PHN must be flexible in presentation style and content to ensure inclusiveness of all group members and optimal knowledge transfer.

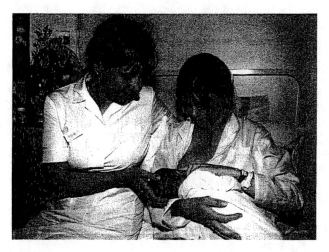

Photo 3.2

Breastfeeding support can be critical in supporting new mothers to exclusively breastfeed until the infant reaches at least six months of age.

Credit: SHOUT / Alamy

CANADIAN RESEARCH BOX

How do nurses work with clients to build capacity for partnership and citizen control?

Aston, M., Meagher-Stewart, D., Edwards, N., & Young, L. M. (2009). Public health nurses' primary health care practice: Strategies for fostering citizen participation. *Journal of Community Health Nursing, 26*(1), 24–34.

This qualitative study examines PHNs' perceptions of their role in engaging citizens to actively participate in control of their health. The study was conducted in a province in Eastern Canada. Forty-three PHNs participated in individual interviews and 31 in focus groups. Several subthemes reflected capacity building for partnership and citizen control:

- working within a population health promotion perspective,
- building trusting relationships and rapport,
- building personal confidence and skills,
- engaging in empowering educational strategies, and
- connecting to a broader social network.

These subthemes all focused on empowerment and accessibility through the lens of social justice and equity, often with marginalized or vulnerable populations. Facilitators and constraints to fostering greater citizen participation evolved around system issues such as manager support to facilitate the work, while lack of resources and fragmented, heavy workloads were some of the constraints. The nursing roles highlighted in the empowerment process include initiators, community planners, collaborators, enablers, educators, and advocates.

Discussion Questions

1. What values and beliefs did these community health nurses demonstrate?
2. What other Canadian Community Health Nursing Standards of Practice apply?
3. What professional responsibility and accountability might you engage in for similar situations?

CASE STUDY

You are a nursing student in your final year of study to obtain your baccalaureate degree in nursing. After writing your registration examination, you will apply for nursing positions in your area. You have enjoyed the community clinical experiences in your nursing education and would like to pursue a career in that area. You are aware of the diversity in practice settings in the community, but the concept of working autonomously, which seems to be a consistent feature in most of them, really appeals to you. You want to make the position a good match for your personality as well as your clinical interests and skills.

Discussion Questions

1. From reading all the descriptions of roles of CHNs in this chapter, assess which one appeals to you the most in terms of the kind of nursing interventions described.
2. What kind of research would you do before submitting an application to a community health nursing agency?
3. How would you prepare for an interview with your employer of choice?

The PHN can also be a key player in policy advocacy within the school setting by working with parent councils and school staff to develop healthy school policies and resulting healthy school environments (see Chapters 4, 6, and 17). The same process can be used within the workplace setting. Comprehensive workplace wellness programs include a combination of education and policy support for a healthy work environment. Community health fairs are another means of engaging the general population in health promoting behaviours. Although it is an education strategy, the target is very broad and awareness of programs and services is the general outcome.

Community as Client A community is viewed as comprising many subgroups or subpopulations. It can be as big as an entire city or a municipal or provincial region serviced by a public health department or regional health authority. It can be very large in geographical size and small in population, such as in a rural outpost region in the more northern parts of Canada. Working with an entire community provides an opportunity for very broad, or macro, health promotion strategies to complement the direct education done with smaller groups or populations. Broad macro strategies are required when working at the community level, such as social marketing, community mobilization, and community development to influence behaviour change and policy development.

Home Health Nursing

The aim of **home health nursing** is to assist individuals experiencing any number of health problems to remain in their home environment and familiar surroundings. Such home care services help to prevent a hospital visit or shorten a hospital stay, thus saving the healthcare system money in the longer term. *Home health nursing* is a specialized area of nursing practice in which the nurse, employed by a home health agency, provides clinical care in the client's home, school, or workplace. HHNs provide the needed resources to promote their clients' optimal level of well-being and functioning and empower their clients and caregivers/families to take charge of their own care. Home health nursing activities include "teaching, curative interventions, end-of-life care, rehabilitation, support and maintenance, social adaptation and integration, and support for the family caregiver" (Canadian Home Care Association, 2008, p. 2).

Although the role of the **home health nurse** (HHN) is commonly categorized as generalist in nature, the trend to well-informed consumers who increasingly expect care from nurses specializing in the relevant clinical area has given rise to numerous specialty roles for HHNs. These include wound ostomy resource nurse, psychogeriatric nurse, continence adviser, diabetes nurse educator, palliative care nurse consultant, respiratory nurse specialist, and many others. These specialty HHNs provide expert client assessment and care and plan guidance that contributes to client care excellence, while augmenting the generalist nurse's knowledge base and competencies.

Home care is not governed by the Canada Health Act, resulting in differences in the kinds of services that are publically funded from one province to the next. Unlike public health, which is government-funded, **home healthcare** is delivered predominantly by private agencies. Some programs receive funding from government(s); however, the remainder is delivered through private insurance coverage, and fundraising initiatives. The Victorian Order of Nurses is an example of a not-for-profit organization that has been providing community healthcare services across Canada for well over 100 years (VON, 2009). There is a mix of not-for-profit and for-profit community healthcare agencies in Canada. Paramed (2008) is the largest for-profit home care agency in Canada, offering service in Alberta and Ontario.

Home healthcare agencies generally have similar philosophies that include the delivery of holistic, evidenced-based healthcare to individuals, families, and groups in community settings. Programs and services vary across agencies and geographical sites since they are dependent upon identified community need and agency resources. Some program areas include community support services (e.g., Meals on Wheels, transportation), health promotion (e.g., immunizations, occupational health), home healthcare services (e.g., wound care, palliative care), home support services (e.g., respite, meal preparation) and workplace wellness (e.g., health and wellness clinics) (Paramed, 2008; VON, 2009).

Individual as Client Client care services are provided within the context of the principles of primary health care, with an emphasis on health promotion and clinical care services. The majority of care is delivered in the client's home, school, workplace, or community clinic.

The HHN's relationship with the client is based on the understanding that the nurse is a "guest in the house." Thus, all care is adapted and mutually agreed upon according to the client's environment and direction. Holistic health assessment skills are critical in order to determine not only the physical and psychosocial needs of the client, but also, as importantly, the role played by the family/caregivers and home environment in supporting or challenging the client's achievement of health goals.

Family as Client Home health nursing views the family as inseparable from the client as focus of care. Assessing the strengths and needs of the family is foundational to maximizing the self-care abilities of the client/family. Accordingly, an understanding of family theory is a prerequisite for HHNs. They mobilize and/or augment the ability of family members to assist the client in meeting the health goals. Where the health support needs of the client are short term, HHNs may teach family members about the particular health alteration and implications (e.g., care considerations for diabetes), specific skills (e.g., wound care), reportable signs and symptoms, and appropriate community supports. Situations where the HHN has a long-term relationship with the family, for example when providing care to a chronically ill child over months or years, requires an in-depth understanding of alterations in the family dynamics arising from the nurse's presence. HHNs need to be knowledgeable and responsive to any indications of child, elder, or spousal abuse (see Chapter 16).

Numerous success indicators provide evidence of the effectiveness of HHNs in caring for clients and families in home and school environments. These indicators include observable improvements in caregivers' confidence and knowledge in providing care, reductions in the stress levels of clients and caregivers, remediation of abusive situations, and the appreciation of clients/caregivers as expressed by verbal and written thanks, often to employers, newspapers, or regulatory colleges.

Group as Client Although opportunities for HHNs to work with groups as the focus of care are limited; they do exist. Examples include an HHN who was contracted to work in a school setting where the student body was composed of children with complex and long-term health needs. The role of the nurse was to provide client-specific care interventions such as medication administration, tube feedings, etc., as well as to consider and provide for the overall health needs of all school children. This latter aspect of the role involved assessing the safety of the school environment, planning activities for the entire school population, and acting as an adviser to the teachers on the intersection of the child's health needs and classroom performance.

Table 3.1 also provides a summary of the characteristics of community health nurses practising in other areas including PHNs and HHNs.

EXPANDING COMMUNITY HEALTH NURSING PRACTICE

Five nursing specialty areas were chosen to illustrate the expansion of community health nursing practice in Canada. The roles, historical perspectives, and/or scope of each specialty practice are described along with the challenges faced by nurses in those practices—namely, nurse practitioners, nurse entrepreneurs, faith community nurses, forensic nurses, and military nurses.

Primary Health Care Nurse Practitioners

A **nurse practitioner** (NP) is an RN with additional education and experience who demonstrates the competencies to autonomously diagnose; order and interpret diagnostic tests; prescribe pharmaceuticals; and perform specific procedures within the legislated scope of practice (Canadian Nurse Practitioner Initiative [CNPI], 2006). NPs work autonomously and in collaboration with an interdisciplinary healthcare team (Canadian Institute for Health Information [CIHI], 2007) to ensure optimal client care. The NP is not a second-level physician or a physician's assistant. NPs complement the roles of other health professionals with their advanced level of clinical skills, in-depth knowledge of nursing theory, and regulatory autonomy (College of Nurses of Ontario [CNO], 2006; CNPI, 2006).

In an attempt to streamline practice expectations, optimize the contribution of NPs, and develop some consistency in advanced nursing practice across the country, the CNA, through federal funding, established the CNPI. The goal of this initiative was to ensure sustained integration of the NP role in the health system. The mandate was to develop recommendations in five broad areas: legislation and regulation; practice and evaluation; human health resource planning; education; and change management, social marketing, and strategic communication (CNPI, 2006).

Major outcomes of the CNPI project evolve around a legislative and regulatory framework that allows for a Canada-wide, consistent, principle-based approach in regulating NP practice, while at the same time giving each provincial and territorial jurisdiction some flexibility in implementation. It also provides a basis for facilitating mobility between jurisdictions and provides clarity for admitting internationally educated NPs (CNPI, 2006). The *Canadian Nurse Practitioner Core Competency Framework* (CNA, 2005b) includes the establishment of core competencies as the basis for NP educational programs and a national NP exam as well as a competency assessment framework for ongoing quality assurance of NP practice. It also recommends title protection for the NP so that only nurses with the defined qualifications would be able to use the title NP. In other words, Canadian NPs have a framework of consistent practice expectations and they must demonstrate specific competencies in the expanded scope of their practice.

Regulatory legislation and standards may vary depending upon the province or territory. As a minimum, NPs can all

TABLE 3.1 Characteristics of Selected Community Health Nurses in Varied Practice Settings

Characteristics / CHNs	Work Settings	Aims	Roles/Function	Client Focus	Funding
Public Health Nurse	Public health units/departments Regional health authorities, client homes, group residences, classrooms, shelters, street outreach	Public Health Nurses are responsible for providing public health programs and services on health protection, promotion, and maintenance; disease and injury prevention; and community participation and development. Public Health Nursing practice is based on the model of primary health prevention and is population focused.	– Performs a variety of functions from home visits to new mothers' class/group educational sessions in various settings – Individual counselling (e.g., sexual health, breastfeeding), – Policy development – Infectious disease follow-up – Program planning and evaluation.	Individual/family, group, or population.	Municipal and/or provincial government funding
Home Health Nurse	Client homes, group residences, classrooms, shelters, street outreach	The focus of home health nursing is the care of individuals and their families throughout the community in settings that include traditional homes, group residences, school classrooms, shelters, and the street. They are often called Visiting Nurses. HHNs are those for whom the scope of practice, in conjunction with the ability to practise holistic nursing, is in the context of a rewarding nurse–client therapeutic relationship.	– Has traditionally been considered a generalist practice, involving the expectation that the nurse demonstrate competence and flexibility in caring for clients across the age and illness continuum – Provides the full spectrum of care, combining critical thinking, comprehensive assessment, and clinical decision-making with expertise in the nursing management of intravenous infusion therapy (often via central venous lines), complex dialysis regimes, medication delivery via ambulatory pumps, and ventilator-dependent clients – Also specialization roles have developed (e.g., wound ostomy resource nurse, psychogeriatric nurse, continence adviser, diabetes nurse educator, palliative care nurse consultant, respiratory nurse specialist, and many others)	Individual and family	Through the facility, which may have both private and public funding sources depending on the program
Community Health Nurse	Community health centre, community location, or the street	A nurse who works in a non-profit organization that provides primary health care and health promotion programs. Community Health Nurses (CHNs) work with individuals, families, and communities to strengthen their capacity to take more responsibility for their health and	– Direct primary health clinical care – Follows client/family from clinic to home	Individual/family, group, or population	Fixed budget from province

TABLE 3.1 Continued

Characteristics

CHNs	Work Settings	Aims	Roles/Function	Client Focus	Funding
		well-being. CHNs work together with others on health promotion initiatives within schools, in housing developments, and in the workplace. They link families with support and self-help groups that offer peer education and support in coping, or are working to address conditions that affect health. As such, CHNs can be seen to be a blend between PHNs and HHNs.			
Occupational Nurse	Workplace	An occupational health nurse is a registered nurse practising in the specialty of occupational health and safety to deliver integrated services to individual workers and worker populations. Occupational health nursing encompasses the promotion, maintenance, and restoration of health and the prevention of illness and injury.	– Direct primary health care. – Addresses health, safety, and well-being of employees – May earn specialty credential from CNA COHN.	Individual or group.	Funded by the employer.
Mental Health Nurse	Community health centres, health authorities, hospitals, various community locations	Psychiatric/Mental Health (P/MH) nurses provide a range of mental health services with a focus on mental health promotion, mental illness prevention, treatment, management, and rehabilitation for individuals with mental illnesses, their caregivers, families, and communities. P/MH nurses recognize the significant impacts the determinants of health (e.g., income, housing, social factors) have on mental health.	– Varies depending on position – Community-based mental health promotion of strategies for client treatment – Requires specialty knowledge of mental health and mental illness, and the factors impacting these – Awareness of the stigma and discrimination associated with mental illness	Individual/family, group, or population.	Through facilities such as CHC, regional health authority.
Outpost/Rural Nurse	Outpost clinic, clients' homes, or other community location	A CHN or PHN who works exclusively in a rural or outpost setting, generally in isolation from a traditional healthcare team support. He/she provides primary health care and makes referrals for more in-depth assessments.	– Primary health care, health education, assessment, and screening – Travels long distances – Adapts to a range of dwellings – Manages a broad spectrum of health needs – Works in isolated communities	Individual, community, group, or population	Provincially or federally funded

TABLE 3.1 Continued

Characteristics

CHNs	Work Settings	Aims	Roles/Function	Client Focus	Funding
PHC–Nurse Practitioner	Family health teams, NP-led clinics, public health units/departments, regional health authorities, post-secondary medical clinics, outposts	Primary Health Care Nurse Practitioners (PHC-NPs) are registered nurses, who are specialists in primary health care, who provide accessible, comprehensive, and effective care to clients of all ages. They are experienced nurses with additional nursing education that enables them to provide individuals, families, groups, and communities with health services in health promotion, disease, and injury prevention, cure, rehabilitation and support. The NP is an advanced practice nurse, functioning within the full scope of nursing practice.	– Provides wellness care, including health screening activities such as Pap smears and monitoring infant growth and development – Diagnoses and treats minor illnesses such as ear and bladder infections – Diagnoses and treats minor injuries such as sprains and lacerations – Screens for the presence of chronic disease, such as diabetes, and monitors people with stable chronic disease, such as hypertension – Works collaboratively with family physicians and other members of the health care team to provide the best care possible by the most appropriate provider.	Individuals, families	Through the agency which is often paid for by the provincial government
Forensic Nurse	Prisons, hospital emergency rooms, police departments, coroners, lawyers	Forensic nurses collect and preserve evidence and DNA from victims of violent crime in order to bring perpetrators to justice.	– Collects evidence and ensures that it is obtained properly at the same time as providing care to the patient – May also collect evidence for victims of domestic or child abuse or homicides – Collects evidence at crime scenes, performs research, and often assists at autopsies to determine the cause of death – Can also work at accident scenes or in labs examining evidence or as a field examiner at the scene of the crime – Can also be hired as an independent consultant by law firms and/or as a trial expert	Individuals, families	Through the facility or privately funded

TABLE 3.1 Continued

Characteristics

CHNs	Work Settings	Aims	Roles/Function	Client Focus	Funding
Nurse Entrepreneur	Nurse entrepreneurs are owners and operators of businesses that offer nursing services to the public	Nurse entrepreneurs are self-employed professionals who organize, manage, and assume the risks of a business enterprise. They work independently and are self-directed and goal focused.	– Is directly accountable to the client – Provides clinical or non-clinical nursing services – Forms partnership, or employs others	Dependent on who is hiring the nurse entrepreneur and the task at hand	Private funding
Military Nurse	Military bases	Nursing Officer is a commissioned member of the Canadian Forces Medical Service (CFMS). Nursing Officer's primary duty is to nurse sick and injured patients, not only in static facilities such as a garrison, base, or wing in a Healthcare Centre, but also in operational facilities such as a Field Hospital. Nursing Officers also provide preventive, occupational and environmental health care services.	– Works at military out-patient facilities that offer in-patient care, or a civilian tertiary-care facility – Serves in operational units (e.g., a Field Ambulance, Field Hospital, or aeromedical staging unit) and may be employed at national headquarters or at a training unit – Can also expect to be deployed overseas on an operational mission	Military personnel and civilians	Federal government

diagnose a common disease, disorder, or condition; order and interpret prescribed diagnostic and screening tests such as X-rays or ultrasounds; and prescribe specific medication. The authority to perform these advanced acts is subject to limits and conditions outlined by the regulatory body and the NP's expertise. The NP seeks consultation with a physician when the diagnosis and/or treatment plan is unclear or beyond the scope of the NP to determine.

Historical Perspectives The road to full development of the NP role has been fraught with difficulties. The movement for an advanced nurse position emerged from the 1960s due to perceptions of physician shortages and a trend toward nursing specialization. In 1971 the Boudreau Report made the implementation of the expanded role of the RN a high priority in Canada's healthcare system. In the 1970s many education programs began graduating NPs, but in the absence of supporting regulatory legislation, these nurses functioned as RNs working under medical directives (Nurse Practitioners' Association of Ontario, 2009). By the 1980s, most NP initiatives had ceased to exist. A small number of NPs continued to function through the 1980s and early 1990s, working mainly in community health centres and in northern or remote outpost nursing stations, with a variety of educational preparations and responsibilities.

Despite the failure of the first initiative, the NP role was consistently cited by many provincial healthcare commissions and task forces as valuable in the delivery of healthcare. During this time, a recognition of the importance of health promotion and the need for more community-based care emerged. Fuelled by limited resources in the 1990s, an enhanced interest and political will to make a shift from a treatment-oriented health care system to a more holistic and upstream approach became a priority. This generated support for a primary health care model of service delivery and ultimately to the creation of formalized NP roles defined in legislation, initially in Ontario and Newfoundland and Labrador (CNPI, 2005). By 2006 in Canada, all but the Yukon Territory had legislation and regulations for NP practice (CIHI, 2006a). In 2008, there were 1026 licensed NPs in Canada with 53.6% in Ontario, 12.9% in Alberta, 6% in Saskatchewan and Newfoundland alike, between 3% to 5.4% in each of Nova Scotia, New Brunswick, Northwest Territories, and Nunavut, and 1.8% in Quebec (CIHI, 2010). The numbers of NPs continues to rise each year.

All jurisdictions in Canada offer licensing for NP practice in primary health care. However, NP education programs and licensing categories vary, and each province or territory identifies NPs who work in community settings differently. For example, Ontario has primary health care NPs while Nova Scotia and Alberta have a licensing stream known as Family/All Ages. Regardless of the category, NPs in community settings have a **primary care** focus, which is a first point of contact for clients, and includes the concept of continuity of care for health services in health promotion, disease and injury prevention, cure, rehabilitation, and support to individuals, families, groups, and communities (CNPI, 2006).

Practice Sites

About 4.1 million Canadians aged 12 and older did not have a family doctor in 2007 (Statistics Canada, 2008). **Primary Health Care Nurse Practitioners (PHCNPs)** provide excellent comprehensive healthcare to people and have the potential to address the significant gap in family practice across the country. As such, the NP role is included in most provincial and territorial plans for primary health care reform (DiCenso et al., 2007) (see Chapter 7).

Community-based NPs in Canada require collaboration with a physician. Although the vast majority of family doctors in Canada are paid through a fee-for-service model, physicians in the NP practice settings are typically paid through capitation or salary. It is difficult to integrate NPs into settings where the physician is paid fee-for-service since the physician loses income when the NP sees the patient. This situation has determined the community settings where NPs in Canada work.

In 2006, 45% of NPs worked in community healthcare and family practice settings, including community health centres, mental health clinics, rural nursing stations, home visiting organizations, public health units, remote and northern communities, and interprofessional family practice settings such as family health teams (DiCenso et al., 2007). The focus of NP care in these settings varies considerably. Some provide care to all ages and stages of life and in settings with a specific health focus such as sexual health, lactation support services, primary health care in secondary schools, or palliative care, etc. Opportunities for NPs in the community continue to expand.

NPs are well suited to palliative care programs and have been an essential part of healthcare delivery in underserviced and rural and remote areas. NP care will become more and more an essential part of primary health care in Canada as barriers to practice are addressed and numbers of NPs increase.

Challenges and Solutions

The full integration of PHCNPs into the primary health care system is an evolving process that has achieved some success in recent years. However, some challenges still exist. There is a lack of a long-term plan, both nationally and in each jurisdiction, to ensure that education of NPs is sufficient to meet the needs of Canadians if NPs are to assume their full scope and appropriate role in Canada's health system (CNPI, 2006). Entry to practice requirements vary from jurisdiction to jurisdiction. The CNPI has recommended that master's degree preparation be required by 2010 or no later than 2015. However, there is a scarcity of data on the use of PHCNPs due to their relatively small numbers and diverse practice areas, and it is therefore difficult to justify with hard evidence requests for more educational opportunities or additional funding for more positions.

Increased public awareness of the NPs' role and their ability to assist with healthcare renewal and access to primary health care is essential to create the policy initiatives to support education and funding needs for a sustained NP workforce. Research on public opinion conducted in conjunction with the CNPI showed that only 60% of Canadians are aware of NPs, but a strong majority (88%) support the integration of

NPs into the healthcare system once the role is explained (Decima Research, 2005). NPs are a valuable resource that can help provide improved and timely access to quality healthcare for Canadians. Further evaluation of outcomes and the evaluation of processes/practices that lead to positive outcomes will be required.

The Nurse Entrepreneur

Nurse entrepreneurs are owners and operators of businesses that offer nursing services to the public. Directly accountable to the client, these nurses are self-employed professionals who organize, manage, and assume the risks of a business enterprise. They may provide the nursing services themselves, form partnerships, or employ others. They work independently and are self-directed and goal-focused. Being in independent practice requires that the nurse develop business expertise in addition to professional knowledge and skills.

Historical Perspectives Nurses in independent practice are not a new phenomenon. Prior to the Second World War, as many as 60% of all RNs in Canada were self-employed in private duty settings for people in their homes (CNA, 1996). Following the war, the demand for hospital nurses escalated with the arrival of universal hospital insurance in the late 1950s. By 1989, very few nurses were still working in private duty as almost 85% of all RNs found employment in hospital settings. The 1990s, however, saw a resurgence of interest in private practice.

Professional Issues More nurses are becoming entrepreneurs as new opportunities for independent practice emerge. In all cases, nurse entrepreneurs are guided by legislation, provincial/territorial standards of nursing practice, and the CNA Code of Ethics for Nursing (CNA, 2008b). The nursing regulatory bodies of each province and territory permit self-employed nurses to offer any service that falls within the defined scope of practice of nursing and does not infringe on the legislated responsibility or the exclusive practice or controlled acts of another health discipline. A nurse who is considering independent practice should begin by reflecting on the competencies required, including personal knowledge, skills, experience, education, and a commitment to continuing education. It is also imperative that the nurse be familiar with the legislated and legal parameters of the profession, both federally and provincially.

The Canadian Nurses Protective Society provides legal services to nurses. They help to determine if the role of the nurse in a situation falls under the legal definition of nurse entrepreneur. Nurses can purchase liability insurance through this organization (Canadian Nurses Protective Society, 2006).

Faith Community Nursing

A **faith community nurse** (FCN) is an RN hired or recognized by a faith community and integrates faith and health in practice. FCNs often have additional training such as Faith Community Nursing courses or a certificate such as the Parish Nursing Certificate. Historically, FCNs have been referred to as parish nurses. The Canadian Association for Parish Nursing Ministry (CAPNM) (2007a) defines a **parish nurse** as a registered nurse with specialized knowledge to promote health, healing, and wholeness for its members. The CAPNM (2007b) has outlined 11 core competencies for education programs and five standards of practice. These standards reflect the values of community health nursing practice but encompass more of the spiritual care elements of holistic nursing.

The term **faith community** refers to a community of people who share similar history, values, and beliefs around their relationship with a higher power and with others in the world. They often gather for purposes of worship and to support one another. **Ministry** refers to one who represents the mission and purposes of a particular faith community, carries out his or her role in accordance with established standards, and is accountable to the public served rather than working in isolation or carrying out a personal agenda.

Historical Perspectives Faith community nursing developed from what is also known as parish nursing. Rev. Granger Westberg (1999) is considered the founder of parish nursing. The idea originated in Chicago, Illinois, in the mid-1980s but rapidly grew throughout the United States. Westberg noticed that the professional knowledge and skills of registered nurses made a significant contribution to the health of people within faith communities. FCNs were prepared to address physical, psychosocial, and spiritual needs, and often served as translators between the faith community and the healthcare system. They function as integrator of faith and health, health educator, personal health counsellor, referral agent, trainer of volunteers, developer of support groups, and health advocate.

Challenges in Practice Education and Research Faith community nursing is relatively new within geographic pockets of Canada. One of the main challenges in practice is the lack of knowledge about the role both within and beyond faith communities. In parts of Alberta, British Columbia, Manitoba, New Brunswick, Ontario, and Saskatchewan, faith community nursing is becoming well established. Early successes have been largely due to continuing education courses for nurses preparing for these roles, various faith groups embracing the idea of nurses on ministry teams, and healthcare organizations partnering to provide start-up funding for beginning faith community nursing programs.

Forensic Nursing

Forensic nursing is a small but growing field in nursing. **Forensic nurses** provide care to victims of crime, collect evidence, and provide healthcare services within the prison system. **Sexual assault nurse examiners** (SANEs) are forensic nurses who are registered nurses educated in the nursing field of forensics. They respond specifically to calls relating to sexual assault or domestic violence in the emergency room setting and provide comprehensive care to sexual assault victims.

SANEs provide primary health care to a variety of victims of sexual assault. Over half (55%) of sexual assaults involve an assailant known by the victim. In the majority of cases the victims are young females between the ages of 15 and 24, and the more serious sexual offences tend to occur in private residences. Although the majority of sexual offences in Canada are of a less severe nature, violations of the person and its impacts on health are of significant importance to the CHN (Brennan & Taylor-Butts, 2008).

Role of Sexual Assault Nurse Examiners In the past, because many survivors often had no visible injuries, they had to wait up to many hours before being seen by emergency room physicians because other, more urgent, clients had priority status. This added unnecessary emotional trauma to the survivors of violence. Today's SANE teams address the specific needs of those survivors of sexual assault and domestic violence at the emergency room immediately following an act of violence. Members of SANE teams are on call around the clock on a daily basis, and they respond quickly to calls from the emergency room for survivors triaged as clinically stable but needing assessment, treatment, and possible referral for matters relating to sexual assault or domestic violence. Response time is usually under one hour, often much less.

Forensic data collection is done for legal purposes. It is neither a prerequisite to nor a replacement for healthcare. The goals of forensic nurses are to provide for healthcare needs and to collect evidence for police in a way that respects clients' dignity, right to choice, and self-determination. The SANE therefore aims to return control to survivors very early in the assessment phase of the interaction and strives to maintain a client-led approach throughout the intervention. (See Photo 3.3.)

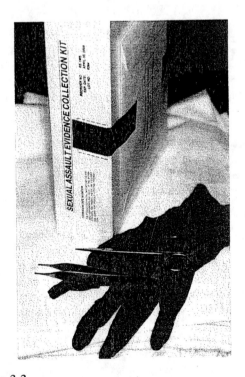

Photo 3.3

Sexual assault evidence collection kit.

Credit: PHOTOTAKE Inc. / Alamy

Domestic violence and sexual assault occur in all cultural, ethnic, and socioeconomic groups at any stage of life. They can occur between male–female dyads and same-sex unions (see Chapter 26). SANEs must be non-judgemental and must be able to explain to the survivors the implications of reporting as this often is the concern of the survivors. Candid discussion of the possible consequences of reporting or not reporting incidents can assist the survivor in making informed decisions. The nurse needs to understand reporting and court procedures; in case prosecution does proceed, the nurse's testimony may be required. Care must be taken to protect evidence, and documentation of assessment findings must be relevant, clear, objective, and, for the physical assessment, detailed.

SANEs must possess knowledge of community resources and work in collaboration with physicians, emergency room staff, social workers, attorneys, police, and crisis intervention workers. They act as initial liaison between survivors and community agencies. They must also possess confidence; knowledge; expert communication, assessment, and treatment skills; and knowledge of legal procedures.

Military Nursing

Military nurses are nursing officers who are commissioned members of the Canadian Forces Medical Service. They are expected to possess leadership skills, and similar to civilian nurses, their primary duty is to care for sick and injured patients. They work not only in static centres, such as hospitals on military bases, but also in operational facilities, such as field hospitals. They form part of a multidisciplinary team with physician and medical technicians. Military nurses exercise leadership skills and are involved in preventive, occupational, and environmental nursing services for their unit. Other career options for military nurses include humanitarian work, education, and administration. Military nursing goes beyond providing healthcare. A nurse working in the Canadian Force needs to be physically fit, socially adaptable, and versatile. Military nursing may not be for everyone but there are many benefits should a nurse be interested in this challenging career (National Defence and the Canadian Forces, 2008).

TRENDS IN COMMUNITY HEALTH NURSING

Established and emerging trends in healthcare and nursing will continue to challenge CHNs to evolve their practice in order to continue to play a central role in the health system and provide effective and relevant care to their clients. Several such trends are described below.

Social Determinants of Health and Health Equity

The **social determinants of health**, as defined by the World Health Organization (2009), "are the conditions in which people are born, grow, live, work, and age, including the health system. These circumstances are shaped by the distribution of money, power, and resources at global, national, and local levels, which are themselves influenced by policy choices" (para 1). When differences in health status are experienced by various groups or populations and result from social conditions that are modifiable and seen to be unjust or unfair, this is termed **health inequities**. Health equity thus implies that everyone, regardless of socially determined circumstances, has an equal opportunity to attain their full health potential without being disadvantaged (Whitehead & Dahlgren, 2006). All nurses need to be aware of the issues that impact health beyond traditional healthcare if they are to make a meaningful difference in people's lives. (See Chapters 5, 6, and 7.)

Technological Advances

Technological innovation continues to advance and nurses need to be ready to embrace the resulting changes. In the community, technology, such as voice mail, email, and wireless devices, has enhanced connectivity. In some settings, nurses document in the client health record by way of laptop or handheld electronic devices. For nurses working in the far North or rural outposts, it is now possible to send test results electronically and receive a diagnosis and treatment order without having to transport a client to a remote medical centre. The emergence of telehealth applications has reduced travel for clients in rural and northern regions by enabling medical and nursing specialists to provide assessment, diagnosis, and treatment protocols via distance technology. Telemonitoring applications are providing new opportunities for remote assessments of wound healing, cardiac and respiratory status, or other health indicators, thus making optimal use of scarce nursing and medical resources. Telephone nursing services are now available in many regions of Canada, and nurses are identifying and evolving telehealth nursing competencies that continue to support a therapeutic nurse–client relationship.

Social networking is the expansion of contacts by making connections through individuals and has been going on for centuries. Yet its full potential as a result of the Internet is starting to be fully recognized. Social networking sites (such as Facebook, Twitter, MySpace, Friendster, and Xanga to name a few), blogging, and video sharing websites (such as YouTube) have become very popular methods of reaching out to a wide variety of audiences. Different sites tend to attract differing age groups. Knowledge of, comfort with, and use of this technology by nurses is inevitable. The challenge will be in keeping up with the trends and having organizational policies that both support and protect staff and the public. (See Chapter 11.)

Evidence-Informed Practice

There is a growing emphasis on an evidence-informed approach to healthcare. Accordingly, best practice guidelines, critical pathways, and care maps will increasingly provide important foundations from which to individualize nursing care and promote consistency and optimal client health outcomes. An excellent example of nursing-led development of best practice guidelines is that of the Registered Nurses Association of Ontario (RNAO). For a list of guidelines, go to www.rnao.org.

Pandemic Planning and Emerging Public Health Threats

Infectious diseases (e.g., SARS and H1N1), bioterrorism (e.g., anthrax post-9/11), and natural disasters (e.g., hurricanes, tsunamis, earthquakes, and oil spills) have galvanized political will to address significant gaps in our public health infrastructure. Following the SARS outbreak in 2003 in Canada, the Naylor report provided many recommendations that have been implemented in public health over the last several years (Health Canada, 2003). These recommendations raised national awareness of the need to be responsive to potential public health threats ranging from bioterrorism threats to pandemic (e.g., H5N1 avian flu, H1N1 swine flu) planning. Nurses are now taking part in emergency preparedness planning and education so that they can be leaders in supporting the community in the event of environmental disasters or pandemics. (See Chapter 30.)

The effect of globalization on health is another critical area of importance. We must consider the impacts of increased economic integration across national borders, enhanced communications as a result of technological change, cultural diffusion, and international travel (e.g., in spreading avian flu and SARS).

TB remains a major public health concern with 9.2 million new cases and 1.7 million deaths worldwide in 2006 (The Lung Association, 2009). Although the incidence in Canada remains relatively low, the clinical presentation and treatment have become increasingly complex, especially when presented with co-morbid conditions such as HIV, as well as being compounded by increasing drug resistance.

SUMMARY

This chapter has described the roles and practice settings of Canada's CHNs, with an emphasis on public health and home health nursing, and highlighted five practice examples. The importance of the growing and expanding roles of CHN and related advocacy cannot be underestimated. As the practice discipline evolves and changes, the national HHNsg and PHNsg competencies provide the foundations and help standardize the required knowledge, skills, and attitudes. CHNs have a unique role within nursing in Canada, epitomizing empowerment at all levels of their varied practice areas, and are key players in promoting evidence-based and equitable client-centred care to improve the health of individuals, groups, communities, and populations across Canada.

CANADIAN RESEARCH BOX

What are the enablers of and barriers to community health nursing practice?

Underwood, J., Baumann, A., Akhtar-Danesh, N., MacDonald-Rencz, & Matthews, S. (2009, March). *National community health nursing study: Comparison of enablers and barriers for nurses working in the community.* (No.14). Hamilton, ON: McMaster University School of Nursing and the Nursing Health Services Research Unit.

This study explored the CHNs' perceptions regarding enablers and barriers to practising their full scope of competencies related to knowledge, skills, and attitudes. Between 2005 and 2007, 6667 questionnaires, representing a 57% response rate, were administered to a random stratified sample of CHNs and LPNs across all provinces and territories. The results identified *work environment* as the most important enabler to support the work of CHNs. In terms of the barriers, CHNs felt that the existing physician/nurse collaboration could be improved; they also felt that ongoing professional development opportunities, updates on changing government policies, and more time/money/access to learning resources were important. Over 50% of the nurses felt that employers and government could be more supportive of CHNs' efforts to address population health needs more effectively. Community groups and workers also need to understand each others' roles and functions.

Discussion Questions

1. What four factors were identified that facilitated nurses to practise to their full scope of competencies? Give examples of each and explain why these might be important to you.
2. Why is research related to community health nursing practice important?
3. Why would organizational support to address the social determinants of health as part of the CHN's scope of practice be important?

KEY TERMS

community health nurses, p. 42
primary prevention, p. 42
secondary prevention, p. 42
tertiary prevention, p. 42
standards, p. 43
competencies, p. 43
health promotion, p. 44
primary health care, p. 44
public health nurse, p. 45
home health nursing, p. 47
home health nurse, p. 47
home healthcare, p. 47
nurse practitioner, p. 48
primary care, p. 53
primary health care nurse practitioner (PHCNP), p. 53

nurse entrepreneur, p. 54
faith community nurse, p. 54
parish nurse, p. 54
faith community, p. 54
ministry, p. 54
forensic nurses, p. 54
sexual assault nurse examiners (SANEs), p. 54
military nurses, p. 55
social determinants of health, p. 55
health inequities, p. 56
social networking, p. 56

REVIEW QUESTIONS

Choose the one alternative that best completes the statement or answers the question.

1. The Canadian Community Health Nursing Standards of Practice were developed to support nursing practice in the community setting. They primarily do this by
   a) defining professional expectations and scope of practice.
   b) describing knowledge, skills, and attitudes.
   c) supporting professional development initiatives.
   d) setting criteria for establishing a community health curriculum.

2. The foundation of nursing practice for Community Health Nurses is based on two major concepts. These are
   a) policy development and program planning.
   b) diversity and inclusiveness.
   c) health promotion and primary health care.
   d) partnership and collaboration.

3. Home Health Nurses mainly work on the principle that
   a) family support is critical to maintaining client care in the home.
   b) holistic assessment and client participation in decision making are key to quality care.
   c) the client must be kept out of the hospital at all costs.
   d) lack of long-term sustainable funding for Home Care agencies makes career planning in this area difficult.

4. Choose the incorrect description of Primary Health Care Nurse Practitioner practice from the following:
   a) grounded in nursing
   b) seen as a second-level physician or physician's assistant
   c) works autonomously and as part of an interdisciplinary team
   d) diagnosing, ordering and interpreting diagnostic tests, prescribing medications, and performing specific procedures within the legislated scope of practice

5. One of the most unique features of Public Health Nursing compared to other community health nursing roles is that
   a) work to influence determinants of health is often not as visible and measurable.
   b) PHNs often do not wear any distinguishable uniform.

c) documentation of interventions can occur in minutes of meetings.

d) PHNs are not involved in tertiary prevention.

6. Community health nursing, with its diversity in practice roles, has had to adapt to societal trends more than institutional nursing because

a) health promotion requires a comprehensive assessment and engagement of the evolving community.

b) technological advances have provided new ways of communicating with clients and the community.

c) emerging infectious diseases are a threat.

d) an aging population will require more services of HHNs, NPs, nurse entrepreneurs, etc.

STUDY QUESTIONS

1. Identify 10 types of practice settings for nurses working in CHNsg.

2. List five broad roles nurses working in CHNsg may perform in the various practice areas discussed in this chapter and explain why each is important.

3. Adult teaching strategies are an important consideration for PHNs. While it may be difficult to know your audience's various learning styles, some strategies can be utilized to enhance success. Identify at least five strategies that can be used in the preparation and delivery of education sessions.

4. How do the HHN, SANE, FCN, and PHCNP incorporate primary health care strategies into their practice?

5. How have trends in community health nursing had an impact on your education?

6. Apply practice examples from any of the CHNsg practice areas discussed in this chapter to the five community health nursing standards.

> *After working through these questions, go to the MyNursingLab at **www.pearsoned.ca/mynursinglab** to check your answers.*

INDIVIDUAL CRITICAL THINKING EXERCISES

1. Which area of community health nursing interests you most and why?

2. Identify five key roles/functions of community health nursing that work toward achieving a healthier community.

3. Describe some examples from your own community where public health has empowered groups to achieve a healthier community.

4. What personal characteristics would draw nurses toward community nursing as opposed to hospital-based nursing?

5. What questions would you ask of a community health nursing organization before accepting employment in that setting? How would you prepare for an interview?

GROUP CRITICAL THINKING EXERCISES

1. Outline a comprehensive plan that a PHN may implement for reducing tobacco use among a school-age population in a low-income neighbourhood. Include the micro and macro strategies your team would employ and describe the collaboration you would need to have with community partners. What challenges might you encounter?

2. Identify strategies to promote an understanding of community health nursing roles among nurses in other sectors.

3. Debate the merits of legislation similar to the Canada Health Act that would provide standardized community healthcare services across Canada.

REFERENCES

Alligood, R. A., & Tomey, A. M. (Eds.). (2006). *Nursing theory utilization and application* (6th ed.). St. Louis, MO: Mosby.

Barstable, S. B. (2008). *Nurse as educator: Principles of teaching and learning for nursing practice* (3rd ed.). Boston, MA: Jones and Barlet.

Brennan, S., & Taylor-Butts, A. (2008). *Sexual assault in Canada 2004 and 2007*. Ottawa, ON: Canadian Centre for Justice Statistics Profile Series, Statistics Canada. Retrieved from http://www.statcan.gc.ca/pub/85f0033m/85f0033m2008019-eng.pdf

Canadian Association for Parish Nursing Ministry. (2007a). *Guide for parish nursing core competencies for basic parish nurse education programs*. Retrieved from http://www.capnm.ca/core_competencies.htm

Canadian Association of Parish Nursing Ministry. (2007b). *Standards of practice: Parish nursing ministry*. Retrieved from http://www.capnm.ca/core_competencies.htm

Canadian Home Care Association. (2008). *Home care: The next essential service: Meeting the needs of our aging population*. Ottawa, ON: Author.

Canadian Institute for Health Information. (2006). *The regulation and supply of nurse practitioners in Canada*. Ottawa, ON: Author.

Canadian Institute for Health Information. (2007). *Canada's health care provider, 2007*. Retrieved from http://secure.cihi.ca/cihiweb/products/HCProviders_07_EN_final.pdf

Canadian Institute for Health Information. (2010). *Regulated nurses in Canada: Trends of registered nurses*. Ottawa, ON: Author. Retrieved from http://secure.cihi.ca/cihiweb/products/regulated_nurses_2004_2008_en.pdf

Canadian Nurses Association. (1996). *Commitment required: Making the right changes to improve the health of Canadians*. Ottawa, ON: Author.

Canadian Nurses Association. (2005a). *Canadian nurse practitioner core competency framework*. Ottawa, ON: Author.

Canadian Nurses Association. (2005b). *List of competencies for the community health nursing certification examination.* Ottawa, ON: Author.

Canadian Nurses Association. (2008a). *2006 Workforce profile of registered nurses in Canada.* Retrieved from http://www.cna-aiic.ca/CNA/documents/pdf/.../2006_RN_Snapshot_e.pdf

Canadian Nurses Association. (2008b). *Code of ethics for registered nurses.* Ottawa: Author.

Canadian Nurses Association. (2009). *Number of RNs with valid CNA certification by year and speciality, 2004–2008.* Retrieved from http://www.cna-aiic.ca/CNA/nursing/certification/stats/default_e.aspx

Canadian Nurse Practitioner Initiative. (2005). *Literature review of nurse practitioner legislation and regulation.* Retrieved from http://206.191.29.104/documents/pdf/Legislation_Regulation_Litertaure_Review_e.pdf

Canadian Nurse Practitioner Initiative. (2006). *Technical report: Nurse practitioners: The time is now.* Retrieved August 9, 2009, from http://www.cpni.ca/cnpe/index.asp.

Canadian Nurses Protective Society. (2006). Collaborative practice: Are nurses employees or self-employed? Retrieved from http://www.cnps.ca/collpract/collpract_e.html

Canadian Public Health Association. (2010). *Public health–community health nursing practice in Canada: Roles and Activities* (4th ed.). Ottawa, ON: Author.

College of Nurses of Ontario. (2006). *Acute care nurse practitioners.* Toronto, ON: Author.

Community Health Nurses Association of Canada and the Public Health Agency of Canada. (2006). *Canadian community health nursing standards of practice toolkit.* Ottawa, ON: Author.

Community Health Nurses Association of Canada. (2008). *Canadian community health nursing standards of practice.* Ottawa, ON: Author.

Community Health Nurses of Canada. (2009a). *Vision and definition of community health nursing in Canada.* Ottawa, ON: Author.

Community Health Nurses of Canada. (2009b). *Public health nursing discipline specific competencies Version 1.0.* Ottawa, ON: Author.

Community Health Nurses of Canada. (2010). *Home health nursing competencies.* Toronto, ON: Author.

Craig, D. (1985). *Standards of nursing practice for community health nurses in Ontario.* Toronto, ON: RNAO.

Decima Research. (2005). *Public opinion research for the Canadian nurse practitioner initiative.* Retrieved from http://www.cnpi.ca/about_the_cnpi/np_final/index.asp?lang=e&

DiCenso, A., Auffrey, L., Bryant-Lukosius, D., Donald, F., Martin-Misener, R., Matthews, S., & Opsteen, J. (2007). Primary health care nurse practitioners in Canada. *Contemporary Nurse, 26* (1), 104–115.

Health Canada. (2003). *Learning from SARS: Renewal of public health in Canada.* Retrieved from http://www.phac-aspc.gc.ca/publicat/sars-sras/naylor/

Health Canada. (2006). *About primary health care.* Retrieved from http://www.hc-sc.gc.ca/hcs-ss/prim/about-apropos/index_e.html

The Lung Association. (2009). *Tuberculosis: Information for health care providers* (4th ed.). Toronto, ON: Author.

National Defence and the Canadian Forces. (2008). *Nursing Officers—Reserve Force.* Retrieved from http://www.forces.gc.ca/health-sante/hp-ps/nur-inf/res-eng.asp

Nurse Practitioners' Association of Ontario. (2009). *History of NP role development in Ontario.* Retrieved from http://www.npao.org/history.aspx

Paramed. (2008). *Paramed get better.* Retrieved from http://www.paramed.ca/homecare/about/

Public Health Agency of Canada. (2007). *Building the public health workforce: Core competencies and skills enhancement programs for public health.* Retrieved from http://www.phac-aspc.gc.ca/php-psp/ccph-cesp/index-eng.php

Raphael, D. (2008). Grasping at straws: A recent history of health promotion in Canada. *Critical Public Health, 18*(4), 483–495.

Statistics Canada. (2008, June 18). Canadian community health survey. *The Daily.* Retrieved from http://www.statcan.gc.ca/daily-quotidien/080618/dq080618a-eng.htm

VON. (2009). *About VON.* Retrieved from http://www.von.ca/en/about/default.aspx

Westberg, G. (1999). A personal historical perspective of whole person health and the congregation. In P. A. Solari-Twadell & M. A. McDermott (Eds.), *Parish nursing: Promoting whole person health within faith communities* (pp. 35–41). Thousand Oaks, CA: Sage.

Whitehead, M., & Dahlgren, G. (2006). *Concepts and principles for tackling social inequities in health: Levelling up Part II.* Europe: World Health Organization. Retrieved from http://www.who.int/social_determinants/resources/leveling_up_part2.pdf

World Health Organization. (1978). *Declaration of Alma-Ata: International conference on primary health care, Alma-Ata, USSR, 6-12.* Europe: Author. Retrieved from http://www.who.int/topics/primary_health_care/en/

World Health Organization. (1984). *Health promotion: A discussion document on the concepts and principles.* Copenhagen, Denmark: WHO Regional Office for Europe.

World Health Organization. (2009). *Social determinants of health.* Retrieved from http://www.who.int/social_determinants/en/

ADDITIONAL RESOURCES

Readings

Canadian Nurses Association. (2006). *Towards 2020—Visions for nursing.* Ottawa, ON: Author. http://www.cna-aiic.ca/CNA/documents/pdf/publications/Toward-2020-e.pdf

Canadian Nurses Association. (2007). Understanding self-regulation. *Nursing Now, 21,* 1–5. http://www.cna-aiic.ca/CNA/documents/pdf/publications/NN_Understanding_Self_Regulation_e.pdf

Canadian Nurses Association. (2008). CNA's preferred future: Health for all. A discussion paper. http://www.cna-aiic.ca/CNA/documents/pdf/publications/Preferred_Future_Webcast_e.pdf

Underwood, J. (2010). *Maximizing community health nursing capacity in Canada: A research summary for decision makers: Report of the national community health nursing study. Canadian Health Services Foundation.* http://www.chsrf.ca/final_research/reiss/pdf/11510_Reiss_report_en_FINAL.pdf

Websites

Association of Ontario Health Centres
http://www.aohc.org

Canadian Association of Sexual Assault Treatment Centres (CASAC)
http://www.casac.ca

Canadian Forces – Nursing (Officer)
http://www.forces.ca

Canadian Nurses Protective Society
http://www.cnps.ca

Community Health Nurses of Canada
http://www.chnc.ca/

International Association of Forensic Nurses
http://www.forensicnurse.org

Video Clips

CNA's Preferred Future: Health For All
http://www.cna-aiic.ca/CNA/documents/pdf/publications/Preferred_Future_Webcast_e.pdf

Vancouver Coastal Health Authority has produced an educational video resource on health inequities. *Population Health: The New Agenda* is a 15-minute video that provides examples of how the social determinants of health impact on various individuals:
http://www.lemongrassmedia.net/lgm/blog/files/pophealth-the-new-agenda.html

National Film Board's film on Inner City Health in Toronto and a mental health nurse partnering with local police:
http://filmmakerinresidence.nfb.ca/

RNAO's Clinical Best Practice Guideline on smoking cessation on YouTube:
http://www.youtube.com/watch?v=L99LxIVJWNM

Community Health Nursing: A Practical View.
This 2009 DVD, from Memorial University, St. John's, Newfoundland, highlights the differences between public health and home health nursing practices in rural and urban settings. It identifies the standards of community health nursing and the various roles of community health nurses.
http://www.ucs.mun.ca/~dwestera/community.html

About the Authors

Claire Warren, RN, BScN, MN, CCHN(c), is Manager of Professional Practice and Development and Community Nurse Specialist at the Sudbury & District Health Unit. She has 15 years experience in public health nursing, has taught community health nursing courses in both French and English at Laurentian University, and is involved in many professional associations such as the RNAO, College of Nurses Community and Public Health Advisory Group, ANDSOOHA: Public Health Nursing Management in Ontario, and the Canadian Evaluation Society.

Roberta Heale, RN (EC), BScN, MN, is an Assistant Professor in the School of Nursing at Laurentian University in Sudbury, Ontario. Prior to taking this position she worked as a primary health care nurse practitioner for 7 years and, before this, as an RN in acute care settings for 11. She is involved with changes in healthcare delivery models through the integration of NPs into community settings, most notably with the development of the Sudbury District Nurse Practitioner Clinics. Roberta is completing a Doctor of Nursing Practice (DNP) degree from Case Western Reserve University in Cleveland, Ohio. Her research interests include the education of NPs and other healthcare providers as well as with their practice in the community.

Liz Haugh, RN, BA, MScN, is the Director of Health Promotion at the Windsor-Essex County Health Unit in Windsor, Ontario, and is also an adjunct professor at the Faculty of Nursing, University of Windsor. She has been involved in Public Health for more than 35 years. She is a past president of the College of Nurses of Ontario, currently President of the Ontario Public Health Association, and member of the board of the Association of Local Public Health Agencies (alPHa) and ANDSOOHA (Public Health Nursing Management in Ontario).

Lucia Yiu, BScN, BA (Psychology, Windsor), BSc (Physiology, Toronto), MScN (Administration, Western Ontario), is an Associate Professor in the Faculty of Nursing, University of Windsor, and an Educational and Training Consultant in community nursing. She has worked overseas and served on various community and social services committees involving local and district health planning.

The authors gratefully acknowledge the input and contributions of the following individuals who assisted with the first and second editions of this chapter: Barb Mildon, Linda Patrick, Lynn J. Anderson, Joanne K. Olson, and Sue LeBeau.

Advocacy, Ethical, and Legal Considerations

Elizabeth Peter, Louise Sweatman, and Kathleen Carlin

OBJECTIVES

After reading this chapter students should be able to:

1. Describe the central values of Canadian nursing and how they relate to community health nursing.
2. Understand the relevance of social justice for community health nursing.
3. Articulate and reflect upon the central ethical and legal issues in community health nursing.
4. Understand the political nature of ethical problems in the community.

INTRODUCTION

Community health nurses (CHNs) encounter ethical issues in all facets of their everyday nursing lives. Ethical nursing practice requires CHNs to be able to reflect critically upon their practice, make sound ethical decisions, and take appropriate action.

TABLE 4.1 CNA Nursing Values and Ethical Responsibilities

Providing Safe, Compassionate, Competent, and Ethical Care
- Nurses provide safe, compassionate, competent, and ethical care.

Promoting Health and Well-Being
- Nurses work with people to enable them to attain their highest possible level of health and well-being.

Promoting and Respecting Informed Decision-Making
- Nurses recognize, respect, and promote a person's right to be informed and make decisions.

Preserving Dignity
- Nurses recognize and respect the intrinsic worth of each person.

Maintaining Privacy and Confidentiality
- Nurses recognize the importance of privacy and confidentiality and safeguard personal, family, and community information obtained in the context of a professional relationship.

Promoting Justice
- Nurses uphold principles of justice by safeguarding human rights, equity, and fairness and by promoting the public good.

Being Accountable
- Nurses are accountable for their actions and answerable for their practice.

Source: "Code of Ethics for Registered Nurses" (June 2008). p. 3. @ Canadian Nurses Association. Reprinted with permission. Further production prohibited.

These capacities must reflect the central values of Canadian nursing expressed in the CNA's (2008) *Code of Ethics for Registered Nurses.* These values are listed in Table 4.1. The CNA Code also recognizes ethical endeavours that address aspects of social justice related to broad societal issues in which nurses are asked to work toward eliminating social inequities.

The term "ethics" has been defined and used in numerous ways. For the purposes of this chapter, **ethics** refers to those values, norms, moral principles, virtues, and traditions that guide human conduct. Often ideas that reflect what is good or right and what we ought, and ought not, to do are associated with ethics. Ethics is also a specialized area of philosophy. Moral philosophers study and reflect upon ethics and have developed formal ethical theories. These theories can be helpful in identifying, articulating, and analyzing ethical issues. The term **bioethics**, also defined as healthcare ethics, refers to the study of ethical issues that are related to health and healthcare. Nursing ethics examines ethical issues in healthcare "from the perspective of nursing theory and practice" (Johnstone, 1999; p. 46).

Bioethics and nursing ethics have made use of a range of ethical theories and approaches, including deontology, utilitarianism, casuistry, principlism, virtue ethics, and feminist ethics. It is beyond the scope of this chapter to describe all these in a meaningful and comprehensive fashion. Instead, several Canadian nursing documents that articulate the central ethical values and concepts used in community health nursing will be used to frame the chapter, including the Canadian Nurses Association's (CNA) *Code of Ethics for Registered Nurses* (2008), *Social Justice . . . a Means to an End, an End in Itself* (CNA 2006a), and the Community Health Nurses Association of Canada's (CHNAC) *Canadian Community Health Nursing Standards of Practice* (2008). Occasionally, insights from other perspectives such as utilitarianism and feminist ethics will be drawn in to add depth to the understanding of the complex issues CHNs face. Ultimately, this chapter, with its emphasis upon social justice and everyday ethical and legal concerns, will assist nurses and nursing students to gain the capacity to reflect critically upon the multiplicity of ethical and legal dimensions inherent in community health nursing.

SOCIAL JUSTICE

Social justice has been defined by the CNA (2006a) as "the fair distribution of society's benefits, responsibilities and their consequences. It focuses on the relative position of one social group in relationship to others in society as well as on the root causes of disparities and what can be done to eliminate them" (p. 7). It assumes that all societies experience broad, systematic oppression and inequities, such as racism, classism, sexism, and heterosexism, which affect some people more than others. Every individual contributes to this inequitable distribution of oppression and inequity, even if unintentionally, and therefore is responsible for contributing to the achievement of social, political, and economic parity. In this way, we are responsible not only for recognizing inequities and oppression, but also for taking responsible action (CNA, 2006a).

The descriptor "social" in social justice places emphasis upon the application of justice to social groups, such as the need to address population health and unjust social institutions and relationships. The experiences of individuals, from this perspective, are embedded within larger political, economic, cultural, and social contexts (Reimer, Kirkham, & Browne, 2006). Fundamental to community health nursing is an understanding of the socio-environmental context of health that recognizes that basic resources and prerequisite conditions are necessary to achieve health (CHNAC, 2008). Powers and Faden (2006) reinforce this notion by stressing that social justice is the foundational moral justification for public health as a social institution. A commitment is needed to address systematic disadvantage that severely limits the potential for well-being of oppressed groups. Well-being involves multiple dimensions, including health, personal security, the ability to reason, respect, human attachment, and self-determination. Social justice strives to achieve sufficiently high levels in all these dimensions for everyone (Powers and Faden, 2006).

Social justice is also important when situating the ethical dimensions of healthcare policy, such as home care policy, within a broad, political understanding of the role of healthcare services within societal structures. Currently, Canadian home care services, because they are not covered by the Canada Health Act (1985), are often not adequately funded, leaving many vulnerable individuals without services. While most home care recipients are frail and elderly, increasingly children with complex medical problems are cared for in the home. This cost-shifting to the home and family has led to excessive demands being placed on unpaid caregivers, especially women (Peter et al., 2007).

Social justice is not just a means to an end or an approach to evaluate current circumstances. It has attributes as a desired result or end. Ten such attributes have been identified. (See Table 4.2.)

TABLE 4.2 Social Justice: Ten Defining Attributes	
Equity (including health equity)	Equity is based on the just treatment of all individuals, which includes equitable access and opportunity to meet health needs.
Human Rights (including the right to health)	These rights are defined by the *United Nations Universal Declaration of Human Rights* and the *Canadian Charter of Rights and Freedoms.*
Democracy and Civil Rights	These are outlined in the Canadian Bill of Rights. Democracy and civil rights exist when all have equal rights and power resides in the people and is not based on hereditary or arbitrary differences in privilege or rank.
Capacity Building	Capacity building refers to giving strength to individual and institutional skills, capabilities, knowledge, and experience through coaching, training, resource networking, and technical support.
Just Institutions	Just institutions engage in just practices and the fair treatment of all individuals in institutions.
Enabling Environments	Enabling environments support positive change, community empowerment, and policy development.
Poverty Reduction	The reduction of poverty though projects, programs, and structural reforms of an economic, social, or political nature increases the standard of living and the social and political participation of the poor.
Ethical Practice	The CNA Code of Ethics for Registered Nurses (2008) and ethics review boards define ethical practice for nurses.
Advocacy	Advocacy involves the active support of individual rights and positive policy or system change.
Partnerships	Partnerships that foster social justice are based on the equitable sharing of roles and responsibilities among institutions and individuals across sectors.

Source: "Social justice . . . a means to an end, an end in itself." (February 2006a). @ Canadian Nurses Association. Reprinted with permission. Further production prohibited.

They include equity (including health equity), human rights (including the right to health), democracy and civil rights, capacity building, just institutions, enabling environments, poverty reduction, ethical practice, advocacy, and partnerships (CNA 2006a). When recognizing and acting on problems of inequity in Canadian society CHNs strive to achieve these attributes in their communities.

It is also important to note three features of social justice approaches that are useful to consider when using social justice as a framework for everyday community nursing practice. These features tend to distinguish this type of approach from principle-focused ones typically used in bioethics. First, social justice approaches tend to be concerned with the ethical use of power in healthcare. Broad political and structural dimensions of problems in healthcare and also the day-to-day use of power by health professionals are examined. Power, in itself, is ethically neutral. How power is used, however, is of ethical significance. Worthley (1997) defines professional **power** as "the influence stemming from the professional position we hold. It is the ability to have an impact on the state of being of a person—physically, mentally, emotionally, psychologically, spiritually—in the context of the professional role" (p. 62). Nurses, and other health professionals, can use their professional influence to improve the health and well-being of individuals, but they can also use this professional power to deny individuals the right to make choices regarding their health. This power can be exercised not only at the level of specific individuals, but can be used to address population-based inequities.

Second, a social justice approach, like feminist bioethics, tends to view persons as unique, connected to others, and interdependent, i.e., vulnerable and unequal in power (Sherwin, 1998). It focuses upon how persons are situated or positioned in society, i.e., the entire context of their lives, including culture, history, politics, and socioeconomic status. This relational definition of persons is appropriate for community health nursing because CHNs often work with vulnerable individuals and groups who are socially disadvantaged. In working with clients, CHNs also emphasize the importance of their relationships with the clients they serve as a means of caring and empowerment.

Third, attending to social justice tends to elicit concern for issues of everyday life, not primarily with crisis issues like euthanasia. Not all ethical issues or problems are ethical/moral dilemmas. **Ethical dilemmas** "arise when there are equally compelling reasons for and against two or more possible courses of action, and where choosing one course of action means that something else is relinquished or let go" (CNA, 2008, p. 6). **Everyday ethics** in nursing refers to "how nurses attend to ethics in carrying out their daily interactions, including how they approach their practice and reflect on their ethical commitment to the people they serve" (CNA, 2008, p. 5). These everyday ethical concerns also can include those related to advocating for clients, working with limited resources, and relieving human suffering. Social justice expands the agenda of bioethics by examining broad healthcare issues that impact on everyday practice, such as the need to examine social inequities in Canada that prevent individuals from acquiring the determinants of health. It also recognizes

CANADIAN RESEARCH BOX

How can clinical education contribute to students' learning about social justice?

Cohen, B. E., & Gregory, D. (2009). Community health clinical education in Canada: Part II—Developing competencies to address social justice, equity, and the social determinants of health. *International Journal of Nursing Education Scholarship*, 6(1), 1–15.

The purpose of this qualitative study was to explore how Canadian nursing programs foster the development of competencies related to social justice/equity and the social determinants of health in their community courses. Course leaders participated in focus groups to identify enabling and challenging factors. Enabling factors included (1) exposing students to concepts of social justice, equity, and the social determinants of health ideally throughout the entire curriculum; (2) using innovative settings that serve the needs of vulnerable populations; (3) involving non-nurse preceptors as mentors; (4) creating learning environments that facilitate student engagement and critical reflective thinking.

Challenges included (1) lack of ideal sites; (2) student concerns with non-traditional placements; (3) inadequate numbers of RN-preceptors in non-traditional settings; (4) lack of time for theory application; and (5) insufficient opportunities to develop traditional public health core competencies.

Discussion Questions

1. How do innovative settings foster learning?
2. How could theory and concepts related to social justice be best taught and applied?

that some perspectives, such as those of clients and nurses, have not been adequately brought into the dialogue and debate on ethical issues nor have they been drawn upon fully in the development of bioethical theory.

ETHICAL AND LEGAL ISSUES ARISING IN COMMUNITY HEALTH NURSING PRACTICE

A number of specific ethical and legal issues can arise in community health nursing practice. These will be identified and addressed using the CHNAC's (2008) Standards of Practice to structure the discussion.

The CHNAC (2008) has identified five interrelated standards of practice that form the foundation of CHN practice (see Table 4.3). Standards of practice are broad descriptions of desired and achievable levels of performance. They are expressions of the minimum knowledge, skills, judgments, and attitudes expected of nurses to deliver safe, effective, and ethical nursing care. As such, they are considered

TABLE 4.3   CHNAC's Five Standards of Practice

1. Promoting health
   - Health promotion
   - Prevention and health protection
   - Health maintenance, restoration, and palliation
2. Building individual/community capacity
3. Building relationships
4. Facilitating access and equity
5. Demonstrating professional responsibility and accountability

Source: Community Health Nurses Association (CHNAC) (2008). Canadian community health nursing standards of practice. p. 10.

authoritative statements that set out the ethical, legal, and professional basis of nursing practice (Keatings & Smith, 2010). Failure to maintain these standards can lead to findings of professional misconduct and incompetence, termination of employment, and exposure to civil and criminal liability.

Standard 1: Promoting Health

CHNs promote health through a) health promotion; b) prevention and health protection; and c) health maintenance, restoration, and palliation (CHNAC, 2008). These strategies can each raise specific ethical and legal concerns that require awareness on behalf of CHNs.

Health Promotion CHNs focus on the health promotion of individuals and communities in a variety of ways. The CHNAC's (2008) Standards state, "Health promotion is a mediating strategy between people and their environments—a positive, dynamic, empowering, and unifying concept that is based in the socio-environmental approach to health. . . . CHNs consider socio-political issues that may be underlying individual/community problems" (p. 10). Interventions can include facilitating community action, assisting in the development of skills, and increasing client knowledge and control over the determinants of health (CHNAC, 2008).

Liaschenko (2002) comments that much of the health promotion work that nurses have engaged in has not focused upon the material and socio-political conditions necessary for health. Instead there has been an overemphasis upon individual behaviour patterns. She explains that this may be the result of nurses working within a biomedical system that primarily values repairing diseased or injured bodies and not the social fabric in which bodies live. CHNs are also not always in a position to directly influence those socio-political factors, such as poverty, that they have identified as moral concerns in their work. There is a collective moral responsibility that goes beyond individual CHNs to bring about broad social and political change.

Nevertheless, there are potential moral harms in health promoting activities that need to be discussed. First, because health is a value-laden concept, CHNs can influence individuals to conform to social norms through health promotion strategies (Liaschenko, 2002). In other words, CHNs can unwittingly become agents of social control and medicalization.

Social control refers "to the social processes by which the behaviour of individuals or group is regulated. Since all societies have norms rules governing conduct all equally have some mechanisms for ensuring conformity to those norms and for dealing with deviance" (Scott & Marshall, 2009). The concept of **medicalization** is "the process of identification of an undesirable social condition or mental state as a medical problem subject to treatment. Studies of medicalization point to the historical and cultural specificity of many "diseases," such as—at different times—alcoholism, homosexuality, juvenile delinquency, and depression" (Calhoun, 2002).

Second, a possible moral harm of health promotion is its potential to create adversarial relationships between those who actively strive to improve their health and those who do not (Liaschenko, 2002). A danger exists that those who are not always trying to enhance their health through such things as diet, exercise, meditation, and so on may be viewed as morally weak and inferior. Taken to an extreme, this type of adversarial relationship, if it existed between CHNs and their clients, could compromise nurses' respect for the **dignity** of those they serve. The requirement for nurses to respect the inherent worth of the persons they serve is a fundamental ethical responsibility of Canadian nurses (CNA, 2008). Ultimately, health promotion activities are powerful tools that must be used with careful reflection as to their consequences for the health and well-being of individuals and communities. CHNs must be mindful of the social and professional power they possess as respected and trusted health professionals. An ethical responsibility exists to reflect upon whose good and whose conception of health is being promoted and why.

Prevention and Health Protection CHNs engage in a variety of strategies that minimize the occurrence of diseases and injuries and their consequences. These activities are often prescribed and regulated by mandated programs and laws and can include education and services regarding such things as birth control and breastfeeding, disease surveillance, immunization, risk reduction, outbreak management, and education about communicable diseases. Social marketing techniques such as media releases and radio interviews may be used to deliver key information to the public (CHNAC, 2008).

While preventive and health protective measures can greatly improve the well-being of populations, they also are not without their potential moral harms. Some of these harms have similarities to those associated with health promotion in that they can further medicalization. Prevention and health protection information can weaken people's confidence and security in their health. Constant surveillance of one's body can be anxiety provoking and could possibly lead to an excess of diagnostic testing as well. These iatrogenic risks are of ethical concern because they can erode a person's sense of well-being (Verweij, 1999). For example, under the current emphasis on obesity, a large body size in women has come to symbolize self-indulgence and moral failure, which in turn may lead women to question their sense of self and right to good healthcare (Wray & Deery, 2008). CHNs must strive to find the right balance of providing information to protect their clients without unduly undermining their self-esteem or alarming them.

TABLE 4.4	Four Ethical Principles for Public Health Interventions

1. Harm principle
2. Least restrictive or coercive means
3. Reciprocity
4. Transparency

Source: Upshur, R.E.G. (2002). Principles for the justification of public health intervention. Canadian Journal of Public Health, 93(2), 101–03.

It is important to recognize that efforts to prevent disease and injury restrict the liberty of individuals, thereby limiting their choice and autonomy. For example, seat belt laws and speed limits restrict the liberty of individuals, but they are needed to protect health. Other strategies such as communicable disease surveillance and reporting not only can restrict liberty; they also can go against the ideals of confidentiality and privacy. Sound ethical reasons and legal authority must exist to impose these liberty-limiting strategies upon clients. In some instances, interventions are targeted to one group of people to protect another group's health, such as mandatory reporting of some communicable diseases. These interventions can be ethically justified if they fairly distribute benefits and burdens and limit burdens to the greatest extent possible.

The CNA (2006b) has adopted four principles developed by Upshur (2002) for ethical decision-making about public health interventions that are a form of social control. These are the **harm principle, least restrictive or coercive means, reciprocity, and transparency**. See Table 4.4. The first, the harm principle, developed by John Stuart Mill (1859/1974), a utilitarian, establishes the initial justification for restricting the liberty of people in a democratic society. He states, "The only purpose for which power can be rightfully exercised over any member of a civilized community, against his will, is to prevent harm to others. His own good, either physical or moral, is not a sufficient warrant" (p. 68). For example, a CHN would only be justified quarantining individuals if they had a harmful communicable disease, such as severe acute respiratory syndrome (SARS).

The second principle, least restrictive or coercive means, stipulates that the full force of governmental authority and power should not be used, unless less coercive methods are unavailable or have failed. Education, negotiation, and discussion should come before regulation and incarceration (Upshur, 2002). The CHN, therefore, would not incarcerate cooperative individuals exposed to SARS, but instead would provide instructions to them regarding quarantining themselves safely at home.

The third, the reciprocity principle, indicates that if a public action is warranted, social entities, such as a public health department, are obligated to assist individuals in meeting their ethical responsibilities. In addition, because complying with the requests of the public health department may impose burdens on individuals, such as time and money, the reciprocity principle demands that compensation be given

(Upshur, 2002). Quarantined individuals, therefore, should be compensated with money for lost income and additional expenses, such as childcare, and be assisted with things such as food while quarantined.

The fourth, the transparency principle, refers to the way in which decisions are made. All relevant stakeholders should participate in decision-making in an accountable and equitable fashion that is free of political interference or coercion (Upshur, 2002). For example, this principle indicates that policy development for controlling infectious diseases, such as SARS, requires that all potentially involved people be involved in the process, such as members of the public, healthcare professionals, hospital representatives, and public health and government officials.

How the prevalence of disease is understood and explained by CHNs also has ethical implications. Krieger and Zierler (1996) describe two distinct theories that explain the interplay between social and biological factors that shape disease susceptibility and the public's health—the lifestyle and social production of disease frameworks. The lifestyle theory suggests that individuals choose ways of living that have health consequences. For example, promiscuity, prostitution, and shared and unclean injection drug use have been posited as lifestyle factors that explain the distribution of HIV/AIDS in a population. In contrast, a framework of social production of disease conceptualizes disease determinants to be economic, social, and political. The relative social and economic positioning of people shapes their behaviours and exposure to disease. With respect to HIV/AIDS, groups that are economically deprived and experience racial discrimination are at increased risk for infection. Gender-based economic inequities, for example, influence a woman's ability to determine the sexual use of her body. Prostitution may offer a woman a strategy for economic survival for herself, and possibly also her children, as opposed to being a lifestyle choice per se.

Without a conscious awareness of these differing perspectives, it is possible that CHNs could too easily blame persons who do not heed health information and acquire a disease. Alternatively, CHNs could view these persons as powerless victims of their socio-political and economic positioning, thereby absolving them from any responsibility for their health and absolving CHNs from any responsibility to provide information or other support to assist them in making health choices. Either extreme would not respect the dignity of these persons and would not promote social justice.

A more helpful perspective would put together these explanatory frameworks in a way that does not eliminate the possibility of choice, but situates it. Sherwin's (1998) notion of relational autonomy is helpful here. She describes how individuals are inherently social and relational beings who are significantly shaped by interpersonal and political relationships. Individuals exercise autonomy and choice within this web of interconnected and sometimes conflicting relationships. Options available to individuals are constrained by circumstances and the availability of resources. Pressure from significant others and social forces can also greatly influence decision-making. For example, a young woman with limited financial means may engage in unprotected sexual intercourse with her male partner who refuses to wear a condom. She may understand the risk of unprotected sex, but "chooses" to have intercourse with him because she is financially dependent upon him and finds it difficult to say no to his requests for sex. While she makes a choice, this choice is limited by her economic dependency and perhaps also by societal expectations upon women to sexually satisfy their male partners. Nevertheless, it is possible that future partners will be more receptive to her request and/or her economic situation may improve. Having health information regarding disease prevention in the latter instance could assist her in making choices that protect her health.

Health Maintenance, Restoration, and Palliation CHNs also provide clinical nursing, palliative care, health teaching, and counselling to individuals and families as they experience illness and life crises, such as the birth or death of a family member. In doing so, CHNs engage in a process of mutual participation with their clients in planning, implementing, and evaluating nursing care while maximizing the capacity of individuals and families to take responsibility for and manage their own care. Nursing interventions are wide ranging and can involve health promotion, disease prevention, and direct clinical care strategies (CHNAC, 2008).

This section of the chapter will address the ethical dimensions of several aspects of this multi-faceted CHN role, including community settings as sites of care, informed consent, family caregiving, and palliative care.

Community Settings as Sites of Care Providing care in the community can be challenging, because unlike hospitals, many community settings were not designed primarily for the purposes of caregiving. Because of the variability of settings, CHNs must often adapt their approaches and procedures and they must often travel significant distances or use technology to reach their clients. For example, CHNs working for the Saskatchewan Cancer Agency provide mammographies for First Nations women, who are an under-screened population for breast cancer, by travelling hundreds of kilometres by gravel road in a mobile mammography bus (Griffin & Layton, 2008). Another example includes a home care program in the Northern Lights Health Region, which serves 20 communities across almost 200 000 square kilometres, within the Alberta Health Services by reaching clients through telemonitoring. The monitoring by nurses of clinical signs and symptoms has reduced ER and primary care visits, hospital admissions, and the number of home care visits (CHCA 2009). The practices of these nurses are working toward social justice because their goals reveal a concern for health equity, the right to health and health services, the development of enabling environments, and advocacy.

Understanding the meaning and impact of various places or settings is central to community health nursing because CHNs deliver nursing services where clients live, work, learn, worship, and play (CHNAC, 2008), not in hospitals. Different places/settings accomplish different kinds of work; have different values, operational codes, and philosophies; and are influenced and structured by different kinds of knowledge and power. These factors combine to influence a person's

agency within a particular place or environment (Peter, 2002). Nurses involved with the Supporting Frail Seniors to Stay Safely at Home Initiative from BC's Northern Health and Interior Health communities understand the importance of home for frail elders. This program has introduced a coordinated, multidisciplinary, planned, and client-centred care approach that has increased the quality of life and independence of frail elders (CHCA, 2008).

Thus, the experience of receiving and providing healthcare services cannot be overtly detached from the place in which it is received or provided (Andrews, 2002). Bioethics, including nursing ethics, has generally assumed that the hospital, not the community, is the setting of healthcare delivery, resulting in the neglect of many issues facing CHNs that are strongly shaped by the uniqueness of the settings/places in which they arise.

Special ethical considerations arise when care is provided in the home because homes are highly significant and idealized places that are imbued with multiple meanings, including personal identity and autonomy, intimacy, normalcy, and security (Peter, et al., 2007). As nursing services increasingly are offered in homes as opposed to hospitals, it is necessary for nurses to become mindful of the social and ethical implications of this change. McKeever (2001) aptly states:

> The devolution of healthcare to the home setting is changing the meanings, material conditions, spatio-temporal orderings, and social relations of both domestic life and health-care work. Unlike institutional settings such as hospitals, homes are idiosyncratic places with aesthetic, physical, and moral dimensions that reflect their occupants' gendered, socioeconomic, and ethnic characteristics. Little is known about the suitability of contemporary homes for providing and receiving extraordinary care, or about the effects of superimposing one major institutional order (healthcare) over another (the family) in light of the changes in structure and function that both have undergone in recent decades. (p. 4)

The potential lack of suitability of homes for the provision and receipt of care raises ethical concerns. Anderson (2001) suggests that assumptions have been made in health policy that we all have homes with family and friends readily available to provide care and that the necessary resources for care are there, such as bedding, laundry facilities, etc. The privileged middle class may possess these things, but many others do not. Poverty and homelessness are increasing in Canada, thereby limiting the access to needed health services for large segments of our population (see Chapter 27). This potential barrier to the receipt of health services is of serious ethical concern. Nurses should aspire to promote social justice to ensure that all persons receive their share of health services and resources in proportion to their needs (CNA, 2008).

Informed Consent As in all areas of nursing practice, CHNs must support and respect the informed choices of their clients (CHNAC, 2008). In order for CHNs to assist clients in making informed choices there are at least two elements that must be considered: the exchange of information between the client and CHN and respect for the client's autonomy. These two elements are often subsumed in the concept of **informed consent**. Consent is a basic principle underlying the provision of care, such that without it, a case for negligence and professional misconduct can be made against the nurse. The process of consent includes CHNs disclosing, unasked, whatever a reasonable person would want to know if he/she were in the position of the client. In other words, the nurse must give the information that the average prudent person in the client's particular position would want to know. CHNs must provide information about the nature of the treatment/procedures they are offering, including benefits and risks, alternative treatments, and consequences if the treatment is not given. The presentation of this information must consider the client's education, language, age, values, culture, disease state, and mental capacity. When clients provide their consent, it must be done voluntarily, i.e., without being coerced and they must have the capacity, i.e., mental competence, to do so. Exceptions exist in which consent for treatment is not needed, such as in emergency situations and as required by law.

Family Caregiving The family's role in caregiving, or informal care, has greatly expanded as responsibility for the provision of healthcare services has progressively shifted from the state to the family or individual. Like formal, i.e., paid, caregiving in the home, women also provide most informal care in the home (CPRN, 2005; Duxbury, Higgins, & Schroeder, 2009). The level of care provision is extraordinary, encompassing both personal and high-tech care. It can include assistance with activities of daily living, e.g., bathing, eating, cooking, laundry, cleaning, and transportation and also the provision and management of medications, injections, IVs, catheterizations, dialysis, tube feeding, and respiratory care. These informal caregivers are often responsible for 24-hour care with little available public support and often with inadequate training for the responsibilities they have been expected to assume (CPRN, 2005) and have been reported to have increased rates of emotional and physical strain (Duxbury, Higgins, & Schroeder, 2009).

The transfer of caregiving responsibilities to family caregivers raises a number of ethical concerns. CHNs have a responsibility to promote and preserve the health and well-being of their clients. Because persons are relational in nature, nurses also have a similar responsibility to a client's family. At times, it may be somewhat difficult to determine who is or should be the focus of care. The evidence cited above illustrates that the health and well-being of clients may be threatened when caregivers are stressed and inadequately educated for their role. Moreover, CHNs, when delegating responsibilities to family caregivers, may be compromising safe, competent, and ethical care in situations where these caregivers do not have adequate support or resources. Choice is also limited because clients may have no other options than to provide and receive care at home. Ultimately, however, the source of these ethical problems lies outside of the nurse–client relationship. It is important to recognize that the situations of both CHNs and their clients are the result of broader political forces and agendas that have limited the availability of resources in order to reduce costs. The CNA Code of Ethics (2008) addresses the importance of nurses to uphold principles of justice and equity to ensure that persons gain access to a fair share of health services and resources that are of their choosing. Advocacy for clients is one way for CHNs to promote justice. Advocating change for clients would also improve the health and well-being of CHNs because it would lessen the frequency of nurses practising in a way that compromises their ethical ideals.

Palliative Care A very special and increasingly frequent part of a CHN's practice is palliative care. Although most deaths occur in institutions, many people are now spending the last days of their lives at home. While advances in Canada have been made, only 37% of dying Canadians have access to appropriate, adequate hospice palliative care, despite the Quality End of Life Care Coalition of Canada (QELCCC) (2008)'s belief that "all Canadians have the right to die with dignity, free of pain, surrounded by their loved ones, in a setting of their choice" (QELCCC, 2008, p. 7).

The philosophy of palliative care is holistic and client-centred. The Canadian Hospice Palliative Care Nursing Standards of Practice (CHPCA, 2002) guide nurses working in palliative care and complement the CNHAC (2008) standards and the CNA (2008) code. The CHPCA standards emphasize "respect for the worth of all humans" and respecting "individual(s) based on recognition of their characteristics and abilities" (p. 11). While performing palliative care is extremely rewarding, it can also be stressful for the CHN, the client, and the family. This intimate area of practice is one in which respecting a client's dignity and right to choice may be difficult for some CHNs. Each CHN may hold his or her own values regarding end of life care practices, such as withholding cardiopulmonary resuscitation (DNR) and other treatments, artificial nutrition and hydration, pain control, and assisted suicide or euthanasia (both illegal in Canada). When these do not accord with the choices made by clients or their families, ethical dilemmas may arise. Clients often have cultural and religious practices or rituals that are important to them around the time of death. For example, a Catholic client may ask for a priest to administer the Sacrament of the Sick and some religions have restrictions on who may care for the body after death. Respecting and facilitating these customs are part of the CHN's care.

One of the most important aspects of palliative care is relief of pain. Promoting the client's health and well-being includes the imperative to provide for the client's comfort. Some CHNs may have moral reservations about advocating for or administering adequate amounts of pain medication. They may worry that they are causing the client's death. Yet, ethically, giving comfort at the end of life is part of effective, dignity-preserving care. The Canadian Senate in its report *Quality End-of-Life Care: The Right of Every Canadian* (2000) recognizes that providing pain control may also shorten life and recommends the clarification of the Criminal Code so that both the public and health professionals can learn that this is an acceptable and legal practice. The Senate also recommends increased training for healthcare professionals in pain control. It is up to CHNs working in this area of practice to keep up to date. Adequate pain control means not only an appropriate dosage of medication, but also having a plan in place so that the client gets the medication when it is needed, e.g., not having to wait for a doctor's order or pharmacy delivery at the last minute.

While clients have the right to make informed choices about their care, as their illnesses progress they often become unable to make decisions (incapable). When a client cannot understand and appreciate the consequences of his or her choices, a substitute decision maker, usually the next of kin, steps in to make decisions for the person. The CHN needs to be aware of the laws in his or her province or territory regarding the process for substitute decision makers. When clients and their families or substitute decision maker have discussed the client's preferences for treatment or withholding treatment, the substitute decision maker is able to make decisions based on what the client has wished. One of the ways that clients can communicate their wishes for care is by means of an **advance directive** (living will). An advance directive contains a person's wishes regarding future healthcare decisions. Advance directives are not only for people who are terminally ill. Anyone may stipulate what medical treatments they will accept or reject in certain situations. It is used only if the person becomes incapable of making choices. The advantage of an advance directive is that it gives a person an opportunity to express wishes about treatments such as cardiopulmonary resuscitation (CPR), artificial feeding, and pain control while he or she is capable of doing so. Advance directives, however, cannot substitute for communication between patients, their families, and their caregivers.

An advance directive contains two sections. The instructional directive sets out wishes for treatment. For example, a person may state that if she becomes terminally ill, she does not want antibiotics for an infection. Another person may stipulate that he does not want to be transferred to hospital in a crisis. The second section, the proxy directive, is a power of attorney for personal care. This means that a person may designate one or more substitute decision makers for healthcare. This could be a family member or a friend, but should be someone who knows the person well and is comfortable carrying out his or her wishes. Each section of an advance directive may exist separately; wishes concerning treatment may be set down without naming a proxy, or a proxy may be named without making any stipulations about treatment.

Standard 2: Building Individual/ Community Capacity

CHNs work collaboratively with individuals/communities when building individual and community capacity. CHNs begin where individuals and communities are, helping them to identify relevant health issues and to assess their strengths and resources. CHNs use strategies that involve advocacy and empowerment (CHNAC, 2008). The CHNAC (2008) has described **empowerment** in the following way: "Community Health Nurses recognize that empowerment is an active, involved process where people, groups, and communities move towards increased individual and community control, political efficacy, improved quality of community life, and social justice" (p. 7).

Schroeder and Gadow (1996) propose an **advocacy** approach to ethics and community health that embraces the character of the CHNAC's (2008) perspective on empowerment. Their ethic of advocacy calls for the development of partnerships between CHNs, other professionals, and community members to enhance community self-determination. In these relationships, CHNs can help a community to discern its values, needs, and strengths in the form of a unique and encompassing health narrative. The goal of the relationship is "improved community health as defined by the members of the community rather than as defined by the professional" (p. 79). Communities are experts regarding their own health. They are not deviants in need of the normalizing efforts of professionals. Advocacy also requires that all persons within a community are heard and represented, not just those with power or authority (Schroeder & Gadow, 1996).

Actions based on empowerment and advocacy foster the everyday ethical practice of CHNs. Empowerment and advocacy enhance the choices and health and well-being of communities because they draw on a community's fundamental strengths and needs without the values of others being imposed upon them. CHNs can exercise their professional power ethically, i.e., in a manner that promotes, rather than restricts, the expression of community choices.

For example, CHNs in a rural community near Edmonton, Alberta, initiated a project that increased the number of community services accessed by pregnant women through advocacy. These women were assessed by public health nurses who referred them to additional services as appropriate. Because prenatal anxiety, low self-esteem, and child care stress have been found to be a predictor of postpartum depression, identifying and supporting women is important during pregnancy (Strass & Billay, 2008). By creating this initiative, these nurses are demonstrating some of the core competencies for public health by building partnerships, collaborating, and advocating for potentially vulnerable pregnant women. These competencies are essential for achieving social justice (Edwards & Davison, 2008).

Advocacy strategies can also involve broader political activities. For example, striving for environmental justice requires political involvement at a governmental level. Currently, disadvantaged communities do not benefit from the production and consumption sectors of society in the same way advantaged communities do in Canada, yet they experience the environmental impact of these sectors to a much greater extent through air and water pollution in the areas in which they live (Buzzelli, 2008). CHNs who are novice to politics can address environmental injustices through voting, serving on a community board, or working on a local election campaign. Nurses can also move on to a more involved phase of political advocacy by running for local political office or becoming the spokesperson of a group dedicated to environmental justice. At the most significant phase, nurses can assume strategic positions in healthcare facilities, professional organizations, and government office. Through these positions, nurses can become engaged with policy development with respect to the health impact of production/consumption practices on disadvantaged groups (Boswell, Cannon, & Miller, 2005).

Standard 3: Building Relationships

The CHNAC's (2008) standards describe how CHNs establish and nurture caring relationships with individuals and communities that promote maximum participation and self-determination. They state,

> Caring involves the development of empowering relationships, which preserve, protect, and enhance human dignity. CHNs build caring relationships based on mutual respect and on an understanding of the power inherent in their position and its potential to impact on relationships and practice. (CHNAC, 2008, p. 13)

CHNs must build a network of relationships with many others including those with clients, groups, communities, and organizations.

CANADIAN RESEARCH BOX

How do CHNs interact with high-risk families?

Browne, A. J., Hartrick Doane, G., Reimer, J., MacLeod, M. L. P., & McLellan, E. (2010). Public health nursing practice with "high priority" families: The significance of contextualizing risk. *Nursing Inquiry, 17*(1), 27–38.

This Canadian study explored how PHNs understand, contextualize, and address risk and how they relate to and interact with at-risk families to promote health and diminish potential harm. Interviews and focus groups were conducted with 32 PHNs to examine how they use relational approaches in their work. Three central features were identified:

1. Contextualizing the complexities of families' lives that involved simultaneously working with risk and capacity, taking a temporal view of families, and being flexible.
2. Working relationally: responding to shifting contexts of risk and capacity that involved working collaboratively, engaging in self-reflexivity, and developing trust through transparency.
3. Working relationally with families under surveillance that involved addressing both safety and vulnerability, and assessing risk within capabilities.

The findings reflect that when PHNs work relationally they can recognize both risk and capacity as intersecting dimensions of at-risk families.

Discussion Questions

1. How do the relational approaches of these PHNs promote social justice?
2. How do the activities of these nurses empower families?

In building relationships, CHNs must recognize the uniqueness of their own attitudes, beliefs, and values regarding health and also those of their clients. They must also maintain professional boundaries while involving and trusting clients as full partners in the caring relationship. Maintaining professional boundaries can become particularly challenging in the home environment where nurse and clients often spend sustained periods of time together in relative isolation (CHNAC, 2008). A **professional boundary** in the nurse–client relationship has been defined as,

> the point at which the relationship changes from professional and therapeutic to non-professional and personal. Crossing a boundary means the care provider is misusing the power in the relationship to meet his/her own personal needs, rather than the needs of the client, or behaving in an unprofessional manner with the client. (CNO, 2009, p. 4)

In other words, the CHN must be cautious that the focus of the relationship remains on meeting the needs of the client and not on his/her own needs. Nevertheless, relationships need not be distant and entirely clinical in nature, given they are often developed in familial setting within home and community.

The caring aspects of the CHN's work reflect some of the fundamental elements of nursing ethics. In recent years, much emphasis has been placed upon the caring nurse–client relationship as foundational to nursing ethics. A caring approach has merit in that it emphasizes the moral importance of reducing human suffering and the relational aspect of nursing practice. Nevertheless, an approach based solely on caring has limitations in that without moral obligation, social justice, and attention to political structures, caring relationships can be exploitative or unfairly partial (Peter & Morgan, 2001). In other words, CHNs require other elements in their moral repertoire beyond caring, such as the promotion of social justice through advocacy, that can assist them in focusing not only upon the health needs of those immediately connected to them, but also upon those who are more distant.

Insite, a supervised injection facility in Vancouver, exemplifies the importance of building relationships that involve caring, trust, and advocacy in the work of CHNs. These nurses work to improve the health of individuals who use injection drugs in a harm reduction setting. Relationship building is central to their activities since their clients experience barriers to accessing mainstream health services because often they face discrimination, and lack financial resources and transportation. Without these nursing relationships, these nurses' roles in promoting health and reducing harm would not be possible. These roles involve a wide range of activities: needle exchange, primary nursing care, harm reduction education, referrals to health and social services, and addiction treatment (Lightfoot et al., 2009).

Standard 4: Facilitating Access and Equity

CHNs collaboratively identify and facilitate universal and equitable access to available healthcare services and the socioeconomic, social, and physical environmental determinants of health. A number of strategies are employed by CHNs, including advocating for appropriate resource allocation, ensuring access through strategies such as home visits, outreach, case finding for vulnerable populations, advocating for healthy public policy by participating in legislative and policy-making activities, and taking action on identified service gaps and accessibility problems (CHNAC, 2008).

It is through the activities of facilitating access and equity that CHNs strive for social justice. CHNs must take into consideration that social factors such as age, sexual orientation, and socioeconomic status restrict equitable access and distribution of health services and determinants of health. Their activities can be at the local or global level and can entail promoting awareness and action regarding human rights, homelessness, poverty, unemployment, stigma, and so on.

Achieving social justice is extremely difficult. While access to healthcare services is highly important, income security, housing, nutrition, education, and the environment are essential in improving the health of vulnerable populations (Lantz, Lichtenstein, & Pollack, 2007). Addressing these concerns requires policy changes and radical social change. Bayer (2000) states, however, that because "public health officials rarely wield the requisite instruments of power, they can only fulfill their mission as advocates for social transformation" (p. 1838). He has termed this perspective " 'public health nihilism" because public health officials can do so little to alter existing patterns of morbidity and mortality in the absence of social change. Bayer's (2000) perspective illustrates well the link between ethics and power. It is important to recognize that small change is nevertheless important in working toward social justice. Two examples of community health professionals facilitating access and equity will be described below to illustrate this possibility.

Lisa Brown, a mental health nurse, is the founder and executive director of Workman Arts (WA) at the Centre for Addiction and Mental Health in Toronto. She was inspired and challenged by the talents of her clients and began to promote their creative expression through theatre. WA employs both professional actors and people who receive mental health services. The mission of Workman Arts (WA) is "to support aspiring, emerging and established artists with mental illness and addiction issues who are committed to developing and refining their art forms, and to promote a greater understanding of mental illness and addiction through film, theatre, visual arts, music, and literary arts" (Workman Arts, 2009). The activities of WA foster social justice because they promote health equity by helping and advocating for people with mental illnesses, an often marginalized group, to access some of the determinants of health, such as employment and income. In doing so, they reduce poverty and build the capacity of vulnerable people.

The LGTB (lesbian, gay, transgender and bisexual) Health Matters Project is another example of CHNs promoting social justice. Because of societal heterosexism and homophobia, LGTB Canadians experience significant health consequences, such as depression, suicide, and substance abuse. Many health and social services providers often lack knowledge or have attitudinal barriers resulting in the lack of consistent provision of accessible and appropriate services. The goal of the project was to ensure that health and social services providers understand the health needs of this group. A curriculum guide was developed based on health theory and research related to LGTB health concerns. In developing this curriculum, the LGTB Health Matters Project recognizes that oppression related to sexual identity is a determinant of health and strives to promote access and equity (Dunn, Wilson, & Tarko, 2007).

Standard 5: Demonstrating Professional Responsibility and Accountability

CHNs work with a high degree of independence and, like all nurses, they are accountable for the quality of their own practice. At times, they are also accountable for the care and services others provide. In demonstrating accountability, CHNs must adhere to regulatory standards, federal and provincial/territorial professional standards, laws, and codes of ethics. They have a responsibility to be knowledgeable and competent and must also help others around them, such as colleagues and students, to develop and maintain competence (CNA, 2008; CHNAC, 2008).

Increasingly, there has been attention given to the legal and ethical responsibility of nurses and other healthcare professionals to keep personal health information private and confidential. At both the federal and provincial/territorial levels privacy legislation has been developed or is in the process of being developed. Because there are some variations across the country both in terms of the specifics of this legislation and its implementation within organizations, readers are urged to examine privacy regulations within their province/territory and employing organization.

A framework, however, has been developed by Health Canada (2005) that can provide CHNs with some guidelines. It summarizes a key principle underlying its provisions in the following way:

> The collection, use and disclosure of health information is to be carried out in the most limited manner, on a need-to-know basis and with the highest degree of anonymity possible in the circumstances. The Framework also recognizes that privacy is a consent-based right and, unless otherwise stated in legislation, the individual's consent must be obtained for any collection, use and disclosure of personal health information. In keeping with current practices within the healthcare sector, an implied knowledgeable consent model is proposed for the collection, use and disclosure of personal health information within the circle of care. (p. 2)

In terms of community nursing practice, CHNs must ensure that utmost care be exercised when disclosing health information. Under usual circumstances, CHNs only share this information with other team members within their organization when needed and must gain the consent of clients to share this information elsewhere.

There are exceptions in which information can be disclosed without consent, however, including court order or subpoena and to prevent serious harm or reduce significant risk to a person or a group of persons, such as in an emergency situation (Health Canada, 2005). The most common exception in the practice of CHNs is the legal requirement to report child abuse and some infectious diseases. There are also less common situations in which CHNs could encounter individuals who disclose information that reveals that a client is a threat to others. In a well-known California case, a psychologist did not warn the intended victim that one of his clients was repeatedly threatening to kill his girlfriend (the intended victim). The court held that the psychologist ought to have warned the girlfriend because he had reasonable grounds to believe that she would be harmed (*Tarasoff* v. *Regents of the University of California*, 1976). In a Canadian case, Mr. Trikha (*Wendan v. Trikha*, 1992), a voluntarily admitted psychiatric patient, ran away from hospital. He drove a car at high speed through a red light, crashing into Ms. Wendan, who suffered severe injuries. In this case, however, the psychiatrist was under no obligation to warn, because there was no way to foresee that Mr. Trikha would pose a threat to himself or others. The general principle is that when nurses are aware that a client represents serious and probable danger to the well-being of another, they owe a duty of care to take reasonable steps to protect such persons, i.e., to warn the third party. This principle is supported by the CNA Code of Ethics (2008) that indicates that nurses may disclose information if there is substantial risk of serious harm to the person or to other persons.

Professional Competence When CHNs do not practise competently there may be allegations of negligence made against them. These situations are very stressful for nurses and it is important to know what comprises negligence in Canadian law. There are four key elements that must be proven to make a finding of negligence: (a) that there was a relationship between the person bringing the claim (i.e., plaintiff, e.g., client, family) and the person being sued (i.e., defendant, e.g., nurse), (b) that the defendant breached the standard of care, (c) that the plaintiff suffered a harm, and (d) that the harm suffered was caused by the defendant's breach of the standard of care.

A nurse–client relationship is usually established from the instant the nurse offers assistance and the client accepts it. A duty of care is established when a nurse owes a duty to another—the nature and extent will depend on the circumstances. The standard of care has been legally defined as bringing a reasonable degree of skill and knowledge and exercising a degree of care that could reasonably be expected of a normal prudent practitioner of the same experience and standing (Keatings & Smith, 2010). The determination of the standard of care is often based on professional standards, such as those set by regulatory bodies and professional associations, e.g., CHNAC. Breaches of standard of care often stem from an action the nurse should have done (i.e., an omission) or an

action that the nurse did negligently (i.e., a commission). The mere breach of the standard of care, however, is insufficient to support a negligence claim. There must be harm suffered from the breach that was reasonably foreseeable and there must be a causal connection between the harm suffered and the nurse's conduct.

CHNs, either individually or in partnership with others, also have the responsibility to take preventive and/or corrective action to protect clients from unsafe or unethical practice or circumstances. This action may entail reporting to appropriate authorities instances of unsafe or unethical care provided by family or others to children or vulnerable adults (CNA, 2008; CHNAC, 2008). In every Canadian jurisdiction there are statutory laws that require nurses to report instances of physical or sexual abuse of persons, situations where a child's welfare is at risk, and information related to communicable and sexually transmitted diseases. These circumstances are supported by a legislated duty to report as the protection of the individual and community take priority over the confidentiality of the client.

CASE STUDY

Jane was recently hired by a visiting nurses agency. She is providing overnight nursing care for five-year-old Anthony who is ventilator-dependent. Anthony lives with his mother, Susan, and two siblings, ages six months and three years. Susan asks Jane if she could care for all three children while she goes to buy groceries at a 24-hour grocery store. Although the children are all sleeping, Jane is reluctant to assume care for Anthony's siblings. She explains to Susan that she cannot. Susan then becomes upset, stating that she cannot afford to pay for a babysitter and that the other nurses have no problem looking after all of the children for short periods of time. Jane does not know what to do.

Discussion Questions

1. What ethical and legal issues are raised by this situation?

2. What socio-political factors situate these issues?

3. How could Jane help Susan in ways that do not violate professional and ethical standards?

SUMMARY

In this chapter, common ethical and legal considerations in community health nursing were discussed. The CNA (2006a) framework on social justice, the CNA (2008) Code of Ethics and the CHNAC (2008) standards were introduced as relevant ethical perspectives and standards to articulate and address these considerations. The unique responsibilities of CHNs and the variable settings in which they work raise particular ethical concerns that must be understood socio-politically. Health promotion and protection activities can enhance the well-being of clients, but they also can be means of social control that can compromise client choice and confidentiality. Legislation can often provide guidance to CHNs in these instances, e.g., legislative requirements regarding the reporting of some communicable diseases. In many instances, CHNs are in a position to advocate for social justice such that the health and well-being of their clients can be protected. Although Canada is a developed nation, many Canadians do not have access to the determinants of health.

The health and well-being of CHNs and clients may be threatened when community settings are not suitable for the provision of care and when informal caregivers do not have the necessary resources to assume responsibility for caregiving. CHNs providing palliative care to clients in their homes must possess an excellent knowledge of the ethical and legal considerations regarding end-of-life care, such as advance directives, pain control, and DNR. Like nurses in all settings, CHNs are required ethically to develop caring relationships with their clients that remain within the limits of professional boundaries. They must also be accountable for their work, and often for the work of others, and must adhere to provincial/territorial and national ethical, legal, and professional standards.

KEY TERMS

ethics, p. 61
bioethics, p. 61
social justice, p. 62
power, p. 63
ethical dilemmas, p. 63
everyday ethics, p. 63
social control, p. 64
medicalization, p. 64
dignity, p. 64
harm principle, p. 65
least restrictive or coercive means, p. 65
reciprocity, p. 65
transparency, p. 65
informed consent, p. 67
advance directive, p. 68
empowerment, p. 68
advocacy, p. 68
professional boundary, p. 69

REVIEW QUESTIONS

1. Which of the following actions should the community nurse engage in to best promote social justice for people who are homeless?

   a) Advocate for affordable housing policies with municipal and provincial/territorial governments.

   b) Provide referrals to homeless shelters.

   c) Spend equal amounts of time with each client visited.

   d) Provide food and clothing to clients as needed.

2. A CHN discovers that women in a particular part of the province receive PAP smears much less frequently than the national average in Canada. How best can she intervene to ensure that access to health services is equitable?

   a) Provide health teaching to these women.

   b) Advocate for better primary health care for women in this area.

   c) Ensure that these women are treated with respect when receiving health services.

   d) Discover what barriers these women experience and plan interventions accordingly

Case

For the last three years a home care nurse has visited a wealthy client, 76-year-old Mrs. Black, twice weekly to help her manage her diabetes. While Mrs. Black is knowledgeable, she tends drink excessively instead of eating regular meals when she becomes socially isolated.

Questions 3 to 5 refer to this case.

3. Mrs. Black and the nurse have a very positive relationship and often talk openly when the nurse is providing care. Mrs. Black becomes aware that the nurse is having financial difficulty supporting her children who are both in university and offers to pay for their tuition. What should the nurse do?

   a) Immediately terminate the relationship with Mrs. Black.

   b) Accept the money to avoid rejecting Mrs. Black's generosity.

   c) Explain to Mrs. Black that taking the money would be crossing a professional boundary and then work toward making the relationship clinically focused.

   d) Thank Mrs. Black but explain to her that taking the money would be crossing a professional boundary.

4. On her way out of the house, Mrs. Black's neighbour asks the nurse whether Mrs. Black's diabetes is still a problem from her and how she can be helpful. Which of the following responses to the neighbour would be best?

   a) "Today Mrs. Black's blood sugar is within the normal range."

   b) "Perhaps you could share your concerns with Mrs. Black. She could best answer your questions."

   c) "Mrs. Black is in need of company. Eating with her on occasion would be helpful."

   d) "It is against the law for me to share Mrs. Black's health information with you."

5. The home care nurse has recently been working with a student who is very critical of Mrs. Black because she does not always eat her meals and drinks alcohol instead despite the health teaching she has received. How should the nurse respond to the student?

   a) Explain that addictions can be difficult to overcome and that it is not helpful to Mrs. Black to view her as a problem.

b) Suggest to the student to learn more about addictions.

c) Suggest to the student that she share her observations with Mrs. Black.

d) Suggest to the student that she explore with Mrs. Black the challenges she is facing with respect to her diet and alcohol intake and help her to seek community supports as needed.

STUDY QUESTIONS

1. Identify and define the seven central ethical values of Canadian nurses.

2. What are the 10 defining attributes of social justice?

3. What are CHNAC's five standards of practice?

4. List and define the four principles for a public health intervention.

5. What does the process of informed consent involve? What information must the CHN provide and what factors must he/she take into consideration?

6. What are the four key elements that must be proven to make a finding of negligence?

*After working through these questions, go to the MyNursingLab at **www.pearsoned.ca/mynursinglab** to check your answers.*

INDIVIDUAL CRITICAL THINKING EXERCISES

1. How are power and ethics related in community health nursing?

2. What aspects of community health nursing bring about social control? Can these be ethically justified? How?

3. How are nurse–client relationships in the community different from those in hospitals? What are the ethical implications of these differences?

4. What ethical responsibilities must the community nurses consider when working with dying clients?

5. How can the CHN promote the health and well-being of family caregivers?

GROUP CRITICAL THINKING EXERCISES

1. Identify a group in your community that experiences inequities that constrain their ability to meet their health needs. Discuss strategies that would promote social justice.

2. Ask each group member to write down his/her definition of health and then share these with the group. How are these definitions similar and different? How do they reflect different values?

3. Identify a nursing leader in your community who is promoting social justice. How is he/she accomplishing this?

REFERENCES

Anderson, J. M. (2001). The politics of home care: Where is "home"? *Canadian Journal of Nursing Research, 33*(2), 5–10.

Andrews, G. J. (2002). Towards a more place-sensitive nursing research: An invitation to medical and health geography. *Nursing Inquiry, 9*(4), 221–238.

Bayer, R. (2000). Editor's note: Public health nihilism revisited. *American Journal of Public Health, 90*(12), 1838.

Boswell, C., Cannon, S., & Miller, J. (2005). Nurses' political involvement: Responsibility versus privilege. *Journal of Professional Nursing, 21*(1), 5–8.

Buzzelli, M. (2008). *Environmental justice in Canada—it matters where you live.* Ottawa, ON: CPRN.

Calhoun, C. (2002). Medicalization. In *Dictionary of the social sciences.* Oxford University Press. Retrieved from http://www.oxfordreference.com.myaccess.library.utoronto.ca

Canada Health Act. 1985, C.6, s.1.

Canadian Home Care Association (CHCA). (2009). *High impact practices.* Ottawa, ON: Author.

Canadian Home Care Association (CHCA). (2008). *High impact practices.* Ottawa, ON: Author.

Canadian Hospice Palliative Care Association (CHPCA). (2002). *Hospice palliative care nursing standards of practice.* Retrieved from http://www.chpca.net

Canadian Hospice Palliative Care Association (CHPCA). (2006). *The Pan-Canadian gold standard for palliative home care.* Retrieved from http://www.chpca.net

Canadian Nurses Association. (2006a). *Social justice . . . a means to an end, an end in itself.* Ottawa, ON: Author.

Canadian Nurses Association. (2006b). *Public health nursing practice and ethical challenges.* Ottawa, ON: Author.

Canadian Nurses Association. (2008). *Code of ethics for Registered Nurses.* Ottawa, ON: Author.

Canadian Policy Research Network (CPRN). (2005). *A healthy balance: Caregiving policy in Canada.* Ottawa, ON: Author.

Canadian Senate Subcommittee to Update *Of Life and Death* (2000). *Quality of end-of-life care: The right of every Canadian.* Retrieved from http://www.parl.gc.ca

College of Nurses of Ontario (CNO). (2009). *Practice standard: The therapeutic nurse–client relationship, revised 2006.* Toronto, ON: Author.

Community Health Nurses Association of Canada (CHNAC). (2008). *Canadian community health nursing standards of practice.* Retrieved from http://www.chnc.ca/documents/chn_standards_of_practice_mar08_english.pdf

Dunn, B., Wilson, S., & Tarko, M. (2007). The LGTB Health Matters Project. *The Canadian Nurse, 103*(8), 8–9.

Duxbury, L., Higgins, C., & Schroeder, B. (2009). *Balancing paid work and caregiving responsibilities: A closer look at family caregivers in Canada.* Ottawa, ON: Canadian Policy Research Networks.

Edwards, N. C. & Davison, C. M. (2008). Social justice and core competencies for public health. *Canadian Journal of Public Health, 99*(2), 130–132.

Griffin, S., & Layton, B. (2008). Bringing care closer to home. *The Canadian Nurse, 104*(6), 12–13.

Health Canada. (2005). *Pan-Canadian health information privacy and confidentiality framework.* Retrieved from http://www.hc-sc.gc.ca

Johnstone, M.-J. (1999). *Bioethics: A nursing perspective.* Sydney, AU: Harcourt Saunders.

Keatings, M., & Smith, O. (2010). *Ethical and legal issues in Canadian nursing* (3rd ed.). Toronto, ON: Elsevier.

Krieger, N., & Zierler, S. (1996). What explains the public's health? A call for epidemiological theory. *Epidemiology, 7*, 107–109.

Lantz, P. M., Lichtenstein, R. L., & Pollack, H. A. (2007). Health policy approaches to population health: The limits of medicalizaton. *Health Affairs, 26*(5), 1253–1257.

Liaschenko, J. (2002). Health promotion, moral harm, and the moral aims of nursing. In L. E. Young & V. E. Hayes (Eds.), *Transforming health promotion practice: Concepts, issues and applications* (pp. 136–147). Philadelphia, PA: F. A. Davis.

Lightfoot, B., Panessa, C., Sargent, H., Thumath, M., Goldstone, I., & Pauly, B. (2009). Gaining Insite: Harm reduction in nursing practice. *Canadian Nurse, 105*(4), 16–22.

McKeever, P. (2001). Home care in Canada: Housing matters. *Canadian Journal of Nursing Research, 33*(2), 3–5.

Mill, J. S. (1974). *On liberty.* London, UK: Penguin Books. (Original work published 1859).

Peter, E. (2002). The history of nursing in the home: Revealing the significance of place in the expression of moral agency. *Nursing Inquiry, 9*(2), 65–72.

Peter, E., & Morgan, K. (2001). Explorations of a trust approach for nursing ethics. *Nursing Inquiry, 8*, 3–10.

Peter, E., Spalding, K., Kenny, N., Conrad, P., McKeever, P., & Macfarlane, A. (2007). Neither seen nor heard: Children and home care policy in Canada. *Social Science & Medicine, 64*, 1624–1635.

Powers, M., & Faden, R. (2006). *Social justice: The moral foundations of public health and health policy.* New York, NY: Oxford University Press.

Quality End of Life Care Coalition of Canada (QELCCC). (2008). *Hospice palliative home care in Canada: A progress report.* Ottawa, ON: QELCCC.

Reimer Kirkham, S., & Browne, A. J. (2006). Toward a critical theoretical interpretation of social justice discourse in nursing. *Advances in Nursing Science, 29*(4), 324–339.

Schroeder, C., & Gadow, S. (1996). An advocacy approach to ethics and community health. In E. T. Anderson & J. McFarlane (Eds.), *Community as partner: Theory and practice in nursing* (pp. 78–91). Philadelphia, PA: Lippincott.

Scott, J., & Marshall, G. (2009). Social control. In *A dictionary of sociology.* Oxford University Press. Retrieved from http://www.oxfordreference.com.myaccess.library.utoronto.ca/views

Sherwin, S. (1998). A relational approach to autonomy in health care. In S. Sherwin (Ed.), *The politics of women's health: Exploring agency and autonomy* (pp. 19–47). Philadelphia, PA: Temple University Press.

Strass, P., & Billay, E. (2008). A public health nursing initiative to promote antenatal health. *Canadian Nurse, 104*(2), 29–33.

Tarasoff v. *Regents of the University of California,* California Supreme Court, 17 California Reports, 3rd Series, 425, decided July 1, 1976.

Upshur, R. E. G. (2002). Principles for the justification of public health intervention. *Canadian Journal of Public Health, 93*(2), 101–103.

Verweij, M. (1999). Medicalization as a moral problem for preventative medicine. *Bioethics, 13*(2), 89–113.

Wendan v. *Trikha* (1992), 124 AR 1 (QB) affd (1993), 135 AR 382 (CA), leave to appeal denied (1993), 149 AR 160n, (1993) SCCA 126.

Workman Arts (WA) (2009). *Workman Arts Project of Ontario.* Retrieved from http://www.camh.net/About_CAMH/Guide_to_CAMH/Communications_ Community/Guide_ASC_Workman.html

Worthley, J. A. (Ed.). (1997). *The ethics of the ordinary in health care: Concepts and cases.* Chicago, IL: Health Administration Press.

Wray, S., & Deery, R. (2008). The medicalization of body size and women's healthcare. *Health Care for Women International, 29*, 227–243.

ADDITIONAL RESOURCES

Websites

Canadian Bioethics Society
http://www.bioethics.ca/

Canadian Nurses Association
http://www.cna-nurses.ca/cna/

Community Health Nurses Association (CHNAC)
http://www.communityhealthnursescanada.org

Dalhousie University, Department of Bioethics
http://bioethics.dal.ca/

McGill University, Biomedical Ethics
http://www.mcgill.ca/biomedicalethicsunit/

Programmes de Bioéthique, University of Montreal
http://www.bioethique.umontreal.ca/

Quality End-of-Life Care Coalition of Canada
http://www.qelccc.ca/Home

University of Alberta, John Dossetor Health Ethics Centre
http://www.ualberta.ca/BIOETHICS/

The W. Maurice Young Centre for Applied Ethics, University of British Columbia
http://www.ethics.ubc.ca/

University of Toronto, Joint Centre for Bioethics
http://www.utoronto.ca/jcb/rsing

About the Authors

Elizabeth Peter, RN, BScN (Windsor), BA (York), MScN (Toronto), PhD (Toronto), is Associate Professor and Associate Dean, Academic Programs at the Lawrence S. Bloomberg Faculty of Nursing, University of Toronto. Dr. Peter's scholarship reflects her interdisciplinary background in nursing, philosophy, and bioethics. She has written extensively in nursing ethics, focusing her work on ethical concerns in community nursing, with a special emphasis upon home care. Theoretically she locates her work in feminist healthcare ethics and has begun to explore the epistemology of nurses' moral knowledge, using the work of Margaret Urban Walker. Elizabeth also is currently the chair of the Ethics Advisory Committee of the Canadian Nurses Association, a member of the Joint Centre for Bioethics, and an expert faculty member on the Nurse Faculty Mentored Leadership Development Program of Sigma Theta Tau International. During her studies, she worked for many years at the Queen Street Mental Health Centre in Toronto as both a staff nurse and a nursing coordinator.

Louise R. Sweatman, RN, BScN, LLB, MSc, is a nurse lawyer. She received her bachelor of nursing and master of science with focus on ethics from the Faculty of Nursing, University of Toronto. She worked as a psychiatric nurse and then went back to school for a law degree from Osgood Hall Law School, York University in Toronto. She has worked in various provincial, national, and international organizations, such as the Ontario Nurses Association, the Canadian Medical Association, the Canadian Nurses Association, and International Council of Nurses. She is the founder and past Chair of the Canadian Network of National Associations of Regulators. She currently is the Chief Operating Officer of Assessment Strategies Inc., Canada's Testing Company (www.asinc.ca).

Kathleen Carlin, RN, MSc (University of Toronto), PhD (University of Toronto), specializes in healthcare ethics. She is currently an Instructor in the Department of Philosophy at Ryerson University. She has been consultant to the Ethics Committee, St. Joseph's Healthcare, Centre for Mountain Health Services (formerly Hamilton Psychiatric Hospital) in Hamilton, Ontario, and has consulted in ethics to community agencies and long-term care institutions. With Louise Sweatman, she co-founded an annual community health ethics workshop day, which ran for several years at the University of Toronto's Victoria College. She was the lead author of the chapter on ethics in *A Guide to End-of-Life Care for Seniors* and has consulted on Ethics in Practice documents for the Canadian Nurses Association. She has given numerous presentations on ethics at conferences and to community and professional groups.

5 Concepts of Health

Lynne E. Young and Joan Wharf Higgins

OBJECTIVES

After studying this chapter, you should be able to:

1. Understand health as discourse—the medical system view of health, the systems view of health, and lay perspectives on health.
2. Understand the concept of the social determinants of health.
3. Understand the relationship between health and the systems in which it is constructed.
4. Examine how these often conflicting yet parallel perspectives on health influence the practice of community health nursing.

INTRODUCTION

I know people who have such low self-esteem that they have allowed themselves to become infected with HIV, and yet they are people visually who would be seen by society and treated by society as very healthy people. They compensate for such low images that they're in the gym four or five days a week so they see themselves as healthy. I have come to know some of them to be very unhappy or very shy socially, they feel inadequate. So to me they are not healthy.

—Glen (pseudonym), a mid-life man (Maxwell, 1997, p. 112)

Health is a ubiquitous but confusing term, as Glen so thoughtfully observed in the above quote. We drink to our health, but some people drink themselves to death. We run for our health, but some people are injured running. Health professionals promote health, but patients/clients may choose to live unhealthfully in spite of these urgings. (In this chapter, "client" is defined as an individual, a family, a community, or a population.) As nurses, we hold to a belief that health is wholeness, but then speak of "heart health" or "breast health." There are health acts, healthcare systems, health management organizations, health fairs, and so on. Health is at the heart of the language of daily living, as expressed when we clink glasses with companions as well as being front and centre in the policy, program, and practice arenas that affect nursing (Rootman & Raeburn, 1994). Thus, the term "health," often used in everyday life as well as in circumstances that shape our nursing world, is a term for which we generally assume a shared meaning. But can we? Should we?

DEFINING HEALTH

Definitions of "health" abound, derived from medicine, nursing, psychology, anthropology, sociology, politics, holism, and lay perspectives (Dubos, 1961; Rootman & Raeburn, 1994; Saylor, 2004). Such definitions portray health as objective and subjective, a state and a process, naturalist and normative. A phenomenon such as health that is portrayed dichotomously is understandably confusing when one attempts to "pin it down." Dubos (1959) captures the nature of health by likening perceptions of health to a receding mirage: from a distance, the health concept is clear, but it is slippery and elusive as one approaches its meaning. While there is little consensus on the definition of health (Saylor, 2004), what is consistent across definitions is that health is desirable because it encompasses positive qualities such as physical strength, emotional stability, and balance.

Health emerged as a central concept for nursing in the writings of Florence Nightingale. In spite of its elusive nature, health as a guiding concept is embraced by the nursing profession (Meleis, 2007). While some theorists posit that the goal of nursing is quality of life (Parse, 1992) or well-being, documents such as the College of Registered Nurses of British Columbia (CRNBC) Scope of Practice document claim healthy and healing to be the focus of nursing (CRNBC, 2009). Because nursing activities comprise a large portion of health expenditures in Canada, the health-related actions of nurses need to be designed to achieve the overall health-related goals of the wider society. With the multitude of definitions of health, what is the relationship between definitions of health and nursing actions?

Reflecting on this in light of numerous scholarly writings on health, what is most important and most interesting to us as chapter authors about the concept of health is not how health is defined, but rather what it means to speak of health in a particular way. Thus, exploring health as discourse, or a patterned way of speaking of something for some purpose, has potential to clear up some of the confusions that nurses face when trying to think about the meaning of the term "health" relative to their nursing work.

Defining Discourse

Discourse is defined in numerous ways (Mills, 2007). Lupton (1992), a nurse theorist, offers a cogent definition of the term. Discourse, she writes, is "a patterned system of texts, messages, talk, dialogue, or conversations which can be identified in these communications and located in social structures" (p. 145). In the philosophical literature (e.g., Foucault, 1972; Habermas, 1973), discourses are commonly understood to play major roles in shaping relations of power—what is valued in society—and subsequently receive attention and resources. Borgman (1992) argues that discourses of prediction and control are characteristic of traditional quantitative science and research, whereas the universal principle of qualitative and naturalistic research in health is to "let everyone speak in the first person, singular and plural" (p. 144). Since traditional science has dominated Western thought from the seventeenth century, with critiques of this approach emerging in the late twentieth century (Borgman, 1992), current discourses of health will have elements of both the traditional and naturalistic ways of thinking.

Discourses of Health

Health is desirable, a social good, and therein lies its power to shape action. What is considered healthy and unhealthy is influenced by cultural context (Capra, 1982). In North America, health is currently conceptualized within two major discourses: the medical model and the systems view. In the medical model, health is conceptualized as the absence of disease, whereas in the systems view, health is understood to be constructed through the interrelatedness and interdependence of all phenomena (Capra, 1982). An emerging sub-discourse on health within the systems view, particularly in Canada, is the **social determinants of health**, wherein health is held to be constructed primarily by social conditions. Finally, lay definitions of health are apparent in scholarly and lay literature.

Medical Model of Health

Health, according to the medical model, is the absence of disease. This definition of health has dominated our culture for the past three centuries (Capra, 1982) and is therefore a deeply entrenched perspective on health. As the dominant health discourse in Western societies (Fox, 1999), the medical model of health has the power to influence massive individual and collective activities and expenditures (Green & Kreuter, 1999).

Current perspectives on medicine can be traced to the seminal work of scholars of the Intellectual Revolution, for example, William Harvey (1578–1657) and Vesalius (1514–1564) (Donahue, 1985). By charting anatomy through investigational procedures with animal and human cadavers, Harvey and Vesalius advanced the view of the body as machine (Donahue, 1985). From these early beginnings, the goal of medicine emerged as primarily to diagnose malfunctions of the "human machine" and to "fix" it. This mechanistic, problem-focused legacy pervades modern medicine. Achieving and maintaining health is a mechanistic, technical process in which physicians play the role of experts on body functioning (Capra, 1982; Ehrenreich & English, 1978). Thus, the body is conceptualized as a machine disconnected from mind, soul, and social and environmental contexts or settings. Health is the state of a perfectly functioning, decontextualized mechanical entity. Health professionals, including nurses, who adopt this view of health are technical experts and, by association, guardians of a "social order" that builds capacities to predict and control health.

Systems View of Health

A competing discourse to the medical model of health is the systems view of health, a shift in understanding health initiated by the World Health Organization (WHO) in 1948 (WHO, 1948). Here, health is "a state of complete physical, mental, and social well-being, not merely the absence of disease and infirmity" (p. 100). Health, then, is more than a physical, mechanistic state; rather, health is conceptualized in terms of dynamic interrelatedness and integration. The systems view of health is embraced by diverse stakeholders: public, population, and community health; health psychology; holism (Larson, 1999); health promotion from an ecological perspective (Green & Ottoson, 1999); holistic nursing models; and proponents of primary health care, to name a few.

This discourse on health began to gain currency in Canada in the mid-1970s with the release of the 1974 report *A New Perspective on the Health of Canadians* (hereafter called the Lalonde Report) (Lalonde, 1974). Signalling the beginning of the current vision for health care in Canada, this report reintroduced lifestyle and environment as key determinants of health, positing that health is tied to overall conditions of living, a long-standing position of the public health tradition (Lalonde, 1974; Raeburn, 1992). The central argument of this report is that health is not achievable solely as a result of medical care, but rather from the interplay of determinants from four health-field elements: human biology, lifestyles, the environment, and health care systems (Labonte, 1994). The Lalonde Report shifted the focus of a vision for the health of a population from illness care to health care and advanced health promotion as a science. Lalonde called this perspective the health-field concept of health.

The Ottawa Charter for Health Promotion (WHO, 1986), written to expand on the 1948 WHO definition of health, stated that, "Health is . . . a resource for everyday living, not the objective of living" (p. 426). The Charter also proposed five major strategies for promoting health: building healthy public policy, creating supportive environments, strengthening community action, developing personal skills, and reorienting health services. Advocating, enabling, and mediating were identified as central strategies for health promotion practice. It also articulated prerequisites for health: peace, shelter, education, food, income, a stable ecosystem, sustainable resources, social justice, and equity, thereby entrenching specific determinants of health into this discourse on health in Canada.

In the same year, the Epp Report, *Achieving Health for All* (Epp, 1986), was introduced by the Canadian government. It built on the Lalonde Report by identifying specific challenges to achieving health for all Canadians: reducing inequities, increasing prevention, and enhancing coping. In addition, the Epp Report postulated that these challenges could be addressed by the health promotion mechanisms of self-care, mutual aid, and healthy environments. Further, this report advanced that central implementation strategies include fostering public participation, strengthening community health services, and coordinating public policy.

In these documents, family plays second fiddle to community as a unit of concern for health professionals, yet the family unit is of particular importance to the development and maintenance of the health of its members (Novilla et al., 2006; Young, 2002). An **ecological perspective** on health promotion reflects a systems view and does much to highlight broad contextual factors (such as family and culture) that influence health (Thompson-Robinson et al., 2006). Ecology is concerned with the relationships between organisms and their environment (Kleffel, 1991), and social ecology is concerned with the nature of the relationships between humans and their social, institutional, and cultural worlds (Stokols, 1992). Health here is the consequence of the interdependence between the individual and the family, community, culture, and the physical and social environments (Green & Kreuter, 1999).

The next wave of thinking in this systems view of health was disseminated in the report entitled *Strategies for Population Health: Investing in the Health of Canadians*, prepared by the Federal, Provincial, and Territorial Advisory Committee on Population Health (FPTACPH, 1994). This report further clarified key factors that influence health: the social and economic environment, the physical environment, personal health practices and coping skills, biology and genetic endowment, and health services. According to the population health approach, health is the capacity of people to adapt to, respond to, or control life's challenges and changes (Frankish et al., 1996). The population health movement in Canada, in collaboration with Health Canada, set out a template to guide action to achieve population health. Key elements of the Population Health Template are depicted in Figure 5.1.

The Canadian Nurses Association led an impressive effort to incorporate these new ideas, beginning with the document *Putting Health into Health Care* (Rodger & Gallagher, 1995). Subsequently, provincial nursing associations across Canada produced position statements and discussion documents that captured these ideas (McDonald, 2002). For example, the Registered Nurses' Association of British Columbia (RNABC) incorporated strategies from the Ottawa Charter (WHO, 1986) in their New Directions for Health Care policies and programs. As well, these ideas were incorporated into a document entitled *Determinants of Health: Empowering Strategies for Nursing Practice* that was a socioenvironmental framework for health promoting nursing practice. It directed nurses' attention to concerns of not only individuals, but also families, small groups, communities, and society (McDonald, 2002). In keeping with the evolution of thinking within the systems view of health, the CRNBC published a position statement on primary health care (CRNBC, 2005) noting that primary health care encompasses prevention, community development, community programs and

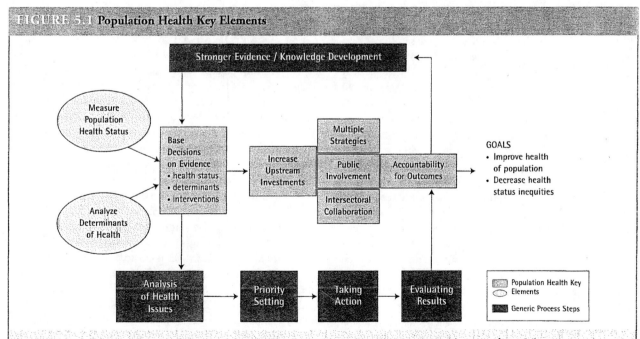

FIGURE 5.1 Population Health Key Elements

Source: The Population Health Template: Key Elements and Actions That Define a Population Health Approach. p. 6 (http://www.phac-aspc.gc.ca/ph-sp/pdf/discussion-eng.pdf), Public Health Agency of Canada, (2001). Reproduced with the permission of the Minister of Public Works and Government Services Canada, 2007.

services, interdisciplinary care, and intersectoral action as this relates to healthy public policy.

According to the systems view, health is envisioned as a dynamic process embedded in a web of relations within which, and as a result of, capacities for conditions of healthful living are constructed. In Canada, the systems view of health has been entrenched in our thinking over the past three decades through a series of government documents, frameworks, and blueprints and their related professional practices. Health professionals, including nurses, who practise from a systems, process-oriented perspective hold to a view that attends carefully to a multitude of capacity-building social and economic relationships, including the relationship between practitioner and client.

Medical Discourse versus Systems Discourse

Following the Second World War and the discovery of penicillin, the medical model of health irrefutably eclipsed other discourses of health. The near-miraculous discoveries emerging from medical science (e.g., the control of and near-eradication of some communicable diseases, procedures such as heart transplantation, and more recently genetic engineering) have captured our money and imagination. Anyone who has witnessed the recovery of a loved one from a near-death traumatic experience because of innovative surgical procedures, or the prolongation and improved quality of life of an aging parent because of newly developed cardiac medications, stands in awe of medical science and practice. While these successes are real and tangible, they are not the whole story.

Critics of the medical model make strong arguments that such an approach to health does not make for a healthy society (Illich, 1975; Raphael, 2001, 2008). In a seminal work, *Medical Nemesis*, published more than 30 years ago, Illich attacked the value of the medical model in producing healthy societies. He opens the book with: "The medical establishment has become a major threat to health" (p. 11), and goes on to argue that a medicalized health care system is a monopoly that serves the interests of medical and paramedical personnel. To this end, he posits that such a health care system obscures the political conditions that render society unhealthy, while seizing the power of individuals to heal themselves.

Heartened by such arguments, consumers have taken steps to regain control over their own health and ensure that medical care and medical science truly serve their interests rather than those of health professionals (Allsop, Jones, & Baggott, 2004; Batt, 1994). Such consumers understand their health to be embedded in a web of social relations. The breast cancer movement is a consumer movement that exemplifies a challenge to the medical model as a dominant discourse on health. Batt, an award-winning Canadian journalist, charts the journey of breast cancer activism in her book *Patient No More*. The idea for the book emerged from her need as a breast cancer survivor to better understand why breast cancer treatments were regarded widely as a medical success when thousands of women die each year in spite of those treatments. At first she was hesitant to take on the experts, but her investigative work revealed themes that pointed to the detrimental influence of vested interests and world views on the medical care of women with breast cancer. She writes, "Our [breast cancer survivors'] central task is precisely to develop and advance a perspective of our own. Our voice must be a counterweight to the medical point of view that dominates discussions of the disease" (Batt, p. xiii). Thus, women began to ask why it is difficult to access accurate information about breast cancer and its treatments and moved on to explore how funding decisions are made. Batt writes, "Many now question the premises of past policies, such as the emphasis on treatment rather than prevention, and the strictly biomedical model of cancer" (p. xiv). Batt notes that the activists have inspired breast cancer specialists to examine the world view that guides their research. She writes, "A new order is forming . . ." (p. xiv).

While the medical view of health as discourse can silence voices and distinguish ideas that do not fit, there are those, such as breast cancer activists, who take issue with the dominance of the medical model and, by their actions, open minds to new ways of thinking about health.

Social Determinants of Health: An Emerging Sub-Discourse

As mentioned earlier, Canadian governments prioritize the funding of health care based on the medical model, and fund interventions aimed at discouraging unhealthy lifestyles to a much lesser extent, a perspective that reflects the health-field concept of health. (This fact exemplifies the power of a dominant discourse to shape social and political action.) Good health comes from a variety of influences, 75% of which are not related to the health-care delivery system (Keon & Pepin, 2009). Fifty percent of the health of the population can be explained from socio-economic factors (Keon & Pepin, 2009). Thus, researchers have begun to explore what constellations of factors that determine health status lie "upstream" of medical treatment (McKinlay & Marceau, 2000; Starfield, Shi, & Macinko, 2005). An emerging body of research on the social determinants of health provides compelling evidence that challenges the dominance of the medical model as a key perspective. Such research indicates that factors with the greatest impact on the development of life-threatening diseases are usually out of an individual's personal control, factors tied to gender, culture, and socio-economic status (Marmot, 2007), as well as conditions of living (Daniel, Moore, & Kestens, 2007).

Indeed, large-scale studies point to poverty, income, place of residence, and education levels, rather than medical and lifestyle factors, as better predictors of individuals' health (Colhoun et al., 2000; Denton, Prus, & Walters, 2004). A study by the Canadian Medical Association (CMA) found that the recent economic downturn has affected how Canadians care for their health (CBC News, 2009). The CMA conducted a telephone and on-line survey with 1200 Canadians and Ipsos-Reid surveyed 1002 Canadian adults between June 7 and 9, 2009.

The study reported that there is a trend in Canadians toward sleeping less, skipping meals, and spending less on recreation and sports programs, dental care, and prescription medications in response to fears about the economy.

Recently, the WHO commissioned a report on the social determinants of health entitled *Closing the gap in a generation: Health equity through action on the social determinants of health* (Commission on the Social Determinants of Health, 2008). This document focuses on the "causes of the causes" and outlines a global agenda to address the social determinants of health, identifying three principles for action: 1) the improvement of daily living conditions; 2) tackling the inequitable distribution of resources; and, 3) increasing the public's awareness of, and health professionals' training in the social determinants of health as foundational to good health and the structural action necessary to address them. Resonant with this WHO report, Raphael (2008) identifies the key social determinants of health as: early life, education, employment and working conditions, food security, health care services, housing, income and its distribution, social safety net, social exclusion, and unemployment and employment security. The WHO document points to the health care system as a determinant of health, calling for a model for health systems that "emphasizes locally appropriate action across the range of social determinants, where prevention and promotion are in balance with investment in curative interventions, and an emphasis is placed on the primary level of care with adequate referral to higher levels of care" (p. 8).

In the United States and Canada, there is on-going lobbying for health care reform (Oberlander, 2008; Picard, 2009; Starfield, 2009). In June 2009, a key document that has potential to turn the tide on this resistant issue is the report: *A healthy productive Canada: A determinants of health approach* (Keon & Pepin, 2009). There are 11 recommendations arising from this report, the first of which is to develop a federal strategy to advance the population health agenda in Canada. The report calls for developing indicators of health disparities and a pan-Canadian strategy for population health. Here, the following health determinants are identified as priorities: clean water, food security, parenting and early childhood learning, education, housing, economic development, health care, and violence against Aboriginal women, children, and elders. If this report is taken up with enthusiasm and commitment by leaders in health care in Canada, it could go some way to moving forward the agenda of population health, thereby influencing action on the social determinants of health. With regard to nursing, the Canadian Nurses Association (CNA) (2005) prepared a background paper addressing the social determinants of health. In this paper, the CNA calls for nurses to orient not only their individual practices toward the social determinants of health but also to participate in reorienting the health system, as well as to advocate for healthy public policy, all decidedly political activities (see also Sparks, 2009).

Shaping environments in support of healthful living and healthy lifestyles and addressing the social determinants of health require a new way of thinking. The **primary health care** model offers such a way and has gained some currency in the discourse on health care in Canada. Primary health care

(PHC) is perceived to be the key to reforming a health care system dominated by the medical model (Green & Ottoson, 1999). PHC was conceived by participants representing 134 nations at the WHO Alma Ata Conference in 1978. They pledged their support for a worldwide effort to shift the emphasis from hospital-based medical treatment to a community-based, participatory model of care (Green & Ottoson, 1999). The catchphrase that emerged from this

CANADIAN RESEARCH BOX

What influences smoking in home environments?

Bottoroff, J. L., Johnson, J. L., Carey, J., Hutchinson, P., Sullivan, D., Mowatt, R., & Wardman, D. (2010). A family affair: Aboriginal women's efforts to limit second-hand smoke exposure at home. *Canadian Journal of Public Health,101*, 32–35.

Bottoroff and Johnson are nurse researchers who have been researching health promotion questions at the interface of smoking and health for almost two decades. In this study they explore issues linking health, lifestyle behaviour, family, community, and culture, a rich site for health promotion research. The objective of the study was to explore what influences smoking in home environments in a Gitxsan community, and women's efforts to minimize exposure to second-hand smoke for their children and themselves. Using a community-based ethnographic study, the researchers interviewed 26 women aged 17 to 35, 15 key informants, 9 elders, 7 middle-aged women, and 6 youths from six reserve communities. Smoking was intricately woven into the family lives of the women in a web of culturally embedded, complex extended family relations. Women negotiated competing demands to protect themselves and their children from second-hand smoke. The competing demands involved preserving relations while respecting others' need to smoke. Women's stories featured not only challenges but also successes in reducing exposure to second-hand smoke. The researchers concluded that reducing exposure to second-hand smoke is a multifaceted challenge for Aboriginal women living in these communities who want to protect their health and the health of their children from the negative health effects of smoking. The researchers propose that these women's efforts to reduce exposure to second hand-smoke could be supported by housing policies, initiatives that foster a social climate of shared responsibility to establishing smoke-free homes, and ongoing efforts to reduce smoking.

Discussion Questions

1. When you read about this research, what personal beliefs, feelings, and values come up for you that may be points of tension in your work with First Nations communities?

2. How would you as a CHN support a pregnant woman in a First Nations community in her efforts to negotiate a smoke-free environment?

conference was "Health for All by the Year 2000." Many influential Canadians who believe that the tenets of PHC will indeed improve the health of Canadians have been in a prolonged, difficult, and often embittered battle to expand the vision for health care in Canada beyond the medical model. Such tensions speak to the power of the medical discourse on health to shape political will. Perhaps the Keon & Pepin (2009) report will go some way towards resolving these tensions, as Keon is a highly esteemed heart surgeon who has now taken up, and is advancing in, highly influential political and medical arenas of the population health/social determinants discourse.

Social Determinants of Health: Heart Health, a Case Example

Low-income, lone mothers are a particular cohort in which operates a constellation of factors detrimental to health. Such women are more likely to live in poverty, to achieve low levels of education, to be on social assistance than are partnered mothers, and to have lower levels of health (Young et al., 2005; Young et al., 2004). In particular, Canadian lone mothers are three to four times more likely to be smokers than are partnered mothers of any income (Young et al., 2004). In a U.S. study, women who had experienced a cardiovascular disease event were 3.28 times more likely to be a lone mother than a partnered mother (Young et al., 2005). In a qualitative study designed to augment the findings of these quantitative studies, Wharf-Higgins et al. (2006) found that low-income lone mothers attribute policies and practices that shape their lives as foundational to their lifestyle patterns. Females across their lifespan, but particularly after age 16, are the least likely to be physically active (FPTACPH, 1999). Women in Canada, when compared to women in the healthiest countries in the world, are gaining more slowly in terms of life expectancy (Fang & Miller, 2009). This is held to be related to smaller mortality reductions in cardiovascular diseases (CVD) and cancer, which are in turn related to smaller reductions in lifestyle risks, obesity, diabetes, and tobacco use (Fang & Miller).

The established approach to promote heart health and prevent heart disease has been, and continues to be, individually focused and behaviourally oriented (Raphael, 2003) despite findings that suggest that only a portion of interindividual variability in CVD incidence can be explained by the major risk factors (Marmot, 1996; Nettleton, 1997). Indeed, Raphael (2001) estimates that 23% of all premature years of life lost prior to age 75 in Canada can be attributed to income differences. Of these premature deaths related to income differences, heart disease and stroke cause the greatest proportion of these years lost: 22%. As such, health policy makers have been encouraged to address issues of poverty, powerlessness, and a lack of social support in addition to the usual care of risk reduction (Marmot & Wilkinson, 1999; Petrasovits, 1992).

Gender is also a critical determinant of heart health. The social determinants of health do not affect women and men in the same way: women are relatively disadvantaged compared to men (Spitzer, 2005). Marked differences exist between men's and women's ability to access, and gender role expectations of accessing, health promoting opportunities (e.g., recreation, continued education, satisfying work). Moreover, the gendered effects of reduced funding to health and social services include fewer jobs for women, more unpaid care work, and reduced access to health care (Kaufert, 1996). As a result, low income is especially concentrated among women. In 1998, 56% of Canadian sole-support mothers lived below the low-income cut-off (Townson, 2000). In an examination of poverty dynamics, lone mothers have a higher entry rate into and lower exit rates from poverty than others (Finnie & Sweetman, 2003). Gender needs to be treated as an important explanatory variable in determining health. As well, more focused efforts are required to ensure that policies and programs take into account existing and new knowledge about women's health. Thus, while the "determinants" model is receiving (deserved) increasing attention for situating lifestyle behaviours and risk factors in the social, cultural, and economic contexts, women continue, in various degrees, to bear an unfair burden of poor health related to gender roles, economic disparities, and other related factors (Spitzer, 2005). A further challenge to the epidemiological tradition of studying heart disease is its ignorance of the lived experience of women (Raphael, 2001).

Lay Definitions of Health: Giving Voice to Our Clients

Before we move on, let's return to the opening scenario in which Glen points to the tension between what "society" defines as healthy and what he observes in his friends. In pointing to what society says about health, Glen refers to society's dominant discourse on health. Reflect on how health is portrayed by society in Canada as a discourse on health. Now, reflect on the difference between what society says is health and how Glen defines health. Reflect on what this difference means to Glen.

Lay perspectives on health are diverse, ranging from popular Western definitions that reflect the medical perspective—health as the absence of disease—to a perspective evident in many non-Western cultures—health as living in harmony with nature (Calnan, 1987; Spector, 1985). In our view, lay perspectives orient nurses to the views on health of those in their care. In this section, an overview of the findings of a qualitative study designed to reveal lay perspectives on health (Maxwell, 1997) is presented and then discussed relative to research in the field. Participants in the study were male and female, ranged in age from 7 to 81, and lived in urban and rural settings. The researcher met with families in their own homes for one or two research interviews that lasted for 1.5–2 hours.

Health was perceived by most to be fundamental to living a functional, meaningful life. As one middle-aged woman put it, "This sounds very cliché but being healthy is . . . if you don't have your health, obviously you don't have anything." Another female participant, a financially strained, married mother of three, elaborates:

> You need your health to have energy to raise your family and everyone wants to raise healthy, happy kids, you know, for the future. (p. 112)

For several people, having energy was an indicator of health. One man observed:

> Healthy is a mental attitude, physically feeling well, and having an energy level to get through the day, and, it's a lifestyle. (p. 111)

Health emerges as an energized state that has physical, mental, and social dimensions, and health is a lifestyle. A male health care professional in his 60s provides a well-thought-through position on his lived experience of health:

> I feel healthy if my back isn't sore or if things don't hurt or my throat is not sore. To me personally, on any given day, whether I feel healthy that day or not is an absence of complaints. But, what does health count as a year? What is a healthy year? Or, what is a healthy decade? Then, we get into that more holistic definition of health. You know the background thing. . . we're comfortable, we have a nice home, we have adequate money and live with it well, and we're not living in fear and this sort of thing. So that background is okay and so that you can sit around and worry about whether or not you've got a sore throat. If you lived in a war-torn country, you really wouldn't give a damn if you had a sore throat or not.
>
> Researcher: So if you had a healthy year, what would that have been like?
>
> Man: I guess free from relatively, well number one, good physical health, free from sort of major worries, free from family worries, that there weren't a lot of things pressing down and adequate rest so that I am not overtired. (p. 113)

This man evaluates his state of health by noting his physical state and the context within which his physical health is experienced, including his family, socioeconomic circumstance, and the political climate of the country. His idea of health counting "as a year" or "decade" is unique.

Not all participants found it easy to speak of health, however. One woman, married with three children under age six and employed full time, observed:

> I've never thought of "I feel healthy." It's either you feel tired or you don't feel tired. I've never said, "Oh I feel healthy today." I wouldn't even know where to start with that one. (p. 115)

A single mother coping with the aftermath of breast cancer treatment and living meagrely with two early teens views health in the following way:

> Gee, I just can't answer that. Isn't that amazing? I don't know. I'm not grasping what health is, being healthy? [pause] Being fit? Is there more? (p. 115)

While most participants openly discussed their views on health, not all found it an easy term to define. Some participants offered thoughtful definitions of, or personal theories about, health. From these interviews, health emerged as an energized, balanced, dynamic, multidimensional state related to self-perception, interpersonal processes, and socioeconomic context, a perspective aligned with a systems view of health but with unique and individualized twists and variations.

A systematic review of 112 qualitative studies that was conducted to develop theory regarding an individual's experience of health and disease was revealing (Jensen & Allen, 1994). These studies involved informants with disease or chronic illness as well as those who considered themselves to be "healthy." Participants ranged in age from early adulthood to very old. The authors identified the following themes to describe the lived experience of health and disease:

- **abiding vitality**, the idea that when one is healthy there is sparkle and animation;
- **transitional harmony**, the idea that, when healthy, one has a sense of harmony and balance, a notion that resonates with the words of participants in the Maxwell (1997) study;
- **rhythmical connectedness**, the idea that, when healthy, one experiences wholeness and an accompanying attachment to the world and that these social connections provide a positive sense of personal contribution or effectiveness as well as positive identity;
- **unfolding fulfillment**, the notion that engaging with life's challenges is meaningful; and
- **active optimism**, the idea that one can cope with life and meet its challenges; that is, one has the attitude and resources to do so.

Two qualitative studies revealed meanings of health similar to but also different from those claimed by the above authors. Maddox's (1999) study of older women and the meaning of health reported that the primary themes arising from research interviews were interactions with a being greater than themselves, acceptance of self, humour, flexibility, and being other-centred. Mexican–American women view health as a compilation of good physical health, sound mental health, and a socially and spiritually satisfying life (Mendelson, 2002). Health for these women exceeded more than these component parts, an embodied experience that transcends illness and is grounded in relationships with family and supported by their spirituality.

The lay perspectives on health presented here mirror each other and resonate with both the medical and systems models of health. A study in Alberta found that survey respondents recognized their health is broadly influenced by social and environmental variables, including issues of social support, supportive environments, and income (Reutter et al., 2001). In an attempt to understand how people arrive at a subjective evaluation of their health, Kaplan and Baron-Epel (2003) surveyed people in three broad age groups (20–40, 41–60, and 61+). When they probed respondents about what factors may have influenced their rating, they found that:

> [H]ealth is a social construction and our beliefs and conceptions of it are rooted in wider socio-cultural contexts. People's perceptions of health are also found to be influenced by biomedicine and by prevailing social and medical ideologies. . . . People's perceptions and judgements about their own health are at once individual and social. (pp. 6–7)

As health professionals, our practice is enriched if we listen carefully to our clients' definitions of health and choose this as a starting point.

DISCOURSES ON HEALTH AND THE ROLE OF THE COMMUNITY HEALTH NURSE

In the previous sections, we discussed health in terms of medical and systems discourses and lay perspectives on health. These are "lenses" on health that CHNs can draw on as they perform their roles. Used in this way, "lens" refers to a particular way of understanding a concept, in this case *health*. One of the primary challenges nurses face is to sort out how each lens on health can be applied to or incorporated into their practice. However, the first step in addressing this dilemma is to understand how and why a particular lens on health shapes health care practice, be it nursing, medicine, or another health care discipline such as physiotherapy, family therapy, or community health promotion.

For purposes of stimulating thinking, discussion, and debate, we suggest that the use of the medical model of health, with its focus on prediction and control, has the potential to engender nurses who enact their role as experts who can predict the causes of, and intervene to control, the health of those in their care. Nurses who fall within this genre take on the role of the expert in identifying problems and catalyzing solutions. When functioning in this role nurses may seem heroic, charging in to instigate a "fix" or solution, or they may act to guard the social order to ensure health: superhero nurses. Society needs nurses who can detect health problems and offer effective solutions, for example when a community experiences the outbreak of a communicable disease.

In contrast, nurses who practise from a systems view, in which health is wholeness, carry out a relational practice in which relationships with clients are paramount to the clients' constructions of health and experiences of wholeness. In such a nursing practice, the nurse builds trusting relationships, collaborates with clients to identify and address their health-related issues, fosters clients' strengths, promotes and protects clients' rights, educates clients about the social determinants of health, practises in an intersectoral manner to address the determinants of health, and strives for a respectful, integrated, accessible system of health care delivery. A metaphor for such a nurse might be nurse as dancer, in which the nurse and client strive to connect across life space—a delicate, gentle act, beautiful in its execution but nonetheless precarious.

CHNs may find themselves caught between the roles of the nurse as superhero and the nurse as dancer, roles that may at times feel untenable. Nurses in British Columbia experienced such tensions and took action to change their practice (Griffiths, 2002). The Public Health Nursing Practice Advisory Committee (PHNPAC), in the South Fraser area of the Fraser Health Authority, received a referral from nursing colleagues concerning dissatisfaction with the problem-oriented recording (POR) system. The POR was incongruent with the philosophy of nursing that the nurses shared. The PHNPAC initiated a series of consultations to assist them in addressing this concern. A presentation by a nursing professor on "The Power of the Text" raised the nurses' awareness of the incompatibility between the way the documentation system

---

CANADIAN RESEARCH BOX

What about disparities in tobacco use?

Reid, J. L., Hammond, D., & Driezen, P. (2010). Socio-economic status and smoking in Canada, 1999–2006: Has there been any progress on disparities in tobacco use? *Canadian Journal of Public Health, 101,* 73–78.

Large databases capture health-related data and are an important tool for health surveillance. In this study, the researchers use data from the Canadian Tobacco Use Monitoring Survey (CTUMS), 1999 to 2006. CTUMS was conducted by Statistics Canada since 1999, and is designed to provide estimates of smoking prevalence. Health promotion is often critiqued on the basis that the outcomes of health promotion interventions, policies, and programs are not evaluated. Such surveys as the CTUMS provide evidence of the effectiveness (or not) of Canadian non-smoking initiatives. In this study, Reid, from the University of Waterloo, who won a student award for this research, and coauthors examined smoking rates across socio-economic groups over a seven-year period in Canada. In this analysis the researchers found that while prevalence rates have declined with equal magnitude across socioeconomic groups, there remain socioeconomic disparities in smoking in Canada, with smoking prevalence higher in less well-educated groups. The researchers note that studies in other Western countries also demonstrate persistent socioeconomic disparities, in spite of declining prevalence across all groups. Researchers concluded that increasing access to current tobacco interventions or designing interventions that target less well-educated Canadians have potential to reduce the disparities in smoking prevalence. What is not captured in survey research such as this are the social processes that underlie the choice to smoke. Qualitative studies such as the study by Bottoroff and colleagues (Box 5.1) have potential to bring to the surface the reasons why those who are less well-educated smoke.

Discussion Questions

1. Identify another source of population-level data in Canada about smoking that a CHN might use when planning programs. How did you find this information?

2. How might a researcher develop a strategy for recognizing gender-related trends in smoking in Canada?

---

was shaping their practice and their philosophy of nursing. More specifically, the POR documentation system, as a problem-oriented practice, shaped their practices to emphasize detecting problems rather than fostering family strengths. Yet, the act of acknowledging and fostering family strengths was what these nurses held to be fundamental to health promotion practice with families.

Tackling this issue head-on, the PHNPAC created its own model for working with high-risk families through a

CASE STUDY

Between 2000 and 2005, the Saanich Peninsula Diabetes Prevention Project explored how community recreation programs and services might prevent or delay the onset of type 2 diabetes in "at-risk" populations. Rather than adhering to a medical model orientation and relying on biomedical variables, such as glucose intolerance, as identifying risk factors, the definition of "at-risk" used in this project was consistent with Health Canada's population health framework and a social determinants view and included low-income citizens, isolated seniors, persons living with disabilities, and Aboriginal populations. Working with recreation professionals, community nutritionists, diabetes educators, social workers, and PHNs, project staff worked to dismantle the barriers to a diabetes-healthy lifestyle for these at-risk groups, as well as to create a supportive community environment. In response to an identified need from these populations, a Diabetes Education and Awareness Fair was held in the fall of 2002. The goal of the fair was to increase the at-risk groups' education and awareness of type 2 diabetes, as well as provide information about, and access to, the resources and supports available in the community for healthy living. The overall focus was to facilitate a change to a diabetes-healthy life while acknowledging the social, economic, and cultural contexts within which lifestyle behaviours occur. The fair consisted of brief seminars on risk factors and conditions, healthy eating, meal preparation, physical activity, and stress management. As well, on-site booths provided information concerning community resources and supports for healthy and active living and access to dietitians, community nurses, kinesiologists, and other health professionals. Participants could also visit booths to have their heart rate, blood pressure, body mass index, and blood glucose levels measured. The fair was held in the local recreation centre, thought to be a more welcoming and non-threatening environment than a health department or hospital.

Despite an emphasis on the broader social determinants of health to the project, the nursing staff at the fair found it difficult to communicate the importance of such factors to visitors, whose questions and search for information reflected a medical model understanding of diabetes. Although the design of the fair and its staff acknowledged and appreciated the population health systems approach, fair participants were mired in the medical model and intent on gathering information concerning physiological and behavioural risks and solutions.

Discussion Questions

1. How might you, as a community health nurse, think about why the nursing staff reported difficulty communicating the importance of the social determinants of health to fair visitors?

2. Is it necessary to emphasize one understanding or discourse of health over the other?

3. How might the fair be reorganized/restructured to encourage a systems understanding of health over a medical one? What different activities, resources, staff, and so on would it be important to include?

---

brainstorming process. Key themes that emerged to inform the development of the model included strengths-based practice, collaboration with clients, and taking steps to increase choices and control for families. As one participant noted, "As nurses, we support people to live in ways that are productive for them" (Griffiths, 2002, p. 16). They linked their work to a systems view of health, citing the Ottawa Charter definition of health promotion, "the process of enabling people to increase control over and improve their own health" (WHO, 1986), as a conceptual and philosophical guide for their newly conceived practice standards.

A **population health** model, offered by McKinlay and Marceau (2000), is a useful framework for thinking about where one's nursing practice fits within the discourses of health. This model suggests that there are three streams to promoting population health:

1. **downstream**, an individual-focused orientation to treatment and cure (e.g., pharmacology, surgery, and rehabilitation);

2. **mid-stream**, support at the community and organization level for creating environments conducive to living healthfully (e.g., opportunities for physical activity, prenatal care programs); and

3. **upstream**, in which healthy public policies, programs, and services deal with macro-level issues of employment, education, and reimbursement mechanisms that affect all in a community (e.g., universal health care).

"Downstream" practice falls within a biomedical view of health, whereas "mid-stream" and "upstream" practices fit within a systems view of health. Where does your usual practice fit?

SUMMARY

In this chapter, we discussed discourses of health, suggesting that there are two primary discourses of health in Canada, the medical model and the systems view on health. Health, a concept of primary importance to CHNs, is not a concrete entity, but rather a concept that has a range of meanings to various groups of health care professionals. What is important about the concept of health for CHNs is to clearly grasp by whom and how health is defined, and for what purposes. Understanding health as a discourse is a first step in grasping who is defining health and for what purposes. CHNs can engage in client-centred care when they can link a particular definition of health to whoever is making claims on the definition, and then determine how well a particular definition aligns with clients' definitions of health in addition to clients' health care needs. Because of their location in the community, CHNs are well-positioned to work in intersectoral relationships to address the social determinants of health—factors that are increasingly held to be the key to health.

KEY TERMS

discourse, p. 77
social determinants of health, p. 77
ecological perspective, p. 78
primary health care, p. 80
abiding vitality, p. 82
transitional harmony, p. 82
rhythmical connectedness, p. 82
unfolding fulfillment, p. 82
active optimism, p. 82
population health, p. 84
downstream, p. 84
mid-stream, p. 84
upstream, p. 84

REVIEW QUESTIONS

1. The social function of discourse is to:
   a) encourage innovative thinking on a topic.
   b) shape relations of power though language.
   c) pattern ideas.
   d) elicit themes.
   e) identify thinking.

2. The systems view of health is:
   a) the health system.
   b) a system adopted by the medical community.
   c) a competing discourse to the medical view.
   d) inadequate when caring for people with heart disease.
   e) one held by all lay people.

3. Research points to the following as key social determinants of health:
   a) genetics, poverty, income, and education levels.
   b) biology, poverty, place of residence, and education levels.
   c) pharmacology, income, place of residence, and education levels.
   d) poverty, income, place of residence, and education levels.
   e) poverty, income, and education levels.

4. Nurses can orient their practice to the social determinants of health by:
   a) educating patients/clients about the social determinants of health; participating in reorienting the health system; advocating for healthy public policy.
   b) educating patients/clients about obesity; participating in reorienting the health system; advocating for healthy public policy.
   c) participating in reorienting the medical system; advocating for healthy public policy.
   d) educating patients/clients about the social determinants of health; participating in reorienting the medical system.
   e) educating the public about lifestyle risk; participating in reorienting the health system; advocating for healthy public policy.

5. Jolene is a 25-year-old single mother who has just had a new baby. You are a community nurse assigned to do the first home visit following the birth of the baby. When you enter the home, you smell cigarette smoke and notice a pile of butts in an ashtray. The mother has a newborn and two toddlers. You are worried about the impact of second-hand smoke on the children and you decide that because this is an urgent matter, you will begin by:
   a) telling Jolene about research that has found that second-hand smoke is a health risk
   b) offering Jolene a pamphlet on the health effects of second-hand smoke on children
   c) asking Jolene if she would like information about a smoking cessation program offered in the health unit
   d) listening while Jolene tells you about her conditions of living
   e) asking Jolene how the economic downturn is affecting her

STUDY QUESTIONS

1. Define "discourse."
2. What are the elements of primary health care?
3. What is the difference between the medical model and the systems view of health?
4. What is the challenge to nurses working within these two views of health?
5. Why was the Lalonde Report important?
6. Why does the ecological perspective on health fit within a systems view of health?
7. What is a relational nursing practice?
8. What has been Canada's role in shaping discourses of health?
9. What are your responses to the metaphors of nursing offered by the authors of this chapter?

*After working through these questions, go to the MyNursingLab at **www.pearsoned.ca/mynursinglab** to check your answers.*

INDIVIDUAL CRITICAL THINKING EXERCISES

1. How do you define your own health?

2. Within which view or discourse of health did you frame your response to the previous question?

3. When you assess clients, what questions would you include to help you understand their perspectives on health?

4. Locate the majority of your nursing work on the McKinlay and Marceau (2000) model and identify distinct tasks that fit on the stream continuum.

5. If you were to move your work more "upstream," what would that look like so that you achieved similar outcomes to your present work?

6. How might you "educate" your patients/clients about the social determinants of health?

GROUP CRITICAL THINKING EXERCISES

1. What are the sources of stress for you as a student? How might you balance study, work, and family to "let go" of stress?

2. As a group, discuss how the economic downturn has affected your health habits.

3. Relative to the above discussions about discourses of health, what does it mean to frame school-related stress as a problem that requires an individual-level solution?

4. How do you as students and the nursing faculty honour the idea of the determinants of health in the everyday life of your school? Brainstorm factors that could be addressed in your school community to make your school a healthier place to be.

REFERENCES

Allsop, J., Jones, K., & Baggott, R. (2004). Health consumer groups in the UK: a new social movement? *Sociology of Health & Illness, 26,* 737–756.

Batt, S. (1994). *Patient no more: The politics of breast cancer.* Charlottetown, PE: Synergy.

Borgman, A. (1992). *Crossing the post-modern divide.* Chicago, IL: University of Chicago Press.

Calnan, M. (1987). *Health and illness: A lay perspective.* London, UK: Tavistock Press.

Canadian Nurses Association. (2005). *Social determinants of health and nursing: A summary of the issues.* Ottawa, ON: Author.

Capra, F. (1982). *The turning point: Science, society, and the rising culture.* New York, NY: Simon and Schuster.

CBC News. (2009). *Economy linked to Canadians' health fears.* Retrieved from http://www.cbc.ca/money/story/2009/08/17/cma-health017.html

Colhoun, H. M., Rubens, M. B., Underwood, S. R., & Fuller, J. H. (2000). Cross-sectional study of differences in coronary artery calcification by socioeconomic status. *British Medical Journal, 18,* 1262–1263.

College of Registered Nurses of British Columbia. (2005). *Primary health care.* Vancouver, BC: Author.

College of Registered Nurses of British Columbia. (2009). *Scope of practice.* Vancouver, BC: Author.

Commission on the Social Determinants of Health. (2008). *Closing the gap in a generation: Health equity through action on the social determinants of health. Final report of the Commission on the Social Determinants of Health.* Geneva, Switzerland: World Health Organization.

Daniel, M., Moore, S., & Kestens, Y. (2007). Framing the biosocial pathways underlying associations between place and cardiometabolic disease. *Health & Place, 14*(2), 117–132.

Denton, M., Prus, S., & Walters, V, (2004). Gender differences in health: A Canadian study of the psychosocial, structural and behavioural determinants of health. *Social Science & Medicine, 58,* 2585–2600.

Donahue, P. (1985). *Nursing: The finest art.* Toronto, ON: C.V. Mosby.

Dubos, R. (1959). *Mirage of health, utopias, progress, and biological change.* New York, NY: Anchor Books.

Dubos, R. (1961). *Mirage of health.* New York, NY: Doubleday.

Ehrenreich, B., & English, D. (1978). *For her own good.* Toronto, ON: Doubleday.

Epp, J. (1986). *Achieving health for all: A framework for health promotion.* Ottawa, ON: Health and Welfare Canada.

Fang, R., & Miller, J. (2009). Canada's global position in life expectancy: A longitudinal comparison with the healthiest countries in the world. *Canadian Journal of Public Health,* 9–13.

Federal, Provincial, and Territorial Advisory Committee on Population Health. (1994). *Strategies for population health: Investing in the health of Canadians.* Ottawa, ON: Minister of Supply and Services.

Federal, Provincial, and Territorial Advisory Committee on Population Health. (1999). *Toward a healthy future: The 2nd report on the health of Canadians.* Ottawa, ON: Health Canada.

Finnie, R., & Sweetman, A. (2003). Poverty dynamics: Empirical evidence for Canada. *The Canadian Journal of Economics/Revue canadienne d'Economique, 36,* 291–325.

Foucault, M. (1972). *The archaeology of knowledge and the discourse on language.* New York, NY: Pantheon Books.

Fox, N. (1999). *Beyond health: Postmodernism and embodiment.* London, UK: Free Association Books.

Frankish, C. J., Green, L. W., Ratner, P. A., Chomik, T., & Larsen, C. (1996). *Health impact assessment as a tool for population health promotion and public policy.* Vancouver, BC: University of British Columbia, Institute of Health Promotion Research.

Green, L., & Ottoson, J. (1999). *Community health and population health.* Toronto, ON: McGraw-Hill.

Green, L. W., & Kreuter, M. W. (1999). *Health promotion planning: An educational and ecological approach* (3rd ed.). Mountain View, CA: Mayfield.

Griffiths, H. (2002). Participatory action research. *Nursing BC, 34,* 15–17.

Habermas, J. (1973). *Theory and practice* (J. Viertel, Trans.). Boston, MA: Beacon Press.

Health Canada. (2001). *Population health template: Key elements and actions that define a population health approach.* Retrieved from http://www.phac-aspc.gc.ca/ph-sp/phdd/pdf/overview_handout_colour.pdf

Illich, I. (1975). *Medical nemesis: The expropriation of health.* Toronto, ON: McClelland & Stewart.

Jensen, L., & Allen, M. N. (1994). A synthesis of qualitative research on wellness-illness. *Qualitative Health Research, 4,* 349–369.

Kaplan, G., & Baron-Epel, O. (2003). What lies behind the subjective evaluation of health status? *Social Science and Medicine, 56*(8), 1669–1676.

Kaufert, P. (1996, August). *Gender as a determinant of health.* Paper presented at the Canada–US Forum on Women's Health, Ottawa. Abstract retrieved from http://www.hc-sc.gc.ca/hl-vs/pubs/women-femmes/can-usa/can-back-promo_12_e.html

Keon, W., & Pepin, L. (2009). *A healthy productive Canada: A determinants of health approach.* Retrieved from http://www.parl.gc.ca/40/2/parl-bus/commbus/senate/Com-e/popu-e/rep-e/rephealthjun09-e.pdf

Kleffel, D. (1991). Rethinking the environment as a domain of nursing knowledge. *Advances in Nursing Science, 14,* 40–51.

Labonte, R. (1994). Death of a program, birth of a metaphor. In A. Pederson, M. O'Neill, & I. Rootman (Eds.), *Health promotion in Canada* (pp. 72–90). Toronto, ON: W. B. Saunders.

Lalonde, M. A. (1974). *A new perspective on the health of Canadians.* Ottawa, ON: Health and Welfare Canada.

Larson, J. S. (1999). The conceptualization of health. *Medical Care and Review, 56,* 123–136.

Lupton, D. (1992). Discourse analysis: A new methodology for understanding the ideologies of health and illness. *Australian Journal of Public Health, 16,* 145–150.

Maddox, M. (1999). Older women and the meaning of health. *Journal of Gerontological Nursing, 25,* 26–33.

Marmot, B. G. (1996). Socio-economic factors in cardiovascular disease. *Journal of Hypertension, 14*(5), S201–S205.

Marmot, M. (2007). Achieving health equity: from root causes to fair outcomes. *Lancet, 370* (9593), 1153–1163.

Marmot, M., & Wilkinson, R. G. (1999). *Social determinants of health.* Oxford, UK: Oxford University Press.

Maxwell, L. (1997). *Family influences on individual health-related decisions in response to heart-health initiatives.* Unpublished dissertation, University of British Columbia, Vancouver.

McDonald, M. (2002). Health promotion: Historical, philosophical and theoretical perspectives. In L. E. Young & V. E. Hayes (Eds.), *Transforming health promotion practice: Concepts, issues, and applications* (pp. 25–42). Philadelphia, PA: F. A. Davis.

McKinlay, J., & Marceau, L. (2000). US public health and the 21st century: Diabetes mellitus. *The Lancet, 356,* 757–761.

Meleis, A. I. (2007). *Theoretical development in nursing: Development and progress* (4th ed.). New York, NY: J. B. Lippincott.

Mendelson, C. (2002). Health perceptions of Mexican American women. *Journal of Transcultural Nursing, 13,* 210–217.

Mills, S. (2007). *Discourse.* New York, NY: Routledge.

Nettleton, S. (1997). Surveillance, health promotion and the formation of a risk identity. In M. Sidell, L. Jones, J. Katz, & A. Peberdy (Eds.), *Debates and dilemmas in promoting health* (pp. 314–324). London, UK: Open University Press.

Oberlander, J. (2008). The partisan divide—the McCain and Obama plans for US health care reform. *New England Journal of Medicine, 359,* 781.

Parse, R. (1992). Theory of human becoming. *Nursing Science Quarterly, 5,* 35–42.

Petrasovits, A. (1992). *Promoting heart health in Canada: A focus on heart health inequities.* Ottawa, ON: Minister Supply and Services.

Picard, A. (2009). 'We have to improve patient care. Period.' Retrieved from http://www.theglobeandmail.com/news/national/we-have-to-improve-patientcareperiod/article1253871/

Raeburn, J. (1992). Health promotion with heart: Keeping a people perspective. *Canadian Journal of Health Promotion, 1,* 3–5.

Raphael, D. (2001). *Inequality is bad for our hearts: Why low income and social exclusion are major causes of heart disease in Canada.* Toronto, ON: North York Heart Health Network.

Raphael, D. (2003). Bridging the gap between knowledge and action on the societal determinants of cardiovascular disease: How one Canadian community effort hit—and hurdled—the lifestyle wall. *Health Education, 103*(3), 177–189.

Raphael, D. (2008). Getting serious about the social determinants of health: new directions for public health workers. *IUHPE-Promotion & Education,15,* 15–20.

Registered Nurses' Association of British Columbia. (2002). Primary health care. *Nursing BC, 34*(4), 13.

Reutter, L., Dennis, D., & Wilson, D. (2001). Young parents' understanding and actions related to the determinants of health. *Canadian Journal of Public Health, 92,* 335–339.

Rodger, G., & Gallagher, S. (1995). The move toward primary health care in Canada: Community health nursing 1985–1995. In M. Stewart (Ed.), *Community nursing: Promoting Canadian's health* (pp. 2–36). Toronto, ON: W. B. Saunders.

Rootman, I., & Raeburn, J. (1994). The concept of health. In A. Pederson, M. O'Neill, & I. Rootman (Eds.), *Health promotion in Canada* (pp. 139–151). Toronto, ON: W. B. Saunders.

Saylor, C. (2004). The circle of health: A health definition model. *Journal of Holistic Health, 22,* 98–115.

Sparks, M. (2009). Acting on the social determinants of health: health promotion needs to get more political. *Health Promotion International, 24,* 199–201.

Spector, R. E. (1985). *Cultural diversity in health and illness.* Norwalk, CT: Appleton-Century-Crofts.

Spitzer, D. L. (2005). Engendering health disparities. *Canadian Journal of Public Health, 96,* S2, S78–96.

Starfield, B. (2009). Toward international primary care reform. *Canadian Medical Association Journal, 180,* 1091–1092.

Starfield, B., Shi, L., & Macinko, J. (2005). Contribution of primary care to health systems and health. *Milbank Quarterly, 83*, 457–502.

Stokols, D. (1992). Establishing and maintaining healthy environments: Toward a social ecology of health promotion. *American Psychologist, 47*, 6–22.

Thompson-Robinson, M., Reininger, B., Sellers, D. B., Suaners, R., Davis, K., & Ureda, J. (2006). Conceptual framework for the provision of culturally competent services in public health settings. *Journal of Cultural Diversity, 13*, 97–104.

Townson, M. (2000). A report card on women and poverty. *Canadian Centre for Policy Alternatives.* Retrieved from http://policyalternatives.ca/documents/National_Office_Pubs/women_poverty.pdf

Wharf-Higgins, J., Young, L. E., Naylor, P. J., & Cunningham, S. (2006). Out of the mainstream: Low-income lone mothers' life experiences and perspectives on heart health. *Health Promotion Practice, 7*(2), 221–233.

Wilkinson, R., & Marmot, M. (1998). *Social determinants of health: The solid facts.* Geneva, Switzerland: World Health Organization, Centre for Urban Health.

World Health Organization. (1948). *Constitution of the World Health Organization as adopted by the International Health Conference* (Official Records of the World Health Organization, No. 2). Geneva, Switzerland: Author.

World Health Organization, Canadian Public Health Association, & Health and Welfare Canada. (1986). *Ottawa Charter for health promotion.* Ottawa, ON: Health and Welfare Canada.

Young, L. E. (2002). Transforming health promotion practice: Moving toward holistic care. In L. E. Young & V. E. Hayes (Eds.), *Transforming health promotion practice: Concepts, issues, and applications* (pp. 1–25). Philadelphia, PA: F. A. Davis.

Young, L. E., Cunningham, S., & Buist, D. (2005). Lone mothers are at higher risk for cardiovascular disease compared to partnered mothers. Data from the National Health and Nutrition Examination Survey III (NHANES III). *Health Care for Women International, 26*, 604–621.

Young, L. E., James, A., & Cunningham, S. (2004). Lone motherhood and risk for cardiovascular disease: The National Population Health Survey, 1998–99. *Canadian Journal of Public Health, 95*, 329–335.

Marmot, M. (2004). *The status syndrome: How social standing affects our health and longevity.* New York, NY: Henry Holt and Co.

Pederson, A., O'Neill, M., & Rootman, I. (2007). *Health promotion in Canada: Provincial, national and international perspectives* (2nd ed.). Toronto, ON: Canadian Scholars' Press.

Raphael, D. (2008). *Social determinants of health: Canadian perspectives* (2nd ed.). Toronto, ON: Canadian Scholars' Press.

Youngkin, E. Q., & Davis, M. S. (Eds.). (2003). *Women's health: A primary care clinical guide* (rev. ed.). Upper Saddle River, NJ: Pearson Prentice Hall.

Websites

B.C. Centre of Excellence for Women's Health
http://www.bccewh.bc.ca/index.htm

Health Canada Publications
http://www.hc-sc.gc.ca/ahc-asc/pubs/index-eng.php

No Easy Task—A General Health Resource Website
http://www.noeasytask.com

HIV/AIDS and Health Determinants: Lessons for Coordinating Policy and Action (Chapter 3. The social Determinants and HIV/AIDS)
http://www.phac-aspc.gc.ca/aids-sida/publication/healthdeterminants/sect3-eng.php

Public Health Agency of Canada
http://www.health.gov.bc.ca/cdms/determinants.html

Women's Breast Cancer Resource Center of Murrieta and Temecula Valley
http://www.michellesplace.org

World Health Organization Publications
http://www.who.int/pub/en/

ADDITIONAL RESOURCES

Readings

Douglas, P. (Ed.). (2002). *Cardiovascular health and disease in women.* Toronto, ON: W. B. Saunders.

Keating, D., & Hertzman, C. (1999). *Developmental health and the wealth of nation: Social biological and educational dynamics.* New York, NY: Guilford Press.

About the Authors

Lynne Young, RN, PhD (University of British Columbia), is an Associate Professor in the School of Nursing, University of Victoria. Her research focuses on health promotion and families in the context of cardiovascular care. Recently, Dr. Young is applying, with others, the grand concepts of health promotion—intersectoral collaboration, mobilizing resources, interdisciplinarity—to address pain care in BC.

Joan Wharf Higgins, PhD (University of British Columbia), is a Professor in the School of Exercise Science, Physical and Health Education, University of Victoria. Her research and teaching interests include the social determinants of health and physical activity and social marketing.

chapter 6

Population Health Promotion Models and Strategies

Benita Cohen

OBJECTIVES

After studying this chapter, you should be able to:

1. Compare and contrast the three approaches to health promotion that have been dominant since the early twentieth century and give examples of how each approach may be utilized by community health nurses.

2. Identify the milestones in the development of health promotion as a multidisciplinary field of policy and practice since the 1970s.

3. Discuss how the concepts of (a) "empowering" strategies for health promotion and (b) a microscopic ("downstream") versus macroscopic ("upstream") approach to health promotion can be applied to community health nursing practice.

4. Describe the population health promotion model and apply it to a typical community health nursing scenario.

5. Describe how CHNs can contribute to the goal of achieving health equity.

6. Discuss guiding principles for a health-promoting community health nursing practice.

INTRODUCTION

Before reading any further, take a minute to think about the following question: "What does the term health promotion mean to you?" If you asked five people that question, you would probably get five different answers. Though one might expect differences in the interpretation of the concept of health promotion between nursing and other disciplines, it might surprise you to know that there is considerable diversity within nursing as well (Maben & MacLeod Clark, 1995). This phenomenon is reflected in the responses of a group of Canadian nursing students in a third-year course on community health promotion, who were asked what the term health promotion meant to them:

- "Health promotion means educating people to make healthy lifestyle choices."
- "Health promotion is a way of being with clients. It's more a philosophy of practice than something specific you do."
- "Health promotion means taking action on the determinants of health—things like poverty, discrimination, marginalization, and so on. It means getting politically active."
- "Everything nurses do is about promoting health. There isn't something specific that is health promotion." (MacDonald, 2002, p. 22)

Is your own description of health promotion similar to one of these responses? Whether it is or not, you may be wondering if there is one interpretation of health promotion that is the correct one. The short answer is no. The purpose of this chapter is to explore the different ways of thinking about the concept of health promotion. The goal is not to provide a step-by-step guide on how to "do" health promotion, but rather to help the reader think critically about the various conceptual and philosophical approaches to health promotion and their implications for community health nursing practice. We will begin by tracing the historical development of health promotion as a multidisciplinary field, including major approaches and key milestones, then explore the historical role of health promotion in community health nursing, and finally end with a few general principles that may guide community health nurses' (CHNs') health promotion practice. It should be noted that although the discussion in this chapter relates primarily to the Canadian context, many of the concepts can be applied to global health promotion issues.

HISTORICAL DEVELOPMENTS IN THE APPROACH TO HEALTH PROMOTION

Labonte (1993) provides a useful way of organizing the discussion by suggesting that there have been three major approaches to health enhancement since the beginning of the twentieth century: biomedical, behavioural (lifestyle), and socio-environmental. In the following sections, each of these approaches will be discussed, highlighting the key concepts, documents, and strategies associated with them—but, even more importantly, highlighting the dominant theories and values that underlie them. Please note that, although these approaches emerged at different points in time, they are all still present to varying degrees in the health field, depending on one's area of practice. Labonte (1993) suggests that all three approaches are useful and that health professionals may find themselves alternating among them at different times and for different purposes. Let's explore these approaches in more detail.

Dominance of the Biomedical Approach

Beginning with the discovery of disease-causing pathogens in the eighteenth and nineteenth centuries, and gaining momentum with the immense expansion of scientific knowledge during the twentieth century, the **biomedical approach** to health enhancement has dominated mainstream thinking in Western society.[1] The key features of this perspective are outlined in the first column of Table 6.1. Essentially, you can think of this approach as synonymous with preventive health care. It is focused on preventing disease or disability in individuals by

TABLE 6.1 Summary of Different Approaches to Health Enhancement

	Biomedical	Behavioural	Socio-environmental
Health concept	• absence of disease or disability	• physical-functional ability; physical-emotional well-being	• goes beyond physical-emotional well-being to include social well-being at individual and community levels; may be viewed as a resource for daily living rather than a "state" that one aspires to
Health determinant	• physiological risk factors (e.g., hypertension)	• behavioural risk factors (e.g., smoking); lifestyle	• psychosocial risk factors (e.g., low self-esteem) • socio-environmental risk conditions (e.g., poverty)
Target	• primarily high-risk individuals (because of above risk factors)	• primarily high-risk groups (because of above risk factors)	• high-risk conditions and environments
Principal strategies	• screening for risk factors • patient education and compliance for behaviour change (e.g., dietary counselling) • immunization	• health education • social marketing • regulatory measures and public policies supporting healthy lifestyle choices (e.g., smoking ban)	• *Ottawa Charter* strategies (strengthening community action, creating supportive environments, developing healthy public policy, developing personal skills, reorienting health systems) • empowerment strategies (personal empowerment, small-group development, community organization/development, advocacy for healthy public policy, political action)
Program development	• professionally managed	• professionally managed, or may be community-based[1]	• community development[2]
Success criteria	• decrease in morbidity and mortality rates • decrease in prevalence of physiological risk factors	• decrease in behavioural risk factors; improved lifestyles • enactment of healthy public policies related to health behaviours	• improved personal perception of health • improved social networks, quality of social support • improved community group actions to create more equitable social distribution of power/resources • enactment of healthy public policies related to social equity and environmental sustainability

1. *Community-based programming: the process of health professionals and/or health agencies defining the health problem, developing strategies to remedy the problem, involving local community members and groups to assist in solving the problem, and working to transfer major responsibility for ongoing programs to local community members and groups.*
2. *Community-development programming: the process of supporting community groups in their identification of important concerns and issues and in their ability to plan and implement strategies to mitigate their concerns and resolve their issues.*

Source: Adapted with permission from Labonte, R. (1993). Health promotion and empowerment: Practice frameworks. *Toronto, ON: University of Toronto, Centre for Health Promotion.*

decreasing their **physiological risk factors** (hypertension, hypercholesterolemia, lack of immunity, etc.). Although the biomedical approach was never the only way that people understood the concept of health, and there have always been areas of overlap with the next approach that we will discuss, this conceptualization of health and health promotion still remains a powerful perspective in our society today. Biomedical strategies, such as immunization and screening tests for early detection and treatment of disease, remain an important part of public health practice.

The Behavioural/Lifestyle Approach

It is generally agreed that the birth of the modern era of health promotion as an organized and distinct multidisciplinary field in health policy and practice occurred in the 1970s. The major turning point in thinking about the concept of health promotion occurred in 1974 with the publication of a discussion paper by the Canadian Department of Health and Welfare entitled *A New Perspective on the Health of Canadians* (Lalonde, 1974). The **Lalonde Report** (as it is commonly referred to) noted that, in spite of a massive expansion of spending on health services during the previous two decades, the health of Canadians was not improving. In fact, morbidity and premature mortality rates for certain chronic or degenerative diseases (such as heart disease, cancer, respiratory disease, sexually transmitted infections) and injuries (especially motor vehicle related) were steadily increasing. Instead of pouring more and more money into services for the sick, the Lalonde Report argued for a "new perspective"— one that paid more attention to the promotion of health.

The Lalonde Report was important for several reasons, one of them being that this was the first time a national government had made such a statement regarding the importance of health promotion as a key strategy for improving the health of a population. Another contribution of the Lalonde Report was that,

although the concept of health was still defined in its most basic form as "freedom from disease and disability" (Lalonde, 1974, p. 8), the added reference to promoting "a state of well-being sufficient to perform at adequate levels of physical, mental and social activity" (p. 8) did allow for a slightly expanded interpretation of health that included the idea of increased functional "ability" and a sense of "wellness" (Labonte, 1993). Perhaps the most important contribution was that the document challenged the dominant thinking of the time, which viewed access to health services as the key to population health. Instead, it suggested that the organization and availability of health services was one of four main categories of factors (or "health fields") that influenced the health of Canadians; the others being human biology, the environment, and lifestyle.

While the Lalonde framework appeared to place equal weight on each of the four fields, a central argument was that a large proportion of the premature mortality and morbidity occurring among the population at the time appeared to be due to individual behaviours or lifestyles that could be modified (smoking and other addictions, poor nutrition, lack of physical activity, risky sexual behaviour, etc.). Therefore, it was argued, the focus of health promotion efforts should be on the use of strategies that encourage the adoption of behaviours or lifestyles that promote functional ability and well-being. This perspective on health and health promotion has come to be known as the **behavioural** or **lifestyle approach** (both terms are commonly used in the literature). The key characteristics of this approach are outlined in the second column of Table 6.1. Essentially, the behavioural approach focuses on the prevention of disease and disability (often expressed in terms of promoting "wellness") in people who are at risk because of their lifestyle or behavioural risk factors such as a high-fat diet, lack of exercise, unsafe sexual practices, or use of tobacco, alcohol, or other drugs. A brief description of strategies that focus on changing behaviour can be found in Table 6.2.

TABLE 6.2 Strategies That Focus on Changing Behaviour/Lifestyle

Health education	Usually refers to activities associated with formal education, including use of audiovisual materials, printed educational materials, teaching strategies for the classroom (e.g., lecture/discussion, case studies, brainstorming), teaching strategies outside the classroom (e.g., health fair). May also refer to one-on-one teaching.
Health communication	Usually refers to the use of the mass media, direct mail, product labels, pamphlets, and posters to communicate a health message to the public. May also refer to health professional–client interaction.
Social marketing	Refers to "a process for influencing human behavior on a large scale, using marketing principles for the purpose of societal benefit rather than commercial profit" (Smith, cited in Kirby, Perkins, & Reizes, 2003, p. 7). The marketing principles are typically described as the "4 Ps," which refer to the product, the price, the place, and the promotion of the product. Additional "Ps" include positioning, partnerships, and politics. Social marketing in public health includes an emphasis on stimulating changes in policy that support voluntary behaviour change (Kirby et al., 2003).
Behaviour modification	Refers to a systematic procedure for changing a specific behaviour by changing the events that precede or result in modification from the behaviour that is to be modified. Most often used to alter smoking, eating, or exercise patterns.
Regulatory measures	Refers to mandated activities (laws, policies, regulations). Examples include laws requiring the use of seatbelts or motorcycle helmets and banning smoking in public places.

The common thread in each of these strategies is the underlying belief that the main determinant of health is individual behaviour or lifestyle, and that information, persuasion, or any other method (including legal coercion) that encourages people to adopt healthier behaviours or lifestyles is the key to health promotion.[2] The behavioural approach to health promotion continues to be very popular. National and provincial governments frequently rely on health communication campaigns to deliver "healthy lifestyle" messages, social marketing techniques have been used in HIV/AIDS prevention initiatives, health education programs based on various theories of behaviour change are commonly used within the school system, and health teaching remains a major part of health care professionals' practice.

The Socio-Environmental Approach to Health Promotion

A number of factors contributed to a new way of thinking about health promotion in the 1980s. The first factor relates to ideological responses to the behavioural approach. Labonte (1993) notes that the 1980s were a time when many of the social movements that emerged in North America in the 1960s and 1970s were maturing. Within these social movements, concepts such as social justice (the belief that all persons are entitled equally to key ends such as health protection and minimum standards of income) and the common good (where the needs of the many have priority over the needs of the individual) (Beauchamp, 1976) were central principles. Many of the activists who took part in these social movements later moved into professional jobs, including those in the health and social services fields. These individuals were critical of the focus on individual behaviour that had come to dominate the field of health promotion in the early 1980s. They argued that health and illness are the result of broad factors such as the socioeconomic and physical environment, the level of social support and social cohesion among individuals and communities, the level of education, working conditions, and so on. They viewed social change (as opposed to individual behaviour change) as the most important goal of health promotion, and social responsibility for health as paramount. From this perspective, approaches that focus solely on individual behaviour change and individual responsibility for health were viewed as a form of victim-blaming, whereby individuals end up being implicitly blamed for being sick because they have "chosen" unhealthy lifestyles or they have unhealthy coping styles when, in fact, their social and economic circumstances have often left them with limited options (Crawford, 1977; Labonte & Penfold, 1981).

At the same time that this ideological critique of the behavioural approach was being articulated, a theoretical perspective emerged from the field of social ecology, which is referred to as an ecological or socio-ecological perspective on health promotion. The central premise of this perspective is that health is a product of the interdependence among the individual and subsystems of the ecosystem (family, community, culture, and physical and social environment). From an ecological perspective, both individual behaviour change and environmental or system change are required elements of health promotion initiatives—neither one on its own is sufficient. This perspective had a major influence on the approach to health promotion that emerged in the mid-1980s.[3]

In addition to the ideological and theoretical critiques of the behavioural approach to health promotion outlined above, two other factors influenced the development of a new way of thinking about it. In the 1980s, several high-profile, population-wide, disease-prevention initiatives to reduce the behaviours that were viewed as major contributors to coronary heart disease (such as smoking, high intake of dietary fat, low levels of physical activity) failed to achieve their intended results (Syme, 1997). Even in cases where disease prevention initiatives did result in reductions in high-risk behaviours, it was primarily the better educated, middle-class members of society who benefited. Many of these programs failed to reach individuals from lower socioeconomic groups who suffered from the poorest social and physical health (Labonte, 1993). As a result, it has been suggested that "effective" health promotion programs that focus on lifestyle change can actually contribute to the increase of social inequalities in health (Armstrong, Waters, & Doyle, 2008; Makara, 1997; NSW Health, 2003; Woodward & Kawachi, 2000).

The final contributing factor to a new way of thinking about health promotion in the 1980s was the epidemiological evidence that could not be ignored. Beginning in the 1970s and escalating in the 1980s and beyond, a substantial body of research emerged suggesting that the distribution of disease in any given society is not the result of individual behaviours, but is the result of the economic, political, and social relationship between individuals and groups in society. In particular, there is now a powerful body of evidence indicating that social and economic inequality is one of the major determinants—some would argue, the major determinant—for disease (Wilkinson & Pickett, 2009; World Health Organization, 2008). There is also a robust body of evidence suggesting that social support (Heaney & Israel, 2002; Richmond, Ross, & Egeland, 2007) and social inclusion/exclusion (Galabuzi, 2009) are major influences on the well-being of individuals and groups within society. Community and neighbourhood characteristics such as social stress (as evidenced by economic deprivation, crowding, family instability, and crime), social cohesion (the flip side of social breakdown), and social capital are also important determinants of health and disease (Patrick & Wickizer, 1995; Sampson, 2003; Stansfeld, 2006; Ziersch, Baum, MacDougall, & Putland, 2005). Together, the various bodies of research suggest that health promotion approaches that focus on individual behaviour change are insufficient to address the key determinants of population health.

Key Milestones in the Development of the Socio-Environmental Approach In addition to the factors previously discussed, several pivotal events and policy statements mark the formal development of a new approach to health promotion. First, it has been noted that the seeds of a social definition of health promotion were sown as early as 1977 when the World Health Organization (WHO) proposed its vision for Health for All by the Year 2000, and in 1978 when the WHO released the Alma Ata Declaration on Primary Health Care (MacDonald, 2002). Primary health care (PHC) was anticipated to be the means of achieving the goals outlined in the Health for All document, and several principles of PHC—especially the importance of community participation and the need for intersectoral collaboration in order to address the broad social and environmental determinants of population health—emerged as key principles in the new approach to health promotion (a more detailed discussion of PHC is available in Chapter 7).

Several Canadian conferences in the early 1980s had an influence on the shift in thinking about health promotion, both in this country and internationally. For example, at the 1984 "Beyond Health Care" conference in Toronto, the concept of healthy cities and the need for healthy public policies that focus on environmental determinants of health such as housing (and other factors contributing to the health of cities) was raised for the first time. This concept challenged the notion of health as an individual characteristic and focused very much on its social and environmental dimensions. The conference is widely recognized as having given birth to a worldwide movement to establish **healthy cities/communities** (Raeburn & Rootman, 1998).

At the international level, 1984 was the year that the WHO released a discussion document that identified five key principles of health promotion:

- Health promotion involves the population as a whole and the context of their everyday life, rather than focusing on people at risk for specific diseases.
- Health promotion is directed toward action on the determinants or causes of health.
- Health promotion combines diverse, but complementary, methods or approaches.
- Health promotion aims particularly at effective and concrete public participation.
- Health professionals, particularly in primary health care, have an important role in nurturing and enabling health promotion. (World Health Organization, 1984)

This idea was elaborated on a couple of years later, when two key events occurred that have contributed to the popular identification of 1986 as the birth date of the "new health promotion." First, the Canadian Minister of National Health and Welfare at the time, Jake Epp, released a document entitled *Achieving Health for All: A Framework for Health Promotion* (Epp, 1986), which clearly distanced itself from the behavioural/lifestyle approach to health promotion. In acknowledgment of the growing body of evidence regarding the social and economic determinants of population health, the Epp Report argued that health promotion was as much a societal responsibility as an individual responsibility. It identified three leading health challenges facing Canadians: the need to reduce inequities in the health of low- versus high-income groups; the need to find new and more effective ways of preventing the occurrence of injuries, illnesses, chronic conditions, and their resulting disabilities; and the need to enhance people's ability to manage and cope with chronic conditions, disabilities, and mental health problems. In order to meet these challenges, three mechanisms for health promotion were identified: self-care, referring to the decisions taken and practices adopted by an individual specifically for the preservation of their health; mutual aid, referring to people's efforts to deal with their health concerns by working together (either through informal social support networks, voluntary organizations, or self-help groups); and the creation of healthy environments at home, school, work, or wherever else Canadians may be. Lastly, three main health promotion strategies were identified as the basis for putting these mechanisms into action: fostering public participation, by helping people assert control over the factors that affect their health; strengthening community health services, by allocating a greater share of resources to those services that have an orientation to health promotion and disease prevention; and coordinating health public policies among sectors (such as income security, employment, education, housing, etc.) that make it easier for people to make healthy choices. It is important to note that the Epp Report clearly stated that a focus on one strategy or mechanism from the framework on its own would be of little significance; it was only by putting the pieces of the framework together that health promotion would be meaningful.

Epp's framework was presented later in 1986 at the first International Health Promotion Conference in Ottawa, where it influenced the development of the **Ottawa Charter for Health Promotion** (World Health Organization, 1986)—a document that was signed by delegates from 38 countries, including Canada. The Ottawa Charter defined health promotion as "the process of enabling people to increase control over, and improve, their health"[4] (p. 5), and it emphasized that achieving **equity in health** was considered to be the main focus of health promotion. A number of essential prerequisites for health were identified (peace, shelter, education, food, income, a stable ecosystem, sustainable resources, social justice, and equity), and the importance of coordinated intersectoral action to ensure these prerequisites for health was underlined. The Ottawa Charter proposed five key strategies for health promotion:

- **Strengthening community action**—Involves supporting those activities that encourage community members to participate in, and take action on, issues that affect their health and the health of others. Community development or community empowerment is viewed as both the means and the end result of this process. Priority is given to those individuals and communities whose living and working conditions place them at greatest risk for poor health.
- **Building healthy public policy**—Involves advocacy for any health, income, environmental, or social policy that fosters greater equity, creates a setting for health, or increases options/resources for health.
- **Creating supportive environments**—Involves generating living, working, and playing conditions that are safe, stimulating, satisfying, and enjoyable and by ensuring that the protection of the natural environment is addressed in any health promotion strategy.

- **Developing personal skills**—Involves supporting personal and social development through the provision of information—education for health and enhancing life skills—in order to increase the options available to people to exercise more control over their own health and environments and to make choices conducive to health.
- **Reorienting health services**—Involves moving beyond the health sector's responsibility for providing clinical and curative services in a health promotion direction that is sensitive to the needs of the community. (World Health Organization, 1986)

An important feature of the new health promotion perspective found in the Ottawa Charter is the link made between the concept of **empowerment** and the promotion of health. Empowerment refers to "an active, involved process where people, groups, and communities move toward increased individual and community control, political efficacy, improved quality of community life, and social justice" (Community Health Nurses Association of Canada [CHNAC], 2008, p. 7). It also refers to the outcome of that process (Vollman, Anderson, & McFarlane, 2008). Individual psychological empowerment involves self-efficacy and motivation to act, while community empowerment involves increased local action, stronger social networks, resource access/equity, transformed conditions, and community competence (Wallerstein, 1992; Zimmerman, 2000). While health care professionals cannot directly empower others—empowerment is something that cannot be given; it must be taken (Vanderplaat, 2002)—they can help people and communities develop, secure, and/or use the resources and skills that promote a sense of control and self-efficacy (Gibson, 1991).

The publication of the Ottawa Charter is widely recognized as marking the transition, at least in theory, from an "old" health promotion practice that focused on medical and behavioural health determinants to a "new" health promotion practice that defined health determinants in psychological, social, environmental, and political terms. See column 3 of Table 6.1 for a summary of the key features of this **socio-environmental approach** to health promotion.

Population Health Promotion

In 1994, the Federal/Provincial/Territorial Advisory Committee on Population Health published a document entitled *Strategies for Population Health: Investing in the Health of Canadians*, which described an approach to public policy that focuses on taking action on the interrelated conditions that influence population health status. These interrelated conditions were identified as income and social status, social support networks, education, employment and working conditions, safe and clean physical environments, biology and genetic makeup, personal health practices and coping skills, early childhood development, and health services. Since that time, the population health perspective has been adopted at the policy level by the federal government, several provincial governments, and some regional health authorities.[5] However, there are a number of characteristics of a population health approach

CANADIAN RESEARCH BOX

Do neighbourhoods contribute to childhood obesity?

Veuglers, P., Sithole, F., Zhang, S., & Muhajarine, N. (2008). Neighborhood characteristics in relation to diet, physical activity and overweight of Canadian children. *International Journal of Pediatric Obesity, 3,* 152–159.

The findings presented in this article are based on an analysis of data collected in the Children's Lifestyle and School-Performance Study (CLASS), a large survey of health, nutrition, and lifestyle factors among Grade 5 students and their parents in Nova Scotia. Students completed a food frequency questionnaire and had their height and weight measured. The parental survey included questions on socioeconomic background; access to shops, playgrounds, parks and recreational facilities; neighbourhood characteristics such as availability of safe places for children to play during the day; and their child's activities. Children residing in neighbourhoods with good access to shops with modestly priced fresh produce and good access to playgrounds, parks, and recreational facilities were less likely to be overweight or obese. The findings add to the evidence that children residing in socioeconomically disadvantaged neighbourhoods are less likely to be physically active and to eat a nutritious diet, and are at increased risk of becoming overweight or obese.

Discussion Questions

1. What roles/activities could CHNs engage in as part of a comprehensive health promotion initiative aimed at improving healthy child development related to nutrition and physical activity among families in low-income neighbourhoods?

2. How would your answer to question 1 differ if you applied each of the approaches to health promotion?

that differ from those of the socio-environmental approach to health promotion outlined earlier. For example, the socio-environmental approach focuses on addressing inequities in health experienced by disadvantaged and marginalized groups; it defines health in its broadest sense as a resource for daily living; and it identifies a wide range of strategies for change that emphasize individual and community empowerment. In contrast, population health is mostly concerned with gradients in health status across all socioeconomic levels; health is defined in terms of traditional epidemiological "sickness" indicators; and the focus is on identifying determinants of disease and death rather than strategies for change.

In an effort to bridge the gap between population health and health promotion, a **population health promotion (PHP) model** was developed by Health Canada (Hamilton & Bhatti, 1996), which attempts to integrate concepts from both perspectives (see Figure 6.1). This three-dimensional model combines the strategies for health promotion outlined in the 1986 Ottawa Charter on one side, the determinants of population health on another side, and various levels of potential intervention on a third side. This model can be used from different

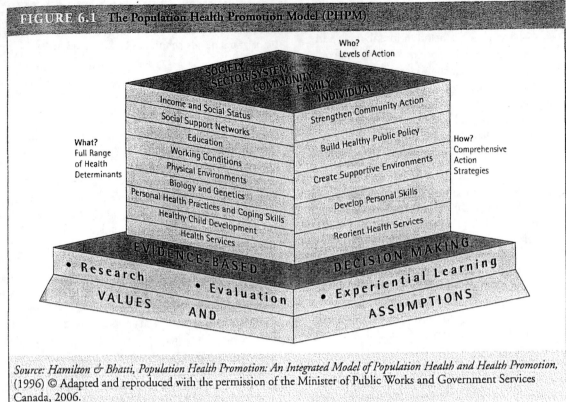

FIGURE 6.1 The Population Health Promotion Model (PHPM)

Source: Hamilton & Bhatti, Population Health Promotion: An Integrated Model of Population Health and Health Promotion, (1996) © Adapted and reproduced with the permission of the Minister of Public Works and Government Services Canada, 2006.

entry points. One can begin with the health determinant that one intends to influence, the action strategy to be used, or the level at which action is to be taken. Or, alternatively, the model can be used to plan a comprehensive range of actions on emerging health issues or issues related to the health of a particular priority group (Hamilton & Bhatti, 1996). Figure 6.2 shows examples of how the model can be used to identify possibilities for influencing various determinants of health. The model can also be used to address the health concerns of groups who are at risk for poor health. The PHPM reflects the socio-environmental perspective. From this perspective we are primarily concerned with social and environmental risk conditions and psychosocial risk factors that are known to affect health status, either directly or indirectly via behaviours. An example of risk conditions would be a deprived neighbourhood where the housing is substandard, there are few recreational facilities, community spirit is weak, and there are feelings of danger and insecurity (Hamilton & Bhatti, 1996).

The positive contribution of the PHPM is that it addresses one of the main criticisms of the population health perspective—that is, that it doesn't provide a model for change (Cohen, 2006a; Labonte, 1995; Raphael & Bryant, 2000). Rather than simply identifying the broad determinants of health, the PHPM proposes strategies for acting on them. Limitations of the PHPM (like the Ottawa Charter itself) include the fact that it does not provide an explanatory model regarding the exact pathways between the determinants of health and health status; the population health determinants don't necessarily include all the prerequisites for health that may be important, and there are few concrete details of how to carry out the PHPM strategies or indicators or tools for evaluating them (leaving each one open to wide interpretation).

SOCIETAL DETERMINANTS OF HEALTH

One of the limitations of the PHPM (and the population health approach in general) is that the list of population health determinants appears to give equal weight to behavioural and socio-environmental determinants, yet there is now substantial evidence that social and economic conditions are the most influential determinants of health (Raphael, 2009). In 2002, a conference of more than 400 Canadian social and health policy experts, community representatives, and health researchers took place at York University in Toronto to consider the state of 10 key **social or societal determinants of health (SDOH)** across Canada (see the box "Social Determinants of Health: The Toronto Charter for a Healthy Canada, 2002") and to outline policy directions to improve the health of

---

Social Determinants of Health: The Toronto Charter for a Healthy Canada, 2002 (Raphael, 2009)

Early child development
Education
Employment and working conditions
Food security
Health care services
Housing shortages
Income and its equitable distribution
Social exclusion
Social safety nets
Unemployment

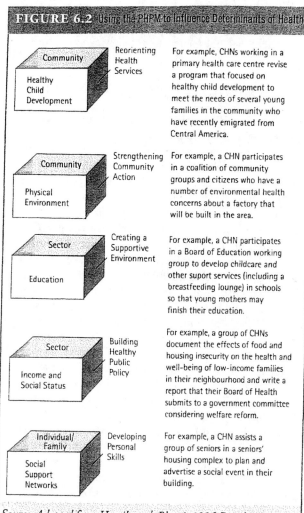

FIGURE 6.2 Using the PHPM to Influence Determinants of Health

Community — Healthy Child Development	Reorienting Health Services	For example, CHNs working in a primary health care centre revise a program that focused on healthy child development to meet the needs of several young families in the community who have recently emigrated from Central America.
Community — Physical Environment	Strengthening Community Action	For example, a CHN participates in a coalition of community groups and citizens who have a number of environmental health concerns about a factory that will be built in the area.
Sector — Education	Creating a Supportive Environment	For example, a CHN participates in a Board of Education working group to develop childcare and other suport services (including a breastfeeding lounge) in schools so that young mothers may finish their education.
Sector — Income and Social Status	Building Healthy Public Policy	For example, a group of CHNs document the effects of food and housing insecurity on the health and well-being of low-income families in their neighbourhood and write a report that their Board of Health submits to a government committee considering welfare reform.
Individual/Family — Social Support Networks	Developing Personal Skills	For example, a CHN assists a group of seniors in a seniors' housing complex to plan and advertise a social event in their building.

Source: Adapted from Hamilton & Bhatti, 1996, Population Health Promotion: An Integrated Model of Population Health and Health Promotion. *Ottawa, ON: Health Canada, Health Promotion and Development Division. Reproduced with the permission of the Minister of Public Works and Government Services Canada, 2010.*

Canadians by influencing the quality of these SDOH (Raphael, 2009). The immediate outcome of the conference was the drafting by conference participants of The Toronto Charter for a Healthy Canada (see Appendix in Raphael, 2009). The Toronto Charter resolved that staff of all health care agencies should be knowledgeable about the SDOH and called for specific immediate and long-term actions to address them. If you look at the list of SDOH, you will see that some of them are very similar to those found in the PHPM, but some are not (e.g., food security, social safety net). If you are interested in addressing one or more of these determinants, they could easily be inserted into the PHPM.

Reducing Inequities in Health

In 2008, two landmark reports reinforced the importance of addressing social determinants of health. Dr. David Butler Jones, Canada's Chief Public Health Officer, released his first *Report on the State of Public Health in Canada* (Public Health Agency of Canada, 2008), which noted that unequal access to the social determinants of health was contributing to unacceptable inequalities in health between the most and least advantaged groups in our society. Soon after the release of Dr. Butler Jones' report, the final report of the World Health Organization's (2008) Commission on the Social Determinants of Health called on all nations to take action on the social determinants of health, with the goal of achieving health equity (the absence of disparities or inequalities in health linked to social disadvantage) within a generation. In order to achieve this goal, it will be essential that population health promotion efforts consider how well they are addressing the needs of the most disadvantaged population groups. Canadian Research Box 6.2 illustrates the importance of understanding the socio-environmental or contextual factors that influence population health.

CANADIAN RESEARCH BOX 6.2

What are the perspectives of First Nations women on smoking in bingo halls?

Bottorff, J., Carey, J., Mowatt, R., Varcoe, C., Johnson, J., Hutchinson, P., . . . Wardman, D. (2009). Bingo halls and smoking: Perspectives of First Nations women. *Health & Place*. doi:10.1016/j.health place.2009.04.005

These findings are based on data collected in a larger ethnographic study to understand how smoke and exposure to second-hand smoke (SHS) influenced the lives of First Nation young mothers (16–35 years of age) and their children in six rural First Nation reserve villages in northwestern British Columbia. The study communities were characterized by high unemployment rates (30–50%) and dependence on social assistance; lack of safe, affordable transportation; lack of daycare services; and limited resources and opportunities for socializing (e.g., no cafes, restaurants, libraries). In addition, the lingering effects of residential schools were widely recognized in the region and evident in experiences of substance use, abuse, and depression to cope with losses. The important role that bingo played in the community emerged as a recurring theme in all study communities. Bingo was positioned as a key source of recreation, an important opportunity for socializing with others and a critical source of revenue for each of the communities. Participating in local bingos took on special significance for women because of their economic situation and need for a safe haven. Unfortunately, in order to be successful, it was viewed as important to attract a large number of people to bingo, so this meant accommodating smokers. During bingos, a thick haze of smoke was commonplace in community halls, putting the health of children, pregnant women, and non-smokers at risk. Many of the women who participated in the study were aware of the health risks of second-hand smoke, but the risk of becoming marginalized from one of the main social activities in their community outweighed the health risk. The economic power attributed to bingos was also a significant barrier to change. Two key factors were identified as having the potential to influence change in these communities: the desire to protect the health of children and the support and influence of elders. The study findings suggest that individual-level health promotion initiatives, such as education about the risks of smoking and support for smoking cessation, are unlikely to be helpful on their own. Instead, the authors state that broad strategies are required that address barriers that lie in the socioeconomic circumstances in First Nation communities.

Discussion Questions

1. Education about smoking risks and support for smoking cessation are obvious health promotion activities in which a CHN working in this type of community could engage in this situation. What are some community-level initiatives to reduce or eliminate health risks related to smoking at bingos that focus on social and economic factors influencing the situation that the CHN could support?

2. Efforts to enact such initiatives should capitalize on the strengths in First Nations communities. How can the two factors that were identified as having the potential to influence change be used?

HEALTH PROMOTION IN COMMUNITY HEALTH NURSING

Now that we have explored the major theoretical developments in the multidisciplinary field of health promotion, let's take a look at the role of health promotion in community health nursing. The idea that nurses are at the heart of the practice of health promotion, are in a position to play a strong leadership role in health promotion, and are the most strategically placed health professionals to accomplish health promotion goals with clients is not uncommon in the nursing literature (MacDonald, 2002). The question is, does everyone use the term "health promotion" in the same way? MacDonald (2002) notes that many nursing authors seem to assume there is a widely shared understanding of the term health promotion, whereas in reality there is considerable diversity in the interpretation and underlying ideologies of health promotion within the nursing profession. In one review of the nursing practice and health promotion literature, the authors identified six different understandings of health promotion: (i) as an umbrella term referring to any activity designed to foster health; (ii) as a synonym for health education; (iii) as the marketing or selling of health; (iv) as a strategy concerned with lifestyle behaviour change; (v) as health education plus environmental and legislative measures designed to facilitate the achievement of health and prevention of disease; and (vi) as an approach that encompasses a set of values including concepts of empowerment, equity, and collaboration (Maben & MacLeod Clark, 1995). The authors note that the first four understandings are in line with a traditional behavioural approach to health promotion, whereas the latter two are synonymous with the socio-environmental approach outlined

in the Ottawa Charter (WHO, 1986). Which understanding of health promotion is the most influential among nurses? This is the question that will be explored in the following sections.

The Behavioural Approach in Nursing

In the early 1980s, Brubaker (1983) found that the primary emphasis of health promotion in the nursing literature of the time was on personal responsibility, lifestyle behaviour change, and high-level wellness. In the 1990s, in spite of the emergence of the socio-environmental perspective in the broader health promotion movement and among certain nursing theorists, the behavioural conceptualization of health promotion remained predominant in nursing practice, including community health nursing practice (Benson & Latter, 1998). In the 2000s, there is evidence that this still remains the case (Whitehead, 2003).

Why have nurses adopted the lifestyle approach to health promotion? It could be argued that this is simply an extension of what they have been doing for years. Healthy lifestyles and behaviours have long been of concern to nurses, and health education has always been a central focus of nursing practice. This is true in the hospital, where nurses provide health teaching to patients and their families, but it has been even more so for nurses working in the community. In the late nineteenth century, Florence Nightingale—widely considered the founder of modern nursing—wrote about the importance of teaching mothers proper sanitation methods and childcare under the supervision of district nurses; by the early twentieth century, advising and instructing people on how to avoid illness through personal hygiene and how to promote healthy child development were primary duties of public health nurses (Novak, 1988). Providing information related to healthy child development and health-promoting behaviours remains a central role of CHNs to this day.

Another reason why the behavioural approach remains influential in nursing practice may have to do with the fact that many of the nursing models used in nursing education and practice since the 1970s have been strongly influenced by concepts and theories from the behavioural sciences, where individual behaviour change is the outcome of interest. For example, Pender's (1996) **Health Promotion Model (HPM)** was the first nursing model to focus explicitly on health promotion. Strongly influenced by the Health Belief Model, which was developed to explain why individuals do or do not take action to prevent disease, the HPM suggests that (a) cognitive factors such as perceived benefits and barriers to action and perceived self-efficacy combine with (b) individual biological, psychological, and socio-cultural characteristics and experience (e.g., prior related behaviour, age, gender, socioeconomic status) and (c) intrapersonal and situational influences (e.g., family, peers, health care providers, environmental cues) to (d) lead the individual to commit to a plan of action that will (e) result in health-promoting behaviour. One of the limitations of this type of health promotion model is that attempting to change someone's health behaviour may be futile if the individual does not have the material or social resources to support the desired behaviour change. Although

Pender's revised HPM (Pender et al., 2005) acknowledges the need for social and environmental change, the nurse's role remains primarily to change perceptions and attitudes that are viewed as non-health enhancing and to assist the client to develop, carry out, and evaluate a behaviour-change plan.[6]

The Socio-Environmental Approach in Nursing

MacDonald (2002) notes that a critique of the lifestyle/behavioural approach to health promotion (which was consistent with the concepts and ideas that were central to the socio-environmental perspective on health promotion) emerged in the mid-1980s, but it never represented more than a marginal position in nursing until the late 1990s. Since that time, many of the foundational concepts in nursing (client, environment, etc.) have expanded to be more congruent with the socio-environmental perspective. For example, "environment" has been challenged to expand from a traditional, narrow focus on the psychosocial environment of the individual to a broader focus on the socio-political context that affects the health of individuals, groups, and communities (MacDonald, 2002). Others have explored the relevance of concepts inherent in the WHO's statements on PHC and the Ottawa Charter—such as empowerment, community participation, community development, and partnerships—to nursing theory and practice in particular settings or with particular client groups (MacDonald, 2002).

One of the most well-known critiques of traditional nursing practice was articulated by Butterfield (1997). Using McKinlay's (1979) famous "upstream–downstream" analogy of people (read: health care providers) being so caught up with rescuing victims (patients) from a swiftly flowing river (representing illness) they have no time to look upstream and see who is pushing these people into the water (the root cause of illness). Butterfield suggested that CHNs needed to adopt a **macroscopic approach** in their practice—more commonly referred to as **thinking upstream**—as opposed to the traditional "downstream" or **microscopic approach** (see Table 6.3). An important aspect of the macroscopic approach in community health nursing is that it is not usually carried out by one nurse alone but often involves the cooperative efforts of nurses and other service providers from school, occupational, and other community settings (Butterfield, 1997), and/or the collective efforts of nurses within organizations or professional associations. Some examples of a macroscopic approach can be found in the box on pages 101–102. Example 2 describes the "upstream" efforts of CHNs in Winnipeg, who successfully worked with their managers to lobby for a change in policy to make condoms available by prescription. Other examples describe cooperative efforts between CHNs and key community stakeholders to engage in community-building activities or to otherwise address the needs of vulnerable or marginalized groups.

The concept of thinking upstream is a valuable contribution to community health nursing practice because it encourages CHNs to address the root causes of health issues in individuals, families, and communities. However, two of the central features of the socio-environmental approach to health promotion—the idea of health promotion as a process of empowerment and the belief that reducing social and economic inequalities in health is a central goal—are not immediately apparent in the macroscopic approach outlined by Butterfield. In contrast, other critiques of traditional approaches to nursing—sometimes referred to as **emancipatory nursing** or **critical social nursing**—have focused specifically on the nurse's role in addressing inequalities in health, and they address the issue of empowerment as well (Carnivale, 2008; Reutter, 2000; Vanderplaat, 2002).

Reutter (2000), a Canadian promoter of a critical social approach to community health nursing, notes that this approach includes asking critical questions to expose inequities, facilitating community involvement by listening to community needs, and assisting in bringing about changes. Rather than presenting solutions and directing lifestyle changes, the nurse's role is facilitative: assisting individuals and groups to reflect on the social and political factors that influence health, sharing expertise, and providing support. More specifically, Reutter suggests that a critical social

---

TABLE 6.3 "Thinking Upstream": Macroscopic vs. Microscopic Approaches in Community Health Nursing

"Downstream" (Microscopic) Approach	"Upstream" (Macroscopic) Approach
• Assessment focuses on individual (and family) responses to health and illness; often emphasizes an individual's behavioural and coping responses to illness or lifestyle patterns	• Assessment focuses on interfamily and intercommunity themes in health and illness • Identifies social, economic, and environmental factors in the community and population that perpetuate the development of illness or foster the development of health
• Nursing interventions are often aimed at modifying an individual's behaviour (including coping behaviours) through changing their perceptions or belief system or providing information	• Nursing interventions may include modifying social or environmental variables (in other words, working to remove barriers to care or improving sanitation or living conditions); this may include social or political action

Source: Community Health Nursing: Promoting the Health of Aggregate, *1997, Butterfield. W. B. Saunders Company, Mosby Churchill Livingstone, Elsevier Science.*

approach to reducing inequities in health would include empowering strategies at the personal, interpersonal (small group), community, and policy levels (see Figure 7.2). At the personal or individual level, Reutter suggests that an empowering nursing strategy would involve not only understanding the psychosocial and socio-environmental context of the individual's concerns and problems and acknowledging these constraints, but also focusing on increasing the capacity of individuals to act upon the roots of their distress and advocating for and with clients to access the resources that they require to change their situation. This level of empowering strategy is similar to the Ottawa Charter strategy of developing personal skills. It may involve the provision of information and advice, but it goes beyond that to building individual capacity for problem solving, decision making, and other life skills. At the interpersonal level, Reutter points out that CHNs can be involved in empowering strategies through facilitating the development of small groups that can decrease the social isolation that often accompanies poverty and providing affirmational, informational, and emotional support. Small groups, therefore, can increase personal empowerment and may foster community action. Small-group development also fits with the Ottawa Charter strategy of creating a supportive environment. At the community level, Reutter suggests that CHNs can use a community development approach to support community groups in identifying important issues related to poverty and in organizing collectively to plan and implement strategies to resolve these issues. This approach fits nicely with the Ottawa Charter strategy of strengthening community action. At the policy level, Reutter notes that CHNs can play an active role in advocating for structural changes that mitigate the effects of or reduce poverty, and/or they can support community groups in their own advocacy efforts to do the same—an approach that Labonte (1993) referred to as "advocacy with." For example, CHNs can serve on intersectoral boards and committees that influence public policy in areas such as housing, unemployment, income security, childcare, and environmental health, or they may get involved with neighbourhood associations, citizens' groups, and advocacy groups such as anti-poverty organizations. This approach is similar to the Ottawa Charter strategy of advocacy for healthy public policy.

One traditional nursing concept that has been given a socio-environmental twist is that of "caring." A Canadian educator and researcher (Falk-Rafael, 2005a) has developed a **critical caring theory** for public health nursing that aims to reincorporate the social justice agenda (characteristic of early public health nursing practice), which has not featured prominently in contemporary nursing theories. One of the core carative processes of PHNs' practice Falk-Rafael identifies is contributing to the creation of supportive and sustainable physical, social, political, and economic environments. The idea that CHNs have a critical role to play in addressing social inequities in health, such as poverty and social exclusion, through advocacy and action for social change is now more common in the literature (Ballou, 2000; Cohen & Reutter, 2007; Falk-Rafael, 2005b; Spenceley et al., 2006; Williamson & Drummond, 2000).

Relatively little has been written about family health promotion compared to individual-level and community-level health promotion (Young, 2002). In Canada, several models have been developed that focus on the family as the unit of nurses' health-promoting interactions (Feeley & Gottlieb, 2000; Hartrick, 2000; Wright & Leahey, 2009). Hartrick's (2000) model of family health promotion is specifically based on an emancipatory approach to nurses' family health promotion practice. Developed at the University of Victoria School of Nursing, this health-promoting family nursing assessment framework suggests that the focus of family assessment is on identifying and resourcing family potential, and facilitating the promotion of client autonomy and empowerment as the family itself identifies courses of action for positive change.

The Socio-Environmental Approach in Canadian Nursing Practice Between 1987 and 1993   In Canada, position statements and discussion documents from national and provincial nurses' associations and the community health nursing section of the Canadian Public Health Association (CPHA) identified health promotion—as defined in the Ottawa Charter (WHO, 1986) and Achieving Health for All (Epp, 1986)—as the primary goal of nursing practice (Canadian Nurses Association, 1992; Canadian Public Health Association, 1990; MacDonald, 2002). In Manitoba, a document entitled *The Role of the Public Health Nurse within the Regional Health Authority* (Manitoba Health, 1998) framed its discussion within the context of the Ottawa Charter strategies for health promotion (see Figure 6.3). At the national level, the Community Health Nurses Association of Canada (2008) developed a new set of standards for practice that identifies the socio-environmental approach to health promotion as the basis for CHNs' practice. The role of the CHN, as outlined in these standards, includes seeking to address root causes of illness and disease and facilitating planned change through the application of Hamilton and Bhatti's (1996) PHPM. The Case Study gives an example of applying the PHPM to a community health nursing scenario.

Recently, the Canadian Nurses Association (CNA) has released two discussion papers that provide strong support for a socio-environmental approach in nursing. *Social Determinants of Health and Nursing: A Summary of the Issues* (Canadian Nurses Association, 2005) summarizes the impact of social and economic factors (such as poverty and economic inequality, low social status, social exclusion, job and food insecurity) on population health. The CNA suggests that nurses can play an important role in addressing these social determinants of health (SDOH) by working on their individual practices (e.g., including SDOH in client assessments and treatment and follow-up plans), helping to reorient the health care system (e.g., ensuring that health promotion programs go beyond lifestyle and behaviour to include SDOH), and advocating for healthy public policies (e.g., using stories from patients to help advocate for policies that address SDOH, making decision-makers aware of the research on the links between socioeconomic factors and health). In *Social Justice: A Means to an End, an End in Itself* (Canadian Nurses Association, 2006) it is proposed that, to put social justice into practice, the nursing

FIGURE 6.3 Role of the PHN within the Regional Health Authority

Build Healthy Public Policy

Goal

Public policy is developed consistent with improvements in the determinants of health.

Services

- Encourage and support community-based advocacy for healthy public policy at all levels and in all sectors (e.g., justice, education, housing, social services, recreation).
- Direct advocacy for healthy public policy.
- Educate and encourage decision makers in all sectors and at all levels to participate in the development of healthy public policy.
- Foster partnership with community decision makers to evaluate public policy.

An Example of Service

PHNs work with communities to advocate for smoke-free public buildings.

Outcome: Ninety percent of public buildings are smoke free.

Create Supportive Environments

Goal

Community members live in healthy social, emotional, spiritual, physical and ecological environments.

Services

- Assess and directly act on the factors affecting health in the community's social, emotional, spiritual, physical and ecological environment.
- Encourage and participate in health-promoting initiatives with other communities and sectors.
- Increase awareness of the ecological and social environments affecting the health of individuals, families, groups, or communities. Encourage and support related action.

An Example of Service

PHNs work with communities to develop strategies to promote safe environments for children.

Outcome: The number of latch-key children under 12 is reduced by 10 percent.

Reorient Health Services

Goal

Responsibility for the determinants of health is shared among individuals, community groups, health professionals, health service institutions, all levels of government, and all sectors, including justice, health, education, business, housing, social services and recreation.

Services

- Primary role in community assessment. Provide consultation with decision makers (e.g., RHA management and board) regarding community strengths and needs as a foundation for health care decisions.
- Promote responsible and effective use of the health care system and community resources.
- Refer individuals, families, groups, and communities for appropriate service.
- Engage other sectors in addressing the determinants of health.

An Example of Service

PHNs work with a community to reorient speech and language services from a facility to accessible community locations based on a partnership among health, education, and community members.

Outcome: A 5 percent increase in early identification and intervention for preschool children with speech and language problems.

Strengthen Community Action

Goal

Community members are actively involved in achieving health.

Services

- Mobilize individuals, families, groups, and communities to take individual and collective action on the determinants of health in the contexts in which they live, learn, work, and play (e.g., schools, workplaces, homes, economic, and social environments).
- Develop and support community-based and self-care services in which community members have ownership and an active role.
- Increase awareness of the ecological and social environments affecting the health of individuals, families, groups or communities. Encourage and support related action.

An Example of Service

PHNs work with a community to identify their assets and needs, determine priority issues, develop strategies, and take action.

Outcome: An active "Healthy Community" network is established.

Develop Personal Skills

Goal

Community members will make effective choices to attain an optimal level of physical, emotional, spiritual, and social development.

Services

- Mobilize individuals to take individual and collective action on the determinants of health.
- Provide information regarding choices.
- Counsel and facilitate healthy choices.

An Example of Service

PHNs facilitate "Nobody's Perfect" parenting sessions for teen mothers and fathers.

Outcome: All parents involved in the parenting program have identified an improved understanding of early childhood development.

Source: Reprinted with permission of Manitoba Health. Prepared by the public health staff of Manitoba Health and Regional Health Authorities. Copyright © 2010, Province of Manitoba.

CASE STUDY

One of the key roles of the CHN working in a public health setting is to support the family in the first year of the life of a new child. This includes assisting parents in their new role(s), promoting optimal child development, and connecting the family with appropriate community resources.

Imagine that you are a CHN who has been given a postpartum referral from the local hospital. The referral contains the following information: first-time mother, 17 years old; newborn male born at 36 weeks' gestation, weighing six pounds; unclear if infant's father is involved; very little contact with the health care system prior to giving birth; receiving social assistance; has no phone. You arrive at the address, which is located in a low-income neighbourhood, and find the mother alone with her infant in a tiny one-bedroom apartment on the third floor of a poorly maintained building without an elevator. You observe that the apartment has very few furnishings, dirty dishes piled in the sink, empty junk food wrappers and containers everywhere, and a strong smell of cigarette smoke. The mother quickly becomes tearful, stating that she doesn't have enough money to pay the rent, and she has no family and few friends in the community.

Using the population health promotion model as a guide, answer the following.

Discussion Questions

1. What information do you already know and what additional information do you need to obtain about the determinants of health affecting this family?

2. Give specific examples of one or more health promotion strategies that you as the CHN could use at the individual/family or community level to address each of the following determinants of health affecting this family. Consider other health professionals or workers in other disciplines/sectors with whom you might collaborate in these strategies:

   a) income and social status
   b) social support networks
   c) personal health practices/coping
   d) healthy child development
   e) access to health services

3. What knowledge/skills/attitudes does the CHN require in order to effectively promote the health of this family?

profession must work toward 10 specific attributes, including "projects, programs and/or structural reforms of an economic, political, or social nature that reduce poverty, increase the overall standard of living, and/or increase the participation of the poor in social and political life" (p. 14).

Challenges of Implementing the Socio-Environmental Approach in Community Health Nursing While the socio-environmental approach to health promotion has been officially adopted by many community health nursing professional associations at the policy level, barriers to putting this approach into action have been identified (Benson & Latter, 1998; Chalmers & Bramadat, 1996; Cohen, 2006b; Reutter & Ford, 1998; Shuster et al., 2001). Some of these barriers originate at the level of the individual CHN (e.g., feeling that they don't have well-developed "upstream" skills or having difficulty in giving up control over the agenda and direction of nurse–client interactions); some originate at the level of the organizations that CHNs are employed in (e.g., lack of organizational culture/policies that value and support this type of approach in CHNs' practice settings). Other barriers originate from the communities where CHNs work (e.g., lack of recognition from the public that this approach is a legitimate part of a CHN's role). In spite of these challenges, there are some excellent examples in Canadian settings of the application of the socio-environmental approach to health promotion in which CHNs have played an active role. See the box "Examples of the Socio-Environmental Approach to Health Promotion" for a description of a few of these initiatives.

Examples of the Socio-Environmental Approach to Health Promotion

Example 1

It was obvious from the heavy utilization of a number of school-based services in a low-income neighbourhood that a larger community service centre would be desirable. CHNs participated in a coalition of agencies to plan for a centre that would meet the needs of the community. Local residents were hired to do a door-to-door survey asking people to list their skills, the strengths of the community, and what they would like to see in a neighbourhood centre. A plan was developed that would build upon these strengths and respond to the dreams of the community. A phased-in plan for local staffing and governance was strictly adhered to. This centre has been functioning very well for many years and is well respected by the community. The role of the CHNs in its development is no longer remembered, but the important thing is that people in this neighbourhood have a place where they can meet and join with others in addressing their needs.

Example 2

When working in a program intended to follow individuals with sexually transmitted infections, CHNs noticed that clients who were receiving social assistance payments could not afford to purchase condoms. Though many drugs were paid for by social assistance when they were given by prescription, condoms were not. The CHNs successfully worked with their managers to lobby for a change in policy to make condoms available by prescription.

→

Example 3

A disadvantaged neighbourhood has an annual "Take Pride Week" that is run primarily by residents but is supported in several ways by local community service providers. "Take Pride Week" provides opportunities for area residents (especially people who are new to the area) to meet their neighbours and become involved in ongoing local activities. CHNs support this community-building event in different ways every year, sometimes helping to plan activities and usually being there to staff some events.

Example 4

Based on data gathered in the community on postpartum visits, district CHNs noticed a high level of isolation among young moms, whether it was their first or subsequent child. The CHNs partnered with the local child and family services agency, which was able to secure funding for a one-year pilot of a moms' group, and with the local church, which provided space and other resources. Personal contact was made with all postpartum moms, inviting them to participate in a planning meeting. The moms, not the CHNs, decided that they wanted the group and determined how they wanted it to function and the weekly agenda. The group has been meeting twice weekly for the past two years and now has plans to expand to an evening session to accommodate working parents. (They have successfully secured additional funding.) The group periodically invites the CHNs to facilitate discussion on topics chosen by the group, but the members now run the group.

Example 5

A CHN is a member of a neighbourhood network that developed in response to several community meetings that identified community needs. The meetings were initiated by a local citizens' group whose original concern was lack of local services and employment opportunities for developmentally delayed students once they became adults. The initial network has expanded to include accessible services related to all areas identified in earlier visioning exercises. The CHN's role is one of consultation, advocacy, and facilitation.

Example 6

The "Families First" program is funded by Healthy Child Manitoba and offered through Public Health. Public health nurses work collaboratively with home visitors, who offer regular home visiting during the first three years of life to families who are identified as requiring assistance to ensure healthy early child development—one of the key determinants of population health. The focus of the program is on building and enhancing family strengths.

Guidelines for Health-Promoting Community Health Nursing Practice

What conclusions can we draw from the preceding discussion? First, it is clear that there can never be one universally accepted definition of health promotion. How one views health promotion will depend on a variety of factors, including one's professional and educational background, the dominant ideology of the time, and one's personal world view. At the level of nursing practice, health promotion appears to be most widely viewed as a set of specific actions or strategies aimed at changing individual behaviours, and with a focus on disease prevention and functional ability. This is in contrast to nursing at the policy and academic levels, where an increasing number of policy and discussion statements have led nursing theorists to adopt a broader view of health promotion—one that is based upon specific values and principles such as social justice, equity, and participation—and focused on modifying the social, political, and economic environment that shapes behaviour (either through direct action or by enabling others to do it for themselves). Second, although a certain percentage of the gap between the rhetoric and reality of nurses' health promotion practice may be due to organizational or societal factors over which they have little control, there is no doubt that much of this gap can be explained by the way that nurses have been socialized—beginning with their educational experiences and continuing in the workplace. How can CHNs narrow the gap between the rhetoric and reality of health promotion in their practice? The following guidelines are offered as a starting point.

Focus on Health and Building Capacity for Health In spite of the fact that nursing theorists have conceptualized health in positive terms such as "self-actualization," "positive adaptation," and "optimal functioning" (Novak, 1988), the truth is that CHNs' health promotion practices have often focused on the negative. For example, most individual, family, and community health assessment models used by nurses focus on the identification of needs, deficits, and problems. If CHNs want to truly help to shift the focus of their services to the promotion of health, then we need to utilize a range of assessment tools and empowering strategies that start by identifying the strengths of individuals, families, and communities, and work with them to build their capacity for health. A focus on capacity building means that the CHN must strive to form collaborative relationships with clients (whether at the individual, family, or community level) and to maximize their involvement in planning, implementing, and evaluating health promotion actions. Remember—every individual, family, or community has some strength that can be capitalized on; your job is to find it and build on it!

Think Upstream It is true that the practice situations of the majority of CHNs involve a lot of work with individuals and families. However, these individuals and families live in communities and societies in which the broader ecological, socioeconomic, political, and cultural environment influences their daily lives. "Thinking upstream" means that, in addition to meeting the immediate needs of individual clients or families (which may involve helping them to cope with their immediate situation or providing information that will assist them to make health-enhancing choices), the CHN should always be (a) assessing the broader socio-environmental determinants of health, (b) thinking about possible strategies that can influence those determinants in a positive manner, and (c) identifying potential partners with whom they might collaborate for maximum effectiveness. (See discussion below.) While the majority of CHNs' health-promoting practice may be "downstream" at the level of personal and small-group empowerment, it is essential to identify all possible opportunities for involvement "upstream" in community empowerment and healthy public policy initiatives. Having said that, whether one works upstream or downstream may not be as important as how one engages in health promotion. That is to say, it is possible to be involved in "upstream" strategies that are disempowering (e.g., taking the initiative to mobilize community action around an issue that the community has not identified as a priority) and "downstream" strategies that are empowering (e.g., working with a single, teenage mother to identify the specific skills she feels are important to improve her chances for success in parenting and finding gainful employment).

Focus on Promoting Equity Some health promotion initiatives (e.g., "healthy living" programs that encourage increased physical activity or other behaviour changes) may be increasing inequities in health because there is greater uptake by socially advantaged groups in society. Be sure to address the needs of socially disadvantaged individuals when planning health promotion initiatives, including ensuring that there are no barriers to participation in health programs and services for disadvantaged people. CHNs can also contribute to the promotion of health equity by monitoring the impact of public policies (e.g., housing, transportation, social assistance) on families and by making decision-makers aware of the research on the links between socioeconomic factors and health inequities.

Look for Partnership Opportunities One of the most challenging aspects of a socio-environmental approach to health promotion for community health practitioners is the recognition that the main determinants of population health—especially social and economic inequalities—lie outside the usual scope of the health system. This has led many CHNs to feel powerless, and has no doubt contributed to a focus in community health nursing practice on helping clients cope with their circumstances, rather than on changing those circumstances. It is imperative that for maximum impact on individual, family, or community health, CHNs identify potential partners with whom they might collaborate. The partners may be from other disciplines within the health sector (e.g., community nutritionists, public health physicians) or they may be from other sectors (e.g., social workers, educators, recreation workers). The key is to leave one's sense of ownership of the issue at the door and to find ways in which each partner can make a unique but complementary contribution to the ultimate goal. It is even more imperative that the partnership should include members from the community who are directly impacted by the initiative. A partnership made up only of service providers can easily lose track of grassroots concerns and will not result in an empowerment process that benefits those who need it most.

Be Patient Perhaps the most challenging aspect of a socio-environmental approach to health promotion is the fact that, unlike many nursing activities, it may take a long time to see positive results. In the case of community development initiatives, this could mean several years. Patience is a virtue in the field of community health nursing. Having to work with multiple partners, follow their lead, and endure frequent delays can leave nurses impatient with the community development process and make them retreat into "safer" direct service work. Constantly sharing and evaluating one's experiences with colleagues and receiving support and encouragement from one's managers may help to alleviate this problem. Ultimately, keep in mind that the empowerment process—as painfully slow and awkward as it may sometimes be—is the most likely way to achieve long-term positive health outcomes.

SUMMARY

We began by exploring the historical development, underlying assumptions, and key characteristics of the three approaches to health promotion—biomedical, behavioural/lifestyle, and socio-environmental—that have been dominant in the twentieth and early twenty-first centuries. While all three of these approaches may be used by health professionals at different times, the biomedical and behavioural/lifestyle approaches have tended to dominate the health promotion practices of nurses and other health professionals. However, the socio-environmental approach has gained momentum within the field of community health nursing in recent years and, in Canada, it has now been formally adopted as the basis for a CHN's practice. Decreasing social and economic inequalities in health, and increasing personal and community empowerment, are at the heart of the socio-environmental approach to health promotion. Educating people regarding healthy behaviours is insufficient to achieve health from this perspective and may actually increase inequities in health. While CHNs who would like to practise from a socio-environmental perspective face some challenges, a few guidelines have been provided that may assist in this process.

KEY TERMS

biomedical approach, p. 90
physiological risk factors, p. 91
Lalonde Report, p. 91
behavioural or lifestyle approach, p. 91
social justice, p. 92
common good, p. 92
social change, p. 92
social responsibility for health, p. 92
victim-blaming, p. 92
ecological or socio-ecological perspective, p. 92

REVIEW QUESTIONS

1. Which one of the following statements about the 1994 Lalonde Report is correct?

   a) It was the first time that a national government had made an official statement regarding the importance of health promotion as a key strategy for improving population health.

   b) It expanded the concept of "health" to include the notion of social well-being at the community level.

   c) It challenged the dominant thinking of the time that a healthy lifestyle was the key to population health.

   d) It argued that the focus of health promotion efforts should be on strategies that would eliminate social inequalities in health.

2. Which one of the following statements about the Ottawa Charter for Health Promotion is correct?

   a) It was signed by delegates from 38 countries, including Canada, in 1974.

   b) It outlined three central strategies for promoting population health.

   c) It emphasized that achieving equity in health was considered to be the main focus of health promotion.

   d) It identified a healthy lifestyle as one of the essential prerequisites for health.

3. Which one of the following statements about health promotion approaches/strategies is correct?

   a) The behavioural approach to health promotion is no longer popular.

   b) The Ottawa Charter for Health Promotion reflects a socio-environmental perspective.

   c) The use of the mass media, direct mail, product labels, pamphlets, or posters to communicate a health message to the public is an example of the Ottawa Charter strategy of developing healthy public policy.

   d) Laws requiring the use of seatbelts or banning smoking in public places are examples of the Ottawa Charter strategy of developing personal skills.

4. Which one of the following statements about promoting health equity is correct?

   a) "Healthy Living" programs that encourage increased physical activity among the population as a whole will likely decrease inequities in health.

   b) It is not part of the CHN's role to make decision makers aware of the research on the links between socioeconomic factors and inequities in health.

   c) The term "health inequities" refers to any disparity or inequality in health between population groups.

   d) CHNs can contribute to the promotion of health equity by monitoring the impact of public policies on families.

5. Which one of the following statements about CHNs' health promotion practices is correct?

   a) According to Falk-Rafael's Critical Caring theory of public health nursing, the PHN's role is primarily to change perceptions and attitudes that are viewed as non-health-enhancing and to assist the client to develop, carry out, and evaluate a behaviour-change plan.

   b) Detailed community assessment that focuses on inter-family and intercommunity themes in health and illness is an example of a microscopic approach in community health nursing.

   c) The Canadian Community Health Nursing Standards of Practice are based on a behavioural perspective of health and health promotion.

   d) The use of a critical social approach to health promotion by CHNs involves the use of empowering strategies at the personal/individual, interpersonal (small group), community, and policy levels.

STUDY QUESTIONS

1. What are the main differences between the three approaches to health promotion in terms of (a) type of health determinant most concerned with, (b) target of the initiative, (c) program management (including the difference between community-based and community development programs), and (d) criteria for success?

2. What is the limitation of using an approach to health promotion that focuses exclusively on behaviour change?

3. What is the central concept that lies at the heart of the socio-environmental approach to health promotion? How would you define this concept and how does it link with health promotion?

4. What are the five key principles of health promotion from a socio-environmental perspective?

5. What are three ways that nurses can play an important role in addressing social determinants of health?

6. What are five guidelines for health-promoting CHN practice?

After working through these questions, go to the MyNursingLab at www.pearsoned.ca/mynursinglab to check your answers.

INDIVIDUAL CRITICAL THINKING EXERCISES

1. Prior to reading this chapter, what did the term "health promotion" mean to you? Has your initial interpretation changed? If so, how?

2. Analyze your personal level of comfort with using the three main approaches to health promotion outlined in this chapter. What factors would increase your comfort in using each one?

3. Think about the community you live in. What are the main issues affecting your community's health or quality of life? Which approach to health promotion would be the most appropriate to deal with these issues? (There may be more than one.) What role could a CHN play in a health promotion initiative that addressed each issue?

4. For each of the examples of the socio-environmental approach to health promotion provided in the box on pages 101–102, identify which of the Ottawa Charter strategies are being implemented. (More than one may apply.)

5. You are a CHN in a community where there appears to be an increasing number of obese children in the elementary school that you visit. Describe a microscopic ("downstream") versus a macroscopic ("upstream") approach to community health promotion in this situation.

GROUP CRITICAL THINKING EXERCISES

1. Discuss your answers to Individual Critical Thinking Exercise 1 with one or more partners. How do your responses compare? What factors influenced your original understanding of health promotion?

2. With a partner, interview a CHN in your community. Ask the following questions: What does the term "health promotion" mean to you? What are the main health promotion issues in your area? Describe some of the health promotion activities in your practice. What are the barriers to engaging in health promotion activities? Analyze the responses with your partner. How would you summarize this CHN's approach to health promotion?

3. With one or more partners, identify examples of each of the behavioural/lifestyle strategies (listed in Table 6.2) that are in use in Canada and/or your region of the country today. Critically assess the strengths and weaknesses of these strategies.

4. With one or more partners, read the Toronto Charter for a Healthy Canada (Raphael, 2009), and identify specific strategies that CHNs could use to address all or some of the SDOH in their practice.

NOTES

1. Of course, other perspectives on health and disease have always existed, both within certain populations in Western societies and among non-Western societies. However, it is beyond the scope of this chapter to explore those perspectives and the approaches to health enhancement that they have generated.

2. Not surprisingly, many of these strategies are based on theories and models—e.g., the health belief model (HBM), the transtheoretical (stages of change) model, and social learning/cognitive theory—that were developed in the field of psychology to explain, predict, and change health behaviours. For a comprehensive discussion of these models, and other theories and models used in the behaviours approach to health promotion, see Glanz, Rimer, & Viswanath (2008).

3. One of the most popular frameworks for health promotion program planning in use today—the "PRECEDE-PROCEED" model (Green & Kreuter, 1999)—is based on the ecological perspective. For further discussion of this and other ecological models, see chapters in Glanz et al. (2008).

4. This original WHO definition is still very popular. However, more recently, it has been expanded as "the process of enabling individuals and communities to increase control over the determinants of health" (Nutbeam, cited in Green, Poland, & Rootman, 2000, p. 6).

5. See the discussion in Chapter 2.

6. This is not to say that there has been no discussion of concepts or models related to the socio-environmental perspective on health promotion in nursing curricula since the 1980s. In fact, one study (Canadian Association of Schools of Nursing Task Force on Public Health Education, 2006) indicated that the vast majority of nursing programs in Canada have done so. The problem may be that discussion of these concepts/models tends to occur in one particular course or in one semester that focuses on population health promotion (often in the final year of the program), rather than being integrated throughout the program (L. L. Stamler, CASN Sub-Committee on Public Health Education, personal communication, April 9, 2007).

REFERENCES

Armstrong, R., Waters, E., & Doyle, J. (Eds). (2008). Reviews in health promotion and public health. Chapter 21 in J. Higgins & S. Green (Eds.), *Cochrane handbook for systematic reviews of interventions*. Version 5.0.1 [updated September 2008]. The Cochrane Collaboration. Retrieved from www.cochrane-handbook.org

Ballou, K. (2000). A historical-philosophical analysis of the professional nurse obligation to participate in sociopolitical activities. *Politics, Policy, & Nursing Practice, 1*(3), 172–184.

Beauchamp, D. (1976). Public health as social justice. *Inquiry, 13*, 3–14.

Benson, A., & Latter, S. (1998). Implementing health promoting nursing: The integration of interpersonal skills and health promotion. *Journal of Advanced Nursing, 27,* 100–107.

Broughton, M. A., Janssen, P. S., Hertzman, C., Innis, S. M., & Frankish, C. J. (2006). Predictors and outcomes of household food insecurity among inner city families with preschool children in Vancouver. *Canadian Journal of Public Health, 97*(3), 214–216.

Brubaker, B. (1983, April). Health promotion: A linguistic analysis. *Advances in Nursing Science, 5*(3), 1–14.

Butterfield, P. (1997). Thinking upstream: Conceptualizing health from a population perspective. In J. Swanson & M. Nies (Eds.), *Community health nursing: Promoting the health of aggregate* (pp. 69–82). Philadelphia, PA: W. B. Saunders.

Canadian Association of Schools of Nursing Task Force on Public Health Education. (2006). *Shaping the future of public health and community health nursing education in Canada.* Presentation to the Pan-Canadian Symposium on Public Health Education, Toronto, ON.

Canadian Nurses Association. (1992). *Policy statement on health promotion.* Ottawa, ON: Author.

Canadian Nurses Association. (2005). *Social determinants of health and nursing: A summary of the issues.* Retrieved from http://cna-aiic.ca/CNA/documents/pdf/publications/BG8_Social_Determinants_e.pdf

Canadian Nurses Association. (2006). *Social justice: A means to an end, an end in itself.* Retrieved from http://cna-aiic.ca/CNA/documents/pdf/publications/Social_Justice_e.pdf

Canadian Public Health Association. (1990). *Community health/public health nursing in Canada: Preparation and practice.* Ottawa, ON: Author.

Carnivale, F. (2008). Editorial: Emancipatory nursing. *Pediatric Intensive Care Nursing, 9*(2), 2.

Chalmers, K., & Bramadat, I. (1996). Community development: Theoretical and practical issues for community health nursing in Canada. *Journal of Advanced Nursing, 24,* 719–726.

Cohen, B. (2006a). Population health as a framework for public health practice: A Canadian perspective. *American Journal of Public Health, 96*(9), 1574–1576.

Cohen, B. (2006b). Barriers to population-focused health promotion: The experience of public health nurses in the province of Manitoba. *Canadian Journal of Nursing Research, 38*(3), 52–67.

Cohen, B., & Reutter, L. (2007). Development of the role of public health nurses in addressing child and family poverty: A framework for action. *Journal of Advanced Nursing,* (electronic version). doi:10.1111/j.1365-2648.2006.04154.x

Community Health Nurses Association of Canada. (2008). *Canadian community health nursing standards of practice.* Retrieved from http://www.chnac.ca /images/downloads/standards/chn_standards_of_practice_mar08_english.pdf

Crawford, R. (1977). You are dangerous to your health: The ideology and politics of victim blaming. *International Journal of Health Services, 7*(4), 663–680.

Epp, J. (1986). *Achieving health for all: A framework for health promotion.* Ottawa, ON: Health and Welfare Canada.

Falk-Rafael, A. (2005a). Advancing nursing theory through theory-guided practice: The emergence of a critical caring perspective. *Advances in Nursing Science, 28*(1), 38–49.

Falk-Rafael, A. (2005b). Speaking truth to power: Nursing's legacy and moral imperative. *Advances in Nursing Science, 28*(3), 212–223.

Federal, Provincial, Territorial Advisory Committee on Population Health. (1994). *Strategies for population health: Investing in the health of Canadians.* Ottawa, ON: Ministry of Supply and Services.

Feeley, N., & Gottlieb, L. (2000). Nursing approaches for working with family strengths and resources. *Journal of Family Nursing, 6*(1), 9–24.

Galabuzi, G-E. (2009). Social exclusion. In D. Raphael (Ed.), *Social determinants of health* (2nd ed., pp. 252–268). Toronto, ON: Canadian Scholars' Press.

Gibson, C. (1991). A concept analysis of empowerment. *Journal of Advanced Nursing, 16,* 354–361.

Glanz, K., Rimer, B., & Viswanath, K. (2008). *Health behaviour and health education: Theory, research and practice* (4th ed.). San Francisco, CA: Jossey-Bass.

Green, L., & Kreuter, M. (2005). *Health Program Planning: An Educational and Ecological Approach* (4th ed.). New York, NY: McGraw-Hill.

Green, L. W., Poland, B. D., & Rootman, I. (2000). The settings approach to health promotion. In B. D. Poland, L. W. Green, & I. Rootman (Eds.), *Settings for health promotion: Linking theory and practice* (pp. 1–43). Thousand Oaks, CA: Sage.

Hamilton, N., & Bhatti, T. (1996). *Population health promotion: An integrated model of population health and health promotion.* Ottawa, ON: Health Canada, Health Promotion and Development Division.

Hartrick, G. (2000). Developing health-promoting practice with families: One pedagogical experience. *Journal of Advanced Nursing, 31*(1), 27–34. doi:10.1046/j.1365-2648.2000.01263.x

Heaney, C., & Israel, B. (2002). Social networks and social support. In K. Glanz, F. Lewis, & B. Rimer (Eds.), *Health behavior and health education: Theory research and practice* (3rd ed., pp. 179–205). San Francisco, CA: Jossey-Bass.

Kirby, S., Perkins, K., & Reizes, T. (2003). *Social marketing and public health: Lessons from the field.* The Social Marketing National Excellence Collaborative. Seattle, WA: University of Washington, Turning Point National Program Office.

Labonte, R. (1993). *Health promotion and empowerment: Practice frameworks.* Toronto, ON: University of Toronto, Centre for Health Promotion & ParticipACTION.

Labonte, R. (1995). Population health and health promotion: What do they have to say to each other? *Canadian Journal of Public Health, 86*(3), 165–188.

Labonte, R., & Penfold, S. (1981). Canadian perspectives in health promotion: A critique. *Health Education, 19*(3/4), 4–9.

Lalonde, M. (1974). *A new perspective on the health of Canadians.* Ottawa, ON: Department of National Health and Welfare.

Maben, J., & MacLeod Clark, J. (1995). Health promotion: A concept analysis. *Journal of Advanced Nursing, 22,* 1158–1165.

MacDonald, M. (2002). Health promotion: Historical, philosophical, and theoretical perspectives. In L. Young & V. Hayes (Eds.), *Transforming health promotion practice:*

Concepts, issues, and applications (pp. 22–45). Philadelphia, PA: F. A. Davis.

Makara, P. (1997). Can we promote equity when we promote health? *Health Promotion International, 12*(2), 97–98.

Manitoba Health. (1998). *The role of the public health nurse within the regional health authority.* Winnipeg, MB: Author.

McKinlay, J. (1979). A case for refocusing upstream: The political economy of illness. In E. Jaco (Ed.), *Patients, physicians, and illness* (pp. 9–25). New York, NY: The Free Press.

Novak, J. (1988). The social mandate and historical basis for nursing's role in health promotion. *Journal of Professional Nursing Practice, 4*(2), 80–87.

NSW Health and Health Promotion Service, South East Health. (2003). *Four steps towards equity: A tool for health promotion practice.* Retrieved from www.health.nsw.gov.au

Nutbeam, D., & Harris, E. (1998). *Theory in a nutshell: A practitioner's guide to commonly used theories and models in health promotion.* Sydney, Australia: National Centre for Health Promotion, Department of Public Health and Community Medicine, University of Sydney, NSW, Australia.

Patrick, D., & Wickizer, T. (1995). Community and health. In B. Amick, S. Levine, A. Tarlov, & D. Chapman Walsh (Eds.), *Society and health* (pp. 46–92). New York, NY: Oxford University Press.

Pender, N. (1996). *Health promotion in nursing practice* (3rd ed.). Stamford, CT: Appleton & Lange.

Pender, N., Murdaugh, C., & Parsons, M. (2005). *Health promotion in nursing practice* (5th ed.). Ann Arbour, MI: Pearson Education.

Public Health Agency of Canada. (2008). *Report on the state of public health in Canada 2008.* Ottawa, ON: Author. Retrieved from http://www.phac-aspc.gc.ca/publicat/2008/cpho-aspc/index-eng.php

Raeburn, J., & Rootman, I. (1998). *People-centred health promotion.* Chichester, UK: John Wiley & Sons.

Raphael, D. (Ed.). (2009). *Social determinants of health: Canadian perspectives* (2nd ed.). Toronto, ON: Canadian Scholars' Press.

Raphael, D., & Bryant, T. (2000). Putting the population into population health. *Canadian Journal of Public Health, 91*(1), 9–12.

Reutter, L. (2000). Socioeconomic determinants of health. In M. Stewart (Ed.), *Community health nursing: Promoting Canadians' health* (2nd ed., pp. 174–193). Toronto, ON: W. B. Saunders.

Reutter, L., & Ford, J. (1998). Perceptions of changes in public health nursing practice: A Canadian perspective. *International Journal of Nursing Studies, 35,* 85–94.

Richmond, C. A., Ross, N. A., & Egeland, G. M. (2007). Social support and thriving health: A new approach to understanding the health of indigenous Canadians. *American Journal of Public Health, 97*(10), 1827–1923.

Sampson, R. (2003). Neighbourhood-level context and health: Lessons from sociology. In I. Kawachi & L. Berkman (Eds.), *Neighbourhoods and health* (pp. 132–146). Oxford, UK: Oxford University Press.

Shuster, S., Ross, S., Bhagat, R., & Johnson, J. (2001). Using community development approaches. *Canadian Nurse, 97*(6), 18–22.

Spenceley, S., Reutter, L., & Allen, M. (2006). The road less traveled: Nursing advocacy at the policy level. *Policy, Politics, and Nursing Practice, 7*(3), 180–194.

Stansfeld, S. (2006). Social support and social cohesion. In M. Marmot & R. Wilkinson (Eds.), *Social determinants of health* (2nd ed., pp. 148–171). Oxford, UK: Oxford University Press.

Syme, S. L. (1997). Individual vs. community interventions in public health practice: Some thoughts about a new approach. *VicHealth, 2,* 2–9.

Vanderplaat, M. (2002). Emancipatory politics and health promotion practice: The health professional as social activist. In L. Young & V. Hayes (Eds.), *Transforming health promotion practice: Concepts, issues and applications* (pp. 87–98). Philadelphia, PA: F. A. Davis.

Vollman, A. R., Anderson, E. T., & McFarlane, J. M. (2008). *Canadian community as partner: Theory and multidisciplinary practice* (2nd ed.). Philadelphia, PA: Lippincott Williams & Wilkins.

Wallerstein, N. (1992). Powerlessness, empowerment, and health: Implications for health promotion programs. *American Journal of Health Promotion, 6*(3), 197–205.

Whitehead, D. (2003). Incorporating socio-political health promotion activities in clinical practice. *Journal of Clinical Nursing, 12*(5), 668–677.

Wilkinson, R., & Pickett, K. (2009). *The spirit level: Why more equal societies almost always do better.* London, UK: Penquin Books.

Williamson, D., & Drummond, J. (2000). Enhancing low-income parents' capacities to promote their children's health: Education is not enough. *Public Health Nursing, 17*(2), 121–131.

Woodward, A., & Kawachi, I. (2000). Why reduce health inequalities? *Journal of Epidemiology and Community Health, 54,* 923–929.

World Health Organization. (1977). *Health for all by the year 2000.* Geneva, Switzerland: Author.

World Health Organization. (1978). *Declaration of Alma Ata.* Retrieved from www.who.int/hpr/archive/docs/almata.html

World Health Organization. (1984). *Health promotion: A discussion document on the concepts and principles.* Copenhagen, Denmark: WHO Regional Office for Europe.

World Health Organization. (1986). *Ottawa Charter for health promotion.* Ottawa, ON: Canadian Public Health Association and Health and Welfare Canada.

World Health Organization. (2008). *Closing the gap in a generation: Health equity through action on the social determinants of health.* Commission on the Social Determinants of Health Final Report. Geneva, Switzerland: Author. Retrieved from http://www.who.int/social_determinants/thecommission/finalreport/en/index.html

Wright, L., & Leahey, M. (2009). *Nurses and families: A guide to family assessment and intervention* (5th ed.). Philadelphia, PA: F. A. Davis.

Young, L. (2002). Transforming health promotion practice: Moving toward holistic care. In L. Young & V. Hayes (Eds.), *Transforming health promotion practice: Concepts, issues and applications* (pp. 3–21). Philadelphia, PA: F. A. Davis.

Ziersch, A., Baum, F., MacDougall, C., & Putland, C. (2005). Neighbourhood life and social capital: The implications for health. *Social Science and Medicine, 60,* 71–86.

Zimmerman, M. (2000). Empowerment theory: Psychological, organizational and community levels of analysis. In J. Rappaport & E. Seidman (Eds.), *Handbook of community psychology* (pp. 43–63). New York, NY: Academic/Plenum.

ADDITIONAL RESOURCES

Readings

Minkler, M. (Ed.). (2004). *Community organizing and community building for health* (2nd ed.). New Brunswick, NJ: Rutgers University Press.

Nutbeam, D., & Harris, E. (2004). *Theory in a nutshell: A practical guide to health promotion theories* (2nd ed.). Sydney, Australia: McGraw-Hill.

O'Neill, M., Pederson, A., Dupéré, S., & Rootman, I. (2007). *Health promotion in Canada: Critical perspectives* (2nd ed.). Toronto, ON: Canadian Scholars' Press.

Poland, B., Green, L., & Rootman, I. (2000). *Settings for health promotion: Linking theory and practice.* Newbury Park, CA: Sage.

Young, L. E., & Hayes, V. (2002). *Transforming health promotion practice: Concepts, issues, and applications.* Philadelphia, PA: F. A. Davis.

The following periodicals are good sources of theoretical and practice-based research articles related to community health nursing and/or health promotion in the community:

Community Health Promotion
Critical Public Health
Global Health Promotion
Health Education Quarterly
Health Education Research
Health Promotion International
Journal of Advanced Nursing
Public Health Nursing

Websites

University of Toronto
http://www.utoronto.ca/chp/who/hpbib.htm

Minnesota Public Health Department: Interventions Manual
http://www.health.state.mn.us/divs/cfh/ophp/resources/docs/phinterventions_manual2001.pdf

Dr. Dennis Raphael, York University
http://www.atkinson.yorku.ca/draphael

Health Promotion: Capacity Checklists
http://www.usask.ca/healthsci/che/prhprc/programs/finalworkbook.pdf

World Health Organization: Health Promotion Glossary
http://www.who.int/hpr/NPH/docs/hp_glossary_en.pdf

World Health Organization: Social Determinants of Health.
http://www.who.int/social_determinants/en/

Health Nexus
http://www.healthnexus.ca

Unnatural Causes: Is Inequality Making Us Sick?
http://www.unnaturalcauses.org/podcasts.php

About the Author

Benita Cohen, RN, PhD (University of Manitoba), is an Associate Professor in the Faculty of Nursing at the University of Manitoba, where she teaches courses in the undergraduate and graduate programs related to prevention of illness and health promotion in the community. She previously worked as a Public Health Nurse in the Toronto area and in the Baffin region of Nunavut. She is currently a member of the Canadian Association of Schools of Nursing Sub-Committee on Public Health Education. Her research program is focused on developing Public Health capacity to reduce health inequities.

The author would like to thank Horst Backe, Bluma Levine, Susan Permut, and Lynda Tjaden—nurses at the Winnipeg Regional Health Authority—for their input into the development of the case study and provision of examples of population health promotion strategies used in their own practice.

Primary Health Care

Dawn Smith, Kim Van Herk, and Zaida Rahaman

OBJECTIVES

After studying this chapter, you should be able to:

1. Describe the concept of primary health care, its values, principles, and elements.
2. Describe current perspectives on primary health care reforms.
3. Describe differences and similarities between primary health care primary care, health promotion, and population health.
4. Describe the central role of social justice in primary health care and give examples of strengths and weaknesses of CHN practice of social justice.
5. Describe community development and empowerment strategies to implement primary health care.
6. Describe nursing's roles in primary health care development and reform in Canada.

INTRODUCTION

Primary health care (PHC) was first described in the landmark document the *Declaration of Alma Ata*, produced at the WHO–UNICEF conference in Alma Ata, Kazakstan in the former Soviet Union in 1978. **Primary health care** was defined as

> essential healthcare based on practical, scientifically sound and acceptable methods and technology made universally accessible to individuals and families in the community through their full participation and at a cost that the community and country can afford to maintain at every stage of their development in the spirit of self-reliance and self-determination. (World Health Organization [WHO], 1978, p. 2)

More specifically, PHC can be summarized as

- evidence-based;
- universally accessible;
- providing for essential health needs at the first level of contact;
- providing a full spectrum of needs, including health promotion, prevention, treatment, and rehabilitation;
- addressing the main determinants of health;
- affordable to community and country;
- relevant to the social, cultural, economic, and political context;
- addressing community priorities;

- multi-sectoral and integral to overall social and economic development;
- requiring and promoting individual and community self-reliance and participation;
- sustaining effective health information systems; and
- relying on a diverse team of appropriately trained and responsive health workers.

The *Declaration of Alma Ata* outlines an intersectoral and community-driven approach to improving health and reducing inequities in health. It outlines eight essential elements to achieve "health for all" (WHO, 1978, p. 2). These include

- education concerning prevailing health problems and the methods of prevention and control;
- promoting an adequate food supply and proper nutrition;
- promoting an adequate supply of safe water and basic sanitation;
- promoting maternal and child health, including family planning;
- immunization against infectious diseases;
- prevention and control of locally endemic diseases;
- promoting appropriate treatment of common diseases and injuries; and
- providing essential drugs.

These guidelines have been used extensively to improve health programming and policy development in developing countries ever since. They have had a tremendous influence on improving health services and national health systems. "It has drawn attention to the needs of the many, and has been a powerful instrument for making governments and their partners recognize that the provision of healthcare cannot be left to the professionals alone . . ."(WHO, 2006, p. 4). Overall improvements in diet, sanitation, disease prevention, and healthcare have increased life expectancy, closing the gap between developed and developing countries respectively.

The political, social, and economic messages of the PHC philosophy have not been applied to the same degree in more developed countries due to the strong biomedical and behavioural approaches to healthcare that predominated during the 1970s and 1980s. However, a recent research study done in Australia strongly encouraged health reform processes to continue to move toward inclusion of all of the elements of PHC within mainstream healthcare services in order to help reduce health disparities (Hurley, Baum, Johns, & Labonte, 2010). PHC remains a vision for improving health that is adaptable across nations, cultures, stage of development, and history. At the heart of PHC are the values and principles for improving health for all, and working in partnership with governments and citizens, and across sectors.

PRIMARY HEALTH CARE VALUES AND PRINCIPLES

Values are the "shared beliefs, ideals and judgments about what is desirable and what is not" (Merriam-Webster, 2010). Values and principles are often implicit in the institutions and practices of governments, organizations, professions, or groups. They guide behaviour, determine directions for policies, and assist in evaluating new ideas and approaches. PHC articulates a set of values that have been ratified across nations, thereby providing guidance for positive change within nations across the globe.

Primary Health Care Values

Achieving "health for all" is a fundamental value of PHC. PHC values are comparable to those of the Canadian Nurses Association's *Code of Ethics for Registered Nurses* (Canadian Nurses Association [CNA], 2008) and the *Standards for Community Health Nursing in Canada* (Community Health Nurses Association of Canada [CHNAC], 2008). *Social justice* and *equity* are two distinctive PHC values.

Social justice refers to the degree of equality of opportunity for health made available by the political, social, and economic structures of a society. The extent to which a society provides opportunities for its citizens to develop socially and economically productive roles influences not only the well-being of individuals, but the health of its entire population (Wilkinson, 1996). One example of the inequities that exist in health status is that the rich are healthier than the poor. It is important, therefore, that Community Health Nurses (CHNs) consider how social justice is enacted in their practice and by the healthcare organization that employs them.

Equity in health "means that people's needs guide the distribution of opportunities for well-being" (WHO, 1998, p. 7). Equity is apolitical concept. It has "normative ethical values that entail fair distribution of resources and access within and among various population groups. . . . Equity efforts include reducing discrimination in access to the benefits of health initiatives" (WHO, 2005, p. 44). An example of equity efforts would be using strategies to improve access of rural/remote clients to specialized health services offered in urban centres. This may require financial support for transportation and housing to facilitate equitable urban access.

Socio-economic inequity is perhaps the biggest factor affecting the health of populations (Navarro, 2009; Public Health Agency of Canada [PHAC], 2003; Raphael, 2002). Unequal societies are plagued by large differences in social support, the social organization of work, predictable patterns of job insecurity and unemployment, and a divisiveness of material wealth (Wilkinson, 1996). Considerable evidence supports that there are relationships between inequality in macro-level social structures, meso-level social processes, and micro-level health effects (Bezruchka, 2002). Usually the term **macro** refers to the "big picture" levels of influence such as policy, and **micro** refers to the very smallest levels of influence, such as the individual person, or even cells. The **meso** level is the "in between," such as family, group, community, and organization. Interventions that take action on the causes of poor health at all levels are fundamental to the PHC approach.

Principles of Primary Health Care

PHC principles describe the nature and scope of action to enact PHC values. The CNA (2000) formulated its position on PHC based on the five principles embodied in the WHO's (1978) original definition. These principles include accessibility, public participation, health promotion, appropriate technology, and intersectoral co-operation, and are described in the box below. Refer to the following Case Study for an example that illustrates the CNA's five principles of PHC.

Canadian Nurses Association's Five Principles of Primary Health Care

Accessibility The five types of healthcare (promotive, preventive, curative, rehabilitative, and supportive/palliative) must be universally accessible to all clients regardless of geographic location. In many cases, the principle of accessibility can best be established by having communities define and manage necessary healthcare services. Distribution of health professionals in rural, remote, and urban communities is key to the principle of accessibility. Accessibility means that clients will receive appropriate care from the appropriate healthcare professional within an appropriate time frame.

Public Participation Clients are encouraged to participate in making decisions about their own health, identifying the health needs of their community, and considering the merits of alternative approaches to addressing those needs. Adoption of the principle of public participation includes respect for diversity. It also means that the design and delivery of healthcare is flexible and responsive. Participation aims to promote effective planning and evaluation of healthcare services in a community.

Health Promotion This refers to efforts aimed at increasing peoples' control over the things that affect their health. Health promotion interventions can include health education, nutrition, sanitation, and prevention and control of endemic disease. Effective health promotion interventions would reduce the demands for curative and rehabilitative care. Through health promotion, individuals and families build an understanding of the determinants of health, and develop skills to improve and maintain their own health and well-being. School health programs are an example of health promotion interventions.

Appropriate Technology Modes of care must be adapted appropriately to the community's social, economic, and cultural development. The principle of appropriate technology recognizes the importance of developing and testing innovative models of healthcare and of disseminating the results of research related to healthcare. However, it also means considering alternatives to high-cost, high-tech services, including the use of low technology in mass media (such as radio) for health education.

Intersectoral Co-operation Health and well-being are linked to both economic and social policy such as in schools, transportation, agriculture, and finance. Intersectoral co-operation is needed to establish and evaluate national and local health goals, and healthy public policy. Inter-sectoral co-operation can also mean having providers from different disciplines collaborate and function interdependently to meet the needs of healthcare consumers and their families. It suggests that services in different sectors, such as housing, health, education. and policing must be designed and delivered in an integrated and congruent fashion.

Source: Adapted with permission from the Canadian Nurses Association. (2000). Fact Sheet on Primary Health Care. www.cna-aiic.ca/CNA/documents/pdf/publications/ FS02_Primary_Health_Care_Approach_June_2000_e.pdf

CASE STUDY: Ottawa Inner City Health: The Five Primary Health Care Principles

The number of homeless people in Ottawa grew from 6572 to 7045 individuals and shelter bed use increased 13% between 2007 and 2008 (Alliance to End Homelessness, 2008). The homeless are exposed to extreme weather, cramped living conditions, and higher rates of violence. As a result, they experience a complex mix of health problems including diabetes, addiction, chronic and debilitating mental health issues, and trauma sustained from violence. Homeless people are frequent visitors to emergency rooms and walk-in clinics. However, mainstream healthcare systems, social service benefits, and housing are not well equipped to address the complex interrelated challenges characterizing this population. As a result, their health concerns are often not adequately addressed. As a response to this gap in health services, Ottawa Inner City Health was formed.

Ottawa Inner City Health Inc. (2009) is a collaboration of expertise and resources comprising the emergency shelter system, healthcare, and services provided through health, social, housing, and legal sector organizations. Services have grown to include:

- Mission Hospice—a partnership with a local shelter where homeless individuals can live out the final stages of life.
- Management of Alcohol—a therapeutic harm reduction setting for homeless people who are addicted to alcohol.
- Special Care Units for Men and Women—care programs for homeless women and men with complex physical and mental health needs.
- Primary Care Clinic—Nurse Practitioner provides healthcare, dental, and HIV treatment services for homeless and street-involved individuals.
- Aging at Home—intensive support services for the elderly homeless or street involved.

Inner City Health's mission, values, and guiding principles reflect the five principles of PHC:

Accessibility—Ottawa Inner City Health's vision is to provide individuals who are chronically homeless equitable access to the supports and services they require to maintain or improve their health. Inner City Health's programs provide homeless individuals with support and services within the shelter system. As a result, they are able to obtain care from a number of different health and social service providers, including registered nurses, physicians, nurse practitioners, mental health workers, and client care workers whom they would otherwise find difficult to approach.

Public Participation—Inner City Health values clients as equal partners and encourages them to participate in making decisions about their own health and in identifying the health needs of their community. For example, clients have been consulted about the changes they would like to see incorporated into a new housing unit.

Health Promotion—Registered nurses ensure that clients are up to date with their immunizations and coordinate with the local public health unit to provide tuberculosis and influenza screening. Clients are also taught life skills, including nutritional cooking on a budget, and engage in group activities that encourage exercise and social integration. A strong harm reduction approach advocates for reducing the negative effects of drug and alcohol use.

Appropriate Technology—Inner City Health uses new technology and the best knowledge and evidence to support innovation, change, and the generation of new ideas. For example, an electronic health record is used by multiple service providers at different locations. This innovation helps to record daily care and communicate client needs among providers.

Intersectoral Co-operation—From the very beginning, Inner City Health has engaged in partnerships with several member organizations to implement their programs and provide the needed services. They also work with the university to conduct research on homelessness and to provide clinical placements to students in medicine and nursing.

Discussion Questions

1. Describe the health issues encountered by CHNs working with homeless populations.

2. Explore the ways organizations from different sectors (e.g., housing, healthcare, social services, and education) can collaborate.

Unfortunately, the *Declaration of Alma Ata*'s explicit attention to the importance of changing structures and policy and enabling socially just values and beliefs to flourish has often been missed. In some countries overall improvements in life expectancy and the health gains of past decades are being reversed by the impact of communicable diseases such as HIV/AIDS. Globalization has also created additional inequities between richer and poorer nations, as demonstrated by increases in food insecurity as a result of bio-fuel production incentives.

PHC REFORM: CHALLENGES AND VISION

Despite enormous progress in health globally, our collective failures to deliver in line with the values [of PHC] are painfully obvious and deserve our greatest attention.

—Dr. Margaret Chan, Director-General, World Health Organization (World Health Organization, 2008, p. viii)

The World Health Organization marked the 30th anniversary of the *Declaration of Alma Ata* with its publication of the 2008 World Health Report entitled, *Primary Health Care: Now More Than Ever*. As outlined, "left to their own devices, health systems do not gravitate naturally towards the goals of health for all, and have develop[ed] in directions that contribute little to equity and social justice" (World Health Organization, 2008, p. xiv).

Examples of challenges faced by a renewed PHC system in this comprehensive document include

- disparities between urban and rural areas within countries, in addition to significant health inequities among diverse social and economic groups within urban areas;
- difficulty responding "equitably and effectively" to the health needs of non-citizen residents such as immigrants, refugees, and displaced persons, and to the linguistic and cultural diversity resulting from migration;
- growing populations in both developed and developing nations who are affected by co-morbidities, including mental health problems, addictions, and violence;
- an oversimplified understanding of PHC, resulting in approaches that are not tailored to specific contexts, populations, or issues—often, PHC is seen as a healthcare delivery program for providing minimal levels of care for poor people;
- the fact that without strong policies and leadership, health systems do not spontaneously gravitate toward PHC values nor respond efficiently to evolving health challenges; and
- health systems as a reflection of a globalizing consumer culture.

Figure 7.1 summarizes the major forces that have contributed to poor progress, and the vision for renewal toward *Health for All*.

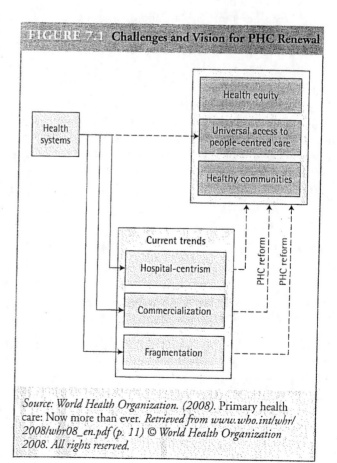

FIGURE 7.1 Challenges and Vision for PHC Renewal

Major forces for PHC renewal are the public's growing expectations regarding societal, community, and individual health issues. Citizens expect their families and communities to be protected from risks and dangers to health. They want to be respected and treated as individuals with rights in a climate of mutual trust. People recognize social inequalities as unjust and support efforts to reduce inequities in health. Increasingly, they do not tolerate social exclusion or disproportionate income distribution (World Health Organization, 2008).

Reflection on the progress over the last 30 years of its core values of social justice and equity, as well as the growing challenges of citizen expectations, led to the formulation of four sets of reforms that articulate a broader vision for PHC in the context of current health system pressures and forces (World Health Organization, 2008). These **primary health care reforms** include

- *universal coverage reforms* that ensure health systems contribute to health equity, social justice, and the end of exclusion in order to move towards universal healthcare access;
- *service delivery reforms* that re-organize health services around people's needs and expectations, so as to make them socially relevant and responsive to the changing world, while producing better outcomes;
- *public policy reforms* that secure healthier communities by integrating public health actions with primary care, by pursuing healthy public policies across sectors, and by strengthening national and transnational public health interventions; and
- *leadership reforms* that "replace disproportionate reliance on command and control on one hand, and laissez-faire disengagement of the state on the other, by inclusive, participatory, and negotiation-based leadership" (World Health Organization, 2008, p. xvi).

Articulation of these reforms by the World Health Organization supports CHN action towards socially just health system change. No longer just a vision at political odds with government agendas of economic restraint, *PHC: Now More Than Ever* provides the direction to support public policy and health system renewal regarding health for all (Figure 7.1).

ACHIEVING A PRIMARY HEALTH CARE SYSTEM IN CANADA

As a signatory to the Alma Ata Declaration in 1978, Canada, like many developed nations, viewed PHC as an approach to address health issues in developing countries. Eight years later, however, the *Ottawa Charter for Health Promotion* (WHO, 1986) was taken up by many developed countries. The Ottawa Charter shared many of the key values and principles of PHC. That same year, for example, the Canadian government's *Achieving Health for All* framework (Epp, 1986) demonstrated its acceptance in Canada.

Despite the endorsement of the *Ottawa Charter's* values and principles, Canada has been slow in implementing the social justice values of PHC. The necessary shift in values was stifled by the structural and ideological legacy of major national policies. For example, the British North America (BNA) Act creating the Dominion of Canada in 1867 gave responsibility for healthcare to the provinces, a significant legislative barrier to *national* healthcare reform.

The Hospital and Diagnostic Services Act of 1957 left a lingering belief system that equates technology and curative intervention with healthcare. The Medical Care Act of 1968 entrenched physicians as the only point of entry into the healthcare system. While midwives and nurse practitioners have been added as points of entry in some Canadian provinces over the last decade, many barriers to their full integration and use remain.

PHC renewal in Canada requires not only greater receptivity to PHC values, but a willingness by key stakeholders to overcome existing legislative barriers and provide additional funding. There has been, however, steady development of these PHC-friendly conditions. In the late 1980s/early 1990s, significant interest in health system change was evident in the numerous commissions on healthcare across the country (Angus, 1995). These resulted in several concerted efforts on behalf of provincial and territorial governments to advance the PHC agenda. For example, in Nova Scotia, the provincial government funded a Task Force on Primary Health Care. From 1994 to 1999, the federal government sponsored the National Forum on Health, a forum of experts and citizens from across the country. This forum produced several reports emphasizing the need for action on the determinants of health, the importance of using evidence to inform health system intervention and change, and the need to shift to more upstream approaches. As a result, the Health Transition Fund was created to support initiatives to test and demonstrate the effectiveness of alternative approaches (Primary Health Care Transition Fund, 2005).

In 2009, the Canadian Senate released a document strengthening the call for action on the determinants of health. In light of the evidence of significant health disparities within Canada, *A Healthy Productive Canada: A Determinant of Health Approach* provided recommendations towards adopting a population health approach (Keon & Pepin, 2009). Emphasizing that 75% of the factors related to health lie outside the healthcare delivery system, the report recommended a more coordinated, cohesive approach in order to address the factors that determine health. Recommendations included intersectoral collaboration between different levels of government, communities, organizations, and various sectors such as education, agriculture, the environment, and the healthcare system. Moreover, it encouraged governments to establish public policies that put people's health, wellness, and quality of life at the forefront.

Nursing Involvement in Primary Health Care Reform

CHNs have been active in promoting PHC since its adoption by the World Health Assembly (Labelle, 1986; Maglacas,

1988). The numerous PHC demonstration projects that have been advocated for by nurses have made significant contributions to advancing the "health for all" agenda in Canada. CHNs' close relationships with individual and community clients enable them to observe the strengths and gaps in the current healthcare system. Their expertise in community development is critical to their success in implementing PHC demonstration projects. For example, nurses in Newfoundland have gained key insights into healthcare reform based on the Danish–Newfoundland PHC Project and other PHC initiatives (Association of Registered Nurses of Newfoundland & Labrador, 2002). In Nova Scotia, nurses were integral to the development and success of the Cheticamp PHC Project, which focused on cultural awareness, economic development, education, general community development, organizational development, self-help, and social support (Downe-Wamboldt, Roland, LeBlanc, & Arsenault, 1994).

The Registered Nurses Association of British Columbia (RNABC) (1998) was at the forefront of developing models for adopting the PHC approach in British Columbia. Their New Directions initiative significantly contributed to the development of a series of background papers, as well as concerted education strategies to inform nurses and the public about PHC. The RNABC advocated for, and achieved, government commitment to launch PHC demonstration projects, and initiated a community-determined process that resulted in establishing a nursing centre in a small rural community on Vancouver Island (Clarke & Mass, 1998). Other provincial nursing associations in Canada have also been active in promoting PHC.

PRIMARY HEALTH CARE: WHAT IT IS AND WHAT IT IS NOT

PHC, primary care, health promotion, and population health: what do these terms mean and how are they related, if at all? CHNs can make significant contributions to PHC by understanding these differing perspectives and developing clear and simple definitions of terms.

The difference between primary care and PHC is often unclear. **Primary care** is narrower in scope than PHC and often is biomedical in focus (Starfield, 1998). It is a person-centred approach to providing care that focuses on the health needs of all individuals within the confines of their communities. The distinctive features of primary care are person-centredness, continuity, comprehensiveness, and integration of services (WHO, 2008). Access to primary care is an essential component of PHC. The distinctions between PHC, health promotion, and population health are less clear. As Lavis (2002) points out, Canadian policy makers and researchers talked about "health fields" in the 1970s, "health promotion" in the 1980s, and "population health" in the 1990s. There is a close relationship between health promotion and PHC in both philosophy and methods. **Health promotion** is "the process of enabling people to increase control over and improve their health" (WHO, 1986, p. 1). However, PHC also involves curative, rehabilitative, and palliative care

methods as a part of provision of first-line contact with the community.

Population health focuses on maintaining and improving the health of entire populations and reducing inequities in health status among population groups. **Population health** "refers to health outcomes and their distribution in the population. The health status of individuals and populations are influenced by the complex interaction of a wide range of determinants over the life course" (Senate Committee on Population Health, 2008, p. 3).

Primary Care is an important component of PHC. One of the major issues facing the Canadian health system is inequitable access to primary care. For example, in 2008, as many as 2 914 557 Ontario citizens reported not having access to a regular primary care physician (Statistics Canada, 2009). Nurse Practitioner [NP]-led clinics were initiated in areas where high numbers of people without a primary care provider were reported.

What are NP-led clinics? **Nurse Practitioner-led clinics** are locally driven family healthcare delivery organizations which include Nurse Practitioners (NPs), Registered Nurses (RNs), family physicians, and a range of other healthcare professionals" (Government of Ontario, 2009, p. 3). The majority of primary care delivered by NP-led clinics is provided by NPs. NPs are RNs in an extended class with expanded functions as primary care providers. Their functions include communicating a diagnosis, prescribing medications, and ordering diagnostic tests. (College of Nurses of Ontario, 2009). NPs provide comprehensive primary care services, including health promotion/disease prevention, treatment of minor injuries, maintenance/monitoring of chronic disease, and palliative care. Most NPs report working with marginalized populations (van Soeren, Hurlock-Chorostecki, Goodwin, & Baker, 2009) in need of comprehensive primary care services. These NPs work to their full scope of practice, ensuring appropriate use of human resources that is affordable to society. NP-led clinics are a part of the Ontario government's "Family Healthcare for All" strategy, to improve timely access to primary care.

Primary care reform in Ontario. Traditionally, physicians have dominated the delivery of primary care services, which in turn influenced major decisions regarding health reform in Ontario. The first NP-led clinic in Sudbury was originally proposed by two NPs living in Sudbury who identified the need for such a model in their community. As the innovators of the Sudbury NP-led clinic, Roberta Heale and Marilyn Butcher played an important role in primary care reform for their community and the province. Since this initial clinic, three additional NP-led clinics in Belle River, Thunder Bay, and Sault Ste. Marie have received funding from the Ontario government. Applications from eight other Ontario communities have submitted additional NP-led clinics. For further information visit http://sdnpc.ca/about-us/welcome-to-our-home-page-bienvenue-chez-nous.html or www.health.gov.on.ca/transformation/np_clinics/np_mn.html.

Possibilities for the future. The introduction and support of NP-led clinics in Ontario is empowering nurses, patients, and other healthcare providers to take on leadership roles to improve access to PHC. NP-led clinics have improved access to primary care services for all citizens, especially disadvantaged populations (Government of Ontario, 2009), and represent an opportunity for nurses to take on community leadership roles to transform and deliver primary care services as a component of health for all.

Discussion Questions

1. Compare CHN and NP roles. How are they similar or different?

2. Describe three different, complementary methods you would use to assess if a community has adequate access to a primary care provider.

Acknowledgement: This Case Study was written by Tammy Armstrong, RN, NP, PhD (c).

COMMUNITY DEVELOPMENT AND EMPOWERMENT

What does community development and empowerment mean to you and why is it an important part of community health nursing? PHC is an approach to healthcare engagement that can be applied across many areas of healthcare. CHNs practise PHC in a variety of roles with individual, family, and population-level clients. The *process* exemplifying PHC values and philosophy has been described as community development (shown in Figure 7.2). **Community development** is a "process based on the philosophical belief that people and communities are entitled to have control over factors that affect their lives. . . . It is grounded in valuing the absolute worth of the individual starting where the individual is. It is a process used frequently (although not exclusively) with disenfranchised groups in society, and involves a community in identifying and reinforcing those aspects of everyday life, culture and political activity conducive to health" (CHNAC, 2008, p. 16). Community development requires an understanding, and careful handling, of community history, resources, and key players.

While the process shown in Figure 7.3 resembles the nursing process of assessment, planning, implementation, and evaluation, there are several key differences. Foremost is the CHN's role as facilitator. Rather than as definer or controller of the process, in a community development approach, CHNs engage with citizens to develop a mutual understanding of issues and priorities, resources, and challenges. Their ability to actively listen to and understand the experiences of

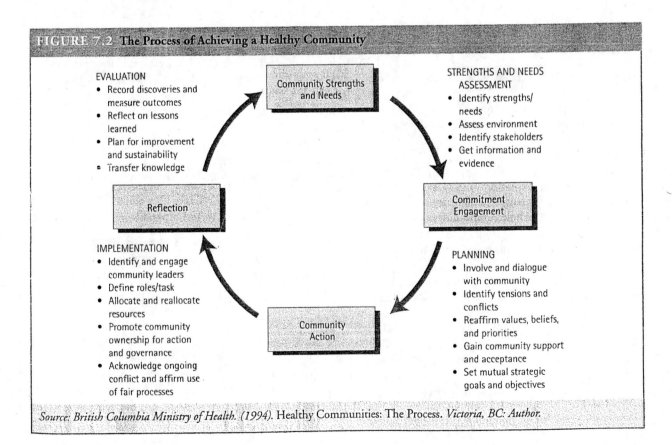

FIGURE 7.2 The Process of Achieving a Healthy Community

Source: British Columbia Ministry of Health. (1994). Healthy Communities: The Process. Victoria, BC: Author.

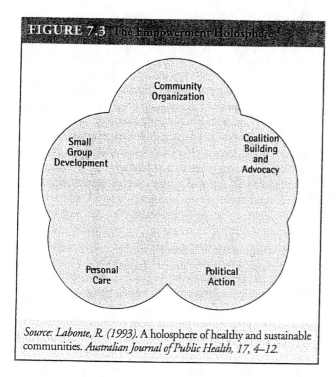

FIGURE 7.3 The Empowerment Holosphere

Source: Labonte, R. (1993). A holosphere of healthy and sustainable communities. Australian Journal of Public Health, 17, 4–12.

people and organizations in a community enables them to effectively promote dialogue and identify similarities and differences among community members. With exploratory dialogue, CHNs facilitate others to question the status quo, providing the basis for a shared vision and plans for action.

PHC values and principles are a community-owned and community-driven process. This approach builds the skills and capacity of those involved in the process, which in turn contributes to sustainability. Community development requires considerable patience, humility, and learning. CHNs using this philosophical and practical approach include themselves as part of the community being "developed," rather than viewing themselves as external controllers of the process.

Essential to CHNs' work in community development is the notion of empowerment. Empowerment is a concept closely related to social justice. "**Empowerment** is an active, involved process where people, groups, and communities move toward increased individual and community control, political efficacy, improved quality of community life, and social justice" (CHNAC, 2008, p. 7). CHNs use empowerment in their work with clients whether they are individuals, families, small groups, or whole communities.

Though dating back to the early 1990s, Labonte's (1993) "empowerment holosphere" (Figure 7.3) is a classic illustration of the complementarity of CHNs' work with individuals, families, small groups, or whole communities as clients (community organization, coalition advocacy, and political action). CHNs engage in all these five roles to implement PHC. For example, in their "individual and family as client" work during postnatal visits, CHNs develop an intimate understanding of the joys and challenges unique to each new mother's experiences. In rapidly growing suburbs, some new mothers may be at home alone with their babies but not yet socially integrated into their new community. Individual and family health promotion is

vital to supporting the woman and her family, to help them develop their capacity to manage the challenges of parenthood in a new community setting. CHNs also use their understanding of the relationships they develop through inter-personal interactions with many new mothers in order to facilitate "women-owned" education, support, and activities. This health promotion strategy builds the capacity of individuals to develop linkages between women who are new to the community. Facilitating the development of small groups in response to community priorities builds linkages, encourages mutual aid and social support between women of similar experiences, and improves access to resources and opportunities from a variety of sectors.

CHNs can also use their understanding of individual and community issues to mobilize interested citizens and organizations to take action. For example, CHNs have often facilitated the opening of Planned Parenthood Services in their communities in response to poor access to relevant reproductive health services. Such initiatives often require full and sensitive engagement in the community development process. CHNs have involved private- and public-sector partners in environmental change that supports heart health, injury prevention, and tobacco-use reduction. This work demonstrates the intersectoral co-operation essential for PHC. The recreation sector has developed walking trails to support a more active lifestyle. Private-sector restaurants are increasingly incorporating "heart healthy" menu choices.

The PHC principles of accessibility, health promotion, and public participation are often used in CHNs' community development work where the community is the client. For example, political action has been used by CHNs to increase access to adequate housing, change legislation to prevent drunk driving, and make bicycle helmets mandatory. A well-known example is the work of Cathy Crowe, a street nurse, educator, and social activist. She co-founded Nurses for Social Responsibility, the Toronto Coalition Against Homelessness, and the Toronto Disaster Relief Committee. The latter organization seeks to have homelessness declared a national disaster (Ward & Piccolo, 2001).

Community development was used to develop Ottawa Inner City Health Inc. (See Case Study, p. 111.) Identifying health and socio-economic inequalities and taking action on their root causes are critical components of practising PHC. The rapid growth of homelessness in Canada has resulted from changes in Canada's social, political, and economic structures that have widened the gap between rich and poor, thereby creating inequities in health. A PHC approach focuses on rectifying those macro-level factors that have enabled homelessness to flourish.

CHN PRACTICE OF SOCIAL JUSTICE: PROGRESS AND CHALLENGES

PHC is an innovative, global approach to healthcare geared towards developing health systems centred on the values of "social justice and the right to better health for all" (WHO, 2008). Nursing has historically acknowledged social justice as a core value (Crigger, Brannigan, & Baird, 2006). Major international nursing organizations, such as Sigma Theta Tau International (STTI), continue to stress the need for nurses to be involved in matters of social justice (Crigger et al.). The Canadian Nursing Association (CNA) also recognizes social justice as a key aspect of nursing ethics—as one of the seven "ethical responsibilities" nurses use to guide their practice, noting "... *nursing ethics is concerned with how broad societal issues affect health and well-being. This means that nurses endeavour to maintain awareness of that effect [on] health and well-being and to advocate for change*" (CNA, 2008).

CHNs often encounter significant social issues in their work including, but not limited to, inadequate housing, poverty, unequal access to healthcare including medication, violence, and lack of opportunities. Boutain (2008) argues that since many of these social issues result in health inequalities, social justice needs to play a more important role in the development of nurses, and particularly CHNs. Yet nursing has not developed a collective, disciplined force to strengthen actions to address the root causes of social, political, and economic inequality (Crigger, 2008). Without a working definition for the meaning of social justice in nursing practice, effective strategies to reduce inequities will remain elusive (Boutain, 2008).

Within the CNA's code of ethics, the prominence placed on fairness in resource distribution, access, and awareness of larger health and social issues reveals a conceptualization of social justice as something that can be achieved without disrupting the current status quo (rather than as a politicized ideal that will require challenging structures and practices that maintain the status quo (Kirkham & Browne, 2006). It is, therefore, important to consider the extent to which foundational nursing discourses support or constrain enacting nursing activities aimed at achieving broader health outcomes in terms of "addressing critical underlying structural barriers limiting the fair distribution of wealth and health in our communities and societies" (p. 331). Canadian Nursing Research Box 7.1 provides an example of the social justice issues related to Aboriginal healthcare services delivery and governance in Canada.

CANADIAN RESEARCH BOX

What is the influence of governance on organizations' experiences of improving care for Aboriginal people: decolonizing possibilities?

Smith, D., Edwards, N., Martens, P. J., Varcoe, C., & Davies, B. (2008). The influence of governance on organizations' experiences of improving care for Aboriginal people: Decolonizing possibilities. *Pimatisiwin: A Journal of Aboriginal and Indigenous Community Health, 6*(1), 1–30.

The governance of healthcare serving First Nations, Inuit, and Métis people is a highly charged issue stemming from a socio-political history of colonization in Canada. This comparative case study included one remote, on-reserve organization and one urban, off-reserve Aboriginal organization that are responsible for preventive and PHC for pregnant and parenting Aboriginal people in British Columbia, Canada. Using a critical postcolonial stance and participatory action principles, experiences in improving care were examined from the perspective of Aboriginal healthcare service delivery organizations and the communities they serve. Data collection included relevant documents, field notes, and in-depth interviews with purposefully selected Aboriginal people, providers, and organizational leaders involved.

Participants in both cases described several dimensions of how governance influenced their organizations' experiences to improve care. These dimensions included the importance of a historically grounded vision, the extent to which Aboriginal community members had a voice in decision making, the autonomy of their organizations, differing views of organizational accountability, and differing approaches to decision making.

These findings suggest that flexible models of governance are required to accommodate diverse views, values, and priorities in complex Aboriginal healthcare contexts. Local Aboriginal healthcare delivery organizations play a crucial mediating role between citizens' and communities' needs, priorities, and broader healthcare decision-making. The results of this study underscore the need for governance models that facilitate, rather than thwart, efforts to decolonize institutions that mediate relationships between Aboriginal clients and organizations, and broader Canadian society.

Discussion Questions

1. What PHC values and principles are reflected in this research box? Why might these be particularly important while working with Aboriginal peoples?

2. Envision interviewing a CHN working in an urban Aboriginal healthcare organization or in a remote or rural setting. Think about the questions you would like to ask him/her about the similarities and differences in their role, the services that their organization provides, as compared to that of community or public health services offered to non-Aboriginal populations. Consider how their role reflects the principles of PHC and how this may differ from other healthcare models.

Within the social justice literature, there is growing criticism towards developed nations and their commitment to maintaining the personal autonomy of the patient. Their approach to social justice has ignored the social and cultural contexts within which people in developing nations live. Crigger (2008) argues that autonomy, as a PHC principle, will need to be embraced "... in view of the extreme poverty and limited resources of the world that a global ethics seeks to encompass" (p. 22).

Our current global economic crisis and healthcare fiscal restraints have made it more difficult for nurses to enact a social justice agenda in healthcare. There continues to be an ongoing "push and pull" struggle between financial spending on the healthcare system and our commitment to equitable healthcare. As Kirkham and Browne (2006) state,

> . . . it has become increasingly difficult for public health nurses (and nurses working elsewhere) to justify socially oriented activities whose outcomes may be viewed as relatively intangible (e.g., community development work aimed at redressing inequities, or lobbying for reforms to health and social policies that exacerbate inequities), particularly in the face of pressures to produce "measurable deliverables" (e.g., shortened lengths of stays, decreased readmissions, decreased waiting times, cost constraint outcomes, etc.). (p. 330)

However, amid these difficulties, social justice continues to hold much promise for how nurses can think about practice, education, and research. For example, within nursing curricula and nursing research, critical theories are beginning to be recognized and used as a means of exploring

> . . . the social, political or historical context (which) does not erase the individual experience . . . but rather makes links between individual experiences and the micro-politics and macrostructures of power that bring about human suffering in its varying forms. (Kirkham & Browne, 2006, p. 336)

The education of nurses presents an opportunity to create a definition of social justice and develop curricula that will teach future nurses how to address the root causes of inequality (Kirkham & Browne, 2006). Canadian Research Box 7.2 is an example of collaborative international nursing research, which puts into real world contexts the possibilities for nurses to participate in global PHC reform. It demonstrates how nurses can use their positions to better address social justice issues. The principles of social justice, such as having accessible services, are a part of CHN's daily practice at a local level of implementation. For example, CHNs in home care working with young children with autism can advocate for families to access local services to support the family to be independent within their community. This example highlights the need for the CHNs to be aware of the resources that were needed by the family and then act as an advocate to support the family to be successful within their local environment. At a different level, example in Canadian Research Box 7.2 demonstrates how CHNs can be engaged in health policy at an international level.

CANADIAN RESEARCH BOX 7.2

How do nurses engage in health policy process?

Edwards, N., & Roelofs, S. *Strengthening nurses' capacity in HIV policy development in Sub-Saharan Africa and the Caribbean* (Year 3 Progress Report, February 1, 2009–January 31, 2010). Ottawa, ON: University of Ottawa.

Nurses are the largest group of health providers in health systems around the world, and have unique health system insights derived from their essential front-line roles; however, they are rarely involved in leading research and policy initiatives. Involving nurses, other frontline health professionals, and community members in research and policy-making processes may support more equitable directions for health policies and programs conceivably tailored to local health priorities and constraints. This is the focus of an international program of research ("Strengthening Nurses' Capacity in HIV Policy Development in Sub-Saharan Africa and the Caribbean"), involving Canada, Kenya, Jamaica, Uganda, and South Africa.

The overall goal of this participatory action research program is to contribute to health systems strengthening for HIV and AIDS in Sub-Saharan Africa and the Caribbean by improving the quality of HIV and AIDS nursing care; supporting the scaling-up of innovative HIV and AIDS programs and practices; and fostering dynamic, sustained engagement of researchers and research users in the policy development process.

Team members have articulated the social justice principles that underlie their work. These include addressing:

- historical factors and gender oppression as root causes for the under engagement of nurses in health systems strengthening; and
- externally designed and imposed HIV/AIDS interventions threatening to displace local innovation and knowledge, thereby reducing local ownership and program sustainability, e.g., internationally funded programs providing anti-retrovirals (ARVs) tend to target training physicians—despite the fact that nurses are typically responsible for administering ARVs and in some cases have introduced successful local community-based initiatives (International Council of Nurses, 2009). Three district/parish-level leadership hubs were established in each of the participating countries. These hubs are intended to act as levers for equitable health systems change. They include members from four stakeholder groups—nurses and nurse managers, researchers, decision makers, and community representatives. The diversity in hub membership is intended to foster collaboration by bringing together different perspectives and strengths in order to create evidence-based strategies to address local health issues. In turn, each hub informs local decision makers on health system priorities, thereby demonstrating the inclusive, participatory, negotiation-based leadership essential to PHC reform.

It is expected that nurses will strengthen their networks for systems change not only with their peers, but also with their colleagues at other system levels, and in other disciplines. Hubs are linked to the National Advisory Committee in each partner country to leverage change vertically through different levels of power and authority within each healthcare system. The local-to-national dimension creates an enabling environment for hub actions by creating venues to bring local experiences and information to decision and policy makers.

Common challenges among the hubs include navigating country-specific political dynamics, managing continuity as hub members are redeployed to other healthcare settings, and dealing with hub members' competing roles and time commitments. Training on how to influence policy has been provided to hub members. Examples of research priorities identified by hub members include exploring gaps in relation to nursing in Ministry of Health human resources policies; examining areas for strengthening workplace policies on issues such as lack of resources (human and financial), patient safety, and quality of nursing care; patient disclosure of HIV status; and, inclusion of nurses in policy making.

Preliminary findings are being introduced to hub members. Workshops on understanding and interpreting both qualitative and quantitative research, using research for decision making, and conducting impact evaluations are planned. Connections among leadership hubs within each country are fostered through initiatives such as joint training sessions. In the longer term, networks among hub members in the participating countries will be supported.

The impact of the leadership hubs will be assessed through several strategies. Hub members will be interviewed to gain insight into the hub process. In the final year of the research program, clinical assessment and management strategies, human resources management, and workplace policies will be re-examined and compared with baseline findings. National and international focus groups will be held with decision makers outside the hubs to learn their perspectives on how hubs have, or have not, been able to leverage change within the health system. Hubs will conduct impact evaluations near the end of the project to examine the program's effect on key local health system issues. Leadership hubs are emerging as a promising approach to engage nurses and other stakeholders in the policy change process.

Discussion Questions

1. Leadership hubs represent an example of nursing research leading the way in PHC reform. Identify how the research described above addresses each of the four types of reform described in the 2008 World Health Report: *PHC, Now More Than Ever.*

2. Identify how CHNs in your province are involved in health policy reform to increase access to essential healthcare for marginalized populations. How can Canadian nurses learn from this example?

3. In small groups, brainstorm various ways nursing students could become involved in international health, on campus, in the community, or abroad.

Acknowledgement: This Canadian Research Box was written by Nancy Edwards, Dan Kaseje, June Webber, Judy Mill, Susan Roelofs, Colleen Davison, Eulalia Kahwa, Hester Klopper, & Mariam Walusimbi.

FUTURE DIRECTIONS OF PHC REFORM IN CANADA

PHC is an area of health services that provides care for diverse populations on micro-level (i.e., individual) to more macro-level interventions (e.g., community coalition building, advocating for healthy provincial policies, international research, and capacity building). CHNs play a large role in providing PHC services, in addressing issues that impact health equity, and in working toward decreasing barriers to care.

CHNs have been effective in implementing innovative approaches to PHC in a variety of settings in Canada. They have been active as care providers, researchers, administrators, and educators in building the capacity needed to implement PHC in both Canadian and international contexts. CHNs have used their organizational base to influence health policy in Canada and abroad. They have also contributed to research informing the design of interventions with special populations in challenging contexts.

As Labelle (1986) stated more than 20 years ago, CHNs have several sources of power, including their presence in multiple settings and at all levels of society, direct and continuous contact with the public, access to and control over massive amounts of information, and access to communication channels with each other through their organizational structures. What Labelle identified then, and what has been validated through research since, is that CHNs' commitment to equity and social justice has made them some of the most trusted members of society (Buresh & Gordon, 2000). While they have demonstrated that they can use these sources of power effectively, they must do so more consistently and strategically in the future.

CHNs actively advocate to address health inequities and work toward change within more local social contexts. At a time of growing inequities in health in Canada and waning political commitment to implementing social and economic interventions to narrow that gap (Raphael, 2002), CHNs must continue to work in multiple roles to create the environments and capacity needed to achieve health for all. Now more than ever, CHNs must expand their participation in community organization, coalition building and advocacy, and political activity to increase awareness and action on the inequities in health. For example, Levesque, Roberge, Hamel, Lamarche, and Haggerty (2009) examined the accessibility and continuity of PHC in Quebec. Their findings supported CHNs' being part of a multi-disciplinary team providing PHC within their community setting in order to improve the accessibility and continuity of care.

CHNs must also add their expertise to address inequities in health internationally (Labonte & Spiegel, 2001) and within their own country. Thus, at various levels, CHNs can contribute to the creation of local and global healthcare delivery systems that exemplify the values and principles of PHC. Similar to the act of recycling to protect the environment, individual CHNs can implement the same values and principles in their practice on a daily basis. Those who participate in action can shape the direction of PHC reform in Canada, and impact the delivery of care to promote health and wellness, address inequities, and advocate for change within communities at their level of involvement.

SUMMARY

The concept and definition of PHC, and a description of its overall approach were described in this chapter. The importance of understanding PHC in its original explication in the *Declaration of Alma Ata* (WHO, 1978) was highlighted. Values and principles of PHC were described, and different types of reforms for PHC renewal were identified and demonstrated through an example of a NP-led clinic. PHC and related terms were defined and compared. CHN's approaches to community development practice to enact PHC values and principles were discussed.

Concepts of social justice and its relationship to addressing health inequities were introduced, as well as challenges CHNs may encounter in practice. The role of PHC in international and global health was reviewed, and examples of Canadian and international organizations working in the field were introduced. Research in Canada and internationally were presented to illustrate social justice issues (e.g., governance) and strategies (e.g., leadership hubs). Finally, CHNs were encouraged to consider ways to contribute to PHC to address micro- to macro-level root causes of inequities in health.

KEY TERMS

primary health care, p. 109
social justice, p. 110
equity in health, p. 110
macro, micro, meso levels, p. 110
accessibility, p. 110
public participation, p. 110
health promotion, p. 111
appropriate technology, p. 111
intersectoral co-operation, p. 111
primary health care reform, p. 113
primary care, p. 114
population health, p. 114
nurse practitioner-led clinics, p. 114
community development, p. 115
empowerment, p. 116

REVIEW QUESTIONS

Choose the one alternative that best completes the statement or answers the question.

1. An outreach team is formed to work with homeless people in a community. Using the principles of PHC, which of the following is an appropriate intervention for the team?
   a) Provide services that are aimed at disease prevention.
   b) Focus on services that are aimed at health promotion.
   c) Manage healthcare needs for the individuals.
   d) Work with other community groups to improve services.

2. A group of CHNs using a population health approach to conduct a community assessment are most likely to
   a) be trying to reduce inequities in health status between population groups.
   b) avoid developing partnerships with other agencies in the area.
   c) be addressing only macro-level or collective factors that determine health.
   d) be working to treat illness in select groups in the population.

3. Identify which of the following descriptions of a project BEST displays the use of the PHC principle of working in collaboration with other disciplines and sectors:
   a) talking with neighbourhood parents to determine how to prevent injuries in the playground
   b) working with other public health nurses to promote flu vaccination among new Canadians
   c) surveying workers in a manufacturing plant on their preference for different types of smoking cessation methods
   d) working with social workers, teachers, and the police to reduce violence in the school playground

4. Community development
   a) is a process where nurses assess needs, and plan, implement and evaluate actions to improve communities.
   b) is a process where nurses consult experts in community planning in order to identify appropriate actions to improve health.
   c) is a process wherein nurses identify priorities and take action to improve the health of marginalized populations.
   d) is a process wherein nurses participate with other community members and groups to identify priorities and take action to improve factors that influence the health of communities.

5. Which of the following is not a structural cause of homelessness?
   a) closure of mental health facilities
   b) high unemployment rates
   c) having friends that are homeless
   d) rising cost of housing

6. Using an empowering approach would require a CHN to
   a) control the environment for the client.
   b) be rigid and inflexible in order to maintain control.
   c) create the client's personal empowerment.
   d) develop actions with the client's active participation.

STUDY QUESTIONS

1. Describe the difference between PHC and primary care.
2. Describe the differences and similarities among PHC, population health, and health promotion.

3. Define the five principles of PHC developed by the Canadian Nurses Association.

4. Homelessness creates issues of inequity in access to care. Name an example of another population or health issue for which CHNs could be involved in improving access to services. Why should social justice be a concern for CHNs within their clinical practice?

5. Outline how a CHN could participate at local, provincial, national, or international levels to reduce inequities in health. Give examples of strategies for each level of involvement and action.

After working through these questions, go to the MyNursingLab at **www.pearsoned.ca/mynursinglab** *to check your answers.*

INDIVIDUAL CRITICAL THINKING EXERCISES

1. Why is it important for CHNs to study and understand the *Declaration of Alma Ata?*

2. Visit the website of your provincial/territorial nursing association. Search for policy or position statements on PHC. Look for descriptions of activities that influence healthcare reform. Discuss the initiative with your peers and colleagues. Identify opportunities for CHNs to participate in the initiative. Reflect on how you can become involved.

3. Relate your own values to the role of CHNs as facilitators of PHC policy and action at local, regional, provincial, or national levels.

4. What social justice issues have you encountered in your clinical placements? What have these issues stemmed from? How do they affect the care you give or are able to give?

5. What social justice actions do you demonstrate in your practice? What social actions have you witnessed other nurses or nursing organizations make? Compare your findings on nursing association policy with those of your provincial ministry.

GROUP CRITICAL THINKING EXERCISES

1. Describe how nursing has contributed and will continue to contribute to reform efforts aimed at the root causes of poor health.

2. As community developers in small communities, how might CHNs apply the "process of achieving a healthy community" (Figure 7.1)?

3. In small groups, brainstorm various ways nursing students could become involved in international health on campus, in the community, or abroad.

REFERENCES

Alliance to End Homelessness. (2008). *Experiencing homelessness: Report card on ending homelessness in Ottawa.* Retrieved from http://www.endhomelessnessottawa.ca/documents/2008ReportCardonEndingHomelessnessinOttawa.pdf

Angus, D. (1995). *Health care reform: Revisiting the review of significant health care commissions and task forces.* Ottawa, ON: Canada Community Health Nurses Association.

Association of Registered Nurses of Newfoundland and Labrador. (2002). Sustaining our public health care system. Submission to the Commission on the Future of Health Care in Canada.

Bezruchka, S. (2002). Foreword. In D. Raphael, *Social justice is good for our hearts: Why societal factors—not lifestyles—are major causes of heart disease in Canada and elsewhere.* Toronto, ON: Centre for Social Justice, Foundation for Research and Education. Retrieved from http://www.cwhn.ca/resources/heart_health/justice2.pdf

Boutain, D. M. (2008). Social justice as a framework for undergraduate community health clinical experiences in the United States. *International Journal of Nursing Education Scholarship 5*(1), 1–12.

Buresh, B., & Gordon, S. (2000). *From silence to voice: What nurses know and must communicate to the public.* Ottawa, ON: Canadian Nurses Association.

Canadian Nurses Association. (2000). *Fact sheet: The primary health care approach.* Ottawa, ON: Author.

Canadian Nurses Association. (2008). *Code of ethics for registered nurses.* Ottawa, ON: Author.

Clarke, H., & Mass, H. (1998). Comox Valley Nursing Centre: From collaboration to empowerment. *Public Health Nursing, 15*(3), 216–224.

College of Nurses of Ontario. (2009). *Practice standard: Nurse practitioners.* Toronto, ON: College of Nurses of Ontario. Retrieved from http://www.cno.org/docs/prac/41038_StrdRnec.pdf

Community Health Nurses Association of Canada. (CHNAC). (2008). *Canadian community health nursing standards of practice.* Ottawa, ON: Author.

Crigger, N. (2008). Towards a viable and just global ethics. *Nursing Ethics 15*(1), 17–27.

Crigger, N. J., Brannigan, M., & Baird, M. (2006). Compassionate nursing professionals as good citizens of the world. *Advances in Nursing Science, 29*(1), 15–26.

Downe-Wamboldt, B., Roland, F., LeBlanc, B., & Arsenault, D. (1994). Cheticamp primary health care project. *Nurse to Nurse, 3,* 14–15.

Epp, J. (1986). *Achieving health for all: A framework for health promotion.* Ottawa, ON: Health and Welfare Canada.

Government of Ontario. (2009). *Introduction to nurse practitioner-led clinics.* Toronto, ON: Author.

Hurley, C., Baum, F., Johns, J., & Labonte, R. (2010). Comprehensive primary health care in Australia: Findings from a narrative review of the literature. *Australasian Medical Journal, 1*(2): 147–152.

International Council of Nurses. (2009). *Delivering quality: Serving communities: Nurses leading care innovations.* Retrieved from http://www.icn.ch/indkit2009.pdf

Keon, W. J., & Pépin, L. (2009). *A healthy, productive Canada: A determinant of health approach. Final report.* Ottawa, ON: Subcommittee on Population Health, The Senate.

Kirkham, S. R., & Browne, A. J. (2006). Towards a critical theoretical interpretation of social justice discourses in nursing. *Advances in Nursing Science, 29*(4), 324–339.

Labelle, H. (1986). Nurses as a social force. *Journal of Advanced Nursing, 11,* 247–253.

Labonte, R. (1993). A holosphere of healthy and sustainable communities. *Australian Journal of Public Health, 17,* 4–12.

Labonte, R., & Spiegel, G. (2003). Setting global health research priorities. *British Medical Journal, 326,* 722–723.

Lavis, J. (2002). Ideas at the margin or marginalized ideas? Non-medical determinants of health in Canada. *Health Affairs, 21*(2), 107–112.

Levesque, J. F., Roberge, D., Hamel, M., Lamarche, P., & Haggerty, J. (2009). *Accessibility and continuity of care: A study of primary health care in Quebec.* Montreal, QC: CIHR and CHSRF. Retrieved from http://www.inspq.qc.ca/pdf/publications/911_ServicesPremLigneANGLAIS.pdf

Maglacas, A. (1988). Health for all: Nursing's role. *Nursing Outlook, 36*(2), 666–671.

Merriam-Webster online dictionary. (2010). Retrieved from http://www.merriam-webster.com/dictionary/value

Navarro, V. (2009). What we mean by the social determinants of health. *International Journal of Health Services, 39*(3), 423–441.

Ottawa Inner City Health Inc. (2009). Inner City Health Inc. Annual report 2008–2009. Unpublished report. Ottawa, ON: Author.

Primary Health Care Transition Fund. (2005). *Primary health care transition fund: Summary of initiatives.* Ottawa, ON: Health Canada.

Public Health Agency of Canada. [PHAC]. (2003, March). *What determines health?* Retrieved from http://www.phac-aspc.gc.ca/ph-sp/determinants/determinants-eng.php

Raphael, D. (2002). *Social justice is good for our hearts: Why societal factors—not lifestyles—are major causes of heart disease in Canada and elsewhere.* Toronto, ON: Centre for Social Justice, Foundation for Research and Education. Retrieved from http://www.cwhn.ca/resources/heart_health/justice2.pdf

Registered Nurses Association of British Columbia. (1998). *The new health care: A nursing perspective.* Vancouver, BC: Author.

Senate Committee on Population Health. (2008). *Population Health Policy: Issues and options.* Ottawa, ON: Author. Retrieved from http://www.parl.gc.ca/39/2/parlbus/commbus/senate/com-e/soci-e/rep-e/rep10apr08-e.pdf

Starfield, B. (1998). *Primary care: Balancing health needs, services and technology.* New York, NY: Oxford University Press.

Statistics Canada. (2009). *Population with a regular medical doctor, by sex, provinces, and territories.* (CANSIM, table 105-0501 and Catalogue no. 82-221-X.). Retrieved from http://www40.statcan.ca/01/cst01/health76a-eng.htm

van Soeren, M., Hurlock-Chorostecki, C., Goodwin, S., & Baker, E. (2009). The primary health care nurse practitioner in Ontario: A workforce study. *Nursing Leadership, 22*(2), 58–72.

Ward, M., & Piccolo, C. (2001, Winter). It's because I am a nurse. *Medhunters,* 1–4. Retrieved from http://www.medhunters.com

Wilkinson, R. (1996). *Unhealthy societies: The afflictions of inequality.* New York, NY: Routledge.

World Health Organization. (1978). *The declaration of Alma Ata.* Geneva, Switzerland: Author. Retrieved from http://www.who.dk/eprise/main/WHO/AboutWHO/Policy/200108271

World Health Organization. (1986). *Ottawa charter for health promotion.* Geneva, Switzerland: Author.

World Health Organization. (1998). *Health promotion glossary.* Geneva, Switzerland: Author. Retrieved from http://www.who.int/healthpromotion/about/HPG/en/

World Health Organization. (2005). *Health for all policy framework for the WHO European region.* Geneva, Switzerland: Author. Regional Office for Europe.

World Health Organization. (2006). *Report prepared for the fifty-seventh World Health Assembly, health systems, including primary health care: Report by the Secretariat.* Geneva, Switzerland: Author.

World Health Organization. (2008). *Primary health care: Now more than ever.* Retrieved from http://www.who.int/whr/2008/whr08_en.pdf

ADDITIONAL RESOURCES

Books

Baumann, A., Valaitis, R., & Kaba, A. (2009). *Primary health care and nursing education in the 21st century: A discussion paper.* Toronto, ON: Nursing Health Services Research Unit.

Health Canada. (2005). *Primary health care transition fund (PHCTF) summary of initiatives.* Ottawa, ON: Health Canada.

Shortt, S., Hwang, S., & Stuart, H. (2005). *Homelessness and health: A policy synthesis on approaches to delivering primary care for homeless persons.* Kingston, ON: Center for Health Services and Policy Research, Queens University.

Wilson, R., Shortt, S. E. D., & Dorland, J. (2004). (Eds.). *Implementing primary care reform—Barriers and facilitators.* Montreal, QC: McGill–Queen's University Press.

Websites

Canadian Council on Social Development
http://www.ccsd.ca

Canadian International Development Agency
http://www.acdi-cida.gc.ca

Canadian Nurses Association
http://www.cna-nurses.ca

The Canadian Health Network
http://www.phac-aspc.gc.ca/chn-rcs/index-eng.php

The Canadian Public Health Association
http://www.cpha.ca

Canadian Population Health Initiative
http://www.cihi.ca/cphi

Canadian Society for International Health
http://www.csih.org

International Society for Equity in Health
http://www.iseqh.org

Network learning (in Primary Health Care)
http://www.networklearning.org/index.html

Pan American Health Organization
http://www.paho.org

Video

School of Nursing, Memorial University, St. John's, Newfoundland (Producer). (2009). *Primary health care in community health nursing* [DVD].

This 29-minute DVD illustrates the interconnection between primary health care and community health nursing. It gives examples of the role of CHNs and their challenges as they apply the principles of primary health care into their practice.

About the Authors

Dawn Smith, BScN (University of British Columbia), MN (Dalhousie University), PhD (University of Ottawa), is an assistant professor at the University of Ottawa, School of Nursing, where she teaches Community Health. She has practised community health nursing in several Canadian provinces as well as overseas.

Kim Van Herk, BScN (McMaster University), MN (University of Ottawa), practises as a CHN working with homeless and street-involved individuals. Her thesis focused on examining Aboriginal women's experiences of accessing care, using an intersectionality analysis.

Zaida Rahaman, BScN (University of Saskatchewan), MN (University of Calgary), Doctoral student in Nursing (University of Ottawa), is interested in integrating community strengths into quality health services delivery for marginalized populations. Zaida has worked in a variety of roles to improve design and implementation of PHC programs in rural and urban communities in Western Canada.

chapter

8

Cultural Diversity

Kathryn Edmunds and Elizabeth Kinnaird Iler

OBJECTIVES

After studying this chapter, you should be able to:

1. Develop a deeper understanding of the assumptions, meanings, and characteristics underlying the concept of culture.

2. Explore the intersections among culture, multiculturalism, diversity, race, and ethnicity.

3. Describe the relationship between culture and health.

4. Evaluate the similarities and differences between cultural competence and cultural safety, and the implications for community health nursing practice.

5. Reflect upon and analyze how cultural beliefs and values shape the interactions between nurses and clients.

6. Describe the needed knowledge, attitudes, sensitivity, processes, and skills to provide culturally competent/culturally safe nursing care.

INTRODUCTION

Canadian nurses have a long history of providing care to all people and communities while adapting to local contexts and resources and advocating for change. This is congruent with nursing's tradition of conceptualizing clients as holistic beings inseparable from their environments, as well as being concerned with issues of individual and collective marginalization, inequity, and social justice. The Canadian Nurses Association (CNA) (2004) recognizes that in order for optimal client outcomes to occur for our increasingly diverse society, nurses must provide care that includes "demonstrating consideration for client diversity; providing culturally sensitive care (e.g., openness, sensitivity, and recognizing culture-based practices and values); and incorporating cultural practices into health promotion activities" (CNA, 2000, p. 1). Valuing multiple ways of knowing, engaging in reflective practice, facilitating access and equity, empowering clients through collaboration, and providing culturally appropriate care in multiple settings are all expectations in the standards of practice of the Community Health Nurses Association of Canada (CHNAC, 2008). Within the category of Diversity and Inclusiveness, CHNAC's Public Health Nursing competencies include

- Recognize how the determinants of health (biological, social, cultural, economic, and physical) influence the health and well-being of specific population groups.

- Address population diversity when planning, implementing, adapting, and evaluating public health programs and policies.

- Apply culturally relevant and appropriate approaches with people from diverse cultural, socioeconomic, and educational backgrounds, and persons of all ages, genders, health status, sexual orientations, and abilities. (CHNAC, 2009, p. 7)

This category is reflective of the CNA's Code of Ethics (2008) in "identifying the competencies required to interact effectively with diverse individuals, families, groups and communities in relation to others in society as well to recognize the root causes of disparities and what can be done to eliminate them. . . . It is the embodiment of attitudes and actions that result in inclusive behaviours, practices, programs and policies" (CHNAC, 2009, p. 7).

In this chapter, we will explore some of the assumptions, meanings, and characteristics of the concept of culture and the intersections among culture, multiculturalism, diversity, race, and ethnicity. The relationship between culture and health will be discussed, as will how constructions of culture shape nurse–client interactions. The knowledge, attitudes, sensitivity, and skills that are needed to provide care and the similarities and differences between cultural competence and cultural safety will be described, including implications for community health nursing practice with all residents of Canada. A variety of client examples will be provided to illustrate "working with culture."

CONCEPT OF CULTURE

"'Culture,' is one of the two or three most complicated words in the English language." (Williams, 1983, p. 87)

Madeline Leininger founded transcultural nursing, which evolved from her work in nursing blended with post-graduate studies in anthropology. For Leininger, care is the central and unifying focus of nursing. Her definition of **culture** is "the learned, shared, and transmitted values, beliefs, norms, and lifeways of a particular culture that guides thinking, decisions, and actions in patterned ways and often intergenerationally" (Leininger, 2006, p. 13). The purpose of her theory of *Culture Care Diversity and Universality* was to discover, explain, and predict factors that influence care meanings and practices from both the client's and nurse's perspectives, and to discover care similarities and differences across cultures in order to guide nursing practice (see Leininger's *Sunrise Enabler to Discover Culture Care* in MyNursingLab). Leininger's transcultural care decisions and actions provide a framework for planning nursing interventions with individuals, families, and communities. These professional decisions and actions are

- cultural care preservation/maintenance,
- cultural care accommodation/negotiation, and
- cultural care repatterning/restructuring.

These actions help clients maintain and preserve relevant healthcare values and practices, accommodate and adapt for beneficial health outcomes, and help clients modify or change existing healthcare patterns while respecting the values of both the client and the nurse. Strengths of Leininger's theoretical approach include the emphases on in-depth assessment, meaning, and care within the context of culture; the inclusion of diverse health contexts; and the generation of nursing knowledge and interventions (Andrews, 2008).

However, Gustafson (2005) contends that transcultural nursing rests on a broadly defined concept of culture that is narrowly applied. The focus is on individual identity within an understanding of culture that essentializes or emphasizes the similarities of experiences and differences. The culture of origin is accentuated and often perceived to be static, rather than recognizing the multiple identities and the relational processes involved in all our encounters. "Commonly drawn-on notions of culture tend to . . . make essential supposed cultural groups as coherent and distinct from mainstream culture, to overlook social positioning and histories of individuals, and, in so doing, often to overlook power operations and inequities" (Reimer Kirkham et al., 2002, p. 225). Transcultural nursing has also been criticized for a lack of clarity in conceptual definitions (such as cultural competence), and for the assumption that knowledge and understanding of other cultures leads to tolerance, respect, and changes in discriminatory behaviours (Andrews, 2008), with little attention as to how to address and reconcile differing perspectives. Gustafson also points out that Leininger's three modes of nursing actions are based on the nurse's assessment of risk to the client—ranging from those cultural practices that the nurse considers "low risk" to health and that can be preserved, to those judged "risky" or potentially harmful that need to be changed. The focus on the individual who is "different" makes it easy to disregard the cultures of healthcare professionals and institutions, and perpetuates existing assumptions, boundaries, and social relations.

Being open to and aware of multiple ways of knowing and experiencing the world leads to the recognition that decisions can take place in different contexts. Identification with a particular culture can lead to **ethnocentrism**, which is the belief that one's own culture is the best or most desirable. Nursing itself is a cultural phenomenon (Dreher, Shapiro, & Asselin, 2006) shaped by societal values and assumptions about health, illness, and caring. Nurses who believe that the culture and practices of nursing are the only or "best" way to interpret what the client is expressing and to achieve improvements in health are being ethnocentric (see the guide *Working with Clients—Questions for Reflection and Building Awareness in Community Practice* in MyNursingLab).

ASSUMPTIONS AND CHARACTERISTICS OF CULTURE

According to the College of Nurses of Ontario's (CNO, 2009) *Practice Guideline for Culturally Sensitive Care*, the following assumptions are the core tenets of providing care that is culturally appropriate:

- *Everyone* has a culture.
- Culture is individual. Individual assessments are necessary to identify relevant cultural factors within the context of each situation for each client.
- An individual's culture is influenced by many factors, such as race, gender, religion, ethnicity, socioeconomic status, sexual orientation, and life experience. The extent to which particular factors influence a person will vary.
- Culture is dynamic. It changes and evolves over time as individuals change over time.
- Reactions to cultural differences are automatic, often subconscious, and influence the dynamics of the nurse–client relationship.
- A nurse's culture is influenced by personal beliefs as well as nursing's professional values. The values of the nursing profession are upheld by all nurses.
- The nurse is responsible for assessing and responding appropriately to the client's cultural expectations and needs. (p. 3)

Yet consider some of the underlying assumptions to the CNO assumptions! The focus on individuals reflects the dominant North American value of individual autonomy, which can deemphasize issues of power and oppressive systems. While nurses do have professional responsibilities for assessment and intervention, assumptions regarding the importance of the relational processes engaged in between the client and the nurse in the development of a plan of care are missing. An almost exclusive focus on the individual has implications for community health nurses (CHNs) providing " . . . little or no guidance for addressing how we act as a community, the duties and obligations, and the mutual and disparate moral interests of individuals, families, and communities" (Shirley, 2007, p. 14). The CHNAC (2008, 2009) standards and competencies related to culture and referred to in the introduction to this chapter reflect a greater emphasis on assumptions regarding the importance of the context of broader structural issues, social justice, and the determinants of health.

Culture is more than beliefs, practices, and values (Aboriginal Nurses Association of Canada [ANAC], 2009). Culture is learned, shared, and changes. It also encompasses all aspects of our lives. What we have learned to value represents our assumptions about how to perceive, think, and behave in acceptable, appropriate, and meaningful ways. There are characteristics shared by all cultures (Allender, Rector, & Warner, 2009) within the fluidity of our individual and collective lives:

- *Culture is socially constructed.* Cultural norms, behaviours, and values are learned through socialization within the family and community. However, culture is interpreted and shaped individually as well as being situated, negotiated, and transformed within social relationships and the broader structural forces that affect us. Behaviours that the nurse may assume are universal will differ across *and within* cultures.
- *Culture is an integrated system* embedded in everyday life. Beliefs and healthcare practices are usually consistent with the overall paradigms that are used to make sense out of the world.
- *Culture is shared.* Beliefs that have meanings and are shared by a group are called cultural values. These values are transmitted within a group and imparted over time. Values shared by people form cultural stability and security. They guide members about what to believe and how to act. However, it is important to remember that individuals may not share all the values of their cultural groups, or their communities (Dreher et al., 2006, p. 25).
- *Culture is largely implicit and tacit.* This means it shapes us at an unconscious level. Most of the time, we do not stop to consider the assumptions and expectations that ground our behaviours and decisions. Culture is one aspect that shapes the way we do things in our everyday lives.
- *Culture is fluid and dynamic.* Culture is always adapting and changing. Consider the changes to Canadian culture that have occurred in the past few decades. Minority cultures have certainly been influenced by the dominant Canadian culture; however, increasing diversity and global interconnectedness have influenced the Canadian culture in return.
- *Culture is expressed and intersects with other social constructs such as race, gender, ethnicity, class, language, and disability.* People with both visible and invisible disabilities may consider themselves to be sharing common cultural identities and experiences, rather than having a "pathological" disorder (Marks, 2007). The historical and current importance of French language rights in Quebec is an outward expression of cultural identity. In particular, culture is often conflated with, or seen to represent, ethnicity and race in ways that reduce very complex situations and ways of being and relating to sets of static behaviours and "cultural" attributes.

INTERSECTIONS

Diversity refers to variety and differences of attributes among, between, and within groups. We all have attributes that give us membership in certain groups, yet we are all diverse and intersect in many ways that are fluid. Diversity can refer to both the preservation and value of traditions, and adaptation leading to creativity and innovation. However, focusing on diversity may have the result of reinforcing differences between groups when diversity is seen as linked to a fixed heritage (Schim, Doorenbos, Benkert, & Miller, 2007). Diversity also includes characteristics and constructs such as gender, language, sexual orientation, and visible and invisible disabilities. Like culture, diversity is a process of change, affecting people is similar and different ways. Cultural diversity has always existed in Canada. However, formal recognition for linguistic duality and different legal systems were restricted to the English and French at the time of Confederation in 1867. Treaty rights, which were negotiated with some First Nations, took place in the context of colonization and were largely motivated by land and resource acquisition.

In 1971, federal multiculturalism policy recognized cultural pluralism and acknowledged this as a contribution to Canadian culture. This was a response to the previous focus on French and English biculturalism (Padolsky, 2000). More recently still, debate about the assumptions, benefits, and barriers of multiculturalism has been articulated as the meaning of multiculturalism in Canada has gone through phases and changes of interpretation. Currently, the focus of **multiculturalism** is the integration of practices of diversity, tolerance, and respect for multiple ways of knowing and being, with issues of equity and social justice (Srivastava, 2007). This is seen to benefit the entire population. The Canadian Multiculturalism Act of 1988 states:

> The Constitution of Canada . . . recognizes the importance of preserving and enhancing the multicultural heritage of Canadians . . . ; [and] the government of Canada recognizes the diversity of Canadians as regards to race, national or ethnic origin, colour and religion as a fundamental characteristic of Canadian society and is committed to a policy of multiculturalism designed to preserve and enhance the multicultural heritage of Canadians while working to achieve the equality of all Canadians in the economic, social, cultural and political life of Canada. (as cited in James, 2003, p. 208)

However, there are issues of power inherent in multiculturalism and CHNs should not assume that all residents of Canada perceive multiculturalism in such a constructive and beneficial light. Power issues are evident when we struggle within and across communities in Canada to reconcile valuing and acceptance of cultural diversity with practices that

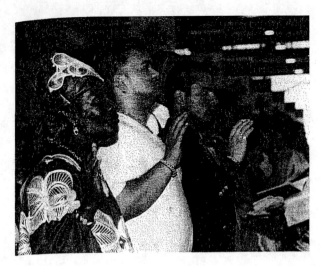

Photo 8.1

New Canadian citizens at a citizenship ceremony in Toronto, Ontario

Credit: CP PHOTO / Aaron Harris

may perpetuate injustice. There have been recent controversies regarding the use of alternative justice systems based on culture and/or religion for that reason. Multiculturalism can be considered to be a state policy that suppresses the need to tackle ingrained inequalities (Varcoe, 2006) and there has been little research that supports cultural sensitivity as a mechanism leading to increased tolerance or respect for ethnic and racialized groups (Yiu Matuk & Ruggirello, 2007).

Ethnicity is a way of describing social identity with a group that is based on a shared history and social structure (James, 2003). However, the dominant culture tends not to define itself in terms of ethnicity; it is usually minority groups that are viewed as ethnic. **Race** is often thought of as an objective biological distinction (usually based on visible differences such as skin colour). Historically, the concept of race has been used to maintain the dominant social order and this continues to occur today. "Race is a socially constructed way of judging, categorizing and creating difference among people. Despite the fact that there are no biological "races", the social construction of race is a powerful force with real consequences for individuals" (Ontario Human Rights Commission [OHRC], 2005, p. 3). **Racism** is interrelated with socioeconomic status, employment opportunities, discrimination, and marginalization. **Racialization** is a term that calls attention to the consequences of assigning racial designations and is defined as "the process by which societies construct races as real, different and unequal in ways that matter to economic, political and social life" (Report of the Commission on Systematic Racism in the Ontario Criminal Justice System as cited in OHRC, 2005, p. 9). The use, significance, and meanings of the concepts of ethnicity and race are inconsistent in nursing research literature, often disregarding the power dynamics involved (Varcoe, 2006).

International movement in immigration means that racial, ethnic, religious, and linguistic diversity will continue to increase and that multiculturalism will continue to dynamically influence the Canadian identity (Padolsky, 2000). As our

understanding of culture broadens to include notions such as workplace cultures and the culture of disabilities, the concept of multiculturalism is becoming increasingly complex. This is reflected in the embeddedness of Canadian society in our interconnected global world, and that people have layered identities and flexible and multiple links within and across socially constructed labels. Open and honest discussion needs to take place regarding which residents of Canada are considered to be multicultural and why, who is considered to be fully Canadian, and the meanings and consequences of these social definitions.

CANADIAN DIVERSITY

More than 200 ethnic origins in the Canadian population were reported in the 2006 Census (Statistics Canada, 2008). Table 8.1 shows the representation of the most frequent ethnic origins, including Aboriginal peoples and those who have immigrated to Canada. All regions of Canada are ethnically diverse, reflected in different ways across the country. In addition, the number of people reporting multiple ethnic ancestries continued to increase in 2006. "An estimated 41.4% of the population reported more than one ethnic origin,

TABLE 8.1	Diversity Across the Nation: Most Frequently Reported Ethnic Origins by Region
Atlantic Provinces Nova Scotia New Brunswick Prince Edward Island Newfoundland and Labrador	Canadian, British Isles, French, Black
Quebec	Canadian, French, Italian, Chinese, Haitian, Spanish
Ontario	English, Canadian, Scottish, Irish, French, German, Italian, Chinese, East Indian, Dutch
Prairie Provinces Manitoba Saskatchewan Alberta	English, German, Scottish, Canadian, Ukrainian, Irish, French, Aboriginal ancestries, Polish, Norwegian, Dutch
British Columbia	English, Scottish, Canadian, Irish, German, Chinese, French, East Indian, Ukrainian, Dutch
Yukon	English, Scottish, Aboriginal ancestries
Northwest Territories	Aboriginal ancestries, British Isles
Nunavut	Inuit, British Isles

Source: Adapted from Statistics Canada (2008). Ethnic Origin and Visible Minorities, 2006 Census. Catalogue No. 97-562-XWE (www12.statcan.ca/english/census06/analysis/ethnicorigin/pdf/97-562-XIE2006001.pdf). Retrieved September 20, 2010.

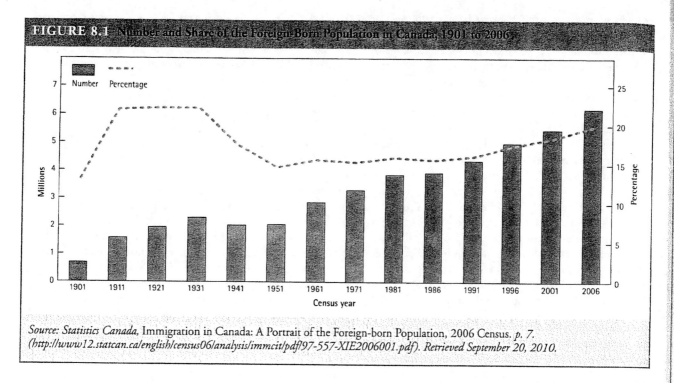

FIGURE 8.1 Number and Share of the Foreign-Born Population in Canada, 1901 to 2006

Source: Statistics Canada, Immigration in Canada: A Portrait of the Foreign-born Population, 2006 Census. p. 7. (http://www12.statcan.ca/english/census06/analysis/immcit/pdf/97-557-XIE2006001.pdf). Retrieved September 20, 2010.

compared with 38.2% in 2001 and 35.8% in 1996" (Statistics Canada, 2008, p. 5). Figure 8.1 shows the number of foreign-born people and their proportion in the total population over the past century.

Newcomers to Canada

Immigration has had a considerable impact on the growth and diversity of Canada's population. Newcomers may share some similarities (e.g., language and cultural barriers, and adjustment and adaptation to Canada); however, there can also be significant differences both within and across cultures. In 2006, Canadian census data showed that 6.2 million people

(19.8% of the total population) were born outside the country, the highest proportion in 75 years (Statistics Canada, 2007a). Between 1900 and 1961, immigrants to Canada were primarily from European countries; since then, most immigrants have been from Asia. Factors that have caused this shift include changes to federal immigration policies and changes in the international movement of immigrants and refugees. The proportion of immigrants born in Asia (including the Middle East) has remained virtually unchanged since the 2001 census (Statistics Canada, 2007a). Table 8.2 shows the top 10 countries of origin for immigrants over the most recent 25-year period.

Between July 1, 2006, and June 30, 2007, Canada received 238 100 immigrants (Statistics Canada, 2007b).

TABLE 8.2 Top 10 Countries of Birth of Recent Immigrants, 1981 to 2006

Order	2006 Census	2001 Census	1996 Census	1991 Census	1981 Census
1	People's Republic of China	People's Republic of China	Hong Kong	Hong Kong	United Kingdom
2	India	India	People's Republic of China	Poland	Viet Nam
3	Philippines	Philippines	India	People's Republic of China	United States of America
4	Pakistan	Pakistan	Philippines	India	India
5	United States of America	Hong Kong	Sri Lanka	Philippines	Philippines
6	South Korea	Iran	Poland	United Kingdom	Jamaica
7	Romania	Taiwan	Taiwan	Viet Nam	Hong Kong
8	Iran	United States of America	Viet Nam	United States of America	Portugal
9	United Kingdom	South Korea	United States of America	Lebanon	Taiwan
10	Colombia	Sri Lanka	United Kingdom	Portugal	People's Republic of China

Note: "Recent immigrants" refers to landed immigrants who arrived in Canada within five years prior to a given census.

Source: Statistics Canada, Immigration in Canada: A Portrait of the Foreign-born Population, 2006 Census. p. 10. (www12.statcan.ca/english/census06/analysis/immcit/pdf/97-557-XIE2006001.pdf). Retrieved September 20, 2010.

Newcomers were younger (57.3% were between the ages of 25–54) as compared to the rest of the population (42.3% were between the ages of 25–54) (Statistics Canada, 2007a). However, since immigrants arrive at an average age of 30, this does not slow our population's overall aging (Statistics Canada, 2007a). Canada's visible minority population is increasing at a faster growth rate than the total population, largely because of the high proportion of recent newcomers (75%) belonging to visible minorities (Statistics Canada, 2008). South Asians (people citing ethnic origins from countries such as India, Pakistan, Sri Lanka, and Bangladesh) became the largest visible minority group in 2006, exceeding Chinese. Canada's largest cities (Toronto, Vancouver, and Montreal) became home to 68.9% of recent immigrants in 2006 (Statistics Canada, 2007a), although the number of newcomers living in metropolitan areas other than Toronto, Vancouver, and Montreal has increased to 28.3%, from 24.7% in 2001 (Statistics Canada, 2007a). In 2006, merely 2.8% of immigrants chose to live in rural areas. (See MyNursingLab for additional immigrant statistics). Quebec controls its own immigration policy and requires commitment to living in a francophone society for acceptance (Blad & Couton, 2009). This reinforces Quebec's sovereignty and is a mechanism to preserve French as the dominant language in that province, while welcoming newcomers. A higher proportion of people from French-speaking countries in Africa and the Middle East immigrate to Quebec compared to the rest of Canada (32% vs. 21%) (Blad & Couton, 2009).

Newcomers bring significant strengths, such as diversity, determination, and resilience, yet they also often experience significant challenges. While most new immigrants have positive opinions about Canada's social and political environment, their most significant difficulties after living in Canada for four years relate to finding appropriate and adequate employment, and learning a new language (Statistics Canada, 2007d).

Language Language acquisition is challenging and is also a significant underlying factor in many aspects of newcomers' lives. English or French as a second language classes are not readily available in all communities and where they are available, child care may not be provided. Statistics Canada's 2003 Adult Education and Training Survey states that financial and time constraints are the barriers to training most frequently cited by all Canadians with unmet training needs (Statistics Canada, 2007d). These reasons were also listed as the biggest challenges by new immigrants seeking language training.

Employment Though the limitations in English or French fluency affect job attainment, there are other factors that also influence newcomers' abilities to secure employment. Newcomer credentials and previous employment may not be recognized in Canada; they may be without a driver's licence, lack Canadian job experience, and frequently do not have business contacts to facilitate job acquisition (Statistics Canada, 2007d). The process for internationally educated nurses to obtain Canadian nursing registration is complex, lengthy, and time consuming.

Food Security Food security is a challenge and is related to limited finances and language barriers. The CHN may suggest the family access a food bank to supplement nutritional needs. Food banks rely on donations and often cannot offer varied food choices. Newcomers may not know how to find the local food bank, may not be familiar with the food available, and may not know how to prepare the food.

Limited Social Support Limited social support, especially for those without extended families, is another challenge for newcomers (Statistics Canada, 2007d). Canadian agencies such as health units frequently encourage families to access supports in the community to assist them in developing a support network. However, newcomers may seem to demonstrate a reluctance to become involved in the community. Reasons for this may be a general lack of trust the individual or family associates with "the government"; the family may never have had their own home and now do not want to leave it; they may dislike the harsh winter climate in some parts of Canada; or there may be cultural, class, or religious differences within newcomer groups from the same countries or regions now living together in Canadian neighbourhoods.

Housing Accessing affordable housing can be problematic. Issues affecting this include lack of credit, and limited knowledge of the area and transportation systems (Statistics Canada, 2007d). If newcomers apply to local housing authorities, the waits can be long because the family must be housed in a dwelling appropriate to the number of people. Since newcomer families can be large, and there are fewer larger subsidized dwellings, the process can be lengthy.

Health All these challenges affect health. There may be waiting periods of up to three months in order to be eligible for provincial health coverage and it is often difficult to find a family doctor, meaning that primary care services may be limited to episodic treatment, rather than comprehensive care. Social isolation, experiences in refugee camps, and awareness of hardships experienced by family members remaining in the country of origin result in the potential for post traumatic stress disorder. Issues such as precarious immigration status, precarious employment, insecure housing, lack of knowledge about the healthcare system, and uncertainty about who to trust are complicated by language barriers and differing cultural meanings regarding health, illness, and care practices. These factors make navigating our complex healthcare system even more complicated and also result in difficulties accessing and understanding Canadian health promotion services, such as screening for breast and cervical cancer (Donnelly, 2008).

The most significant barriers to healthcare cited by recent immigrations are language, not knowing where to go, long waiting lists, and being unable to find a physician accepting new patients (Statistics Canada, 2007d). Building trust is an essential first step to building a relationship, and often interpreters are necessary. The resources *Working with Interpreters* and *Strategies for Working Effectively with Interpreters* can be found in MyNursingLab. The CHN working with the newcomer population must be aware of the needs of this group related to immigration and settlement. However, while there are certainly unique challenges for newcomers, nurses must also be aware that many of the issues faced by newcomers vary little from issues faced by the general Canadian-born population. Nurses also need to remember that despite the preceding emphasis on challenges, newcomers have considerable and important skills and strengths; they have demonstrated resiliency through the act of immigration itself. Recent immigrants are healthier than resident Canadians (Beiser, 2005), highly educated, and have many positive and health promoting cultural values and practices. As with all clients, effective CHN care builds on collaboration in the context of existing resiliencies, strengths, and supports.

CANADIAN RESEARCH BOX

What are the meanings of cancer care and end of life experiences?

Maddalena, V. J., Bernard, W. T., Etowa, J., Murdoch, S. D., Smith, D., & Jarvis, P. M. (2010). Cancer care experiences and use of complementary and alternative medicine at end of life in Nova Scotia's Black communities. *Journal of Transcultural Nursing, 21*(2), 114–122. doi:10.1177/1043659609357634

The aim of this research was to explore the meanings and experiences of African-Canadian caregivers related to cancer and end-of-life care, including the use of complementary and alternative medicine (CAM). A qualitative case study methodology was used to focus on the cancer care experiences of three decedents and their caregivers from one rural family (African-Nova Scotian, or those whose families had immigrated to Nova Scotia prior to 1815), one urban family (African-Nova Scotian), and one recent immigrant family (Caribbean). All participants were African-Canadian residents of Nova Scotia and either the primary caregiver for a family member who had died of cancer in the preceding three years, or identified by the primary caregiver as someone who was involved in the care, for a total of seven participants. While recognizing the diversity of African-Canadian history, migration and current experiences, the authors state that there is a shared cultural identity among many African-Canadians that influences meanings of illness, pain, and death.

Four themes were identified from the participants' interview data through thematic and discourse analysis: roles and expectations of caregivers, lack of knowledge of both the health system and the disease, the importance of spirituality during illness and death, and complementary and alternative healing practices. Participants emphasized the strong expectation that family members, usually women, would adopt a primary caregiving role during illness, and that care at home was preferable to care in an institution. Yet caregivers assumed multiple responsibilities for the ill person, as well as their own families, and were not always aware of the services available. The

importance of spirituality and common use of CAM and home remedies were also highlighted.

Discussion Questions

1. How would you provide care that balances your awareness of the diversity of individual and family experiences within any group and your knowledge of shared cultural characteristics?

2. "Preference for caring for loved ones at home may render many African-Canadian families 'invisible' to the palliative care network of services" (p. 121). What steps would you take to counteract this, and at what levels?

Temporary Migrant Workers

The term **temporary migrant worker** applies to different types of employees, who have differing prospects and experiences, and who come from other countries (Sharma, 2006). Most of the skilled temporary workers entering Canada are from the United States and Europe; low-skilled workers come from countries such as Mexico, the Caribbean (mainly men), and the Philippines (mainly women), and compete for jobs that are poorly paid and considered to be less desirable (Boyd & Pikkow, 2008). Women temporary migrants are more likely to be streamed into the low-skilled category compared to men. The number of temporary foreign workers relative to permanent immigrants who were admitted as workers has shifted toward non-permanent admittance and is currently at a ratio of 2:1. In 2004, Canada admitted 113 945 skilled/independent workers for permanent immigration; in that same year, 238 093 non-immigrant temporary workers were admitted, including both skilled and low-skilled workers (Sharma, 2006). In 2007, a total of 439 100 non-permanent residents were living in Canada (Statistics Canada, 2007b).

As countries in the developed world have become increasingly protectionist, opportunities for the permanent immigration of low-skilled workers and their families have been reduced (Sharma, 2006). Recurring migration for employment, reflecting the intersection of economic globalization and local necessity, is becoming progressively widespread. At the same time that increasing numbers of Canadian citizens are migrating internally in search of work, there is growing dependence on temporary foreign workers in sectors where it is difficult to find local people who will work for low wages in often isolated and hazardous circumstances, and where the work is not mobile, such as agriculture, construction, and hospitality services (Preibisch, 2007).

CULTURE, COMMUNITY, AND HEALTH

Considering culture in the context of diversity and multiple intersections also means being aware of the relationship among the social determinants of health, and culture and health. As described by the World Health Organization

(WHO), "the structural determinants and [social] conditions of daily life constitute the social determinants of health and are responsible for a major part of health inequities between and within countries" (2008, p. 1). These determinants of health, such as culture, income, education, social support, and access to healthcare, are significant for all individuals, families, and communities. According to Allendar et al. (2009), culture is possibly the most relevant social determinant of community health. The underlying premise for culture as a determinant of health is defined by the Public Health Agency of Canada (2003) as "Some persons or groups may face additional health risks due to a socioeconomic environment, which is largely determined by dominant cultural values that contribute to the perpetuation of conditions such as marginalization, stigmatization, loss or devaluation of language and culture, and lack of access to culturally appropriate healthcare and services." The emphasis in this statement is on the role of the dominant culture in maintaining conditions damaging to those who are different from the mainstream. Yet this emphasis remains largely ignored in how we demonstrate being culturally aware and sensitive in our day-to-day practice, where the focus becomes helping those who are different integrate into systems and structures that may be detrimental to their health.

As culture is individually and collectively defined and expressed, so is health. Many newcomers and residents of Canada define health, healthcare, and health promotion very differently from the dominant culture. This can lead to the perception on the part of healthcare providers that people "don't care" about their health or the health of their families. Newcomers and temporary migrant workers will continue to utilize healthcare practices from within their cultures of origin and may have little reason to trust that the Canadian healthcare system will be understanding or responsive in ways that are meaningful to them (Waxler-Morrison & Anderson, 2005).

Yet many of the needs of newcomers and temporary workers are the same as for other Canadians. Determinants influencing health such as precarious employment, literacy, lack of housing, and food security affect many residents of Canada. Newcomers and those with language barriers may need more assistance with very practical strategies in their daily lives; however, CHNs need to be assessing the values, beliefs, and needs of all their clients in order to probe further in their assessments; provide more comprehensive, anticipatory, and preventive care; and to advocate for and collaborate with all people.

Culture is not a problem to be solved and "cultural barriers" often have more to do with the limitations of our organizations, systems, and focus on a disease orientation, than the "different" cultural values, beliefs, and practices of our clients! Diverse perspectives and insights can enhance community action and change. "Capacity-building, civic engagement, inclusion, and participation are keys to health promotion and social transformation within communities. The [cultural] lens through which individuals, organizations, and communities see each other informs their response to health and social problems as well as their action in building community" (Racher & Annis, 2008, p. 187).

CULTURAL COMPETENCE AND CULTURAL SAFETY

First described by Leininger, **cultural competence** was seen as the mechanism to address culturally specific health needs. The concept of cultural competence integrates the knowledge, attitudes, and skills that the nurse would utilize in order to plan effective and appropriate interventions. It is also a process that "includes a genuine passion to be open and flexible with others, to accept differences and build on similarities, and to be willing to learn from others as cultural informants" (Camphina-Bacote, 2002, p. 183). Becoming a culturally competent CHN requires reflection of oneself, openness to the discovery of different realities, and the opportunity to practise assessment and collaborative skills. Camphina-Bacote describes five constructs, the intersections of which informs the process of cultural competence: cultural awareness (self-examination), cultural knowledge, cultural skill (collecting and assessing data), cultural encounters (the process of relationships), and cultural desire (motivation of the healthcare provider).

Critiques of cultural competency centre on the abstract nature and lack of understanding of the concept (Engebretson, Mahoney, & Carlson, 2008); that it is the providers who mostly define cultural competency (not the clients), leading to the focus on the attributes of providers in many current evaluation tools rather than a focus on client outcomes (Schim et al., 2007); and that cultural competency obscures power relations and de-emphasizes disparities by concentrating on the activities of the individual nurse and the cultural "specifics" of an individual client (Gustafson, 2005).

Current conceptualizations of cultural competence acknowledge that is a life-long process of approaching relationships with openness and humility rather than focusing on "knowing" specific cultures. "Abandoning a desire for certainty, closure, and control in relationships and replacing it with efforts to be tentative, experimental, and open-ended is useful in community practice.... Building bridges to connect diverse worlds is not merely a set of strategies but is an all encompassing 'way of being' that comes from an ethic of care ... " (Racher & Annis, 2008, p. 184). The CHN is the learner, and the course of culturally competent care emerges from the interaction between providers and recipients (Schim et al., 2007).

In addition to individual resources and skills, it is also important to recognize the role of institutional resources (such as interpreters, continuing education, and policies), which support culturally competent practices (Srivastrava, 2007), and the importance of the social determinants of health in shaping people's lives. As affirmed by Ludwig-Beymer (2008), "cultural competency cannot live in one or two nurses; it must be systematic. It must involve all layers of the organization: the policy-making level, the administrative level, the management level, and the provider level. In addition, an organization must have a mutually beneficial relationship with the community it serves to achieve cultural competency" (p. 222). Thriving community health development ". . . and examples of real cultural competence are community-based programs that are targeted to specific social groups, engage community leaders, work through local institutions, and use culturally established channels of communication" (Dreher et al., 2006, p. 8).

The concept of cultural safety arose in New Zealand in response to issues raised by Maori nurses. It has some elements in common with cultural competence; however, cultural safety makes explicit issues of power. **Cultural safety** is defined as effective nursing practice with a client from another culture, as determined by that client. "Unsafe cultural practice comprises any action which diminishes, demeans or disempowers the cultural identity and wellbeing of an individual" (Nursing Council of New Zealand, 2005, p. 4). The emphasis is on the experience of the client receiving nursing care, the capacity of clients to shape and contribute to their health experiences and outcomes, and the recognition of the context of power relations.

Strengths of a cultural safety approach include drawing our attention more explicitly to addressing inequities, supporting CHNs to

- improve healthcare access for patients, aggregates, and populations
- acknowledge that we are all bearers of culture
- expose the social, political, and historical contexts of healthcare
- enable practitioners to consider difficult concepts such as racism, discrimination, and prejudice
- understand that cultural safety is determined by those to whom nurses provide care
- understand the limitations of "culture" in terms of having people access and safely move through healthcare systems and encounters with care providers, and
- challenge unequal power relations (ANAC, 2009, p. 24)

Proponents of cultural safety consider cultural awareness, sensitivity, and competence as providing a starting place for comprehending cultural complexities, and that cultural safety is particularly congruent with advocacy (ANAC). However, similar to cultural competence, the concept of cultural safety has been criticized for being inadequately understood and utilized in practice, and lacking research with regard to patient outcomes (Johnstone & Kanitsaki, 2007).

IMPLICATIONS FOR COMMUNITY HEALTH NURSING PRACTICE

Knowledge of every culture is impossible and unnecessary (Waxler-Morrison & Anderson, 2005). CHNs need to have the assessment, interviewing, and collaborative skills in order to be open to the processes of discovery and reflection required for providing effective care with every client. These skills are not only needed with clients but also with other healthcare providers, and community agencies and organizations. CHNs work with unique individuals within complex and changing families and communities for the mutual construction of actualized and potential solutions at downstream

and upstream levels of care. Planning and implementing nursing care is not based on how different (or similar) someone might seem; it is based on bringing assessment and relational skills to every encounter so that values and beliefs can be discovered and strengths supported.

Both nurses and clients bring multiple cultures to their interactions. Their personal culture(s), the culture of nursing, and the culture of their institution shape nurses. Clients (individuals, families, communities, populations) are shaped by their personal cultures, professional values, and unique life experiences as well. While discovering the client's values, beliefs, and assumptions, nurses need to avoid focusing on the clients' cultures in a way that promotes stereotyping and excludes reflection regarding issues of power, professional and organizational cultures, and personal self-awareness (see the guide *Working with Clients—Questions for Reflection and Building Awareness in Community Practice* in MyNursingLab). The keys to understanding and providing effective care lie in approaching relationships with humility, appreciating the diversity within all of us, and acknowledging influences such as the effects of dominant cultures and the social determinants of health.

CANADIAN RESEARCH BOX 8.2

How to enhance nursing students' cultural competence?

Koskinen, L., Campbell, B., Aarts, C., Chassé, F., Hemingway, A., Juhansoo, T., & Nordstrom, P. M. (2009). Enhancing cultural competence: Trans-Atlantic experiences of European and Canadian nursing students. *International Journal of Nursing Practice, 15*, 502–509. doi:10.1111/j.1440-172X.2009.01776.x

The purpose of this exchange experience was to develop and strengthen nursing students' sensitivities to community determinants of health related to cultural and social health inequalities. Trans-Atlantic student exchange projects were conducted in rural community placements for 8–16 weeks among 48 senior nursing students from Canada, England, Estonia, Finland, and Sweden. The purpose of the study was to explore the cultural competence, understandings, and growth of the student nurse participants. Cultural competence was considered to be ". . . an ongoing personal maturation process that includes increasing self-awareness, ability to see through others' eyes when conflicting values and expectations occur in interaction, willingness to negotiate mutually acceptable solutions and capacity to act in culturally diverse contexts" (p. 503).

The students described their cultural experiences through journal writing using critical incident technique (CIT), whereby an incident that either positively or negatively affected a clinical situation was reflected upon. Qualitative content analysis was used to analyze 134 critical incidents. Five student reflective learning categories were identified: cross-cultural ethical issues, cultural and social differences, health-care inequalities, population health concerns, and personal and professional awareness. Four cultural perspectives related to health also emerged from the students' reflections: health promotion realm, sensitivity to social and cultural aspects of people's lives, channels between the health sector and society, and cultural language and stories of local people. The students gained insight into the need and value of these perspectives in order to work more effectively with communities, especially when numerous and significant challenges to health existed.

Discussion Questions

1. The authors state "Cultural experiences can be provided to learners through diverse experiential methods in real or simulated cultural contexts, but learning cultural competence requires an extended cultural immersion including encounters with culturally different people" (p. 503). Do you agree or disagree with this statement, or elements of this statement? Why or why not?

2. Is it possible or desirable to work with communities experiencing detrimental or negative determinants of health without considering the nature of existing power relations (i.e., a more culturally safe approach)?

Cultural Assessments

A variety of cultural assessment guides for individuals and families have been developed (Andrews & Boyle, 2008; Giger & Davidhizar, 2008; Leininger, 2006; Spector, 2009). Useful guides need to provide a format with open-ended questions that facilitate descriptive responses and build a relationship between the client and the nurse. Yiu and Edmunds (2009) have developed A Guide to Transcultural Assessment, which is located in MyNursingLab. Cultural assessment guides share the classification and identification of important cultural domains in order for the provision of culturally appropriate care to take place. The limitations of current assessment guides are shared as well, comprising ". . . the tendency to include too much cultural content ultimately negating the "heart of the matter," which is the process itself, [and the difficulty of separating] client-specific data from normative data" (Giger & Davidhizar, 2008, p. 4).

When participating in cultural assessments, the CHN must be careful not to focus on how the client differs from the nurse (which we often assume to be the "norm"). Knowledge of shared cultural characteristics and patterns can be useful as a beginning; however, individual experiences and meanings vary as everyone participates in multiple cultures, has many layers of identity, and is influenced by the dominant social order. Generalizations can be useful in providing background information about meanings of care and health practices, but must be used with caution and sensitivity. Clients, whether

individuals, families, or communities, may or may not share or value generalizations about their culture that are known to the nurse. There is always continuous interplay between making use of background information the nurse may have and checking that information with every client. Background information that is never checked with the client and assumed to be true for all becomes a **stereotype**.

Most often, cultural assessments are conducted with individuals and families. Yet individual clients are always embedded in and influenced by their larger society. CHNs are aware of the interaction between the cultural assessments of individuals, families, and the group focus necessary for a community assessment. Questions relating to culture need to be integrated within the community assessment (see Chapter 13). Other valuable considerations can be found in MyNursingLab in Touchstones for Working with Diverse Communities. Adding a cultural component to a community nursing assessment strengthens the base upon which everything follows, as ". . . it is often the characteristics [determined by shared cultural experiences] of people that give every community its uniqueness" (Boyle, 2008, p. 279).

CASE STUDY

You are a CHN in a rural town of 15 000 people. In recent years there has been an increase in the number of both newcomers who are permanent residents and temporary migrant workers who are "visibly" different. Prior to this, the population of the community had remained fairly constant. You are aware of comments circulating in the community such as "These people are changing our town, it doesn't look the same anymore" and "Why should we be providing services to newcomers and people who are only here to work? Our grandparents started from nothing when they came to Canada."

You have been asked to join a community committee sponsored by the local social planning council to assess and address settlement needs such as translation services and improving available resources, as well as concerns regarding isolation and work safety of the temporary workers. The social planning council has the mandate to assess needs, provide services, and make recommendations for the entire community.

Discussion Questions

1. Which people representing which groups should be on the committee? Why?

2. How would you contribute to constructive discussion, exploring viewpoints and perspectives?

3. What could be some achievable outcomes from the committee work? How long would this take?

Community Cultural Assessment

- How would you define or describe what culture means to your community?
- With which culture(s) do you identify?
- Are there some shared cultural values for your community?
- Are there any aspects of your community's culture that are beneficial to your life and health?
- Are there any aspects of your community's culture that "get in the way" of your health?
- What are some of the other forces or areas of your everyday life that enhance or create barriers for your health?
- What would you like nurses to know about your community's culture(s)?
- How would you like nurses to work with you in order to improve health in your community?

SUMMARY

This chapter has explored the concept of culture, and the intersections among culture, multiculturalism, diversity, race, and ethnicity. Canadian experiences of diversity and multiculturalism were discussed, as were the relationships among culture, health, and the social determinants of health. The culturally competent and culturally safe sensitivities and skills that are needed to provide care during nurse–client interactions were described, including implications for community health nursing practice with all residents of Canada.

A culturally competent/culturally safe approach requires commitment to personal reflection and growth, an understanding of the layers of cultural identity that shape us all, and the development of knowledge and relationship-building skills. This is so that in every interaction the nurse strives to discover the values and meanings of health for the client in the context of structural forces and power relations. "Working with culture" means working with communities to identify and strengthen their cultural capital so that effective action can be taken (Dreher et al., 2006). As CHNs, we must nurture our common humanity and social responsibilities while also addressing systemic inequities. This means listening for history and context, not only to understand our clients, but in order to comprehensively change policy and practice (Hrycak & Jakubec, 2006). Culturally relevant community-based services are developed through ". . . collaboration and partnerships between community leaders, health consumers, and healthcare providers. When community residents or health consumers are involved as partners, community-based services are more likely to be responsive to locally defined needs, are better used, and are sustained through local action" (Boyle, 2008, p. 262).

KEY TERMS

culture, p. 125
ethnocentrism, p. 125
diversity, p. 126
multiculturalism, p. 126
ethnicity, p. 127
race, p. 127
racism, p. 127
racialization, p. 127
temporary migrant workers, p. 130
cultural competence, p. 131
cultural safety, p. 132
stereotype, p. 133

REVIEW QUESTIONS

Choose the one alternative that best completes the statement or answers the question.

1. Based on his or her conclusions after assessing a client, a CHN has formulated a plan of care. The nurse believes that through the application of nursing expertise the "correct" plan has been determined. This is an example of

   a) stereotyping.   c) a useful generalization.

   b) ethnocentrism.   d) cultural competence.

2. A CHN is a member on a committee planning a community health day. One suggestion is to have healthy foods representing the diverse cultures within that community. Some committee members express disagreement stating "cultural foods" would perpetuate stereotyping of certain groups. The nurse realizes that

   a) the solution would be to promote total integration of all cultures through assimilation.

   b) the committee needs to reach unanimous agreement on all suggestions in order to have a successful community health day.

   c) issues of perception and how people are portrayed are not inherent in multiculturalism.

   d) values and beliefs regarding positive expressions of multiculturalism are diverse.

3. A new CHN discovers that a section for racial designation is included in an agency's client assessment form. The categories are: White, Black, and Asian. The nurse questions the usefulness of this racial categorization because

   a) the concept of race is not objective and has been used create and sustain subordinate groups.

   b) the nurse believes that there are more than three racial groups.

   c) the nurse is aware that different racial categories are used in the United States.

   d) the nurse does not know how someone who is biracial would be categorized.

4. A CHN is working with a newcomer family who is experiencing language barriers, unemployment, and precarious housing. Many of the family's traditions and values from their culture of origin remain helpful. Which statement best describes the family's situation?

   a) The family's traditions and values are strengths in a situation currently shared by many Canadians.

   b) The family is not at risk for poor health because their traditions will keep them healthy.

   c) All values and beliefs from their culture of origin will remain intact after immigration.

   d) Once family members attend English language training they will successfully adapt to Canadian life.

5. A major difference between cultural competence and cultural safety is that

   a) a culturally competent approach explicitly addresses all the characteristics of culture; a culturally safe approach does not.

   b) a culturally safe approach explicitly addresses all the characteristics of culture; a culturally competent approach does not.

   c) a culturally competent approach explicitly addresses issues of power; a culturally safe approach does not.

   d) a culturally safe approach explicitly addresses issues of power; a culturally competent approach does not.

6. A CHN conducting a community assessment should be demonstrating

   a) a focus on how the community's culture(s) differ(s) from the culture(s) of the nurse.

   b) an exclusive focus on the culture(s) of origin of community members.

   c) comprehensive and complete knowledge about all cultures in the community prior to starting the assessment.

   d) awareness of the intersections of the community's cultural values and the social determinants of health throughout the assessment.

STUDY QUESTIONS

1. Describe the characteristics of culture.
2. Define and describe the links among culture, multiculturalism, diversity, race, and ethnicity.
3. What is the relationship between culture and health?
4. Describe the similarities and differences between cultural competence and cultural safety.
5. Describe how cultural beliefs and values shape the interactions between nurses and clients.
6. Describe the knowledge, attitudes, sensitivity, and skills needed to provide nursing care framed by culture to all residents of Canada.

After working through these questions, go to the MyNursingLab at www.pearsoned.ca/mynursinglab to check your answers.

INDIVIDUAL CRITICAL THINKING EXERCISES

1. What implications does the Canadian Charter of Rights (1982) have on nursing practice when working with culturally diverse families?

2. In your work as a public health nurse you meet a family with school age children seeking immunization to prepare for school registration. Communicating using very limited English the family tells you that money is very scarce, the mother is pregnant with her fifth child, the family does not have permanent residence status in Canada, and they are uncertain whether they will be allowed to stay. They are worried they will be deported to their country of origin. With what community supports and services would you assist this family to access in order of priority and why?

3. What are the key differences between healthy cultural identification and ethnocentrism?

4. How would you assess whether the nursing model or theory you are using is helping you deliver culturally competent and/or culturally safe care?

5. How does culture influence health and illness within diverse communities?

GROUP CRITICAL THINKING EXERCISES

1. How would you go about gaining and demonstrating the skills and behaviours needed for culturally competent and/or culturally safe practice?

2. In pairs, do a cultural assessment (*A Guide to Transcultural Nursing Assessment* can be found in MyNursingLab). What have you learned about your own culture? What have you learned about your partner's culture? What did you discover about the process?

3. Are the members of your nursing class representative of your community's population? Why or why not?

4. Discuss as a group the similarities and differences between your understandings of diversity and multiculturalism.

REFERENCES

Aboriginal Nurses Association of Canada. (2009). *Cultural competence and cultural safety in First Nations, Inuit and Métis nursing education: An integrated review of the literature.* Ottawa, ON: Author. Retrieved from http://www.cna-nurses.ca/CNA/documents/pdf/publications/Review_of_Literature_e.pdf

Allender, J. A., Rector, C., & Warner, K. (2009). *Community health nursing: Promoting and protecting the public's health* (7th ed.). Philadelphia, PA: Lippincott, Williams & Wilkins.

Andrews, M. (2008). Theoretical foundations of transcultural nursing. In M. Andrews & J. Boyle (Eds.), *Transcultural concepts in nursing care* (5th ed., pp. 3–14). Philadelphia, PA: Wolters Kluwer/Lippincott Williams & Wilkins.

Andrews, M. M., & Boyle, J. S. (2008). *Transcultural concepts in nursing care* (5th ed.). Philadelphia, PA: Wolters Kluwer/Lippincott Williams & Wilkins.

Beiser, M. (2005). The health of immigrants and refugees in Canada. *Canadian Journal of Public Health, 96* (Supplement 2), S30–S44.

Blad, C., & Couton, P. (2009). The rise of an intercultural nation: Immigration, diversity and nationhood in Quebec. *Journal of Ethnic and Migration Studies, 35*(4), 645–667. doi:10.1080/13691830902765277

Boyle, J. (2008). Culture, family, and community. In M. Andrews & J. Boyle (Eds.), *Transcultural concepts in nursing care* (5th ed., pp. 261–296). Philadelphia, PA: Wolters Kluwer/ Lippincott Williams & Wilkins.

Boyd, M., & Pikkow, D. (2008). Finding place in stratified structures: Migrant women in North America. In N. Piper (Ed.), *New perspectives on gender and migration: Livelihood, rights and entitlements* (pp. 19–58). New York, NY: Routledge.

Camphina-Bacote, J. (2002). The process of cultural competence in the delivery of healthcare services: A model of care. *Journal of Transcultural Nursing, 13*(3), 181–184. Retrieved from http://tcn.sagepub.com.proxy1. lib.uwo .ca:2048/cgi/reprint/13/3/181

Canadian Nurses Association. (2000). Cultural diversity— changes and challenges. *Nursing Now: Issues and Trends in Canadian Nursing, February, 7*, 1–6.

Canadian Nurses Association. (2004). *Position statement: Promoting culturally competent care.* Ottawa, ON: Author.

Canadian Nurses Association. (2008). *Code of ethics for registered nurses.* Ottawa, ON: Author. Retrieved from www.cna-aiic.ca/CNA/documents/pdf/ publications/ Code_of_Ethics_2008_e.pdf

College of Nurses of Ontario. (2009). *Practice guideline: Culturally sensitive care.* Toronto, ON: Author. Retrieved from www.cno.org/docs/prac/41040_CulturallySens.pdf

Community Health Nurses Association of Canada. (2008). *Canadian community health nursing standards of practice.* Ottawa, ON: Author. Retrieved from www.chnac.ca/ images/downloads/standards/chn_standards_of_practice_ mar08_english.pdf

Community Health Nurses Association of Canada. (2009). *Public health nursing discipline specific competencies version 1.0.* Ottawa, ON: Author. Retrieved from www.chnac.ca/ images/downloads/competencies/competencies_june_2009_ english.pdf

Donnelly, T. T. (2008). Challenges in providing breast and cervical cancer screening services to Vietnamese Canadian women: The healthcare providers' perspective. *Nursing Inquiry, 15*(2), 158–168. Retrieved from http://journals2 .scholarsportal.info.proxy1.lib.uwo.ca:2048/tmp/ 15314015660646451218.pdf

Dreher, M., Shapiro, D., & Asselin, M. (2006). *Healthy places healthy people: A handbook for culturally competent community nursing practice.* Indianapolis, IN: Sigma Theta Tau International.

Engebretson, J., Mahoney, J., & Carlson, E. (2008). Cultural competence in the era of evidence-based practice. *Journal of Professional Nursing, 24*, 172–178. doi:10.1016/ j.profnurs.2007.10.012

Giger, R., & Davidhizar, R. (2008). *Transcultural nursing: Assessment and interventions* (5th ed.). St. Louis, MO: Mosby Elsevier.

Gustafson, D. L. (2005). Transcultural nursing theory from a critical cultural perspective. *Advances in Nursing Science, 28*(1), 2–16.

Hrycak, N., & Jakubec, S. (2006). Listening to different voices. *Canadian Nurse, 102*(6), 24–28. Retrieved from http://proquest.umi.com.proxy1.lib.uwo.ca:2048/ pqdweb?index=8&did=1079310661&SrchMode=1&sid=1 &Fmt=6&VInst=PROD&VType=PQD&RQT=309&VN ame=PQD&TS=1275240450&clientId=11263

James, C. E. (2003). *Seeing ourselves: Exploring race, ethnicity and culture* (3rd ed.). Toronto, ON: Thompson Educational Publishing.

Johnstone, M-J., & Kanitsaki, O. (2007). An exploration of the notion and nature of the construct of cultural safety and its applicability to the Australian health care context. *Journal of Transcultural Nursing, 18*(3), 247–256. doi:10.1177/1043659607301304

Leininger, M. (2006). Culture care diversity and universality theory and evolution of the ethnonursing method. In M. Leininger & M. R. McFarland (Eds.), *Culture care diversity and universality: A worldwide nursing theory* (2nd ed., pp. 1–41). Boston, MA: Jones and Bartlett.

Ludwig-Beymer, P. (2008). Creating culturally competent organization. In M. Andrews & J. Boyle (Eds.), *Transcultural concepts in nursing care* (5th ed., pp. 197–225). Philadelphia, PA: Wolters Kluwer/ Lippincott Williams & Wilkins.

Marks, B. (2007). Cultural competence revisited: Nursing students with disabilities. *Journal of Nursing Education, 46*(2), 70–74. Retrieved from http://proquest.umi.com. proxy1.lib.uwo.ca:2048/pqdweb?index=106&did= 1210832281&SrchMode=1&sid=4&Fmt=6&VInst= PROD&VType=PQD&RQT=309&VName=PQD&TS= 1275240821&clientId=11263

Nursing Council of New Zealand. (2005). *Guidelines for cultural safety, the Treaty of Waitangi and Maori health in nursing education and practice.* Wellington, NZ: Author. Retrieved from www.nursingcouncil.org.nz/ Cultural%20Safety.pdf

Ontario Human Rights Commission. (2005). *Policy and guidelines on racism and racial discrimination.* Toronto, ON: Author. Retrieved from www.ohrc.on.ca/en/resources/ Policies/RacismPolicy/pdf

Padolsky, E. (2000). Multiculturalism at the Millennium. *Journal of Canadian Studies, 35*(1), 138–160. Retrieved from http://gateway.proquest.com.proxy1.lib.uwo.ca:2048/ openurl?ctx_ver=Z39.882003&xri:pqil:res_ver=0.2&res_ id=xri:lion-us&rft_id=xri:lion:ft:abell:R04236049:0

Preibisch, K. L. (2007). Local produce, foreign labor: Labor mobility programs and global trade competitiveness in Canada. *Rural Sociology, 72*(3), 418–449. Retrieved from http://web.ebscohost.com.proxy1.lib.uwo.ca:2048/ehost/

pdfviewer/pdfviewer?vid=2&hid=8&sid=5ca5dabc-e87e-44bb-b394-3be4b2bc593d%40sessionmgr10

Public Health Agency of Canada (2003). *Underlying premises and evidence table.* Retrieved from www.phac-aspc.gc.ca/ph-sp/determinants/determinants-eng.php#culture

Racher, F., & Annis, R. (2008). Honouring culture and diversity in community practice. In A. Vollman, E. Anderson, & J. McFarlane (Eds.), *Canadian community as partner: Theory and multidisciplinary practice* (2nd ed., pp. 164–189). Philadelphia, PA: Wolters Kluwer/Lippincott Williams & Wilkins.

Reimer Kirkham, S., Smye, V., Tang, S., Anderson, J., Blue, C., Browne, A., et al. (2002). Rethinking cultural safety while waiting to do fieldwork: Methodological implications for nursing research. *Research in Nursing & Health, 25,* 222–232.

Schim, S., Doorenbos, A., Benkert, R., & Miller, J. (2007). Culturally congruent care: Putting the puzzle together. *Journal of Transcultural Nursing, 18*(2), 103–110. doi:10.1177/1043659606298613

Sharma, N. (2006). *Home economics: Nationalism and the making of 'migrant workers' in Canada.* Toronto, ON: University of Toronto Press.

Shirley, J. (2007). Limits of autonomy in nursing's moral discourse. *Advances in Nursing Science, 30*(1), 14–25.

Spector, R. (2009). *Cultural diversity in health and illness* (7th ed.). Upper Saddle River, NJ: Pearson Prentice Hall.

Srivastava, R. (2007). *The health care professional's guide to clinical cultural competence.* Toronto, ON: Mosby.

Statistics Canada. (2007a). *Immigration in Canada: A portrait of the foreign-born population, 2006 census.* Ottawa, ON: Author. Retrieved from http://www12.statcan.ca/english/census06/analysis/immcit/pdf/97-557-XIE2006001.pdf

Statistics Canada. (2007b). *The daily: Canada's population estimates.* Ottawa, ON: Author. Retrieved from www.statcan.ca/Daily/English/070927/d070927a.htm

Statistics Canada. (2007c). *Portrait of the Canadian population in 2006, by age and sex, 2006 census.* Ottawa, ON: Author. Retrieved from http://www12.statcan.ca/english/census06/analysis/agesex/pdf/97-551-XIE2006001.pdf

Statistics Canada. (2007d). *Canadian social trends. Immigrants' perspectives on their first four years in Canada: Highlights from three waves of the longitudinal survey of immigrants to Canada.* Ottawa, ON: Author. Retrieved from www.statcan.ca/english/freepub/11-008-XIE/2007000/pdf/11-008-XIE20070009627.pdf

Statistics Canada. (2008). *Canada's ethnocultural mosaic: Census year 2006.* Ottawa, ON. Author. Retrieved from http://www12.statcan.ca/english/census06/analysis/ethnicorigin/pdf/97-562-XIE2006001.pdf

Varcoe, C. (2006). Doing participatory action research in a racist world. *Western Journal of Nursing Research, 28*(5), 525–540. doi:10.1177/0193945906287706

Waxler-Morrison, N., & Anderson, J. (2005). Introduction: The need for culturally sensitive care. In N. Waxler-Morrison, J. Anderson, E. Richardson, & N. Chambers (Eds.), *Cross-cultural caring: A handbook for health professionals* (2nd ed., pp. 1–10). Vancouver, BC: UBC Press.

Williams, R. (1983). *Keywords.* Oxford: Oxford University Press.

World Health Organization. (2008). *Closing the gap in a generation: Health equity through action on the social determinants of health.* Geneva, Switzerland: Author. Retrieved from http://whqlibdoc.who.int/publications/2008/9789241563703_eng.pdf

Yiu Matuck, L., & Ruggirello, T. (2007). Culture connection project: Promoting multiculturalism in elementary schools. *Canadian Journal of Public Health, 98*(1), 26–29. Retrieved from http://find.galegroup.com.proxy1.lib.uwo.ca:2048/gtx/infomark.do?&contentSet=IACDocuments&type=retrieve&tabID=T002&prodId=CPI&docId=A159919542&source=gale&srcprod=CPI&userGroupName=lond95336&version=1.0

FURTHER READING

Allen, D. G. (2006). Whiteness and difference in nursing. *Nursing Philosophy, 7,* 65–78.

Cooper Brathwaite, A., & Majumdar, B. (2006). Evaluation of a cultural competence educational programme. *Journal of Advanced Nursing, 53*(4), 470–479.

Gray, D. P., & Thomas, D. (2005). Critical analysis of "culture" in nursing literature: Implications for nursing education in the United States. *Annual Review of Nursing Education, 3,* 249–270.

Johnston, M., & Herzig, R. (2006). The interpretation of "culture": Diverging perspectives on medical provision in rural Montana. *Social Science & Medicine, 63,* 2500–2511. doi:10.1016/j.socscimed.2006.06.013

ADDITIONAL RESOURCES

Websites

Cultural Diversity in Nursing
http://www.culturediversity.org

Government of Canada: Multiculturalism
http://www.cic.gc.ca/english/information/faq/multiculturalism/index.asp#multi

Transcultural Nursing Society
http://www.tcns.org

Nova Scotia Department of Health. (2005). A cultural competence guide for primary health care professionals in Nova Scotia.
http://healthteamnovascotia.ca/cultural_competence/Cultural_Competence_guide_for_Primary_Health_Care_Professionals.pdf

Registered Nurses' Association of Ontario (2007). Healthy work environments best practice guideline. Embracing cultural diversity in healthcare: Developing cultural competence.
http://www.rnao.org/Storage/29/2336_BPG_Embracing_Cultural_Diversity.pdf

Films

Hangin On (2006). National Film Board of Canada.

Between: Living in the Hyphen (2005). National Film Board of Canada.

About the Authors

Kathryn Edmunds, RN, BN (University of Manitoba), MSN (Wayne State University, with a specialization in transcultural nursing), PhD (c) is currently a Doctoral Candidate in the Arthur Labatt Family School of Nursing at the University of Western Ontario. She has been a faculty member in Nursing at the University of Windsor and has extensive experience as a public health nurse with the Windsor-Essex County Health Unit working in rural southwestern Ontario. Current theoretical and research interests include the relationships among uprootedness, displacement, gendered migration, culture, and health, and the current critiques in the nursing literature of the concept of culture from critical theoretical perspectives.

Elizabeth Kinnaird-Iler, RN, BScN, and MSc (University of Windsor) is a manager in the Healthy Babies Healthy Children program at the Windsor-Essex County Health Unit. She provides direct supervision to public health nurses and family home visitors who visit new mothers and young families from a variety of cultural backgrounds. Her interests include the areas of women's health, program evaluation, health promotion, and transcultural health.

chapter 9

Epidemiology

Lynnette Leeseberg Stamler

OBJECTIVES

After studying this chapter, you should be able to:

1. Describe the theoretical underpinnings of the epidemiologic process and its historical and present value to CHNs.

2. Differentiate between association and causality and explain some of the criteria that suggest a causal relationship.

3. Understand the various measurements used in epidemiologic research and reports and their meaning for CHNs.

4. Describe the research study designs commonly used in epidemiologic research and link the research question with the appropriate design.

5. Discuss how epidemiology has expanded to the study of disease and health promotion.

INTRODUCTION

Throughout history, humans have ascribed different causes for disease. During the religious era, disease was thought to be a consequence of divine intervention. The environment was the next general cause of disease, which was attributed to miasmas (vaporous atmospheres) or other physical forces. It was not until the 1870s that specific bacteria were recognized as causing disease. During the past century, health professionals have come to understand that there are multiple factors or influences on many diseases and health challenges. In addition to learning the many causes of disease, health researchers are working to discover the factors that promote health.

In this chapter, you will learn the basics of the science of epidemiology, understand the types of data used in community health nursing, and begin to acquire the skills to identify and ask questions, using epidemiologic data to find some of the answers.

WHAT IS EPIDEMIOLOGY?

Epidemiology is defined as "the study of the occurrence and distribution of health-related states or events in specified populations, including the study of the determinants influencing such states and the application of this knowledge to control the health problem" (Porta, 2008, p. 81). While the most well-known of these would be public health epidemiology (or infectious disease epidemiology), these authors go on to note that the sub-disciplines can be divided into two streams: the exposure-oriented sub-disciplines (e.g., nutritional, social, environmental) and the disease-oriented sub-disciplines (e.g., cancer, injury, perinatal). Some sub-disciplines have less clear categorizations, such as occupational epidemiology or molecular epidemiology.

Friis and Sellers (2009) note that the purpose of epidemiology is to describe, explain, predict, and control challenges to population health. Epidemiologists first seek to describe health-related events by answering the questions who, what, when, and where, and by following trends in the population. Further explorations expand descriptions by answering the questions how and why, and by examining causality and modes of transmission. From this information come predictions that guide interventions and the use of healthcare resources. Finally, controls are implemented to prevent new illness, cure, if possible, those who are ill, and rehabilitate or prevent complications for those with a chronic disease.

Historical Background of Epidemiology

Though large-scale, focused epidemiologic studies are a relatively new phenomenon, the basis of understanding for such studies has been noted throughout history. Hippocrates is credited with being the first to notice and record a possible relationship between the environment and the health or disease of people.

He suggested that physicians study "the mode in which the inhabitants live and what are their pursuits, whether they are fond of eating and drinking to excess, and given to indolence, or are fond of exercise and labour, and not given to excess in eating and drinking" (Hippocrates, 400 BCE).

Though history has recorded the existence and duration of epidemics such as the plague or the Black Death, few large-scale efforts were made to accurately record data that would increase the understanding of these epidemics. By the 1600s, statistics such as numbers of births and deaths were being recorded in London, England, and a haberdasher, John Graunt, was the first to study these statistics. He noted, for instance, gender differences in births (more males than females), seasonal variations in deaths, and high levels of infant deaths.

It was not until 1839 that Dr. William Farr initiated a more complete gathering of statistical data in England. With these data he was able (among other things) to compare death rates among workers in different types of jobs, and between prison inmates and the rest of the population. During a cholera epidemic in the mid-1850s, Dr. John Snow noticed an apparent relationship between the number of cholera deaths in various neighbourhoods and the source of the drinking water. He clearly demonstrated that people who lived in areas/homes served by particular water companies had much higher death rates from cholera than those in neighbourhoods served by other water companies.

Florence Nightingale, a contemporary of Snow and Farr, was also convinced of the effect of the environment on disease and death. When she arrived at Scutari during the Crimean War, she discovered horrendous conditions and a lax method of recording deaths and their causes. She stressed accurate recording of these statistics and used them to explain and publicize the reality of the situation. Her polar diagrams, for instance, clearly demonstrated that in January 1855, 2761 soldiers died from contagious diseases, 83 from wounds, and 324 from other causes. It became clear that without ongoing recruitment, the entire army could have been wiped out from disease alone (Cohen, 1984). It was through her influence and her record-keeping that she was able to persuade authorities to allow her to implement sanitation practices that significantly decreased the death rates during and after the war.

In the 1900s, it became evident that although vital statistics of death and illness were important, following populations for a period of time to ascertain the progression of various diseases and their treatments was also important. As well, new research methodologies were developed to gather and compare data appropriately. As medical scientists discovered and implemented new treatments, the primary causes of death changed over time from predominantly contagious diseases to chronic diseases that were influenced by lifestyle behaviours. For instance, between the 1920s and the 1970s, death rates from health challenges such as cardiovascular and renal diseases rose, while death rates for diseases such as tuberculosis and influenza decreased (see Figure 9.1). In 1949, the first cohort study—the Framingham Heart Study—was begun, followed in 1950 by the publication of the first case-control studies of smoking and lung disease. Four years later, the Salk polio vaccine field trial was conducted. Modern

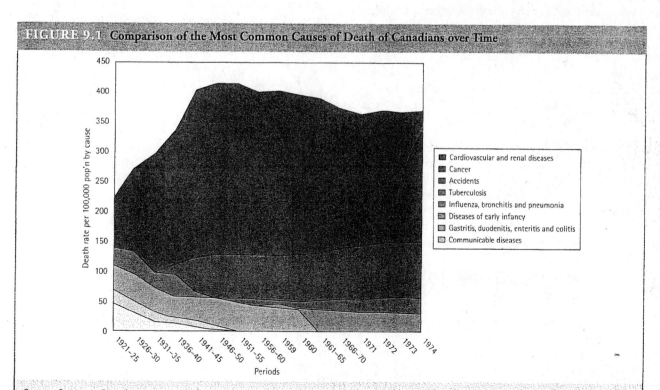

FIGURE 9.1 Comparison of the Most Common Causes of Death of Canadians over Time

Source: Statistics Canada, www.statcan.ca/english/free[in/11-516-XIE/sectionb/sectionb.htm. Reproduced with permission.

Adapted from Table B35-50 Average annual number of deaths and death rates for leading causes of death, Canada, for five-year periods, 1921 to 1974. Available from http://www.statcan.gc.ca/pub/11-516-x/sectionb/b35-50-eng.csv

Fraser, R. D. (1983). Section B: Vital Statistics and Health, In Statistics Canada, Historical statistics of Canada (2nd ed.). Available from http://www.statcan.gc.ca/pub/11-516-x/11-516-x1983001-eng.htm

epidemiological studies have all been developed from these pioneering works.

Basic Building Blocks in Epidemiology

Several concepts and processes are the basic building blocks of the science of epidemiology. These include the epidemiologic model, the concept of susceptibility, modes of transmission, the natural history/progress of disease, association and causation, and the web of causation. These concepts and processes arose from early epidemiologic observations and analyses and were developed to help scientists understand the hows and whys of disease. Modern CHNs use these same concepts and processes to determine and test appropriate interventions.

Epidemiologic Model The classic epidemiologic model contains the elements of host, agent, and environment. The model is frequently presented as a triangle (see Figure 9.2). The **host** is the human being in which the disease occurs. The **agent** is the contagious or non-contagious force that can begin or prolong a health problem. Agents include bacteria and viruses, as well as "stimuli" such as smoking or the absence of vitamin C. The **environment** is the context that promotes the *exposure* of the host to the agent. The **epidemiologic model** posits that disease is the result of the interaction among these three elements.

Some authors have included other elements in the epidemiologic model. For example, Gordis (2000) included the vector as an additional concept. He defined **vector** as a factor (such as a deer tick) that moves between the agent and the host, assisting the movement of the disease between the other two elements. Timmreck (1998), on the other hand, added the concept of time to the model. Harkness (1995) noted that using a **Venn diagram** instead of the classic triangle emphasized the interrelatedness within the model. With the Venn diagram overlaps do exist (see Figure 9.3)

Epidemiologic Variables In order to completely and accurately describe the patterns of health challenges, the descriptive variables of epidemiology are used. These are named person, place, and time (Friis & Sellers, 2009). Within each variable are factors or characteristics that further describe the event. For instance, under the variable of person, one might look at age differences, sex, ethnicity, genetic predisposition, immune

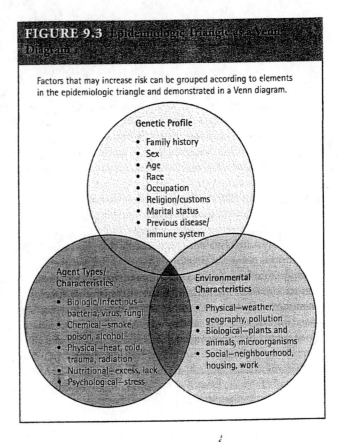

FIGURE 9.3 Epidemiologic Triangle as a Venn Diagram

Factors that may increase risk can be grouped according to elements in the epidemiologic triangle and demonstrated in a Venn diagram.

Genetic Profile
- Family history
- Sex
- Age
- Race
- Occupation
- Religion/customs
- Marital status
- Previous disease/immune system

Agent Types/Characteristics
- Biologic/Infectious—bacteria, virus, fungi
- Chemical—smoke, poison, alcohol
- Physical—heat, cold, trauma, radiation
- Nutritional—excess, lack
- Psychological—stress

Environmental Characteristics
- Physical—weather, geography, pollution
- Biological—plants and animals, microorganisms
- Social—neighbourhood, housing, work

status, marital status, place of birth, and immigration. Other environmental influences for the person such as education level, socio-economic status, and occupation are also important pieces of information. Lastly, individual lifestyle characteristics such as dietary practices, use of alcohol or tobacco, and physical activity may be helpful.

The variable of time considers such characteristics as cyclic or seasonal variation of a health event, health challenges following specific events (such as postpartum depression), or time trends (increase of chronic disease over time) (Friis & Sellers, 2009). The variable of place can include variation between regions, countries, or continents; population density; rural/urban; or specific geographical characteristics such as working in a particular building or living close to a cataclysmic event such as Chernobyl (Friis & Sellers). During the beginning identification of AIDS, careful documentation of person, time, and place assisted health professionals to accurately describe the health challenge.

Susceptibility One might think that if a group of people were all exposed in the same manner to the same disease, all would get the disease to the same degree. However, the combination of characteristics of each individual within that host group, interacting with the factors present or absent in the other elements of the epidemiologic triangle, determines the risk (or degree of susceptibility) of each person to a particular agent. **Susceptibility** and **risk** can also be described as vulnerability, which determines the individual host response. The answers to the person/place/time questions, while pointing to group susceptibility, can also point to group protection. For

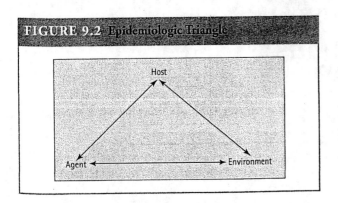

FIGURE 9.2 Epidemiologic Triangle

Host

Agent

Environment

instance, we may discover that one or more of the characteristics studied (such as age or physical activity) may in fact mitigate some of the effects of other characteristics.

Within each element of the epidemiologic triangle are factors or characteristics that may increase or decrease the risk or susceptibility of the host to the disease. Figure 9.3 identifies some of these factors/characteristics. It is evident that some factors (e.g., lifestyle behaviours) may be changed or modified by the individual, while others (e.g., age, gender, genetic makeup) are not under the control of the individual.

Modes of Disease Transmission A mode of transmission is one way in which a disease moves to a new host. There are two main modes of transmission: direct and indirect. **Direct transmission** involves contact between the person with the disease and another person. This may be accomplished through touching with contaminated hands, skin-to-skin contact, or sexual intercourse. **Indirect transmission** involves a common vehicle or vector that moves the disease to the new host. An example of a common vehicle is a contaminated water supply or lake. A mosquito can also function as a common vector in disease transmission. Indirect transmission may be airborne (droplets or dust), water-borne, vector-borne, or vehicle-borne (contaminated utensils, hygiene articles, or clothing). Different **pathogens** (microorganisms or other substances that cause disease) are viable under different conditions; therefore, one needs to ascertain the potential mode of transmission for each disease.

Because a given disease may have more than one mode of transmission, understanding those modes is central to controlling the disease. For example, when AIDS first became recognized as a threat to public health, the mode of transmission was greatly misunderstood: it was not known whether the disease could be contracted through everyday contact, such as by using a toilet seat used by someone with AIDS or by shaking that person's hand. It soon became clear that such minimal contact did not result in disease transmission. However, the fear of AIDS greatly increased the use of universal precautions by health professionals—a positive outcome.

Natural History/Progression of a Disease A disease in a human host should be seen as a process rather than as a single incident. In 1965, Leavell and Clark plotted the natural progression of the disease process and identified prevention and health promotion strategies that could be employed at each stage. As illustrated in Figure 9.4, the first stage in the disease

FIGURE 9.4 Natural History of a Disease

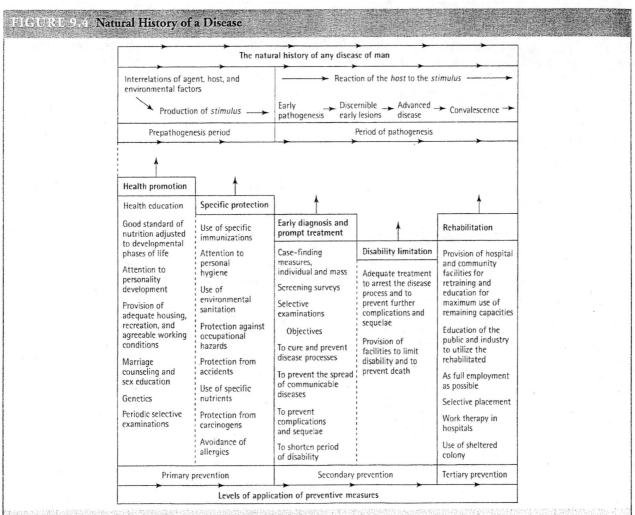

Source: Leavell, H. F., & Clark, E.G., Preventive Medicine for the Doctor in His Community. 1965, McGraw-Hill, p. 21.
Reproduced with permission of The McGraw-Hill Companies.

process is the **prepathogenesis** period. During prepathogenesis, the human host may be exposed to a variety of agents through several modes of transmission. Depending on the unique characteristics of the prospective host, repeated exposure or a combination of additional stressors may be required for the host to become susceptible to the agent and the disease to begin. **Stressors** are events or situations that cause discomfort to a person, such as chronic fatigue or a poor diet. During the prepathogenesis period (also called the incubation period), **primary prevention** activities, or "measures designed to promote general optimum health" (Leavell & Clark, p. 20) are used by health professionals and the general public alike.

When the human host begins to react to the agent (or stimulus), the period of **pathogenesis** begins. Depending on the disease, the host may or may not experience symptoms, but microscopic changes take place that indicate the presence of the disease. Pathogenesis ends with recovery, disability, or death. Two categories of health promotion activities are used during the period of pathogenesis. The first category is early diagnosis and treatment, which occurs early in the pathogenesis period. For instance, screening mammography is used for early detection of breast cancer, and the Pap test screens for cervical cancer. The second category, disability limitation, occurs later in the pathogenesis period, when the disease is active or there are recognizable symptoms. During this period, health promotion activities are aimed at preventing complications: for example, ongoing examination and care of the feet in persons living with diabetes. Early diagnosis and disability limitation may also be called **secondary prevention**. Screening is a tool for early diagnosis and is the application of a specific test to detect the presence of a disease.

Tertiary prevention is the term given to the last health promotion category and occurs during the latter phases of the pathogenesis period. At this stage, health promotion activities might include client/family education to understand the chronicity of the disease, to adapt to sequelae of the disease process, or to maximize the health of the individual through use of aids such as a walker or adapted eating utensils. Figure 9.4 identifies this period as rehabilitation, but it may also be the time when palliative care and assistance for the individual and family to move toward a dignified death would also be appropriate. It is important to recognize that the presence of chronic diseases/health challenges in individuals also increases their vulnerability or susceptibility to additional health challenges. This has become increasingly evident as more and more of our population live longer due to enhanced medical care and health practices. Disease processes that would have ensured a speedy death only a few decades ago are now managed with little ongoing medical care. CHNs can use their knowledge of the progression of a disease and the levels of prevention to plan and implement interventions at the individual, family, aggregate, and population levels.

Association and Causation Before planning interventions that prevent or ameliorate a disease or health problem, one has to clearly understand the how and why of the disease or health problem. Two terms are used to describe the relationship between a stressor and a disease: association and causation. An **association** occurs when there is reasonable evidence that a connection exists between a stressor or environmental factor and a disease or health challenge. For example, a CHN might notice that many patients who exhibit a certain condition spent their childhoods in a particular geographic location. Thus, the relationship is first noticed through observation. Based on these observations, the CHN or epidemiologist examines the data to see if the relationship or association is strong or weak—is it all patients or just a few? If the association appears strong from the limited data sample, then a larger, more comprehensive exploration might be conducted. Such investigations often generate data from several sources.

When a relationship or association has been confirmed beyond doubt, **causation** (or causality) is said to be present. In other words, causality occurs when one can state that there is a definite, statistical, cause-and-effect relationship between a particular stimulus and the occurrence of a specific disease or health challenge, or that the occurrence could not happen by chance alone.

In some ways, causation was simpler when the majority of diseases were infectious, as they were more likely to have only one cause. For example, streptococcus bacteria produce strep infection. Two important concepts in establishing causality are "necessary" and "sufficient." "Necessary" refers to the notion that a particular stressor *must* be present before a given effect can occur. For example, exposure to *Mycobacterium tuberculosis* is required before a person becomes ill with tuberculosis. "Sufficient" refers to the amount of exposure required to result in the disease. For instance, some people exposed to *Mycobacterium tuberculosis* only once (minimal dose) become ill, and some do not become ill unless exposed several times (larger dose).

In the past 40 years, several authors have identified factors or criteria that researchers and practitioners could use to assess a causal relationship between a stimulus and the occurrence of a disease (Hill, 1965). The most commonly cited criteria of causation are summarized in Table 9.1 (Bhopal, 2008; Gordis, 2009; Merrill and Timmrick, 2006). The criteria may be used for individual health challenges as well as population events.

Though strict adherence to these criteria is perhaps the purview of researchers, CHNs can use them as well. When reading research that examines a particular nursing practice or new intervention, it is prudent to examine the presented results/recommendations in light of the criteria in Table 9.1. Similarly, when CHNs observe a recurring phenomenon that appears to have a relationship with a human or environmental factor, a close examination of the data in light of the criteria may assist them in planning subsequent observations.

Web of Causation Previous chapters have introduced the concept of determinants of health. In contrast to the time when each illness was thought to have a unique and specific cause, it is now recognized that many health problems have multiple causal factors, both direct and indirect. For instance, issues of

TABLE 9.1 Illustrations of Causation Criteria

Temporal relationship	A person does not get the disease until after exposure to the cause
Strength of association	Exposure to a specific stressor or cause is most likely to bring on the disease
Dose-response	Persons who are most exposed to the contaminated food (e.g., ate the most) are the most ill
Specificity	The cause is linked to a specific disease, e.g., *Mycobacterium tuberculosis* does not result in chickenpox
Consistency	Everyone who eats contaminated food gets the illness. If other food in another time and place is contaminated with the same bacteria, the same illness occurs
Biologic plausibility	Consistent with the biologic/medical knowledge that is known (new discoveries may precede biologic plausibility)
Experimental replication	Several studies done by different scientists in different places produce the same or similar results

poverty, education, and environment (e.g., pollution) have been shown to be influential in many health challenges. It is in looking for the causes of today's health challenges and assessing for the presence or absence of particular determinants of health that the CHN is well served by partnering with practitioners from a variety of disciplines. For instance, in addition to other health professionals, the CHN looking at population influences might look to the disciplines of sociology, anthropology, genetics, psychology, geography, and economics. As well, working with experts in social trends and public policy could bring additional understanding to the specific issue at hand.

A model called a **web of causation** can be helpful to CHNs in visualizing the relationships among the many causes or influences of a given health challenge. Within that model, the relationship between the direct and indirect causes can be hypothesized, at which point research studies can be designed to test the hypotheses suggested by the web of causation.

Figure 9.5 illustrates a web of causation for adolescent tobacco use. Obviously, the most direct causes or factors of adolescent tobacco use are the decision to use tobacco and the actual purchase or acquisition of tobacco. However, behind those primary causes are several other causal factors possessing various levels of influence. For instance, the decision to use

FIGURE 9.5 Web of Causation for Adolescent Tobacco Use

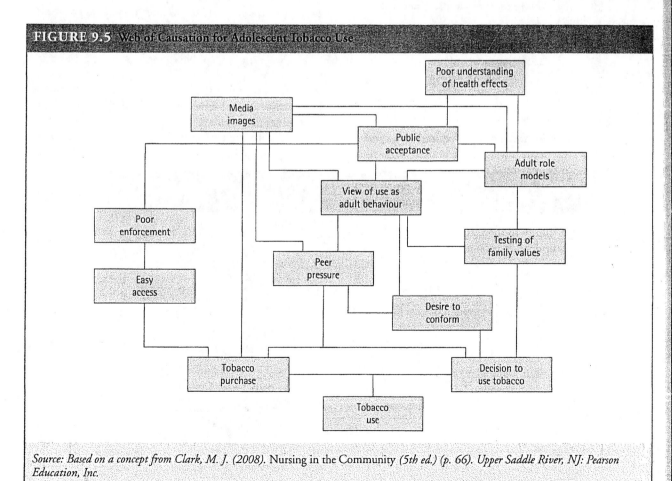

Source: Based on a concept from Clark, M. J. (2008). Nursing in the Community (5th ed.) (p. 66). Upper Saddle River, NJ: Pearson Education, Inc.

tobacco can be influenced both by peer pressure and the testing of family values.

At any one time, each individual is subjected to multiple agents delivered through many modes of transmission. If one compared webs of causation for several common health challenges, some specific health promotion activities would appear to serve more than one purpose. Conversely, there may be a health promotion activity that is helpful for one challenge, but contributes to susceptibility for another challenge. CHNs must examine all possible benefits and consequences of an intervention.

MEASUREMENT IN EPIDEMIOLOGY

To determine the extent of a disease process or health challenge and its final effects on a population, data must be collected and analyzed. However, for the resulting measurements to be useful to the CHN, the raw data or crude numbers must be presented in conjunction with other factors, such as population, time frame, or human characteristic (e.g., gender, race, age). These numbers, expressed as fractions, are known as **rates**. The numerator of each fraction is generally the crude count of the disease in question, and the denominator is generally the size of the population in question. In each case, the population or subpopulation of the numerator and denominator of the fraction are the same. For example, a rate of teen pregnancies might look like this:

$$\text{Rate} = \frac{\text{Number of live births delivered to teen mothers in the population}}{\text{Total number of teen women in the population}}$$

This fraction, or rate, is usually expressed for a set number of the population (e.g., per 100 000 people, per 100 cases, or per 1000 births) so that different-sized populations can be compared.

Table 9.2 presents the formulae for commonly used rates, and the following section describes these rates and shows how they are calculated and how they might be used by CHNs.

Mortality (Death) Rates

Physicians are legally required to complete death certificates for all deaths and file them with the government authorities. Thus, death or **mortality rates** are generally complete and easily obtainable. Mortality rates can be crude or specific in nature. **Crude mortality rates** compare the number of deaths from a specific cause within the entire population, while **specific mortality rates** compare the number of deaths from a specific cause in a particular subgroup with that whole subgroup. For example, if one examined all deaths from motor vehicle collisions and compared them with the total population, one would have a crude mortality rate. However, if one examined only teenage male deaths from motor vehicle collisions, one would compare that with the number of male teens driving at that time, a specific mortality rate. Mortality rates from a specific cause are often different when different subgroups (e.g., teenage males, children aged 4–8, elderly persons) are examined. For example, Figure 9.6 illustrates the age-specific suicide rates for Canada for 2005, stratified (divided) by gender. Note the line that represents the specific total mortality rate for each age group. If only these data were presented, it would be statistically correct, but would fail to inform the reader that the rate for males is significantly higher than for females in each age group. These stratified data would lead one to conclude that males are more susceptible (or at least more successful) than females to death by suicide.

Proportional mortality rates can be used to stratify crude mortality rates. The number of deaths from a specific cause in a given population for a particular time period is compared with the total number of deaths in that same

Rate	Formula
Crude mortality rate	$\dfrac{\text{Total deaths from any cause in a given year in a population}}{\text{Average total population for the same year}}$
Specific mortality rate	$\dfrac{\text{Total deaths from a specific cause in a given year in a population (subgroup)}}{\text{Average number of population (subgroup) for the same year}}$
Infant death rate	$\dfrac{\text{Total deaths of infants in given year in population}}{\text{Total number of live births in same year in population}}$
Prevalence rate	$\dfrac{\text{Number of people with given disease in given population at one point in time}}{\text{Total in given population at same point in time}}$
Incidence rate	$\dfrac{\text{Number of new cases of given disease in population in given time (1 year)}}{\text{Average total population in same time}}$
Relative risk	$\dfrac{\text{Incidence rate of disease in exposed population}}{\text{Incidence of disease in unexposed population}}$

TABLE 9.2 Commonly Used Rates in Epidemiology

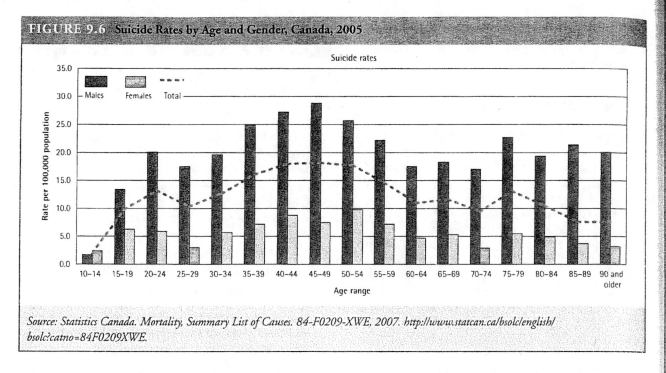

FIGURE 9.6 Suicide Rates by Age and Gender, Canada, 2005

Source: Statistics Canada. Mortality, Summary List of Causes. 84-F0209-XWE, 2007. http://www.statcan.ca/bsolc/english/bsolc?catno=84F0209XWE.

population and time period. A common use of proportional mortality rates is to state that x % of the deaths in a given year were due to breast cancer or motor vehicle collisions (see Figure 9.7). Note that two causes of death, cancers and diseases of the heart, account for over half the deaths.

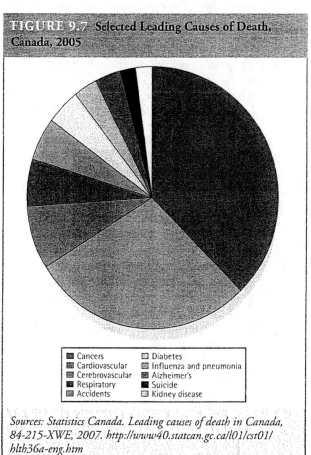

FIGURE 9.7 Selected Leading Causes of Death, Canada, 2005

Legend:
- Cancers
- Cardiovascular
- Cerebrovascular
- Respiratory
- Accidents
- Diabetes
- Influenza and pneumonia
- Alzheimer's
- Suicide
- Kidney disease

Sources: Statistics Canada. Leading causes of death in Canada, 84-215-XWE, 2007. http://www40.statcan.gc.ca/l01/cst01/hlth36a-eng.htm

Historically, the health of a population has been exemplified by maternal and infant mortality rates. Families used to have many children, partly because few were expected to live past the first years of life (assuming the mother and child survived the birth and neonatal period). With the advent of better hygiene as well as prenatal and postnatal care, maternal and infant mortality rates decreased. CHNs often compare infant mortality rates across developing and developed countries, the assumption being that lower maternal and infant mortality rates are indicative of a healthier population. When looking at these statistics, it is particularly important to determine the stage (e.g., perinatal vs. infant) that has been studied so that the comparisons are accurate. The following definitions are used in maternal and infant mortality statistics. In all but the perinatal rate, the denominator is the number of live births in that year in that population.

- Maternal or puerperal death rate: any deaths of the mother resulting from pregnancy-related causes.
- Perinatal death rate: fetal deaths occurring during the last few months of pregnancy and during the first seven days of life. Here the denominator includes both live births and fetal deaths.
- Neonatal death rate: deaths occurring in infants in their first 28 days of life.
- Infant death rate: deaths occurring in the first year of life.

A more recent way of presenting mortality statistics is in terms of **potential years of life lost** (PYLL). This has arisen from the assumption that a person who dies early in life has lost greater potential than has a person who dies much later in life. PYLL statistics give CHNs additional information on which health challenges or diseases result in the greatest lost potential to the population. While this may raise some ethical issues in terms of where a society or country chooses to place its resources, PYLL statistics are certainly a part of the picture that must be heeded.

Survival (Prognosis) Rates

Survival rates are often used to describe the effect of a given disease (e.g., cancer) and are also referred to as prognosis rates. Survival rates partially answer the common client question, "How bad is it?" Survival rates can also be used to compare the efficacy of various treatments for a specific disease. For diseases such as cancer, and its treatments, the prognosis or survival rate most frequently used is the five-year survival rate. This is determined by calculating the percentage of persons with the disease who are alive five years after diagnosis. While five years is a convenient time period to use for comparing the effect of various treatments, it is easy for clients and health professionals alike to fall into the trap of somehow equating five-year survival with a decreased risk of future mortality from that disease. One of the arguments presented in favour of widespread breast screening is early detection of the disease. While it is hoped that early detection coupled with prompt treatment will increase the survival time, there is still conflicting evidence that these actions in fact contribute to decreased mortality rates from breast cancer.

The **case-fatality rate** is calculated by dividing the number of people who die from a disease by the number of people who have the disease, answering the question, "How likely is it that I will die from this disease?" For instance, while recent advances have greatly increased the length of time between the diagnosis of a person with a positive HIV test and that person's death, the case-fatality rate for HIV/AIDS remains very high, as most people will die from the complications of the disease. The case-fatality rate for a person with arthritis, for instance, is much lower.

Morbidity (Illness) Rates

Illness or morbidity rates are valuable for the CHN. **Morbidity rates** give a picture of a population and a disease or health challenge over time, suggesting questions about the susceptibility of the population or subpopulation and the effectiveness of either health promotion or treatment strategies. Two types of rate are commonly used to describe morbidity in a population. The first is **prevalence,** which provides a picture of a specific disease process in a population at one given point in time. The second is **incidence,** which describes the identification of new cases of a disease in a population over time. Together with mortality rates and survival rates, they present a fairly complete picture of the population's response to a disease or health challenge.

If the disease is short-lived, such as measles or the flu, the prevalence does not reveal much. However, CHNs might use this rate in epidemic situations to plan for extra staff to deal with increased inquiries or clinic visits from concerned clients, for example during the H1N1 crisis. If the disease is short-lived, resulting in few deaths, the incidence and prevalence

CASE STUDY

Recently, the whole world was caught up in the issue of H1N1 and the vaccination for this disease. The lay press was full of stories discussing the severity of the threat, as well as the efficacy of the vaccine in preventing it. One of the popular topics was who was at risk and who should get the vaccine, and in what order. For example, which age segments of the population should be vaccinated first, or were there special groups who should be treated differently because of their perceived importance to society? This decision was approached in diverse ways in different sections of the country. From the viewpoint of the committee charged with implementing the rollout of a vaccine for a given health challenge like H1N1, consider the following questions.

Discussion Questions

1. How would the committee use epidemiological data to inform them about the health challenge? What other data might the committee consider?

2. What sources of information would the committee consult to inform them and why?

3. What information would it be important to share with the media to inform the public about the health challenge and the committee's plans?

rates are very similar. If, on the other hand, the health challenge is chronic in nature, the incidence rate (number of new cases) stays fairly static over time, while the prevalence rate increases as more people live with the disease. If the disease is long-term with complications, such as diabetes or multiple sclerosis, the prevalence rate over time informs CHNs about the need for community and institutional support for the future. This is very important in terms of public and community health planning.

The population in question is usually the population at risk for the disease. For instance, when calculating the incidence of prostate cancer, the number of cases is compared with the population of males, rather than with the whole population. Incidence rates, when calculated within the same population over several years, show whether the population seems more or less susceptible to the disease in question. For example, the number of motor vehicle collisions in a given year involving teenage drivers might change over time in response to changes in the legal drinking age.

When CHNs test for a specific cause of a health challenge, they compare the incidence of that health challenge in a population exposed to the identified cause with the incidence of the same health challenge in a population not exposed to the same cause. If the suspected cause was indeed a factor, one would expect the incidence rates to be quite different. For example, one would expect the incidence of lung cancer to be much greater in smokers than in non-smokers. If the cause being examined is not the *only* cause of the disease (e.g., lung cancer), one might find that the incidence rates are more similar than expected. Such results might lead the CHN to explore other factors (e.g., second-hand smoke) to explain the incidence rates.

One frequently asked question is, "Are some populations more at risk of or vulnerable to a specific disease than others?" To find the answer to that question, a statistic known as **relative risk** is used. This measure divides the incidence of a given problem or disease in a population exposed to a given risk factor by the incidence of the same problem in a population not exposed to the same risk. For example, CHNs might compare the incidence of childhood asthma in a population exposed to a certain air pollutant with the incidence in a population not exposed to that pollutant. If the resulting number is 1.0, it means that both groups have the same risk of the health problem, and most likely the risk factor in question makes little or no difference. If the resulting number is >1.0, it indicates that the risk in the exposed group is higher than the risk in the unexposed group, and the risk factor in question is at least one of the significant risk factors for the problem or disease. Should the relative risk ratio be <1.0, the given risk factor is probably not significant for the problem or disease. However, such results may indicate that the factor in question has a protective effect; for example, a population where the physical activity is high may have a low relative risk for diabetes.

Incidence and prevalence rates can be further stratified to increase the descriptiveness of the statistic. Data are frequently obtained through interviewing members of the population, also known as self-reporting. For instance, the question, "Do you currently smoke?" elicits data that could contribute to a **point prevalence** statistic of smokers in the population. This statistic describes the situation only for that particular point in time. The question, "Have you smoked within the last six months?" gives us data that could be useful for **period prevalence** statistics. However, asking, "Have you ever smoked?" gives the researcher data that could be used for **cumulative** or **lifetime incidence** statistics. This demonstrates why it is important for researchers to clearly state their methods and sources of data in journal articles and reports, and why it is equally important for CHNs reading those articles to critically examine the evidence presented.

RESEARCH IN EPIDEMIOLOGY

Sources of Epidemiologic Data

Surveillance is the constant watching or monitoring of diseases to assess patterns and quickly identify events that do not fit the pattern. In the case of infectious diseases, surveillance may also include the monitoring of people with the disease, and their contacts. In the case of diseases with a genetic component, data may be collected to track the disease through extended family relationships.

Surveillance and other epidemiological analyses and research are only as good as the data on which they are based. Thus, CHNs need to ensure that they use consistent and accurate sources of data. One of the largest sources of epidemiologic

data is the government. Canada has several sources of government or government-funded data such as the Public Health Agency of Canada, Health Canada, Statistics Canada, and the provincial government health ministries. As birth and death statistics are required by law to be filed with the appropriate government agency, they are generally very accurate. Birth and death statistics can be teamed with the census data reported by Statistics Canada for further detail. Statistics Canada data can be found in their daily newsletter (*The Daily*), which reports on recent data and analysis and often provides a historical trend analysis for the disease (e.g., breast cancer) or issue (e.g., family structure in Canada). Statistics Canada also has a website where more detailed information such as profiles of individual communities and archived newsletters can be found.

In the wake of Walkerton and SARS, it was recognized that a stronger emphasis on public health by the government was required. In response, the Public Health Agency of Canada (PHAC) was formed. Many of the reports and statistics previously reported by Health Canada may now be found at the PHAC website. These include information on surveillance of **reportable diseases** (diseases that are required to be reported by law, for example, tuberculosis, sexually transmitted infections, AIDS) as well as surveillance data on cancer, chronic disease, and cardiovascular diseases. Health Canada remains a source of information on many disease states, including epidemiological data and links to other sites. All provinces also maintain health websites that provide information for the province in question. Specifically, many of the provincial health ministry websites provide birth and infant mortality statistics.

The Canadian Institute for Health Information (CIHI) is also an excellent source for data. A non-governmental organization, CIHI collects and collates information from many sources to provide analyses that can inform policy. The epidemiological data that it reports includes data from hospital sources and from the various provincial health plans. Thus, this organization may provide information on incidence and prevalence of non-reportable diseases.

In addition, there are agencies that focus solely on specific disease issues. For example, the Canadian Diabetes Association or the Heart and Stroke Foundation of Canada are sources for statistics relative to those diseases. When using information found on the Internet, the CHN needs to examine the source of the data to ensure it is from a reputable organization.

For the CHN wanting to compare data between Canada and the United States, the Centers for Disease Control and Prevention website is a valuable resource. For international data, the World Health Organization's website is very helpful. These and other selected websites are listed at the end of this chapter. In addition to websites, many organizations produce a variety of reports that are frequently found in university and college libraries or are available for download or purchase in print.

The final source of data is to gather data oneself. Although this can result in accurate data that deal with the specific question being asked, the cost of creating a survey instrument that is clear and understood by all respondents, choosing an appropriate sample (especially a national sample), and gathering the data often is beyond the financial reach of most researchers. If this is the case, researchers may be able to add questions to a survey being conducted by a community healthcare centre or agency.

Types of Epidemiological Research

Research is one method of finding answers to questions. It is critical that CHNs have a clear understanding of research methodologies in order to understand, participate in, and conduct research. This is because the study design is strongly linked to the research question: if an inappropriate study design is chosen, the results will not provide answers.

Different authors categorize types of epidemiologic research in different ways. For example, Grobbee and Hoes (2009) viewed it from a medical perspective and categorized in terms of diagnostic, etiologic, prognostic, and intervention research—each contributing different kinds of evidence to use in clinical practice. Conversely, Bhopal (2008) used the types of research designs as the categories—case series/population case, cross-sectional, case-control, cohort, and trial. The first four can also be termed observational or descriptive research, because they are concerned with the variables of time, person, and place and answer the basic questions of who, when, and where. Analytic observational research adds the techniques of comparison and attempts to answer the questions of how and why. Trial or intervention research is considered experimental research, where the researcher manipulates selected variables and, for example, examines the efficacy of a new treatment, tests for causality, or compares communities in terms of a public health intervention. In the following section, each of the research designs will be considered.

Case series studies are counts of selected variables within a specific population. Through this data collection the researcher determines morbidity and mortality rates, and through analysis of the various factors, looks for evidence of association and causality. Case series studies are often the basis of higher level studies—and provide the researcher with data to generate hypotheses to be tested. Examples of research questions that could be answered include: "Are mortality rates for cardiac disease higher for men than for women," "Does age at diagnosis or geographic residence affect survival rates for persons with multiple sclerosis," and "What are the current incidence rates for HIV in young homosexual males compared with 5, 10, or 20 years ago?" Frequently, factors that increase risk may be used as a variable of interest; for example, gender may be considered to be a risk factor for heart disease.

Cross-sectional studies are snapshots of the present and may also be called prevalence studies. Cross-sectional data may be collected as baseline data for planning and implementing interventions, or to measure change. For example, CHNs may be concerned about the age of initiation of smoking behaviours relative to a specific planned health curriculum. The CHNs may work with the community to develop an anonymous survey that asks about smoking behaviours and administer it to students in various grade levels within the

school district. The results of the survey may indicate that more than one-third of students in Grade 6 have already tried smoking, suggesting that beginning health education about smoking in Grade 6 is too late. The CHNs and teachers decide to move their initial anti-smoking education to Grades 1 and 2, in which fewer than 3% of the students have tried to smoke. A time series of cross-sectional studies could also be used with a particular group of students to assess the effectiveness of the intervention. After implementing the new curriculum in Grades 1 and 2, Grade 6 classes would be tested in subsequent years. The data would be compared with those from the present Grade 6 students, who did not receive the intervention, to ascertain if the program made a difference in the future smoking behaviours of students.

CANADIAN RESEARCH BOX

Can e-communication assist in social support for mothers of infants and toddlers?

Hall, W., & Irvine, V. (2009). E-communication among mothers of infants and toddlers in a community-based cohort: A content analysis. *Journal of Advanced Nursing, 65*(1), 175–183.

In this research, the use of e-communication was examined as a health-promoting activity for mothers of infants and toddlers. Preliminary assumptions included noting that mothers within this cohort who are also working may feel somewhat isolated in terms of finding support. Forty middle-class Canadian mothers who were already involved in an online support group completed a quantitative survey and gave permission for the researchers to analyze the online communication within the group. Researchers found that the women "used the e-cohort to develop community connections, request and provide emotional support, share information and facilitate learning, and normalize infants' development and mothers' parenting experiences" (p. 178).

Discussion Questions

1. What other community cohorts may experience isolation in terms of health issues within their families?

2. How could the CHN use this study to examine alternate ways to provide support or other health promotion activities in a community?

In **case-control** studies, the individuals in the group with the disease are matched with individuals who are similar in some characteristics (e.g., age, gender, time, geographic residence) but who have not manifested the disease in question. The health histories or characteristics of the individuals in both groups are then obtained. These data are compared and the common factors/differences are identified between the two populations.

A case-control study of children with type 2 diabetes would include children with the disease in one group and children without the disease in the other group. The two groups would be matched for age and geographic location. The epidemiologist might search for common and different factors such as amount of physical activity, obesity, and family

TABLE 9.3   Calculation of Odds Ratio

Risk Factor	Persons with Lung Cancer	Persons without Lung Cancer	Total
Smokers	35 (a)	15 (b)	55
Non-smokers	15 (c)	135 (d)	145
Total	50	150	200

$$\text{Odds ratio} = \frac{\text{Exposed persons with the disease/unexposed persons with the disease}}{\text{Exposed persons without the disease/unexposed persons without the disease}}$$

$$OR = \frac{a/c}{b/d} = \frac{ad}{bc} = \frac{(35)(135)}{(15)(15)} = \frac{4725}{225} = 21$$

The odds ratio for these data is 21. As with the relative risk ratio, a number >1.0 means that the persons exposed to the risk factor are more likely to develop the disease than those who are not exposed. In this example, male smokers are 21 times as likely to develop lung cancer as men who do not smoke.

history of diabetes. In each case, the researcher would expect to find some similarities and differences between the two groups that could contribute to theories of causality.

The relative risk ratio compares the risk for a particular disease between two populations: one exposed to a stressor and one not exposed to the stressor. Case-control studies also involve two groups: one group composed of individuals who have the disease and one of individuals who do not have the disease. Relative risk cannot be calculated here because neither the incidence nor the prevalence is known. The **odds ratio** provides epidemiologists with an estimate of the relative risk factor. To demonstrate the calculation of this statistic, consider the following example. A hypothetical community health centre practice has 200 male patients between the ages of 45 and 65; 50 of them have lung cancer and 150 do not. Thirty-five of the patients with lung cancer are smokers, while 15 patients without lung cancer are smokers. Table 9.3 illustrates the calculation of the odds ratio for this example.

In **cohort studies**, the researcher examines the individual histories of a group of people manifesting a particular disease to find out what common factors they share and what differences can be discerned. Cohort studies may be retrospective or prospective. **Retrospective studies** are studies that begin in the present and search the past for information to explain the present **Prospective studies** (or longitudinal studies) begin in the present and follow the subjects into the future or make predictions about the future that can be tested at a later date. These studies focus on individuals exposed to a particular health problem or potential stressor over time. For a prospective study, it is important to measure the incidence of the problem at various times. For instance, a group of people with high exposure to a stressor (e.g., occupational stress) may be matched with a group of people with low exposure to the problem, and both are followed for a period of time. The incidence levels of the health problem being studied (e.g., hypertension or myocardial infarction) in the two groups are compared at each measuring time.

CANADIAN RESEARCH BOX 9.2

Are there gender differences in community-based persons with a history of mental illness?

Forchuk, D., Jensen, E., Csiernik, R., Ward-Griffin, C., Ray, S., Montgomery, P., & Wan, L. (2009). Exploring differences between community-based women and men with a history of mental illness. *Issues in Mental Health Nursing, 30,* 495–502.

In this study, the researchers wanted to explore the relationship between gender and indicators of health status. Secondary analysis of data gathered as part of a longitudinal study on housing situations for psychiatric consumers/survivors was examined in light of gender. A total of 1503 community clients completed part of the study; all participants were offered the opportunity to participate in subsequent years. Factors where gender provided significant differences included that more women than men were diagnosed with a mood disorder, while more men were diagnosed with schizophrenia. More men had substance abuse issues compounding their mental health issues. More women were likely to suffer from post-traumatic stress disorder. No significant differences in levels of functioning were noted, but more women identified support people present in their lives. Finally, more women than men were housed rather than homeless. It was noted that some findings (e.g., age, demographic characteristics, and degree of severity of illness) were not statistically significant according to gender, nor varied across the five years of data collection.

Discussion Questions

1. How could the CHN use this study to influence the type of interview questions he/she used with clients with mental illness?

2. How might the CHN use this study to implement housing services in a community while paying attention to gender differences noted?

Prospective studies have several problems:

- The sample size must be very large at the beginning to allow for attrition as people move, die, or lose interest.
- It is evident that health problems generally increase with increased age. By its very nature, a longitudinal study follows a group of people who are aging. Thus, a method to control for the effects of aging must be applied to any results.
- Outside factors may affect the different groups differently. For instance, researchers may decide to compare hypertension in Canadian and U.S. executives who live in large cities and experience long commutes to work. The cities chosen are Toronto, Montreal, Chicago, and New York. The time frame is 1990–2010. Might the events of September 11, 2001, have an effect on the data and results?

In trials or experimental studies, the researcher manipulates some of the variables in order to ascertain the effect of the manipulation. **Manipulation** means to change something that is happening to some or all of the subjects within the study, rather than only observing what is present. In healthcare, the manipulation usually involves a new treatment or the encouragement of a new behaviour. The researcher believes that the new treatment or behaviour will positively affect the health of the subjects and uses the research to test that belief or hypothesis.

The "gold standard" of experimental study design is the **randomized controlled trial** (RCT). In fact, some scientists consider this the only valid form of experimental design. In an RCT design, individuals are assigned randomly either to a group that receives the new treatment or to a group that does not receive the new treatment. The latter is known as the control group. After a period of time, specific variables are measured in each group and compared. Frequently, neither the researchers nor the subjects are aware of which group they are part of until the end of the study. This is known as a blind RCT.

In community nursing and health promotion, the treatment or intervention studied may be a new health education or social marketing protocol (e.g., new advertisements for breast screening) or a change in policy (e.g., adding fluoride to drinking water for a community). In the example of new marketing for screening, the outcome examined could be the increase or decrease in the number of persons participating in the screening. In the case of adding fluoride to the drinking water, the outcome measured might be the number of dental cavities found in six-year-olds.

In the examples above, randomized control groups would be almost impossible. One variation of this might be that several communities may be compared, with one or more serving as treatment groups and the others serving as control groups. Another variation may be that the community might serve as its own control group—measuring the outcome of interest (e.g., participation in screening) before and after the treatment (e.g., advertising for breast screening clinics).

Ethical Concerns Ethical concerns during observational studies such as case, cross-sectional, case-control, or cohort are rare but possible because of the nature of those studies. The researcher is not manipulating the variables, but is systematically collecting and analyzing observations to make inferences and predictions. However, CHNs must always remember that most people are interested in participating in any study that they perceive will help someone else with a health problem. If a researcher has no intention of *using* the data (e.g., to plan interventions that are intended to be carried out), it is unethical to collect them. Ethics approval must be sought for any study where data are collected about or from humans. In any trial or experimental study, the competing issues of strong scientific experimental design and ethical considerations must be addressed. The first ethical concern is how the human subjects are approached. Most healthcare agencies and university research centres have an ethics committee that reviews research proposals to ensure that humans are treated fairly, the information is gathered and used in a confidential manner, and the privacy of the subjects is protected. However, ethical questions also arise about the design of the research. For instance, is it ethical to withhold a treatment that is felt to be beneficial from people who need it because a research design with a control group would be more scientific? Researchers must consider these questions and consult with appropriate sources for advice when designing scientific and ethical research studies.

SUMMARY

In this chapter, the science of epidemiology, its historical influences, and the evolution of its theoretical underpinnings were examined. The theories have been presented with modern examples, illustrating how the historical continues to have influence in the present. The notions of agent, host, and environment have been discussed, as well as modes of transmission and the natural history of disease.

Measurement is an important concept in epidemiology, and mortality, morbidity, and survival rates were each presented. The notion of risk or susceptibility was examined both theoretically and statistically. The importance of accurate sources for epidemiologic data was noted, as well as sources for Canadian data. Observational and experimental research designs were presented, with the caution that it is very important that the research design should fit the research question. Causality as a societal belief as well as a statistical conclusion was noted, and causality criteria that the CHN can use to examine observations as well as published research were included. The notion of the web of causation was presented to coincide with the current belief in multiple direct and indirect causes for most health challenges.

The science of epidemiology is an important one for the CHN. Community health professionals are confronted with increasingly complex health challenges that were unheard of just a few short decades ago, such as type 2 diabetes in children. It is becoming increasingly evident that Hippocrates had it right more than two millennia ago: nurses must look at what the person eats, what the person does, and what the person's habits are. Health practitioners face the task of using the results of epidemiologic research to influence citizens to change or enhance their activities of daily living to actively promote maximum health, while recognizing that the individual and group environment may well influence people in other directions.

Modern CHNs, while facing more complex challenges, also have the advantages of access to strong data, government and societal interest in health, and a better-educated populace. The science of epidemiology is but one of their tools.

KEY TERMS

epidemiology, p. 139
host, p. 141
agent, p. 141
environment, p. 141
epidemiologic model, p. 141
vector, p. 141
Venn diagram, p. 141
susceptibility, p. 141
risk, p. 141
mode of transmission, p. 142
direct transmission, p. 142
indirect transmission, p. 142
pathogen, p. 142
prepathogenesis, p. 143
stressors, p. 143
incubation, p. 143
primary prevention, p. 143
pathogenesis, p. 143
secondary prevention, p. 143
screening, p. 143
tertiary prevention, p. 143
association, p. 143
causation, p. 143
web of causation, p. 144
rates, p. 145
mortality rates, p. 145
crude mortality rates, p. 145
specific mortality rates, p. 145
proportional mortality rates, p. 145
potential years of life lost (PYLL), p. 146
survival rates, p. 147
case-fatality rate, p. 147
morbidity rate, p. 147
prevalence, p. 147
incidence, p. 147
relative risk, p. 148
point prevalence, p. 148
period prevalence, p. 148
cumulative or lifetime incidence, p. 148
surveillance, p. 148
reportable diseases, p. 148
case series, p. 149
cross-sectional studies, p. 149
case control, p. 149
odds ratio, p. 150
cohort studies, p. 150

retrospective studies, p. 150
prospective studies, p. 150
manipulation, p. 151
randomized controlled trial, p. 151

REVIEW QUESTIONS

Choose the one alternative that best completes the statement or answers the question.

1. Statistics that assist the CHN to understand the ultimate threat (death) to a population from a specific health challenge are
   a) morbidity.   c) mortality.
   b) survival.   d) stratified prevalence.

2. A group of CHNs want to discover the knowledge and sexual activity within the school district. The research design that they use would most likely be
   a) cohort.
   b) cross sectional.
   c) case control.
   d) trial.

3. Tuberculosis and STIs are examples of
   a) infectious diseases.
   b) case studies.
   c) reportable diseases.
   d) census statistics.

4. Risk is an important concept in epidemiology because
   a) different segments of the population respond to stressors in different ways.
   b) it represents the threat of a health challenge to the professionals working in the population.
   c) the ultimate goal of a CHN is to remove all sources of risk in a population.
   d) it assists the CHN to understand the survival rates of a given health challenge.

5. The most important reason that experimental research (trials) may be difficult in population healthcare is
   a) it is too complicated to get more than one segment of the population to participate.
   b) experimental population health research is very costly and labour intensive.
   c) the results take such a long time to achieve that finding funding is impossible.
   d) it is often unethical to withhold a helpful treatment or innovation from one segment of the population.

STUDY QUESTIONS

1. Identify and define five criteria for causality.

2. Differentiate between mortality and morbidity rates. How does each inform the CHN?

3. Name and define three types of observational studies relating to CHN practice. Using different examples from those in the chapter, suggest two research questions that might be answered with each of the types.

4. Identify the three elements of the epidemiologic triangle and define each.

5. Differentiate between incidence and prevalence. What does it mean when the incidence and prevalence rates for a given health problem are very different? What does it mean when they are very similar?

6. Describe prospective and retrospective studies and give two examples of research questions that could be answered with each.

After working through these questions, go to the MyNursingLab at **www.pearsoned.ca/mynursinglab** *to check your answers.*

INDIVIDUAL CRITICAL THINKING EXERCISES

1. Select a health problem. Using Figure 9.3 as a guide, suggest five CHN actions for each level of prevention. Include actions for individuals as well as populations. How might CHNs collaborate with other health professionals to implement the actions?

2. Discuss the pros and cons of having national registries for disease process such as tumours, diabetes, and HIV/AIDS. Did your discussion differ according to the statistics available regarding incidence and prevalence? What about possible social stigma?

3. One of the more recent mortality statistics is PYLL. Suicide is one health problem that is examined in terms of PYLL. Using the data in Figure 9.6, at what age group would you target your prevention interventions? Why? How did the concept of PYLL influence your decision?

4. How might CHNs use their knowledge of surveillance and epidemiological data for their community to influence their practice? How can CHNs be involved in epidemiological research and/or the collection and analysis of epidemiological data?

5. Why are infant and child mortality rates used as a measure of the health of a population? Using the national and provincial infant mortality rates (www40.statcan.gc.ca/l01/cst01/health21a-eng.htm), what do you discern about provincial disparities? Are you surprised? What factors might influence the rates noted? Where might you go to find further evidence?

GROUP CRITICAL THINKING EXERCISES

1. Select a condition that you are familiar with (e.g., type 2 diabetes, asthma, heart attack). From two different provinces' health websites and the Public Health Agency of Canada website, compare the mortality and morbidity rates for that condition. Are they similar or different? What factors might influence the rates in those jurisdictions?

2. As a group, discuss the pros and cons of using an epidemiological approach to planning CHN actions.

3. Physical activity is recognized as a protector of health for all humans, regardless of age and current health status. Using the table found at http://www40.statcan.gc.ca/l01/cst01/health78b-eng.htm and http://www40.statcan.gc.ca/l01/cst01/health46-eng.htm, consider how you might design a national campaign aimed at increasing physical activity. Which groups would be most important to target? Why?

REFERENCES

Bhopal, R. (2008). *Concepts of epidemiology: Integrating the ideas, theories, principles and methods of epidemiology.* New York, NY: Oxford University Press.

Cohen, I. B. (1984). Florence Nightingale. *Scientific American, 3,* 128–137.

Friis, R. H., & Sellers, T. A. (2009). *Epidemiology for public health practice* (4th ed.). Sudbury, MA: Jones and Bartlett.

Gordis, L. (2009). *Epidemiology* (4th ed.). Philadelphia, PA: W. B. Saunders.

Grobbee, D. E., & Hoes, A. W. (2009). *Clinical epidemiology: Principles, methods and applications for clinical research.* Sudbury, MA: Jones and Bartlett.

Harkness, G. A. (1995). *Epidemiology in nursing practice.* St. Louis, MO: Mosby.

Hill, A. B. (1965). The environment and disease: Association or causation? *Proceedings of the Royal Society of Medicine, 58,* 295–300.

Hippocrates. (400 BCE). *On airs, waters and places.* The Internet Classics Archive. Retrieved from http://classics.mit.edu/Hippocrates/airwatpl.1.1.html

Leavell, H. F., & Clark, E. G. (1965). *Preventive medicine for the doctor in his community: An epidemiologic approach.* New York, NY: McGraw-Hill.

Merril, R. M., & Timmreck, T. C. (2006). *An introduction to epidemiology.* Sudbury, MA: Jones and Bartlett.

Porta, M. S., & the International Epidemiological Association. (2008). *A dictionary of epidemiology* (5th ed.). Oxford, UK: Oxford University Press.

Timmreck, T. C. (1998). *An introduction to epidemiology.* Sudbury, MA: Jones and Bartlett.

Timmreck, T. C. (2002). *An introduction to epidemiology* (2nd ed.). Sudbury, MA: Jones and Bartlett.

ADDITIONAL RESOURCES

Websites

B.C. Ministry of Health Services
http://www.vs.gov.bc.ca/stats/

Alberta Health Ministry
http://www.health.gov.ab.ca

Saskatchewan Ministry of Health
http://www.health.gov.sk.ca/

Manitoba Health, Public Health
http://www.gov.mb.ca/health/publichealth/

Ontario Ministry of Health and Long-Term Care
http://www.health.gov.on.ca

Quebec—Santé et services sociaux
http://www.msss.gouv.qc.ca/en/

New Brunswick Health
http://www.gnb.ca/0051/index-e.asp

Nova Scotia, Department of Health
http://www.gov.ns.ca/health/

Prince Edward Island Health and Social Services
http://www.gov.pe.ca/hss/index.php3

Newfoundland and Labrador Health Information System
http://www.nlchi.nf.ca/

Nunavut Health and Social Services
http://www.gov.nu.ca/health/

Northwest Territories Health and Social Services
http://www.hlthss.gov.nt.ca/

Canadian Institute of Health Information
http://www.cihi.ca

CCDR (Canada Communicable Disease Report)
http://www.phac-aspc.gc.ca/publicat/ccdr-rmtc/

Centers for Disease Control and Prevention (U.S.)
http://www.cdc.gov

CDC Morbidity and Mortality Weekly Report (CDC—U.S.)
http://www.cdc.gov/mmwr/

CDC National Center for Health Statistics (U.S.)
http://www.cdc.gov/nchs

Health Canada
http://www.hc-sc.gc.ca

Public Health Agency of Canada
http://www.phac-aspc.gc.ca

PHAC Notifiable Disease Report
http://www.phac-aspc.gc.ca/bid-bmi/dsd-dsm/ndmr-rmmdo/index.html

Statistics Canada
http://www.statcan.ca

World Health Organization Weekly Epidemiological Record
http://www.who.int/wer

About the Author

Lynnette Leeseberg Stamler, RN, PhD, is Professor and Assistant Dean at the College of Nursing, University of Saskatchewan. She completed her BSN at St. Olaf College, Minnesota; her MEd at the University of Manitoba; and her PhD at the University of Cincinnati. Her research interests include patient/health education, diabetes education, nursing education, and quality care. She was a VON nurse for four years prior to her teaching career. She is active in national and international nursing organizations, including Sigma Theta Tau International, the Nursing Honor Society, and was President of the Canadian Association of Schools of Nursing from 2008–2010.

Research

Donna Ciliska and Rebecca Ganann

OBJECTIVES

After studying this chapter, you should be able to:

1. Describe evidence-based practice as it relates to community health nursing.
2. Critically appraise research articles reporting on the effectiveness of treatment, prevention, or qualitative research to judge whether they should be utilized in practice, management, or policy decisions.
3. Understand the barriers to utilizing research to change practice, management, and policy making.
4. Define how one might be involved in future community health research.

INTRODUCTION

Community health nurses (CHNs) continuously participate in research and have opportunities, frequently unrecognized, for improving their care by utilizing high-quality research. For example:

- Maternal-child CHNs provide breastfeeding support as part of their role, but they are not sure about the effectiveness. Are there any interventions that have been shown to increase the duration and exclusivity of breastfeeding? Can peer telephone support increase the duration of breastfeeding in new mothers (Dennis et al., 2002)?
- The local school board is concerned that there is too little time to teach the required curriculum, so they are considering reducing the time spent in physical activity. At the same time, the region is concerned about the increasing numbers of overweight children. Are school-based physical activity programs effective in improving activity duration in children (Dobbins et al., 2009)?
- Parents of developmentally delayed children experience considerable stress. Can parenting programs reduce their psychological distress (Singer et al., 2007)?

Every day, questions like these face CHNs. After graduation, how can nurses continue to be educated critical thinkers whose practice is based on high-quality research evidence? How can busy nurses keep current with the research findings? How can nurses meet the provincial nursing standards for using evidence in practice, the national public health Core Competencies (Public Health Agency of Canada, 2008), or the national Community Health Nursing Standards of Practice

(Community Health Nurses Association of Canada (2008)? This chapter highlights strategies that CHNs can use to develop and sustain evidence-based nursing practice.

WHAT IS EVIDENCE-BASED NURSING?

The term **evidence-based nursing** (EBN) has evolved from the initial work done in evidence-based medicine and is defined as the conscientious, explicit, and judicious use of current best evidence in making decisions about the care of individual patients. The practice of evidence-based medicine means integrating individual clinical expertise with the best available external clinical evidence from systematic research (Sackett et al., 1996). We have conceptualized "evidence-based nursing" as broader in context than research utilization. The practice of EBN involves the following steps:

- formulation of an answerable question to address a specific patient problem or situation (Flemming, 1998);
- systematic search for research evidence that could be used to answer the question (McKibbon & Marks, 1998a; 1998b);
- appraisal of the validity, relevance, and applicability of research evidence;
- decision making regarding a change in practice;
- implementation of the evidence-based practice decision; and
- evaluation of the outcome of the decision.

In evidence-based practice, research utilization is integrated with other information that might influence the management of health issues and problems, such as clinical expertise, client preference for alternative forms of care, and available resources (DiCenso et al., 1998). In Figure 10.1, elements in evidence-based decision making are presented. In the figure they all have equal weight; however, this is unlikely in reality. For example, peer breastfeeding supporters have the skills to teach and support breastfeeding, have employers who encourage them to utilize work time doing the intervention, and know from the research evidence that the breastfeeding intervention is effective (Dennis et al., 2002). However, some new mothers may see the peer support person as intrusive and be unwilling to allow it to occur, even by telephone. Similarly, you tell your clients with osteoarthritis that glucosamine can be effective (Towheed et al., 2005), but some of your patients do not have the money to purchase it.

Historically, some people have misunderstood evidence-based practice to mean the application of research findings to a decision, regardless of the context or patient preferences. In an effort to overcome some of that connotation, some authors now call the process "evidence-informed practice," particularly in relation to the use of evidence in policy making (Canadian Health Services Research Foundation, 2004). What difference does the use of research make? Heater et al. (1988) conducted a meta-analysis to determine the contribution of research-based practice to client outcomes. They found 84 nurse-conducted studies involving 4146 patients and reported that clients who received research-based nursing care made "sizeable gains" in behavioural knowledge and physiological and psychosocial outcomes compared with those receiving routine nursing care. The same review would be a massive undertaking today, as there are so many more studies that would need to be included.

So why don't all nurses base their practice on evidence? Luker and Kenrick (1992) used qualitative techniques in an exploratory study of CHN decision making in the United Kingdom and determined that the nurses had an awareness of research but did not perceive it as informing their practice. Bostrom and Suter (1993) found that only 21% of 1200 practising nurses had implemented a new research finding in the previous six months. Nurses have reported difficulty in accessing and appraising published research, either because they do not have access to journals and libraries or because they have not been taught how to find and appraise research (Blythe & Royle, 1993; Pearcey, 1995).

Estabrooks (1998) surveyed staff nurses about their use of various sources of knowledge. Those most frequently used were found to be experiential, intuition, workplace sources, nursing school (even though the average length of time since completing their basic nursing education program was 18 years), physician sources, and past usual practice. Literature (whether in textbook or journal form) was rated in the bottom five sources of information for frequency of use. The nurses were also asked to identify the one most common source from which they learned about research findings. Though 39% identified nursing journals, additional analyses revealed that the primary journals the nurses were reading were not research journals, but rather trade magazines published by nursing professional organizations. The more current research has switched focus from general use and measurement of use of research to specific instances of understanding the factors that determine specific research utilization (Dobbins, Davies, Danseco, Edwards, & Virani, 2005; Farmer et al., 2008; Graham et al., 2006; Légaré, Turcot, Grimshaw, Harvey, McGowan, & Wolf, 2008.

The sheer volume of research is more than any nurse can manage. Nurses working individually could only hope to find and read a small proportion of the research that is published each year. This is compounded by the fact that much of the research relevant to community health nursing is published in non-nursing journals.

There is a substantial time lag of 8 to 15 years between the time technical information is generated and the time it is used in actual practice (Lomas, 1991; Utterback, 1974). In addition to barriers faced by individual nurses, multiple political, cultural, economic, and other environmental barriers must be overcome in order to practise in an evidence-based way. However, this chapter will focus more on the abilities and strategies of individual nurses and teams of nurses to implement evidence-based practice.

FIGURE 10.1 Evidence-Based Decision Making

Clinical state and circumstances

Patient preferences and actions

Clinical Expertise

Research evidence

Health care resources

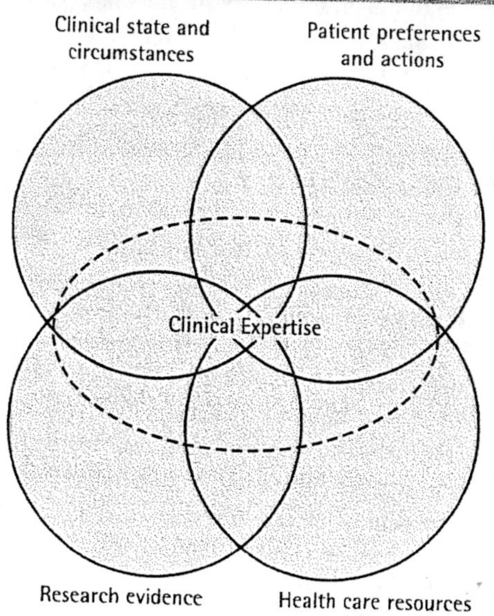

Source: Based on model by DiCenso, A., Cullum, N., & Ciliska, D. (2008). Implementing evidence-based nursing: Some misconceptions. In N. Cullum, D. Ciliska, R. B. Haynes, & S. Marks (Eds.), Evidence-based nursing: An introduction. Oxford, UK: Blackwell.

THE PROCESS OF EVIDENCE-BASED NURSING

Asking Clinical Questions

Nurses need to maintain inquiring minds in order to evaluate interventions and consider options for other interventions. In order to find relevant research, **clinical questions** (also called **structured questions**) need to be structured, usually to consist of the situation, the intervention, and the outcomes (Flemming, 1998). The **situation** is the patient, client, population, or problem being addressed; the **intervention** is the action that is under consideration for some health promotion, disease prevention, or treatment effect; and the **outcome** is the result of interest from the client or clinical perspective. To return to some of the questions in the "What Is EBN?" section, above, the phrasing of the questions might be:

- For new mothers (situation), does a structured breastfeeding support program delivered by a CHN (intervention) affect duration and exclusivity of breastfeeding, and gastrointestinal infections or eczema in the infants (outcomes)?
- Is glucosamine (intervention) effective in reducing pain and increasing functional ability (outcomes) in people with osteoarthritis (situation)?

Conducting an Efficient Search of the Literature

When you conduct a search, you can consider synonymous terms for the situations, interventions, and outcomes. For example, for the patient or population, new mothers might be found under other search terms such as postpartum, maternal, primipara, or multipara. The same process is followed for the interventions and outcomes. This will allow you to find all the possible search terms for an efficient search. The most efficient search is done with the help of a health sciences librarian, taking the original question, the list of synonyms for each component of the question, and any articles already found on the subject. The latter will allow the librarian to see how this type of article is indexed in the relevant databases. It is also important to be clear about the purpose in finding this literature. Is the goal to find a systematic review (which would give direction regarding management or policy and procedure decisions; see the section "What Is a Systematic Review?" below), or are the details of the interventions and their effectiveness needed (in which case the review would give the references for the studies, but one would likely want the individual primary studies as well)?

But what if you don't have access to a librarian? The most time-efficient sources of good data are the websites that give you "pre-appraised" research, meaning they have selected the best articles through critically appraising, rating, and summarizing the research, and just giving you the good quality research, or the "gold nuggets." For nurses in Canada in community health, the first "go-to" place for pre-appraised research is Health-Evidence (www.health-evidence.ca). This service searches broadly (Medline, Embase, Cochrane Library, Campbell Collaboration Library, and others), on a quarterly basis, for systematic reviews that are relevant to community health in Canada. Any relevant reviews are entered into the Health-Evidence database and rated for quality, on a scale of 1–10, independently by two different raters. You can search by free text, or by the narrowed categories or strategies they offer for

different populations, different intervention types, and different intervention locations. Some of the high quality reviews have a three- to four-page structured abstract that has a brief description of the background to the issue, results of the review, and level of evidence for different outcomes, and implications for practice and policy. This is a huge bonus since reviews (particularly Cochrane reviews) may be 60 pages or more in length. The summary statements give you a quick assessment about whether or not there is an "actionable message"—in other words, whether it is worthwhile to read the entire document.

Some other examples of pre-processed research include journals like *Evidence-Based Nursing, ACP Journal Club, Evidence-Based Medicine,* and *Evidence-Based Mental Health.* These journals are similar in format in that they select high-quality research from published journals using explicit quality criteria. Articles that report studies and reviews that warrant immediate attention from nurses attempting to keep pace with important advances are summarized in structured abstracts and commented on by clinical experts. The evidence-based journals are valuable resources that overcome the barriers of time (for example, the time to read all the issues of the more than 150 journals that are read for *Evidence-Based Nursing*), search skills, physical access to the original journals, and critical appraisal skills. While each issue of an evidence-based journal may contain only a few articles relevant to community health nursing, searchable online databases of abstracts and web-based updates for a specific user profile of clinical interests are available.

Yet another source of pre-processed information is *Clinical Evidence* (http://clinicalevidence.bmj.com). It is an evidence-based tool organized around common primary care or hospital-based problems. It provides concise accounts of the current state of knowledge, ignorance, and uncertainty about the prevention and treatment of a wide range of clinical conditions based on thorough searches of the literature. *Clinical Evidence* uses information from the Cochrane Library (see below) and the abstraction journals. However, it starts not with the journals, but with clinical questions such as prevention and treatment of pressure sores or management of acute stroke or acute myocardial infarction.

The Cochrane Collaboration is an international organization that aims to help people make informed decisions about health by preparing, maintaining, and ensuring the accessibility of rigorous, systematic, and up-to-date reviews (including meta-analyses where appropriate) of the benefits and risks of health care interventions (Jadad & Haynes, 1998). Examples of the Cochrane Collaboration's relevance to community health include smoking cessation in the workplace, parent training for improving maternal psychosocial health, and prevention of falls in the elderly. The Cochrane Library is the product of the Collaboration's work and includes reports and protocols; 4000 systematic reviews produced within the Collaboration; abstracts of more than 11 000 reviews summarized and critically appraised by the Centre for Reviews and Dissemination at the University of York, UK; and citations for more than 600 000 randomized controlled trials. One can search the Cochrane Library on-line, without charge, for abstracts of reviews, and through subscription. At the time of this writing, the Public Health Agency of Canada was supporting a pilot trial of paying for free access to the Cochrane Library for all Canadians.

Much smaller than Cochrane, the Effective Public Health Practice Project (www.ephpp.ca) is a review group for community health content. They produce reviews under contract and some are in conjunction with the Cochrane Public Health Review Group. Some of their reviews are on-line. It is important to remember, however, that all reviews by the Effective Public Health Practice Project, the Cochrane Collaboration, and the Campbell Collaboration are also in Health-Evidence, if they are of relevance to public health in Canada, reinforcing the effective search strategy of going to Health-Evidence first.

If no answer is found to the structured question within the pre-appraised literature, it is necessary to go to other databases. Free online access is available for PubMed, which can be searched with key words, setting limits for type of publication, year of publication, language, a nursing subset of journals, and so on. Another useful place to search is Cumulative Index of Nursing and Allied Health Literature (CINAHL), but it is not free unless there is access through an academic centre. Similar to PubMed, it allows for limits to be set and to search by author or key word. In all cases, there is a mixture of free access and pay-per-view access to full-text articles, unless you have access through an established library consortium.

Critically Appraising Retrieved Articles

Once the articles are found and retrieved, one must decide if their quality is sufficient that one can be confident in using them. Some health care research is too poor in quality to be used in decision making regarding clinical practice. As stated above, this is less critical with some of the pre-appraised sources of research. Several checklists for quality (validity) have been developed (Ciliska, Thomas, & Buffett, 2008) to help people develop **critical appraisal skills**; that is, the ability to decide if an article is of sufficient methodological quality that it warrants attention for decision making. With a little practice, these skills become easier and quicker to apply.

Outcomes or intervention research answers questions about effectiveness or harm and has a quantitative design. As stated in Chapter 9 on epidemiology, different research designs are best for answering particular types of questions. For example, questions about effectiveness or harms of certain interventions and prevention are best answered by **randomized controlled trials** in which the investigators have no control over who is placed in the intervention group versus the control group. The most efficient way to access evidence of this type that may inform your practice is a systematic review of randomized trials. However, randomized trials may be unethical, such as randomizing mothers to breastfeed or not to see if breastfeeding is associated with eczema, or randomizing preteens to smoke to see if it causes lung cancer. Also, trials are very expensive. If a trial cannot be done (ethically or financially), the next best design to answer the question

is a cohort design, where at least two groups are compared before and after one group receives an intervention. (See Chapter 9 or a basic nursing research text for more information on study designs.)

Questions exploring perceptions, feelings, and experiences are best answered through a qualitative design such as phenomenology or grounded theory. Questions and interventions that evolve through partnerships between researchers and participants are best dealt with through participatory action research. **Participatory action research** is action-oriented research in which the researchers and participants are partners in developing the question, intervention, and evaluation. It may be quantitative or qualitative and may involve triangulation of data from multiple sources (Burns & Groves, 2001).

One principle when critically appraising articles is to ensure that the appropriate design was used to answer the question. More recently, researchers are realizing that healthcare topics are very complex and that mixed methods research may be most appropriate. Mixed methods include both quantitative and qualitative methods, either concurrently or sequentially. For example, a randomized trial of the effectiveness of different forms of birth control for teens would be enhanced by an understanding of their preferences for type of birth control.

The Additional Research Boxes in MyNursingLab discuss criteria for critical appraisal of systematic reviews, single intervention studies, and qualitative research and demonstrate the application of the criteria to actual research studies.

Critical Appraisal of Studies of Interventions

The decision to use a study of intervention (usually a treatment or prevention) depends on the findings and the quality of the study design. The quality determines the level of confidence in the findings of the study. The major questions used to evaluate primary studies of interventions or prevention are

- Are the results valid?
- What are the results?
- Will the results help me in improving the health of clients? (Ciliska et al., 2001; Sackett et al., 2000)

The following section discusses more specific critical appraisal criteria that help to answer these questions. See MyNursingLab, Additional Research Box 10.1, for an example of application of the critical appraisal criteria to an article (Ratner et al., 2004).

Are the Results Valid? This question considers whether the reported results are likely to reflect the true size and direction of the treatment effect. Was the research designed to minimize bias and lead to accurate findings?

Was the assignment of participants to treatment groups randomized, and was the randomization concealed? The purpose of randomization is to remove any control over who is assigned to an intervention or control group. As well, groups should be similar in all respects except for exposure to the intervention. Known and unknown factors (age, gender, socioeconomic status, disease severity) that could influence the outcome of the study are evenly distributed among the groups. Different methods, such as a table of random numbers or computer-generated random numbers, ensure that all participants have an equal chance of being in each of the study groups. The methods section of the article should tell if and how participants were randomized.

The person recruiting the participants into the study should not know to which group each person is allocated. This is called *allocation concealment*. Concealment could happen through a process of calling a central office to get the allocation of the participant or through the use of numbered, opaque, sealed envelopes. In this way, the recruiter does not know until after participants are registered to which group they will be assigned, and the participant does not know at all. This prevents the recruiter from exercising bias in recruitment.

Was follow-up sufficiently long and complete? The first of these two criteria has to be judged by the clinician reading the paper. The definition of appropriate length of follow-up varies with different clinical questions. For example, success in weight loss measured at six months after a year-long intervention does not give a true picture of how many people are able to maintain the weight loss. A minimum expectation would be a one-year follow-up. Similarly, with early childhood interventions, follow-up for only two years may mean that some important outcomes that occur later in life for the child or family are missed.

The second part of these criteria relates to completeness of follow-up. Seldom are studies able to retain all participants until the end of the follow-up. If large numbers are lost, it reduces the confidence one can have in the results. To continue with the weight-loss example, large dropouts are usual during treatment and follow-up. If the author reports on only those who remained in the study, those participants are more likely to be doing well in terms of their weight loss. Participants who were unsuccessful with the intervention are more likely to drop out, making the intervention look far more effective than it is in reality. A retention rate of 80% is considered good; however, this is somewhat topic dependent, as one would expect the dropout rates of a transient population to be much higher.

Were participants analyzed in groups to which they were assigned? This criterion relates to the fact that participants should be analyzed in the group to which they were randomized, regardless of whether or not they actually received the treatment or completed treatment as assigned. This is called **intention-to-treat analysis.** If the participants who discontinued treatment, for example, due to unpleasant side effects, were omitted from analysis, we would be left only with participants who had better outcomes, making the treatment look more effective than it actually was.

Were participants, clinicians, outcome assessors, and data analysts unaware of (blinded to or masked from) participant allocation? Several of the groups involved in a trial have the potential to bias the outcomes if they know whether a participant is in the intervention or control group. **Bias** means any systematic tendency to produce an outcome that differs from

CANADIAN RESEARCH BOX

What is the evidence for school-based activity programs?

Dobbins, M., DeCorby, K., Robeson, P., Husson, H., and Tirilis, D. School-based physical activity programs for promoting physical activity and fitness in children and adolescents aged 6–18. *Cochrane Database of Systematic Reviews, 2009*, Issue 1. Art. No.: CD007651.

The purpose of this systematic review was to summarize the evidence of the effectiveness of school-based interventions in promoting physical activity and fitness in children and adolescents.

13 841 titles were identified and screened and 482 articles were retrieved; 104 were relevant and of those, four were assessed as having strong methodological quality, 22 were of moderate quality, and 78 were considered weak. In total, 26 studies were included in the review. The authors conclude that there is good evidence that school-based physical activity interventions have a positive impact on four of the nine outcome measures (duration of physical activity, television viewing, VO^2 max, and blood cholesterol). At a minimum, a combination of printed educational materials and changes to the school curriculum that promote physical activity result in positive effects.

Discussion Questions

1. Some people naively look at systematic reviews and see that many titles were discarded; in the example above, they found 104 of the initial 13 841 titles. They then claim that not all studies get used; large numbers get thrown out, making a systematic review not really a look at all the available research. How would you respond?

2. Is this conclusion convincing—that school-based interventions can improve physical activity, VO^2 max, and blood cholesterol, and reduce television viewing? Are these meaningful changes? Are they worth putting resources into school-based interventions?

the truth. It includes the tendency to look more carefully for particular outcomes or to probe more deeply for outcomes in one group and not the other, as well as for participants to more likely recall an event or exposure that could have an impact if they have an adverse outcome than if they do not have an adverse outcome (Oxman et al., 2002). Studies can be labelled single, double, or triple blinded depending on how many of the groups were unaware of the allocation of the participants. Authors should clearly state which groups were blinded or masked. For example, if participants know they are in the intervention group, they may have a sensitivity to the good or bad effects of the treatment. Participant blinding is easier to do in drug trials where placebos can be made to look identical to the active drug. However, it is far more difficult in community nursing to blind participants to a nurse coming to their home or delivering a physical versus a primarily psychosocial intervention. It is often possible to minimize the potential bias by assuring that the participant does not know

How to Critically Appraise Studies of Treatment or Prevention

1. Are the results of this study valid?
   a) Was the assignment of participants to treatment groups randomized, and was the randomization concealed?
   b) Was follow-up sufficiently long and complete?
   c) Were participants analyzed in the groups to which they were assigned?
   d) Were participants, clinicians, outcome assessors, and data analysts unaware of (blinded to or masked from) participant allocation?
   e) Were participants in each group treated equally except for the intervention being evaluated?
   f) Were the groups similar at the start of the trial?
2. What were the results?
   a) How large is the effect? Is it clinically important?
   b) How precise is the treatment effect?
3. Will the results help me in caring for my clients?
   a) Are my clients so different from those in the study that the results do not apply?
   b) Is the treatment feasible in our setting?
   c) Were all the clinically important outcomes (harms as well as benefits) considered?
   d) What are my clients' values and preferences for both the outcomes we are trying to prevent and the side effects that may arise?

Source: Adapted from Cullum, 2001.

the specific outcome. Similarly, clinicians who care for the participants and know the allocation may unconsciously alter the way they give care and may have a heightened awareness of positive outcomes or adverse outcomes in a way that biases the evaluation.

The most important group to be blinded is the one that measures the outcomes. Ideally, clinicians providing care are not assessing outcomes. The measurement of key outcomes can be unconsciously distorted by the clinicians' beliefs about the intervention and its side effects. Objective outcome measures, such as glycated hemoglobin, are less subject to outcome assessor bias. Similarly, data analyses should be done with coded data that do not allow for identification of treatment groups.

Consequently, readers of randomized trials should look for reports of which groups were and were not blinded to the participant allocation. If blinding is not possible, the authors should report on steps taken to minimize possible biases.

Were participants in each group treated equally except for the intervention being evaluated? Randomization should ensure that the only difference between study groups is the treatment being evaluated. An important principle is that additional treatments, or extra care, should not be given. Readers of

randomized trials should look carefully at the descriptions of interventions received by all groups, especially if the clinicians are not blinded to allocation.

Were the groups similar at the start of the trial? Randomization should ensure that the groups of study participants were similar at the beginning. Usually a table of baseline characteristics is prepared and some analysis is done to check that randomization actually "worked." If the groups show statistically significant differences at the beginning, the impact of the intervention may be altered, which can affect the validity of the result. If imbalances do exist at baseline, adjustment in the analysis can be done with statistical techniques.

What Were the Results? Once one has determined that the results are valid, it important to understand what the results really mean.

How large is the effect? Is it clinically important? How precise is the treatment effect? The effects of treatment are measured using one or more outcome measures. They can be dichotomous (yes/no; alive/dead; pregnant/not pregnant) or continuous (weight, adjustment score, blood pressure, self-esteem). Different statistical tests are used for different types of data. Often statistical test results are reported as *p* values. The convention is that any *p* value less than 0.05 is considered statistically significant and means that the intervention has an effect on the outcome. More information may be gained about the extent of that difference by the use of other statistical tests such as relative risk reduction (RRR) and absolute risk reduction (ARR).

The **relative risk reduction** is the proportional reduction in rates of poor outcomes (e.g., death or readmission) between the experimental (better outcomes) and control (greater poor outcomes) participants. It is calculated as:

$$\text{Relative risk reduction} = \frac{\text{Event rate in control group} - \text{Event rate in experimental group}}{\text{Event rate in the control group}}$$

For example, an RRR of 50% means that there were 50% fewer deaths in the experimental group compared with the control group.

Relative risk (RR) is the proportion of participants experiencing an outcome in the intervention group divided by the proportion experiencing the outcome in the control group. However, RR does not take into account the number of people in the study who would have died anyway without the intervention.

This is called the **absolute risk reduction** and is calculated as:

$$\text{Absolute risk reduction} = \text{Event rate in control group} - \text{Event rate in experimental group}$$

For example, an ARR of 2% means that there were 2% fewer deaths in the experimental group than the control group.

Yet another approach is to report the **number needed to treat (NNT)**. This describes the number of people who must be treated with the intervention in order to prevent one additional negative outcome (e.g., death) or promote one additional positive outcome (e.g., smoking cessation). The NNT is calculated as:

$$NNT = \frac{1}{\text{Absolute risk reduction}}$$

When researchers report statistical significance, it is imperative to ask if this is clinically important or meaningful. It is quite possible for results to be statistically significant but clinically unimportant. In a hypothetical example studying weight-loss interventions for obese women, the group with a more intensive intervention lost a mean of 5 kg more than the group in the less intensive intervention. Though the researchers found this statistically significant ($p = 0.03$), it did not meet the preset goal of a 10% weight loss in order to be a meaningful difference; that is, to be associated with health risk reduction. It also was not personally meaningful to the morbidly obese women.

Precision of the results can never be absolute but is estimated by calculating **confidence intervals** around the RRR or ARR. Confidence intervals (CI) are a range of values with a specified probability (usually 95%) of including the true effect, which can never be known absolutely. Wide confidence intervals indicate less precision in the estimated effect of the intervention. Precision increases with larger sample sizes.

Will the Results Help Me in Caring for My Clients?

- Are my clients so different from those in the study that the results do not apply?
- Is the treatment feasible in our setting?
- Were all the clinically important outcomes (harms as well as benefits) considered?
- What are my clients' values and preferences for both the outcome we are trying to prevent and the side effects that may arise?

In order to use the findings of a study, one needs to consider these questions and make judgments in relation to one's own client population. Consider how similar the characteristics of the study participants are to your own clients. Think about reasons why you should *not* apply the study results to your clients, rather than the looking for evidence that the clients are exactly the same as yours. Feasibility in your setting depends on factors such as cost, organizational resources, nursing skills, availability of special equipment, and acceptability to clients. Harms and benefits should be included in the reports by various obvious outcomes such as health but also other outcomes like quality of life and economics. In particular, negative effects or side effects should be included. Once again, for application of these criteria, see MyNursingLab, Additional Research Box 10.1.

Critical Appraisal of Systematic Reviews

What Is a Systematic Review? A systematic review is a summary of research evidence that relates to a specific question. It could involve causation, diagnosis, or prognosis, but more frequently involves **effectiveness** of an intervention. The terms "systematic review" and "overview" are often used interchangeably. Basing a clinical decision on a single study may be a mistake, as the study may have an inadequate sample size to detect clinically important differences between treatments, leading to a false negative conclusion. Discrepant findings across studies of the same question may occur due to chance or subtle differences in study design or participants. Therefore, it is useful to look at a summary of all the research related to a single clinical question.

In a narrative review, authors may selectively pick articles that support their viewpoint and ignore those that do not, so that the conclusion is set before the articles are selected. Systematic reviews differ from an unsystematic narrative review in that they attempt to overcome possible biases by following a rigorous methodology of search, retrieval, relevance and validity (quality) rating, data extraction, synthesis, and report writing. Explicit pre-set criteria are used for relevance and validity. Two people conduct each stage independently, then compare results and discuss discrepancies before moving on to the next stage. Details of the methods used at every stage are recorded.

A **meta-analysis** is the quantitative combination of results of several studies to get an overall summary statistic that represents the combined effect of the intervention across different study populations. The reviewers must decide whether the statistical combination (meta-analysis) is appropriate by using both clinical judgment and a statistical test for heterogeneity. The clinical judgment requires the reviewers to examine the methodologies and statistical tests completed in the studies under review and ascertain if it is reasonable to combine them in a meta-analysis. The statistical tests determine the extent to which the differences between results of individual studies are greater than one would expect if all studies were measuring the same underlying effect and the observed differences were due only to chance. The more significant the test of heterogeneity, the less likely that the observed differences are from chance alone and that some other factor, such as design, participants, intervention, or outcome, is responsible for the differences in the treatment effect across studies (Sackett et al., 2000). Readers must use their own expertise to decide whether the statistical combination is reasonable in terms of clinical and methodological sense.

Systematic reviews help to answer clinical questions without having to access large numbers of research reports; they overcome the obstacles of lack of time and, sometimes, lack of skills necessary to conduct the critical appraisal. But can one be confident in using all reviews? A search may easily yield more than 200 reviews—are they all of equal value? What does one do if they give conflicting results?

Common misconceptions of systematic reviews are that many readers think they include *only* randomized trials, that they must adopt a biomedical model, and that they have to have some statistical synthesis (Petticrew, 2001). If these were true, there would be few reviews of interest in community health, as many community health questions have not been or cannot be addressed by randomized trials. Fortunately, review methods are improving to include non-randomized studies, such as cohort studies, to use a population health model, and to synthesize without necessarily including meta-analysis. The Cochrane Public Health Review Group (previously the Health Promotion/Public Health Field) has been a leader in promoting the methods, conduct, and use of systematic reviews and meta-analyses in community health care. Many websites contain high-quality systematic reviews relevant to community health and resources for skill building in critical appraisal of reviews. (See Additional Resources.)

Appraising Systematic Reviews In this section, we look at how to critically appraise systematic reviews to decide if the methods have sufficient rigour that the results may be applied to client or management decisions. The same major questions used for evaluation of intervention studies can be used to evaluate systematic reviews. (See the box "How to Critically Appraise Review Articles.") For an example of application, see Additional Research Box 10.2 in MyNursingLab.

Are the Results Valid? *Is this a systematic review of randomized trials?* Questions about the effectiveness of treatment or prevention are best answered by randomized controlled trials if it is ethically possible to do so, whereas questions about harm or prognosis are best answered by cohort studies (Roberts & DiCenso, 1999). The reader of systematic reviews should look to see if the authors used randomized trials (if ethically possible) or the next most rigorous design that included a comparison group (quasi-experimental or cohort analytic designs).

Does the systematic review include a description of the strategies used to find all relevant studies? A thorough search for both published and unpublished studies should be done for a systematic review. The publication of research in a journal is more likely to occur in studies that have statistically significant results. Studies in which a new intervention is not found to be effective are frequently not published, a phenomenon known as publication bias (Dickersin, 1990). Systematic reviews that do not include unpublished studies may overestimate the effect of an intervention; that is, it will appear that the intervention is more effective than it really is. Therefore, in addition to searching through relevant databases such as CINAHL, MEDLINE, PsycINFO, ERIC, or Cochrane Library, researchers should hand-search relevant journals; review reference lists from retrieved articles; contact experts, authors, and relevant manufacturing companies; and review abstracts presented at relevant scientific meetings. Unless the authors of the reviews tell us what they did to locate relevant studies, it is difficult to know if any were missed.

Every systematic review grows from a focused question, through the development of the search strategies and search terms for each database, to retrieval of studies. Explicit inclusion/exclusion criteria are predetermined, and the review should state that two people independently reviewed each article for inclusion.

Does the systematic review include a description of how the validity of individual studies was assessed? A narrative review often reports on study findings without considering the methodological strengths of the studies. Differences in study quality often explain differences in results across studies, with

---

How to Critically Appraise Review Articles

1. Are the results of this systematic review valid?
   a) Is this a systematic review of randomized trials?
   b) Does the systematic review include a description of the strategies used to find all the relevant trials?
   c) Does the systematic review include a description of how the validity of individual studies was assessed?
   d) Were the results consistent from study to study?
2. What were the results?
   a) How large was the treatment effect?
   b) How precise was the estimate of treatment effect?
3. Will the results help me in caring for my clients?
   a) Are my clients so different from those in the study that the results do not apply?
   b) Is the treatment feasible in our setting?
   c) Were all the clinically important outcomes (harms as well as benefits) considered?
   d) What are my clients' values and preferences for both the outcomes we are trying to prevent and the side effects that may arise?

Source: Adapted from Ciliska, Cullum, & Marks, 2001, and Sackett et al., 2000.

---

those of poorer quality tending to overestimate the effectiveness of the interventions (Kunz & Oxman, 1998). Quality ratings are sometimes used in the analysis to compare outcomes across studies by study strength. Or, if there are many studies to consider, the authors may choose to apply a quality rating threshold for inclusion or give greater attention and weight to the stronger studies.

The predefined quality checklist minimizes reviewer bias by helping to ensure that reviewers appraise each study consistently and thoroughly. Having two or more raters helps to reduce mistakes and bias and increases the reader's confidence in the systematic review. The quality rating tools usually include criteria such as those presented for evaluating interventions.

Were the results consistent from study to study? The reader would be most confident using the results of a review if the results were similar in all included studies; that is, showing the same direction of effect, all being positive, all negative, or all showing no effect. But what if the direction of effect differs across studies? Differences may be due to types of clients included; the timing, duration, and intensity of the intervention; the outcomes measured; and/or the ways in which the outcomes were measured.

What Were the Results? *How large was the treatment effect? How precise is the estimate of treatment effect?* Comparing a simple count of studies that helped, harmed, or showed no difference in treatments would assume that all studies had equal validity, power of the sample size to detect a difference, and duration and intensity of interventions and follow-up. Meta-analysis, when appropriate, can assign different weights to individual studies so that those with greater precision or higher quality make a greater contribution to the summary statistic. Summary statistics usually used include odds ratio, relative risk (RR, defined earlier), and weighted mean difference. The **odds ratio (OR)** describes the odds of a participant in the experimental group having an event (e.g., pregnancy) divided by the odds of a participant in the control group having the event. In a study such as prevention of pregnancy, one would consider that an RR or OR of less than 1 represents a beneficial treatment. **Weighted mean difference** is the mean of the difference found between control and intervention groups across studies entered into a meta-analysis. Both OR and RR are used for dichotomous data (dead/alive, pregnant/not pregnant), while weighted mean difference is used for continuous data (blood pressure, blood glucose, stress measurement scale). (For more information on OR and RR, see Chapter 9.)

The precision of the results is estimated by calculating confidence intervals (CI, defined earlier) around the summary statistic. The CI is useful for decision making because we can look at both extremes of the effect. If the lower extreme is 1 or close to it, the effect of the intervention is quite small and probably not worthwhile. A hypothetical display is shown in Figure 10.2 to demonstrate how output tables are read. The summary odds ratio of the three studies in Figure 10.2 is 0.69 (95% CI: 0.51–0.90), which indicates that the treatment was effective in producing the desired outcome.

Will the Results Help Me in Caring for My Clients?

- Are my clients so different from those in the study that the study results do not apply?
- Is the treatment feasible in our setting?

FIGURE 10.2 Example of Meta-Analysis Display

Each study is shown as a horizontal line with the OR for that study as the point on the line. The ends of the line show the 95% CIs. The numbers of participants are shown to the left of the line, and to the right are the numerical OR and 95% CIs. If a CI touches or crosses the vertical line of 1, that result is not statistically significant. The horizontal line just above the x-axis is the summary of the studies (the meta-analysis) that shows the combined impact of the intervention.

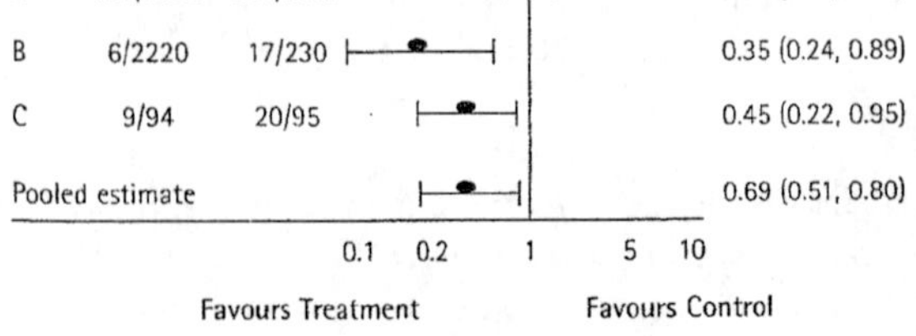

Study	Expt n/N	Ctrl n/N		OR
A	188/2160	201/2170		0.92 (0.77, 1.21)
B	6/2220	17/230		0.35 (0.24, 0.89)
C	9/94	20/95		0.45 (0.22, 0.95)
Pooled estimate				0.69 (0.51, 0.80)

0.1 0.2 1 5 10

Favours Treatment   Favours Control

- Were all the clinically important outcomes (harms as well as benefits) considered?
- What are my clients' values and preferences for both the outcome we are trying to prevent and the side effects that may arise?

These questions have to be answered by the readers in the context of their own work and client-encounter situations. For example, feasibility in a multi-faceted sexual health program intervention would relate not only to the skills of the nurses and resources of the health department to complete such an intervention, but also to the ability of the school board to withstand the parental pressures for abstinence programs.

Researchers try to look for all outcomes of interventions, both positive and negative, that might affect the participants and the health care system. Outcomes might include mortality, morbidity, costs, quality of life, and participant satisfaction. Participant and family values must be considered. If, in the example above, families are unwilling to have their children exposed to multi-faceted sexual health education programs, the students must be given an alternative during that school time.

Critical Appraisal of Qualitative Research

Qualitative research is important for the development of nursing knowledge. **Qualitative research** describes, explores, and explains phenomena and is concerned with the process or experience rather than outcomes. Done for the purpose of obtaining rich data, sampling is purposive as opposed to the random or probability sampling in quantitative research. Data collection is done in many ways, but the most common are observation and group or individual interviews. Data analysis is by codes, themes, and patterns, not by statistical techniques, and it produces rich, deep descriptions rather than numbers. Qualitative research does not allow inference to a population as a whole, but allows the researcher to generalize to a theoretical understanding of the phenomena being studied (Ploeg, 1999).

Major types of qualitative research used in nursing include phenomenology, grounded theory, and ethnography. **Phenomenology** seeks to describe the lived experiences of people, such as the experience of people returning home after a stroke. **Grounded theory** generates theories or models of the phenomena being studied, such as the development of a model of coping used by family caregivers of people who have HIV. **Ethnography** describes a culture and answers questions such as what it is like to be a pregnant teen trying to continue with school. Reading qualitative research deepens our understanding of the potential and actual experiences of people we work with and has the potential to enrich our interactions and care.

Once again, the same major questions used to evaluate primary treatment studies or systematic reviews can be used to evaluate qualitative research. (See the box "How to Critically Appraise Qualitative Research Reports.") For application of

How to Critically Appraise Qualitative Research Reports

1. Are the findings valid?
   a) Is the research question clear and adequately substantiated?
   b) Is the design appropriate for the research question?
   c) Was the method of sampling appropriate for the research question?
   d) Were data collected and managed systematically?
   e) Were the data analyzed appropriately?
2. What are the findings?
   a) Is the description of findings thorough?
3. How can I apply the findings to patient care?
   a) What meaning and relevance does the study have for my practice?
   b) Does the study help me understand the context of my practice?
   c) Does the study enhance my knowledge about my practice?

Source: Russell, C. K., and Gregory, D. M. (2003). Evaluation of qualitative research reports. Evidence-Based Nursing, 6, 36–40. Reproduced with permission of the BMJ Publishing Group.

these criteria to Canadian studies, see Additional Research Boxes about a grounded theory study (Box 10.3) and participatory action study (Box 10.4) in MyNursingLab.

Are the Findings Valid? *Is the research question clear and adequately substantiated?* This question will determine whether the qualitative study will be read or not. The article should clearly establish the question and what is already known about the topic.

Is the design appropriate for the research question? On a grand level, it is important to determine that the authors used the appropriate method that fits the purpose of the study (e.g., that phenomenology is used to explore experience and meaning for clients following colostomy, rather than using an ethnographic approach). A more sophisticated appraisal considers the fit of the philosophical background of a particular perspective with the purpose of the study.

Was the method of sampling appropriate for the research question? The study should report on how participants were selected. Many different types of sampling are used in qualitative research, including purposeful sampling for maximum variation, typical cases, extreme cases, or critical cases.

Were data collected and managed systematically? The study should try to define the breadth (variation, multiple perspectives) and depth (numbers and types of data collected). Also, has each investigator kept track of the process, hunches, data collection, decision making, and data collection procedures through the use of journaling and memos?

Were the data analyzed appropriately? The researcher should report on how the data were organized and reduced in order to identify patterns. Often the analysis identifies further areas for data collection and analysis. Usually, the researcher uses other team members to assist in the analysis, providing various interpretations of the data. Member checking (taking the results back to the participants or people associated with the issue under study) is often done to validate the findings, assess for resonance of findings with participant experience, and to gather alternative interpretations of the analysis.

What Are the Findings? *Is the description of findings thorough?* Qualitative research is difficult to write within the word limit of standard journals. It is difficult to fit the rich description and analysis into one publication. It is expected that authors have used direct quotations of the participants to illustrate the descriptions and conceptualizations.

How Can I Apply the Findings to Patient Care?

■ What meaning and relevance does the study have for my practice?
■ Does the study help me understand the context of my practice?
■ Does the study enhance my knowledge about my practice?

The authors should establish the need and relevance of the research while both arguing why they conducted the research as well as discussing the results. Readers must use their critique of the study as well as the information presented in the report to decide if any parts of the research findings are potentially transferable to their own practice.

Making the Decision about Implementation

Each Additional Research Box in MyNursingLab shows high-quality evidence around the clinical scenario and clinical question. In community health nursing, many decisions to implement a change in practice are probably beyond the individual; they are decided by a team. In every case, the decision involves all of the four aspects of Figure 10.1: the research evidence, available resources, skills of the practitioners, and the client values and choices. Furthermore, if the decision goes beyond individual clients or small groups, political and organizational elements become involved. This is particularly evident in the final decision of the example of an intervention around sexual health education. The students, parents, and high school would all have to be involved in the decision if there is any chance for a school-based intervention for sexual health to be successful.

What does one do if no research evidence is found during the database search? Or if the research that comes up is of consistently poor quality? In those cases, expert opinion or usual practice is the standard for decision making. One may be able to find practice guidelines on the topic. These depend on a thorough literature review, then consensus meetings with expert panels in order to make practice decisions, particularly where research evidence does not exist (Registered Nurses Association of Ontario, 2010; U.S. Department of Health and Human Services, Agency for Healthcare Research and Quality, 2010). Similarly, "best practice" documents describe programs or interventions that seem to be effective, but may not yet have been rigorously evaluated.

Caution must be exercised when implementing interventions for which there is no good evaluation. CHNs must be particularly vigilant in observing for effects, both positive and negative, then charting them. Unfortunately, many effects are not evident until years after the intervention when no one is observing any longer! Areas of clinical interest where evaluation does not exist are prime research questions that should receive priority attention from funding agencies.

Planning for Dissemination and Implementation

Once a decision is made to change practice and organizational support is achieved, a comprehensive plan has to address how the others who work within the organization will be informed of the proposed change. Changing the practice of healthcare professionals has been studied extensively with mixed and unclear results. The "Effective Practice and Organization of Care" review group (www.epoc.cochrane.org/en/index.html) within the Cochrane Collaboration conducts systematic reviews of educational, behavioural, organizational, financial, and regulatory interventions related to changing practice of healthcare professionals or the organization of health care. One review studied strategies for guideline dissemination and implementation (Grimshaw et al., 2004). This review included 235 studies of 309 comparisons. They found median absolute improvements in performance across interventions was 14.1% in comparisons of reminders, 8.1% in comparisons of dissemination of educational materials, 7.0% in comparisons of audit and feedback, and 6.0% in comparisons of multifaceted interventions involving educational outreach. This is somewhat surprising, as you might expect that there would be enhanced performance improvements with multiple interventions.

It is recommended that a "diagnostic analysis" be done to identify factors likely to help and hinder the proposed change (University of York, NHS Centre for Reviews and Dissemination, 1999). For example, opinion leaders have been shown to be effective in some studies with physicians, but not other studies (University of York, NHS Centre for Reviews and Dissemination, 1999), and they were not successful as an intervention with nurses (Hodnett et al., 1996). Thus, evidence of the use of opinion leaders as a strategy of change has been inconclusive.

The diagnostic analysis (environmental scan) must consider barriers and supports in relation to the characteristics of the innovation (the change being introduced), individual clients and practitioners, the organization, and the environment so that barriers can be reduced and supports strengthened. It is important to consider characteristics of the innovation such as the resources it will require (will it cost more or actually be time/resource saving?) and how different it is from current practice. Relevant characteristics of individual practitioners include such issues as level of education, years of experience, and general acceptance or resistance to change. Organizational characteristics include affiliation with an academic setting, size, level of care, funding sources, organizational structure, research participation, research orientation, and usual valuing of research findings. The environment includes factors such as rural/urban, economic status of the community, and health issues valued by the community (Dobbins et al., 2002).

Important stakeholders must be identified. They may include the nurses, medical staff, clients, and accounting staff. Each group should attend a different meeting to hear a tailored message about the proposed change, rationale, and timelines. The goal of each meeting is to get support for the practice change from each stakeholder group. A champion may be needed with the enthusiasm and energy to push for this practice change. Identifying opinion leaders and influencing their understanding and attitudes about the proposed practice change is another strategy worth pursuing, despite the inconclusiveness (mentioned above) that this strategy is effective. Interventions to promote dissemination, uptake, and utilization of research results is an area that requires further focused research in order to complete the cycle of evidence-based practice from question identification to implementation and evaluation.

Evaluation

After implementing a practice or policy change, an evaluation period is needed to see if it is working in the organization with the new population and staff. This does not mean replicating the original study that was used as a basis for the practice change. It does, however, mean a period of data collection or chart review to ensure that the desired outcomes are similar to the rates of those in the original study and that the client acceptability and negative outcomes are also similar.

USING RESEARCH FOR MANAGEMENT DECISIONS AND POLICY DEVELOPMENT

While research evidence is useful for individual practitioners working with individual clients, it is also important that management decisions be evidence based. Decisions regarding the implementation of a new intensive intervention in a community are usually made where there is no additional funding coming to an agency for the new program. Therefore, if the organization wishes to begin such a program, it needs to find the resources within what currently exists. This may mean taking staff away from some other programs or activities. Reviewing the research evidence for both the proposed activity and any existing programs helps managers to make those decisions. For example, following a string of four adolescent

CANADIAN RESEARCH BOX

How can participatory action research change primary health care?

Hills, M., Mullett, J., and Carroll, S. (2007). Community-based participatory action research: Transforming multidisciplinary practice in primary health care. *Revista Panamericana de Salud Pública, 21* (2–3), 125–135.

In a small community (population 11 000) in Canada, the researchers studied multidisciplinary practice within a primary health care centre using a participatory action research method. Community members who had received care at the centre and practitioners who worked there participated in critical incident technique and a community forum. Community members focused on a broad concept of health (more than medical care) and valued the different disciplines. Practitioners felt a need to move away from physician-driven care, which would involve changing underlying values, power relationships, and roles within the health care system and the broader community.

Discussion Question

1. As a nurse working in a primary health care centre, how would you use this information in practice? What value can it add to your work?

suicides, one school requested that the health department offer suicide prevention interventions at the school the following fall. During the summer, the health department conducted a systematic review of the effectiveness of school-based suicide prevention programs for teens. They found that the available research was of poor quality and no evidence supported the decision to implement the suicide prevention programs; furthermore, some studies indicated that there was harm to adolescent males who experienced such a program in that they were more likely to engage in negative coping behaviours and to commit suicide (Ploeg, 1999). The management decided to present this information to the school and to offer instead a comprehensive "healthy school" initiative, which would also be evaluated.

Similarly, people working at institutional or government policy levels are increasingly aware of and value the need for research evidence, yet they face other competing factors (public opinion and pressures, fiscal restraints) when making policy decisions.

The actual conduct (as opposed to the search and discovery) of systematic reviews has contributed to their use by clinicians and policy-level decision makers. From the chapter authors' experiences with the Effective Public Health Practice Project (www.ephpp.ca), potential review questions are sought from the policy, management, and frontline clinician perspectives. The groups that conducted the reviews included the methodological experts along with the community practitioners who were chosen for their content expertise and their understanding of the context and relevance to community

health. They assisted in identifying and refining the priority questions, rating articles for relevance to the question, reviewing drafts, and helping to write clinical, management, and policy implications. This process has also been used in Alberta by the Alberta Heritage Foundation for Medical Research.

Participating in Community Health Research

CHNs are involved in many different types of research, the most common being program evaluation using process outcomes such as numbers of clients, numbers of groups, hours spent, and reasons for home visits. These types of data are important for tracking uses of services and how resources are spent within the agency. Client outcome measurement is the next most likely information collected, such as client mortality, morbidity, immunization status or coverage, communicable disease outbreak, goals met, or adolescent pregnancies after a school program. Nurses are usually asked to log these data, at least in formal records. They also may be required to report it in other formats, or the agency may conduct periodic chart reviews or database summaries. These local data often feed into provincial and national databases and registries of statistics. Some of these databases are available to regions within the provinces so that local rates can be followed.

Especially if associated with an academic setting, CHNs may also be involved in effectiveness research; that is, testing an alternate intervention against usual or no intervention. They might deliver interventions such as a falls prevention program for the elderly or a child abuse prevention intervention for families already identified as abusers or at high risk for abuse. CHNs may also collect the data for an effectiveness study, such as assessing functional status in people who have suffered a stroke and who have received the specialist nurse home intervention. Initiation and maintenance of relationships with academic settings is beneficial from the perspective of agencies and the universities. The agency can gain consultation on research utilization and program evaluation, and the nursing faculty can be kept current on clinical issues in the community and priority research needs.

CHNs may also be involved in participatory action research, where the community group of interest identifies the question and is involved in every phase of planning and conducting the study.

SUMMARY

In this chapter, we reviewed evidence-based practice as it relates to community health nursing. While evidence can be observations made by the nurse, expert "gut hunches," or advice of colleagues, we too often ignore the evidence from research (Estabrooks, 1998). Therefore, this chapter focused on research evidence—finding, critiquing, and using it. Particular detail was presented in relation to critical appraisal of research articles on effectiveness questions (primary studies or systematic reviews) or qualitative research to judge whether they should be utilized in practice, management, or policy decisions.

The process of using quality research evidence does not end with the critical appraisal and individual decisions to implement with clients. In community nursing, it more often involves getting organizational "buy-in" and changing policies and procedures or care maps. Thus, we presented information about understanding the barriers to utilizing research to change practice, management, and policy making.

Research, in the form of process evaluation, currently takes place daily in every community organization in Canada. Therefore, CHNs can never avoid involvement in research. Further, as the valuing of research evidence increases in community health nursing, the critical attitude to practice will increase so that clinicians will more frequently ask relevant clinical questions. Since there is not a research-based answer for every clinical question within community health, the need to conduct research in community health will continue. CHNs will find they are asked to participate in research by collecting data, providing interventions, or developing research proposals.

KEY TERMS

evidence-based nursing (EBN), p. 155
clinical questions, p. 157
structured questions, p. 157
situation, p. 157
intervention, p. 157
outcome, p. 157
critical appraisal skills, p. 158
randomized controlled trials, p. 158
participatory action research, p. 158
intention-to-treat analysis, p. 159
bias, p. 159
p values, p. 160
relative risk reduction, p. 160
relative risk (RR), p. 160
absolute risk reduction, p. 160
number needed to treat (NNT), p. 160
confidence intervals, p. 161
systematic review, p. 161
effectiveness, p. 161
meta-analysis, p. 161
odds ratio (OR), p. 163
weighted mean difference, p. 163
qualitative research, p. 163
phenomenology, p. 163
grounded theory, p. 163
ethnography, p. 163

REVIEW QUESTIONS

1. Which of the following is an example of a source of primary studies as opposed to pre-appraised evidence?
   a) health-evidence.ca
   b) the Cochrane Library
   c) Evidence-Based Nursing
   d) Canadian Nurse
   e) Clinical Evidence

2. Which characteristic most influences the design that a researcher chooses when developing a research proposal?
   a) population
   b) research question
   c) study outcomes
   d) sample size
   e) type of data to be collected

3. You have a clinical question about the effectiveness of school-based interventions to prevent obesity. You find studies that include all the following designs. In which design would you have the most confidence in the results?
   a) randomized controlled trial
   b) grounded theory
   c) cohort analytic study
   d) case-control study
   e) cross-sectional study

4. Including drop-outs in the final analysis of any intervention study is called:
   a) sensitivity analysis
   b) specificity analysis
   c) number needed to treat analysis
   d) intention to treat analysis
   e) reliability analysis

STUDY QUESTIONS

1. Identify four factors to consider for evidence-based decision making.
2. What is the most critical attitude for a nurse in order to practise in an evidence-based way?
3. In what ways might you conduct research as part of your daily role in community health nursing?
4. Why would you seek out systematic reviews to answer clinical questions?
5. Name the four major categories of factors to consider when planning to implement a clinical practice or policy change. Give a few examples under each category.
6. Give examples of patient-related questions that would most appropriately be answered by phenomenology, grounded theory, and ethnography.

*After working through these questions, go to the MyNursingLab at **www.pearsoned.ca/mynursinglab** to check your answers.*

INDIVIDUAL CRITICAL THINKING EXERCISES

1. Pick an intervention that has been shown to be effective and discuss how you would plan to implement that practice change in a nursing agency. What factors would you assess? What processes would you use?

2. Answer the following using Figure 10.3.

   a) How many studies were involved in this meta-analysis?

   b) Which of those studies had statistically significant findings?

   c) How would you interpret the result? Is the intervention effective? Is it statistically significant? Is it precise?

FIGURE 10.3 Results of Meta-Analysis

Study	Expt n/N	Ctrl n/N		RR
A	24/130	43/120		0.55 (0.36, 0.85)
B	170/500	230/490		0.75 (0.63, 0.89)
C	250/300	260/300		0.98 (0.90, 1.05)
D	25/80	600/1050		0.89 (0.50, 1.56)
Pooled estimate				0.88 (0.71, 1.19)

Favours Treatment   Favours Control

3. In a randomized trial about physical activity for obese middle-aged women, the intervention group (diet and exercise) lost 2.4% of their original weight, versus the control group who lost 1% of their original weight. This was statistically significant ($p < 0.05$). Is this a clinically important outcome? Would you use this study to advocate for diet and exercise for weight loss?

4. In a study of an intervention to increase school students' use of helmets when in-line skating, the intervention consisted of in-school educational video plus free helmets, versus the video alone. The odds ratio for observed helmet use was 3.85 in favour of the video plus free helmets (CI 3.05 to 4.11). Was this a statistically significant result? Put the results into words using the odds ratio.

GROUP CRITICAL THINKING EXERCISES

1. Select an article that evaluates an intervention relevant to community health nursing. Use the criteria in the first text box to critically appraise the article and come to a decision about using the intervention in your own practice.

2. As in question 1, critically appraise a systematic review article using the criteria in the second text box.

3. As in question 1, critically appraise an article on qualitative research using the criteria in the third text box. If it is a valid study, discuss what the study findings contribute to your understanding of the issue that was explored.

REFERENCES

American College of Physicians. (2001). *Best evidence* [CD-ROM]. Philadelphia, PA: Author.

Arthur, H. M., Wright, D. M., & Smith, K. M. (2001). Women and heart disease: The treatment may end but the suffering continues. *Canadian Journal of Nursing Research, 33*, 17–29.

Blythe, J., & Royle, J. A. (1993). Assessing nurses' information needs in the work environment. *Bulletin of the Medical Librarians Association, 81*, 433–435.

Bostrom, J., & Suter, W. N. (1993). Research utilisation: Making the link to practice. *Journal of Nursing Staff Development, 9*, 28–34.

Burns, N., & Groves, S. K. (2001). *The practice of nursing research: Conduct, critique and utilization*. Philadelphia, PA: W. B. Saunders.

Canadian Health Services Research Foundation (CHSRF). (2004). *What counts? Interpreting evidence-based decision-making for management and policy*. Report of the 6th CHSRF Annual Invitational Workshop. Retrieved from http://www.chsrf.ca/knowledge_transfer/pdf/2004_workshop_report_e.pdf

Ciliska, D., Cullum, N., & Marks, S. (2001). Evaluation of systematic reviews of treatment or prevention interventions. *Evidence-Based Nursing, 4*(4), 100–104.

Ciliska, D., Thomas, H., & Buffett, C. (2008). *A compendium of critical appraisal tools for public health practice*. Hamilton, Ontario, National Collaborating Centre for Methods and Tools. Retrieved from http://www.nccmt.ca/tools/index-eng.html

Community Health Nurses Association of Canada (2008). *Community health nurses standards of practice*. Retrieved from http://www.chnac.ca/index.php?option=com_content&task=view&id=19&Itemid=35

Cullum, N. (2000). Evaluation of studies of treatment or prevention interventions. *Evidence-Based Nursing, 3*(4), 100–102.

Cullum, N. (2001). Evaluation of studies of treatment or prevention interventions, part 2: Applying the results of studies to your patients. *Evidence-Based Nursing, 4*(1), 7–8.

Dennis, C. L., Hodnett, E., Gallop, R., & Chalmers, B. (2002). The effect of peer support on breast-feeding duration among primiparous women: A randomized controlled trial. *Canadian Medical Association Journal, 166*(1), 21–28.

DiCenso, A., Cullum, N., & Ciliska, D. (1998). Implementing evidence-based nursing: Some misconceptions. *Evidence-Based Nursing, 1*, 38–40.

Dickersin, K. (1990). The existence of publication bias and risk factors for its occurrence. *JAMA: The Journal of the American Medical Association, 263*, 1385–1389.

Dobbins, M., Ciliska, D., Cockerill, R., Barnsley, J., & DiCenso, A. (2002). A framework for the dissemination and utilization of research for health care policy and practice.

Online Journal of Knowledge Synthesis in Nursing,
9(7). Retrieved from http://www.sttedu/
VirginiaHendersonLibrary/articles/090007.pdf

Dobbins, M., Davies, B., Danseco, E., Edwards, N., & Virani,
T. (2005). Changing nursing practice: Evaluating the
usefulness of a best-practice guideline implementation
toolkit. *Nursing Leadership, 18*(1), 34–45.

Dobbins, M., DeCorby, K., Robeson, P., Husson, H., &
Tirilis, D. (2009). School-based physical activity programs
for promoting physical activity and fitness in children and
adolescents aged 6–18. Cochrane Database of Systematic
Reviews Art. No.: CD007651. doi:10.1002/
14651858.CD007651

Estabrooks, C. A. (1998). Will evidence-based nursing practice
make practice perfect? *Canadian Journal of Nursing
Research, 30,* 15–36.

Flemming, K. (1998). Asking answerable questions. *Evidence-
Based Nursing, 1,* 36–37.

Farmer, A. P., Légaré, F., Turcot, L., Grimshaw, J., Harvey, E.,
McGowan, J. L., & Wolf, F. (2008, July). Printed
educational materials: Effect on professional practice and
health care outcomes. *Cochrane Database Systematic
Reviews, 16,* (3): CD004398.

Friere, P. (1972). *Pedagogy of the oppressed.* New York, NY:
Herder & Herder.

Graham, I. D., Logan, J., Harrison, M. B., Straus, S. E.,
Tetroe, J., Caswell, W., et al. (2006). Lost in knowledge
translation: Time for a map? *Journal of Continuing
Education in the Health Professions, 26,* 13–24.

Grimshaw, J. M., Thomas, R. E., MacLennan, G., Fraser, C.,
Ramsay, C. R., Vale, L., Whitty, P., Eccles, M. P., et al.
(2004). Effectiveness and efficiency of guideline
dissemination and implementation strategies. *Health
Technology Assessment, 8*(6). doi:10.3310/hta8060

Heater, B. S., Becker, A. M., & Olson, R. (1988). Nursing
interventions and patient outcomes. A meta-analysis of
studies. *Nursing Research, 37,* 303–307.

Hodnett, E. D., Kaufman, K., O'Brien-Pallas, L., Chipman,
M., Watson-MacDonell, J., & Hunsburger, W. (1996). A
strategy to promote research-based nursing care: Effects on
childbirth outcomes. *Research in Nursing and Health, 19*
(1), 13–20.

Jadad, A. R., & Haynes, R. B. (1998). The Cochrane
collaboration: Advances and challenges in improving
evidence-based decision making. *Medical Decision Making,
18,* 2–9.

Kunz, R., & Oxman, A. (1998). The unpredictability paradox:
Review of empirical comparisons of randomized and non-
randomized clinical trials. *British Medical Journal, 317,*
1185–1190.

Lomas, J. (1991). Words without action? The production,
dissemination, and impact of consensus recommendations.
Annual Review of Public Health, 12, 41–65.

Luker, K. A., & Kenrick, M. (1992). An exploratory study of
the sources of influence on the clinical decisions of
community nurses. *Journal of Advanced Nursing, 17,*
457–466.

McKibbon, A., & Marks, S. (1998a). Searching for the best
evidence, part 1: Where to look. *Evidence-Based Nursing, 1,*
68–70.

McKibbon, A., & Marks, S. (1998b). Searching for the best
evidence, part 2: Searching CINAHL and Medline.
Evidence-Based Nursing, 1, 105–107.

Oxman, A., Guyatt, G., Cook, D., & Montori, V. (2002).
Summarising the evidence. In G. Guyatt & D. Rennie
(Eds.), *Users' guides to the medical literature: A manual for
evidence-based clinical practice* (pp. 155–173). Chicago, IL:
AMA Press.

Pearcey, P. A. (1995). Achieving research-based nursing
practice. *Journal of Advanced Nursing, 22,* 33–39.

Petticrew, M. (2001). Systematic reviews from astronomy to
zoology: Myths and misconceptions. *British Medical
Journal, 322,* 98–101.

Ploeg, J. (1999). Identifying the best research design to fit the
questions, part 2: Qualitative designs. *Evidence-Based
Nursing, 2,* 36–37.

Public Health Agency of Canada (2008). *Core Competencies for
Public Health. 1.0.* Retrieved from http://www.phac-aspc
.gc.ca/ccph-cesp/index-eng.php

Ratner, P. A., Johnson, J. L., Richardson, C. G., Bottorff, J. L.,
Moffat, B., Mackay, M., . . . Budz, B. (2004). Efficacy of a
smoking-cessation intervention for elective-surgical
patients. *Research in Nursing and Health, 27*(3), 148–161.

Registered Nurses Association of Ontario. (2010). *Best practice
guidelines.* Retrieved from www.rnao.org

Roberts, J., & DiCenso, A. (1999). Identifying the best
research design to fit the question, part 1: Quantitative
designs. *Evidence-Based Nursing, 2,* 4–6.

Russell, C. K., & Gregory, D. M. (2003). Evaluation of
qualitative research reports. *Evidence-Based Nursing, 6,*
36–40.

Sackett, D. L., Rosenberg, W., Gray, J. A. M., & Haynes, R. B.
(1996). Evidence-based medicine: What it is and what it
isn't. *British Medical Journal, 312,* 71–72.

Sackett, D. L., Strauss, S. E., Richardson, W. S., Rosenberg,
W., & Haynes, R. B. (2000). *Evidence based medicine: How
to practice and teach EBM.* London, England: Churchill
Livingstone.

Sandberg, J., Lundh, U., & Nolan, M. R. (2001a). Placing a
spouse in a care home: The importance of keeping. *Journal
of Clinical Nursing, 10,* 406–416.

Sandberg, J., Lundh, U., & Nolan, M. R. (2001b).
Randomised controlled trial of specialist nurse intervention
in heart failure. Placing a spouse in a care home: The
importance of keeping. *Journal of Clinical Nursing,
10,* 406–416. Abstract obtained from *Evidence-Based
Nursing, 2002, 5,* 32.

Singer, G. H. S., Ethridge, B. L., & Aldana, S. I. (2007).
Primary and secondary effects of parenting and stress
management interventions for parents of children with
developmental disabilities: A meta-analysis. *Mental
Retardation and Developmental Disabilities Research Reviews,
13,* 357–369.

Towheed, T., Maxwell, L., Anastassiades, T. P., Shea, B.,
Houpt, J. B., Welch, V., Hochberg, M. C., & Wells, G. A.
(2005). Glucosamine therapy for treating osteoarthritis.
Cochrane Database of Systematic Reviews. Art. No.:
CD002946. doi:10.1002/14651858.CD002946.pub2

University of York, NHS Centre for Reviews and Dissemination. (1999). Getting evidence into practice. *Effective Health Care, 5*(1). Retrieved from http://www.york.ac.uk/inst/crd/ehc51.pdf

U.S. Department of Health and Human Services, Agency for Healthcare Research and Quality. (2010). *National guideline clearinghouse.* Retrieved from www.ahrq.gov

Utterback, J. M. (1974). Innovation in industry and the diffusion of technology. *Science, 183,* 620–626.

ADDITIONAL RESOURCES

Books

Cullum, N., Ciliska, D., Haynes, R. B., & Marks, S. (Eds.). (2008). *Evidence-based nursing: An introduction.* Oxford, England: Blackwell.

Journals of Pre-Appraised Research

Evidence-Based Nursing
http://www.ebn.bmjjournals.com

Evidence-Based Mental Health
http://www.ebmh.bmjjournals.com

Evidence-Based Medicine
http://www.ebm.bmjjournals.com

Other Useful Websites

BMJ Journals Online
http://www.bmjjournals.com

BMJ *Clinical Evidence*
http://www.clinicalevidence.org

Cochrane Collaboration Health Promotion/Public Health Field
http://www.vichealth.vic.gov.au/cochrane

Cochrane Library
http://www.thecochranelibrary.com

Evidence-Based Nursing
http://www.evidencebasednursing.com

Health-evidence.ca
http://www.health-evidence.ca

National Collaborating Centre for Methods and Tools
http://www.nccmt.ca

National Guideline Clearinghouse
http://www.guideline.gov

Teaching/Learning Evidence-based Practice
http://www.mdx.ac.uk/www/rctsh/ebp/main.htm

U.K. National Health Service, Health Development Agency (formerly the Health Education Authority)
http://www.hda.nhs.uk

Users' Guides Interactive
http://www.usersguides.org

About the Authors

Donna Ciliska, RN, PhD, is a Professor at the School of Nursing, McMaster University, and has an appointment as Nursing Consultant with Hamilton Public Health and Community Services. Dr. Ciliska is an editor of the journal *Evidence-Based Nursing.* Her research interests include community health, obesity, eating disorders, and research dissemination and utilization.

Rebecca Ganann, RN, MSc, is an Instructor and doctoral student in the School of Nursing, McMaster University, and a Research Coordinator of the Canadian Community Health Nursing Study and the Effective Public Health Practice Project. She is Secretary of the Community Health Nurses Initiatives Group. Her research interests include community health, knowledge translation, immigrant women's perinatal health, and service accessibility.

Information Technology

Ruta Valaitis, Linda Ferguson, and Jane Sparkes

OBJECTIVES

After studying this chapter, you should be able to:

1. Identify basic informatics competencies for community health nurses.

2. Describe the use of the Internet to access health information by various Canadian population groups.

3. Evaluate the quality of a health website.

4. Describe a variety of Internet technology applications with potential to support health promotion, disease prevention, and chronic disease management.

5. Identify ways to increase accessibility to health information on the Internet for the public.

6. Describe emerging technology tools that can support community health nursing practice, professional development, and knowledge exchange in community health nursing.

INTRODUCTION

Exponential growth has occurred in the use of Internet-based **information and communication technologies (ICTs)** by health professionals and the public. The term ICT represents a variety of computer-based technology systems that support gathering, analyzing, archiving, retrieving, processing, and transmitting information and communication. ICTs can support people to increase control over their health through access to health information, provide social support, facilitate behaviour change, and support community mobilization. Primary health care nursing service delivery can be improved through the use of innovative, interactive **e-health** interventions that are tailored to individual needs. Eysenbach (2001) defined e-health as

> . . . an emerging field in the intersection of medical informatics, public health and business, referring to health services and information delivered or enhanced through the Internet and related technologies. In a broader sense, the term characterizes not only a technical development, but also a state-of-mind, a way of thinking, an attitude, and a commitment for networked, global thinking, to improve healthcare locally, regionally, and worldwide by using information and communication technology. (p. 1)

Community health nurses (CHNs) can support the effective use of ICTs to promote health, prevent illness, and manage chronic disease using e-health interventions.

CHNs are expected to meet the Canadian Community Health Nursing Standards of Practice (CHNAC, 2008),

which include specific standards related to nursing informatics (see Appendix A). Nursing informatics (Staggers & Bagley Thompson, 2002) has been defined as

> . . . a specialty that integrates nursing science, computer science, and information science to manage and communicate data, information, and knowledge in nursing practice. Nursing informatics facilitates the integration of data, information, and knowledge to support patients, nurses, and other providers in their decision making in all roles and settings. This support is accomplished through the use of information structures, information processes, and information technology. (p. 262)

In this chapter, you will learn about CHN competencies as they relate to **nursing informatics** and gain an overview of current research on accessing and using the Internet for health information and communication. You will explore innovations in technology that have shown potential to support health promotion, disease prevention, and chronic disease management. Finally, you will be introduced to ICTs that support professional development and knowledge exchange in community health nursing.

NURSING INFORMATICS COMPETENCIES

Public health informatics is defined as "the systematic application of information and computer sciences and technology to public health practice, research and learning" (Yasnoff,

O'Carroll, Koo, Linkins, & Kilbourne, 2000, p 68). The Canadian Community Health Nursing Standards of Practice are based on the principles of primary health care that include the appropriate use of technology and resources. Specifically, the Standards state that CHNs are expected to use "nursing informatics (information and communication technology) to generate, manage and process relevant data to support nursing practice" (CHNAC, 2008, p. 15). Complementary to these standards is a set of public health informatics competencies developed in the United States for front-line staff, senior-level technical staff, and supervisory and management staff (Centers for Disease Control and Prevention and University of Washington's Center for Public Health Informatics, 2009). The Canadian Nursing Informatics Association (CNIA) has also made recommendations concerning basic Internet and computer competencies of nursing graduates (CNIA, 2003). CNIA identified a need to build strong links between nursing informatics and evidence-based practice; increase informatics skills of educators, clinicians, and students; identify how informatics is covered in curricula; build stronger human, material, and financial infrastructure for ICT in clinical and academic settings; and strengthen partnerships with the private sector.

USE OF THE INTERNET TO ACCESS HEALTH INFORMATION

Rapid growth has occurred in Canadians' use of the Internet to access health information. According to The Internet Use Survey (Figure 11.1), in 2009, 69.9% of individuals searched for medical or health information at home using the Internet;

(Statistics Canada, 2009). The use of the Internet for health information in the United States continues to grow also; Pew Internet surveys conducted between 2002 and 2008 showed that between 75 and 83% of Internet users searched for health information online (Fox & Jones, 2009).

Underhill and McKeown reported that Internet searches for health information are more likely to be done by women with higher income and education (2008), while young men were least likely to perform this type of search. Health-related Internet searches focused on specific diseases, healthy lifestyle, symptoms, drugs or medications, and alternative therapies. About 38% of those who searched for health information online discussed their findings with a healthcare provider (Fox & Jones, 2009).

Although study participants viewed physicians as the most credible source of health information, 48.6% of respondents reported using the Internet first, while 10.9% reported going to their physicians first (Hesse et al., 2005). Kivits (2006) noted similar trends in the United Kingdom, where Internet users indicate needing Internet health resources to prepare for consultations with physicians or to follow up on limited information from their healthcare provider.

A random survey of 2038 adults in the Pew Internet Project found that although sick or disabled adults were less likely to use the Internet, they did search for online health information more than their healthier counterparts (Goldner, 2006). Another trend noted by Hesse et al. (2005) was increasing Internet use for personal health maintenance, with a corresponding increase in Internet users (approximately 9%) who purchased pharmaceuticals online. Approximately 7% communicated with physicians via email—a phenomenon that will have significant management issues for physicians—and

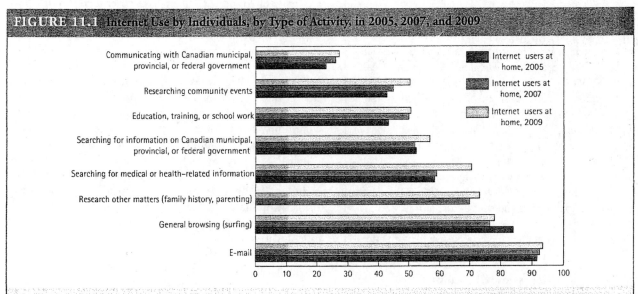

FIGURE 11.1 Internet Use by Individuals, by Type of Activity, in 2005, 2007, and 2009

Source: Statistics Canada. (2010). Internet use by individuals, by type of activity. Summary Tables, CANSIM Table 358-0130 (http://www40.statcan.gc.ca/l01/cst01/comm29a-eng.htm?sdi=internet).

Note: The target population for the Canadian Internet Use Survey has changed from individuals 18 years of age and older in 2005 to individuals 16 years of age and older in 2007 and beyond. (Internet users at home are individuals who responded that they had used the Internet from home in the past twelve months.)

4% participated in online support groups. In addition, incidental online health information acquisition was positively correlated with increased Internet use and seeking online health information for self or others (Tian & Robinson, 2009).

Personal empowerment, defined as the development of personal involvement and responsibility, is enhanced by the use of online health resources (Lemire, Sicotte, & Paré, 2008). Through self-report, Internet users identified three aspects of empowerment: compliance with expert advice; self-reliance through individual choice; and social inclusion through the development of collective support. Internet users perceived that all three aspects were enhanced by access to online health information (Lemire et al., 2008).

Khechine, Pascot, and Prémont (2008) demonstrated that persons with long-term illnesses were more likely to access websites that were scientific in nature (medical, electronic library, government websites, or foundations). They often accessed online health information at two points in the medical decisional process: identification of possible treatments and treatment follow-up. In this study, only about 25% of respondents frequently used online discussion forums for information even though Hoffman-Goetz, Donelle, and Thomson (2009) demonstrated that 91% of the advice provided in the forums was congruent with best practice guidelines.

CANADIAN RESEARCH BOX

Can the Internet be used as a health promotion marketing tool?

Gosselin, P., & Poitras, P. (2008). Use of an Internet "viral" marketing software platform in health promotion. *Journal of Medical Internet Research, 10,* e47.

An online health promotion game named the "The Crazy Race" was promoted through the use of viral marketing with the aim of increasing traffic to a Canadian government health promotion website (Canadian Health Network). Viral marketing relies on person-to-person electronic communications about a topic, which are self-generating—an electronic version of "word-of-mouth" communication. The aim is to target whole populations or segments of a population. In this study, an initial group of 215 people were sent invitations to participate in the campaign. After 15 days, and with no media support, the campaign generated itself. A total of 110 200 Web users registered to participate and sent a total of 439 275 invitations to others. This represented 2% of the Canadian Web user population. Viral marketing was shown to be an affordable mass marketing tool for public health campaigns.

Discussion Questions

1. How could you use a viral marketing approach to develop a health campaign for university students?
2. What do you think motivates people to forward information from the Internet to others? What advantages does this have for health promotion interventions?

Although patients bring their search results to discuss with their physicians (Underhill & McKeown, 2008), it is worrying that nurses and doctors are rarely asked for advice regarding where to search for health information online (Rice, 2006). This finding highlights an important health education role for CHNs, especially when working with Internet users. Nurses are cautioned that online health information is only one approach to delivering health messages within myriad other communications media (Kivits, 2006).

Internet Access Issues

Although many populations use the Internet for health information, not everyone has access. Tapscott (1998) first identified the **digital divide** as information "haves" and "have-nots," which divided society into knowers and know-nots, and doers and do-nots. The digital divide refers to the division of population groups who have and do not have access to—and/or the capability to use—information technology. A new digital divide was proposed differentiating three classes of access, including people with no access (22%), modest connections (such as dial-up) (40%), and the broadband elite (33%) (Fox, 2005). Further, Lenhart et al. (2003, p. 3) described four main types of Internet non-users. "Net-evaders" constitute 20% of non-users, who live in connected households and use family members as proxies to send and receive email and search the Web. "Net dropouts" make up 17% of non-users (overlapping with "net-evaders"), who used the Internet in the past but stopped because of technical problems or because they did not like it. Many of them think they may return to the Internet someday. "Intermittent users" are made up of 27 to 44% of Internet users who dropped out and have now returned to the Internet. The last group is made up of 69% of non-users who are "truly disconnected." They have never used the Internet and do not live with or know many Internet users. Despite these access limitations, Goldner (2006) warned health professionals to provide education to the sick about the quality of online health information despite their low Internet use because they will likely search the Internet for health information in the future. Low-income communities in the United States have long been shown to use and benefit from community-based Internet access to empower and build healthier neighbourhoods (Milio, 1996; Schon, Sanyal, & Mitchell, 1999). However, the Internet has also been found to be a poor source of health information for some groups, including the Chinese immigrant population of Vancouver, British Columbia and Seattle, Washington (Woodall et al., 2009). Therefore, nurses should not assume that all clients can, or will, access the Internet for health information.

Youth are early adopters of technology; therefore, technology has the significant potential to enhance youth's health decision making. Their access issues differ from those of others. Skinner, Biscope and Poland (2003) studied 210 Ontario youth to explore their perceptions of the Internet for health information and resources. The quality of Internet access was significantly impacted by four factors. *Privacy* referred to youths' ability to search for information on sensitive topics without being observed by others; *gate-keeping* referred to blocks put on certain websites or limits to types of use; *timeliness* was related to the ability to have access to information for as long as needed (e.g., access limited during school hours or limitations from parents on Internet time); *functionality* referred to technical issues such as speed of access and functions such as ICQ ("I Seek You"—an instant messaging program). The latter was strongly related to socioeconomic status and geographic location. Health and education professionals should support interventions to address the "access quality divide" for more vulnerable populations (Skinner et al., 2003).

Access for Disabled Populations

CHNs often work with disabled populations. The Canadian Council on Social Development reported that more than half a million adult Canadians have some form of vision loss, more than a million have some form of hearing loss, and a fair number have both (2005). People with disabilities can benefit from using ICTs, since they can reduce isolation by helping them reach people with similar experiences (Seymour & Lupton, 2004), become better informed, increase communication, and enhance access to health information. The next section will review accessibility standards that guide the design of health information websites, and provide a basic overview of technology tools to enhance disabled clients' Internet access.

The World Wide Web Consortium (W3C) (www.w3.org) is an international organization that oversees the standardization and operation of the Web. In 1997, to ensure equitable and universal access to information for all populations including people with disabilities, W3C launched the **Web Accessibility Initiative (WAI)** (W3C, 2009). Under this initiative, accessibility standards for Web content designers and developers were created. The **Web Content Accessibility Guidelines (WCAG)** document was updated in 2008 (Caldwell, Slatin & Vanderheiden, 2008). These guidelines define **accessible** as "usable to a wide range of people with disabilities, including blindness and low vision, deafness and hearing loss, learning difficulties, cognitive limitations, limited movement, speech difficulties, photosensitivity, and combinations of these." Standards were grouped into different priority levels. Disability advocates recommend that websites at a minimum meet the Priority Level One standard.

Priority Level One design standards are relatively simple to meet. For example, Web page images need clear text descriptions. Html code should include alt tags (alternative text tags) so that when a user rolls over the image, a text description appears. When browser preferences are set for "text only," the option for viewing images is turned off. This option is useful for the visually impaired. Screen readers turn screen text to speech and can read text programmed in the alt tag codes, thereby informing visitors what images are on the page. Another Priority One standard includes the use of contrasting background and text colours. Such standards help to ensure that Web documents are navigable. The Treasury Board of Canada Secretariat has also identified a set of guidelines for all federal government department websites called the "Common Look and Feel for the Internet" (2007). These

guidelines incorporate Priority One and Priority Two W3C checkpoints and should be used to ensure accessibility.

Health information websites generally get failing grades with respect to accessibility. Lüchtenberg, Kuhli-Hattenbach, Sinangin, Ohrloff,, & Schalnus (2008) report that 82% of 139 evaluated health information sites were not fully accessible to the visually impaired. More accessible sites are likely visited more often and may even be preferred by the non-disabled consumer. An evaluation of U.S. State Health Department websites indicated that public agencies "fall short of fair and equitable e-health accessibility and confidentiality" (West & Miller, 2006, p. 656). There was also limited access to translations to meet the public's needs.

Numerous software and hardware devices are available to assist disabled populations. Some commonly used devices for the visually impaired include screen readers, screen magnifiers, Braille displays, voice recognition technologies, data extraction tools that filter content from overly busy Web pages, and OCR software to turn a printed page into electronic text for screen reading. Portable note-taking devices can help people with speech communication disorders, and ergonomic adapters, dictation programs, and voice controlled software can assist the mobility impaired (Fichten et al., 2003). Simple adjustments can be made with most operating systems to enhance accessibility. For example, explore the "Accessibility Options" folder in the Control Panel of your own computer to adjust settings for hearing, vision, and mobility.

QUALITY OF HEALTH INFORMATION ON THE INTERNET

Access to good-quality health information can empower clients to address their health issues; however, increased public access to health information on the Internet has introduced

TABLE 11.1 Recommended Nursing Actions with Respect to Health Information on the Internet

Develop skills in online health information retrieval and evaluation to identify and recommend the best online sites for health information.

Assess clients' Internet access, computer competencies, health literacy, online activity, desired role in decision making, and need for assistive devices to access the Internet.

Identify local community resources for Internet access.

Invite clients to discuss the health information they have found online.

Consider client–provider online communication options (email, bulletin boards, instant messaging), and develop guidelines for email triage in practice settings similar to telephone triage protocols.

When using Internet-based communications with clients, learn about the security of the site and ramifications for client privacy.

Consider gender and culture preferences when developing Web-based health promotion interventions.

Teach clients how to evaluate quality and appropriateness of health information on the Web.

Source: Adapted from Dickerson, S. S. (2006). Women's use of the internet: What Nurses need to know. Journal of Obstetric, Gynecologic, & Neonatal Nursing, 35(1), 151–156. doi:10.1111/J.1552-6909.2006.00004.x with permission.

both risks and opportunities. The quality of health information on the Internet is highly variable. The public is challenged to determine the quality and trustworthiness of the health information provided. Health information on the Internet includes health promotion information, screening tests, personal accounts of illness, patient testimonials about treatment effectiveness, patient opinions or perspectives on their illness experiences, product advertisers, treatment providers, patient/client discussion and support groups, peer-reviewed articles, and decision-making aids. A goal for CHNs includes assisting clients to become knowledgeable consumers of information available to them in this medium (Lemire, Sicotte, & Paré, 2008). Recommendations for nurses are listed in Table 11.1.

Many Internet users have expressed concern about the credibility of Internet-based health information. They have also indicated interest in accessing a variety of Internet-based health information resources, including scientific and medical information and patient testimonials about the illness experience (Kivits, 2009). Unfortunately, even though Internet users may indicate they use criteria such as source credibility, language, and transparency to determine the value of online health information, they have tended to disregard these criteria when actually conducting a search. In addition, Internet users have tended to rely on common sense or personal experience to judge the usefulness of the information (Eysenbach, 2007), and used correspondence with the content of other websites to judge its accuracy (Kivits, 2009). Users have tended to develop a practical knowledge based on their experience to

determine what information and sources of knowledge to select (Kivits, 2009). Norman & Skinner (2006) developed a reliable and valid scale to measure consumer's e-health literacy, which is based on a consumer's knowledge, comfort, and perceived skills at finding, evaluating, and applying health information. The complete scale is available at www.jmir.org/2006/4/e27.

Comfort and familiarity with the Internet does not guarantee the ability to obtain credible online health information. An Internet behaviour and preference study of 60 English-speaking Caribbean immigrant women in New York City revealed that although Internet use was high in this group, many participants did not know the differences among websites with domain names of .edu, .gov, .com, or .net (Changrani & Gany, 2005). When searching for health information on the Internet, participants used links from the first screen of results displayed by the search engine and rarely refined their search terms or repeated the search. Most searches were concluded within five minutes. If participants repeated a search, they stated it was because they did not trust the source or understand the information. Eysenbach and Kohler (2002) and Kivits (2009) have reported similar findings.

Tools Available for Rating Health Information on the Internet

There are many tools available to consumers and healthcare providers that rate the quality of health information on the Internet. Various dimensions of Internet resources can be evaluated, including content, journalistic value, targeted audience, website design, readability/usability, and ethical issues of privacy. These dimensions have changed over time as **Web 2.0** technologies, including collaborative, adaptive, and interactive sites have emerged (O'Grady et al., 2009). Unfortunately, consumers may have difficulties determining the value of the ratings provided on the health information websites.

Providing clients with clear criteria of credible online information is the best means of enabling them to assess its quality. Using the **HON Code** (Health on the Net Foundation, 2009) to examine online information with clients is an effective way of teaching the criteria while simultaneously critiquing the online information. In Table 11.2, eight principles are listed and described.

Although healthcare professionals may be adept at applying HON criteria, most laypersons will not be.

Table 11.3 illustrates questions that clients may use in assessing the health information they have accessed on the Internet. Assisting clients to interpret and apply these criteria will empower them to use Internet health information with greater confidence. HON (Health on the Net Foundation, 2009) also supports a service where health information consumers may submit a URL to the "WRAPIN" service (http://www.wrapin.org) to determine if the site is accredited or trustworthy (WRAPIN, 2007). Sites are searched in various languages. In addition, clients can be encouraged to download the HON code toolbar into their browser, which helps them search for HON-approved sites (http://www.hon.ch/HONcode/Plugin/Plugins.html).

TABLE 11.2   HON Code of Conduct for Medical and Health Websites

1. Authority	Any medical or health advice provided and hosted on this site will only be given by medically trained and qualified health professionals unless a clear statement is made that a piece of advice offered is from a non-medically qualified individual or organisation.
2. Complementarity	The information provided on this site is designed to support, not replace, the relationship that exists between a patient/site visitor and his/her existing physician.
3. Privacy	Confidentiality of data relating to individual patients and visitors to a medical/health Web site, including their identity, is respected by this Web site. The Web site owners undertake to honour or exceed the legal requirements of medical/health information privacy that apply in the country and state where the Web site and mirror sites are located.
4. Attribution	Where appropriate, information contained on this site will be supported by clear references to source data and, where possible, have specific HTML links to that data. The date when a clinical page was last modified will be clearly displayed (e.g. at the bottom of the page).
5. Justifiability	Any claims relating to the benefits/performance of a specific treatment, commercial product, or service will be supported by appropriate balanced evidence in the manner outlined above in Principle 4.
6. Transparency	The designers of this Web site will seek to provide information in the clearest possible manner and provide contact addresses for visitors that seek further information or support. The webmaster will display his/her email address clearly throughout the Web site.
7. Financial disclosure	Support for this Web site will be clearly identified, including the identities of commercial and non-commercial organizations that have contributed funding, services or material for the site.
8. Honesty in advertising & editorial policy	If advertising is a source of funding, it will be clearly stated. A brief description of the advertising policy adopted by the Web site owners will be displayed on the site. Advertising and other promotional material will be presented to viewers in a manner and context that facilitates differentiation between it and the original material created by the institution operating the site.

Source: © *Health on the Net Foundation, http://www.hon.ch/HONcode/Pro/Conduct.html. Reproduced with permission.*

TABLE 11.3   Questions for Clients to Use in Assessing Internet Health Information

1. Is the health information provided by a qualified medical practitioner or an organization that is committed to the public's health?
2. Does the website encourage you to discuss the health information with your physician or another health care professional?
3. Is your identity protected on this website?
4. Does the website indicate sources or references for the information provided? Are these sources credible?
5. Are claims of effectiveness of treatments supported by credible evidence?
6. Is the authorship of this website clear to you? Can you contact the webmaster for more information?
7. Is the sponsorship of the website clearly apparent to you?
8. Are the commercial advertisements clearly separated from the health information presented on the website? Is the advertising policy stated on the website?
9. Is there a link to the homepage of the sponsoring organization from the health information webpages?
10. Does the homepage explain the mission, purpose and objectives, sources of funding, and governance of the organization?

Assessment of Health Information Websites

The usability of health information websites may relate to more than the accuracy of the information provided. The Health Information Technology Institute provided another set of criteria that evaluate health information websites on their usability for consumers (Health Summit Working Group, 2010). These criteria include credibility, content, disclosures, links, design, interactivity, and caveats (Table 11.4) and relate to the presentation of information and ease of use.

Readability of text is an important design aspect of every Web page. Readability is a measure of how easily and comfortably text can be read. People with lower reading skills also use the Internet. For websites intended for laypersons, reading levels should be focused approximately at a Grade 9 level. Reading experts suggest that the majority of the population prefers written materials three grades below the last grade attended at school (Gottlieb & Rogers, 2004). Although this level seems low, it may still be higher than the reading comprehension level of the general population, which is on average Grade 5–6 level (Gottlieb & Rogers, 2004). Within the Canadian population, 7% of anglophones and 18% of francophones have not completed Grade 9 (Statistics Canada, 2006), and a 42% of the working-age population scored

TABLE 11.4   HITI Criteria for Assessing Health Information Websites

1. Credibility	Source: Sponsoring agency logo and information are displayed, along with relevant personal or financial associations. Disclosure of sponsorship is clear. Currency: Including date of posting and the date of the document on which information is based. Relevance: Content corresponds to intended purpose of website. Site evaluation: Editorial/content review process.
2. Content	Accuracy and completeness of content, with source identified Disclaimer: Statement that content is general health information and not medical advice.
3. Disclosures	Clear statement of the purpose of the site. Collection of user information: Indicating any user information collected from site and its intended purpose.
4. Links	Selection: Appropriate links are selected. Architecture: Ease of navigation to sites and back to original page. Content of links: Relevant to original website, accurate, external sites clearly identified.
5. Design	Accessibility: For lowest-level browser technology, use by hearing or visually impaired. Logical organization: Including design and layout, readability, language, balance of text and graphics. Navigability: Simple, internally consistent, and easy to use. Internal search capability: Highly desirable.
6. Interactivity	Feedback mechanisms: Feedback mechanisms and exchange of information among users.
7. Caveats	Clarification of the site's function to market products or services.

Source: Adapted from the Health on the Net Foundation. (2009). HON Code of Conduct (HONcode) for medical and health websites. Health on the Net Foundation. Retrieved from http://www.hon.ch/HONcode/Guidelines/guidelines.html

TABLE 11.5   SMOG Readability Assessment Tool: Document Assessment for Approximate Grade Level of Reading Skills

Step 1 Sample selection	Select 30 sentences from the text material: 10 consecutive sentences from the start, the middle, and the end of the material. A sentence is a complete idea with a period, question mark, or exclamation mark, a bulleted point, or both parts of a sentence with a colon included.
Step 2 Word count	Count the number of words with more than three syllables (polysyllabic) in the 30-sentence sample. Include all repetitions of a word, proper nouns, the full text of abbreviations, and hyphenated words as one word.
Step 3 Short text conversion	For documents of fewer than 30 sentences, multiply the number of polysyllabic words by a factor to simulate a sample of 30 sentences. For example, if the document contained 15 sentences, the factor would be 30 divided by 15 to equal a factor of 2. For documents of 24 sentences, the factor would be 30 divided by 24 to equal 1.25.
Step 4 Calculate	Determine the nearest square root of the number of words in the sample. A square root is a number multiplied by itself to equal a perfect square. For example, 8 multiplied by 8 (square root) equals 64 (perfect square). The number that is a square root is usually between 3 and 15.
Add the constant "3" to the square root obtained in step 4.	Example: A sample is assessed as having 86 polysyllabic words in 30 sentences. The nearest square root is 9 (9 times 9 equals 81). The constant of 3 is added to give an approximate reading level of 12, or more appropriately described as a reading level requiring the reading skills approximately at the Grade 12 reading level.

The result is the approximate grade level of reading skills required to read the document. The resultant grade level is correct within 1.5 grades in 68% of cases.

Source: SMOG (Simple Measure of Gobbledygook) Readability Test: Adapted from an article by McLaughlin, G. H. (1969). SMOG-grading: A new readability formula. Journal of Reading, 12, 639–646.

TABLE 11.6 Examples of Different Reading Levels

Grade 13 reading level*	Include exercise such as walking, biking, swimming, jogging, and active sports, according to your individual preferences. Consider other means of transportation or use stairs instead of elevators. Incorporate physical activities into your interactions with your children. The recommended amount of activity per week is 20 minutes of activity daily, on at least 5 separate occasions per week. Monitor your pulse rate, keeping it within the recommended target level during your activity. To stay physically fit, keep active and have fun.
Grade 9 reading level*	Include exercise such as walking, biking, swimming, jogging, and active sports, as you prefer. Consider walking to the store or using the stairs instead of elevators. Be active with your children. We recommend 20 minutes of activity daily, at least 5 times per week. Monitor your pulse rate, keeping it within the target level during your activity. To stay physically fit, keep active and have fun.
Grade 6 reading level*	Include walking, biking, swimming, jogging, and active sports in your daily life. Choose other ways of being active. Take the stairs. Walk to the store. Play with your kids. We suggest at least 20 minutes of exercise per day, 5 times per week. Include more time as you wish. Learn how to take your own pulse rate. Keep your pulse rate within the target level. Stay fit. Keep active. Have fun.

Source: SMOG (Simple Measure of Gobbledygook) Readability Test: Adapted from an article by McLaughlin, G. H. (1969). SMOG-grading: A New Readability Formula. Journal of Reading, 12, 639–646.

*Approximate reading levels based on SMOG assessment

below the functional level in prose literacy scales (Statistics Canada, 2008). Unfortunately, websites have much higher reading levels. Ache & Wallace (2009) found that Internet-based patient education materials were generally written at the Grade 7 to 12 levels, with a mean of Grade 11.

Health professionals who are recommending or creating websites for clients can assess the readability of written or Internet text using a relatively simple tool, the SMOG (Simple Measure of Gobbledygook) Readability Test (McLaughlin, 1969) (Table 11.5). SMOG reading levels correlate well with grade levels identified by other tests of readability (Gottlieb & Rogers, 2004). Because these tests are based on two variables of reading comprehension, word length and sentence length, the reading level of text materials can be reduced by using simple words and shorter sentences (Table 11.6). The Canadian Public Health Association [CPHA] (1999), in its National Literacy and Health Program, published the Directory of Plain Language Health Information to assist health educators in publishing clear and easily understood written materials. Key points are summarized in Table 11.7. CPHA also offers a Plain Language service for the assessment and clarification of health resources (CPHA, 2010).

Healthcare professionals may refer clients to well-developed websites specific to their needs. Factors to be considered when judging the utility of online health information include ease of navigation and ease of accessing Web pages within the site (Bensley, Brusk, Rivas, & Anderson, 2006). Internal links for ease of access are beneficial to users. External links should be assessed for their relatedness and ease of return to the original website. Use of graphics to illustrate concepts enhances usability; however, advertising on the website and irritating pop-ups may interfere. Users also find a pleasing appearance and the opportunity for interactivity, such as calculations of body mass index (BMI),

daily calorie counters, or self-report progress charts, to be beneficial (Ferney & Marshall, 2006). Ease of usage enhances a user's ability to read and use information contained on a website. Clients can also be referred to government-sponsored health information websites.

Targeting Specific Users of Online Health Information

Online health information should be designed for specific users. A combination of health messaging with individual-level participant information permits better **targeting**. Targeting is "the development of a single intervention approach for a defined population sub-group that takes into account characteristics shared by sub-group's members" (Kreuter & Skinner, 2000, p.1). The concept comes from advertising principles that are related to market segmentation.

Although immigrant women use the Internet at the same rate as the general population, only 6% used the Internet for health information, compared to 63% of the general population of Internet users (Changrani & Gany, 2005). Many of these immigrant women indicated a preference for simple navigation sites, simple language, and simple URLs. They preferred soft, soothing colours, images congruent with their culture, "not too much information," and interactive tools such as question-and-answer forums and video and slide show illustrations. They also valued information tailored to their health beliefs and specific needs.

Because scrolling through a website presents challenges for some seniors, designing websites or recommending those that present one paragraph per Web page is a better alternative (Roush, 2006). The U.S. National Institute on Aging maintains a website (http://www.nihseniorhealth.gov) with common health concerns, where text can be enlarged and a "talking function"

TABLE 11.7 Plain Language Strategies

- Use active voice by stating the subject of the action first, e.g., "You should eat 5 to 10 fruits and vegetables per day," instead of "5 to 10 fruits and vegetables should be eaten every day."
- Write directly to the reader, using "you" or implying "you" as the subject of the sentence, e.g., "Take this medication once per day," instead of "This medication should be taken once per day."
- Maintain a positive tone, stating actions as positive behaviours rather than avoidance behaviours, e.g., "Contact your doctor as soon as you feel sick," instead of "Avoid waiting too long to contact your doctor."
- Use common simple terms rather than technical jargon, e.g., "Medicine will relieve your child's pain," instead of "An analgesic will relieve your child's pain."
- Use short words and short sentences.
- Replace more difficult words with simpler words:
  — *drug* or *medicine* in place of *medication*
  — *heart* in place of *cardiac*
  — *doctor* in place of *physician*
  — *take part in* rather than *participate*
  — *problems* in place of *difficulties*
- When in doubt, ask your learners what words are most meaningful.
- Don't change verbs into nouns. The action word is a stronger depiction; e.g., "Decide when to involve your children in meal planning," instead of "Make decisions about your children's involvement in meal planning."
- List important points separate from the text.
  — Use bullets to highlight important points.
  — Keep bullets short.
  — Use boxes to highlight important information.
- Write instructions in the order that you want them to be carried out.
- List items in parallel form such as nouns or actions.
- Keep your writing in a conversational form.
- Test whatever you write with learners before you formalize it.

Source: Adapted from the Plain Language Service of the Canadian Public Health Association (1999) http://www.pls.cpha.ca/english/english.pdf.

can be activated as needed. The site provides links to other credible websites to assist seniors in making decisions about the value of the information they have accessed. Websites with these characteristics will be more useful to seniors.

Tailoring E-Health Messages

The integration of features that enhance **interactivity** has long been known to enhance learning (Stout, Villegas, & Kim, 2001). Interactivity refers to a process where a user is an active participant in using technology and information exchange occurs (i.e., chat rooms, calorie calculators, links). For example, computer programs that integrate social cognitive theory to promote behaviour change for management of weight and physical activity have shown positive results (Winett, Tate, Anderson, Wojcik, & Winett, 2005). Features in programs that generate personalized responses can increase positive attitudes and learning about health issues and have been shown to result in positive health outcomes (Kypri & McAnally, 2005; Strecher, Shiffman, & West, 2005; Suggs & McIntyre, 2009; Winett et al., 2005) For example, generation of clear and understandable tailored

messages that include the user's name and provide specific information addressing individual health needs is important when designing computer-based health promotion interventions (Eakin, Brady & Lusk, 2001). Compared to the concept of targeting, which focuses on interventions for groups, **tailoring** has been referred to as a "process of creating individualized intervention materials or strategies" (Kreuter & Skinner, 2000 p.1). Tailored messages are typically "pushed" to the user, as opposed to sites where users "pull" or search for information from fact sheets, booklets, videos, and images. Tailored messages are typically presented with self-comparison and recommendations based on authoritative research (Figure 11.2). Suggs and McIntyre (2009) found that only 13 of 497 English language online health resources were tailored messages, in spite of the identified efficiencies of such websites. However, a study of tailored versus targeted computer-based interventions to promote hearing protection use among construction workers showed that a targeted intervention was preferred and was more cost effective (Kerr, Savik, Monsen, & Lusk, 2007). Overall, tailoring on individual characteristics (age, gender, readiness) has been shown to outperform static health information (Bennett, & Glasgow, 2009).

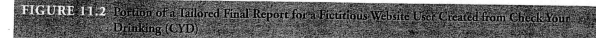

FIGURE 11.2 Portion of a Tailored Final Report for a Fictitious Website User Created from Check Your Drinking (CYD)

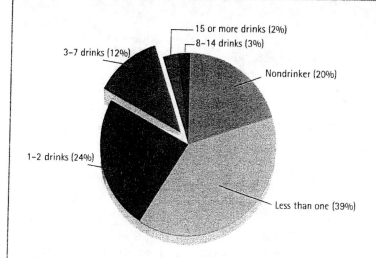

- 15 or more drinks (2%)
- 8–14 drinks (3%)
- 3–7 drinks (12%)
- Nondrinker (20%)
- 1–2 drinks (24%)
- Less than one (39%)

The average number of drinks you reported consuming per week was 6. How do you compare to females your age from Canada? The highlighted slice of the pie chart is where your drinking fits compared to other females in your age range from Canada.

Within the last 12 months:

- You reported drinking on approximately 42.7% of days in the last year.
- You reported that you drank a total of 312 drinks in the last year.

This also means that:

- You spent approximately $1248 in the last year, depending on where you drank (at home, in a bar, etc.)
- You consumed (on average) 200 calories from alcohol on days you drank. Based on the total amount of drinking you had enough alcohol to add roughly 9 pounds to your weight in the past year. Note: One drink has about 100 calories and 3500 calories roughly equals 1 extra pound of weight . . .

Average drinks per week for females age 35–44 from Canada

Source: V-AlcoholHelpCentre.net, http://www.alcoholhelpcentre.net/cyd. Reprinted with permission.

TECHNOLOGY TO SUPPORT HEALTH PROMOTION, DISEASE PREVENTION, AND CHRONIC DISEASE MANAGEMENT

The use of ICTs to support e-health promotion interventions has grown. Evers (2006) attributed this growth to increased Internet use by the public, the low cost of delivery, and public willingness to actively manage their health. It has been argued that e-health promotion interventions can be effective (Evers, 2006). Online interventions for weight management (Bennett & Glasgow, 2009), mental health interventions (Ybarra & Eaton, 2005), cancer care (Donelle & Hoffman-Goetz, 2009), and smoking-cessation programs (Etter, 2005), among others have shown promise. Online counselling interventions can be helpful for people who live in remote areas, value anonymity, belong to a special interest group (Donelle & Hoffman-Goetz, 2008), or have access problems (transportation, scheduling). A systematic review of randomized controlled trials of consumer health informatics interventions (Gibbons et al., 2009) showed that many applications that addressed diet, exercise, physical activity, alcohol abuse, smoking cessation, breast cancer, diabetes, mental health, asthma/chronic obstructive pulmonary disease, and menopause/hormone replacement therapy studies had significant positive impact on at least one intermediate health outcome. No studies identified harm attributed to health informatics interventions. A review of the Internet as a delivery platform for public health interventions showed potential for broad population dissemination of primary and secondary

prevention interventions, many of which showed positive results (Bennett & Glasgow, 2009). The authors concluded that although the reach of Internet interventions is low, there is great potential for growth. They also stressed the importance of intervention designs and components. For example, the most effective weight loss interventions were highly structured, focused on tailored materials, included a counsellor and promoted frequent Web logins. Table 11.8 lists rationale for and drawbacks to delivering health interventions using the Internet (Griffiths, Lindenmeyer, Powell, Lowe, & Thorogood, 2006). Web 2.0 technologies and socially oriented sites such as YouTube, Twitter, Facebook, and MySpace have gained popularity, especially among youth. Research on the use of these technologies to promote health and provide support is still at a stage of infancy, although potential benefits are becoming more evident. Web 2.0 emphasizes the social and participatory nature of Web services, empowering users as well as focusing on content generation and the phenomenon of inclusion (Randeree, 2009). Although these features are well aligned to enhance health promotion and prevention, they have been underutilized for this purpose (Vance, Howe, & Dellavalle, 2009). A study reviewing human papillomavirus (HPV) information found on YouTube showed that 146 videoclips on HPV were available on February 8, 2008 (Ache & Wallace, 2008); most clips were sourced from television clips. About 75% portrayed the vaccination in a positive light and a third generated comments from viewers. On December 29, 2009, a search of the term human papillomavirus on YouTube resulted in 4320 videoclips, illustrating the growth and potential power of this medium for health information and misinformation.

TABLE 11.8   Summary of Findings from Systematic Review of Rationale and Drawbacks for Delivering Health Interventions using the Internet

Reasons for Internet delivery	■ reducing cost and increasing convenience for users ■ reduction of health services costs ■ reduction of isolation of users ■ the need for timely information ■ reduction of stigma ■ increased user and supplier control of the intervention
Possible drawbacks of Internet interventions	■ potential for reinforcing the problems the intervention was designed to help ■ may overcome isolation of time, mobility, and geography, but may be no substitute for face-to-face contact
Elements of future evaluations	■ incorporate the cost; not just the cost to the health service, but also to users and their social networks ■ be alert to unintended effects of Internet delivery of health interventions, and include a comparison with more traditional modes of delivery

Source: Griffiths F., Lindenmeyer A., Powell J., Lowe P., Thorogood M. Why Are Health Care Interventions Delivered Over the Internet? A Systematic Review of the Published Literature. J. Med Internet Res 2006;8(2):e10 (http://www.jmir.org/2006/2/e10/). *Except where otherwise noted, articles published in the Journal of Medical Internet Research are distributed under the terms of the Creative Commons Attribution License* (http://www.creativecommons.org/licenses/by/2.0/).

Computer programs that include interactive components are thought to be more effective. Examples of interactive components are calculators that estimate the cost of smoking, online social support groups where participants communicate with ex-smokers, features that permit posting of personal stories, and email follow-ups before and after quit dates for added support. Such programs can supplement face-to-face programs. It is important for online intervention programs to aim to minimize attrition. Many suffer high attrition over time and the intensity of interventions is also typically low (Bennett & Glasgow, 2009). Newer technologies are also being studied. A Cochrane review of mobile phone-based interventions, using text messaging in particular, showed short-term positive effects on smoking cessation, although no long-term effects were found (Whittaker, Borland, & Bullen, 2009).

CANADIAN RESEARCH BOX

What kinds of health activities can be found on Second Life?

Beard, L., Wilson, K., Morra, D., & Keelan, J. (2009). A survey of health-related activities on Second Life. *Journal of Medical Internet Research, 11*(2): e17.

Second Life is a Web 2.0 interactive communication strategy that incorporates simulated 3-D environments, where users create virtual selves (avatars) in a virtual world where they can meet others, shop, join groups, and create new objects and spaces. Content is generated by users where anonymity and interactivity are encouraged. Users can also access and learn about health issues and discuss health topics. Canadian researchers reviewed and classified the types of health activities on Second Life. Of 68 sites, 34 focused on education and awareness, such as discussion groups and lectures, on topics such as sexual health, training for emergencies, and experiencing schizophrenic hallucinations. One-to-one support with doctors, therapists, or nurses was found on 14 sites related to specific illnesses. Group support was also available (e.g., for sexual transmitted diseases and transgendered persons). Eleven sites provided training of people in healthcare, and marketing and promotion of health services, were found at six sites. Early research results indicate that such applications have potential to impact behaviours in real life.

Discussion Questions

1. What advice would you offer to someone wishing to visit such sites to get health information?

2. What types of health applications do you think could be effective in a Web 2.0 environment like Second Life? Why?

Tailored messages are particularly appropriate for online screening. Online screening interventions have been implemented with varying degrees of success, including screening for mental health (Farvolden, McBride, Bagby, & Ravitz, 2003), chlamydia (Gaydos et al., 2006), fruit and vegetable consumption, fitness levels (Kypri & McAnally, 2005), and alcohol intake (Cunningham, Humphreys, Kypri, & van Mierlo, 2006). U.S. researchers (Saitz et al., 2004) found that screening and management of alcohol problems was a successful Internet health-promotion intervention. Many users were women reporting hazardous amounts of alcohol intake who might not have otherwise looked for help. Gaydos et al. (2006) promoted women in Maryland to obtain home chlamydia screening kits through a website. Of the women who used the site, 97.2% requested the kit by email rather than by phone. Infection rates were 10.3%, indicating that the service was valuable, and users reported high satisfaction.

Online Social Support Groups

Nine percent of people in the United States who used the Internet for health information used an online social support group (Rice, 2006). In February 2010, Yahoo! listed over 12 000 online groups under the fitness and nutrition topic and Google groups listed over 12 500 English-speaking health groups (Figure 11.3). A systematic review (Eysenbach, Powell, Englesakis, Rizo & Stern, 2004) of online support groups found 35 relevant studies. In addition to peer-to-peer support, most studies provided multiple interventions, such as online communication with a professional, and psychoeducation

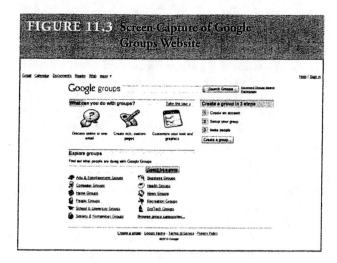

FIGURE 11.3 Screen Capture of Google Groups Website

programs. Because of this, conclusions about the impact of peer-to-peer social support online as a single intervention cannot be drawn. Studies tended to measure outcomes related to social support and depression, and often reported no effects. Despite this, such groups appear to be growing, and no reported cases of harm were found. Barak, Bonniel-Nissim, and Suler (2008, p. 1867) contend that online support groups foster "well-being, a sense of control, self-confidence, feelings of more independence, social interactions, and improved feelings"—all non-specific but highly important psychological factors.

The growth of online groups for new parents has been rapid. The Internet can provide social support to parents who feel psychologically or geographically isolated, and can meet the needs of parents with unique interests (i.e., adoption, bereavement, multiple births). A review of Internet use by parents showed that many parents turn to the Internet for information and support as a result of weaker supports from family and friends (Plantin & Daneback, 2009). Problems identified by parents in using online information and supports included usability problems of a technical nature, a lack of confidence in Internet use, large volumes of off-topic chatter, and occasional disagreements in discussion groups. Although some reports of rude or disrespectful communication exist, the opposite has also been reported, possibly related to the application of Internet etiquette or "netiquette" rules.

POPULATION HEALTH AND TECHNOLOGY

Many Internet technologies can support population health interventions. Computer and Internet technologies have long been used to support community empowerment and capacity building (Korp, 2006; Mehra, Merkel, & Bishop, 2004; Milio, 1996; Schon et al., 1999). An evaluation of the use of an interactive website to involve local citizens in driving policy related to a smoking bylaw in Calgary was very successful (Grierson, van Dijk, Dozios, & Mascher. 2006). The website sparked public debate about the issue, provided citizens with

information about smoking, suggested messages to communicate to city councillors, and updated citizens on how council voted on the issue. Public response was very positive. The website was an effective community capacity-building tool and mobilization strategy that increased citizen participation in building local policy for a healthier community.

Numerous population-based surveillance systems exist within the public health system, which provide valuable data for program planning and evaluation. The Canadian Integrated Public Health Information System (CPHIS), which is being adopted across Canada, combines iPHIS—a client health-reporting surveillance system that supports tracking, follow-up, reporting, and management of cases related to immunization, communicable disease, and population health surveillance—with a Laboratory Data Management System. Panorama, developed by Canada Health Infoway, is being rolled out to support outbreaks with tools to support outbreak identification, vaccine inventory management, case management, and notifications (Mowat & Butler-Jones, 2007). CANSIM (Canadian Socioeconomic Information Management System) tables report social trends impacting the lives of Canadians that can be accessed through E-STAT, which also provides access to Canadian census data. It is available at no cost to students and educators through educational institutions (http://www.statcan.gc.ca/english/Estat/intro.htm). These data are essential for program planners.

ELECTRONIC DOCUMENTATION FOR COMMUNITY HEALTH NURSING

The use of technology to support electronic documentation systems has been growing across Canada, including community health organizations. Three types of electronic documentation systems that have been developed are the *electronic medical record (EMR)*, the *electronic patient record (EPR)*, and the *electronic health record (EHR)*. Nagle (2007) differentiated these terms with respect to access to information, scope of the information included in the documentation, and custodianship of the record. Typically, EMRs are found in primary health care settings and clinics, whereas EPRs are maintained by healthcare organizations. Access to both of these records is limited to authorized caregivers, and the content typically reflects information that used to be recorded in paper-based systems. The EHR is a more comprehensive record that includes contents from the EPR and EMR. It typically includes most information gathered from encounters with the healthcare system, such as primary care, pharmacies, laboratories, and diagnostic imaging units. The client controls access to his or her record, which is "owned" by the client but is hosted by a jurisdiction (Nagle, 2007, p. 2). The EHR, which provides a longitudinal record of an individual's health history and care, is currently being tested in numerous provinces by Canada Health Infoway. Urowitz et al. (2008) indicate that there is a trend to move to EHRs, although the goal to have a pan-Canadian EHR by 2010 is still at a stage of infancy.

TECHNOLOGIES THAT SUPPORT KNOWLEDGE EXCHANGE AND PROFESSIONAL DEVELOPMENT

ICTs can greatly benefit CHNs through the provision of access to supports for professional development and evidence-based decision making. These technologies include online communities of practice, portals, and repositories of evidence-based community health literature. A community of practice refers to groups of people who share common interests, values, and problems about a topic and interact together to deepen their knowledge (Wenger, McDermott, & Snyder, 2002). Canadian nursing researchers investigated networking needs of community health nursing researchers and decision makers (Edwards & Kothari, 2004; Kothari et al., 2005). They identified a need for a formal community health network to assist decision makers, researchers, and practitioners to debate the management of complex community health problems supported by relevant research. Although face-to-face networks were preferred, there was willingness to try online networks. Findings resulted in an online networking project, CHNET-Works! Nurses are encouraged to join the asynchronous communication boards and web-enhanced teleconferences on current community health topics (www.chnet-works.ca).

NurseONE/INF-Fusion developed by the Canadian Nurses Association is a personalized interactive Web 2.0 resource designed to assist nurses in Canada to manage their professional development, connect with colleagues, and gain access to current, credible, reliable information resources and tools to support evidence-based nursing practice (www.nurseone.ca; see Figure 11.4). The Public Health Agency of Canada (PHAC) (2006) has developed a portal for knowledge exchange: the Canadian Best Practices Portal for Health Promotion and Chronic Disease Prevention (http://cbpp-pcpe .phac-aspc.gc.ca). It aims to enhance knowledge exchange in best practices and provides a central access point for best practices approaches. PHAC also provides practitioners with online learning modules to enhance skills in public health practice (www.phac-aspc.gc.ca/sehs-acss/index-eng.phpl). Practitioners in public health can register to take the skills enhancement online modules. A reliable source of evidence-based materials relevant to CHNs includes the fully searchable online service Health-Evidence.ca (http://health-evidence.ca). The Effective Public Health Practice Program also provides links to numerous systematic literature reviews and summaries (www. ephpp.ca/). The National Collaborating Centre of Methods and Tools (NCCMT) (www.nccmt.ca) provides information and resources about knowledge translation methods and tools relevant for community health students and practitioners. In particular, the NCCMT has collaborated with The Health Communication Unit to develop and disseminate the Online Health Program Planner (www.thcu.ca/ohpp/), which is an interactive, flexible, and intuitive tool to assist with the development of evidence-informed program plans (Ciliska et al., 2009).

SUMMARY

ICTs have the potential to provide information, communication, and other supports to empower individuals, groups, and communities. The rapid growth of Internet use by the public to access health information cannot be ignored. CHNs need to incorporate this into their plan of care and take a leadership role in enabling the public to use this health information resource in a safe and effective manner. CHNs can also help ensure accessibility to quality health information for the populations that they serve. Although research into the use of ICTs to support health promotion, disease prevention, and chronic disease management is relatively new, it shows great promise. ICTs can also foster professional development for CHNs by providing access to communities of practice, online learning modules, and evidence-based materials to support practice.

KEY TERMS

information and communication technologies (ICTs), p. 171
e-health, p. 171
nursing informatics, p. 171
public health informatics, p. 171
digital divide, p. 173
Web Accessibility Initiative (WAI), p. 174
Web Content Accessibility Guidelines (WCAG), p. 174
accessible, p. 174
Web 2.0, p. 175
HON code, p. 175
readability, p. 176
SMOG (Simple Measure of Gobbledygook) Readability Test, p. 178
targeting, p. 178
interactivity, p. 179
tailoring, p. 179

FIGURE 11.4 Screen Capture of NurseONE/INF-Fusion

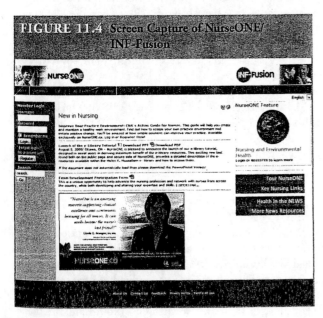

Source: @ Canadian Nurses Association. Reprinted with permission. Further production prohibited.

REVIEW QUESTIONS

1. Which statement is true about viral marketing?

    a) It relies on person-to-person electronic communications about a topic that is self-generating—an electronic version of "word of mouth" communication.

    b) It is caused by computer viruses that are spread when searching for information on the Internet.

    c) It is online marketing of pharmaceuticals for the treatment of common viruses.

    d) It is an issue when a site gets overloaded and is unable to cope.

2. Which are recommended ways to check the quality of the information of a consumer health information website?

    a) Run the URL through a website accessibility checker.

    b) Ignore any sites with a HON code logo.

    c) Assess the site using the HITI criteria.

    d) Use the SMOG criteria.

3. What should nurses consider with respect to educating their clients about the quality of health information on the Internet?

    a) Nurses should provide education to the sick about the quality of online health information despite their low Internet use.

    b) Nurses should not bother providing education to seniors because they generally do not have access to the Internet.

    c) Nurses should not educate visually disabled individuals because sites are not accessible to them.

    d) Nurses should encourage their clients to only use government websites to ensure that they access quality health information.

4. Which feature of health information websites is useful to enhance health promotion?

    a) websites that foster interactivity

    b) tailored messages that do not contain self-comparisons

    c) websites that are written at a Grade 11 reading level

    d) websites that consist of positive personal testimonials

5. Which is correct?

    a) The electronic medical record (EMR) can be found in primary care and other clinic settings.

    b) The electronic patient record (EPR) is found primarily in home care.

    c) The electronic health record (EHR) (which includes contents from the EPR and EMR) has not yet been implemented in Canada.

    d) Electronic computer records will be obsolete in favour of microchips embedded in identity cards.

6. Which statement is true about informatics competencies?

    a) Although it is useful for community health nurses to apply nursing informatics in practice, there is no national standard that relates to this topic.

    b) The Canadian Nursing Informatics Association has made specific recommendations concerning basic Internet and computer competencies of nursing graduates.

    c) Public Health Informatics competencies have been developed in the United States, but they are aimed only at senior-level technical staff.

    d) Informatics standards are covered in the Community Nurses Association of Canada Nursing Practice Standards.

STUDY QUESTIONS

1. Identify different ways that the "digital divide" has been conceptualized since the term first appeared.

2. Describe three tools that can be used to enhance Internet accessibility for disabled populations.

3. What is HON code and what is its purpose?

4. Describe three online health promotion interventions that show promise.

5. Where can community health nurses get access to evidence-based information on the Web to guide their decision making in practice?

6. What is the nursing role with respect to health information on the Internet?

> *After working through these questions, go to the MyNursingLab at **www.pearsoned.ca/mynursinglab** to check your answers.*

INDIVIDUAL CRITICAL THINKING EXERCISES

1. What criteria would you use to evaluate a health promotion intervention, such as a smoking-cessation website?

2. What would you need to consider when working as a community health nurse with a client who is visually impaired and wants to use the Internet?

3. Discuss the merits and drawbacks of the HON code. Review the editorial and the response to it found in the *Journal of Medical Internet Research* by Eysenbach (2000).

4. What would you need to take into account when designing a Web-based intervention for a senior?

5. How can technology help to empower individuals and communities?

GROUP CRITICAL THINKING EXERCISES

1. Discuss the informatics core competencies you think a new graduate working in community health is required to have at a high level of proficiency. Use the Community Health Nurses Standards of Practice (Appendix A) to help you.

2. What trends do you anticipate in the use of the Internet to promote health by youth, senior, new immigrant, and disabled populations? What role could Web 2.0 technologies have in promoting health and preventing disease?

3. Should nurses encourage their clients to join online social support groups? Why or why not?

REFERENCES

Ache, K., & Wallace, L. (2008). Human papillomavirus vaccination coverage on YouTube. *American Journal of Preventive Medicine, 35*, 389–392.

Ache, K. A., & Wallace, L. S. (2009). Are end-of-life patient education materials readable? *Palliative Medicine, 23*, 545–548.

Adaptech Research Network. (2010). *Adaptec, Dawson College*. Retrieved from http://adaptech.dawsoncollege.qc.ca/prdes_e.php

Barak, A., Boniel-Nissim, M., & Suler, J. (2008) Fostering empowerment in online support groups. *Computers in Human Behavior, 24*(5), 1867–1883.

Bennett, G. G., & Glasgow, R. E. (2009). The delivery of public health interventions via the Internet: Actualizing their potential. *Annual review of Public Health, 30*, 273–292.

Bensley, R., Brusk, J. J., Rivas, J., & Anderson, J. V. (2006). Impact of menu sequencing on internet-based education module selection. *International Electronic Journal of Health Education, 9*, 73–80.

Caldwell, B., Slatin, J., & Vanderheiden, G. (2008). Web content accessibility guidelines 2.0. *World Wide Web Consortium W3C*. Retrieved from http://www.w3.org/TR/WCAG20/

Canadian Council on Social Development. (2005). *Disability information sheet number 19* (Rep. No. 19).

Canadian Nurses Association. (2006). *NurseONE, the Canadian nurses portal*. Retrieved from http://www.cna-nurses.ca/CNA/nursing/portal/about/default_e.aspx

Canadian Nursing Informatics Association. (2003). *Educating tomorrow's nurses: Where's nursing informatics?* (Rep. No. G3-6B-DP1-0054).

Canadian Public Health Association. (1999). *Directory of plain language health information*. Retrieved from http://www.cpha.ca/en/portals/h-l/resources.aspx

Canadian Public Health Association. (2010). Plain language service. *Canadian Public Health Association*. Retrieved from http://www.cpha.ca/en/pls.aspx

Centres for Disease Control and Prevention and University of Washington's Centre for Public Health Informatics. (2009). *Competencies for public health informaticians, 2009*. Atlanta, GA: U.S. Department of Health and Human Services, Centres for Disease Control and Prevention. Retrieved from http://www.cdc.gov/InformaticsCompetencies

Changrani, J., & Gany, F. (2005). Online cancer education and immigrants: Effecting culturally appropriate websites. *Journal of Cancer Education, 20*, 183–186.

Ciliska, D., Clark, K., Hershfield, L., Jetha, N., Mackintosh, J., & Finkle, D. (2009). *Using an Online Health Program Planner: What's in it for you?* Ottawa, ON: Canadian Public Health Association; 8 pp.

Community Health Nurses Association of Canada. (2008). *Canadian community health nursing standards of practice*. Toronto, ON: Author.

Cunningham, J. A., Humphreys, K., Kypri, K., & van Mierlo, T. (2006). Formative evaluation and three-month follow-up of an online personalized assessment feedback intervention for problem drinkers. *Journal of Medical Internet Research, 8*(2), e5.

Daneback, K., & Plantin, L. (2008). Research on parenthood and the internet: Themes and trends. *Cyberpsychology: Journal of Psychosocial Research on Cyberspace, 2*(2), article 1. Retrieved from http://cyberpsychology.eu/view.php?cisloclanku=2008110701&article=1

Dickerson, S. S. (2006). Women's use of the internet: What nurses need to know. *Journal of Obstetric Gynecologic and Neonatal Nursing, 35*, 151–156.

Donelle, L., & Hoffman-Goetz, L. (2008). An exploratory study of Canadian Aboriginal online health care forums. *Health Communications, 23*(3), 270–281.

Donelle, L., & Hoffman-Goetz, L. (2009). Functional health literacy and cancer care conversations in online forums for retired persons. *Informatics for Health and Social Care, 34*(1), 59–72.

Eakin, B. L., Brady, J. S., & Lusk, S. L. (2001). Creating a tailored, multimedia, computer-based intervention. *Computers in Nursing, 19*, 152–160.

Edwards, N., & Kothari, A. (2004). CHNET-Works! A networking infrastructure for community health nurse researchers and decision-makers. *Canadian Journal of Nursing Research, 36*(4), 203–207.

Etter, J. F. (2005). Comparing the efficacy of two internet-based, computer-tailored smoking cessation programs: A randomized trial. *Journal of Medical Internet Research, 7*, e2.

Etter, J. F. (2006). The internet and the industrial revolution in smoking cessation counselling. *Drug and Alcohol Review, 25*(1), 79–84.

Evers, K. E. (2006). eHealth promotion: The use of the internet for health promotion. *American Journal of Health Promotion, 20*, 1–7.

Eysenbach, G. (2001). What is e-health? *Journal of Medical Internet Research, 3*, e20.

Eysenbach, G. (2007). From intermediation to disintermediation and apomediation: New models for consumers to access and assess the credibility of health information in the age of Web2.0. *Studies in Health Technology and Informatics, 129*(1), 162–166.

Eysenbach, G., & Kohler, C. (2002). How do consumers search for and appraise health information on the world wide web? Qualitative study using focus groups, usability tests, and in-depth interviews. *British Medical Journal, 324*, 573–577.

Eysenbach, G., Powell, J., Englesakis, M., Rizo, C., & Stern, A. (2004). Health related virtual communities and electronic support groups: Systematic review of the effects of online peer to peer interactions. *British Medical Journal, 328,* 1166.

Farvolden, P., McBride, C., Bagby, R. M., & Ravitz, P. (2003). A Web-based screening instrument for depression and anxiety disorders in primary care. *Journal of Medical Internet Research, 5*(3), e23.

Ferney, S. L., & Marshall, A. L. (2006). Website physical activity interventions: Preferences of potential users. *Health Education Research: Theory and Practice, 21,* 560–566.

Fichten, C. S., Barile, M., & Asuncion, J. (2003). Computer technologies and postsecondary students with disabilities: Implications of recent research for rehabilitation psychologists. *Rehabilitation Psychology, 48,* 207–214.

Fox, S. (2005). Digital divisions: There are clear differences among those with broadband connections, dial-up connections, and no connections at all to the internet. *Pew Internet and American Life Project.* Retrieved from http://www.pewinternet.org/PPF/r/165/report_display.asp

Fox, S., & Jones, S. (2009). *The social life of health information: Americans' pursuit of health takes place within a widening network of both online and offline resources* (Rep. No. 202-149-4500). Washington, DC: Pew Internet and American Life Project.

Gaydos, C. A., Dwyer, K., Barnes, M., RizzoPrice, P. A., Wood, B. J., Flemming, T., et al. (2006). Internet-based screening for Chlamydia trachomatis to reach non-clinic populations with mailed self-administered vaginal swabs. *Sexually Transmitted Diseases, 33,* 451–457.

Gibbons, M. C., Wilson, R. F., Samal, L., Lehmann C. U., Dickersin, K., Lehmann, H. P., . . . Bass, E. B. (2009, October). *Impact of consumer health informatics applications* (Evidence Report/Technology Assessment No. 188). (Prepared by Johns Hopkins University Evidence-based Practice Center under contract No. HHSA 290-2007-10061-I). AHRQ Publication No. 09(10)-E019. Rockville, MD: Agency for Healthcare Research and Quality.

Goldner, M. (2006). Using the internet and email for health purposes: The impact of health status. *Social Science Quarterly, 87,* 690–710.

Gosselin, P., & Poitras, P. (2008). Use of an Internet "viral" marketing software platform in health promotion. *Journal of Medical Internet Research, 10,* e47.

Gottlieb, R., & Rogers, J. L. (2004). Readability of health sites on the internet. *International Electronic Journal of Health Education, 7,* 38–42.

Grierson, T., van Dijk, M. W., Dozois, E., & Mascher, J. (2006). Policy and politics. Using the internet to build community capacity for healthy public policy. *Health Promotion Practice, 7,* 13–22.

Griffiths, F., Lindenmeyer, A., Powell, J., Lowe, P., & Thorogood, M. (2006). Why are health care interventions delivered over the internet? A systematic review of the published literature. *Journal of Medical Internet Research, 8,* e10.

Health on the Net Foundation. (2009). HON code of conduct (HONcode) for medical and health Web sites. *Health on the Net Foundation.* Retrieved from http://www.hon.ch/HONcode/Guidelines/guidelines.html

Health Summit Working Group. (2010). *Information quality tool. Mitretek Systems.* Retrieved from http://www.ieee.org/organizations/pubs/newsletters/npss/march2000/health.htm

Hesse, B. W., Nelson, D. E., Kreps, G. L., Croyle, R. T., Arora, N. K., Rimer, B. K., et al. (2005). Trust and sources of health information. *Archives of Internal Medicine, 165,* 2618–2624.

Hoffman-Goetz, L., Donelle, L., & Thomson, M. D. (2009). Clinical guidelines about diabetes and the accuracy of peer information in an unmoderated online health forum for retired persons. *Informatics for Health and Social Care, 34*(2), 91–99.

Kerr, M., Savik, K., Monsen, K. A., Lusk, S. L. (2007). Effectiveness of computer-based tailoring versus targeting to promote use of hearing protection. *Canadian Journal of Nursing Research, 39*(1), 80–97.

Khechine, H., Pascot, D., & Prémont, P. (2008). Use of health-related information from the Internet by English-speaking patients, *Health Informatics, 14,* 17–28.

Kivits, J. (2009). Everyday health and the internet: A mediated health perspective on health information seeking. *Sociology of Health and Illness, 31*(5), 673–687.

Korp, P. (2006). Health on the internet: Implications for health promotion. *Health Education Research, 21,* 78–86.

Kothari, A., Edwards, N., Brajtman, S., Campbell, B., Hamel, N., Legault, F., et al. (2005). Fostering interactions: The networking needs of community health nursing researchers and decision-makers. *Evidence and Policy, 1,* 291–304.

Kreuter, M. W., & Skinner, H. (2000). Tailoring: What's in a name? *Health Education Research, 15,* 4.

Kypri, K., & McAnally, H. M. (2005). Randomized controlled trial of a web-based primary care intervention for multiple health risk behaviors. *Preventive Medicine, 41,* 761–766.

Lemire, M., Sicotte, C., & Paré, G. (2008). Internet use and the logics of personal empowerment in health. *Health Policy, 88,* 130–140.

Lenhart, A., Horrigan, J., Rainie, L., Boyce, A., Madden, M., & O'Grady, E. (2003). *The ever-shifting internet population: A new look at internet access and the digital divide.* Washington, DC: The Pew Internet and American Life Project.

Lüchtenberg, M., Kuhli-Hattenbach, C., Sinangin, Y., Ohrloff, C., & Schalnus, R. (2008). Accessibility of health information on the Internet to the visually impaired user. *Opthalmologica, 222*(3), 187–193.

McLaughlin, G. H. (1969). SMOG-grading: A new readability formula. *Journal of Reading, 12,* 639–646.

Mehra, B., Merkel, C., & Bishop, A. P. (2004). The internet for empowerment of minority and marginalized users. *New Media and Society, 66,* 781–802.

Milio, N. (1996). *Engines of empowerment: Using information technology to create healthy communities and challenge public policies.* Chicago, IL: Health Administration Press.

Mowat, D., & Butler-Jones, D. (2007). Public health in Canada: A difficult history. *Healthcare Papers, 7,* 31–36.

Nagle, L. (2007). Informatics: Emerging concepts and issues. *Nursing Leadership, 20,* 30–32.

National Institute on Aging. (2002). *Making your website senior friendly.* Retrieved from http://www.nlm.nih.gov/pubs/checklist.pdf

Norman, C. D., & Skinner, H. A. (2006). eHealth Literacy: Essential skills for consumer health in a networked world. *Journal of Medical Internet Research, 8*(2):e9. doi:10.2196/jmir.8.2.e9

O'Grady, L., Witteman, H., Bender, J. L., Urowitz, S., Wiljer, D., & Jadad, A. (2009). Measuring the impact of a moving target: Towards a dynamic framework for evaluating collaborative adaptive interactive technologies. *Journal of Medical Internet Research, 11*, e20.

Public Health Agency of Canada. (2006). *The Canadian Best Practices Portal for health promotion and chronic disease prevention: About the portal.* Retrieved from http://cbpp-pcpe.phac-aspc.gc.ca/

Randeree, E. (2009). Exploring technology impacts of healthcare 2.0 initiatives. *Telemedicine Journal and e-Health, 15*, 255–260.

Rice, R. E. (2006). Influences, usage, and outcomes of internet health information searching: Multivariate results from the Pew surveys. *International Journal of Medical Informatics, 75*, 8–28.

Roush, K. (2006). Two NIH Web sites on aging: One is for providers and the other is for older adults. *American Journal of Nursing, 106*, 17.

Saitz, R., Helmuth, E. D., Aromaa, S. E., Guard, A., Belanger, M., & Rosenbloom, D. L. (2004). Web-based screening and brief intervention for the spectrum of alcohol problems. *Preventive Medicine, 39*(5), 969–975.

Schon, D., Sanyal, B., & Mitchell, W. (1999). *High technology and low-income communities.* Cambridge, MA: MIT Press.

Seymour, W., & Lupton, D. (2004). Holding the line online: Exploring wired relationships for people with disabilities. *Disability and Society, 19*, 291–305.

Skinner, H., Biscope, S., & Poland, B. (2003). Quality of internet access: Barrier behind internet use statistics. *Social Science and Medicine, 57*, 875–880.

Staggers, N., & Bagley Thompson, C. (2002). The evolution of definitions for nursing informatics: A critical analysis and revised definition. *Journal of the American Medical Informatics Association, 9*, 255–262.

Statistics Canada. (2006). *Literacy and the official languages minority.* Retrieved from http://www.statcan.gc.ca/daily-quotidien/080109/dq080109a-eng.htm

Statistics Canada. (2007). *Canadian Internet use survey.* Retrieved from http://www.statcan.gc.ca/daily-quotidien/080612/dq080612b-eng.htm

Statistics Canada. (2008). *International survey of reading skills.* Retrieved from http://www.statcan.gc.ca/daily-quotidien/080109/dq080109a-eng.htm

Statistics Canada. (2009). *Internet use by individuals, by type of activity.* Retrieved from http://www40.statcan.gc.ca/l01/cst01/comm29a-eng.htm?sdi=internet

Stout, P. A., Villegas, J., & Kim, H. (2001). Enhancing learning through the use of interactive tools on health-related websites. *Health Education Research, 16*, 721–733.

Strecher, V., Shiffman, S., & West, R. (2005). Randomized controlled trial of a Web-based computer-tailored smoking cessation program as supplement to nicotine patch therapy. *Addiction, 100*, 682–688.

Suggs, L. S., & McIntyre, C. (2009). Are we there yet? An examination of online tailored health communication. *Health Education and Behavior, 36*, 278–288.

Tapscott, D. (1998). The digital divide. In *Growing up digital: The rise of the net generation* (pp. 255–279). New York, NY: McGraw-Hill.

Tian, Y., & Robinson, J. D. (2009). Incidental health information use on the Internet. *Health Communication, 24*, 41–49.

Treasury Board of Canada Secretariat. (2007). Common look and feel standards for the internet (CLF 2.0). *Treasury Board of Canada Secretariat.* Retrieved from http://www.tbs-sct.gc.ca/clf-nsi/index-eng.asp

Underhill, C., & McKeown, L. (2008). Getting a second opinion: Health information and the internet. *Health Report, 19*, 65–69.

Urowitz, S., Wiljer, D., Apatu, E., Eysenbach, G., DeLenardo, C., Harth, T., . . . Leonard, K. (2008). Is Canada ready for patient accessible electronic health records? A national scan. *BMC Medical Informatics and Decision Making, 8*(33).

U.S. Centers for Disease Control and Prevention and University of Washington's Center for Public Health Informatics. (2009). *Competencies for public health informaticians.* Atlanta, GA: Author.

U.S. Department of Health and Human Services, Centers for Disease Control and Prevention. (2009). *Informatics competencies.* Retrieved from http://www.cdc.gov/InformaticsCompetencies

Vance, K., Howe, W., & Dellavalle, R. P. (2009). Social internet sites as a source of public health information. *Dermatologic Clinics: Epidemiology and Public Health, 27*(2), 133–36. doi:10.1016/j.det.2008.11.010

W3C. (2009). Web accessibility initiative (WAI). *World Wide Web Consortium W3C.* Retrieved from http://www.w3.org/WAI/

Wenger, E., McDermott, R., & Snyder, W. (2002). *A guide to managing knowledge: Cultivating communities of practice.* Boston, MA: Harvard Business School Press.

West, D. M., & Miller, E. A. (2006). The digital divide in public e-health: Barriers to accessibility and privacy in state health department websites. *Journal of Health Care for the Poor and Underserved, 17*(3), 652–667.

Whittaker, R., Borland, R., Bullen, C., et al. (2009). Mobile phone-based interventions for smoking cessation. *Cochrane Database of Systematic Reviews* Oct. 7 (4):CD006611.

Winett, R. A., Tate, D. F., Anderson, E. S., Wojcik, J. R., & Winett, S. G. (2005). Long-term weight gain prevention: A theoretically based internet approach. *Preventive Medicine, 41*(2), 629–641.

WRAPIN. (2007). *Worldwide online Reliable Advice to Patients and Individuals.* European Project-IST-2001-33260. Retrieved from http://www.wrapin.org

Woodall, J., Taylor, V. M., Chong T., Li, L., Acorda, E., Tu, S., . . . Hislpo, G. (2009). Sources of health information among Chinese immigrants to the Pacific Northwest. *Journal of Cancer Education, 24*(4), 334–340.

Yasnoff, W., O'Carroll, P., Koo, D., Linkins, R., & Kilbourne, E. (2000). Public health informatics: Improving and transforming public health in the information age. *Journal of Public Health Management Practice, 6*, 67–75.

Ybarra, M. L., & Eaton, W. W. (2005). Internet-based mental health interventions. *Mental Health Services Research, 7*(2), 75–87.

WEBSITES

The websites for this chapter have been cited in the text.

About the Authors

Ruta Valaitis, RN, PhD, is an Associate Professor in the School of Nursing at McMaster University and was awarded the Dorothy C. Hall Chair in Primary Health Care Nursing in 2007. She has worked as a visiting nurse and a public health nurse and has had extensive experience as a clinical consultant for the Ontario Public Health Research Education and Development Program. Some of her past research has focused on the use of communication technologies to support health sciences education and public health nursing practice, e-health promotion for teen parents and rural youth, and online communities of practice to support nursing and knowledge transfer. Currently, she is leading a national program of research exploring primary care and public health collaboration.

Linda Ferguson, RN, PhD, is a Full Professor in the College of Nursing, University of Saskatchewan. Her undergraduate, master's, and PhD are in the field of nursing, and she has a Post-Graduate Diploma in Continuing Education. She has worked extensively in the field of faculty development within the College of Nursing and the University of Saskatchewan. She has taught educational methods courses at the undergraduate (nursing and physical therapy), post-registration, and master's levels for the past 19 years. Her research has focused on the continuing education needs of registered nurses in practice, mentoring and precepting nurses, teaching excellence, inter-professional education, podcasting and nursing education; and the process of developing clinical judgment in nursing practice. She is currently the Director of the Centre for the Advancement of the Study of Nursing Education and Inter-professional Education (CASNIE) within the College of Nursing at the University of Saskatchewan.

Jane Sparkes, RN, BSN, M.Sc.eHealth received her Bachelor of Science in Nursing Degree from the University of Victoria, British Columbia, and her M.Sc.eHealth from McMaster University. She has practised as staff nurse working on general surgery and orthopaedics wards for over 20 years. Her areas of interest include nursing informatics and mobile health technology in particular remote patient monitoring. Her thesis work investigated the usability of remote cardiac monitoring and smartphone devices in the field.

Communicable Diseases

Sheila Marchant-Short and Leeann Whitney

OBJECTIVES

After studying this chapter, you should be able to:

1. Discuss the evolving perspectives on communicable diseases in the global community.

2. Explain the nature and types of communicable diseases: vaccine-preventable diseases, foodborne and waterborne infections, vector-borne diseases, zoonotic infections, and parasitic infections.

3. Describe surveillance, contact tracing, and the use of vaccines in the control and management of communicable diseases.

4. Describe the roles of international, national, provincial/territorial, and local authorities in the management and reporting of communicable diseases.

5. Describe the role of the community health nurse in the control and management of communicable diseases.

INTRODUCTION

As long as humans have inhabited the earth, communicable diseases have been a part of their lives. Communicable diseases occur in every society, from rural areas to urban cities, from country to country, and without discrimination between rich and poor. With advances in technology and modern medicine, the severity of the illnesses associated with many of these diseases has been reduced. However, with increasing population mobility due to efficient transportation systems, and with lifestyle and environment changes, communicable diseases know no boundaries and are now seen in previously untouched areas across the world. Community health nurses (CHNs) must have a sound knowledge base of communicable diseases in order to prevent or limit the transmission of these diseases and protect the health of the public. This chapter will describe general concepts related to communicable disease and its impact on the global community, discuss the role of CHNs in communicable disease control, and discuss management in relation to the legislative mandate locally, provincially/territorially, and federally.

EVOLVING PERSPECTIVES ON COMMUNICABLE DISEASES

For many centuries, communicable diseases such as tuberculosis (TB), smallpox, leprosy, cholera, scarlet fever, typhoid fever, diphtheria, and poliomyelitis have caused many casualties and threatened the health of humankind. The first recorded worldwide threat from a communicable disease was bubonic plague, which killed about one-third of the population in Europe in the thirteenth century. More recently, the influenza pandemic (Spanish flu) in 1918–1919 was a major global threat, resulting in at least 20 million deaths worldwide (Heymann, 2008). Many communicable diseases were brought to Canada with the arrival and migration of early settlers in the 16th century. Since aboriginals had not had exposure to these diseases, and therefore had not had an opportunity to develop natural immunity, they had little or no resistance to these diseases. Aboriginal people were decimated by the infectious and parasitic diseases carried by the settlers.

Since the mid-1800s, advances in scientific and medical knowledge and in public health measures have contributed to the declining mortality and morbidity among Canadians from communicable diseases. The development of microscopes, germ theories, vaccines, and the improvement of nutrition, sanitation, and living conditions have been instrumental in this decline (see Chapter 1). Additionally, the 1974 World Health Organization's (WHO) Expanded Program on Immunization initiative led to the vaccination of 85% of children around the world against measles, mumps, rubella, tetanus, pertussis, diphtheria, and poliomyelitis by 1985, and the eradication of smallpox in 1977 (WHO, 1998). Public health professionals continue their efforts to combat infectious diseases such as malaria, TB, and parasitic diseases, which can cause life-long disabilities and have socioeconomic consequences (WHO, 2009a).

As a result of recent developments in vaccine production and disease control, infectious diseases such as TB and influenza now cause less threat and impact on morbidity and mortality in Canada. However, new emerging and re-emerging infectious diseases are increasingly challenging the public health system worldwide. The most recent infectious diseases in Canada are Creutzfeldt-Jakob disease (CJD), severe acute respiratory syndrome (SARS), and West Nile virus (WNV). Increasing public awareness of CJD and reporting by healthcare professionals through the CJD federal surveillance program are vital in creating disease data to demonstrate the prevalence and incidence of this emerging infection (Public Health Agency of Canada [PHAC], 2009a).

When treatment protocols to cure TB were developed in 1948, it was anticipated that the disease would be eradicated by 2000. Ironically, TB has now re-emerged as an increased public health threat because of multi-drug-resistant strains and clients' non-compliance with chemoprophylaxis. It affects vulnerable populations such as older adults, those with immune deficiencies, and the poor. Today's global travel and trade, climate change, poverty, inconsistent healthcare resources, the challenges of vector control programs, overuse of antibiotics, and changing lifestyle practices can lead to rapid transmission of infectious diseases. Determinants of health, such as income, education, and housing, have been shown to globally affect the incidence of TB, such as in the First Nations and homeless populations where the incidence of TB is higher than in the general population.

Although existing diseases such as influenza create less threat than was true historically due to the availability of vaccines and antiviral drugs, the advent of new strains of influenza, such as pandemic influenza H1N1 2009, also tax the healthcare system during the vaccine development period, with the medical system waiting to obtain strain-specific vaccine for primary prevention. The WHO has become increasingly vigilant with mechanisms for international disease surveillance, which has reduced the delay in recognizing global communicable disease threats. One of the very positive outcomes of increased vigilance has been demonstrated in Pandemic (H1N1) 2009. Unlike SARS, there was a relatively short period between the first cases of Pandemic (H1N1) 2009 influenza in Mexico and notification of international public health agencies about the potential threat.

In Canada, in part as a response to the SARS outbreak in 2003, the Government of Canada recognized the need to strengthen Canada's capacity to protect Canadians from infectious diseases and other threats to their health. The Public Health Agency of Canada was established in September 2004, and was confirmed as a legal entity in December 2006 by the Public Health Agency of Canada Act (PHAC, 2008).

COMMUNICABLE DISEASES

Communicable diseases are illnesses caused by a "specific infectious agent, or its toxic products that arise through transmission of that agent, or its products from an infected person, animal or inanimate source to a susceptible host; either directly or indirectly through an intermediate plant or animal host, vector or the inanimate environment" (Heymann, 2008, p. 704). There are four main categories of infectious agents that can cause diseases: bacteria, fungi, parasites, and viruses. Some communicable diseases are passed on by direct or indirect contact with infected hosts or with their excretions. Most diseases are transmitted or spread through contact or close proximity because the causative bacterium or virus is airborne (see Chapter 9).

A communicable disease may occur as an individual case or a group of cases, known as an outbreak. An **outbreak** occurs when the new cases of a disease exceed the normal occurrence during a given period of time. For example, TB and invasive pneumococcal disease are common outbreaks in underhoused populations in winter/spring seasons in Canada. **Endemic** refers to the steady presence of a disease in a defined geographic area or population group (e.g., TB among foreign-born residents of Canada). Occasionally, the occurrence of a disease is higher than what would be expected normally; this is called an **epidemic** (e.g., influenza). More rarely, a **pandemic** occurs when a disease spreads and affects a large number of populations worldwide (e.g., Pandemic [H1N1] 2009 influenza, SARS, and acquired immune deficiency syndrome [AIDS]).

"Communicable diseases kill more that 14 million people each year mainly in the developing world. In these countries, approximately 46% of all deaths are due to communicable diseases, and 90% of these deaths are attributed to acute diarrhoeal and respiratory infections of children, AIDS, tuberculosis, malaria, and measles" (Heymann, 2008, p. 12). Preventing transmission is key to controlling the number of people infected with an organism. Understanding the infectious agent's characteristics is paramount to assisting healthcare personnel diagnose, control, and manage a communicable disease. Table 12.1 summarizes several of the communicable diseases present in Canada. Communicable diseases may be examined in the categories described below.

Vaccine-Preventable Diseases

"The impact of vaccination on the health of the world's people is hard to exaggerate. With the exception of safe water, no other modality, not even antibiotics, has had such a major effect on mortality reduction and population growth" (Plotkin & Orenstein, 2008, p. 1). The goal of the immunization program in Canada is the elimination of vaccine-preventable diseases (Public Health Agency of Canada, 2006). Smallpox (globally) and poliomyelitis (in developed countries) have been eradicated through successful immunization programs. Measles, mumps, and rubella have been dramatically reduced in some countries. Diphtheria, haemophilus influenzae type b, hepatitis B, human papillomavirus (HPV), influenza, measles, meningococcal disease, mumps, pertussis, streptococcus pneumoniae (pneumococcus), poliomyelitis, rubella, tetanus, and varicella are vaccine-preventable diseases. An age-specific schedule of immunizations (see Table 12.2) aims at providing optimum protection throughout life. Depending

TABLE 12.1 Selected Communicable Diseases in Canada

Disease	Infectious Agent	Mode of Transmission	Incubation Period	Clinical Presentation	Period of Communicability	Control Measures
Acquired immuno-deficiency syndrome (AIDS)	Human immuno-deficiency virus (HIV, types 1 and 2) (retrovirus)	Unprotected intercourse with an infected person; inoculation with or exposure to infected blood, other body fluids, needle stick injuries/sharing; from infected woman to the fetus during pregnancy or breastfeeding	3 weeks to 20 years+ (average 10 years)	Initially, mononucleosis-like illness for a week or two; may then be free of clinical signs or symptoms for months or years before developing Pneumocystis carinii pneumonia, opportunistic infections, and cancers. Infants and young children present with failure to thrive, inherited immuno-deficiencies and other childhood health problems.	From onset of infection and persists for life. Infectivity is high during first few months of infection.	■ Contact tracing and HIV testing ■ Public education ■ Zidovudine (AZT), dideoxycytidine (DDC), and dideoxyinosine (DDI) treatment, including prophylaxis for the opportunistic infectious diseases that result from HIV infection ■ AZT treatment to pregnant mother and newborn can reduce risk of perinatal transmission ■ Recommendations for HIV post-exposure prophylaxis include a basic four-week regimen of two drugs (zidovudine plus lamivudine, stavudine plus lamivudine, or stavudine plus didanosine) for most HIV exposures and an expanded regimen that includes the addition of a third antiretroviral drug for HIV exposures that pose an increased risk of transmission
Chickenpox/ Herpes Zoster (varicella)	Varicella-zoster virus	Airborne through respiratory secretions or direct or indirect contact from vesicle fluid of person with varicella-zoster	10–21 days	Low-grade fever, maculopapular rash on trunk, face, scalp, mucous membrane of mouth, then changed to vesicular for 3–4 days. Herpes zoster is a local manifestation of reactivation of latent varicella infection in the dorsal root ganglia.	2–5 days before onset of rash and until all skin lesions have crusted	■ Exclude from childcare, school, work, and public places at least 5 days until all vesicles become crusted ■ Avoid contact with immunosuppressed persons ■ Varicella-zoster immunoglobulin (IG) within 96 hours of exposure in susceptible close contacts of cases
Diphtheria	Corynebacterium diphtheriae	Droplet spread through direct contact with a patient or carrier, or indirect contact with articles soiled with nasopharyngeal secretions	2–5 days	Greyish spots on tonsils; sore throat, enlarged and tender cervical lymph nodes; marked swelling and edema of the neck in severe cases.	If untreated, 2 weeks to several months Treated, 2–4 weeks	■ Offer needed immunization to contacts surveillance for 7 days ■ Throat culture ■ Antitoxin and Benzathine penicillin or Erythromycin treatment for infected persons ■ Isolate until two cultures taken more than 24–48 hours apart are negative after the cessation of antibiotics; or isolate for 14 days if no culture available ■ Disinfect contact articles ■ Quarantine adult contacts with food-handling occupations.

TABLE 12.1 Continued

Disease	Infectious Agent	Mode of Transmission	Incubation Period	Clinical Presentation	Period of Communicability	Control Measures
Enterohemorrhagic Escherichia coli infection (EHEC)	E. coli O157:H7	Mainly through ingestion of contaminated water or food (beef, produce, unpasteurized dairy). Direct person-to-person transmission may also occur in families, child care, and health settings.	2–10 days, with the median of 3–4 days	Diarrhea may range from mild and non-bloody to stools that are virtually all blood. Lack of fever in most patients can help to differentiate this infection from that due to other enteric pathogens. Hemolytic uraemic syndrome (HUS) is the most severe clinical manifestation, found in 8% of persons with this infection.	Duration of excretion is typically 1 week or less in adults, and 3 weeks in children. Prolonged carriage is uncommon	■ Isolation during acute illness utilizing enteric precautions ■ Small infective dose, therefore infected clients should not be employed to handle food, or provide child or patient care until 2 successive negative fecal samples or recall swabs (collected 24 hours apart and not sooner than 48 hours after the last dose of antimicrobials) ■ Concurrent disinfection of feces and contaminated articles/structures (i.e., wells) ■ Contacts with diarrhea should be excluded from health, childcare, and food service employment until 2 negative stool samples are obtained ■ All cases and contacts must be educated at first opportunity about thorough handwashing after defecation and before handling food or caring for children or patients
Hemophilus influenza type B	H. influenza type B (Hib)	Droplet infection and discharges from nasopharyngeal discharges	Unknown, probably short, 2–4 days	Upper respiratory obstruction, vomiting, fever, bulging fontanelle in infants, stiff back and neck in older children, epiglottitis, meningitis, bacteremia, septic arthritis, cellulitis.	Most infectious in the week prior to onset of illness and during the illness until treated, usually 24–48 hours after treatment started	■ Early surveillance on children under six to prompt early medical treatment as needed ■ Provide needed immunization and antibiotic prophylaxis
Hepatitis A	Hepatitis A virus (HAV)	Direct or indirect contact through fecal–oral route transmission, through contaminated water, or non-cooked food contaminated by infectious food handlers.	15–50 days, range is 28–30 days	Acute febrile, nausea, anorexia, diarrhea, lethargy, abdominal discomfort, jaundice. Infants and young children may not exhibit jaundice.	2 weeks before onset of symptoms to 1 week after onset of jaundice	■ Exclude from school or work for 1 week following onset of illness ■ Health education, immunoglobulin treatment, contact tracing ■ Sanitary disposal of feces, urine and blood
Hepatitis B	Hepatitis B virus (HBV)	Sexual, perinatal, and percutaneous exposure through blood, serum, and vaginal fluids	Usually 60–90 days, range 45–180 days	Insidious onset of symptoms, nausea, vomiting, anorexia, lethargy, abdominal discomfort, jaundice	Many weeks before onset of symptoms, may persist for life	■ Pre-exposure vaccination to at-risk populations; vaccination to susceptible sexual contacts ■ Give HBIG treatment to contacts as needed ■ Universal precautions to prevent exposure to blood and blood products
Hepatitis C	Hepatitis C virus (HCV)	Parenterally; less frequently are sexual and mother to child	6–9 weeks	Insidious, with anorexia, nausea, vomiting, lethargy, abdominal discomfort, jaundice. Progression to jaundice less frequent than Hep B (90% asymptomatic)	From 1 or more weeks before onset of symptoms. Persists in most people indefinitely.	■ No available vaccine ■ Routinely screen blood products ■ Education ■ Interferon treatment for active disease

TABLE 12.1 Continued

Disease	Infectious Agent	Mode of Transmission	Incubation Period	Clinical Presentation	Period of Communicability	Control Measures
Influenza	Influenza A and B virus	Airborne spread and direct contact in crowded populations in enclosed spaces	1–3 days	Fever, headache, prostration, coryza, sore throat, and cough. Nausea, vomiting, and diarrhea are uncommon, but may accompany respiratory phase, usually in children	From 24 hours before onset of symptoms to 5 days in adults; up to 7 days in children	■ Education about basic personal hygiene (hand hygiene) ■ Yearly immunization for the immunocompromised, those with chronic conditions, the elderly, and those who might spread infection (health personnel) ■ Antivirals available to the unimmunized and to residents in institutions ■ Cohort ill persons from well persons in institutions and at home, if possible
Listeriosis	Listeria monocytogenes	Ingestion of raw or contaminated mild, soft cheeses, vegetables, and ready to eat meats Organisms can be transmitted from mother to fetus in utero or during passage through infected birth canal	Cases have occurred 3–70 days following a single exposure to an implicated product. Estimated median incubation period is 3 weeks	This bacterial disease usually manifests as meningoencephalitis and/or septicaemia in newborns and adults. In pregnant women, as fever and abortion. Onset can be sudden with fever, intense headache, nausea, vomiting, and signs of meningeal irritation	Mothers of infected newborn infants can shed the infectious agent in vaginal discharges and urine for 7–10 days after delivery, rarely longer Infected individuals can shed the organisms in their stools for several months	■ Pregnant and immune-compromised individuals should avoid ready-to-eat foods, smoked fish, and soft cheeses made with unpasteurized milk ■ Cook leftovers or hot dogs until steaming hot ■ Thoroughly wash raw vegetables before eating ■ Thoroughly cook raw food from animal sources such as beef, pork, or poultry ■ Ensure safety of foods of animal origin and pasteurize all dairy products ■ Wash hands, knives, and cutting boards after handling uncooked foods ■ Avoid the use of untreated manure on vegetable crops ■ Re-call any processed foods contaminated by Listeria monocytogenes
Measles	Measles virus (morbillivirus)	Airborne by droplet spread or by direct contact with infected nasal or throat secretions	7–18 days	Fever ≥ 38°C, cough, coryza, conjunctivitis, Koplik's spots on buccal mucosa, red blotching rash appearing on 3rd to 7th day, beginning on face then generalizing to body	1/2 day before onset of symptoms to 4 days after appearance of rash	■ Exclude from childcare or school for at least 4 days after first appearance of rash ■ Check immunization of all close contacts and offer vaccination within 72 h of contact for non-immune persons
Meningo-coccal infections	Neisseria meningitides	Direct contact including respiratory droplets from nose and throat of infected persons	2–10 days	Acute onset of meningitis and septicaemia with fever, intense headache, nausea, vomiting, stiff neck, purpuric rash on trunk, limbs and body, joint pain.	Until 24 hours of effective therapy has been received	■ Prompt treatment with parenteral penicillin followed by 24 hr respiratory isolation ■ Close surveillance of all close contacts and exclusion from school or work until at least 2 days after chemotherapy.

TABLE 12.1 Continued

Disease	Infectious Agent	Mode of Transmission	Incubation Period	Clinical Presentation	Period of Communicability	Control Measures
Mumps	Paramyxovirus	Droplet spread; airborne transmission and contact with saliva of an infected person.	14–25 days	Swelling of salivary glands (usually parotid), orchitis, fever.	2 days before to 4 days after onset	■ Exclude susceptibles from childcare, school, or workplace. ■ Respiratory isolation for 9 days from onset of parotitis.
Pertussis	*Bordetella pertussis*	Direct contact via airborne or droplet spread from respiratory discharges of infected persons	6–20 days, usually 9–10 days	Whooping cough, slight fever, non-specific respiratory tract infection in infants. Paroxysms frequently end in vomiting with adults.	To three weeks after onset of paroxysms if not treated	■ Exclude from childcare or school until at least 5 days after a minimum of the 14-day erythromycin treatment ■ Immunize non-immune infants, children, and young adults.
Pulmonary Tuberculosis (TB)	Mycobacterium tuberculosis	Exposure to tubercle bacilli in airborne nuclei, 1–5 microns in diameter, produced by people with pulmonary or respiratory tract tuberculosis during expiratory efforts (coughing, singing, or sneezing) and inhaled by a vulnerable contact.	From infection to a primary lesion or significant tuberculin reaction, about 2–10 weeks. Latent infection may persist for a lifetime. Tuberculin reactivity persists regardless of treatment	Most children (less than 5 years) with TB are asymptomatic at presentation. Older children and adolescents are more likely to experience adult-type disease and often present with a classic triad of fever, night sweats, and weight loss. Physical findings are often minimal relative to chest x-ray abnormalities, including lung infiltrates, typically but not always in the upper zone(s), that may be cavitated. Delay in diagnosis of adolescents is common and may reflect lack of suspicion by clinician.	Untreated or inadequately treated clients may be intermittently sputum-positive for years. Degree of communicability depends on number of bacilli discharged, virulence of bacilli, and adequacy of ventilation, exposure of bacilli to sun or UV light, and opportunities for aerosolization through coughing, sneezing, talking or singing or during aerosolized procedures. Effective antimicrobial chemoprophylaxis usually eliminates communicability within 2–4 weeks	■ Isolation until antibiotic treatment of a minimum of 2 weeks has been completed ■ Contact tracing and TB skin testing of all vulnerable contacts ■ Screening with tuberculin testing/x-rays amongst the at-risk populations ■ Provide adequate anti-TB chemotherapy and prophylactic treatments ■ Encourage compliance to follow prescribed treatments. Utilize Directly Observed Therapy (DOT)

TABLE 12.1 Continued

Disease	Infectious Agent	Mode of Transmission	Incubation Period	Clinical Presentation	Period of Communicability	Control Measures
Poliomyelitis	Poliovirus, types 1, 2, and 3 (enterovirus)	Direct contact via fecal-oral route where sanitation is poor; pharyngeal spread more common during epidemics and when sanitation is good.	3–21 days	Fever, malaise, headache, nausea and vomiting, muscle pain, stiffness of the neck and back with or without flaccid paralysis.	Greatest for 7–10 days after onset of symptoms, and up to six weeks or longer	▪ Isolate ▪ Exclude from school for at least 14 days after onset of illness ▪ Disinfect throat discharges and fecal soiled articles ▪ Vaccinate all non-immunized close contacts
Rubella	Rubella virus	Droplet or direct spread with infected persons through pharyngeal secretions	14–21 days	Fever (≤38.3°C) diffuse, punctate maculopapular skin rash. Malaise, headache, coryza, and conjunctivitis more common in adults.	7 days before to 4 days after onset of rash	▪ Contact should avoid pregnant women ▪ Exclude from school and work at least 5 days after onset of rash ▪ Routine MMR immunization as preventive measure
Severe Acute Respiratory Syndrome (SARS)	Corona virus	Direct or indirect transmission of respiratory secretions via droplet or airborne through close contact with a symptomatic person	2–10 days	Sudden onset of high fever (≥40°C), malaise, headache, cough, shortness of breath, sore throat, diarrhea.	Early symptoms up to 10 days after fever subsides.	▪ Wear mask; isolation; hand washing ▪ Active daily surveillance for 10 days ▪ Quarantine of close contacts for 10 days ▪ Public education and traveller advisory and screening
Tetanus	*Clostridium tetani*	Bacterial spores may be introduced through contaminated puncture wounds, lacerations, burns, trivial wounds or injected contaminated street drugs	2 days–2 months; average 10 days	Painful muscular contractions generalized from: site of injury to back muscles; lockjaw; respiratory and laryngeal spasm.	Not transmitted from person to person. Spores enter and devitalize tissues in infected wound	▪ Use IV tetanus immune globulin (TIG) and penicillin in large doses for 14 days ▪ Adequate wound adequately

Sources: Heymann, D. L. (Ed.). (2008). Control of communicable diseases manual (19th ed.). Washington, DC: American Public Health Association. Health Canada. (1999). Routine practices and additional precautions for preventing the transmission of infection in health care: Revision of isolation and precaution techniques. Canada Communicable Disease Report, 25S4. Pickering, L. K. (Ed.). (2009). Red book: 2009 report of the Committee on Infectious Diseases (28th ed.). Elk Grove Village, IL: American Academy of Pediatrics. Government of Victoria, Australia. (2009). The blue book: Guidelines for the control of infectious disease. Retrieved from http://www.health.vic.gov.au/ideas/downloads/bluebook.pdf.

TABLE 12.2 Publicly Funded Immunization Programs in Canada—Routine Schedule for Infants and Children (including special programs and catch-up programs)

Province/ Territory	DTaP-IPV-Hib	DTaP-IPV	Td, Tdap or Td-IPV	HB	MMR	Var	MMRV	Men-C	Men-C-A, C, Y, W-135	Pneu-C-7	Pneu-C-10	Pneu-C-13	Inf	HPV	Rot
NACI recommendation	2, 4, 6, 18 mths	4–6 yrs	14–16 yrs	Infancy (3 doses) OR Pre-teen/teen (2–3 doses)	12 mths AND 18 mths OR 4–6 yrs	12–18 mths (1 dose)	12 mths AND 18 mths OR 4–6 yrs	Infancy (1–4 doses)[1] AND Pre-teen (1 dose)[1]	Pre-teen (1 dose)[1]	2, 4, 6, 12–15 mths	2, 4, 6, 12–15 mths	2, 4, 6, 12–15 mths	6–23 mths (1–2 doses)	Females 9–13 yrs (3 doses at 0, 2, 6 mths)[2]	2, 4, 6 mths
BC	2, 4, 6 (DTaP-HB-IPV-Hib); 18 mths (DTaP-IPV-Hib)	4–6 yrs	Tdap, Gr. 9	2, 4, 6 mths (DTaP-HB-IPV-Hib); Catch-up Gr. 6 (HB)	12, 18 mths	12 mths; Catch-up 4–6 yrs, Gr. 6		2, 12 mths; Gr. 6				2, 4, (6 HR), 12 mths	6–23 mths	Females GR. 6, 9	
AB	2, 4, 6, 18 mths	4–6 yrs	Tdap, Gr. 9	Gr. 5	12 mths, 4–6 yrs	12 mths		2, 4, 12 mths		2, 4, 6, 18 mths			6–59 mths	Females Gr. 5; Catch-up Gr. 9 in 2009–12	
SK	2, 4, 6, 18 mths	4–6 yrs	Tdap, Gr. 8	Gr. 6	18 mths; Catch-up Gr. 8, 12	12 mths; Catch-up Gr. 6	October 2010: 12 mths	12 mths; 4–6 yrs; Catch-up Gr. 6				2, 4, 6, 18 mths	6–59 mths	Females Gr. 6	
MB	2, 4, 6, 18 mths	4–6 yrs	Tdap, 14–16 yrs	Gr. 4	12 mths; 4–6 yrs	12 mths; Catch-up 4–6 yrs, Gr. 4		12 mths, Catch-up Gr. 4				2, 4, 6, 18 mths	2010– 11 ≥ 6 mths	Females Gr. 6	
ON	2, 4, 6, 18 mths	4–6 yrs	Tdap, 14–16 yrs	Gr. 7	12, 18 mths	15 mths or 4–6 yrs		12 mths; Catch-up Gr. 7, 14–16 yrs	Gr. 7		2, 4, 6, 15 mths		≥ 6 mths	Females Gr. 8	

TABLE 12.2 Continued

Province/ Territory	DTaP-IPV-Hib	DTaP-IPV	Td, Tdap or Td-IPV	HB	MMR	Var	MMRV	Men-C	Men-C-A, C, Y, W-135	Pneu-C-7	Pneu-C-10	Pneu-C-13	Inf	HPV	Rot
QC	2, 4, 6, 18 mths	4–6 yrs	Tdap, Gr. 9	Gr. 4	12, 18 mths	12 mths; Catch-up 4–6 yrs, Gr. 4, 3rd year of high school, all non-immune individuals		12 mths; Catch-up < 18 yrs		2, 4, 12 mths; Catch-up < 5 yrs	2, 4, 12 mths		6–23 mths	Females Gr. 4; Catch-up 3rd year of high school until 2013; offers to the 9–17 years	
NB	2, 4, 6, 18 mths	4–6 yrs	Tdap, Gr. 9 if not received in Gr. 6	0, 2, 6 mths	12, 18 mths, Catch-up Gr. 12 2007–13	12 mths		12 mths	Gr. 9			2, 4, 6, 12 mths; Catch-up children born between July 2nd, 2008 and June 30th, 2009 (1 dose)	6 mths–18 yrs	Females Gr. 7	
NS	2, 4, 6, 18 mths	4–6 yrs	Tdap, Gr. 7, and 8 for 2010–11 only	Gr. 7	12 mths, 4–6 yrs	12 mths; Catch-up 1–6 yrs;		12 mths; Catch-up Gr. 7				2, 4, 6, 18 mths	≥ 6 mths	Females Gr. 7, and 8 for 2010–11 only	
PE	2, 4, 6, 18 mths	4–6 yrs	Tdap, Gr. 9	2, 4, 15 mths	15, 18 mths	12 mths		12 mths	Gr. 9	2, 4, 6, 18 mths				Females Gr. 6	
NL	2, 4, 6, 18 mths	4–6 yrs	Tdap, Gr. 9	Gr. 4 (3 doses)	12, 18 mths	12 mths		12 mths	Catch-up Gr. 4		2, 4, 6, 18 mths		6–23 mths	Females Gr. 6,	
NT	2, 4, 6, 18 mths	4–6 yrs	Tdap, Gr. 9	0, 1, 6 mths	12, 18 mths, Post secondary students attending schools outside NT	12 mths; Catch-up <5 yrs		2, 12 mths; Catch-up <5 yrs, Gr. 9	Post secondary students attending schools outside NT			2, 4, 6, 18 mths	6–23 mths	Females Gr. 4; Catch-up Gr. 9–12 2009–14	

TABLE 12.2 Continued

Province/ Territory	DTaP-IPV-Hib	DTaP-IPV	Td, Tdap or Td-IPV	HB	MMR	Var	MMRV	Men-C	Men-C-A, C, Y, W-135	Pneu-C-7	Pneu-C-10	Pneu-C-13	Inf	HPV	Rot
YT	2, 4, 6, 18 mths	4–6 yrs	Tdap, Gr. 9	2, 4, 12 mths; Catch-up ≤19 yrs	12, 18 mths	12 mths		2, 12 mths; Catch-up Gr. 9, post-secondary students not previously immunized		2, 4, 6, 18 mths			> 6 mths	Females Gr. 6 Catch-up Gr. 7, 8	
NU	2, 4, 6, 18 mths	4–6 yrs	Tdap, Gr. 9	0, 1, 9 mths	12, 18 mths; Catch-up Gr. 12	15 mths		12 mths; Catch-up 14–16 yrs		2, 4, 6, 15 mths			≥ 6 mths	March 2010, Females Gr. 6 (≥ 9 yrs)	

DTaP: Diphtheria, Tetanus, Acellular Pertussis
HB: Hepatitis B
Hib: Haemophilus Influenzae Tybe b
HPV: Human Papillomavirus
Inf: Influenza
IPV: Inactivated Polio
Men-C: Meningococcal conjugate
MMR: Measles, Mumps, Rubella
MMRV: Measles, Mumps, Rubella, and Varicella
Pneu-C-7, Pneu-C-10, Pneu-C-13: Pneumococcal conjugate 7, 10, and 13 valent
Rot: Rotavirus
Var: Varicella

Recommended use:
1. If meningococcal C conjugate vaccine is given to infants < 12 months of age, a booster dose should be given in the second year of life (from 12 to 23 months of age). The early adolescent dose may be given using either meningococcal C conjugate (Men-C) vaccine or quadrivalent conjugate meningococcal vaccine (Men-C-ACYW), depending on the burden of illness from serogroups A, Y, and W135 and the age distribution of cases by serogroup in individual Provinces/territories. Updated Invasive Meningococcal Vaccine Conjugate Recommendations can be found at: http://www.phac-aspc.gc.ca/publicat/ccdr-rmtc/09pdf/acs-dcc-3.pdf

2. The HPV vaccine is recommended for females between 9 and 13 years of age, as this is before the onset of sexual intercourse for most females in Canada and the efficacy would be greatest. Females between the ages of 14 and 26 years would benefit from the HPV vaccine, even if they are already sexually active, as they may not yet have HPV infection, and are very unlikely to have been infected with all four HPV types in the vaccine. Females between the ages of 14 and 26 years who have had previous Pap abnormalities, including cervical cancer, or have had genital warts or known HPV infection, would still benefit from the HPV vaccine.

Source: Routine immunization schedules, Recommendations from the National Advisory Committee on Immunization (NACI) provided by the Public Health Agency of Canada. Retrieved from http://www.phac-aspc.gc.ca/im/ptimprog-progimpt/table-1-eng.php

on resources and the burden of illness in the specific province, this schedule, developed by Health Canada, can be modified by individual provinces and territories.

Between 2000 and 8000 Canadians die of influenza and its complications annually, depending on the severity of the season (PHAC, 2009b) *Human influenza* is a respiratory infection caused by influenza virus, and is spread by droplets through coughing or sneezing. Vaccination against influenza lasts four to six months, and is routinely given on an annual basis at the onset of the influenza season, typically starting in October or November. Each year, influenza vaccine contains three influenza strains, predicted by WHO to be the most common circulating strains, in any particular season. Due to the significant morbidity, mortality, and societal costs associated with influenza, it is recommended that everyone 6 months or older be vaccinated, especially those with chronic illness, people aged 65 and over, residents in chronic care and nursing homes, healthcare service providers, and pregnant women (PHAC). The spread of *avian influenza H5N1* (or bird flu) throughout Southeast Asia and Europe had generated much discussion on the implications for human health, however in April 2009 a novel strain of influenza H1N1 was recognized in Mexico, causing a cluster of illness with the potential to become a pandemic. On June 11, 2009, the WHO raised the pandemic alert level to 6, indicating that a novel strain of influenza was rapidly spreading from human to human and across international jurisdictions (see Figure 12.1 and MyNursingLab). Globally, many nations declared an influenza pandemic. This event moved public health activity from the planning phase to action at local, provincial, and federal levels throughout Canada.

New vaccines licensed in Canada since June 2006 include the *human papillomavirus (HPV)* vaccine and the rotavirus vaccine. HPV is mainly transmitted by sexual contact, and the vaccine is available to prevent an infection that occurs years before but is associated with the appearance of cervical cancer. The rotavirus vaccine would decrease rotaviruses consistently involved in acute gastrointestinal illnesses in children. Vaccines against West Nile virus (Drebot & Artsob, 2006) and malaria are also in development. The National Advisory Committee on Immunization (NACI) is instrumental in developing guidelines for any newly licensed vaccines in

Canada. It also provides general guidelines for the most desirable immunization practices to assist CHNs and other healthcare providers in critically examining their standards of practice related to immunization (see MyNursingLab).

Blood Borne Pathogens

Blood borne pathogens are those that can be spread by exposure to contaminated blood, either by direct or indirect exposure. The most common examples are HIV, hepatitis B, hepatitis C, and viral haemorrhagic fevers. Diseases that are not usually transmitted directly by blood contact, but rather by insect or some other vector, are more usefully classified as vector-borne diseases, even though the causative agent can be found in blood. Vector-borne diseases will be discussed as a separate category in this chapter and blood borne pathogens will be discussed in Chapter 29.

As our scientific knowledge and surveillance abilities have increased, potential indirect contact modes of transmission in some diseases have been identified, such as donor organs and blood products that are transplanted/transfused. Changes to screening practices were subsequently made to organ and blood donor screening and testing practices as well as the clinical use of donated organs and blood. Canadian Blood Services (2009) now screens all blood products for known infectious diseases, such as HIV, syphilis, hepatitis B and C, and WNV.

Foodborne Infections

Foodborne infection and **foodborne intoxication** are illnesses acquired through the consumption of contaminated food. Riemann and Cliver (2006) noted that *infections* occur when people consume food containing pathogenic microorganisms, which multiply in the gastrointestinal tract; *intoxications* occur when bacteria multiply in food and produce a toxin that is poisonous to the person ingesting the food. The most common causes of foodborne illnesses include

- toxins released by bacterial growth in food before consumption (e.g., clostridium botulism, staphylococcus aureus, and bacillus cereus) or in the intestines (clostridium perfringens);

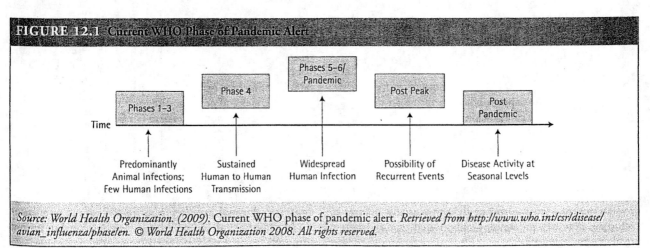

FIGURE 12.1 Current WHO Phase of Pandemic Alert

Time

Phases 1–3 → Predominantly Animal Infections; Few Human Infections

Phase 4 → Sustained Human to Human Transmission

Phases 5–6/ Pandemic → Widespread Human Infection

Post Peak → Possibility of Recurrent Events

Post Pandemic → Disease Activity at Seasonal Levels

- bacterial, viral, or parasitic infections (brucellosis, campylobacter enteritis, diarrhea caused by Escherichia coli, hepatitis A, listeriosis, salmonellosis, shigellosis, toxoplasmosis, viral gastroenteritis, trichinosis); and
- toxins produced by harmful algal species (shellfish poisoning).

Foodborne infections can usually be recognized by illness that occurs within a variable but usually short time frame after a meal. **Foodborne outbreaks** are recognized when illness presents among individuals who have consumed common foods. For example, a community foodborne outbreak of E. coli O157:H7 was identified in 2008 in Ontario, when over 350 persons who all consumed food from the same fast-food establishment became ill. Fifty persons in this outbreak had lab-confirmed disease (North Bay Parry Sound District Health Unit, 2009). Foodborne outbreaks can be community-based or have a much more widespread impact depending on food distribution patterns. For example, a foodborne outbreak with national impact occurred in 2008 when listeria was associated with contaminated meat. Another foodborne outbreak with provincial impact occurred in 2005 in Ontario when bean sprouts were found to be associated with salmonella disease. Thorough and prompt collection and testing of implicated foods is essential, as is laboratory testing of stool samples obtained from cases. Many cases are often unreported to health authorities, and outbreaks are often unrecognized.

Foodborne diseases can be prevented and controlled by (a) avoiding food contamination, (b) destroying contaminants (e.g., meat irradiation is one option), and (c) eliminating spread or multiplication of the contaminants. Ultimately, prevention rests on educating food handlers about proper practices in cooking and storage of food and personal hygiene. This includes (a) keeping clean, (b) separating raw and cooked, (c) cooking thoroughly, (d) keeping food at safe temperatures, and (e) using safe water and raw materials (WHO, 2009b).

Waterborne Zoonoses

Waterborne pathogens usually enter water supplies through fecal contamination from animals or humans to cause enteric illnesses (e.g., cholera, typhoid fever, dysentery, some types of salmonella, shigellosis, vibrio, and various coliform bacteria including E. coli O157:H7). Municipal water systems that have appropriate filtration and chlorination have decreased diseases such as amebic dysentery and giardiasis. Control of protozoa requires effective filtration devices, as they do not respond to traditional chlorine treatment like enteric and coliform bacteria. Outbreaks of cryptosporidium in North Battleford, Saskatchewan (PHAC, 2001) and E. coli in Walkerton, Ontario (PHAC, 2000) have raised awareness of the importance of safe municipal water systems across Canada.

An **outbreak of waterborne disease** is usually defined as two cases that are epidemiologically linked that experience similar symptoms after consuming water from a common source. Public health inspectors and public health nurses work closely with the local medical officer of health to investigate, track, and determine linkages between cases. Provincial databases such as the integrated Public Health Information System (PHAC, 2007a) allow tracking of disease occurrence and its source, if known.

Vector-Borne Diseases

Vector-borne diseases are illnesses for which the infectious agent is transmitted by a carrier, or vector, which is usually a mosquito, tick, or fly. Climate change has a potential impact on the distribution of various diseases. Vector-borne diseases most commonly seen in Canada include Eastern equine encephalitis, Lyme disease, and West Nile virus.

Lyme disease, for example, is transmitted by black-legged ticks carried by migratory birds, mice, squirrels, rodents, and other small animals that can carry the bacterium. Black-legged ticks (also called deer ticks) can be found in all areas of Canada; however, only about 10% are infected with Lyme disease. Areas of concern include parts of southern Ontario; Lunenburg County in Nova Scotia; and parts of southern British Columbia. Lyme disease is not a nationally reportable disease in Canada (PHAC, 2009c), although provincial surveillance and reporting is common. Malaria and dengue fever, also vector-borne diseases, are seen in travellers who have contracted these diseases in other countries from the bite of an infected mosquito.

West Nile virus (WNV) is carried and spread by mosquitoes. WNV can cause severe neurological complications. Personal protection against this vector and reducing areas where mosquitoes breed are important in its control.

Zoonotic Infections

Zoonotic infections are diseases transmissible between animals and humans; however, they do not need humans to maintain their life cycles. Transmission is by bites, inhalation, ingestion, direct contact, and arthropod intermediaries. Rabies, hantavirus pulmonary syndrome, salmonellosis, listeriosis, and brucellosis are zoonotic diseases.

Rabies has the highest case fatality rate of any known human infection, considered essentially 100%. The major carriers of rabies in Canada include bats, foxes, raccoons, and skunks. The virus is transmitted through a bite, scratch, or pre-existing open wound, and attacks the central nervous system. The best prevention is the vaccination of animals against rabies and pre-exposure vaccination of animal workers. Post-exposure prophylaxis (PEP) is available after an exposure, done in consultation with public health officials. Determination of the need for follow-up by a CHN requires critical assessment of the endemic rates; for example, an animal exposure in Newfoundland would require further investigation to determine the history of the animal's habitation, since rabies is not usually present in the animal population in Newfoundland but could be introduced by an animal brought from or who migrated from an endemic area. An exposure in Eastern Ontario, where raccoon rabies is prevalent, would require follow-up. Often CHNs recommend or administer rabies immune globulin (RIG) with the dosage calculation based on client weight, with a series of rabies vaccine. The animal, if located, should be kept in a confined area for a period of 10 days, in order to determine if the animal was infectious with rabies at the time of the exposure. Most infected animals will succumb to rabies within a five-day period, but 10 days is used to avoid any possible exceptions. If the animal exhibits signs and symptoms of rabies or dies during the isolation period, the exposed person is started on PEP as soon as possible. If the animal is deceased immediately following the exposure, rabies testing of brain tissue is conducted at a national laboratory and the exposed individual is offered PEP based on the findings. If a client is started on PEP and animal testing indicates that the rabies virus was not present, the PEP can be stopped prior to completion (PHAC, 2006).

Hantavirus is a viral disease carried by deer mice (in Canada) that can be transmitted through direct or indirect contact. Mice shed the virus in urine, feces, or saliva. Humans can inhale the virus, which may lead to hantavirus pulmonary syndrome (HPS). The earliest documented case of HPS in Canada was contracted in Alberta in 1989. Since then, there have been over 70 confirmed cases. Most of the cases occurred in western Canada (Manitoba, Saskatchewan, Alberta, and British Columbia). Hantavirus infections contracted by Canadians outside the country have also been recognized, including two fatal cases from South America (PHAC, 2009d). HPS is extremely serious since approximately 30–40% of cases are fatal (PHAC). Prevention strategies taken by those at risk, such as workers in agricultural or rural settings or hikers/campers, include keeping woodpiles away from dwellings, keeping items off the floor to prevent rodent nesting, trapping rodents, wet-mopping areas where droppings are located to prevent aeration of feces, and not camping near rodent-infected areas.

Parasitic Diseases

Often found in developing countries, parasites are generally not considered important in Canada, although international travel, immigration, and recent outbreaks remind us that we are not immune. *Pinworm infections* are seen most often in children and are common in crowded and institutional settings. Another common parasite is *giardia*. Control of both parasites is available with effective drug treatment. Unlike *cryptosporidium*, which is another intestinal protozoa that can cause diarrheal illness and is transmitted by fecal–oral contact, there is no treatment other than rehydration. Correct identification of parasites is essential to providing appropriate treatment and prevention education. Diagnosis is dependent on an accurate travel history, clinical signs and symptoms, and appropriate specimen and laboratory testing. Safe sexual practices, effective sanitation, and personal hygiene practices, including hand washing, are paramount in controlling parasitic disease.

Diseases with Multiple Transmission Modes

CHNs often are challenged with the need to manage cases of disease that do not fit one specific mode of transmission and therefore make case and contact follow-up complex and multifaceted. For example, hepatitis A can be transmitted through contaminated food and water or through sexual contact. Therefore, the CHN must identify contacts and recommend post-exposure prophylaxis based on all possible modes of transmission, and prevent further transmission by providing comprehensive education and exclusion.

Nosocomial Infections

Nosocomial infections, such as hospital-associated methicillin-resistant staphylococcus aureus (HA-MRSA), are acquired during a hospital stay and may involve patients, visitors, or staff. Community-associated staphylococcus aureus (CA-MRSA) emerges in community settings among children in daycare, soldiers, athletes, incarcerated populations, homosexuals, and Native populations (Allen, 2006). Effective surveillance systems and infection control education for nurses in hospitals and community settings, including long-term care homes, are essential in controlling the spread of infections to vulnerable clients. Infections of a bacterial nature may be treated with antibiotics; however, often the clients with nosocomial infections are the most prone to opportunistic infections, which may contribute to the development of antibiotic-resistant organisms. Hand hygiene is the most effective way of preventing the spread of nosocomial infections by direct contact with hands, surfaces, or objects that have been contaminated by the feces of an infected person. Enterococci bacteria are naturally present in our intestinal tract; healthy individuals usually are not at risk of this infection. However, some strains of enterococci can become resistant to vancomycin. Hospitalized patients with cancer, blood disorders, or immune deficiencies are particularly vulnerable, and the infections can be life-threatening to them. The significant rise in the incident rate for VRE patient admissions in Canada is alarming. It rose from 5.34/100 000 in 1999 to 15.52/100 000 in 2005 (PHAC, 2007b). Healthcare providers can help halt the transmission of nosocomial infections by practising infection-control precautions such as thorough hand hygiene.

REPORTABLE/NOTIFIABLE DISEASES

The terms *reportable* and *notifiable* diseases are commonly used interchangeably. A communicable disease is identified as a **notifiable disease** through the collaboration and consensus of experts in infectious disease. These experts from around the world study the impact of an identified disease by analyzing morbidity and mortality and then recommend the need for notification. The morbidity and mortality impact may be in a small defined area, or on a worldwide scale. As a result, reporting of some communicable diseases is required within provinces and territories, within Canada, and, in some instances, internationally to the WHO.

In Canada, the list of notifiable diseases at the federal level is agreed upon by consensus among provincial, territorial, and federal health authorities. This *National Notifiable Diseases* list helps to ensure uniformity among provincial/territorial efforts and conformity with international reporting requirements and to facilitate both tracking and required control efforts by public health personnel (PHAC, 2009e). Because the epidemiology of infectious diseases changes, this necessitates a periodic review of and modification to the *National Notifiable Diseases* list (see Table 12.3).

TABLE 12.3   Diseases Under National Surveillance, as of January 2009

Acquired Immunodeficiency Syndrome (AIDS)	Hepatitis B	Poliomyelitis
Acute Flaccid Paralysis (AFP)	Hepatitis C	Rabies
Anthrax	Human Immunodeficiency Virus (HIV)	Rubella
Botulism	Influenza, laboratory-confirmed	Salmonellosis
Brucellosis	Invasive *Haemophilus influenzae* type b (Hib) and non-b Disease	Severe Acute Respiratory Syndrome (SARS)
Campylobacteriosis		Shigellosis
Chlamydia	Invasive Group A Streptococcal Disease	Smallpox
Cholera	Invasive Listeriosis	Syphilis
Clostridium difficile Associated Diarrhea	Invasive Meningococcal Disease	Tetanus
Congenital Rubella Syndrome (CRS)	Invasive Pneumococcal Disease	Tuberculosis
Creutzfeldt-Jakob Disease (CJD), Classic and New Variant	Legionellosis	Tularemia
	Leprosy (Hansen's Disease)	Typhoid
Cryptosporidiosis	Lyme Disease	Varicella (Chickenpox)
Cyclosporiasis	Malaria	Verotoxigenic *Escherichia coli* Infection
Diphtheria	Measles	Viral Hemorrhagic Fevers
Giardiasis	Mumps	West Nile virus Infection
Gonorrhea	Norovirus infection	Yellow Fever
Group B Streptococcal Disease of the Newborn	Paralytic Shellfish Poisoning	
Hantavirus Pulmonary Syndrome (HPS)	Pertussis	
Hepatitis A	Plague	

Source: Public Health Agency of Canada. (2010). Diseases under national surveillance *(as of January 2009). Retrieved from* http://www.phac-aspc.gc.ca/bid-bmi/dsd-dsm/duns-eng.php

Non-Reportable Diseases

Some communicable diseases are **non-reportable**. They commonly occur in the population and the burden of illness to the community is not considered great. Examples include the common cold, herpes, pediculosis, bed bugs, conjunctivitis, and scabies. The role of the CHN with regard to non-reportable diseases is usually an educational and supportive one. For example, in daycare outbreaks of non-reportable diseases, the CHN is often called upon to educate daycare staff and parents about transmission and management to prevent further occurrences.

Reporting of Communicable Diseases

In Canada, both provincial/territorial and national guidelines and legislation dictate which diseases must be reported, who is responsible for reporting them, and what the reporting format and the mechanism for reporting are to the national surveillance system. The list of reportable diseases is mandated by provincial/territorial legislation and therefore differs by province/territory, although the recommendations are provided by PHAC. Currently, some provinces and territories report within iPHIS (PHAC, 2007a). If there is a requirement for international health reporting, the PHAC reports to WHO. The *International Health Regulations* (IHR) (WHO, 2009c) are the only legally binding instrument requiring the reporting of communicable diseases at the international level, currently limited to cholera, plague, and yellow fever (Heymann, 2008). The WHO updates and revises the IHR to address the threat of new and re-emerging infections and to accommodate new reporting sources. A number of diseases *under surveillance* by WHO (e.g., H5N1 and AIDS) are required to be reported at varied frequency, depending on the disease and the geographic area in which it has occurred.

While some infectious diseases are common and mild (such as the common cold or pediculosis), others are serious enough to be defined as notifiable diseases (such as hepatitis C and HIV/AIDS) and must be reported to the local health authority. Local public health personnel are mandated by the provinces and territories to report all notifiable disease to their respective Ministry of Health; in addition, some diseases are also required to be reported at the federal level.

CONTROL AND MANAGEMENT OF COMMUNICABLE DISEASES

The successful control and management of communicable diseases is integrally tied to using sound principles of epidemiology (see Chapter 9). Surveillance of a disease consists of "the process of systematic collection, orderly consolidation, analysis and evaluation of pertinent data with prompt dissemination of the results to those who need to know, particularly those who are in a position to take action" (Heymann, 2008, p. 713). Through data analysis, the investigator may uncover the cause or source of the disease (e.g., investigation of a case of salmonella infection may uncover a contaminated food item in a restaurant).

Active Surveillance

Monitoring of diseases, investigation of disease outbreaks, and observation of patterns of disease are responsibilities of the local health authorities. **Active surveillance** is the collection of data utilizing screening tools, interviews, and sentinel systems to identify disease occurrence in the community when individuals present with suggestive symptoms. Such surveillance depends on the creation of surveillance screening tools that heighten the awareness of healthcare practitioners in relation to a specific disease.

Active surveillance may be best illustrated by the screening created in response to the increasing risk across Canada of West Nile virus (WNV), first recognized as a threat in North America in 1999. When WNV was first reported, provincial and federal health authorities applied public health measures to identify the spread of this new communicable disease. WNV was detected for the first time in Canada in 2001, in birds and mosquitoes. In 2002, Canadian health authorities documented human WNV illness activity in five provinces: Nova Scotia, Quebec, Ontario, Manitoba, and Saskatchewan. In 2007, more than 2200 human cases were identified in Canada (PHAC, 2009f). The active surveillance activities during the early days of WNV infections in Canada were conducted partly through the availability of a screening tool. Similarly, a screening tool (see the box "Screening Tool for Influenza-Like Illness [ILI] in Healthcare Settings") has been developed by the Ontario Ministry of Health and Long-Term Care for active surveillance of influenza-like illnesses (ILI). The ILI screening tool is utilized in emergency rooms and other acute care settings to provide consistent and early identification of respiratory illnesses such as influenza and SARS, in order to facilitate the necessary control activities to decrease transmission risks in hospitals and other settings. It is also utilized to quickly detect and contain clusters and outbreaks, and helps to identify any new or virulent microorganism-caused respiratory infections (Ontario Ministry of Health and Long-Term Care, 2009).

Passive Surveillance

Passive surveillance relies on the healthcare provider to notify the local health authority of clients with signs and symptoms associated with a reportable disease. It also relies on laboratory test results if the disease or infectious agent is on the reportable disease list for the respective province/territory. Completeness of the notification report depends on the healthcare workers' ability to recognize the signs and symptoms, their attention to the necessity for surveillance, and their interest in providing a detailed and comprehensive report. A report must include all the necessary demographics of the person, the symptoms and date of onset of the presenting illness, and travel history, and may include social history, sexual history, diagnostic tests done to date, and prescribed treatment.

Screening Tool for Influenza-Like Illness (ILI) in Healthcare Settings

1. Do you have new/worse cough or shortness of breath? If "no," no further action is required If "yes," ask patient to follow directions and continue with next question. If the answer is "yes," patient should perform hand hygiene using alcohol-based hand rub and put on a mask covering their nose and mouth.

2. Are you feeling feverish,* or have you had shakes or chills in the last 24 hours? If "no," no further questions. If "yes," nurse to take temperature as part of clinical assessment

Note: Some people, such as the elderly, and people who are immunocompromised, may not develop fever.

If the answer is "yes," move patient to a separate area if possible.

Source: Ontario Ministry of Health and Long-Term Care. (2009). Screening tool for influenza-like illness in health care settings. *Retrieved from http://www.health.gov.on.ca/english/ providers/program/emu/health_notices/screening_tool_20090519.pdf*

Surveillance, whether active, passive, or both, does not end with the notification of the disease case to the local health authority; rather, it initiates the next steps toward the control and management of the disease. Surveillance also plays a significant role in the management of reports of suspected cases of disease. CHNs provide guidelines to institutions, healthcare professionals, and others in relation to diagnostic tests and control measures to identify and manage a *suspected* case of disease in terms of transmission risk and potential community impact.

Contact Tracing

Contact tracing is a response to a communicable disease report. After a notifiable communicable disease is reported to the local health authority, the infected person is interviewed by a CHN regarding **contacts**, people exposed to the client during the incubation of the disease. The CHN must know the mode of transmission, incubation period, and infectious period of the particular disease in order to determine what constitutes a contact in each individual situation. The *initial contact definition* must be formulated based on signs and symptoms and place and time of exposure. A list of contacts must be collected from the first identified case. With this list, the local health authority proceeds with further assessment and investigation and follows up with recommendations for treatment or post-exposure chemoprophylaxis as deemed necessary.

Contacts are identified based on the possibility of transmission, where the window of risk can be very short or quite long. For example, when investigating a case of measles, the CHN would include in the contact list those people who were in contact with the infectious individual seven days prior to the onset of the rash; whereas, while investigating a case of TB, the CHN may identify not just recent contacts but

contacts as far back as three months ago. The **degree of exposure** (the time spent with the infected person) and where the exposure took place are included in the collected data. Not all reportable diseases warrant the same type of contact tracing, because of varying degrees of burden of illness (e.g., varicella), and/or because the nature of the communicability (e.g., TB).

The ease with which public health professionals are provided with comprehensive and inclusive lists of contacts will depend on how the individual or community comprehends the scope of the issue, or an individual's or community's experience with the disease in the past. For example, obtaining contacts from those who have had an experience with an adolescent dying from meningococcal disease is easier than obtaining a comprehensive list of contacts from an infected food service worker whose perception is that hepatitis A infection is not a serious disease. The report is only as reliable and accurate as the person relaying the information and the parameters required for reporting. That is, if the physician or nurse is unsure of the signs and symptoms of the disease, the need for reporting will go unrecognized and the surveillance and contact tracing may be delayed.

Ongoing education of healthcare professionals helps to ensure detailed disease reporting. The **integrated Public Health Information System** (iPHIS) (PHAC, 2007a) is an electronic system of reporting that allows jurisdictions within a province to communicate disease patterns and contacts with one another. As well, the **Canadian Integrated Outbreak Surveillance Centre** (CIOSC) (2009), an outbreak-specific electronic system, has been developed for healthcare professionals to communicate outbreaks of respiratory or enteric illnesses interprovincially. It enables public health professionals to make links in person, place, and time for clients with similar presentation.

Contact tracing requires a confidential approach, since much of the information is disease- and client-specific. An exception to the confidential necessity and practice of contact tracing is occasionally required. During the SARS outbreak that occurred in Toronto during March through May of 2003, quarantine acts of the federal and Ontario Ministries of Health allowed health and safety authorities to conduct contact tracing in a public forum by naming those with SARS in the public media. Their purpose was to protect the public as well as to notify the contacts of those first infected persons in order to allow the contacts to self-identify and come forward for health assessment. Although contact tracing might be viewed as an infringement of a person's right to privacy, it is necessary to contain the spread of disease while providing ethically competent care (see Chapter 4).

Effective contact tracing requires comprehensive assessment of the infected individual and accurate disease reporting. While facilitating this process, the CHN is also assessing the individual as part of the community where they live, work, and play. For example, contact tracing conducted during an outbreak of TB in a homeless shelter required the local public health unit to become cognizant of the community defined by this unique population. This involved learning about the soup kitchens, drop-in centres, parks, and other areas where these individuals congregated. Local public health personnel could not achieve this task without the assistance of the ill individual (who provided information about the likely first case) and the community partners (who work closely with this population). These partners are not limited to healthcare providers but include all community agencies that provide services to the homeless. The result of the partnership was to develop a more focused and targeted screening of contacts. CHNs who work with marginalized populations, such as in Street Nursing programs across Canada, develop trusting relationships that facilitate contact tracing in these populations.

Contact tracing can involve identification of individuals who have not had any proximal contact with the case, and these individuals are called **indirect contacts**. In order to effectively manage cases of blood borne disease with possible indirect contact modes of transmission, it is important in contact tracing to recognize that an individual infected with a disease may not be able to provide all contact information as some contacts may be unknown to them. As noted earlier, blood products and solid organ implantation is now recognized as a significant disease transmission risk for recipients. For example, West Nile virus (WNV) was identified in four clients receiving organs from an asymptomatic donor in 2002 (Centers for Disease Control and Prevention, 2002). Other emerging diseases such as Creutzfeldt-Jakob disease (CJD) necessitate that the CHN thoroughly understand modes of transmission in order to perform thorough history taking in contact tracing. It would be important to know, for example, if instruments used in invasive procedures involving brain or neural tissue on a client diagnosed with CJD may have been contaminated.

Response to Outbreaks

An *outbreak* can be identified when expected symptoms in the population exist at an increased level. These symptoms may exist in the general population or in institutions such as hospitals, long-term care homes, or daycares. An outbreak may not necessarily be a reportable disease, but may initially be of unknown etiology, suggestive of a communicable disease. An outbreak can be identified when a group of persons present with similar signs and symptoms—such as fever, coughing, and malaise in the case of an outbreak of influenza-like illness. Generally, *outbreak reports* are communicated to public health authorities as soon as possible to allow investigation for a

cause of illness. In addition, early notification facilitates early institution of appropriate control methods, such as cohorting (separation) of well and ill clients into separate areas.

The terms "case" and "index case" are used throughout any discussion of outbreaks. A **case** refers to a single ill individual. When an individual person is identified as the likely first case in an outbreak, this person is referred to as the **index case**. Often, the index case in an outbreak is identified after other persons become ill and all surveillance data indicates that the outbreak began with the identified individual. The purpose in identifying a common source (contaminated food) or an index case (infectious person) is two-fold: (a) to interrupt further transmission of the disease by identifying the route of transmission, and (b) to understand the cause of the outbreak by identifying the origin of the pathogen. The information that a CHN gathers to understand and define an outbreak is often like pieces of a puzzle, and requires the CHN to possess critical-thinking and analytic skills.

Steps in Managing an Outbreak The initial investigation of an outbreak includes review of the signs and symptoms the ill clients share in common, the onset, and whether some clients are recovering, the usual course of the illness, and the source of the outbreak (e.g., source of outbreak can be a contaminated air conditioning unit in a legionella outbreak or an infected person in the case of a pertussis, measles, or mumps outbreak). Heymann (2008) outlines six general steps in the management of an outbreak: verifying the diagnosis, confirming the existence of an outbreak, identifying affected persons and characteristics, defining and investigating the population at risk, generating a hypothesis, and containing the outbreak (see MyNursingLab).

Generally, an outbreak report is generated after the outbreak is determined to be over, although in large outbreaks reporting may occur throughout the course of the outbreak. Scientific study and learning is generated after each outbreak as each outbreak presents differently. Debriefing sessions with all those involved in any aspect of the outbreak is an important and often missed learning opportunity. Efforts should be made to approach debriefing sessions with a structured format to avoid placing blame on individuals and to ensure behaviour change occurs to prevent similar outbreaks from happening again.

CASE STUDY: Outbreak Investigation

In a pertussis outbreak, the CHN initially gathered the following information: seven ill children, all in elementary schools, only two children in the same school, all children in the same city; there appeared to be no other common links—they did not know each other, had no common social events or travel, and no shared activities. The CHN could not identify a common source. Then an adult was diagnosed with pertussis and, on investigation, the CHN found that the adult was a teacher's spouse who had been ill for several weeks with pertussis-like

symptoms. The teacher was a special education teacher who travelled throughout the city to elementary schools. This teacher had been in every school that the ill children attended.

Discussion Questions

1. Who is the index case?

2. Would you do active surveillance or passive surveillance? Why?

3. Outline the steps to control and manage the pertussis outbreak.

PREPAREDNESS FOR DELIBERATELY CAUSED OUTBREAKS OF INFECTIOUS DISEASE

The *natural occurrence of disease* in populations helps us identify when an unusual event may be occurring, if a disease occurrence is suspicious, and if it should be investigated. **Bioterrorism** can be defined as the deliberate act of using microorganisms such as bacteria or viruses with the intent of causing infection and harm to achieve certain goals or gains (Shah, 2003). Agents considered to be a bioterrorism concern include anthrax, botulism, hemorrhagic fevers, plague, smallpox, and tularemia. For example, in 2001, anthrax spores were discovered in the U.S. postal system, causing 22 infections and 5 deaths (Centers for Disease Control and Prevention, 2008). More than 32 000 contacts of those who may have come into contact with anthrax-contaminated mail envelopes were provided antibiotics. Smallpox, although considered eradicated in 1977 (Heymann, 2008), is still considered a concern because of the belief that a stockpile exists somewhere in the world and that terrorists may access these sources.

It is expected that in deliberately caused outbreaks, the demand for acute care and public health services would be great and the demand for active surveillance and contact tracing would greatly increase. The agent used would determine the risk of person-to-person transmission and communicability. A strong public health infrastructure would be required to deal with rapid and effective detection and response mechanisms through emergency preparedness and funding activities such as stockpiling drugs, vaccines, and equipment. Strategies that have helped public health deal with infectious disease outbreaks such as SARS should be considered in preparation for a bioterrorist event. Special training may include basic emergency management, communicating within the Incident Management System, infection control, dealing safely with specimens, and decontamination procedures.

ROLE OF THE COMMUNITY HEALTH NURSE

History has shown that communicable diseases are controlled through changes in practice or environment. Typhoid and cholera are two communicable diseases that can be transmitted via contaminated water. The sanitation of water is one of the public health triumphs that occurred in the early 1900s. Improved sanitation and the development of vaccines for typhoid and cholera have virtually eliminated these diseases from the developed world. These diseases still continue to plague developing countries where water sanitation and vaccination programs are limited or not available (Heymann, 2008).

CHNs broke the chain of infection at the mode of transmission link by educating the public on personal hygiene and the importance of clean drinking water. Today, breaking the chain of infection is achieved through various methods, each one targeted at different links. For example, immunization programs (especially for children) modify the susceptible host into a resistant host, whereas prophylaxis can diminish or reduce the ability of the infectious agent to multiply after entry into the susceptible host. Sterilization of instruments, proper cleaning of food in restaurants, and harm-reduction methods are strategies targeted at the reservoir, thereby altering the ability of the infectious agent to transmit from one host to another.

Mounting immunization campaigns, screening, ensuring that quarantine requirements are met, instituting isolation, providing prophylaxis, and acting as consultants on communicable disease to community groups are some of CHNs' service delivery activities. CHNs working with the medical officer of health are responsible for monitoring and reporting communicable disease occurrences in the community as reported by other healthcare providers, schools, childcare agencies, laboratories, the general public, and healthcare institutions.

Levels of Preventive Measures

CHNs use the nursing process to implement primary, secondary, and tertiary prevention activities in controlling communicable diseases. *Primary prevention* attempts to prevent the disease from occurring. *Secondary prevention* detects a disease or condition in a certain population, usually by screening or testing for the disease. *Tertiary prevention* involves the reduction of the extent and severity of the health problem in order to minimize the disability.

The main **primary prevention measures** for controlling communicable disease include

- promoting and implementing immunization programs, notifying contacts, and making referrals for follow-up diagnosis;
- providing chemoprophylaxis and antitoxins for prevention of disease;
- working with public health authorities and community partners concerning protective and control measures for communicable diseases; and
- educating the public on safe sexual practices, optimal nutrition, healthy environments for better air quality and sanitation, and use of preventive measures such as universal precautions.

Secondary prevention measures include

- screening, which includes case finding, referral, and mass screening for early detection;
- early diagnosis, which includes interpretation of diagnositic results;
- early treatment, which includes provision of antimicrobial medications for newly diagnosed contacts;
- teaching for medication and treatment compliance, including provision of supportive care such as diet, rest, and exercise, and teaching for side effects of medications; and
- advocacy for accessible diagnostic and treatment services for socially disadvantaged groups such the poor, the underhoused, and people with language and cultural barriers.

Screening There are two reasons to test or screen for a communicable disease. The first is in response to the disease being identified in the community. Epidemiological reports can reveal or identify a population that is at risk for disease. CHNs screen the population to validate these reports and to identify the at-risk individuals. The persons being tested have not been identified in the contact screening but are part of the population at risk. For example, a student is diagnosed with TB; all students in his/her school, and not just those with close contact to the index student, may be tested for TB. The list of exposures of the case must be analyzed to also identify the *index* or *first case*. As well, the history of the cases may help to determine the *index case*; that is, who first presented with the disease symptoms. The second and a more general strategy is testing and screening after broad immunization campaigns, which are done as a standard of practice (e.g., titres following a hepatitis B vaccination series). The **titres** check the efficacy of the immunization to ensure that those who received the vaccine now have antibodies to the disease. A random sample of those immunized is used as a strategy by pharmaceutical companies to demonstrate efficacy of vaccine by using *seroconversion rates*.

Isolation and Quarantine Isolation and quarantine are also secondary preventive measures. Treatment or management of some infectious agents includes isolation or quarantine to reduce the transmission and break the chain of infection. **Isolation** refers to separation of an *infectious person* for a period of time to prevent or limit the direct or indirect transmission of the infectious agent. **Quarantine** is the restriction of activities for a *well person* who has been exposed to an infectious agent. Generally, communicable diseases that are transmitted by direct or airborne routes require that the contacts be separated from other people and possibly placed in quarantine. The length of the isolation or quarantine period is specific to the incubation and communicable period of each disease (Heymann, 2008). For example, varicella is considered to be most infectious two days before the onset of the rash, remaining infectious until all lesions are dried and crusted, whereas hepatitis A is most infectious during the two weeks before onset of symptoms until one week after the appearance of jaundice. The communicable period is not always known for every disease, especially emerging diseases. SARS is considered to have an incubation period of up to 10 days (Heymann, 2008). During the SARS outbreak, it was uncertain when the infected person was most contagious or when the symptoms displayed by the patient equated to communicability. For this reason, contacts were placed in quarantine for a minimum of 10 days.

Prophylaxis Prophylaxis, a secondary preventive measure, is the utilization of chemoprophylaxic or immunoprophylaxic agents to prevent illness from a pathogen or infectious agent following a known or possible exposure. Prophylaxic agents may be prescribed for exposed vulnerable hosts such as pregnant women, infants, people who have an immune disorder or transplant, or anyone who had contact with a disease that has high morbidity and mortality rates or a disease that has significant long-term effects.

Immunoprophylaxic agents are inclusive of both active and passive immunizing agents. **Active immunizing agents** are vaccines that stimulate the immune system to create antibodies. **Passive immunizing agents** include immune serum globulin, which is of human origin, and immune globulins that contain specific antibodies to a particular organism, such as hepatitis B immune globulin (HBIG) or rabies immune globulin (RIG).

Prophylaxis provides protection to the vulnerable hosts in the general population. The role of the CHN is to identify the vulnerable hosts, monitor the therapy if it is long term, and possibly administer or facilitate the administration of one-time prophylaxis. An example of the use of *chemoprophylaxis* includes the administration of Isoniazid (INH) to children younger than six years of age who are identified as contacts in a TB outbreak despite having a negative response to the tuberculin skin test. These children are given this medication daily for three months. It is recognized that young children may not have the ability to fight the TB organism as well as an older child or adult. The medication provides the child with the ability to fight the organism, reduces bacterial load, and reduces the possibility of disseminated disease. A tuberculin skin test is repeated after three months, and if the result continues to be negative and no other immune disorder appears to exist, the INH can be discontinued. *Immunoprophylaxis* can be an appropriate choice if, for example, during an outbreak of varicella in the community, contact tracing reveals that one of the contacts is a pregnant woman; she may be a candidate for varicella-zoster immune globulin (VZIG). The VZIG will either protect the woman from acquiring varicella or lessen the symptoms if the disease occurs, thereby protecting the fetus.

Tertiary prevention measures aim to reduce the extent and severity of the health problems in order to minimize the complications by

- educating and monitoring treatment compliance to prevent complications, and
- monitoring effectiveness of treatment and identifying and referring for adverse effects.

Education of the public may be carried out at the individual, family, and community levels through community-based programs. Education is not directed at a single stage in the chain of infection; rather, it targets the whole chain and teaches measures that can be adopted into the individual's personal health habits. The goal is to help the client and the community return to baseline functioning, or a new state of health. Examples include the administration of **direct observed therapy (DOT)**, which is a mechanism used to ensure TB clients takes their prescribed medications. The nurse observes the clients taking the medications on a pre-set schedule. This is to prevent the risk of non-compliance and thereby reduce the possibility of drug-resistant TB, which could place communities at risk.

Through various levels of prevention activities, CHNs play major roles in education, health promotion, direct care, community development and mobilization, liaison, research, advocacy, program planning and evaluation, and policy formulation. All are essential skills in epidemiologic investigation for successful management and control of communicable diseases. Utilizing these skills is essential as was shown by the role of CHNs in the H1N1 pandemic of 2009. Although the 2009 pandemic was considered to be mild, Canada was one of the few countries that had a pandemic plan in place well in advance of the H1N1 influenza virus outbreak. The overall goals of the Canadian Pandemic Influenza Plan were to minimize serious illness and overall deaths, and to minimize societal disruption caused by the pandemic. In the 2009 pandemic, there were 428 deaths and 8678 hospitalizations in Canada due to influenza A/H1N1 (PHAC, 2010). Across Canada, recommendations for healthcare workers that were made by PHAC were followed by acute and community health workers on issues like infection control and occupational health, resource management, clinical care, and the distribution of antivirals and vaccines. Guidelines were followed by CHNs on addressing the outbreak, reinforcing the recommended infection control practices, and public health measures. As a result, minimal illness occurred and societal disruption was kept to a minimum. Effective pandemic preparedness is essential to mitigate the effects of a pandemic, particularly if it becomes severe. CHNs play a pivotal role in planning with community partners to create policies, to enhance environmental supports, and to provide educational resources.

WHO PRIORITIES IN CONTROLLING COMMUNICABLE DISEASES

Like other nations, Canada works in partnership with the WHO to reduce the incidence and impact of communicable diseases on its population. The role of the WHO in communicable disease control is to lead global efforts in surveillance, prevention, control, and research. What continues to be a challenge for all nations can be seen in the following priorities set by the WHO (2000, 2006):

- to reduce the negative consequences of malaria, TB, HIV/AIDS;
- to strengthen prevention, surveillance, monitoring, and response to control communicable disease with established policies;
- to strengthen international partnership and communication between governments and to provide resources and technical assistance when needed; and
- to generate new knowledge through research for development of tools and intervention methods.

Control of communicable disease must be a national and international effort. With increasing international cooperation in managing diseases and knowledge exchange, infrastructures for protecting public health become a priority for both developing and developed countries. Examples can be seen in the 2009 Canadian Pandemic Preparedness Meeting in Toronto and studies conducted regarding the impact of international travel (see Canadian Research Box 12.2).

CANADIAN RESEARCH BOX

What is the research agenda for a pandemic situation?

Canadian Institutes of Health Research, Rx & D Health Research Foundation, & Canadian Food Inspection Agency. (2009, July 8). *Canadian pandemic preparedness meeting: H1N1 outbreak research response.* Toronto, ON. Retrieved from http://www.cihr-irsc.gc.ca/e/documents/iii_cppm_report_2009_e.pdf

In April 2009, the first deaths from a novel strain of H1N1 influenza A virus were reported in Mexico and the United States. The virus quickly spread to other countries including Canada. As of July 2009, the WHO reported almost 100 000 confirmed cases of human infection worldwide and almost 500 deaths, including 25 in Canada.

Healthcare providers and policymakers were under significant pressure to make informed healthcare and public health decisions based on scientific information. To facilitate this process, the Canadian Institutes of Health Research (CIHR), Research-Based Pharmaceutical Companies (Rx & D), Health Research Foundation, and Canadian Food Inspection Agency (CFIA) sponsored a one-day research meeting of more than 180 influenza and pandemic experts from across Canada on July 8, 2009, in Toronto. The goals of the meeting were:

- to facilitate information sharing among researchers and other influenza experts;
- to network and develop collaborations in order to focus the Canadian research response to the pandemic; and
- to discuss gaps in research knowledge about the pandemic H1N1/09 virus.

Discussion Questions

1. Which possible disciplines/professionals would you most likely invite to participate in this multidisciplinary team to derive a research agenda on response to H1N1 outbreak?

2. Why is it important for healthcare providers and policy makers to collaborate in a research agenda?

SUMMARY

This chapter has discussed the basic principles of communicable disease control, including vaccine-preventable diseases and the role of the CHN in dealing with them. The topic of communicable disease control is broad, and each day the world faces a new disease that may or may not find its way into any community. CHNs must be prepared to respond to the unexpected. They must work in partnership with the local, national, and global communities to develop effective surveillance methods and screening tools, to enhance emergency response mechanisms, and to implement public health measures in primary, secondary, and tertiary prevention for communicable disease control. It is imperative that CHNs possess a strong relationship with their community partners, a solid knowledge base of epidemiology and current information on communicable diseases, knowledge of available resources, and strong decision-making and research skills. Integration of these skills will help the CHN to be successful in the role of protecting and promoting the health of Canadians.

KEY TERMS

communicable diseases, p. 190
outbreak, p. 190
endemic, p. 190
epidemic, p. 190
pandemic, p. 190
blood borne pathogens, p. 199
foodborne infection, p. 199
foodborne intoxication, p. 199
foodborne outbreaks, p. 200
waterborne pathgens, p. 200
outbreak of waterborne disease, p. 200
vector-borne disease, p. 200
zoonotic infections, p. 200
nosocomial infections, p. 202
notifiable diseases, p. 202
non-reportable diseases, p. 203
surveillance, p. 203
active surveillance, p. 203
passive surveillance, p. 203
contact tracing, p. 204
contacts, p. 204
degree of exposure, p. 204
integrated Public Health Information System, p. 204
Canadian Integrated Outbreak Surveillance Centre, p. 204
indirect contacts, p. 205
case, p. 205
index case, p. 205
bioterrorism, p. 206
primary prevention measures, p. 206
secondary prevention measures, p. 206
titres, p. 207
isolation, p. 207
quarantine, p. 207
prophylaxis, p. 207
active immunizing agents, p. 207
passive immunizing agents, p. 207
tertiary prevention measures, p. 207
direct observed therapy (DOT), p. 207

REVIEW QUESTIONS

Choose the one alternative that best completes the statement or answers the question.

1. The first recorded worldwide threat from a communicable disease, which killed about one-third of the population in Europe in the 13th century, was
   a) typhoid.
   b) tuberculosis.
   c) bubonic plague.
   d) leprosy.

2. Which of the following are vital in creating disease data to demonstrate the prevalence and incidence of an emerging infection?
   a) healthcare professional awareness
   b) reporting by the public
   c) surveillance program
   d) immunization uptake rates

3. Communicable diseases are
   a) caused by infectious toxins.
   b) transmitted from a vulnerable person, an animal, or an inanimate source.
   c) transmitted by indirect exposure to toxic products.
   d) passed on by infected hosts or with their excretions.

4. Which of the following is accurate regarding influenza and influenza prevention programs?
   a) Between 2000 and 4000 Canadians can die of influenza and its complications annually.
   b) Human influenza is a respiratory infection caused by a coronavirus.
   c) Influenza is spread by droplets through coughing, sneezing, or singing.
   d) Vaccination against influenza is routinely given on an annual basis starting at the onset of the influenza season, typically in January.

5. Which of the following vaccines has not been licensed for use in Canada since June 2006?
   a) human papillomavirus (HPV)
   b) pandemic influenza H1N1
   c) rotavirus vaccine
   d) West Nile virus vaccine

6. Which of the following bacteria caused a large community outbreak in Walkerton, Ontario, in 2000, when the town's water supply became contaminated?
   a) Escherichia coli
   b) listeria monocytogenes
   c) cryptosporidium
   d) legionellae

7. Which of the following is a vector-borne disease?
   a) rabies
   b) pertussis
   c) Lyme disease
   d) hantavirus

STUDY QUESTIONS

1. What is the link between epidemiology and control of communicable diseases?

2. What are the modes of transmission of communicable diseases?

3. A high school student is diagnosed with tuberculosis. How would you conduct contact tracing?

4. A daycare centre has just notified you, a new CHN, that a child in its care has meningitis. The staff and parents of other children are very anxious. Describe your nursing interventions.

5. The local health authority has just hired you to work on hepatitis A management and control. Being new to the region, what would be your priority tasks?

6. What information would you need from the infectious individual and about his or her disease (e.g., HIV) to conduct comprehensive contact tracing?

---

*After working through these questions, go to the MyNursingLab at **www.pearsoned.ca/mynursinglab** to check your answers.*

INDIVIDUAL CRITICAL THINKING EXERCISES

1. You receive several laboratory reports for the same disease from the same geographical area. What steps are needed to differentiate between an increased incidence as opposed to a usual occurrence of the disease?

2. In question 1 above, what would be your sources of information for the investigation?

3. You are working in a downtown clinic that provides services to marginalized/vulnerable persons. A client presents to the clinic with non-specific ailments. You are collecting the history. The client reveals a history of addictions to crack cocaine and other substances and that he has multiple sexual partners. Your recommendation is to have a full work-up for sexually transmitted infections. The client refuses. Discuss your nursing responsibilities.

4. Refer to question 3 above; the client's HIV test shows a positive result. What should be your next steps?

5. You have been assigned a client who has active tuberculosis, and who has been on treatment in his or her home country and has just arrived in Canada and does not understand English or the purpose of the treatment. How would you ensure an accurate nursing assessment for this client and how would you facilitate a supportive treatment environment for this client?

GROUP CRITICAL THINKING EXERCISES

1. Large numbers of immigrants come from regions where the prevalence of tuberculosis is high. This has resulted in the importation of a large burden of latent infection that can be expected to generate future active cases in aging immigrant populations. Discuss the implications for caring for the future active cases. Healthy public policy should be included in the discussion as opposed to local health authority policy.

2. AIDS can manifest after years of HIV-positive status; a positive HIV test may not occur until three months after the contact. Similarly, in tuberculosis, the skin test can be negative up to 12 weeks post-exposure, and the manifestations of the disease may occur sometime in the person's lifetime. Discuss the implications of contact tracing for these two diseases.

3. Emerging diseases, changes in antibiotic resistance, and threats of terrorism with biological agents have heightened the awareness of surveillance needs worldwide. Since September 11, 2001, the threat of smallpox and anthrax has been in the media. Discuss the information needed to control the spread of smallpox.

REFERENCES

Allen, U. A. (2006). Public health implications of MRSA in Canada. *Canadian Medical Association Journal, 175*(2), 161–162.

Canadian Blood Services. (2009). *Testing.* Retrieved from http://www.bloodservices.ca/centreapps/internet/uw_v502_mainengine.nsf/page/testing?OpenDocument

Canadian Integrated Outbreak Surveillance Centre: Enteric Alerts. (2009). *Enteric alerts.* Retrieved from http://www.hc-sc.gc.ca/hc-ps/ed-ud/respond/food-aliment/fiorp-priti_11-eng.php

Centers for Disease Control and Prevention. (2002, September 6). Public health dispatch: West Nile virus infection in organ donor and transplant recipients—Georgia and Florida, 2002. *Morbidity and Mortality Weekly Report, 51*(35), 790. Retrieved from http://www.cdc.gov/mmwr/preview/mmwrhtml/mm5135a5.htm

Centers for Disease Control and Prevention. (2008). *Questions and answers about Anthrax.* Retrieved from http://emergency.cdc.gov/agent/anthrax/faq

Drebot, M. A., & Artsob, H. (2006). West Nile virus: A pathogen of concern for older adults. *Geriatrics and Aging, 9*(7), 465–471.

Heymann, D. L. (2008). *Control of communicable diseases manual: An official report of the American Public Health Association* (19th ed.). Washington, DC: American Public Health Association.

North Bay Parry Sound District Health Unit. (2009). *Investigative summary of the escherichia coli outbreak associated with a restaurant in North Bay, Ontario: October to November 2008* (North Bay: NBPSDHU, June 2009). Retrieved from http://www.healthunit.biz/docs/Ecoli%20Outbreak/2008%20NBPSDHU%20Ecoli%20Report_June%202009_Formatted.pdf

Plotkin, S. A., & Orenstein, W. A. (2008). *Vaccines* (5th ed.). Philadelphia, PA: W. B. Saunders.

Pubic Health Agency of Canada. (2000). *Waterborne outbreak of gastroenteritis associated with a contaminated* municipal water supply, Walkerton, Ontario. Communicable Disease Report (CCDR). Retrieved from http://www.phac-aspc.gc.ca/publicat/ccdr-rmtc/00vol26/dr2620eb.html

Public Health Agency of Canada. (2001). Waterborne Cryptosporidiosis outbreak, North Battleford, Saskatchewan. Canada Communicable Disease Report (CCDR). Retrieved from http://www.phac-aspc.gc.ca/publicat/ccdr-rmtc/01vol27/dr2722ea.html

Public Health Agency of Canada. (2006). Canadian immunization guide (7th ed.). Ottawa, ON: Government Services Canada.

Public Health Agency of Canada. (2007a). Canadian Integrated Public Health Surveillance (CIPHS). Retrieved from http://www.phac-aspc.gc.ca/php-psp/ciphs-eng.php#wiphis

Public Health Agency of Canada. (2007b). The Canadian nosocomial infection surveillance program. Retrieved from http://www.phac-aspc.gc.ca/nois-sinp/survprog-eng.php

Public Health Agency of Canada. (2008). Who we are. Retrieved from http://www.phac-aspc.gc.ca/about_apropos/who-eng.php?option=print

Public Health Agency of Canada. (2009a). Creutzfeldt-Jakob disease (CJD). Retrieved from http://www.phac-aspc.gc.ca/hcai-iamss/cjd-mcj/cjdss-ssmcj/stats_e.html#canada

Public Health Agency of Canada. (2009b). Influenza. Retrieved from http://www.phac-aspc.gc.ca/influenza/index-eng.php

Public Health Agency of Canada. (2009c). Number of cases of Lyme disease. Retrieved from http://www.phac-aspc.gc.ca/id-mi/lyme-eng.php

Public Health Agency of Canada. (2009d). Hantaviruses. Retrieved from http://www.hc-sc.gc.ca/hl-vs/iyh-vsv/diseases-maladies/hantavirus-eng.php

Public Health Agency of Canada. (2009e). National notifiable diseases. Retrieved from http://dsol-smed.phac-aspc.gc.ca/dsol-smed/ndis/list_e.html

Public Health Agency of Canada. (2009f). West Nile virus MONITOR: Human surveillance (2002–2008). Retrieved from http://www.phac-aspc.gc.ca/wnv-vwn/index-eng.php

Public Health Agency of Canada. (2010). Surveillance: Deaths associated with H1N1 flu virus in Canada. Retrieved from http://www.phac-aspc.gc.ca/alert-alerte/h1n1/surveillance-archive/20100128-eng.php

Riemann, C., & Cliver, D. (Eds.). (2006). Foodborne infections and intoxications (3rd ed.). New York, NY: Academic Press.

Shah, C. P. (2003). Public health and preventative medicine in Canada (5th ed.). Toronto, ON: Elsevier Canada.

World Health Organization. (1998). Report of the director-general. 1998 world health report: Health in the 21st century: A vision for all. Geneva, Switzerland: Author.

World Health Organization. (2000). Communicable diseases: 2000 highlights of activities in 1999 and major challenges for the future. Retrieved from http://www.who.int/infectious-disease-news/CDS2000/PDF/cd2000-e.pdf

World Health Organization. (2006). Speeches/statements—striving for better health in South-East Asia. Selected speeches by Dr Uton Muchtar Rafei regional director, WHO South-East Asia region. Volume II: 1997–2000. Retrieved from http://www.searo.who.int/EN/Section980/Section1162/Section1167/Section1171_4747.htm

World Health Organization. (2009a). Communicable diseases: Highlights of communicable disease activities, major recent achievements. Retrieved from http://www.searo.who.int/EN/Section10.htm

World Health Organization. (2009b). Five keys to safer food. Retrieved from http://www.who.int/foodsafety/consumer/5keys/en/

World Health Organization. (2009c). International health regulations. Retrieved from http://www.who.int/csr/ihr/en/

ADDITIONAL RESOURCES

Readings

The Chief Public Health Officer's Report on the state of public health in Canada. (2009). Growing up well—priorities for a healthy future. (Also available at http://publichealth.gc.ca/CPHOreport)

Ellis, E., Gallant, V., Scholten, D., Dawson, K., & Saunders, A. (2007). Tuberculosis in Canada, 2007. Ottawa, ON: Public Health Agency of Canada. (Also available at http://www.publichealth.gc.ca/tuberculosis)

Liverman, C. T., Harris, T. A., Rogers, M. E. B., & Shine, K. I. (2009). Respiratory protection for healthcare workers in the workplace against novel H1N1 Influenza A. Washington, DC: The National Academies Press. (Also available at http://www.nap.edu/catalog/12748.html)

Public Health Agency of Canada. (2007, December). Recommendations on a human papillomavirus immunization program. Canadian Immunization Committee. (Also available at http://www.phac-aspc.gc.ca/publicat/2008/papillomavirus-papillome/papillomavirus-papillome-2-eng.php)

Videos

Tuberculosis, The Silent Killer
http://www.youtube.com/watch?v=149H13ocPqw
Award-Winning Photos Highlight Drug-Resistant Tuberculosis
http://www.youtube.com/watch?v=QgVchBERVng&feature=related
Malaria: No Ordinary Mosquito Bite
http://www.youtube.com/watch?v=IVbq2yQH52g&NR=1
Malaria in the 21st century
http://www.youtube.com/watch?v=iwAEsOpvHn0&feature=related
The Fight Against Infectious Diseases: Partnership in Health
http://www.youtube.com/watch?v=VIxoGdtZB3k

Websites

Centers for Disease Control and Prevention (CDC):
MMWR: Morbidity and Mortality Weekly Report
http://www.cdc.gov/mmwr/

Community and Hospital Infection Control Association
Canada (CICA)
http://www.chica.org

Government of Australia
http://www.health.vic.gov.au/ideas/bluebook

Pan American Health Organization
http://new.paho.org/hq/index.php?lang=en

Public Health Agency of Canada (PHAC)
http://www.phac-aspc.gc.ca/publicat/ccdr-rmtc/

World Health Organization: Integrated Disease Surveillance
Programme
http://www.afro.who.int/en/clusters-a-programmes/
dpc/integrated-disease-surveillance/programme-
components/integrated-disease-surveillance-including-
data-management-ids.html

World Health Organization: Briefing Note on five keys to
safer food
http://www.who.int/foodsafety/consumer/Briefing_keys.pdf

Public Health Agency of Canada: Listeria Outbreak
http://www.phac-aspc.gc.ca/alert-alerte/listeria/archive/
listeria_2008-eng.php

Ontario Ministry of Health and Long-Term Care:
Salmonella associated with bean sprouts
http://www.health.gov.on.ca/english/media/news_releases/
archives/nr_05/nr_112505.pdf

About the Authors

Sheila Marchant-Short, Diploma (Seneca College), BScN (University of Western Ontario), MScN (University of British Columbia), is a Regional Manager of Communicable Disease Control Programs with Community Health Services and Public Health, Eastern Health, St. John's, NL. She has an extensive background in nursing, including acute care, nursing education, and public health. Ms. Marchant-Short has been working in the area of Communicable Disease Control for many years, including at the Epidemiology and Disease Control Centre in Victoria, BC, with the BC Ministry of Health, with North Bay Parry Sound District Health Unit, ON and currently with Eastern Health. She has been involved in communicable disease prevention efforts locally, provincially, and nationally. She has been a keynote speaker on topics such as immunization decision-making, influenza, pandemic planning, and the role of nurses in communicable disease control.

Leeann Whitney, BScN (Laurentian University), MAEd (Central Michigan), formerly the Director of Infectious Disease at the North Bay Parry Sound District Health Unit, she is currently involved in private consulting for nursing and public health locally and provincially including the nursing education sector. Ms. Whitney's background includes nursing in acute care and teaching settings throughout Ontario, and in community nursing in the control of infectious disease, vaccine preventable diseases, sexual health and family health programs. She is formerly a member of the College of Nurses of Ontario Leadership Advisory Committee and the Community Health Nurses Interest Group (RNAO).

chapter 13

Community Care

Lucia Yiu

OBJECTIVES

After studying this chapter, you should be able to:

1. Discuss the concept of community, community functions, and community dynamics.
2. Describe the selected common models and frameworks used in community health nursing practice.
3. Explain the application of community health nursing process in caring for community clients.
4. Discuss the purposes and use of selected participatory tools in community assessment, planning, and intervention.
5. Explain the importance of population health promotion, risk assessment, community engagement, community governance, capacity building, and community development.
6. Discuss the role of the nurse in caring for clients in the community.

INTRODUCTION

Community health nurses (CHNs) care for people where they live, learn, play, and work. Their goal is to improve the health of the community by promoting, preserving, and protecting the health of individuals, families, aggregates, and populations. Their practice includes promoting health, building individual/community capacity, connecting and caring, facilitating access and equity, and demonstrating professional responsibility and accountability (Community Health Nurses Association of Canada, 2008). When entering the practice of community health nursing, novice nurses often ask, "What does caring for a community mean?" "Where and how do I begin?" and "What is a healthy community?"

Unlike having clients in hospitals or acute care settings, who actively seek episodic care for their presenting problems, CHNs must determine who and where their clients are—and when, why, what, and how best to promote their health in the community. They must understand the complexity and needs of their diverse populations and the relationship of environment and health, and must work autonomously to build community partnerships that are based on a philosophy of primary healthcare. This chapter provides an overview of the community health nursing process including community assessment, selected community health practice models, population health promotion, community development, and community participatory tools.

COMMUNITY DEFINED

CHNs have always cared for the community as their clients. The earliest form of visiting nurses cared for the sick and the destitute families. Florence Nightingale cared for the soldiers in the Crimean War and advocated for improved sanitation and hygiene conditions to reduce infections and deaths among them. Lillian Wald established the Henry Street Settlement in New York to improve housing, nutrition, and sanitation for impoverished mothers and children (Stanhope & Lancaster, 2006). Today, Cathy Crowe advocates for improved access for the homeless population in Toronto, Ontario, Canada. She demanded all governments commit an additional 1% of their budgets to an affordable social housing program (Stamler & Yiu, 2008). These nurses understood their communities' and clients' needs. They worked with politicians and community partners to advocate and help improve their clients' health and well-being.

Developing an understanding of a community, its functions and dynamics, and the relationships between these and the health of the people is fundamental to providing competent community care. A **community** may be defined as a group of people who live, learn, work, and play in an environment at a given time. They share common characteristics and interests and function in a social system that meets their needs within a larger social system such as an organization, a region, a province, or a nation.

The core of any community is its people, who are characterized by their age, sex, socioeconomic status, education level, occupation, ethnicity, and religion. A community may be defined by its place or geopolitical boundaries, which often are used to determine the location of service delivery (Vollman et al., 2008). **Geopolitical boundaries** refer to both geographic boundaries such as mountains, rivers, or lakes, and political boundaries such as program or agency service districts. **Aggregate communities** refer to groups of people with common interests, culture, beliefs, or goals. More recently, CHNs also have begun to examine **virtual communities**, where members meet in various Internet communities—such as chat rooms, MySpace, blog, Twitter, widget, and Facebook—to share their common interests.

Community Functions

All communities carry out various functions to sustain the day-to-day livelihood of their residents. These **community functions** include provision of:

- space and infrastructure for housing, schools, recreation, government, and health and social service;
- employment and income including productivity and distribution through consumption of goods, trading, and economic growth;
- security, protection, and law enforcement to protect the public from crime;
- participation, socialization, and networking for all community members; and
- linkages with other community systems for opportunities for growth and capacity building.

Community Dynamics

Community functions are supported by three interactive **community dynamics**: effective communication, leadership, and decision making (Clemen-Stone et al., 2002).

Communication Competent communities possess strong and cohesive vertical, horizontal, and diagonal patterns of communication among the community key partners. *Vertical communication* enables communities to link to larger communities or to those with higher decision-making power. *Horizontal communication* allows the community to connect to and work collaboratively with its own members, environment, and other service systems. *Diagonal communication* reinforces the cohesiveness and communication of all system components, both horizontally and vertically, and helps reduce the silo effects that occur when communication is done only vertically and horizontally.

Leadership Formal and informal leaders lead their members by influencing the decision-making process, using their status and position in the community. *Formal leaders* are elected official politicians such as mayors, members of parliament, or the prime minister. *Informal leaders* are those with prominent positions in the community, such as religious leaders, executives or representatives of community organizations or professionals, elders of community groups, philanthropists, or local heroes.

Decision Making Formal leaders use government policies to guide their decision making for the community, while informal leaders use their status to influence community groups and to effect change. Based on community needs, these leaders collaborate and negotiate with community groups to advocate for optimal change.

Competent community dynamics foster public participation, mutual support, and community action to promote community growth and ultimately healthy communities. What, then, does a healthy community look like? See the box "A Healthy Community Process and Characteristics of Healthy Communities."

A Healthy Community Process

A healthy community process involves:

- Wide community participation
- Broad involvement of all sectors of the community
- Local government commitment
- Creation of healthy public policies

Characteristics of Healthy Communities

- Clean and safe physical environment
- Peace, equity, and social justice
- Adequate access to food, water, shelter, income, safety, work, and recreation for all
- Adequate access to healthcare services
- Opportunities for learning and skill development
- Strong, mutually supportive relationships and networks
- Workplaces that are supportive of individual and family well-being
- Wide participation of residents in decision making
- Strong local cultural and spiritual heritage
- Diverse and vital economy
- Protection of the natural environment
- Responsible use of resources to ensure long-term sustainability

Source: Ontario Healthy Communities Coalition. (2010). What makes a community healthy? Retrieved from http://www.ohcc-ccso.ca/en/what-makes-a-healthy-community

---

SELECTED MODELS AND FRAMEWORKS OF COMMUNITY HEALTH NURSING PRACTICE

CHNs use models and frameworks to systematically collect data and analyze the relationships of various data components. The selected model or framework for practice must be easy to use and reflect one's practice philosophy. A number of existing nursing models and frameworks focus only on individual and not community care. This section briefly describes those frameworks commonly used in community nursing practice.

Community-as-Partner Model

Vollman et al. (2008) described community and nursing process as the two main attributes in their community-as-partner model. The *community attribute* is the **community assessment wheel**, which depicts that a community comprises eight interacting subsystems: physical environment, education, safety and transportation, politics and government, health and social services, communication, economy, and recreation. At the core of this community assessment wheel are the community residents, who have their unique history, demographics, values, and beliefs.

The *nursing attribute* reflects Betty Neuman's stress adaptation model, which is derived from the general systems theory. Within the community are the *lines of resistance* or strengths that protect the community from harm or threats. Surrounding the community are the *normal lines of defence* that reflect the normal state of health attained by the community. *Flexible lines of defence* form the outer layer around the community. They serve as a buffer zone that represents the community's temporary health response to stressors. These stressors create tension-producing stimuli and may, in turn, penetrate the various lines of defence surrounding the community, affecting the system equilibrium. CHNs assess and analyze the degree of reaction to the stressors experienced by the community and implement purposeful primary, secondary, and tertiary interventions to promote client optimal health.

Epidemiologic Framework

CHNs may use the *epidemiologic triangle* (host–environment–agent) to examine the frequency and distribution of a disease or health condition in the population being studied. They determine *what* the community is, *who* is affected (host), *where* and *when* the condition occurred (environment), and *why* and *how* (agent) it occurred. They may also use the "web of causation" to study the chains of causation and their effects on a health problem. (See Chapter 9.)

Community Capacity Approach

Capacity building is a process that strengthens the ability of an individual, an organization, a community, or a health system to develop and implement health promotion initiatives and sustain positive health outcomes over time. It involves individual and organizational skills development, human resource development, leadership, partnership, resource allocation, and policy formulation (Centers for Disease Control and Prevention, 2009). Optimal capacity building builds on community strengths, not deficits. It is realized when the community is committed and empowered to change, has resources to

draw from, and has a strong infrastructure to support its functions and dynamics (Minkler, 2005; Sahay, 2004).

A **community assets map** may be used to outline the assets and capacity of the community and identify strengths and potential resources for interventions. Data for creating the community assets map include skills and experiences of individuals and organizations, services, and physical and financial resources within and outside the community. (See MyNursingLab for Community Assets Mapping.)

Community Health Promotion Model

Evidence from health promotion research has supported that approximately 25% of the health of the population is attributed to the healthcare system and the remaining 75% is determined by a multiplicity of factors that include social and economic environments (50%), biological and genetic endowment (15%), and physical environments (10%) (Kirby, 2002; Senate of Canada, 2009). The **community health promotion model** (Figure 13.1) therefore incorporates the four health fields (Lalonde, 1974) and determinants of health (Public Health Agency of Canada [PHAC], 2010) to assess the health of the community. It then uses Epp's (1986) health promotion strategies, the Ottawa Charter of Health Promotion (World Health Organization [WHO], Canadian Public Health Association, & Health and Welfare Canada, 1986), and primary healthcare principles (WHO, 1978) to guide community planning, intervention, and evaluation. (See Chapters 5, 6, 7, and 14.) The goal of the community health promotion model (CHPM) is to apply community health promotion strategies to achieve collaborative community actions and to improve sustainable health outcomes of the community.

Nursing process is an integral part of the CHPM and is used to systematically assess, plan for, intervene in, and evaluate the health of the community. The model applies primary health concepts through purposeful community assessment, planning, implementation, and evaluation. The CHPM supports community development and community engagement. The CHPM provides a holistic approach to promoting the health of the population so that a higher quality of community life and equity in health can be attained. It recognizes that a community's health is impacted by more than just genetics, healthcare services, and lifestyle risk factors such as poor nutrition, lack of physical activity, and tobacco use. It emphasizes the importance of social determinants of health in influencing the health of the community. These factors include employment, housing, food, education, childhood years, workplace safety, social inclusion, and access to health systems. They impact how people cope with their environment and thereby influence health inequities among people of various social positions within and between communities and countries (PHAC, 2004; Raphael, 2008; WHO, 2010). For example, a young single mother's decision to feed a high-carbohydrate diet to her children may not be her poor lifestyle choice, but rather her inability to meet her family's nutritional needs because of her low education and income and lack of family support and resources. Community health nursing process using the CHPM is described below.

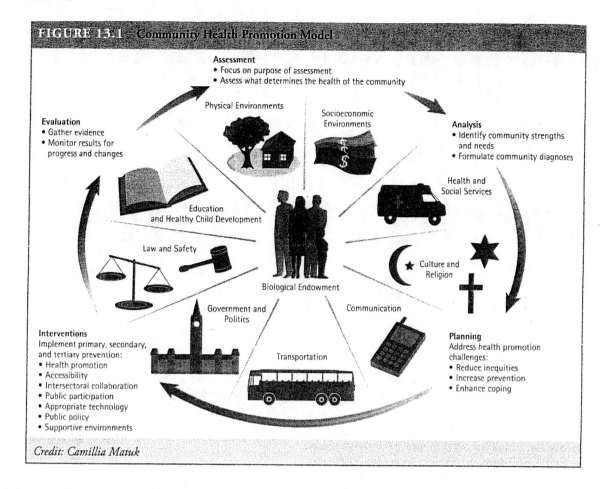

FIGURE 13.1 Community Health Promotion Model

Assessment
• Focus on purpose of assessment
• Assess what determines the health of the community

Physical Environments

Socioeconomic Environments

Evaluation
• Gather evidence
• Monitor results for progress and changes

Analysis
• Identify community strengths and needs
• Formulate community diagnoses

Health and Social Services

Education and Healthy Child Development

Law and Safety

Culture and Religion

Biological Endowment

Government and Politics

Communication

Interventions
Implement primary, secondary, and tertiary prevention:
• Health promotion
• Accessibility
• Intersectoral collaboration
• Public participation
• Appropriate technology
• Public policy
• Supportive environments

Transportation

Planning
Address health promotion challenges:
• Reduce inequities
• Increase prevention
• Enhance coping

Credit: Camillia Matuk

COMMUNITY HEALTH NURSING PROCESS

The process of community health nursing is continuous and cyclical; it consists of four phases: assessment, planning, implementation, and evaluation. CHNs may enter at any of these phases, but must first determine the purpose or goal of their nursing involvement. This goal-oriented activity enables CHNs to critically analyze the problem or issue, make inferences on the implications and consequences of the problems or issues, formulate community nursing diagnoses, plan and implement the interventions, and evaluate the outcomes. This chapter focuses on community assessment and related tools. Community planning, intervention, and evaluation are further elaborated in Chapter 14.

Community Assessment

Community assessment is an ongoing quantitative and qualitative systematic appraisal of the community. It can be a comprehensive process because of the complexity of community functions and dynamics. Some key questions that guide the beginning steps of community assessment are:

■ What is the purpose of my community assessment? Why is it needed? Which social determinants of health are being affected?

■ Who, where, and what are the characteristics of my community?

■ Who, where, and what are the characteristics of my target population? How is my population different from others in the region?

■ What information about the community do I need to know and where can I obtain this information?

■ What would be the best approaches or techniques to collect my community data? How will I engage the community in choosing the approaches?

■ What are my resources or constraints to complete this community assessment (e.g., time, political environment, expertise, labour, and cost)?

Purpose of Community Assessment

Community assessment must be purposeful and evidence-based. The following describes reasons for community assessment that may be used alone or in a combination. These are environmental scan, needs assessment, problem investigation, and/or resource evaluation. See Tables 13.1A and 13.1B for examples of how evidence-based PISO purpose statements or questions are formulated (Albert & Herrera, 2009). In this PISO case example, a CHN wants to address risky drinking on university campus by applying a harm reduction strategy. The aim is to decrease the incidence of negative consequences associated with excessive alcohol consumption.

TABLE 13.1A   Formulating a Focus–Evidence–Purpose Statement/Question

PISO* statement: What **harm reduction strategies** are effective in **decreasing risky drinking** and negative consequences among **campus students** at the **University of Windsor**?

Population	undergraduate students
Intervention	harm reduction strategies
Setting	University of Windsor
Outcome	decreasing risky drinking and negative consequences

TABLE 13.1B   Examples of PISO* Focus Evidence Questions

Type of Community Assessment	Population	Intervention/Strategy	Setting	Outcome	Focus Evidence Question
Problem investigation	Grades 4–12 students	Prevention activities	Grade schools and high schools	Smoking prevention	What strategies are effective in engaging **children in Grades 4–12** in smoking prevention activities in schools?
Problem investigation	Campus students (17–22 yrs)	Harm reduction strategy	University of Windsor	Decrease risky drinking behaviour	What **harm reduction strategies** are effective in decreasing risky drinking and negative consequences among **campus students** at the **University of Windsor**?
Resource evaluation	Expectant teen parents	Program evaluation	Windsor-Essex County	Healthy pregnancy through the Health Unit's prenatal education program	Did the **Health Unit's prenatal education program improve pregnancy outcomes** for expectant teen parents in Windsor-Essex County?
Resource evaluation	Clients with low income	Program evaluation	Downtown area in Windsor	Use of Methadone clinic from January to June	How well do **low-income clients** living in the **downtown core of Windsor** use the **Methadone clinic** from Jan–June?
Environmental scan	Clients with disabilities	Community mapping and surveys	Windsor-Essex County	Transportation service for individuals with disabilities	Based on **community mapping and surveys,** how available are the transportation services for **rural clients with disabilities** living in Windsor-Essex county?
Needs assessment	Newcomers	Focus groups	Windsor-Essex County	Challenges and barriers to assessing breast health services	Through **focus groups** discussions, what are the **challenges and barriers to accessing breast health services** as experienced by **newcomers** living in Windsor-Essex County?

*PISO is a term used in Albert, D., & Herrera, C. (2009, November 20). Getting lost in the evidence? Part 1: Developing an evidence question and search srategy. *Fireside Chat Presentation*. Ottawa, ON: University of Ottawa.

Environmental Scan The most preliminary and fundamental assessment of the community is an **environmental scan**, in which one scans the overall environment through a **windshield survey**. CHNs can drive around the neighbourhood or take a walking tour, and use their senses of sight, touch, hearing, and smell to collect information and form their preliminary assessment of their community. They can see the people, the housing conditions, the geography, and the physical layout of various services in the community. During a walking tour, CHNs can listen to what languages people speak to one another and what concerns them during their daily conversations in their neighbourhood cafés or markets. They can smell the air quality or taste the water, and they can feel the oppression or friendliness of the people. By scanning the environment, CHNs can familiarize themselves with their work environment and connect people to the resources and environment in which they live. Windshield surveys are best done at two different times of day and on different days of the week for data comparison purposes.

Needs Assessment Appropriate and cost-effective services that meet the health needs of the population are based on the community's needs or deficits, not on its unrealistic wants or desires. **Needs** are what the community perceives as the gap between its current situation and desired situation. To perform a needs assessment, CHNs must (a) investigate the nature of the needs, (b) determine if the expressed needs represent the opinions of the community, and (c) determine whether the community is willing and has the resources to take action.

Problem Investigation Problem investigations are done specifically in response to a problem or concern. For example, with an outbreak of E. coli, tuberculosis, or sexually transmitted infections in a community, CHNs investigate the occurrence and distribution of the disease, explore the roots or causes of the problems and their effects, and develop plans to respond appropriately.

Resource Evaluation Service providers aim to provide cost-effective, efficient, and seamless services through resource allocation and re-allocation. **Resource evaluation** involves the assessment and evaluation of existing community resources and services. This includes an examination of the adequacy of human, financial, and physical resources, community partnerships, service utilization, gaps and duplications, affordability, and accessibility to the target populations.

Components in Community Assessment

Various community health nursing practice models may view the community differently, but they all study the basic community components or subsystems as follows:

Community History and Perception Understanding the past allows the CHN to build on existing strengths and avoid repeating the same failures. Areas for examination include the history of the issues of concern and community actions taken in the past. The perceptions of the residents on the community issues; the attitudes of officials and local politicians; and the community's attitudes, beliefs, and felt needs for health, education, and healthcare services should be specifically explored.

Population The very core of any community is people. A **population** is a diverse group of people or aggregates residing within the boundaries of a community. A **group** refers to two or more people, while an **aggregate** is a group of people based on shared common interests, demographics, cultural heritages, and socioeconomic and education levels. Population and aggregates are terms commonly used interchangeably. A **target population** refers to the population for whom nursing intervention is intended. **Population at risk** refers to a group of individuals who have a high probability of developing illness. People who are susceptible to inequity, injury, disease, or premature death are described as a **vulnerable or indigent population**. Personal characteristics and health behaviours of the aggregates or populations may have positive or negative impacts on their own health status and that of the community. For example, employees may encourage their peers to attain a healthy weight by joining a weight-loss or walk-fit program in their workplace; communities with a high number of smokers may not reject the anti-smoking by-law despite the rising rates of chronic respiratory diseases and cancer.

In addition to biology and genetic endowment, an understanding of the composition of the population by age distribution, sex, marital status, social class, occupation, birth rate, employment, religion, education level, family size, and other factors enables CHNs to assess who their population is in terms of their developmental and situational needs. Health status data of the community, such as trends in mortality rates (especially maternal and infant death rates), morbidity rates (e.g., common infectious diseases and chronic conditions), and life expectancy give indications regarding the health of the population. Studying the rate of population growth or decline also allows the CHN to examine the population trends and anticipate needed services (e.g., chronic health conditions in the aging population put more demands on home care services). A scenario is to note the aging Canadian population in Figure 13.2 and the most recent hospital admission statistics, where about 62% of the fall-related hospital admissions were for people over 65 years of age (Canadian Institute for Health Information [CIHI], 2004). Such community data should alert the CHN to consider fall prevention programs as priority interventions especially for frail elderly clients living alone in their homes.

People tend to reside in areas for a variety of reasons: proximity to their employment and extended family, accessibility to education, amenities, recreational facilities, crime rate, political reasons, and climate. The *density* of the population may shift with time and demographic makeup. For example, an influx of refugees or unemployed workers into a community may be driven by economic or political changes.

Communities are not static. The needs, characteristics, makeup, and health status of the population also change over

FIGURE 13.2 Age Pyramid of the Population

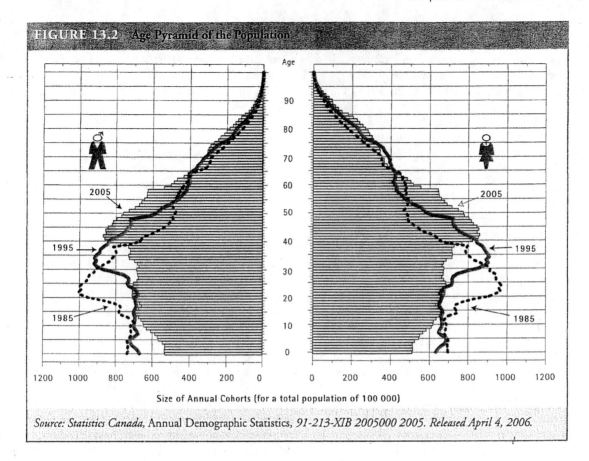

Size of Annual Cohorts (for a total population of 100 000)

Source: Statistics Canada, Annual Demographic Statistics, 91-213-XIB 2005000 2005. Released April 4, 2006.

time within its physical and social environments. For example, a surge in a community's unemployment rate may result in high family stress, a poor economy, and the relocation of many young people to other communities for work; strengthening community and social services for these communities would then become a health priority (Canadian Institute of Health Information [CIHI], 2008). Similarly, promoting healthy lifestyles and community support to combat social isolation and poverty is much needed in the remote northern communities because of their higher rates of smoking, obesity, suicide, and alcohol use compared to the nation's averages (Statistics Canada, 2002). CHNs must clearly identify the target population in relation to the scale of the problem experienced by the community as a whole; collect relevant population data; and examine, compare, and estimate the health outcomes and risk factors within the community or at the regional, provincial, and/or national conditions.

Boundaries The boundary of the community refers to where the target population lives, works, plays, and learns. Healthy communities do not exist in isolation. They are separated from or connected to other communities by physical or artificial boundaries. **Physical boundaries** include geographic boundaries, such as mountains, valleys, roads, lakes, rivers, or oceans. **Artificial boundaries** include (a) *political boundaries*, which depict governance of various townships, counties, cities, and provinces; and (b) *situational boundaries*, which are governed by specific circumstances such as zoning for school

children, traffic patterns, or smoking areas. Healthy communities have permeable boundaries for the exchange of services among communities.

Physical Environments Physical, chemical, biological, social, and psychosocial factors in the environment contribute to our quality of life (WHO, 2007). Air and water pollution in our physical environment may cause respiratory problems, digestive problems, cancer, and birth defects; geographic isolation may lead to poor access to health services and subsequent inequity in health status (PHAC, 2004) (see Chapter 24). Physical environments that affect community health include the following factors:

- Biological and chemical characteristics: vegetation and forestry, animals and insects, bacteria and other microorganisms, food and water supply, chemicals, and toxic substances.
- Physical characteristics: geography, climate, and natural resources such as soil, mountains, valleys, rivers, lakes, oceans, water, air, oil, and designs of communities, buildings, and roads.

Socioeconomic Environments The interaction between social and economic conditions of the community affects the health and well-being of individuals and populations. High employment rates, new housing, and business developments are common signs for communities with a healthy economy.

In poor economic times, a community must have resources such as social services, housing, and food banks to assist those in need.

In 2007, the national child poverty rate was 11.5%. Canadians living in poverty are more pronounced in racialized, First Nations, and recent immigrant communities. In 2008, 37% of food bank users were children. The unemployment rate was at 8.2% early in 2010. Many low-income families are working poor; they are in and out of poverty depending on job and housing availability and whether they have health issues. The income gap between the rich and the poor is wider than ever. Low-income families pay between 30% and 50% of their income toward rent. Income equality, employment, housing, and food security all affect people's health and their sense of well-being (BC Campaign 2000, 2009; Statistics Canada, 2010).

Income and Social Status Income and social status are positively associated with education level, good health, and quality of life (PHAC, 2010). Canadians in lower socioeconomic groups were at least two times more likely to be hospitalized than those in higher socioeconomic groups (CIHI, 2008). The reasons for hospital admissions ranged from mental illness, diabetes, and substance-related disorders to chronic obstructive pulmonary disease. Hospitalization rates for children from low SES groups were 56% more than those from high SES groups.

Income and education are the most important determinants of health (Senate of Canada, 2009). People with low income tend to have low education and reside in geared-to-income housing. They are in poorer health than those who are well educated and whose income level allows them to live in middle- to upper-class locales. However, upward or downward mobility can be seen in various social classes during economic turmoil.

Employment and Working Conditions Employment and working conditions significantly affect one's physical, mental, and social health and general well-being. People who are employed and work in a safe workplace experience less stress, live longer, and have fewer health problems (PHAC, 2010).

Social Supports and Networks Early hospital discharge, an aging population, and rising chronic diseases have led to the need for strong formal and informal social supports and networks in communities. Research shows that there is a positive relationship between social support and health status and perceived health (Colbert, Kim, Sereika, & Erlen, 2010; PHAC, 2010).

Diversity and Social Inclusion Healthy communities embrace harmony, safety, and diversity as the social norm. For example, schools instill cultural awareness and sensitivity in young children, thereby reducing racism or bullying; service agencies provide classes to strengthen parenting skills and promote family relationships, which indirectly prevents family violence; and neighbourhood watches reduce crime rates. Social inclusion by gender, age, ability, sexual orientation, race, ethnicity, and

religion will create a community where people feel they belong and so strive to reach their full potential as members (Nishii & Mayer, 2009; PHAC, 2010).

Recreation Recreation provides a form of socialization and a means for healthy physical and mental activity for people outside of their family, school, and work life. CHNs can assess where and how people spend their time together after school or work, whether local recreational facilities/activities are appropriate to people of all ages, and whether these activities are accessible and affordable to the public.

Education and Healthy Child Development Health status is directly associated with levels of education and socioeconomic status (Victorino & Gauthier, 2009). Education provides people the life skills needed for their day-to-day living and the technical skills for their career advancement. Canadians with low literacy skills are more likely to be poor and unemployed, suffer from poor health, have low self-esteem, and miss opportunities for learning and community participation than those with higher levels of education (Human Resources and Skills Development Canada, 2005; PHAC, 2010).

Schools are ideal settings in which children can learn to adopt societal norms and health behaviours in their early years. Youth with positive assets such as parental nurturing and monitoring, school engagement, volunteerism, and peer connections are more likely to report high self-worth and healthy lifestyles (CIHI, 2010) (see Chapters 15 and 17).

Healthy physical, cognitive, and emotional development in children is determined by effects ranging from preconception health and prenatal care to the quality of parental nurturing and supervision. Disadvantaged children tend to not perform well in school. Low-income children are at greater risk for poor health. Poor early childhood developmental characteristics, such as low birth weight or poor nutrition, can delay language or brain development and compromise physical and mental health through to adulthood (CIHI, 2010).

With over two-thirds of Canadian mothers working in dual-income families, limited childcare spaces, poverty, and wider income gaps (Townson, 2009), CHNs must attend to more than just teaching parenting skills when caring for families in community settings. They must be responsive to the adequacy of social policy surrounding issues such as parental leaves, national childcare policy, unemployment benefits, and social assistance, and to the impact of these factors on the health and social needs of families and children.

Culture and Religion Canada has a vast number of people of different races or ethnic groups, colours, and religions; and one in every five Canadians belongs to a visible minority group (Statistics Canada, 2008). Culture is the way we think, live, act, and feel. Various ethnocultural groups in many Canadian communities strive to preserve their heritages through their own social events, language classes, and educational programs. Visible minorities or new Canadians with language and cultural barriers are often alienated from the mainstream society and experience inequities in health from poverty, social isolation, bullying, and poor access to care (e.g., high unemployment rate in newcomers and high incidence of suicide and diabetes in Aboriginal people) (Craig, 2004; Gilmore, 2009). Despite efforts from the government to promote multiculturalism, many ethnic groups tend to live and work in their own ethnic communities to avoid marginalization. CHNs can address the diversity and health needs of the community population and how the various cultural practices may affect its health beliefs and practices. (See Chapter 8.)

Religion offers a form of spiritual support for many people, especially those in crisis. Some religions can affect the healthcare practices of various members of the population. For example, Jehovah's Witnesses refuse blood transfusions, and Muslims need adjustment of family, school, and work routines during their religious celebrations and prayers.

Health and Social Services Most people, whether sick or healthy, seek health services at some time in their lives. *Health services* include primary, secondary, and tertiary care, ranging from promotion and protection of health to hospital, rehabilitative, and palliative care services. *Social services*, including welfare, unemployment benefits, mothers' allowance, and disability pensions, are examples of assistance for those who are single parents, unemployed, or have physical and/or mental disabilities. An infrastructure of a wide range of health and social services can help people emerge from their crises. CHNs can refer and coordinate services as availability alone will not improve the health status of the community.

Territorialism and unwillingness to share information or resources among community agencies for fear of losing funding to support their own programs often result in fragmentation and/or duplication of services. CHNs assess what and how health and social services are used and delivered to their communities, and whether service gaps, unmet needs, duplications, and strengths exist. They work with the community to make these services better coordinated, accessible, affordable, and known to the people in need. Assessment of service needs also includes examining individual lifestyle choices such as physical activity; healthy eating; healthy weights; tobacco, alcohol, and drug use; workplace safety; gambling; safe sex; HIV testing; and multiple risk behaviours. Adoption of personal health practices and coping skills can prevent disease and promote personal health. How these skills are practised is influenced by individuals' culture, social relationships, sense of belonging, and the socioeconomic environments in which they live, work, learn, and play (PHAC, 2010).

Transportation A reliable and affordable transportation system is essential to ensure that community members have access to all the services they need. CHNs must particularly assess the transportation needs for rural clients, the poor, the frail elderly, and those with physical limitations, and seek ways to mobilize local resources to meet their needs (e.g., reduced taxi fare or volunteer drivers for seniors).

Communication Effective and efficient communication is crucial for building supportive and collaborative relationships and thereby the delivery of quality care to community members. In addition to conveying clear messages, the methods, location, and timing of communication are also pivotal in the communication process. The common modes of formal and informal communication for community members are usually the local newspapers, newsletters, emails, radio, television, flyers, and community forums.

Governments and Politics Governments provide an organized structure that sets policies to ensure all essential services are in place and will meet the basic needs and goals of the community. They provide formal leadership to work with communities and reinforce compliance to their policies (e.g., smoke-free regulations). While formal leaders hold authority in making decisions, informal leaders and community members often have the power to influence change. CHNs must examine the extent to which a community engages and empowers its members in making decisions on issues that affect their health.

CHNs must be aware of the existing government policies, work with both formal and informal leaders, and be involved in the decision-making process. They can also assess evidence of community development, relationships between the community and other agencies, the degree of cooperation or conflict between agencies and decision-making bodies, and the effectiveness of the decisions made.

Law and Safety Governments set rules and regulations as law. Crimes such as homicides, assaults, and thefts are symptoms of family and community response to stress (e.g., family violence, unemployment, and drug use). Safety is a prerequisite to quality of life. Communities grow and prosper economically in peaceful times. Peace is achieved when society has law and order. CHNs can assess whether residents are feeling safe in their community by examining the occurrences of crimes (i.e., types, rates, and locations) and collaborating with the police in crime prevention to create a safe place for people to live.

Sources of Community Data

Because communities have multi-system components, data concerning them can be abundant and complex. Therefore, the data collected must be applicable to the purpose of the community assessment, and credible sources and appropriate data collection techniques must be used to ensure the validity of the assessment. There are two main types of community data:

- *quantitative data*, such as facts and figures that are commonly found in population statistics or health status reports, and
- *qualitative data*, such as statements or opinions gathered from windshield surveys, focus groups, open forums, key informants, or public meetings.

Generally, existing data should be examined before gathering new data. New data can be gathered from surveys and meetings with community residents and leaders. With today's information technology, data are easily accessible on the Internet.

CASE STUDY: What Does Health Mean to People Living in a Slum Area?

Study the community scene illustrated in Figure 13.3. List and rank what you think the people in this community would say was needed to improve their health. In a group of four to six students, compare the individual rankings and discuss the following questions.

Discussion Questions

1. Who are the experts in identifying the local needs of a community? By priority, rank the areas that you feel would improve the health of this community and relate them to the determinants of health.

2. If you were a resident of this community, how would you feel if someone made judgments about your living situation? Why? What do you see as the priority area to improve the health of your community?

3. What data sources and data collection methods would you use to establish a community profile as depicted in this figure?

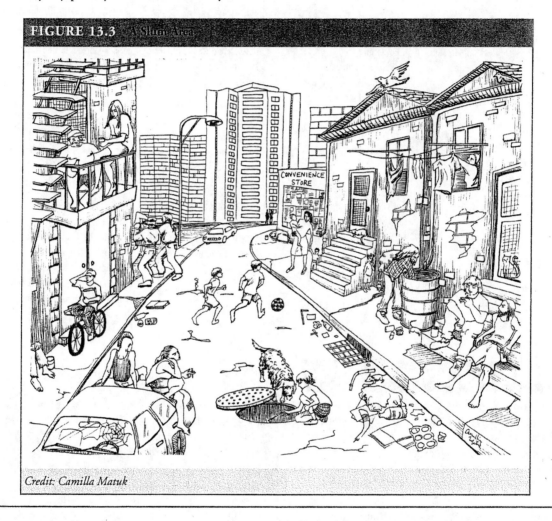

FIGURE 13.3 A Slum Area

Credit: Camilla Matuk

Community nursing diagnoses and nursing diagnoses are similar. They differ in that community nursing diagnoses are broad, addressing a community or aggregate, whereas nursing diagnoses address individuals or families. All communities have strengths as well as problems. Community health nursing diagnoses should therefore include both problem and wellness diagnoses, with statements consisting of the following components:

- the specific aggregate or target group;
- the actual or potential unhealthy or healthy response/ situation that a nurse can change;

- the etiology or cause for the unhealthy or healthy response/situation; and
- the characteristics (i.e., signs and symptoms) or evidence that describe the response or situation.

There is no classification or taxonomy for community-oriented diagnoses to date, but this should not deter CHNs from developing their own community diagnoses. Their community analysis will help develop and organize nursing knowledge and further the continued development of nursing diagnoses. Table 13.3 illustrates examples of nursing diagnoses formulation.

TABLE 13.3 Examples of Community Health Nursing Diagnosis

Components of Nursing Diagnosis	Focus Population	Problem or Wellness Diagnosis	Etiology	Characteristics
What do the components mean?	Who is your target group or community?	What is the potential/actual community issue, concern, situation, or response you need to manage or intervene?	Why is there this community issue, concern, situation, or response? Identify the causation factors.	How did you make this etiologic inference? Give supporting community data/evidence or manifestations (signs or symptoms)
Example 1	Students in high school	Potential for healthy lifestyles	Related to their desire to learn about nutrition and physical activities	As evidenced by integrated school curriculum with an emphasis on healthy lifestyle components
Example 2	Residents in Kent community	Potential dysfunction in value–belief pattern: ethical conflicts between the public and government	Related to introducing users' fees for the healthcare system	As evidenced by debates and public demonstrations over the need for a two-tiered healthcare system
Example 3	West end community	Optimal waste disposal	Related to effective management of the community recycling system	As evidenced by 98% of utilization of the recycling programs, and 25% reduction of rodents in the city area
Example 4	Newcomers	Inadequate income and resources and high family stress level (aggregate energy deficit)	Related to inadequate language and skilled trades program to prepare newcomers to be employable	As evidenced by high unemployment rates at 25%, unable to find work because of lack of language skills and Canadian work experience/requirements, high anxiety, and stress expressed by family

CANADIAN RESEARCH BOX

Are women with low incomes at higher risk to have low-birthweight (LBW) babies than those with higher incomes?

Canning, P. M., Frizzell, L. M., & Courage, M. L. (2010). Birth outcomes associated with prenatal participation in a government support programme for mothers with low incomes. *Canadian Journal of Nursing Leadership, 22*(4), 24–39.

The Newfoundland and Labrador Mother-Baby Nutrition Supplement (MBNS) prenatal program provides low-income women with a monthly financial supplement, prenatal/infant health education, and referral to public health nursing services. This study examined and compared the birth outcomes (e.g., birth weight, weeks of gestation), timeliness of enrolment, and rates of full-term low-birth-weight (LBW) infants of the 1599 women who participated in the MBNS program to those in Canada between August 2002 and December 2004. Of these mothers, 862 were parity zero. The results showed that the MBNS participants were more often single, younger, and less educated than the average woman who gave birth in the province or Canada in 2004. Mothers enrolled early in the program were less likely to have a full-term LBW baby than those enrolled late. Those who enrolled late had a higher rate of full-term LBW than those in the province and Canada and those who enrolled earlier. This study concluded that the MBNS is an effective intervention for improving birth outcomes in at-risk prenatal women. CHNs face the challenge of identifying pregnant women for early prenatal education.

Discussion Questions

1. List the risk factors for the mothers who attended the MBNS program. Refer to Table 13.2 and relate the risk factor data sources to the relevant population health indicators.

2. Why is it important to identify at-risk population?

3. Refer to Appendix 13A, Population Health Key Elements, and describe how you would use a population approach to improve the birth outcomes of the at-risk prenatal mothers in your community.

CANADIAN RESEARCH BOX

What are the hindering factors for youth to access STI testing?

Shoveller, J., Johnson, J. M., Greaves, L., Patrick, D. M., Oliffe, J. L., & Knight, R. (2009). Youth's experiences with STI testing in four communities in British Columbia, Canada. *Sexually Transmitted Infections, 85*(5), 397–401.

The purpose of this qualitative study is to analyze the experiences of youths accessing sexually transmitted infection (STI) services and to examine the perspectives of service providers in four British Columbia communities. A total of 70 men and women (15–24 years) and 22 service providers at 11 clinic sites (e.g., youth clinics, doctors' offices, public health units, and a STI testing clinic) were interviewed about their experiences providing STI testing services. STI testing policies and practice guidelines were also examined. Data from the in-depth interviews revealed five barriers to accessing and/or providing youth-friendly STI testing:

1. Privacy concerns isolated many youths, particularly those from rural communities, from testing services.
2. Services were perceived to be tailored to women because of the feminine decor and the fact that the clinic was staffed mainly by female service providers.
3. Difficulty was expressed in disclosing risky sexual behaviour to clinicians, especially for lesbian, gay, bisexual, and transgender youths because of stereotyping.
4. Women thought that Pap smears included STI testing.
5. Men avoided STI testing thinking that they needed the urethral swab and were unaware of other methods of specimen collection.

The study concluded that STI testing is hindered by structural and socio-cultural barriers.

Discussion Questions

1. List the possible the barriers for the youths to access STI testing in this study.
2. Give examples of determinants that affect the youths' access to STI testing.
3. Formulate the most likely nursing diagnosis based on the findings in this study.

Planning, Implementation, and Evaluation

Once the community needs are prioritized, nursing interventions will be devised to resolve those needs. The intervention plan must address the challenges to achieving health for all: reducing inequalities, increasing prevention, and enhancing community coping (Epp, 1986). (See Chapter 6.) The goals and objectives for intervention are derived from the community nursing diagnoses. Nursing interventions include primary, secondary, and tertiary preventive services that reflect the five principles of primary health care: accessibility, promotion and prevention, inter-sectoral cooperation, appropriate technology, and public participation (WHO, 1978). (See Chapter 7.) To provide population-focused health promotion, strategies used may include but are not limited to advocacy for healthy public policy, the strengthening of community action, and the creation of supportive environments (CHNAC, 2008; Epp, 1986). See also Appendix 13A for population health key elements and actions.

Though some CHNs, such as home health nurses, may focus on direct-care services to individuals and families, PHNs apply a different set of skills for population-focused care. Specific interventions include consultation, counselling, health teaching, case management, referral and follow-up, screening, outreach, disease surveillance, policy development and enforcement, social marketing, advocacy, community organizing, coalition building, and collaboration (CHNAC, 2008). (See Chapter 3.)

Nursing interventions will be successful when the community is fully engaged and empowered throughout the nursing process. CHNs must feel empowered to challenge the expectations of the top-down approaches to planning and management. To truly advocate for bottom-up planning, CHNs must possess competent knowledge, skills, critical judgment, and confidence in their practice.

Subjective and objective data collected during the community assessment help form the needed indicators for evaluation of any evidence of success. Community planning and interventions will be effective when public policy and supportive environments are addressed. Above all, there needs to be commitment from the community to work on the identified need or issue. See Chapter 14 for details regarding program monitoring and evaluation. The following section describes common planning and evaluation tools used in community settings.

Community Participatory Tools for Community Planning

A **community participatory approach** is key to community planning. Through dialogue with stakeholders in the process, the community decides what makes a need into a priority; who is to take the action; what the action will be; when and how it is to be done; and who, when, and how to do what. Community participatory tools help quantify and qualify the health issues, needs, or concerns that they identify. Active participation and sharing of experiences can empower people to take responsibility and ownership in health and to effect change (Yiu, Matuk, & Ruggirello, 2007). (See MyNursingLab for assessment tools.)

Community Needs Matrix Tool Participants may use this tool to discuss, identify, rate, or explain what they perceive to be the

Identified Health Need	Not a Concern	Somewhat Concerned	A Concern	Very Concerned
TABLE 13.4 Example of the Results of a Community Needs Matrix Tool				
Accidents	*	***	***	****
Nutrition	*	**	**	****
Pneumonia	*	**	***	*
STIs	*	***	***	*

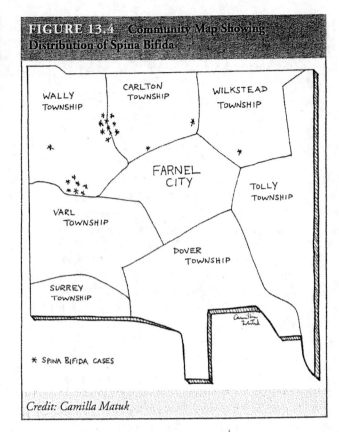

FIGURE 13.4 Community Map Showing Distribution of Spina Bifida

* SPINA BIFIDA CASES

Credit: Camilla Matuk

most important health problems or the most feasible interventions in their community. The degree of concern about each issue is tallied on a blank chart similar to that in Table 13.4. Table 13.4 indicates that this community is most concerned about accidents. CHNs use good listening and facilitation skills to learn what the community has to say about their lived experiences. Through mutual planning, they can also validate the data collected, educate the community, and increase their awareness of their choices of action.

Community Mapping Community mapping is a schematic map of the community indicating the distribution and occurrence of illness, disease, and health; major resources; environmental conditions; and accessibility and barriers to various services. CHNs may ask the community members to look at their accessibility and the resources in their living environment as part of the intervention plan. The participants could use community mapping to express their perceptions and experiences. Figure 13.4 illustrates an example of community map on the case distribution of spina bifida.

Present–Future Drawing The community clients may draw a present–future drawing (Figure 13.5) to reflect upon their present situation and what resources and constraints contributed to it, and to visualize how the future might appear. This tool allows the nurse to see where the community wants to go and, hence, to formulate mutual intervention goals and objectives.

Community Engagement and Community Governance

Community engagement and community governance are keys to achieving sustainable programs and program accountability, as well as to building community capacity and ownership (Ktpatzer Consulting, 2006). **Community engagement** is "a process involving citizens at various levels of participation based on interpersonal communication and trust and a common understanding and purpose" (p. 4). Local community members or representative aggregates start

by receiving the information from the healthcare providers or government, and through consultation, involvement, collaboration, and partnerships they eventually are empowered with the authority to make decisions on issues that affect the health of their own communities. **Community governance** is a "method of community engagement that ensures effective involvement and empowerment of local community representatives in the planning, direction setting and monitoring of health organizations to meet the health needs and priorities of the populations within local neighbourhood communities" (p. 4).

The Senate of Canada (2009) endorses a new style of governance in which the federal, provincial, territorial, and local governments must take a leadership role to implement population health policies with clear program goals and targets. Local government must create healthy and inclusive communities by engaging the community and reinforcing the citizen's capacity and expertise. Thus while the coordination is from top down, it is also implemented from bottom up.

Community Development

Community development is the "process of involving a community in the identification and reinforcement of those aspects of everyday life, culture and political activity which are conducive to health. This might include support for

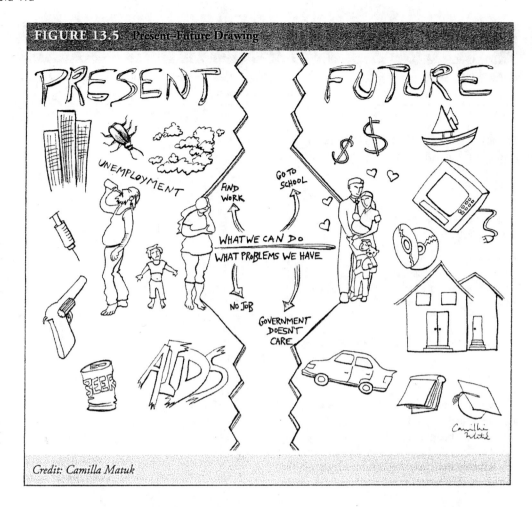

FIGURE 13.5 Present-Future Drawing

Credit: *Camilla Matuk*

political action to modify the total environment and strengthen resources for healthy living, as well as reinforcing social networks and social support within a community and developing the material resources and economic base available to the community" (Canadian Public Health Association, 1990, p. 19). The community begins with a need or a vision for change. CHNs work in partnership with their communities as they define their own goals, mobilize resources, and develop action plans for collectively identified issues or problems. All the stakeholders are engaged in this consensus-building process. Community development focuses on improving, strengthening, and sustaining community life and local conditions and to enable people, particularly those in disadvantaged situations, to engage in decision making and to achieve control over their circumstances. One example can be seen in groups in various urban communities working with governments on health and social issues to provide safe and affordable housing for those who are homeless. Another example is with rural residents, addressing suicide as a community problem and through consensus building and resource mobilization with their stakeholders finding solutions to strengthen community social support and improve mental health for the residents.

Community interventions must be evaluated to measure whether the expected results were achieved and where the successes and problems lie. The steps involved in **community program evaluation** are (a) determining what needs to be evaluated and the evaluation criteria; (b) engaging stakeholders and assessing resources; (c) determining the appropriate methods of measurement; (d) developing data collection instruments, budget, and timeline for evaluation; (e) collecting and analyzing data; (f) reporting and disseminating the results; and (g) making decisions for action. (See MyNursingLab for program evaluation tool kits and Chapter 14.)

Successes should be shared with the community so that the work can be sustained within the community and become a model to benefit other communities. Lessons learned from challenges or barriers can teach others to avoid making the same mistakes. Plans should be made for any future changes needed in the community. Interventions should be evaluated and documented to support evidence-based practice. Table 13.5 provides a summary guide that CHNs may use to assess the general health of a community and develop a community intervention plan.

TABLE 13.5 Guide to Community Health Nursing Process

AREAS FOR COMMUNITY ASSESSMENT (Modify these general questions to reflect the specific purpose of the community assessment)	DATA/OBSERVATIONS
A. ASSESSMENT	
1. Purpose of Community Assessment, Target Group, and Location – Purpose of assessment (e.g., environmental scan, needs assessment, problem investigation, or resource evaluation)? – Rationale for the assessment? – Who is the target group? What are their characteristics? – Boundaries where target group resides? – Supportive evidence for the health needs of the target group?	
2. Community Historical and Perception – Previous history of community actions by local groups or government? – Perceptions of the residents on the community issues, problems, attitudes, beliefs, felt needs?	
3. Population – Total composition and characteristics of the population in the community (e.g., age group distribution, gender, marital status, birth rate, family size)? – Density and rate of population growth, increased or decreased? – Health status • Mortality and morbidity rates for age-specific diseases or causes, their incidence and prevalence? • Comparison of mortality and morbidity rates with previous years, with regional, provincial, and national rates? • Life expectancy and trends? • Biologic and genetic endowment? • Health status: indicators and influencing factors related to purpose of assessment (e.g., nutrition; immunization; lifestyles; stress; sexually transmitted infections; unplanned pregnancy; prenatal care; emergency care; primary, secondary, and tertiary care)?	
4. Physical Environments – Location: boundaries, geography, climate, plants, and animals posing threats to health, percentage of urban or rural area? – Housing: type, condition, slum areas, sanitation, adequacy, crowding? – Shopping facilities: types, location, and accessibility? – Safety: crime rates, types, and where? Feeling safe? Police and relationships with the community? – Water supply: quality and adequacy? – Sanitation: sewage and waste disposal?	
5. Socioeconomic Environments – Income: income levels, poverty rate, number receiving social assistance? – Social status and mobility • Percentages for each social class? • Patterns and impact of mobility on health needs and health service planning? – Employment and working conditions • Major industries and business establishments? • Employment rate, primary occupations? • Occupational hazards? • Safe and supportive work life? – Social supports and networks: support groups and community group involvement? – Social inclusion: embrace diversity and share social experience by gender, sex, sexual orientation, race, ethnicity, and religion? – Recreation: facilities, affordability, accessibility, and appropriateness for all ages?	

TABLE 13.5 Continued

AREAS FOR COMMUNITY ASSESSMENT (Modify these questions to reflect the purpose of the assessment)	DATA/OBSERVATIONS

6. Education and Healthy Child Development
  – Education: literacy rates, attitudes, and facilities/programs for life skills and technical skills?
    • Peer connection and engagement in school?
    • Relationships to health status and employment?
  – Healthy child development: preconception health, prenatal and parenting class, and daycare?	

7. Culture and Religion
  – Ethnic and racial group composition and subcultures, culture, and languages spoken?
  – Cultural diversity and tolerance, positive and negative influence on health practices?
  – Cultural adaptation, perceptions of health?
  – Religious affiliations and spiritual support and influence on health practices?	

8. Health and Social Services
  – Services and community organizations
    • Location, ratios of health workers to rural and urban populations?
    • Number of beds available and type, health service utilization?
      Health budgets priority, amount per capita and spending?
    • Provision of primary, secondary, and tertiary care?
    • Service coordination, gaps, and duplications?
    • Evidence of community engagement and community governance (e.g., intersectoral cooperation, health promotion, public participation, and appropriate technology used in service delivery)?
    • Available and adequate social assistance to meet community needs?
  – Personal health practices and coping skills (e.g., healthy lifestyle practices, effective or maladaptive coping)?	

9. Transportation – Type, availability, accessibility, affordability, and usage?	

10. Governance and Politics
  – Communications
    • Methods, timing, and locations of verbal and nonverbal communication (e.g., newspapers, radio, television, flyers, and forums)?
    • Relationships with other organizations, degree of conflict and collaboration?
    • Evidence of interpersonal relationships, commitment, and partnerships?
  – Leadership
    • Formal and informal leaders, visions for the community?
    • Power structure, delegations, politics?
  – Decision making: effective and efficient process of decision making (e.g., policy formulation, human resources)?	

B. ANALYSIS	

1. Wellness Nursing Diagnoses
  – Potential and actual community strengths?
2. Problem Nursing Diagnoses
  – Potential and actual community needs and gaps?	

C. PLANNED INTERVENTIONS	

– Implementation of primary, secondary, and tertiary preventive care focusing on health promotion challenges such as reducing inequities, increasing prevention, and enhancing coping?
  – Evidence of incorporation of primary health care principles, public policy, and supportive environments in nursing care planning?
  – Expected outcomes and target dates clearly defined?	

D. EVALUATION	
– Monitoring of progress and gathering of evidence of success based on outcomes objectives? – Lessons learned, decision for action, and knowledge transfer?	

SUMMARY

CHNs work in complex social, political, and economic environments. Their political activism work may be invisible, yet their commitment to implement their primary healthcare roles to social justice to address health inequities for the marginalized populations remain a focus of their care (Paterson, Duffett-Leger, & Cruttenden, 2009). When promoting the health of communities, CHNs use a population approach to work with individuals, families, aggregates, populations, and the community. Problems identified at the individual and family levels (such as poverty and teen pregnancy) may call for further actions at the system or community level. CHNs must be able to conduct accurate community assessment before they can provide community health promotion.

An understanding of the community makeup and dynamics will guide the implementation of the community nursing process. Sound community assessment requires that CHNs know the purpose of the assessment, what techniques to use to collect evidence-based data, and where to collect them. The use of a population health approach to community health promotion allows the nurse to look beyond the traditional delivery of health services and to examine various determinants of health, including how social and political environments impact community health. Community analysis requires CHNs to work with the community to analyze the data and devise a mutual plan for community action and evaluation. Throughout this community health nursing process, CHNs may use various community participatory tools to interact with community stakeholders and population groups to address the community's health needs. They must understand the importance of community engagement, community governance, and community development to advocate positive change. If CHNs are to improve the health of the community and achieve social justice and health for all, they must take an evidence-based approach to seek research evidence and display competent leadership in community health promotion.

KEY TERMS

community, p. 213
geopolitical boundaries, p. 214
aggregate communities, p. 214
virtual communities, p. 214
community functions, p. 214
community dynamics, p. 214
community assessment wheel, p. 215
capacity building, p. 215
community assets map, p. 215
community health promotion model, p. 215
community assessment, p. 216
environmental scan, p. 218
windshield survey, p. 218
needs, p. 218
resource evaluation, p. 218
population, p. 218
group, p. 218
aggregate, p. 218

target population, p. 218
population at risk, p. 218
vulnerable or indigent population, p. 218
physical boundaries, p. 219
artificial boundaries, p. 219
culture, p. 220
religion, p. 221
community surveys, p. 222
community forums, p. 222
focus groups, p. 222
population health, p. 222
population health template, p. 222
risk, p. 223
risk factors, p. 223
risk assessment, p. 223
community analysis, p. 223
community nursing diagnoses, p. 223
community participatory approach, p. 226
community engagement, p. 227
community governance, p. 227
community development, p. 227
community program evaluation, p. 228

REVIEW QUESTIONS

Choose the one alternative that best completes the statement or answers the question.

1. Which of the following is a population health indicator for community characteristic?
   a) number of visible minority population
   b) patient satisfactory
   c) exposure to air pollution
   d) number of low-birth-weight babies

2. Which of the following is the most important social determinant of health to allow people to receive various healthcare services in the community?
   a) transportation
   b) government and policies
   c) education
   d) culture

3. The main goal of a population health approach is to
   a) eliminate unemployment rates in the community.
   b) reduce the infant mortality rate in the community.
   c) mobilize the community to make participatory healthcare decisions.
   d) reduce inequities and maintain and improve the health status of the entire population.

4. There is an increased hospital admission rate for postpartum depression in your community. In order to identify who are the women at risk so that you can provide the needed interventions, which of the following approach would you take?
   a) Assess and interview all prenatal and postnatal women.
   b) Assess and interview prenatal and postnatal women who are at risk for postpartum depression.
   c) Assess and interview postnatal women after they have been diagnosed for postpartum depression.
   d) Conduct a focus group for newly diagnosed postpartum women to discuss what services they need.

5A. Your assigned task is to find out how best to deliver a seamless and integrated home care service system in your community. Who would be your most likely target population requiring home care services?
   a) children
   b) adults
   c) older adults
   d) families

5B. Referring to question 5A, which of the following is the best method to gather your community response?
   a) community survey
   b) community forum
   c) focus group
   d) census data

6. Who is responsible to set population health policies with clear program goals and targets?
   a) federal, provincial, and local governments
   b) local governments
   c) healthcare providers
   d) consumers

7. Which of the following is an example of community development?
   a) A community marathon run event to raise money for cancer research
   b) A food bank program
   c) A community health survey
   d) Construction of a sport centre in the community

STUDY QUESTIONS

1. Name four community settings where CHNs work, and describe their role and functions.

2. What are the characteristics of a healthy community?

3. What nursing process skills will you use to promote the health of the community?

4. What assessment components are used when assessing community health?

5. Define population health, community engagement, community governance, community development, and capacity building.

6. Discuss the benefits of community dialogue between community health nurses and Aboriginal communities or any other population groups.

After working through these questions, go to the MyNursingLab at www.pearsoned.ca/mynursinglab to check your answers.

INDIVIDUAL CRITICAL THINKING EXERCISES

1. Why is it important for the nurse to provide care to the community?

2. How does the community health nursing process differ from the individual nursing process?

3. How would you work with your community to identify their health needs and share their community experiences?

4. In developing a health profile for a community, what assessment questions would you ask for each category of the community components? Where and how would you collect the needed data?

5. Why is it important to use participatory tools for community planning?

GROUP CRITICAL THINKING EXERCISES

1. Based on the community needs matrix tool (Table 13.4), what are some of the questions you would want to ask the community about their ratings? What would be the next steps?

2. In a group of two to four, spend about an hour visiting and talking to people in your local neighbourhood. Describe your community visit and explain your impression about the felt needs, real needs, and wants of the community. Formulate your nursing diagnoses and propose your actions.

3. Discuss possible ways to engage your community to meet the identified health needs in question 2.

REFERENCES

Albert, D., & Herrera, C. (2009, November 20). *Getting lost in the evidence? Part 1: Developing an evidence question and search srategy.* Fireside Chat presentation. Ottawa, ON: University of Ottawa.

Almey, M. (2007). *Women in Canada: Work chapter updates.* Statistics Canada, Catalogue no. 89F0133XIE. Ottawa, ON: Ministry of Industry.

Campaign 2000. (2009). *2009 report card on child and family poverty in Canada: 1989–2009.* Retrieved from http://www.nwac-hq.org/en/documents/Campaign20002009NationalReportCard.pdf

Canadian Institute for Health Information (CIHI). (2004). *National trauma registry 2004 report: Injury hospitalizations (includes 2002–2003 data).* Ottawa, ON: Author.

Canadian Institute for Health Information. (2008). *Reducing gaps in health: A focus on socio-economic status in urban Canada.* Ottawa, ON: Author.

Canadian Institute for Health Information (CIHI). (2010). *Improving the health of young Canadians, 2005–2006 report series.* Retrieved from http://secure.cihi.ca/cihiweb/dispPage.jsp?cw_page=AP_1217_E

Canadian Public Health Association. (1990). *Community health–public health nursing in Canada: Preparation and practice.* Ottawa, ON: Author.

Centers for Disease Control and Prevention. (2009). *Capacity building.* Retrieved from http://www.cdc.gov/hiv/topics/cba/

Clemen-Stone, S., Eigsti, D., & McGuire, S. (2002). *Comprehensive community health nursing* (6th ed.). Toronto, ON: Mosby.

Cohen, B. (2006). Barriers to population-focused health promotion: The experience of public health nurses in the province of Manitoba. *Canadian Journal of Nursing Research, 38*(3), 52–67.

Colbert, A. M., Kim, K. H., Sereika, S. M., & Erlen, J. A. (2010). An examination of the relationships among gender, health status, social support, and HIV-related stigma. *Journal of the Association of Nurses in AIDS Care, 21*(8), 1007–1013.

Community Health Nurses Association of Canada. (2008). *Community health nursing standards of practice.* Ottawa, ON: Author.

Craig, W. (2004). Bullying and fighting. In W. Boyce (Ed.), *Young people in Canada: Their health and well-being* (pp. 87–96). Ottawa, ON: Health Canada.

Epp, J. (1986). *Health for all: A framework for health promotion.* Ottawa, ON: Health and Welfare Canada.

Gilmore, J. (2009). *The 2008 Canadian Immigrant Labour Market: Analysis of Quality of Employment.* The Immigrant Labour Force Analysis Series, Statistics Canada. Ottawa, ON: Minister of Industry. Retrieved from http://www.statcan.gc.ca/pub/71-606-x/2009001/beforetoc-avanttdm1-eng.htm

Human Resources and Skills Development Canada. (2005). *Health literacy in Canada.* Retrieved from http://www.servicecanada.gc.ca/eng/hip/lld/nls/Resources/10_fact.shtml

Kirby, M. (2002). *The health of Canadians—The federal role final report, Vol. 6: Recommendations for reform.* Part VI: Health promotion and disease prevention. The Standing Senate Committee on Social Affairs, Science and Technology. Retrieved from http://www.parl.gc.ca/37/2/parlbus/commbus/senate/Com-e/soci-e/rep-e/repoct02vol6-e.htm

Ktpatzer Consulting. (June 2006). *Trends and benefits of community engagement and local community governance in health care.* Toronto, ON: Association of Ontario Community Health Centres. Retrieved from http://www.aohc.org/app/wa/doc?docId=157

Lalonde, M. (1974). *A new perspective on the health of Canadians.* Ottawa, ON: Government of Canada.

Minkler, M. (Ed.). *Community organizing and community building for health* (2nd ed.). New Brunswick, NJ: Rutgers University Press.

Nishii, L. H., & Mayer, D. M. (2009). Do inclusive leaders help to reduce turnover in diverse groups? The moderating role of leader-member exchange in the diversity to turnover relationship. *Journal of Applied Psychology, 94*(6), 1412–1426.

Paterson, B. L., Duffett-Leger, L., & Cruttenden, K. (2009). Contextual factors influencing the evolution of nurses' roles in a primary health care clinic. *Public Health Nursing, 26*(5), 421–429.

Public Health Agency of Canada [PHAC]. (2002). *Summary table of population health key elements.* Retrieved from http://www.phac-aspc.gc.ca/ph-sp/approach-approche/pdf/summary_table.pdf

Public Health Agency of Canada [PHAC]. (2004). *The social determinants of health: An overview of the implications for policy and the role of the health sector.* Retrieved from http://www.phac-aspc.gc.ca/ph-sp/oi-ar/01_overview-eng.php

Public Health Agency of Canada [PHAC]. (2005). *Population health: What is population health approach?* Retrieved from http://www.phac-aspc.gc.ca/ph-sp/index-eng.php

Public Health Agency of Canada [PHAC]. (2010). *What determines health?* Retrieved from http://www.phac-aspc.gc.ca/ph-sp/determinants/index-eng.php

Raphael, D. (Ed.). (2008). *Social determinants of health: Canadian perspectives* (2nd ed.). Toronto, ON: Canadian Scholars' Press.

Sahay, T. (2004). *A review of the literature on the links between health promotion capacity building and health outcomes.* Toronto, ON: Ontario Health Promotion Resource System. Retrieved from http://www.ohprs.ca/resources/tina_finalreport_27dec2004.pdf

Senate of Canada. (2009). *A healthy, productive Canada: A determinant of health approach.* The Standing Senate Committee on Social Affairs, Science and Technology Final Report of Senate Subcommittee on Population Health. Retrieved from http://www.parl.gc.ca/40/2/parlbus/commbus/senate/Com-e/popu-e/rep-e/rephealthjun09-e.pdf

Stamler, L. L., & Yiu, L. (2008). *Community nursing: A Canadian perspective* (2nd ed.). Toronto, ON: Pearson Education Canada.

Stanhope, M., & Lancaster, J. (2006). *Foundations of nursing in the community: Community-oriented practice* (2nd ed.). St.Louis, MO: Mosby Elsevier.

Statistics Canada. (2002). *Health reports: How healthy are Canadians? 2002 Annual report.* Retrieved from http://www.statcan.gc.ca/pub/82-003-s/2002001/pdf/4195132-eng.pdf

Statistics Canada. (2008). *Canada's Ethnocultural Mosaic, 2006 Census.* Catalogue no. 97-562-X. Ottawa, ON: Minister of Industry.

Statistics Canada. (2010). *The Daily: Latest release from the Labour Force Survey.* Retrieved from http://www.statcan.gc.ca/subjects-sujets/labour-travail/lfs-epa/lfs-epa-eng.htm

Townson, M. (2009). *Women's poverty and the recession.* Ottawa, ON: Canadian Centres for Policy Alternatives.

Victorino, C. C., & Gauthier, A. H. (2009). The social determinants of child health: Variations across health outcomes – a population-based cross-sectional analysis. *BMC Pediatrics, 9*(53), doi:10.1186/1471-2431-9-53

Vollman, A., Anderson, E., & McFarlane, J. (2008). *Community as partner: Theory and practice in nursing* (Canadian 2nd ed.). Philadelphia, PA: Lippincott, Williams & Wilkins.

World Health Organization. (1978). *Primary health care: Report on the International Conference on Primary Health Care,* Alma Ata, USSR, 6–12, September 1978. Geneva, Switzerland: Author.

World Health Organization (WHO), Canadian Public Health Association, & Health and Welfare Canada. (1986). *Ottawa Charter of health promotion.* Ottawa, ON: Health and Welfare Canada.

World Health Organization. (2007). *Public health and environment.* Retrieved from http://www.who.int/phe/en/

World Health Organization. (2010). *Social determinants of health*. Retrieved from http://www.who.int/social_determinants/en/

Yiu Matuk, L., & Ruggirello, T. (2007). Culture connection project: Promoting multiculturalism in elementary schools. *Canadian Journal of Public Health, 98*(1), 26–29.

ADDITIONAL RESOURCES

Readings

Diem, E., & Moyer, A. (2005). *Community health nursing projects: Making a difference.* Toronto, ON: Lippincott Williams & Wilkins.

Health Goals for Canada. (2010). http://www.phac-aspc.gc.ca/hgc-osc/new-1-eng.html

Senate of Canada. (2009). *A healthy, productive Canada: A determinant of health approach.* The Standing Senate Committee on Social Affairs, Science and Technology Final Report of Senate Subcommittee on Population Health. http://www.parl.gc.ca/40/2/parlbus/commbus/senate/Com-e/popu-e/rep-e/rephealthjun09-e.pdf

Statistics Canada. (2009). *Canadian community health survey, 2008.* http://www.viha.ca/mho/stats_and_maps/Canadian+Community+Health+Survey.htm

The Conference Board of Canada. (2010). *A report card on Canada: Health.* http://www.conferenceboard.ca/HCP/Details/Health.aspx

Websites

Canadian Public Health Association
http://www.cpha.ca

Canadian Institute for Health Information (CIHI)
http://www.cihi.ca

Public Health Agency of Canada
http://www.phac-aspc.gc.ca

Videos

Community and Aggregate Assessment, Memorial University, 2009 (Length: 24 minutes)

This video presents the process and issues related to assessing a geographic community and various aggregates using a partnership approach. It describes the concept and methods of community/aggregate assessment and the role of the nurse in the process.

Community Development in Community Health Nursing, Memorial University, 2009 (Length: 25 minutes)

This video illustrates the experiences of community health nurses and community members while engaging in the community development process. It highlights the concept and principles of community development and the outcomes and challenges faced in the community nursing process.

About the Author

Lucia Yiu, BScN, BA (Psychology, University of Windsor), BSc (Physiology, University of Toronto), MScN (Administration, University of Western Ontario), is an Associate Professor in the Faculty of Nursing, University of Windsor, and an Educational and Training Consultant in community nursing. She has worked overseas and served on various community and social services committees involving local and district health planning.

Appendix 13A
Summary Table of Population Health Key Elements

The goals of a population health approach are to maintain and improve the health status of the entire population and to reduce inequities in health status between population groups.

Key Element	Actions
1. Focus on the Health of Populations	1.1 Determine indicators for measuring health status 1.2 Measure and analyze population health status and health status inequities to identify health issues 1.3 Assess contextual conditions, characteristics, and trends
2. Address the Determinants of Health and Their Interactions	2.1 Determine indicators for measuring the determinants of health 2.2 Measure and analyze the determinants of health, and their interactions, to link health issues to their determinants
3. Base Decisions on Evidence	3.1 Use best evidence available at all stages of policy and program development 3.2 Explain criteria for including or excluding evidence 3.3 Draw on a variety of data 3.4 Generate data through mixed research methods 3.5 Identify and assess effective interventions 3.6 Disseminate research findings and facilitate policy uptake
4. Increase Upstream Investments	4.1 Apply criteria to select priorities for investment 4.2 Balance short- and long-term investments 4.3 Influence investments in other sectors
5. Apply Multiple Strategies	5.1 Identify scope of action for interventions 5.2 Take action on the determinants of health and their interactions 5.3 Implement strategies to reduce inequities in health status between population groups 5.4 Apply a comprehensive mix of interventions and strategies 5.5 Apply interventions that address health issues in an integrated way 5.6 Apply methods to improve health over the life span 5.7 Act in multiple settings 5.8 Establish a coordinating mechanism to guide interventions
6. Collaborate Across Sectors and Levels	6.1 Engage partners early on to establish shared values and alignment of purpose 6.2 Establish concrete objectives and focus on visible results 6.3 Identify and support a champion 6.4 Invest in the alliance building process 6.5 Generate political support and build on positive factors in the policy environment 6.6 Share leadership, accountability, and rewards among partners
7. Employ Mechanisms for Public Involvement	7.1 Capture the public's interest 7.2 Contribute to health literacy 7.3 Apply public involvement strategies that link to overarching purpose
8. Demonstrate Accountability for Health Outcomes	8.1 Construct a results-based accountability framework 8.2 Ascertain baseline measures and set targets for health improvement 8.3 Institutionalize effective evaluation systems 8.4 Promote the use of health impact assessment tools 8.5 Publicly report results

Source: Public Health Agency of Canada. (2002). The population health template: Key elements and actions that define a population health approach. © Reproduced with the permission of the Minister of Public Works and Government Services Canada, 2010. (Available from http://www.phac-aspc.gc.ca/ph-sp/approach-approche/pdf/summary_table.pdf)

14

Community Health Planning, Monitoring, and Evaluation

Nancy C. Edwards, Josephine Etowa, Wendy E. Peterson, and Margaret Ann Kennedy

OBJECTIVES

After studying this chapter, you should be able to:

1. Describe the importance of program planning, monitoring, and evaluation in the practice of community health nursing.

2. Describe how the socioecological determinants of health can be reflected in our approach to planning, monitoring, and evaluation.

3. Describe components of the assessment–planning–evaluation cycle and the involvement of community stakeholders in this process.

4. Develop a planning–implementation–evaluation plan using a logic model.

5. Describe elements of the multiple interventions framework and its application to a complex community health issue.

6. Explain how commonly used evaluation models and the choice of indicators may be structured to address program accountability.

INTRODUCTION

Planning, monitoring, and evaluating community health programs are fundamental processes used by community health nurses (CHNs) as they work in partnership with the community (Community Health Nurses Association of Canada [CHNAC], 2008). With more scrutiny of how public funds are being expended, increased demands for evidence-based programs, standards of practice, and national and international interest in population health intervention research, these processes have become even more critical (Commission on Social Determinants of Health [CSDH], 2008; Senate Subcommittee on Population Health, 2009). The Canadian Community Health Nursing Standards of Practice (CHNAC, 2008) describe how nurses are expected to plan new programs, redesign existing services, monitor the implementation of programs, and evaluate their impact. Nurses often make important contributions to these processes with the substantial involvement of community representatives, key stakeholders from a variety of service sectors, and colleagues from multiple disciplines.

There are many tools available to assist CHNs in program planning, but their utility will be diminished if underlying determinants of health are ignored, and programs are developed without considering social justice issues. Bringing evidence and theory to bear on complex community health problems is a necessary, yet insufficient, approach to

planning. The authentic engagement of the community in planning, monitoring, and evaluating community health programs is essential to address underlying social determinants of health.

PROGRAM PLANNING AND EVALUATION

The planning–evaluation cycle involves several key components. Although various planning frameworks are in common use, all contain similar elements. A classic **planning–implementation–evaluation cycle** (see Figure 14.1) involves the following steps:

- conducting a situational analysis or community assessment;
- identifying the problems or issues of concern;
- considering possible solutions or actions to address the problem;
- selecting the best alternative(s);
- designing and implementing the program;
- monitoring and evaluating the program;
- analyzing and interpreting results of the monitoring and evaluation process; and
- using the results to make modifications to the program or to inform decisions about other programs.

FIGURE 14.1 Planning–Implementation–Evaluation Cycle

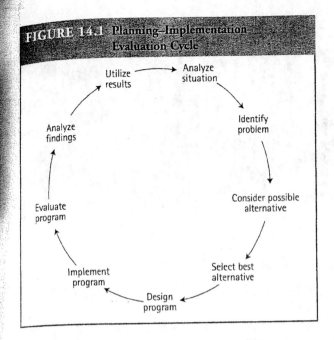

The steps in this cycle may need to be repeated as one develops a better understanding of an issue and obtains additional input from partners. It may be necessary to go back to other steps in the planning cycle and try to develop a more complete picture of the factors that are affecting the problem and the potential solutions that need to be considered.

Selecting a Program Planning and Evaluation Framework

There are many program planning and evaluation frameworks available. Frameworks provide a guide for the types of information that need to be assembled and the organization of this information into a coherent plan. Several factors should be considered in selecting a framework for use. First, most community health agencies will have a standard planning framework that is used across departments. Use of a common framework allows for a coherent and consistent approach to planning within an organization. Second, the use of a particular framework may be a requirement of those who fund programs, as this allows them to compare results across funded programs. Third, a framework may be chosen because it helps detail a particular aspect of the planning process that is vexing or challenging. For instance, a framework may be chosen because it is particularly useful in defining the underlying socioecological determinants of a problem, it guides the choice of theory that will help define program elements, or it is more appropriate for addressing the needs of marginalized populations. Finally, the selection of a framework may be influenced by a set of underlying values or principles such as participatory development or social justice (Edwards & Davison, 2008).

The **program logic model** is used extensively in many public health agencies in Canada, both at regional and municipal levels, and by provincial and federal government agencies (Porteous, Sheldrick, & Stewart, 2002). Logic models provide

a coherent structure for complex health programs, help to expose gaps, and yield an overview of programs with appealing visual clarity. As a support to planning, analysis, and program evaluation preparation, the logic model provides a diagram of "what the program is supposed to do, with whom, and why" (Porteous et al., p. 116).

Cooksy, Gill, and Kelly (2001) note that the logic model is unique among tools for its simplicity in demonstrating program interrelationships and linkages. Logic models should be developed in collaboration with community and academic partners. In this way, both experiential learning and research findings can inform model development. Joint preparation of a logic model will help build consensus about program priorities among the planning team. In using a logic model, one should avoid positioning it as a rigid guideline, which prevents iterative evolution or lateral exploration of the program under review. (See sample Logic Model in MyNursingLab.)

Development of a logic model consists of two planning stages, referred to as CAT (**Components, Activities, and Target groups**) and SOLO (**Short-term Outcomes and Long-term Outcomes**). For the CAT stage, activities are first clustered thematically into components for the program under review. For example, a suicide prevention program for youth might include the components of risk assessment, crisis intervention, and peer support. Activities are the specific intervention strategies to be used for each component. Using the suicide prevention example, the crisis intervention component may include training youth workers in crisis management, developing community supports for youth in crisis, and establishing better communication among social and health services organizations about youth in crisis. Target groups are the intended recipients of a program. In this example, this might be homeless youth, youth having difficulty in school and the front-line workers for youth in schools, homeless shelters, and other health and social service organizations.

The purpose of the SOLO stage is to identify program outcomes. **Short-term outcomes** are the immediate and direct results of the program, while **long-term outcomes** reflect the ultimate goals of the program. Building the knowledge and skills of youth workers to identify and support youth in crisis would be a short-term outcome, while reducing youth suicide rates would be longer-term. Many extraneous factors may influence the achievement of long-term outcomes. Thus, they are more difficult to directly and exclusively attribute to the program.

The Program Evaluation Tool Kit (Figure 14.2) incorporates the use of a logic model and identifies which evaluation processes may be used to inform decision making during program planning and implementation (Public Health Agency of Canada, 2008). **Evaluation** is an ongoing, dynamic process that supports further refinement of program activities and helps to identify gaps or flaws in the original program design. It is critical to involve community partners in the evaluation process. They can play key roles in helping with data interpretation and identifying recommendations emerging from program evaluation. (See MyNursingLab, use of Program Evaluation Tool Kit to evaluate H1N1 pandemic planning.)

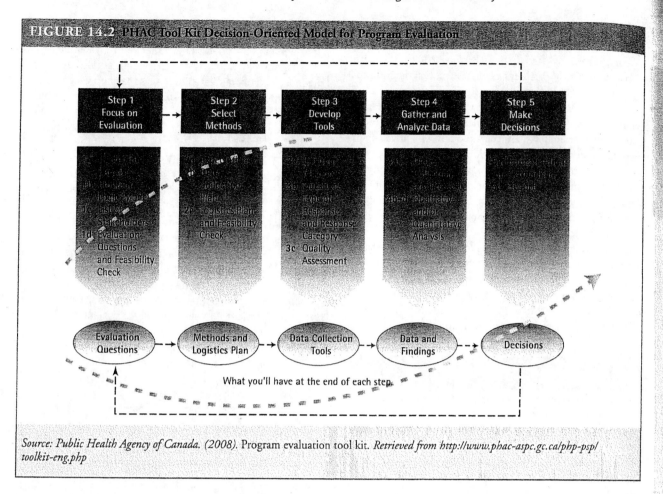

FIGURE 14.2 PHAC Tool Kit Decision-Oriented Model for Program Evaluation

Source: Public Health Agency of Canada. (2008). Program evaluation tool kit. *Retrieved from http://www.phac-aspc.gc.ca/php-psp/toolkit-eng.php*

Tools and Processes to Support Planning and Evaluation Processes

Many tools and processes may be used in combination with an organizing framework. However, these tools must be used in conjunction with approaches that build relationships and create opportunities to hear the voices of disadvantaged groups. The efficient involvement of community partners is important because those working in service delivery sectors have many demands on their time. Involving them in the planning process helps build commitment to the program and aids the design of a program that reflects the dynamic realities and strengths of the community.

Gathering Information about Community Needs and Priorities

Environmental scans are conducted to gather information about community needs and priorities. There are practical tools available to help with this process of gathering information. Examples of methods that can engage partners in a planning process are assessment of strengths, weaknesses, opportunities, and threats; key informant interviews; and/or focus groups. (See Chapter 13.)

SWOT (Strengths, Weaknesses, Opportunities, and Threats)

A **SWOT analysis** identifies internal strengths and weaknesses of the organization or program, along with external opportunities

and threats. A SWOT analysis may involve document and policy reviews, community meetings, key informant interviews, and focus groups. It helps those planning a program to customize the fit between the organizations (or in this case the program) to its environment (Fraser & Stupak, 2002). A SWOT may also assist in determining the feasibility of initiating or continuing a program and may help identify service gaps. SWOT analyses are frequently used as part of a strategic planning process when managers are developing long-term plans for the organization.

Assessing Needs through Qualitative Interviews and Focus Groups

The use of qualitative research strategies such as individual interviews and focus groups elaborates those issues and experiences that are not readily understood through quantitative and statistical tools (Pope & Mays, 2000). For example, although quantitative evaluation tools may demonstrate that a particular subpopulation is less likely than another to use community health services, they may not be able to explain why and how. Similarly, quantitative data may not shed light on the perceived appropriateness of community health services and programs (Dana, 2002). Qualitative research tools not only address these gaps, but also can be used to assess the meanings of health and care (Sofaer, 1999). Qualitative data can increase the relevance and interpretability of quantitative data generated during a needs assessment.

Individual interviews allow for exploration of first-person experiences and prompt interactive discussions that centre on the perspectives of participants (Patton, 2002). In-depth interviews may yield pertinent examples and rich descriptions of experiences (Rubin & Rubin, 2005). **Focus groups** are used "to elicit and validate collective testimonies" (Kamberelis & Dimitriadis, 2005, p. 897). The composition of focus groups must be carefully planned. Although some diversity of viewpoints is important, one should try to assemble a group where there is not an underlying power structure among its members that may discourage some participants from openly sharing their viewpoints. For example, it may not be appropriate to have a focus group consisting of both front-line workers and their managers because front-line workers may hesitate to discuss issues concerning organizational leadership or working conditions when their managers are present. Focus groups provide opportunities for members to share and validate their individual experiences. The discussion may stimulate participant ownership of the program under development and may prompt participants toward action.

CANADIAN RESEARCH BOX

How is stigma experienced by Aboriginal and non-Aboriginal persons living with HIV and AIDS and their healthcare providers?

Mill, J., Edwards, N., Jackson, R., & MacLean, L. (2010). Stigmatization as a social control mechanism for persons living with HIV and AIDS. *Qualitative Health Research, 11,* 1469–1483.

Mill, J., Edwards, N., Jackson, R., Austin, W., MacLean, L., & Reintjes, F. (2009). Accessing health services while living with HIV: Intersections of stigma. *Canadian Journal of Nursing Research, 41*(3), 168–185.

Mill, J., Austin, W., Chaw-Kant, J., Dumont-Smith, C., Edwards, N., et al. (2007). *The influence of stigma on access to health services by persons with HIV illness: Final report.* Edmonton, AB: University of Alberta, Faculty of Nursing.

Stigma has both individual and social dimensions. Although it is experienced by individuals, it is influenced by social, political, institutional, and symbolic contexts. Several authors have described the layering of stigma that may occur, particularly among marginalized populations.

Funded by the Canadian Institutes of Health Research, this participatory action research study used a descriptive design. The principles of ownership, control, access, and possession for the conduct of research with Aboriginal communities were followed. Community advisory committees were formed at both project sites (Ottawa and Edmonton). Focus groups and interviews were undertaken with health care providers and in-depth interviews were completed with Aboriginal and non-Aboriginal individuals living with HIV.

Thirty-three individuals, all HIV positive, agreed to an in-depth interview. Among the 27 healthcare providers, seven participated in a focus group and 20 in an interview. Participants described the experience of layered stigma, that is, stigma related to their HIV status that was compounded by stigma related to their behaviour, gender, sexual orientation, culture, or social class. They described how organizational policies such as universal precautions and models of care, and the physical layout of clinics could worsen stigma.

Both those living with HIV and healthcare providers described passive and active social control mechanisms that were applied either overtly or in more subtle ways. These mechanisms included labelling, shunning, and ostracizing, and disempowering healthcare practices. Participants identified a number of strategies to manage, resist, or weaken the social control that exacerbated stigma. These included consistently practising universal precautions, bending the rules, and relaxing institutional policies to accommodate client preferences, shifting or expanding services to meet client needs, balancing disclosure to family and healthcare providers, forgiving discriminatory behaviour, and reducing "HIV-positive" labelling.

Following analysis, community consultation workshops were held in three Canadian cities. These were attended by 97 Aboriginal and non-Aboriginal community partners. This input was used to develop recommendations for best practices to reduce HIV and AIDS stigma.

Discussion Questions

1. How would you assess stigma in a community needs assessment?
2. How might you apply the principles of ownership, control, access, and possession for the conduct of research with Aboriginal communities in a community needs assessment?

Organizing Information and Setting Priorities

The second set of tools help with organizing and understanding data and information, and guide priority-setting. See Chapters 9, 10, and 13 for additional examples.

Qualitative Data Analysis and Representation Analyzing qualitative data involves describing, classifying, and connecting the data. Content analysis is frequently used for planning purposes. It is a systematic, replicable technique for compressing large volumes of text data into fewer content categories based on explicit rules of coding. This involves assigning codes or labels to the text data. Data are then grouped into categories to reflect emerging patterns of responses. Systematic counting and recording techniques may also be used to help identify patterns of responses such as the predominant use of certain kinds of phrases by some respondents but not others (Stemler, 2001).

Analyzed qualitative data can be packaged in text, matrix, or figure formats. A text format involves the use of illustrative quotes. Matrices are used to compare major categories of data and highlight differences and similarities among sub-groups. For example, a matrix of needs assessment information may be used to compare responses from homeless men and shelter staff regarding the fairness of the shelter rules; or to compare the perspectives of teachers, parents, and students regarding the acceptability and need for school sexual health clinics. Figures may be a useful visual tool to reflect emerging relationships amongst categories of coded data.

Using Quantitative Data

Many sources of quantitative data may be accessed as you plan a program. These include local and provincial data documenting the magnitude of the problem and contributing factors. These data are often obtained through sources such as special surveys (e.g., school surveys to document patterns of smoking among youth), routinely collected information (e.g., police and ambulance reports), and surveillance data (e.g., reports of communicable diseases). There are many excellent examples of reporting formats that have been developed to display quantitative data. A useful starting point is to examine existing reports (e.g., health status reports) and to enlist the assistance of someone with epidemiological training.

A second use of quantitative data is to help with estimating program costs and the potential return on investments. Various methods and tools may be of relevance here, including the use of the balanced score card (Woodward, Manuel, & Goel, 2004) and the application of health economics methods (Shiell, Hawe, & Gold, 2008).

Interpreting systematic reviews is a third use of quantitative data. Systematic reviews assemble findings from studies with a common research objective (e.g., to examine the effectiveness of exercise and balance programs to reduce the risk of falls among seniors). Those undertaking systematic reviews use a thorough and rigorous set of methods to both identify all potentially relevant studies and to review the methodological quality of these studies. Studies deemed to be relevant and of adequate quality are included in the review. Outcome data are extracted using standard procedures. When possible, the quantitative findings from two or more studies are collapsed into a single estimate of effect. This is done using statistical techniques and the review process is then called a meta-analysis.

Figure 14.3 summarizes the results from 15 studies on the effectiveness of fall prevention interventions. There are three important things to understand in this diagram. First, the relative risk is used to indicate whether or not the study group that received the intervention has a lower rate of falls than the study group that did not receive the intervention. If there is no difference between the groups, the relative risk is one. If the intervention group has a lower rate of falls than the control group, the relative risk will be less than one (indicating a protective effect). Fourteen of the 15 studies had a relative risk less than one (range 0.34 to 0.97). Second, if this intervention effect is statistically significant (indicating that if we repeated the experiment, we are 95% certain that we would again find a difference between groups), then the confidence interval around the relative risk will also be less than one. In Figure 14.3, the

---

FIGURE 14.3   Assessment Followed by Multifactorial Intervention vs. Control

Review: Interventions for preventing falls in older people living in the community
Comparison: 16 Multifactorial intervention after assessment vs control

Outcome: 1 Rate of falls

Study or subgroup	Intervention N	Control N	log [Rate ratio] (SE)	Rate ratio IV, Random, 95% CI	Weight	Rate ratio IV, Random, 95% CI
Carpenter 1990	181	186	−1.08 (0.33)		3.0%	0.34 [0.18, 0.65]
Close 1999	141	163	−0.89 (0.09)		7.8%	0.41 [0.34, 0.49]
Davison 2005	144	149	−0.45 (0.17)		5.9%	0.64 [0.46, 0.89]
Elley 2008	155	157	−0.04 (0.17)		5.9%	0.96 [0.69, 1.34]
Gallagher 1996	50	50	−0.21 (0.15)		6.4%	0.81 [0.60, 1.09]
Hogan 2001	75	77	−0.3 (0.09)		7.8%	0.74 [0.62, 0.88]
Hombrook 1994	1611	1571	−0.17 (0.03)		8.8%	0.84 [0.80, 0.89]
Lightbody 2002	155	159	−0.16 (0.11)		7.4%	0.85 [0.69, 1.06]
Lord 2005	396	201	−0.03 (0.09)		7.8%	0.97 [0.81, 1.16]
Mahoney 2007	174	175	−0.21 (0.18)		5.7%	0.81 [0.57, 1.15]
Nikolaus 2003	181	179	−0.37 (0.16)		6.2%	0.69 [0.50, 0.95]
Rubenstein 2007	327	352	−0.17 (0.14)		6.6%	1.19 [0.90, 1.56]
Salminen 2008	292	297	−0.08 (0.09)		7.8%	0.92 [0.77, 1.10]
Tinetti 1994	147	144	−0.58 (0.15)		6.4%	0.56 [0.42, 0.75]
Wyman 2005	126	126	−0.33 (0.15)		6.4%	0.72 [0.54, 0.96]
Total (95% CI)					100.0%	0.75 [0.65, 0.86]

Heterogeneity: Tau^2 = 0.06, Chi^2 = 90.82, df = 14 (P<0.00001), I^2 = 85%
Test for overall effect: Z = 4.03 (P = 0.000057)

0.2   0.5   1   2   5
Favours intervention   Favours control

Source: Gillespie, L. D., Robertson, M. C., Gillespie, W. J., Lamb, S. E., Gates, S., Cumming, R. G., & Rowe B. H. (2009). Interventions for preventing falls in older people living in the community. Cochrane Database of Systematic Reviews, Issue 2. Art. No.: CD007146. doi:10.1002/14651858.CD007146.pub2.

confidence interval is shown as a horizontal line on the diagram and listed in the right-hand column. We can see that only eight of the 15 studies found statistically significant protective effects of the intervention. Third, results are then pooled across the 15 (the meta-analysis part of the exercise). A weighting factor is used in making this calculation so that studies with small sample sizes will contribute less weight to the pooled estimate than studies with large sample sizes. In this example, the pooled relative risk is 0.75 and the result is statistically significant—test for overall effect yields a p value < 0.000057. Thus, it follows that the recommendation in the abstract for this review concludes that "assessment and multifactorial intervention reduced rate of falls (RR 0.75, 95% CI 0.65 to 0.86)" (Gillespie et al., 2009, p. 1).

Priority Setting

Setting priorities is a vital step in the planning process. An in-depth examination of a problem in the community may leave one overwhelmed at the thought of narrowing down the possibilities for action. The guiding principles for priority-setting are buy-in, transparency, and communication. Setting priorities inevitably means that one can neither address all the identified needs nor operationalize all the proposed interventions. Engaging community members and key stakeholders in discussing the problem may initially help with *buy-in* but runs the risk of backfiring if the priorities selected suggest that their input and ideas were not considered. Thus, it is also important to look at ways to engage the community in the process of setting priorities as one begins to more clearly define program components and activities. While it may not be realistic to involve a large community in a priority-setting exercise, one can invite input on the selection of criteria to inform priority-setting. Agreement among senior managers on a common priority-setting process for an organization will help ensure managerial support for the priorities identified.

The second principle is *transparency,* whereby the process for selecting priorities is made apparent to those who were not directly involved in the process. In other words, key stakeholders are able to understand how you got from point A (understanding the problem and considering possible intervention strategies) to point B (priority definition of the problem and strategies). Both objective and subjective criteria are important to identify priority interventions. **Objective criteria** are measurable facets of a problem and its solutions. For example, what is the magnitude (prevalence or incidence) of a problem, what are the short- and long-term consequences of the problem (e.g., mortality or morbidity), are there effective strategies to address the problem, and how cost-effective are the strategies relative to other approaches? **Subjective criteria** require judgment calls that are based on underlying values about the issue and the implementing organization. For instance, will working on the problem lead to new and stronger partnerships with other community agencies? Is tackling the problem within the mandate of our organization? Is there community readiness and political will to address this problem both in the short and long terms?

The third principle is *communication.* A clear communication strategy needs to accompany efforts to set priorities. Both internal and external communication processes are vital. Internally, the identification of priorities should be directly linked to the approval mechanisms for program funding. Externally, one needs to communicate priorities to partners who have provided input on the program. This will help to ensure more buy-in for program implementation.

Planning, Monitoring, and Evaluating Programs

There are various resources available to assist nurses and other public health professionals to plan, monitor, and evaluate programs. (See MyNursingLab, The Online Health Program Planner.) **Gantt charts**, depicted in a tabular format, are a commonly used tool to present the sequence and timing of activities that must take place in order to accomplish the specific objectives of the program or project. These charts are particularly helpful when one is planning activities for a complex program with many components. The Gantt chart provides a good starting point for identifying these main components. The timelines for particular sets of activities, which activities precede other critical tasks, and details about the activities are then elaborated. For instance, permission must be obtained for the use of space before focus groups can be held and focus groups must take place before a meeting is convened. One example of a Gantt chart is provided in Figure 14.4. Software packages such as Microsoft Project and Excel can also be used to help develop planning and managing timelines with Gantt charts.

THE SHIFT TO MULTIPLE INTERVENTIONS

Increasingly, community health programs are targeting the complexity and root causes of problems. This requires a socioecological examination of the issue of interest and a planning–intervention–evaluation cycle that addresses these underlying determinants. Raphael (2008) defines **social determinants of health** as "the economic and social conditions that influence the health of individuals, communities and jurisdictions as a whole" (p. 1). Several key features of these social determinants are shaping contemporary community health programs. The determinants do not reside in isolation from each other. Rather, determinants are nested; that is, they are inter-related and as one determinant changes, another may also shift. Some determinants are deeply embedded, following from historical inequities such as the oppression that Aboriginal populations have experienced (Smith, Varcoe, & Edwards, 2005), and stigma faced by marginalized groups (Friedman, Cooper, & Osborne, 2009). This notion that health is largely influenced by multiple factors beyond biology, genetics, and the healthcare system provides the foundation for a population health approach. A **population**

FIGURE 14.4 Example of a Gantt Chart

Activity	Year 1				Year 2		
	Q1	Q2	Q3	Q4	Q1	Q2	Q3
Develop Focus Group Interview Schedule	■						
Obtain Permission to Hold Focus Group in Community Centre	■						
Recruit Participants		■					
Hold Focus Group with Co-moderator		■					
Analyze Data			■				
Prepare Initial Version of Report for Community Consultation			■				
Present Findings to Community Stakeholders					■		
Integrate Feedback from Community into Final Report						■	
Circulate Final Report to Health Department Managers							■

health approach addresses the health of groups of people and disparities among groups by influencing a range of social, economic, personal, and health service factors that are well recognized as having an impact on our health (Health Canada, 2001). There have been both national and global calls for a "determinants of health approach" that addresses coherent, multi-level policies in health and other sectors with a specific focus on reducing health disparities (Senate Subcommittee on Population Health, 2009; Commission on Social Determinants, 2008). A **health impact assessment** can be used to examine the potential effects of a policy including its anticipated impact on health disparities (Taylor & Blair-Stevens, 2002). This determinants of health approach recognizes the need to implement population health interventions at multiple levels of the system (individual, community, municipal, provincial, and federal).

The **Multiple Intervention Program (MIP) framework** arises from earlier work by Edwards and Moyer (1999). In Ontario, in the late 1980s, there was a shift away from public health programs that predominantly involved home visits and clinically-oriented services in schools and workplaces. As evidence on socioecological determinants increased, and as considerations of how best to distribute scarce resources in public health were debated, programs increasingly began to focus on interventions targeting multiple layers of the system. Nurses were being asked to expand their repertoire of interventions to include not only those appropriate for individuals and families (such as home visits and primary care clinics), but also those targeted at community, organizational, and policy levels (such as community action, environment change, and policy strengthening and enforcement). With the input of front-line public health nurses and managers in Ottawa, a program framework was developed to reflect the integration of self-care capacity and action, collective care capacity and action, and environmental supports (Edwards & Moyer, 1999).

The next generation of this framework was developed 10 years later (Edwards, Mill, & Kothari, 2004). Its evolution arose from the observations and reflections of practitioners and from research. Managers identified the challenges of trying to plan and evaluate multiple intervention programs. Research findings were shedding light on a related set of issues. Through the 1990s, results from some well-designed experimental studies of multiple intervention programs were yielding unexpected and disappointing findings (Bauman, Suchindran, & Murray, 1999; Merzel & D'Afflitti, 2003; Sorenson, Emmons, Hunt & Johnston, 1998). For instance, the COMMIT trial (COMMIT Research Group 1995a) was a four-year multiple intervention study that targeted tobacco cessation and compared 11 matched-pairs of communities in the United States and Canada. Eleven communities were in the control group and received no intervention. Eleven communities received a theory-based intervention that aimed to increase cessation rates amongst heavy smokers. The intervention program that was designed was considered "state-of-the-art-and-science." It included over 50 strategies that were aimed at various levels of the system including individual behaviour change strategies, community mobilization, and organizational and policy change. However, the goal of reducing smoking rates among heavy smokers was not reached (COMMIT Research Group, 1995b). Authors have attempted to describe reasons for the failures of the COMMIT trial and other multiple interventions to achieve their expected outcomes (Zanna et al., 1994). Common reasons include the failure to involve the community in the planning process, the short duration of programs that does not allow enough time for policy change, failure to plan for long-term sustainability, and inadequate funding (Edwards, MacLean, et al., 2006; Merzel & D'Afflitti, 2003).

Yet, in apparent contradiction to some of the research on multiple intervention programs, there have been compelling examples of significant multiple intervention program successes in fields such as tobacco control and injury prevention. Prolonged efforts (often over more than a decade) have yielded substantial improvements in health outcomes from multi-strategy, multi-level, and multi-sector interventions. In the case of injury prevention, for example, multiple intervention programs have included a combination of strategies aimed at raising awareness (e.g., public media campaigns); supporting behaviour change (e.g., infant car seat clinics); changing social norms (e.g., a generation of children now think that wearing a seatbelt is the norm; it is no longer socially acceptable to drink and drive); and developing regulations or passing legislation and setting up enforcement approaches (e.g., using traffic calming strategies, and police checkpoints for seat belt use and drunk driving).

THE MULTIPLE INTERVENTION PROGRAM FRAMEWORK

The MIP framework consists of five main elements (see Figure 14.5). Use of the framework involves an iterative cycle whereby emerging lessons from program implementation and new research findings continuously inform program adjustments. Optimal application of the framework should be based on in-depth knowledge of the local community (tacit knowledge), expertise with relevant theories, and up-to-date

familiarity with good quality research evidence (both primary studies and systematic and integrative reviews). We describe each element of the framework, using illustrative examples for the problem of preventing falls among seniors. Table 14.1 provides a summary of the types of research studies that are relevant to each element of the model. These are described in more detail below. (See MyNursingLab for MIP examples and interactive exercises.)

Identification of Community Health Issue

The first element is the identification of a community health issue that is the program focus. It is important to identify population subgroups that may be disadvantaged because they bear an unequal or inequitable burden of the health problem.

Describe Socioecological Determinants

The second element involves describing the socioecological determinants of the problem. Here, a socioecological perspective helps to expose the factors that may be contributing to and/or causing the problem. Similarly, strengths and capacities at different levels of the system may reveal potential solutions to the problem.

Several types of research inform this element of the framework. Etiological research examines putative causes of health problems. Both qualitative and quantitative studies may reveal the complex relationships among determinants. Laboratory studies may yield insights into biological or

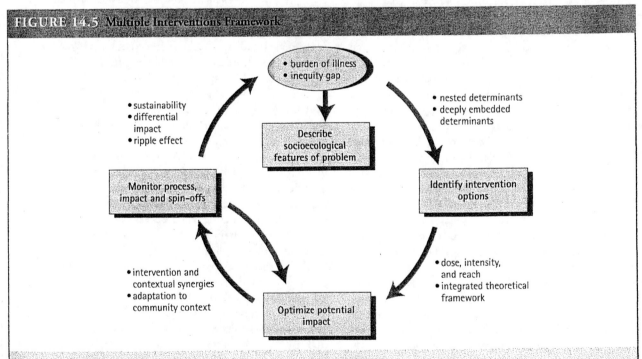

FIGURE 14.5 Multiple Interventions Framework

Source: Adapted from Edwards, N., Mill, J., & Kothari, A. (2004). Multiple Intervention Framework, 36(1), 40–54, p. 44. Reprinted by permission of CJNR.

TABLE 14.1 Assembling the Research Evidence

Element of Framework	Description of Relevant Research Studies and Data	Examples from Research on Preventing Falls
Burden of illness and inequities	Prevalence and incidence of disease burden Age- and gender-specific rates of disease Policy coverage for sub-populations	*Burden of Illness:* One in three seniors falls each year. Approximately 25% of all falls result in injuries. Falls are the sixth leading cause of death among seniors in Canada. *Inequities:* Although seniors living in publicly subsidized apartment buildings have worse health status than seniors living in privately owned apartment buildings, they are significantly more likely to have universal access to grab bars (Edwards, Birkett, Nair et al., 2006).
Socioecological determinants of problem	Etiological studies, laboratory studies, integrative reviews, qualitative and quantitative studies of determinants	Findings from individual studies and reviews (Gill, Williams, & Tinetti, 2000; O'Loughlin, Robitaille, Boivin, & Suissa, 1993; Rawski, 1998) indicate that major risk factors for falls among community-dwelling seniors are: ■ Use of benzodiazepine sedative hyponotics ■ Polypharmacy (using four or more drugs) ■ Problems with balance and peripheral neuromuscular dysfunction ■ Environmental hazards Qualitative and quantitative studies identify the perspectives of seniors on risk factors for falls and identify the outcomes that are most important to them (e.g., loss of independence) (Aminzadeh & Edwards, 1998). Laboratory studies identify specific features of the built environment (e.g., configuration of grab bars, height of stairs, dimensions of handrails) that may interact with personal variables (e.g., chronic illness, balance, hand grip strength, cognition) to increase the risk of falls (Maki, Perry, Scovil, Mihailidis, & Fernie, 2006; Sveistrup, Lockett, Edwards, & Aminzadeh, 2006). Policy studies examine policy gaps and the influence of the policy environment on the risk of falls (Perdue, Stone, & Gostin, 2003).
Intervention options	Efficacy and effectiveness studies, cost-effectiveness or cost–benefit studies, program evaluation, systematic reviews, best practice guideline documents, theories	Cochrane reviews and primary studies provide evidence of effectiveness on strategies to prevent falls and fall-related injuries (Gillespie et al., 2003; McClure et al., 2005; Parker, Gillespie, & Gillespie, 2006). Best practice guidelines for preventing falls (Scott, Dukeshire, Gallagher, & Scanlan, 2001) are informed by effectiveness studies. Community health evaluation studies yield promising strategies from fall prevention programs (Gallagher & Scott, 1997).
Optimal blend of strategies	Effectiveness studies of multi-strategy and multi-level interventions Studies informed by integrated theories Studies that examine contextual influences on intervention strategies	Evidence that exercise programs are effective when used in combination with modifications to the built environment (Gillespie et al., 2009). Evidence that multifactor approaches are more effective in reducing falls than single strategies (Tinetti et al., 1994). Sociobehavioural factors explain underutilization of efficacious interventions (Edwards, Lockett, Aminzadeh, & Nair, 2003; Fisher, Li, Michael, & Cleveland, 2004; George, Binns, Clayden, & Mulley, 1988; Naik & Gill, 2005). Studies examining the application of theory to fall prevention (Sampson & Morenoff, 2000)
Monitoring and evaluating process, impact, spin-offs, and sustainability	Identification of potential indicators, ways of assembling data to support decision making	The Ontario Public Health Standards 2008 (Ministry of Health and Long-term Care, 2008) include societal outcomes for injury prevention programs.

TABLE 14.2 Socioecological Determinants of Falls Among the Elderly

Level of Socioecological Model	Example and Reference to Supporting Empirical Literature
Individual	Patterns and type of exercise (Benjamin, Edwards, & Bharti, 2005)
	Seniors' perceptions of barriers to physical activity (Lockett, Willis, & Edwards, 2005)
Interpersonal	Buddy systems in apartment buildings where neighbours check on each other to see if anyone has had an injurious fall
Community	Coalitions or other organized collectives taking action on preventing falls by raising awareness and addressing policy change (Edwards, 1999)
Built/physical environment	Presence of grab bars in bathrooms (Aminzadeh, Edwards, Lockett, & Nair, 2001)
	Features of safe stairs (Maki et al., 2006)
Social environment	Accessibility of esthetically pleasing and safe walking areas near seniors' housing (Giles-Corti & Donovan, 2003)
Organizational policy (e.g., workplace, places of worship, housing)	Skilled volunteers organized in the community to make home modifications such as installing handrails on indoor and outdoor stairs (Edwards, Benjamin, & Lockett, 2006)
Municipal policy	Policies regarding the marking of cracks in public sidewalks and length of time to fix these cracks (Gallagher & Scott, 1997)
Provincial policy	Provincial building codes for private and public housing (Edwards, Birkett, et al., 2006)
National policy	Recommendations for building codes provided by National Research Council and uptake of empirical evidence in modifications to building codes (Edwards, 2008)

environmental factors that are at play; while organizational and policy studies may reveal determinants that operate at a macro level. While individual primary studies may be useful, systematic or integrative reviews that identify causal factors from a synthesis of the best available evidence are more informative. Integrative reviews use findings from both qualitative and quantitative studies (Mays, Pope, & Popay, 2005). The phases of an integrative review process include (1) problem formulation, (2) data collection or literature search, (3) evaluation of data from diverse research designs, (4) data analysis, and (5) interpretation and presentation of results (Whittemore & Knafl, 2005). Integrative reviews may also contribute to the identification of theoretical insights to guide program strategies. Evidence on socioecological determinants is lined up with relevant levels of the socioecological model (see Table 14.2). In consultation with the community, priority levels for action are then selected based on community characteristics and knowledge of the policy context.

The nature or scope of different health issues may render various levels of the model more relevant than others. For instance, in the case of injury prevention, features of the built environment are likely to be a central concern; whereas with tobacco control, the accessibility of tobacco products, addiction, and social norms are particularly important. Furthermore, the level(s) of government (municipal, provincial, federal) to target is determined by who has budgetary and policy jurisdiction over the problem. Community partners will provide much-needed input on the joint action on

determinants that is required in their setting and opportunities for same.

Intervention Options

The third element of the framework specifies intervention options. Here, one considers strategies that have demonstrated effectiveness and are theoretically sound. This knowledge must be coupled with community input on the feasibility of implementing interventions in their setting and the need to adapt interventions to ensure cultural and geographic relevance. For instance, while there is strong evidence of efficacy from laboratory studies and some evidence of effectiveness from studies with nursing home residents that hip protectors will reduce the risk of a hip fracture when a fall occurs, problems with compliance in using hip protectors have been reported (Parker, Gillespie, & Gillespie, 2006). Reasons for non-compliance include inconvenience when: busy nursing staff in long-term care settings have to help residents with dressing, seniors try hip protectors but find them to be bulky under regular clothing, and seniors accidentally soil their hip protector garments due to urge incontinence. These factors reduce the effectiveness of hip protectors as an injury-prevention strategy.

A mix of studies is required to inform intervention choices. For example, etiological studies indicate that the use of benzodiazepine sedative hypnotics is consistently a risk factor for falls. This suggests that minimizing use of these medications would be a useful fall prevention strategy. For those planning a program, however, the question that arises is: who is the most effective target, the seniors or physicians who prescribe the medication? Studies from the field of addictions indicate that it is difficult to wean an individual off this class of drugs following long-term use. However, studies that have targeted changes in prescribing practice suggest that academic detailers (e.g., representatives from pharmaceutical companies who directly market new drugs to physicians), and audit and feedback strategies are effective in modifying physician prescribing (Foy et al., 2002). This combination of evidence indicates that a public health strategy targeting individual counselling for those who are taking benzodiazepines may be less likely to have a population impact than a public health strategy that targets prescribing patterns among family physicians.

When selecting intervention options, planning teams also need to pay close attention to the reach, dose, and intensity of strategies that are required (Jilcott, Ammerman, Sommers, & Glasgow, 2007) to have their intended effect. The **reach** of an intervention concerns what proportion and which particular segments of an intended target population receive the interventions. For example, a public service advertisement, intended for all seniors, will only reach those who are watching television or listening to the radio when the advertisement is run. The **dose** is the amount of intervention required to have an effect. Multiple exposures to a public service announcement are required to change awareness. The **intensity** of the intervention refers to its quality and whether it is tailored to the targeted population subgroup. For instance, a media campaign about the importance of walking regularly may have adequate intensity for seniors who have good functional status but is unlikely to provide suitable messages for very frail seniors who are not independently mobile. A note of caution is important here. If strategies that appear promising are watered down due to funding constraints or other limitations on program delivery capacity, the dose and intensity required for the intervention to make a difference may be diluted and the expected outcome is unlikely to be achieved.

Choosing strategies requires in-depth knowledge of the community characteristics that may influence uptake and effectiveness of the intervention strategies. The readiness and capacity of the community for the intended change is an important consideration that can best be gauged by community partners. The identification of policy windows and policy levers is also important (Kingdon, 1995). **Policy windows** are periods of opportunity to get an issue on the policy agenda. Policy windows may open because of a community crisis; mounting concern about a growing problem among the public and substantial press coverage on this issue; or a period of planned change such as the amalgamation of municipalities. These policy windows can create the momentum and public support required for policy change. Identifying **policy levers** requires an understanding of the ways in which different kinds of policies (e.g., community health nursing standards, National Research Council building code recommendations, and legislation) can be introduced or changed. It is important to involve those with expertise in policy change processes such as individuals with political science,

public administration, or legal backgrounds in content-specific areas on your planning team.

In addition to evidence on what works and knowledge of the community, theoretical considerations should also drive the planning process. We are often inclined to apply those theories most familiar to us, rather than those theories most pertinent for the problem at hand. Since a multiple intervention program approach tackles more than one level of the socioecological system (Stokols, 1996), a mix of theories is required to guide the program. This involves integrating theories from various disciplines and is likely to require the expertise of individuals from different disciplines who know the theories well. Identifying a range of relevant theories may expand the intervention options to be considered.

Optimizing Intervention Strategies

The fourth framework element focuses on optimizing intervention strategies. That is, how can we increase the likelihood that the combination of interventions works in a well-orchestrated fashion and how can we adapt our interventions to a dynamic context? Sorting this out requires that we attend to the sequence and combination of strategies and to the ways in which the political, social, organizational, and policy environments (contexts) are changing. The integrated theory that guides our program should inform decisions on how to optimize intervention strategies. Since intervention strategies may work together either positively or negatively, questions to consider when discussing how to optimize them include the following:

- What is a particular program trying to achieve and how can we combine intervention strategies to potentiate this?
- Are there ways in which a particular combination of interventions might nullify each other's effects?
- What is going on in the community that might enhance or reduce the impact of the intervention?

Two examples of how selected interventions might be optimized are provided in Table 14.3. The first example, which involves using the media and a risk counselling approach, illustrates how intervention strategies can be combined to potentiate their effect. The second example shows how a planned intervention strategy can be successfully combined with a contextual influence. Although programs have no direct control over contextual influences, anticipating those that may arise and making program adjustments to reflect contextual influences that do emerge may either optimize the planned intervention strategies or mitigate the negative influences of contextual changes.

Monitoring and Evaluating Impacts, Spin-offs, and Sustainability

In the final element, monitoring and evaluating program outputs, outcomes, impacts, spin-offs, and sustainability are the central concern. **Outputs** indicate that a program is being

TABLE 14.3   Optimizing Interventions

Examples of intervention strategies and intended effect	Underlying theory and research to support plan for intervention strategies	Optimizing the intervention
Media campaign to raise awareness about the risk of hazardous stairs, and volunteer program to encourage seniors to take action to improve safety of home stairs.	Social marketing theory, media communication studies, and stages of change theory (Prochaska & Velicer, 1997) indicate that a media campaign can shift a segment of the population from precontemplation to contemplation in a short interval (days or weeks).	Media campaign should be timed to coincide with accessible options for action, such as a help line for seniors to call to obtain volunteer assistance to make modifications to stairs (e.g., installation of handrails).
Collective action by a fall prevention coalition to increase community awareness of the importance of bathroom grab bars in combination with providing input to technical review committee for five-year review process of building codes.	Kingdon's (1995) theory indicates that public opinion is a critical influence in the policy change process, both with respect to creating a demand for the change and the support necessary for introducing a new policy or modifying one that already exists. Kingdon's theory also identifies the importance of policy windows, periods of time when a particular policy change is more likely to happen.	Because the process of changing the National Research Council's building code recommendations, and subsequently provincial building code legislation, involves an extended period, coalitions must be ready to mobilize public support for changes to the building codes at several time points. Effective and strategic application of Kingdon's (1995) theory by a coalition requires an understanding of how the building code revision process works and how public input on proposed changes is obtained, and knowledge of whether other key stakeholders such as the home building industry are supporting or opposing proposed changes to the building codes. The action by fall prevention coalitions through this process will require timely interventions to (a) mobilize public awareness and support, (b) work with key stakeholders to mobilize action by them, and (c) network with other coalitions.

implemented as planned. Identifying output indicators involves looking at the critical steps that are required for the program. For instance, initiating partnerships with other community organizations, engaging community members on a coalition, and getting a health issue on a political agenda would be relevant indicators to assess progress toward ultimately achieving policy change. **Outcomes** are medium-term changes that can be attributed to the program. Changes in knowledge, attitudes, and behaviours among the target population would be anticipated at several levels. In the case of fall prevention, these outcomes would be assessed among the elderly, among health professionals (e.g., prescribing practices, assessing patients' risk profile for falls), and among those responsible for policy change (e.g., awareness of existing policies that increase risk for falls). **Impacts** are the longer-term results of a program, often taking some years to achieve. As with outputs and outcomes, impacts may be assessed at various levels of the socioecological model. Thus, one might expect to see impact indicators of individual health status changes, shifts in social norms, changes to the built environment, or policy change, all depending on the original intent of the program.

The selection of impact indicators should be guided by what we know about effective interventions and the "dose" of intervention expected to achieve a particular effect. Programs that are overly-ambitious may appear ineffective because their resources are spread too thinly. When program managers cannot demonstrate an improvement in program outputs or outcomes, ongoing funding for the program may be threatened.

Spin-offs are unintended effects of a program. They may be positive or negative. One rarely sees formalized plans to assess spinoffs. They may, however, be identified through reflective approaches such as the maintenance of field notes during program implementation or team meeting discussions regarding observed spinoffs, and via mid- or end-of-program interviews with key informants and others who have participated in the program.

Sustainability concerns the longer-term viability of the program interventions. Evidence of sustainability at an organizational level may occur when an intervention becomes part of the routine. For instance, the introduction of a new assessment form during a program may become routinized when this form becomes part of standard data collection within the agency. Sustainability at a policy level may occur when the policy is established and enforcement strategies are routinely put in place. Sustainability does not necessarily refer to the ongoing funding of a program nor does it infer that a program will be organized the way it started out nor run by the same organization. Rather, the intent of sustainability is to continue addressing the problem and to evolve strategies to match how the problem is changing.

CANADIAN RESEARCH BOX

What are the short-term effects of a two-generation preschool program on parenting stress, self-esteem, life skills, and children's receptive language?

Benzies, K., Tough, S., Edwards, N., Nagan, K., Nowicki, B., Mychasiuk, R., & Donnelly, C. (2009). Effects of a two-generation Canadian preschool program on parenting stress, self-esteem, and life skills. *Early Childhood Services: An Interdisciplinary Journal of Effectiveness, 3*(1), 19–32. First published online January 2010.

Poverty and its sequelae are important determinants of health and their impact is perhaps most deleterious for young children and their families. Lack of school readiness and parenting stress may be associated with poverty, inadequate housing, and unemployment. Early interventions can offset these health effects.

This two-generation program is aimed at the needs of both the preschool children and their parents. Program interventions included early childhood education (20 hours per week provided by the Centre), parenting and life skills education (designed and implemented on-site by program staff), and family support provided by a registered social worker during home visits. This multiple intervention program was offered to families at no cost. A pretest/post-test was used to evaluate outcomes. Socioecological theory guided the evaluation. Fifty-five caregivers of 76 children participated in the portion of the study examining the impact of the program on parents. These caregivers were asked to complete a parenting stress index, community life skills scale, and self-esteem scale. Measures were self-completed at the outset of their enrolment in the program and following program completion. In the portion of the study examining child outcomes, 112 children participated. A research assistant assessed their receptive language skills using the Peabody Picture Vocabulary Test.

Parents reported significantly decreased parental distress and defensive responding, decreased total stress, increased self-esteem, and increased daily life management skills. Findings suggest that appropriate and timely supports and services for low-income families can reduce the negative impact of their economic pressures. Overall, the preschool children demonstrated a statistically significant improvement in receptive language skills. For Aboriginal children, a longer duration of time in the program was associated with stronger gains in language skills.

Discussion Questions

1. How does poverty affect children living in low-income families?

2. What are the strengths and limitations of the research design used to assess the impact of this program?

3. Were the evaluation measures used examples of output, outcome or impact indicators?

SUMMARY

CHNs are key players in health program delivery, and must also be integral to the dynamic process of program planning and evaluation. Familiarity with the tools and processes described in this chapter will help you contribute fully as a member of a program planning and evaluation team. As our examples have illustrated, community health programs are often aimed at community issues with a complex set of underlying determinants. It is not surprising that the planning process needs to be informed by a diverse set of data and evidence. Planning and evaluation should not occur in isolation. Rather, one must pull together an interdisciplinary team with a wide range of experience to help with different facets of this process. By working together, CHNs with program planning experience, academic researchers who are familiar with the theoretical and empirical literature, and community partners who bring important insights and essential experiential learning can substantially strengthen the design and evaluation of multiple intervention programs in community health. This in turn will help us meet the complex needs of populations, while demonstrating better accountability for the public funds used when programs are delivered.

KEY TERMS

REVIEW QUESTIONS

Choose the one alternative that best completes the statement or answers the question.

1. A classic planning–implementation–evaluation cycle
   a) is a linear set of eight sequential steps.
   b) should be completed before obtaining additional input from partners.
   c) allows for "cycling back" to previous steps in the process.
   d) should identify the single best alternative to address the issue of concern.

2. A logic model
   a) is a written summary of what the program is supposed to do.
   b) demonstrates program interrelationships and linkages.
   c) should be developed prior to collaboration with academic partners.
   d) is a guideline that all partners should agree to follow.

3. One component of a suicide prevention program for youth is crisis intervention. An example of a short-term outcome of a suicide prevention program for youth is
   a) training youth workers in crisis management.
   b) reducing suicide rates among youth.
   c) increasing knowledge of youth workers.
   d) identifying the target group.

4. Setting priorities is a vital step in the planning process. A guiding principle for priority-setting is
   a) ensuring that all identified interventions can be implemented.
   b) ensuring that key stakeholders understand how and why specific priorities have been selected.
   c) using objective (measurable) criteria to determine priorities.
   d) involving the large community in a priority-setting exercise.

5. Buddy systems located in apartment buildings where neighbours check on each other to see if anyone has had an injurious fall are an example of
   a) an individual level determinant of falls among the elderly.
   b) an interpersonal level determinant of falls among the elderly.
   c) a social environment level determinant of falls among the elderly.
   d) a community-level determinant of falls among the elderly.

6. A public health nurse is developing a program to prevent elementary school-yard injuries. Which of the following strategies is most appropriate for successful implementation?
   a) Offer to visit classrooms to teach preventive strategies to the children.
   b) Involve parents, teachers, and children in program development.
   c) Ask the school board to replace outdated play structures.
   d) Initiate a structured program for children during recess.

STUDY QUESTIONS

1. Are the steps in the planning–implementation–evaluation cycle always followed in a linear fashion? Explain.
2. List four factors that influence the choice of a program planning and evaluation framework.
3. Identify some tools commonly used in planning programs.
4. List three uses of quantitative data in planning and evaluating a program.
5. Identify the three principles of priority setting.
6. List the five main elements of the Multiple Intervention Program framework.

After working through these questions, go to the MyNursingLab at www.pearsoned.ca/mynursinglab to check your answers.

INDIVIDUAL CRITICAL THINKING EXERCISES

1. Your healthcare agency is collaborating with a community advocacy group to address escalating substance use among youth ages 12 to 17. What are some of the underlying socioecological determinants of substance abuse in this age group?
2. Using the substance abuse problem above, what types of evidence would you assemble to support the development of the program plan and why?
3. What are the strengths and weaknesses of each type of evidence you have selected for the substance abuse problem?
4. What are some examples of indicators you can use to assess the impact of the substance abuse program at the individual, organization, community, and policy levels?
5. Identify a community health issue of interest. What are some examples of synergies that might be expected to occur between program strategies and community context?

GROUP CRITICAL THINKING EXERCISES

1. You are part of a team evaluating a childhood obesity program delivered through the local schools. What information would you need to develop a logic model for this initiative? Describe to the members of your team why it is important to spend time developing the logic model.

2. Locate a good example of a community health program plan that illustrates the integration of several different theories. Do these theories reflect different levels of socioecological determinants?

3. You have been asked to develop a multiple intervention program and evaluation plan to address homelessness among older adults. What community partners would you involve in this process and why? How would you get community partners involved?

REFERENCES

Aminzadeh, F., Edwards, N., Lockett, D., & Nair, R. C. (2001). Utilization of bathroom safety devices, patterns of bathing and toileting, and bathroom falls in a sample of community living older adults. *Technology and Disability, 13*(2), 95–103.

Bauman, K. E., Suchindran, C. M., & Murray, D. M. (1999). The paucity of effects in community trials: Is secular trend the culprit? *Preventive Medicine, 28*(4), 426–429.

Benjamin, K., Edwards, N., & Bharti, V. (2005). Attitudinal, perceptual, and normative beliefs influencing the exercise decision of community-dwelling physically frail seniors: An application of the theory of planned behaviour. *Journal of Aging and Physical Activity 13*(3), 276–293.

Commission on Social Determinants of Health (CSDH). (2008). *Closing the gap in a generation: Health equity through action on the social determinants of health. Final report of the Commission of Social Determinants on Health.* Geneva, Switzerland: World Health Organization.

COMMIT Research Group. (1995a). Community Intervention Trial for Smoking Cessation. (COMMIT). I: Cohort results from a four-year community intervention. *American Journal of Public Health, 85*(2), 183–192.

COMMIT Research Group. (1995b). Community Intervention Trial for Smoking Cessation. (COMMIT). II: Changes in adult cigarette smoking prevalence. *American Journal of Public Health, 85*(2), 193–200.

Community Health Nurses Association of Canada [CHNAC]. (2008). *Canadian community health nursing standards of practice.* Retrieved from http://www.chnc.ca/documents/chn_standards_of_practice_mar08_english.pdf

Cooksy, L. J., Gill, P., & Kelly, P. A. (2001). The program logic model as an integrative framework for a multimethod evaluation. *Evaluation and Program Planning, 24,* 119–128.

Dana, R. H. (2002). Mental health services for African Americans: A cultural/racial perspective. *Cultural Diversity and Ethnic Minority Psychology, 8*(1), 3–18.

Edwards, N. (1999). Prevention of falls among seniors in the community. In M. Stewart (Ed.), *Community nursing: Promoting Canadians' health* (2nd ed., pp. 296–316). Toronto, ON: W. B. Saunders.

Edwards, N. (2008). Performance-based building codes: A call for injury prevention indicators that bridge health and building sectors. *Injury Prevention, 14,* 329–332.

Edwards, N., & Aminzadeh, F. (1998). Exploring seniors' views on the use of assistive devices in fall prevention. *Public Health Nursing, 15*(4), 297–304.

Edwards, N., Benjamin, K., & Lockett, D. (2006, September 25–27). *Environmental hazards and falls prevention: Defining a new research agenda.* Poster presented at the 2006 Australian Public Health Association conference, Sydney, Australia.

Edwards, N., Birkett, N., Nair, R., Murphy, M., Roberge, G., & Lockett, D. (2006). Access to bathtub grab bars: Evidence of a policy gap. *Canadian Journal on Aging, 25*(3), 295–304.

Edwards, N., & Davison, C. (2008). Social justice and core competencies for public health: Improving the fit. *Canadian Journal of Public Health, 99*(2), 130–132.

Edwards, N., Lockett, D., Aminzadeh, F., & Nair, R. (2003). Predictors of bath grab-bar use among community-living older adults. *Canadian Journal on Aging, 22*(2), 217–227.

Edwards, N., MacLean, L., Estable, A., & Meyer, M. (2006). *Multiple intervention program recommendations for Mandatory Health Program and Services Guidelines Technical Review Committees.* Ottawa, ON: Community Health Research Unit, University of Ottawa.

Edwards, N., Mill, J., & Kothari, A. (2004). Multiple intervention research programs in community health. *Canadian Journal of Nursing Research, 36*(1), 40–54.

Edwards, N., & Moyer, A. (1999). Community needs and capacity assessment: Critical component of program planning. In M. Stewart (Ed.), *Community nursing: Promoting Canadian's health* (2nd ed., pp. 420–442). Toronto, ON: W. B. Saunders.

Fisher, K. J., Li, F., Michael, Y., & Cleveland M. (2004). Neighborhood-level influences on physical activity among older adults: A multilevel analysis. *Journal of Aging and Physical Activity, 12*(1), 45–63.

Foy, R., Penney, G. C., Maclennan, G., Grimshaw, J., Campbell, M., & Grol, R. (2002). Attribute of clinical recommendations that influence change in practice following audit and feedback. *Journal of Clinical Epidemiology, 55*(7), 717–722.

Fraser, D. L., & Stupak, R. J. (2002). A synthesis of the strategic learning planning process with the principles of andragogy: Learning, leading and linking. *International Journal of Public Administration, 25*(9), 1199–1220.

Friedman, S. R., Cooper, H. F. L., & Osborne, A. H. (2009). Structural and social contexts of HIV risk among African Americans. *American Journal of Public Health, 99*(6), 1002–1008.

Gallagher, E. M., & Scott, V. J. (1997). The Steps Project: Participatory action research to reduce falls in public places among seniors and persons with disabilities. *Canadian Journal of Public Health, 88*(2), 129–133.

George, J., Binns, V., Clayden, A., & Mulley, G. (1998). Aids and adaptations for the elderly at home: Underprovided, underused, and undermaintained. *British Medical Journal, 296,* 1365–1366.

Giles-Corti, B., & Donovan, R. J. (2003). Relative influences of individual, social environmental, and physical environmental correlates of walking. *American Journal of Public Health, 93*(9), 1583–1589.

Gill, T., Williams, C., & Tinetti, M. (2000). Environmental hazards and the risk of nonsyncopal falls in the homes of community-living older persons. *Medical Care, 38*(12), 1174–1183.

Gillespie, L. D., Robertson, M. C., Gillespie, W. J., Lamb, S. E., Gates, S., Cumming, R. G., & Rowe B. H. (2009). *Interventions for preventing falls in older people living in the community.* Cochrane Database of Systematic Reviews, Issue 2. Art. No.: CD007146. doi:10.1002/14651858. CD007146.pub2.

Health Canada. (2001). *The population health template: Key elements and actions that define a population health approach.* Strategic Policy Directorate of the Population and Public Health Branch, Health Canada. Retrieved from http://www.phac-aspc.gc.ca/ph-sp/pdf/discussion-eng.pdf

Jilcott, S., Ammerman, A., Sommers, J., & Glasgow, R. E. (2007). Applying the RE-AIM framework to assess the public health impact of policy change. *Annals of Behavioural Medicine, 34,* 105–114.

Kamberelis, G., & Dimitriadis, G. (2005). Focus groups: Strategic articulations of pedagogy, politics and inquiry. In N. K. Denzin & Y. S. Lincoln (Eds.), *The Sage handbook of qualitative research* (3rd ed., pp. 887–907). Thousand Oaks, CA: Sage.

Kingdon, J. W. (1995). *Agendas, alternatives, and public policies* (2nd ed.). New York, NY: Addison-Wesley.

Lockett, D., Willis, A., & Edwards, N. (2005). Through seniors' eyes: An exploratory qualitative study to identify environmental barriers to and facilitators of walking. *Canadian Journal of Nursing Research, 37*(3), 48–65.

Maki, B. E., Perry, S. D., Scovil, C. Y., Mihailidis, A., & Fernie, G. R. (2006). Getting a grip on stairs: Research to optimize effectiveness of handrails. In R. N. Pikaar, E. A. P. Koningsveld, & P. J. M. Settels (Eds.), *Proceedings IEA 2006 Congress* (pp. 4669–4674). Amsterdam, The Netherlands: Elsevier.

Mays, N., Pope, C., & Popay, J. (2005). Systematically reviewing qualitative and quantitative evidence to inform management and policy-making in the health field. *Journal of Health Services Research & Policy, 10*(S1), 6–20.

McClure, R., Turner, C., Peel, N., Spinks, A., Eakin, E., & Hughes K. (2005). *Population-based interventions for the prevention of fall-related injuries in older people.* Cochrane Database of Systematic Reviews, 1, Art. No.: CD004441. doi:10.1002/14651858.CD004441.pub2.

Merzel, D., & D'Afflitti, J. (2003). Reconsidering community-based health promotion: Promise, performance, and potential. *American Journal of Public Health, 93*(4), 557–574.

Ministry of Health and Long-Term Care, (2008). *Ontario Public Health standards 2008.* Retrieved from http://www.health.gov.on.ca/english/providers /program/pubhealth/oph_standards/ophs/progstds/pdfs /ophs_2008.pdf

Naik, A. D., & Gill, T. M. (2005). Underutilization of environmental adaptations for bathing in community-living older persons. *Journal of the American Geriatrics Society, 53*(9), 1497–1503.

O'Loughlin, J., Robitaille, Y., Boivin, J. F., & Suissa, S. (1993). Incidence of and risk factors for falls and injurious falls among the community-dwelling elderly. *American Journal of Epidemiology, 137,* 342–354.

Parker, M. J., Gillespie, W. J., & Gillespie, L. D. (2006). Effectiveness of hip protectors for preventing hip fractures in elderly people: Systematic review. *British Medical Journal, 332,* 571–574.

Patton, M. Q. (2002). *Qualitative research and evaluation methods* (3rd ed.). Thousand Oaks, CA: Sage.

Perdue, W. C., Stone, L. A., & Gostin, L. O. (2003). The built environment and its relation to the public's health: The legal perspective. *American Journal of Public Health, 93*(9), 1390–1394.

Pope, C., & Mays, N. (2000). Qualitative research: Reaching the parts other methods cannot reach: An introduction to qualitative methods in health and health services. *British Medical Journal, 311,* 42–45.

Porteous, N., Sheldrick, B., & Stewart, P. (2002). Introducing program teams to logic models: Facilitating the learning process. *The Canadian Journal of Program Evaluation, 17*(3), 113–141.

Prochaska, J. O., & Velicer, W. F. (1997). The transtheoretical model of health behaviour change. *American Journal of Health Promotion, 12,* 38–48.

Public Health Agency of Canada. (2008). *Program evaluation tool kit.* Retrieved from http://www.phac-aspc.gc.ca/php-psp/toolkit-eng.php

Raphael, D. (Ed.). (2008). *Social determinants of health: Canadian perspectives* (2nd ed.). Toronto, ON: Canadian Scholars' Press.

Rawski, E. (1998). Review of the literature on falls among the elderly. *Journal of Nursing Scholarship, 30*(1), 47–52.

Rubin, J. H., & Rubin, I. S. (2005). Listening, hearing and sharing social experiences. In *Qualitative interviewing: The art of hearing data* (pp. 1–18). Thousand Oaks, CA: Sage.

Sampson, R. J., & Morenoff, J. (2000). Listening, hearing and sharing social experiences. In *Qualitative interviewing: The art of hearing data* (2nd ed., pp. 1–18). Toronto, ON: Sage.

Scott, V., Dukeshire, S., Gallagher, E., & Scanlan, A. (2001). *A best practice guide for the prevention of falls among seniors living in the community.* Ottawa, ON: Federal/Provincial/Territorial Ministers of Health and Ministers Responsible for Seniors.

Senate Subcommittee on Population Health. (2009). *A healthy, productive Canada: A determinant of health approach.* The Standing Senate Committee on Social Affairs, Science and Technology. Retrieved from http://www.parl.gc.ca/40 /2/parlbus/commbus/senate/com-e/popu-e/rep-e /rephealth1jun09-e.pdf

Shiell, A., Hawe, P., & Gold, L. (2008). Complex interventions or complex systems? Implications for health economic evaluation. *British Medical Journal, 336,* 1281–1283.

Smith, D., Varcoe, C., & Edwards, N. (2005). Turning around the intergenerational impact of residential schools on Aboriginal people: Implications for health policy and practice. *Canadian Journal of Nursing Research, 37*(4), 38–60.

Sofaer, S. (1999). Qualitative methods: What are they and why use them? *Health Services Research, 34,* 1101–1118.

Sorenson, G., Emmons, K., Hunt, J. K., & Johnston, D. (1998). Implications of the results of community intervention trials. *Annual Review of Public Health, 19,* 379–416.

Stemler, S. (2001). An overview of content analysis. *Practical Assessment, Research & Evaluation, 7*(17). Retrieved from http://PAREonline.net/getvn. asp?v=7&n=17

Stokols, D. (1996). Translating social ecological theory into guidelines for community health promotion. *American Journal of Health Promotion, 10*(4), 282–298.

Sveistrup, H., Lockett, D., Edwards, N., & Aminzadeh, F. (2006). Evaluation of bath grab bar placement for older adults. *Technology and Disability, 18,* 1–11.

Taylor, L., & Blair-Stevens, C. (Eds.). (2002). *Introducing health impact assessment (HIA): Informing the decision-making process.* National Health Services Health Development Agency, UK. Retrieved from http://www.nice.org.uk/niceMedia/documents/hia.pdf

Tinetti, M. E., Baker, D. I., McAvay, G., Claus, E. B., Garrett, P., Gottschalk, M., . . . Horwitz, R. I. (1994). A multifactorial intervention to reduce the risk of falling among elderly people living in the community. *The New England Journal of Medicine, 331*(13), 821–827.

Whittemore, R., & Knafl, K. (2005). The integrative review: Updated methodology. *Journal of Advanced Nursing, 52*(5), 546–553.

Woodward, G., Manuel, D., & Goel, V. (2004). *Developing a balanced score card for public health.* Institute for Clinical Evaluative Sciences, Toronto, ON. Retrieved from http://www.ices.on.ca/file/Scorecard_report_final.pdf

Zanna, M., Cameron, R., Goldsmith, C. H., Poland, B., Lindsay, E., & Walker, R. (1994). Critique of the COMMIT study based on the Brantford experience. *Health and Canadian Society, 2*(2), 319–336.

ADDITIONAL RESOURCES

Readings

Galea, S. (Ed.). (2007). *Macrosocial determinants of population health.* New York, NY: Springer Science.

Riley, B., & Edwards, N. (2009). *A primer on multiple intervention programs and some implications for a research agenda.* CHRU & NBPRU Publication No. M2009-1.

Websites

Health Canada. (2004). Canadian Handbook on Health Impact Assessment.

http://www.hc-sc.gc.ca/fniah-spnia/pubs/promotion/_environ/handbook-guide2004/index-eng.php

Child Welfare Information Gateway. (2010). Logic model builder.

http://toolkit.childwelfare.gov/toolkit/

About the Authors

Nancy Edwards, RN, PhD, is a Full Professor at the University of Ottawa, School of Nursing and Department of Epidemiology and Community Medicine. She holds a Nursing Chair in multiple interventions for community health nursing, funded by the Canadian Health Services Research Foundation, the Canadian Institutes of Health Research, and the Government of Ontario. Nancy is Scientific Director, Canadian Institutes of Health Research, Institute of Population and Public Health.

Josephine Etowa, RN, PHD, is an Associate Professor at the University of Ottawa, School of Nursing, and a founding member, and past president of the Health Association of African Canadians. Her research is grounded in over 24 years of clinical practice and is in the area of inequity in health and healthcare including diversity in nursing.

Wendy Peterson, RN, PhD, is an Assistant Professor at the University of Ottawa, School of Nursing. Wendy's research focuses on access and utilization of perinatal health services by marginalized groups.

Margaret Ann Kennedy, RN, PhD, is a Director of Standards at the Standards Collaborative, Canada Health Infoway. She is the President-Elect for the Canadian Nursing Informatics Association, Past President for the Nova Scotia Nursing Informatics Group, an educator, and a consultant.

Our thanks to Sabrina Farmer, Alex Budgell, and Diana Ehlers, who provided assistance with this manuscript.

chapter
15

Maternal and Child Health

Helen Brown and Gladys McPherson

OBJECTIVES

After studying this chapter, you should be able to:

1. Understand foundational concepts of maternal and child health in a Canadian context.
2. Explore key issues and challenges related to maternal and child health promotion within the broader context of health and healthcare in Canada.
3. Examine how the social determinants of health influence health indicators, health risks, health experiences, and health outcomes for infants, children, and women/mothers.
4. Use a relational approach to promote women and children's health within families, communities, and populations.

INTRODUCTION

The health of childbearing women, infants, children, and families is considered a key indicator of human flourishing and the health status of communities, nations, and societies. Created to mark the inception of the World Health Organization (WHO) in 1948, World Health Day in 2005 was themed *Make every mother and child count* (WHO, 2010a). The objective was to raise awareness and promote action on a set of tragic global facts that are not unlike similar estimates around the world in 2010: More than half a million women die from pregnancy-related causes every year; 10.6 million children under 5 also die each year, 40% of them in the first month after birth. Many of these deaths could be prevented with available interventions and population health promotion initiatives. The intent of the event was to initiate and sustain policy makers, service providers, governmental bodies, and healthcare organization to work together to address this critical situation to save lives and reduce the burden of suffering.

In Canada, we have good maternal and child health overall. However, there are women and children in this country who do not share these good outcomes and who face health risks and considerable challenges (Public Health Agency of Canada, 2008). Although we are considered to be a wealthy nation, child and family poverty rates are increasing. We know that poverty is associated with poorer health outcomes for mothers and children (Campaign 2000, 2009). This chapter focuses on community health nursing practice and the health of mothers and children, and, in particular, how maternal and child health is socially, politically, and economically structured (WHO, 2010b)—in other words, how poverty, social exclusion, unemployment, poor working conditions, and gender inequalities act to determine to a large extent the health of maternal and child populations in Canada.

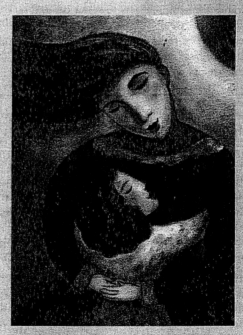

Source: © imageZoo / Alamy

MATERNAL HEALTH PROMOTION IN CANADA

The term **maternal health** generally refers to the health of women during pregnancy, childbirth, and the postpartum period. In Canada, the concept of **maternal healthcare** encompasses family planning, preconception, prenatal, and postnatal care and is therefore closely related to reproductive health. Within the framework of WHO's definition of health as a state of complete physical, mental, and social well-being, and not merely the absence of disease or infirmity;

reproductive health addresses the reproductive processes, functions, and system at all stages of life. *Reproductive health*, therefore, implies that people have the capability to reproduce and the freedom to decide if, when, and how often to do so. Implicit in this definition is the right of men and women to be informed of and to have access to safe, effective, affordable, and acceptable methods of fertility regulation of their choice; and the right of access to appropriate healthcare services that will enable women to go safely through pregnancy and childbirth and provide couples with the best chance of having a healthy infant. While this chapter focuses on maternal health, the topic is located within the fields of reproductive health in Canada and is shaped by the concepts of *reproductive justice* and *reproductive rights*.

Reproductive justice is a concept linking reproductive health with social justice recognizing that women's reproductive health is connected to and affected by conditions in their lives, for example, their socioeconomic status, human rights violations, race, sexuality, and nationality (Silliman, Fried, Ross, & Gutierrez, 2004). Those advocating for reproductive justice argue that women cannot have full control over their reproductive lives unless issues such as socioeconomic disadvantage, racial discrimination, inequalities in wealth and power, and differential access to resources and services are addressed (Ross, 2006).

Reproductive rights are a series of legal rights and freedoms relating to reproduction and reproductive health. Reproductive rights can be defined as follows:

> Reproductive rights rest on the recognition of the basic right of all couples and individuals to decide freely and responsibly the number, spacing and timing of their children and to have the information and means to do so, and the right to attain the highest standard of sexual and reproductive health. (Amnesty Internation USA, 2005, para. 2)

They also include the right of all to make decisions concerning reproduction free of discrimination, coercion, and violence.

Maternal Health within the Context of Women's Health

Definitions of **women's health** have always focused primarily on reproduction. Yet, women's lives are about more than reproduction and childbearing. The tendency to conflate women's health with maternal health arises from the fact that, for many women, the first time they encounter the healthcare system is when they are confronted with fertility challenges, are seeking preconception care, or when they first become pregnant. The historical and contemporary factors shaping women's lives in Canadian society are diverse, and filled with experiences influenced by culture, societal expectations, as well as political, economic, historical, and environmental factors. While women's and maternal–child healthcare share key practice and policies issues and actions, women's healthcare is more than a euphemism for maternal–child healthcare.

Women's reproductive health, in part because it has been ignored or poorly understood, has concentrated on women's biology and reproductive process, overlooking cultural, political and environmental influences ... that have lead to pathologizing and over-medicalization of normal processes. (Varcoe, Hankivsky, & Morrow, 2007, p. 15)

Seeing reproductive health as a biomedical process has also been shaped by the values of **liberal individualism**, further impacting women's access to effective and responsive care. Individualism is a central feature of liberalism and promotes the idea that people are rational, self-interested, autonomous actors who can be known and understood separately from their economic, historical, cultural, political, and social context (Browne, 2001). Such ideologies permeate the Canadian healthcare context and run counter to understanding the complexity of women's lives, and their interrelationships with others and their environments as shaping in all aspects of childbearing. The values of liberal individualism locate women's individual responsibility for their reproductive health within their own hands, thereby obscuring how multiple contexts and relations are influential. The health of childbearing women and mothers must therefore be understood in relation to multiple intersecting axes such as race, class, geography, ability, sexual orientation, and poverty, among other forces shaping women's lives. (See Chapter 18.)

Comprehensive Reproductive Health

Over the last four decades, **total fertility rates** (TFRs), or the number of children each woman bears on average, have decreased worldwide and particularly in developed countries such as Canada. The Canadian fertility rate has decreased by more than 60%, from 3.90 per woman in 1960 to 1.49 in 2000, below the replacement level of 2.1 children per woman. This reduction is attributed to some of the obvious improvements in women's maternal and reproductive health in this period, including significant decreases in the rates of maternal mortality and other pregnancy complications. However, beyond these obvious consequences, not many data are available about the impact on women's health of reduced fertility rates, delayed fertility, and more births to unmarried women (Public Health Agency of Canada, 2008). Optimal maternal health cannot be achieved without a comprehensive approach to reproductive health, which includes assisted human reproduction, reproductive technologies, preconception health assessment and screening, contraception and family planning, and access to legal, safe abortion.

Reclaiming the Normalcy of Pregnancy and Birth

A key feature of maternal health and childbearing continues to be how pregnancy and childbirth are shaped by biomedical conceptions of health. The tendency to see a normal healthy pregnancy and childbirth process as pathological underlies the medicalization of childbirth and reproduction (De Koninck, 1998; Oakley, 1984). Medicalization implies that a normal process is brought under the purview of medicine. The normal process of pregnancy and childbirth when viewed from a biomedical perspective is evident in the uptake of certain ideologies in maternity care delivery and approaches to practice. Childbearing becomes viewed through particularly narrow understandings that create stereotypical and biomedical approaches to childbirth. While the introduction of technologies to monitor progress in labour has improved perinatal outcomes within certain circumstances, there is also evidence to suggest that increased fetal surveillance has contributed to increased cesarean section rates, creating new risks that can increase risks for mothers and newborns (Alfirevic, Devane, & Gyte, 2007).

While medicalization and the use of technology is a prominent feature of pregnancy and childbirth in Canada, maternity care and women's experiences are also shaped by ongoing efforts to restore the normalcy of birth. The regulation and publically funded practice of midwives—albeit not consistent in all provinces—illustrate the historical and cultural importance of traditional birth attendants in Canadian society. In many cultures, women experienced in childbirth have traditionally attended births, and such caregivers generally gained their knowledge through apprenticeships with older, more experienced midwives. A trained **midwife** provides the necessary supervision, care, and advice to women during pregnancy, labour, and the postpartum period, conducts deliveries on her own responsibility, and cares for the newborn and the infant (Canadian Association of Midwives, 2010). Care given by midwives includes preventive measures, the detection of abnormal conditions in mother and child, the procurement of medical assistance, and the execution of emergency measures in the absence of medical help. Midwives also play a role in maternal, family, and community education. They may practise in hospitals, clinics, birth centres, or private homes, depending on the jurisdiction in which they practice. (See MyNursingLab—Keeping Birthing Close to Home: "The Maternity.")

"Risk" Discourses and Childbearing

A consequence of the medicalization of pregnancy and birth in Canada is the tendency to conceptualize health in pregnancy based on an analysis of risk rather than based on an understanding of the normalcy of birth. Kaufert and O'Neil (1993) describe how with increasing technology and better access to transportation in the 1970s, obstetric policy changed to transporting Inuit women to southern communities to give birth. Policy makers and maternity service providers used comparisons of infant and perinatal mortality as an indicator of well-being and as a benchmark for measuring the health of Inuit people. The intervention of evacuation became justified to reduce "risk"; however, Inuit women became disconnected from their own culture and birthing traditions, which undermined connections to their families and communities. Perceptions of greater "risk" for Inuit women worsened the effect of the trend toward urbanization and evacuation, and little attention was paid to the connection between increased

pregnancy and birth risks that followed colonization, loss of traditional occupations and natural resources, reliance on "white" food, and the erosion of traditional care.

The higher risks for adverse birth outcomes for First Nations women in British Columbia have also been linked to risks associated with a lack of attendance for prenatal care, a high incidence of adolescent pregnancy, more high- and low-birth-weight babies, more pregnancy-associated diabetes, poorer nutrition during pregnancy, and higher rates of multiple birth than the rest of the Canadian population. The mechanism of colonization, however, as a major determinant of health is often overlooked (Brown, Varcoe, & Calam, in press; Kelm, 1998) and explanatory models appear to "blame the victim," for example, for not having better nutrition and not accessing prenatal care. Browne (2005) describes how nurses who seek to move beyond a racializing explanation of differences in maternal–infant birth outcomes consider how Aboriginal women's experiences of healthcare pose considerable barriers to care. Rural women also identify barriers to receiving maternity care consonant with their needs due to geographic realities, financial costs of leaving their home communities to give birth, and availability of local healthcare resources (Kornelsen & Grzybowski, 2006). All these factors constitute the broader context for interpreting maternal and newborn population health indicators and, more importantly, preventing adverse birth outcomes in specific communities and populations.

Mothering: A Nexus of Discourses

Women's experiences of mothering are shaped by multiple social and structural forces in Canada, as are their personal resources and capacities. Therefore, becoming a mother affects women's health in diverse ways. While for many women mothering can have positive effects on health, for a significant number of women, mothering can create vulnerability to health risks. Varcoe and Hatrick Doane (2007) describe how women often face increased workloads, poverty, and violence when becoming mothers. For example, the 2006 census data shows that 83% of lone-parent families were female headed and 56% of lone-parent mothers had incomes that fell below the low-income cutoffs (Statistics Canada, 2007). Being a single mother creates the conditions for poor health if a woman cannot access the necessary social and economic resources that are known to be linked to optimal health. For these reasons, it is ineffectual to understand a mother's parenting capacities, self-efficacy, and maternal competence solely on the basis of personal attributes or coping styles.

Effective parenting and a satisfying mothering experience become possible through social support, connections to a community that values social determinants of health, and access to local maternity care that is respectful, responsive, and culturally safe (Brown et al., in press). Optimizing infant health and parent–infant relationships can be best served by tailoring postnatal education and support to women's individual needs. Educational interventions that impact maternal knowledge, infant health, and parent–infant relationships are infant sleep enhancement, behaviour, general safety issues and safe sleeping, post-birth health, partner/father involvement/ skills with infants, and breastfeeding support (Bryanton & Beck, 2010).

MATERNAL HEALTH RISKS AND CHALLENGES IN CANADA

Maternal, Fetal, and Infant Health: Health Determinants and Outcomes

Infant mortality has been considered one of several comprehensive measure of health in society. Caution must be used when interpreting indicators for underrepresentation of particular populations (see Chapters 9 and 10). *Determinants of maternal, fetal, and infant health* in Canada are clustered for measurement purposes into two categories: (a) maternal behaviours and practices, and (b) health services. Behaviours and practices considered to determine maternal, fetal, and infant health at a population level are rates of maternal smoking, exposure to second-hand smoke, consumption of alcohol, breastfeeding initiation and maintenance, folic acid supplementation, maternal education level, live birth to teenage mothers, and older mothers (aged 35–49). At present, the central contributing factors to *disparities in reproductive health* have been identified as reproductive choice, nutritional and social status, co-incidental infectious diseases, information needs, access to health system and services, and the training and skill of health workers. For pregnant women, the most prominent risks to life are identified as those directly associated with pregnancy: childbirth, haemorrhage, infection, unsafe abortion, pregnancy-related illness, and complications of childbirth. In relation to health service, maternal, fetal, and infant health is also determined by rates of labour induction, cesarean delivery, operative vaginal delivery, rates of maternal discharge from hospital following childbirth, and rates of neonatal discharge from hospital after birth (Public Health Agency of Canada, 2008).

Maternal, fetal, and infant health outcomes in Canada are determined on the basis of maternal mortality ratios, severe maternal morbidity rate, induced abortion ratio, rate of ectopic pregnancy, and rate of maternal readmission after discharge following childbirth. Fetal and infant health outcomes are documented by measuring the rates for preterm birth (less than 37 weeks' gestation), post-term birth (more than 42 weeks' gestation), small-for-gestational-age, large-for-gestational-age, fetal mortality, infant mortality rate, severe neonatal morbidity, multiple births, prevalence of congenital anomalies, and neonatal hospital readmission after discharge following birth.

According to the Canadian Perinatal Health Report (Public Health Agency of Canada, 2008), several measures have generated attention:

- The *preterm birth rate* has increased from 7.0 per 100 live births in 1995 to 8.3 per 100 live births in 2004. Explanations include an increase in obstetrical interventions,

multiple birth, older maternal age, and increased ultrasound use. The provincial/territorial preterm birth rates varied widely, from 7.4 per 100 in Saskatchewan to 12.2 per 100 in Nunavit.

- *Large-for-gestational-age rate* has also increased from 1995 to 2004 and is associated with risks to both fetus and mother (fetal macrosomia and birth injury and maternal postpartum hemorrhage).

- *Fetal mortality rates* have decreased from 6.3 per 1000 live birth in 1995 to 5.1 per 1000 in 2004.

Maternal and Infant Health Inequities

Unlike inequity, the terms "inequality" and "disparity" are generally used to describe differences of any sort in health and access to healthcare within a population. Despite improvements in health in general, significant inequities in health persist in Canada (Raphael, 2006). Within the context of childbearing, differences in birth outcomes are associated with the social determinants of health; specifically, a lack of social support and life stress have been linked to psychological impacts that result in adverse birth outcomes (Geronimus, 2001).

Preterm birth is the leading cause of infant mortality in industrialized countries. Despite several decades of investigation, an understanding of the etiologic pathways remains largely unknown and few effective prevention strategies have been identified. In fact, preterm birth rates continue to rise throughout the developed world (Kramer et al., 2009). Low birth weight (LBW)[1] and preterm birth (PTB)[2] are purported to be central antecedents to inequities in infant health and infant mortality[3] (Dominguez, 2008). In particular, preterm birth has been identified as one of the most important perinatal health problems in industrialized nations and accounts for 75–85% of all perinatal mortality in Canada (Public Health Agency of Canada, 2007). According to the Institute of Health Economics (2007), both LBW and PTB arise within a complex combination of individual and social factors that have profound short- and long-term consequences for individual women, infants, families, and society. Both PTB and LBW infants are more likely than those born of normal weight and at term to experience significant adverse and developmental outcomes, factors that have social and economic costs on multiple levels simultaneously. Access to perinatal and neonatal specialists and advanced technology have been of positive benefit for women experiencing difficult pregnancies, achievements that have significantly contributed to the survival and long-term health of preterm and low-birth-weight infants.

For women who are disadvantaged through a lack of access to adequate housing and nutrition and who live with the intersecting risks of poverty, violence, addiction, and HIV, pregnancy and birth outcomes are considerably worse. Deprivation of such social determinants of health leads to poorer health status in pregnancy. For many women, ensuring optimal pregnancy, fetal, and infant outcomes involves providing primary maternal health services suited to the social, cultural, historical, geographical, and demographic features of specific locales, while also acting upon the structural inequities that impact maternal health.

The Complexity of Access to Maternity Care

Within Canada, it is assumed that women have equal access to contraception, antenatal care, safe facilities in which to give birth, and trained staff to provide pregnancy, delivery, and postpartum care; the diagnosis and treatment of sexually transmitted infections (STIs), including HIV; infertility treatment; and care for unsafe or unintended pregnancy. Many reproductive health initiatives aim to address the complex interplay of economic, sociodemographic factors, health status, and health service factors associated with elevated risk of morbidity and mortality related to reproductive events during the life course. Access to care, however, is also shaped by geography, local healthcare, maternity practices and policies, health human resources, and availability of culturally safe services.

From a population health perspective, access to comprehensive and culturally relevant care is a key determinant of maternal health. For example, in many First Nations communities, historic emphasis on supposedly necessary modern medical interventions by doctors spread to Aboriginal health services. The impact was that many ancient birthing and midwifery practices were eroded and few Aboriginal midwives were left to pass along indigenous knowledge and traditional practices. The removal of births from many Aboriginal communities has had profound spiritual and cultural consequences, which are difficult to quantify (National Aboriginal Health Organization, 2004). While "access" to care is available for women transferred to urban centres, significant social and economic costs are incurred that create risks for mothers and families when leaving home (Smith, 2002). When women are separated from the support of families and friends, there is an increase in small, premature infants, as well as maternal and newborn complications, even though the majority of women have come to maternity centres providing a good standard of care (Klein, Johnston, Christilaw, & Carty, 2002).

Reproductive Mental Health

Women are approximately twice as likely as men to experience depression. The effects of stress, violence, poverty, inequality, and low self-esteem likely increase women's vulnerability to depression (Bowen, Stewart, Baetz, & Muhajarine, 2009). The highest rates of depression are seen among women of reproductive age. Approximately 10–20% of pregnant women suffer from depression, and any life situation that creates social disadvantage increases risks for depression (Bowen et al., 2009). Women living in poverty and experiencing significant social and health inequities are at a higher risk for perinatal depression.

Perinatal depression, which occurs from the time of conception to one year after birth, is a significant health issue in Canada. Perinatal depression can be experienced during the antenatal or postnatal period, described as *antenatal* or *postpartum depression*; both are potentially deleterious to the mother and fetus/infant. Perinatal depression is different from the "**baby blues**"—a feeling of distress and tearfulness that can affect mothers of newborns and usually disappears within the first few weeks of their baby's birth. **Perinatal depression** covers a spectrum of illnesses affecting women, from depressive symptoms to a major depressive episode occurring at any time between conception and one year following the birth of their child. Five or more of the following symptoms

---

CASE STUDY: The Economic and Health Consequences of Leaving Home to Give Birth

The economic burden of costs to family members is extremely stressful for pregnant mothers. It is not uncommon for the expectant mothers from rural Aboriginal communities to travel significant distances for childbirth. A woman from Alert Bay, BC, spoke of having to wait for a month or longer "down island" until it was time to give birth. Without financial support, families are unable to live "down island" for four to six weeks with the expectant mother. "It only seems reasonable that if women are expected to go down island because we can't have a delivery facility here, then the government should pay for the costs of housing us down there. Either build us the capability to deliver babies here or pay for our expenses to go to where those facilities are located." Another woman from the same First Nations community on Vancouver Island stated: "The hardships the mom faces being away from home are loneliness, being scared, and worrying about the well-being of the other children left at home. Everyone worries and it is a long time to be away" (Calam, Varcoe, & Brown, 2008, p. 39).

Discussion Questions

1. How does the geographic context of women's lives impact the economic burden of their birthing experiences?

2. Imagine that local maternity care policies do not allow for low-risk birthing facilities in a rural and remote community. What role can the CHN play to facilitate a positive birthing experience away from home? What actions could be taken to minimize negative economic and social consequences for the parent/family–infant relationship?

3. What population health promotion strategies can mitigate the negative impacts of birthing away from home?

experienced most of the day, nearly every day, for two weeks or more contribute to a diagnosis:

- Feelings of sadness, emptiness, and helplessness
- Extreme feelings of guilt, worthlessness, and hopelessness
- Loss of interest and pleasure in activities enjoyed in the past, including sex
- Decreased energy, feeling of fatigue
- Changes in sleep or appetite
- Restlessness and irritability
- Difficulty concentrating or remembering
- Thoughts of death or suicide (BC Reproductive Mental Health Program, 2006).

Maternal depression affects approximately 10% of mothers, but up to 50% of women who experience depression during pregnancy or postpartum depression are undiagnosed, since the condition can mimic the mood changes associated with normal pregnancy (Public Health Agency of Canada, 2010). The greatest challenge lies in the complexity of association between maternal depression and other issues, including poverty, teen pregnancy, isolation, and family violence. The impact of perinatal depression, however, is not borne by mothers alone. The babies of perinatally depressed women are at increased risk for low birth weight and preterm birth, and a mother's experience of depression influences her ability to create a healthy attachment relationship with her infant. Children of mothers who experience perinatal depression exhibit deficiencies in cognitive, behavioural, and social skills (Grace, Evindar, & Stewart, 2003). In British Columbia, the BC Reproductive Mental Health Program (2006) created an "upstream approach" framework for addressing perinatal depression for outlining a Four Pillar approach:

1. Education and prevention
2. Screening and diagnosis
3. Treatment and self-management
4. Coping and support networks

Violence and Maternal Health Violence against women remains an endemic problem that has a tremendous impact on the health of mothers and of their children (Status of Women Canada, 2010). Intimate partner violence is a real or threatened physical, sexual, emotional, or physical abuse perpetrated against a spouse or life partner. The impacts include unwanted pregnancies and miscarriages, sexually transmitted diseases including HIV/AIDS, psychological trauma, and poor mental health. These place pregnant women experiencing violence at greater risk for adverse birth outcomes and postnatal depression. Poverty, homelessness, lost educational/employment opportunities, loss of self-esteem, and loss of safety create compounding social impacts that also contribute to health risks in pregnancy and poor maternal, fetal, and infant outcomes. Violence against women has been recognized as a violation of human rights, an important health policy issue, and a problem with alarming socioeconomic costs to society (Hankivsky & Varcoe, 2007). (See Chapter 26.)

Violence in the lives of childbearing women and mothers is not experienced equally by all women in Canada. Different

CANADIAN RESEARCH BOX

What are maternal perceptions of a postpartum depression peer support intervention?

Dennis, C. L. (2010). Postpartum depression peer support: Maternal perceptions from a randomized controlled trial. *International Journal of Nursing Studies, 47*(5), 560–568.

In this randomized controlled trial, the effectiveness of a peer support intervention for high-risk women is examined. Women from seven health regions in Ontario who were determined to be at risk for postnatal depression were randomly assigned to receive usual postpartum care or usual postpartum care plus telephone-based peer support. Emotional, informational, and appraisal support was reported by 80.5% of mothers as the reason they were satisfied with their peer support experience. In particular, the mothers reported trust and acceptance are increasing their satisfaction. Nursing implications include the enhancement of existing postpartum support to include peer-based relationships matched with mothers' desire for support, age, parity, and breastfeeding status as a prevention strategy for postpartum depression.

Discussion Questions

1. Describe the relevance of the study findings for postpartum support resources provided by CHNs. How can peer support and peer volunteer experience mitigate the risks for postpartum depression?

2. Taking into account how social inclusion and exclusion are social determinants of health, how can the findings of this study inform CHN practice aimed toward the prevention of postpartum depression?

sources of subjugation and oppression manifest in the context of women's lives and produce different vulnerabilities. Aboriginal women, women of colour, lesbians, immigrant women, women living with disabilities, young women, and older women face greater risks for violence (Day & McMullen, 2005), and the impacts of violence on childbearing women's lives intersect with the social determinants of health to increase risk throughout the childbearing years. Physical and emotional violence threatens women's health during pregnancy and can place a fetus at risk for low birth weight and other detrimental conditions, such as brain damage and broken limbs (Boy & Salihu, 2004).

Mental Health and Addictions in Pregnancy Use of alcohol, drugs, or both during pregnancy creates risks such as premature labour, abruptio placentae, still birth, and other complications (Bhuvaneswar & Chang, 2009). Specific substances are correlated with specific effects on the pregnancy and fetal health. For example, alcohol-related effects put the fetus at risk for various disorders such as fetal alcohol spectrum disorder, while heroin has been linked to Sudden Infant Death Syndrome. Because maternal cocaine use restricts uterine blood flow and placental function, it has been linked to numerous adverse fetal outcomes such as intrauterine growth restriction and organ malformations. Subtle effects on the growth and development of young children warrant attention and early identification, and community health nurses (CHNs) are well positioned to identify infants and young children experiencing these effects and to begin processes of early intervention. Withdrawal symptoms for mothers, infants, or both include irritability, poor feeding, respiratory complications, tremors, and other neuropsychological challenges.

Nursing practice with these women and their families goes beyond simply providing education about the adverse effects of substance use on their fetus, to considerations of the complex causes of the connections among mental health, substance use, and addiction. *Harm reduction* approaches to substance use in pregnancy are emerging to mitigate the harmful effects on both mothers and fetuses. Women can be treated with methadone during pregnancy and have been shown to achieve a better chance of a positive pregnancy outcome than women who are not treated. (See Chapter 28.)

HEALTH PROMOTION AND YOUNG CHILDREN'S HEALTH IN CANADA

As a prosperous country, Canada has a universal healthcare system and a variety of services and programs, many of which are directed toward the health and development of infants and preschool children. Despite this, among Organization for Economic Co-operation and Development (OECD) nations, Canada ranks 22nd when it comes to preventable childhood injuries and deaths, 27th in childhood obesity, and 21st in overall child well-being (UNICEF Innocenti Research Centre, 2007). These and other health indicators suggest that there is much to do to improve infant and child health in Canada and CHNs have many opportunities to contribute to these efforts (Leitch, 2007).

CHNs encounter infants and preschool children in a variety of community settings: homes, daycare centres, preschools, and community health centres. They have diverse opportunities to work with infants, children, and their families toward optimizing their health in ways that have far-reaching effects on children's later well-being. CHNs can create programs with nursing activities related to fostering the social, emotional, and physical growth and development of infants and children, while paying particular attention to the complex contexts of their young lives. Infants and young children are also particularly vulnerable to certain specific illnesses (both acute and chronic) and injuries (both accidental and non-accidental). Understanding these vulnerabilities provides direction to CHNs as they develop individual and population-based approaches promoting the health and well-being of this group.

The term **child health** is generally used to refer to the broad range of physical, social, cognitive, and emotional

indicators of child well-being. Health and development during the early years of life have profound consequences for well-being in later life. Research shows that individuals' physical, socioemotional, and cognitive potential are profoundly shaped by the experiences of infancy and the preschool years (Kershaw, Anderson, Warburton, & Hertzman, 2009; National Scientific Council on the Developing Child, 2007a). Therefore, efforts to promote young children's health, including fostering growth and development, have profound implications for the children themselves, their families, and our communities. CHNs are well positioned to assess children's growth and development and to assist families to provide the kind of supportive and nurturing environments that maximize children's opportunities. This section focuses on areas of concern related to Aboriginal children's health and the health of infants and young children, in particular, growth and development during infancy and the preschool years, diet and nutrition, and parenting practices.

Aboriginal Children's Health

One in four children living in First Nations communities lives in poverty. This is in contrast with the overall rate of poverty among Canadian children (one in nine) (United Nations Children's Fund [UNICEF], 2009). The health of aboriginal children is far worse than in the general Canadian population. The problems include higher infant mortality rates and greater incidence of conditions such as obesity, asthma, and fetal alcohol spectrum disorder.

Discussion of young children's health requires consideration of the issue of *children's rights*. The United Nations Convention on the Rights of the Child (UNICEF, 1989) document guarantees all children various rights related to protection, participation, and survival and development. These rights are summarized in Table 15.1.

TABLE 15.1	Children's Rights under the United Nations Convention on the Rights of the Child (UNICEF, 1989)
Rights	These rights include
Survival and development rights	■ adequate food, water, and shelter ■ formal education ■ primary health care ■ leisure and recreation ■ information about their rights
Protection	■ protection from all forms of child abuse, neglect, and exploitation ■ special protection during times of war ■ special protection within the judicial system
Participation	■ freedom to express opinions and to have a say in the important matters of their lives ■ right to information and freedom of association

The Importance of Relationships The core concepts of development listed in "Core Concepts of Development" highlight the importance of relationships for ensuring the well-being of infants and young children. Children's development is profoundly influenced by relationships with the important people in their lives. The very architecture of a child's brain is shaped by the establishment and sustenance of these relationships. CHNs are often faced with questions about infants' and children's relationships with siblings, parents, other children, and caretakers. Secure, stable attachments contribute to infants' and young children's sense of safety and security in the world, to their evolving sense of self, and to their capacity to develop and sustain meaningful relationships throughout their lives. The National Scientific Council on the Developing Child (2007b) summarized the following research evidence that may guide CHNs working with infants and young children and their families:

- The emotional connection between an infant and mother (or other primary caregiver) shapes the infant's brain architecture and creates the conditions wherein learning and engagement with the world can be fostered and affirmed.
- Young children benefit from relationships with other children. They learn important skills for engaging with others and begin the lifelong process of participating in social life.
- Sustained stable relationships with caring adults are essential for infants and young children because it is in these relationships that adults assure that young children's needs are met—including needs for nutrition; for protection from injury, illness, and excessive stress; and for various health promotion activities.
- Parent–child relationships can be strengthened although successful interventions in this area are more difficult to achieve in families experiencing violence or serious disruption.
- Infants and young children are very vulnerable to negative effects arising from parental mental health problems and family violence.

This research evidence provides justification of CHNs work not only to assess and support the physical, social, emotional, and cognitive growth and development of infants and young children, but also to pay particular attention to the primary relationships in the child's life. Supporting families in their efforts to care for their children, and creating or advocating for policies that ease the stress on the parents of young children (particular those families who are particularly vulnerable) will go a long way toward promoting optimal growth and development among infants and preschool children.

Negative Effects of Excess Stress Excess stress has a detrimental effect on brain development (National Scientific Council on the Developing Child, 2005). **Toxic stress** refers to excessive and frequent activations of the body's stress management

Core Concepts of Development

Child development is a foundation for community development and prosperity, as capable children are crucial to a prosperous and sustainable society.

Brains are built over time.

The interaction between genes and experience shapes the architecture of the developing brain. The key ingredient to healthy development is the nature of children's relationships with parents and other care-givers.

Both brain architecture and developing abilities are built "from the bottom up," with simple abilities and skills providing the scaffolding for more advanced learning.

Toxic stress in infancy and early childhood has persistent effects on the nervous system and stress systems that can damage developing brain architecture and lead to lifelong problems in learning, behaviour, and both physical and mental health.

Creating the right conditions for development in infancy and early child hood is likely more effective and cost-efficient than addressing established problems in later years.

Adapted from National Scientific Council on the Developing Child. (2007a). The science of early childhood development: Closing the gap between what we know and what we do. Cambridge, MA: Author.

systems. When these systems are overloaded for a prolonged period of time, the young child's brain is affected and the stress system may be shifted so that it responds significantly to events that may not be stressful to other infants or young children. Because the neural circuits for dealing with stress are particularly sensitive during the early childhood years, prolonged toxic stress may result in heightened vulnerability to a range of physical and psychological courses through the lifespan (National Scientific Council on the Developing Child). Not surprisingly, the relationships children have with their parents and other caregivers play important roles in regulating the young child's stress responses during the early years of life. This knowledge is important for CHNs, as various family situations, including economic hardship, family violence, or child maltreatment, and the availability of affordable, quality child care, all have consequences for the young child's lifelong well-being.

Nutrition in Infancy and the Preschool Years Nutrition is crucial to the growth and development of infants and young children, and diet and nutrition are usually a central concern of parents and other caregivers. For these reasons, CHNs need to have a sense of general principles related to eating patterns and nutrition for infants and young children, as well as access to resources addressing the many issues presented by the various caregivers among this group of children. Assessing an infant's or young child's nutritional status involves obtaining detailed information about the child's usual 24-hour intake, obtaining comprehensive medical histories from the parents and other caregivers, and measuring the infant or young child's height (or length) and weight. CHNs may be involved in a variety of interventions intended to support optimal nutrition. These may include counselling families or parent groups about nutrition for young children, referral of infants and young children with their families for medical or nutritional follow-up, and screening for nutritional challenges such as failure to thrive, lactose intolerance, and obesity.

Nutrition in Infancy Nutrition is vital in the first year of life—this is a time of rapid growth, with birth weight generally doubling in the first six months of life and tripling by the end of the first year. Infants born at low birth weights or prematurely are particularly vulnerable to inadequate nutrition in the first months of life. When loss of weight, developmental delay, symptoms of malnourishment, or failure to thrive (FTT) occur, the possibility of nutritional deficits must be explored and, if identified, intervention is necessary. Many factors may contribute to inadequate nutrition during infancy. Lack of financial resources, substance misuse, insufficient family support, lack of knowledge, difficulty breastfeeding, and a variety of physiological conditions may contribute to inadequate nutrition in infancy. Based on the CHN's assessment, intervention may be warranted. These interventions may include education, assisting parents to access resources, referral to dietary experts, or referral for medical assessment.

Failure to thrive occurs when an infant falls below the third percentile for both weight and height on standard growth charts. There are three categories of FTT: organic, non-organic, and idiopathic. *Non-organic FTT* is generally caused by factors related to parents' ability to provide adequate nutrition for their infant (Reifsnider, 2007), while *organic FTT* is caused by physical problems such as cardiac or respiratory illness. When no cause is identified, *idiopathic FTT* may be diagnosed. Failure to thrive may have significant long-term consequences, so early identification is ideal. Assessment of the infant's growth and development, including height and weight, as well as observation of various aspects of the familial and social situation of the child and family, will assist in addressing this significant problem.

Nutrition in the Preschool Years Nutrition during the early years of life has implications for the child's well-being throughout the lifespan. Currently, substantial attention has been drawn to the growing problem of obesity among children and adults, with growing evidence that adult obesity has its roots in early childhood dietary patterns (Ben-Sefer, BenNaten, & Ehrenfeld, 2009). In attempting to provide proper diets for their young child, parents are often faced with young children with decreased appetite and strong preferences regarding food. CHNs need to work with these families and reassure parents that the swings in children's preferences is usual, while assessing for potential nutritional deficits or dietary patterns. Generally, preschool children like small portions of food, and are drawn to finger foods. There are many guides for parents as they grapple with the fickle appetites and food preferences of young children. (See Additional Resources at the end of this chapter.)

Not all families have access to the food necessary to meet the dietary needs of their children. The goal of community nursing practice would be more about assisting families to access the resources needed to provide for their children than simply about education regarding nutritional practices in the home. Each community is different on this front, and CHNs require knowledge about emergency funding for families, social services support, food banks, and other potential resources.

Child Abuse and Neglect Although the guidelines for child abuse or neglect reporting differ, in all provinces in Canada, nurses and all other professionals are legally required to intervene and report suspected incidents of the abuse or neglect of an infant or child. Most health agencies have specific guidelines for assessing and reporting concerns about child abuse or neglect. (See MyNursingLab for "Hook &Hub" Approach to Community-Based and Community-Paced Early Childhood Health Promotion.)

A RELATIONAL APPROACH TO MATERNAL AND CHILD HEALTH PROMOTION

Maternal and child health are dynamic experiences that are personally and contextually constructed. A *relational approach* to maternal and child health promotion is based on the assumption that people are contextual beings who live their lives in relation with others and with social, cultural, political, and historical processes and communities (Thayer-Bacon, 2003). Doane and Varcoe (2005) note that because people are relational beings, their experiences of health, their health status, and their health needs are complex and multifaceted. They outline the following processes and skills of relational practice relevant for CHNs engaged in promoting women and children's health *within* families, communities, and populations:

- A socioenvironmental approach to health promotion assumes women and children have strengths and resources that can be enlisted during nursing assessments and interventions. While women and children will clearly have health needs and problems that require servicing, an overriding emphasis on deficiency can disempower women, children, and families. The expertise, proficiency, and techniques of CHNs are not the single source of knowledge and authority for solving health problems; rather, the nurse's skills are enlisted not to "do for" but to "do with," such that women and children's capacities are realized.

- Assessment frameworks and tools are useful for gathering information; however, there is potential that the tool itself may mean that the nurses' questions and approaches for collecting information override those of individual women, children, and families. For example, the Edinburg Postnatal Depression Scale (Cox, Holden, & Sagovsky, 1987) provides effective screening for women at risk; however, it cannot replace conversation and discussion between CHNs and new mothers to reveal the broader context of women's lives within which depression is manifested.

- Inquiring into what is meaningful for women and children creates the chance for CHNs to "follow the lead" of individual women/children, families, groups, and communities. Through being curious, tuning into women's and children's capacities and resources, and by being cautious about assuming the stance of an expert, CHNs, women, and children can work together to put in place the conditions for optimal health.

A relational approach to CHN practice with women/mothers and children involves engaging in action to promote population health promotion and policy that facilitates health equity. CHNs have an important role to play for recognizing, naming, and addressing inequities and structural conditions, taking a critical stance toward discourses that marginalize women and children (i.e., good mothers stay at home to raise their children), and developing a critical approach to healthcare practice and policies that facilitate access to effective programs and services aimed to enhance maternal and child health.

CANADIAN RESEARCH BOX

How do public health nurses promote health for high priority families?

Browne, A. J., Hartrick Doane, G., Reimer, J., MacLeod, M. L. P., & McLelland, E. (2010). Public health nursing practice with "high priority" families: The significance of contextualizing "risk." *Nursing Inquiry, 17*(1), 27–38.

This study explored how public health nurses engage with and promote health for "high priority" families. The findings from focus groups with 32 PHNs indicate how they use relational approaches to understand and account for the contextual complexities that shape families' lives, while also supporting families who are under "surveillance." Nursing implications from this study indicate the importance of contextualizing risk and capacity within the context of families' lives as the basis for creating and sustaining effective working relationships with families.

Discussion Questions

1. How can reconceptualizing "risk" tap the strengths, resources, and capacities of socially complex women, children, and families?

2. What actions strategies can CHNs champion that can mitigate the conditions for risk in women's/mothers' and children's lives?

SUMMARY

With maternal and child health now dominating the international political agenda, and given its central position during the G8 Summit in Canada in June of 2010, the need for effective primary health care strategies occupies the attention of Canadians and health leaders around the world. CHNs who engage with women and children as individuals, and within families, groups, communities, and populations, make a significant contribution to their everyday health and well-being. As CHNs integrate population health promotion approaches with socioenvironmental perspectives on maternal and child health, significant advances can be made towards redressing health inequities that shape the lives and health of women and children in Canada. By integrating principles of relational practice, CHNs can also act upon the contexts of women's and children's lives while also engaging in health promotion actions that address the complex interplay of a range of factors that are genetic, environmental, and behavioural. The ethical and professional commitments of CHN practice will uphold the legacy of *Making every mother and child count* in Canada now and into the future.

KEY TERMS

maternal health, p. 253
maternal healthcare, p. 253
reproductive health, p. 254
reproductive justice, p. 254
reproductive rights, p. 254
women's health, p. 254
liberal individualism, p. 254
total fertility rate, p. 254
midwife, p. 255
baby blues, p. 257
perinatal depression, p. 257
child health, p. 259
toxic stress, p. 260
failure to thrive, p. 261

REVIEW QUESTIONS

1. Women's health can best understood as shaped by
   a) genetic endowment.
   b) biology.
   c) behaviour.
   d) an interplay of personal and environmental factors.

2. Mothering, when intertwined with poverty,
   a) impacts childhood nutrition.
   b) cannot be considered a political issue.
   c) is not a health policy issue.
   d) is only relevant during the preschool years.

3. Living with more than one source of material deprivation (i.e., inadequate housing, food insecurity)

a) creates positive birth outcomes.

b) does not impact access to prenatal care.

c) is not a healthcare issue.

d) exacerbates poor health status in pregnancy.

4. Screening for antenatal depression is important because

a) it can enhance postpartum support and access to resources.

b) it can prevent postpartum depression.

c) it cannot be treated in pregnancy.

d) it is unresponsive to non-pharmacological treatment.

5. The most important ingredient in a child's healthy development is

a) access to material resources.

b) genetic predisposition.

c) access to health and sustained relationships with caring adults.

d) freedom from stress.

6. Toxic stress has a negative effect on child development and children's long-term health. It affects child development primarily through

a) altering brain structure and function.

b) disrupting relationships with adults.

c) the resulting physical injuries.

d) preventing the development of relationships with other children.

7. Which of the following is the CHN's primary responsibility when child abuse or neglect is suspected?

a) to assess the family structure and function and seek to bolster parental coping mechanisms

b) to report the potential incidence of abuse or neglect to the relevant provincial regulatory body

c) to question the child about the source of the injury or the extent of the neglect

d) to inquire about past incidents of abuse or neglect within the specific family

STUDY QUESTIONS

1. Describe how maternal health has been shaped by the sociopolitical context of women's health in Canada.

2. Name one strategy for enhancing the health of new mothers.

3. Outline two critical periods for healthy child development.

4. Define the difference between the terms *health inequality* and *health inequity* and name one strategy for reducing each for mothers and children.

5. Describe how a social determinants of maternal and child health perspective and a relational approach can help CHNs identify the adversities that might constrain women/children's power, choice, and ability to achieve optimal health.

6. Considering current concerns about "food security," describe one population health intervention that can enhance prenatal nutrition for mothers living in rural and remote communities.

> After working through these questions, go to the MyNursingLab at *www.pearsoned.ca/mynursinglab* to check your answers.

INDIVIDUAL CRITICAL THINKING EXERCISES

1. Why is it important for CHNs to know about maternal and child health in a global context?

2. Visit the website of your territorial/provincial nursing association or regulatory body and consider how policy, position, or best practice guidelines can facilitate primary health care for mothers and children.

3. What is the relationship between the CNA Code of Ethics and the CHN's role in reducing inequities in maternal and child health?

4. What threats to child rights are amenable to CHN action?

GROUP CRITICAL THINKING EXERCISES

1. Select one infant health outcome reported in the Canadian Perinatal Health Report (2008), http://www.publichealth.gc.ca/cphr/. Describe how a social determinants of health approach to CHN practice can promote population health for infants in Canada.

2. Assume that your student group is a team of researchers preparing to submit a proposal to develop test the efficacy of two interventions to (1) reduce postpartum depression and (2) increase breastfeeding rates and duration for the specific population of young mothers living in an urban context. What intervention(s) will you propose for this investigation and how can the findings be integrated into CHN practice?

3. Daycare staff ask you for a presentation about nutrition for children ages 2–5. What key principles will you integrate into your presentation plan?

NOTES

1. LBW: an infant born with a birth weight of less than 2500 grams.

2. PTB: an infant born prior to 37 weeks' gestation.

3. Infant mortality rate: number of deaths of live-born infants within the first year of life per total infants born in a given year.

REFERENCES

Alfirevic, Z., Devane, D., & Gyte, G. (2007). Continuous cardiotocography (CTG) as a form of electronic fetal monitoring (EFM) for fetal assessment during labour. *The Cochrane Library, 3:* CD006066.

Amnesty International USA. (2005, July 20). *Reproductive rights: A fact sheet.* Retrieved from http://www.amnestyusa .org/women/pdf/reproductiverights.pdf

BC Reproductive Mental Health Program. (2006, July). *Addressing perinatal depression: A framework for BC's health authorities* (Brochure). Retrieved from http://www .bcwomens.ca/NR/rdonlyres/483927DE-698E-42A7-89E5-6E7080D6ABA9/18624/Perinatal _Brochure. pdf%29

Ben-Sefer, E., Ben-Natan, M., & Ehrenfeld, M. (2009). Childhood obesity: Current literature, policy and implications for practice. *International Nursing Review, 56*(2), 166–173.

Bhuvaneswar, C., & Change, G. (2009). Substance use in pregnancy. In K. T. Brady, S. E. Back, & S. F. Greenfield (Eds.), *Women and addiction* (pp. 432–525). New York, NY: The Guilford Press.

Bowen, A., Stewart, N., Baetz, M., & Muhajrine, N. (2009). Antenatal depression in socially high-risk women in Canada. *Journal of Epidemiology and Community Health, 63,* 414–416.

Boy, A., & Salihu, H. (2004). Intimate partner violence and birth outcomes: A systematic review. *International journal of fertility and women's medicine, 49*(4), 159–164.

Brown, H., Varcoe, C., & Calam, B. (in press). Rural Aboriginal women's birthing experiences in context: Implications for practice. *Canadian Journal of Nursing Research.* Accepted for publication, December 2009.

Browne, A. J. (2001). The influence of liberal political ideology on nursing science. *Nursing Inquiry, 8*(2), 118–129.

Browne, A. J. (2005). Discourses influencing nurses' perceptions of First Nations patients. *Canadian Journal of Nursing Research, 37,* 62–87.

Browne, A. J., Hartrick Doane, G., Reimer, J., MacLeod, M. L. P., & McLelland, E. (2010). Public health nursing practice with "high priority" families: The significance of contextualizing "risk." *Nursing Inquiry, 17*(1), 27–38.

Bryanton, J., & Beck, C. T. (2010, January 20). Postnatal education for optimizing infant general health and parent–infant relationships. *Cochrane Database of Systematic Reviews,* 1.

Calam, B., Varcoe, C., & Brown, H. (2008). *Rural Aboriginal maternity care report.* Final report submitted to CIHR.

Campaign 2000. (2009). *2009 report card on child and family poverty in Canada: 1989–2009.* Retrieved from www.campaign2000.ca

Canadian Association of Midwives. (2010). *What is a Canadian registered midwife?* Retrieved from http:// www.canadianmidwives.org/what-is-a-midwife.html

Cox, L., Holden, J. M., & Sagovsky, R. (1987) Detection of postnatal depression: Development of the 10-item Edinburgh Postnatal Depression Scale. *British Journal of Psychiatry,150,* 782–786.

Day, S., & McMullen, N. (2005). *A decade of going backwards: Canada in the post-Beijing era.* Canadian Feminist Alliance for International Action. Retrieved from http://fafia-afai.org/images/pdf/B10_0105.pdf

De Koninck, M. D. (1998). Reflections on the transfer of "progress": The case of reproduction. In S. Sherwin (Ed.), *The politics of women's health: Exploring agency and autonomy* (pp. 150–177). Philadelphia, PA: Temple University Press.

Doane, G. H., & Varcoe, C. (2005). *Family nursing as relational inquiry: Developing health promoting practices.* Philadelphia, PA: Lippincott, Williams & Wilkins.

Dominguez, T. P. (2008). Race, racism, and racial disparities in adverse birth outcomes. *Clinical Obstetrics and Gynecology, 51*(2), 360–370.

Geronimus, A. T. (2001). Understanding and eliminating racial inequalities in women's health in the United States: The role of the weathering framework. *Journal of the American Medical Women's Association, 56*(4), 133–136.

Grace, S. L., Evindar A., & Stewart, D. E. (2003). The effect of postpartum depression on child cognitive development and behavior: A review and critical analysis of the literature. *Archive of Women's Mental Health, 6*(4), 263–274.

Hankivsky, O., & Varcoe, C. (2007). From global to local and over the rainbow. In M. Morrow, O. Hankivsky, & C. Varcoe (Eds.), *Women's health in Canada: Critical perspectives on theory and policy* (pp. 477–506). Toronto, ON: University of Toronto Press.

Institute of Health Economics. (2007, May 23–25). Healthy mothers–healthy babies: How to prevent low birth weight consensus statement. *Institute of Health Economics Consensus Statements, 2.*

Kaufert, P. A., & O'Neil, J. (1993). Analysis of a dialogue on risks in childbirth: Clinician, epidemiologists and Inuit women. In S. Lindenbaum & M. Lock (Eds.), *Knowledge, power and practice: The anthropology of medicine in everyday life* (pp. 32–54). Los Angeles, CA: University of California Press.

Kelm, M.-E. (1998). *Colonizing bodies: Aboriginal health and healing in British Columbia 1900–50.* Vancouver, BC: UBC Press.

Kershaw, P., Anderson, L., Warburton, B., & Hertzman, C. (2009). *15 by 15: A comprehensive policy framework for early human capital investment in BC.* Vancouver, BC: Human Early Learning Partnership.

Klein, M., Johnston S., Christilaw, J., & Carty, E. (2002). Mothers, babies and communities: Centralizing maternity care exposes mothers and babies to complications and endangers community sustainability. *Canadian Family Physician / Medecin De Famille Canadien, 28,* 1177–1179.

Kornelsen, J., & Grzybowski, S. (2006). The reality of resistence: The experiences of rural parturient women. *Journal of Midwifery and Women's Health, 51*(4), 260–265.

Kramer, M. S., Lydon, J., Séguin, L., Goulet, L., Kahn, S. R., McNamara, H., . . . Platt, R. W. (2009). Stress pathways to spontaneous preterm birth: The role of stressors, psychological distress, and stress hormones. *American Journal of Epidemiology, 169,* 1319–1326.

Leitch, K. K. (2007). *Reaching for the top: A report by the advisory on healthy children and youth.* Ottawa, ON: Health Canada.

National Aboriginal Health Organization (NAHO). (2004). *Position paper on midwifery and aboriginal midwifery in Canada.* Ottawa, ON: Author.

National Scientific Council on the Developing Child. (2005). *Excessive stress disrupts the architecture of the developing brain.* Cambridge, MA: Harvard University.

National Scientific Council on the Developing Child. (2007a). *The science of early childhood development: Closing the gap between what we know and what we do.* Cambridge, MA: Author.

National Scientific Council on the Developing Child. (2007b). *Working paper #1. Young children develop in an environment of relationships.* Retrieved from http://www .developingchild.net/pubs/wp/Young_Children_Environment_ Relationships.pdf

Oakley, A. (1984). *The captured womb: A history of medical care of pregnant women.* Oxford, UK: Basil Blackwell.

Public Health Agency of Canada. (2007). *Measuring up: A health surveillance update on Canadian children and youth. Preterm birth.* Retrieved from http://www.phac-aspc.gc.ca/ publicat/meas-haut/mu_d_e.html

Public Health Agency of Canada. (2008). *Canadian perinatal health report.* Ottawa, ON: Author.

Public Health Agency of Canada. (2010). *Government of Canada helping mothers deal with maternal depression: Kitchener-based national program to increase awareness and aid detection.* Retrieved from http://www.phac-aspc.gc.ca/ media/nr-rp/2010/2010_0126-eng.php

Raphael, D. (2006). Social determinants of health: An overview. In D. Raphael, M. H. Rioux, & T. Bryant (Eds.), *Staying alive: Critical perspectives on health, illness and health care* (pp. 115–138). Toronto, ON: Canadian Scholars' Press.

Reifsnider, E. (2007). The use of human ecology and epidemiology in nonorganic failure to thrive. *Public Health Nursing, 12*(4), 262–268.

Ross, L (2006). *Understanding reproductive justice.* Retrieved from http://www.sistersong.net

Royal Commission on Aboriginal People. (1996). *Gathering strength, Vol. 1 & 3, final report.* Retrieved from http:// www.ainc-inac.gc.ca/ch/rcap/sg/sim2_e.html

Silliman, J., Fried, M. G., Ross, L., & Gutierrez, E. R. (2004). *Undivided rights: Women of color organize for reproductive justice.* Cambridge, MA: South End Press.

Smith, D. (2002). *Comprehensive maternal childcare in First Nations and Inuit communities.* Unpublished document. Ottawa, ON: First Nations and Inuit Health Programs Branch, Health Canada.

Statistics Canada. (2007). *2006 census.* Ottawa, ON: Author.

Status of Women Canada: (2010). *National Day of Remembrance and Action on Violence Against Women.* Retrieved from http://www.swc-cfc.gc.ca/dates/vaw-vff/ index-eng.html

Thayer-Bacon, B. (2003). *Relational (e)pistemologies.* New York, NY: Peter Lang.

UNICEF. (2009). *Canadian supplement to The State of the World's Children 2009. Aboriginal children's health: Leaving no child behind.* Toronto, ON: Author.

UNICEF Innocenti Research Centre. (2007). *Child poverty in perspective: An overview of child well-being in rich countries. Report card 7.* Geneva, Switzerland: UNICEF.

United Nations Children's Fund. (1989). *Convention on the rights of the child.* Geneva, Switzerland: Author.

Varcoe, C., Hankivsky, O., & Morrow, M. (2007). Introduction: Beyond gender matters. In M. Marrow, O. Hankivsky, & C. Varcoe (Eds.), *Women's health in Canada* (pp. 3–30). Toronto, ON: University of Toronto Press.

Varcoe, C., & Hartrick Doane, G. (2007). Mothering and women's health. In M. Marrow, O. Hankivsky, & C. Varcoe (Eds.), *Women's health in Canada* (pp. 297–326). Toronto, ON: University of Toronto Press.

World Health Organization. (WHO). (2010a). *2005: Make every mother and child count.* Retrieved from http://www .who.int/world-health-day/previous/2005/en/

World Health Organization. (WHO). (2010b). *Sexual and reproductive health.* Retrieved from http://www.who.int/ reproductivehealth/en/

ADDITIONAL RESOURCES

Readings

Keon, W. J. (2009). Cuba's system of maternal health and early childhood development: Lessons for Canada. *Canadian Medical Association Journal, 180*(3), 314–316.

Marrow, M., Hankivsky, O., & Varcoe, C. (Eds.). (2007). *Women's health in Canada.* Toronto, ON: University of Toronto Press.

Video

National Aboriginal Health Organization (NAHO). (2009). *Celebrating birth: First Nations and Metis approaches to mother and child care* [Video recording]. Ottawa, ON: Author.

Websites

BC Women's Hospital and Health Centre—Reproductive Mental Health
http://www.bcwomens.ca/Services/HealthServices/ ReproductiveMentalHealth/default.htm

Dietitions of Canada—Advancing health through food and nutrition
http://www.dietitians.ca/

Health Canada—Canada's Food Guide: Children
http://www.hc-sc.gc.ca/fn-an/food-guide-aliment/ choose-choix/advice-conseil/child-enfant-eng.php

Health Canada—Women's Health Surveillance Report
http://secure.cihi.ca/cihiweb/products/ CPHI_WomensHealth_e.pdf

Human Early Learning Partnership, UBC
http://www.earlylearning.ubc.ca/

National Aboriginal Health Organization (NAHO)—
Report: Midwifery and Aboriginal midwifery in Canada
http://www.naho.ca/documents/naho/english/
midwifery/podcast01_transcript.pdf

Public Health Agency of Canada—Government of Canada
helping mothers deal with maternal depression
http://www.phac-aspc.gc.ca/media/nr-rp/2010/2010_
0126-eng.php

Public Health Agency of Canada—Depression in Pregnancy
http://www.phac-aspc.gc.ca/mh-sm/preg_dep-eng.php

Public Health Agency of Canada—Canada Prenatal
Nutrition Program (CPNP)
http://www.phac-aspc.gc.ca/dca-dea/programs-mes/
cpnp_goals-eng.php

University of Victoria, Early Childhood Development
Intercultural Partnerships: Hook and hub: Coordinating
program to support indigenous children's early learning and
development
http://www.ecdip.org/docs/pdf/WIPCE%20Hook%20
and%20Hub.pdf

About the Authors

Helen Brown, PhD, RN, is an Assistant Professor in the School of Nursing at the University of British Columbia. Her nursing career spans maternal–infant care in both acute and community contexts, in addition to teaching and research in the area of neonatal care. She is also involved in investigating inequities in maternal–infant health with a particular focus on the social context of adverse birth outcomes. Her involvement in research on maternity care in a rural Aboriginal context provided the impetus for a current study on First Nations culture as a health promotion strategy to enhance equity and health policy processes.

Gladys McPherson, PhD, RN, is an Assistant Professor in the School of Nursing at the University of British Columbia. Her passion is for the nursing care of children, with particular interest in children's rights and children's participation in healthcare decision making. She is currently involved in research projects exploring policy processes relevant to the care of infants and young children, and in another project (with Helen Brown), exploring the relationship between culture and health in Aboriginal communities.

Family Health

Patricia A. Sealy and Julia O. Smith

OBJECTIVES

After studying this chapter, you should be able to:

1. Define family and its basic purposes.
2. Describe the theoretical underpinnings of family healthcare nursing.
3. Discuss the components and basic characteristics of family assessment.
4. Relate family home visits to the Canadian Community Health Nursing Standards and Public Health Core Competencies in practice.
5. Discuss case management and family-centred care.
6. Discuss the opportunities and challenges, including future research, for community health nurses who provide family healthcare nursing.

INTRODUCTION

We all begin life as daughters or sons to our natural and/or adopted parents. We become sisters or brothers, grandchildren, nieces or nephews, and/or cousins within the traditional view of the family. For many, our friends and pets may feel like family members. We assume many different roles in our life and play many different roles in the lives of our family members and friends. Thus, families can be a major source of functional, emotional, psychological, and informational support.

As nurses, our clients also have families and significant others who can make a difference to their lives. It can be perilous for clients if nurses neglect their clients' families and focus solely on treating the individual. Being a family nurse can have personal rewards. Family nurses feel satisfied knowing that they have made a difference in promoting health or reducing suffering in the lives of their clients.

Family health nursing has evolved considerably over the past 20 years to become a specialty area in nursing (Rowe Kaakinen, Gedaly-Duff, Padgett Coehlo, & Harmon Hanson, 2010). Since the family can be a major source of support and influence, community health nurses (CHNs) recognize that "improving the health of families is one way to improve the health of communities" (Cooley, 2009, p. 341).

In this chapter, you will begin to understand the social and cultural context of the family. You will also learn nursing theory to guide the assessment, intervention, and evaluation of family care within the context of the Canadian Community Health Nursing (CCHN) Standards (Community Health Nurses Association of Canada, 2008) and the Public Health Core Competencies (Public Health Agency of Canada, 2007). You will also understand the goals of family case management and family-centred care.

WHY STUDY FAMILY NURSING?

Society tends to romanticize or stigmatize families; the media reflect and reinforce these beliefs (Rank, 2009). The **romanticized family** is a nuclear one with two loving heterosexual parents and two well-accomplished children (typically a son and a daughter). The family lives in a middle-class neighbourhood; the children attend school, have at least above average grades, and play sports and music; the parents have successful careers; and the family attends religious services regularly. The family has a wide network of support through their extended family and friends. Overall, the family is predominantly healthy and easily copes with whatever crisis ensues.

In contrast, the **stigmatized family** has a litany of problems. Typically, these problems include poverty, substance abuse, violence, and learning difficulties. Same-sex couples and single-parent families can be viewed as abhorrent behaviour. Society typifies these families as chaotic and dysfunctional. Many of the family members experience several, often severe, health problems. Some believe that these families deserve or "bring on" their problems, as a result of their poor decisions. It is important for CHNs to consider the impact of their own values and beliefs about family and how these may shape the approach that they take in collaborating with families in the community.

WHAT IS FAMILY?

A **family** is "a social group whose members share common values and interact with each other over time" (Hunt, 2009, p. 81). It is central to society by providing core ingredients that determine the quality of life for its members at all ages (Bomar, 2004). The Vanier Institute of the Family (2010) defines family as "any combination of two or more persons who are bound together over time by ties of mutual consent, birth and/or adoption or placement" (p. xii).

    Family forms include nuclear families, extended families, single-parent families, blended families, and homosexual families. In Canada, same-sex marriage has been legalized across Canada by the *Civil Marriage Act* enacted on July 20, 2005 (Department of Justice Canada, 2009). A pet may even be considered a valued family member for the person, especially if he/she lives alone. Best practice guidelines published by the Registered Nurses Association of Ontario (RNAO) (2006) reinforce that the CHN who works with families should respect each family as being unique and assess individuals in the context of the family as they define it.

    Denham (2005) describes **family function** as "the individual and cooperative processes used by developing persons as to dynamically engage one another and their diverse environments over the life course" (p. 277). The Vanier Institute of the Family (2010) described the following functions or responsibilities assumed by a family:

- physical maintenance and care of group members;
- addition of new members through procreation or adoption;
- socialization of children;
- social control of members;
- production, consumption, distribution of goods and services; and
- affective nurturance—love. (p. xii)

CHNs can address a family's functional processes, as identified above, during healthcare visits. Families may benefit from intervention by CHNs during times of family transitions and/or a health crisis or when setting goals to improve the family's health capacity.

Societal Changes Affecting the Canadian Family

According to the 2006 census (Statistics Canada, 2009), the proportion of traditional families is declining. Statistics Canada (2007a) reports that married couples are now in the minority in Canada with over half of Canadian adults falling into a cohort of never having married; living common-law; or being divorced, separated, or widowed. The number of childless couples is now surpassing those with children. Specifically, "since 1986, the proportion of married couples with children has declined from 49.4 to 34.6%" (p. 1) (Figure 16.1). During this same time period, the percentage of common-law couples with children increased from 3 to 7% and common-law couples without children increased from 4.5 to 9%. It is interesting to note however, that the percentage of common-law couples in Quebec increased 20.3% (Statistics Canada, 2007a), representing one-third of all couples in the province (national average, 13.4%) (Statistics Canada, 2009).

    Other significant demographic changes that are impacting the composition of the family are related to the aging of the Canada population along with increasing life expectancy (Statistics Canada, 2007b). The large cohort of baby-boomers (born between 1946 and 1964) is now moving into their senior years. Younger adults, sometimes referred to as "baby busters," are fewer in numbers. Baby busters tend to have lower fertility rates, leading to the increasing numbers of couples without children. There are also increasing trends for young adults, aged 20 to 29, staying at home with their parents instead of moving into separate dwellings, and for seniors living with their children as part of a three-generation household.

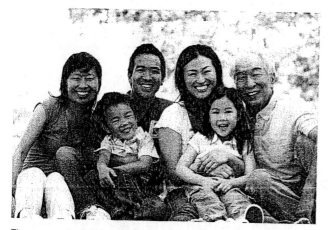

Three-generation households are becoming increasingly common in Canada.

Credit: Monkey Business Images / Shutterstock

FAMILY HEALTH NURSING PRACTICE

Family health nursing is defined in the literature in different ways, and though there is no one overall theory, family nursing is based on theory guided by evidence-based knowledge (Rowe Kaakinen & Harmon Hanson, 2004). Harmon Hanson, (2005a) defined **family healthcare nursing** as

> a process of providing for the health care needs of families that are within the scope of nursing practice. This nursing care can be aimed toward the family as context, the family as a whole, the family as a system, or the family as a component of society. (p. 9)

Nurses in community settings who have the family as client must take a broader and more comprehensive approach to nursing care. In order for the care to be most effective, the

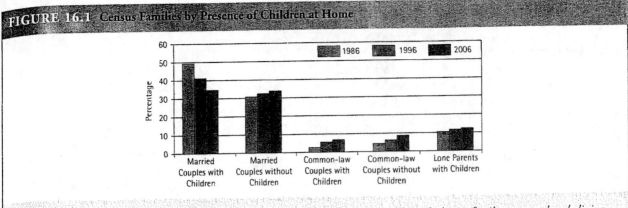

FIGURE 16.1 Census Families by Presence of Children at Home

Source: Statistics Canada. (2009). Married-couple families with children aged 24 and under is the largest family structure, but declining (97-553-XIE). Retrieved from http://www12.statcan.gc.ca/census-recensement/2006/as-sa/97-553/figures/c1-eng.cfm

CHN works within the family's context. The following points are essential to consider when caring for individuals within the context of family (Hunt, 2009):

- "One part of the family cannot be understood in isolation from the rest of the system.
- A family's structure and organization cannot be understood in isolation from the rest of the system.
- Communication patterns between family members are essential in the functioning of the family." (p. 90)

Family as Context

The CHN focuses on either the individual within the context of his or her family or on the family with the individual as context. Viewing the family as context is the traditional focus of nursing, in which the individual is the foreground and the family is in the background (Friedman, Bowden, & Jones, 2003; Harmon Hanson, 2005a). The nurse who interviews a newly married woman with cancer and her husband concerning the woman's experience with the life-threatening illness is an example of concentrating on the individual within the context of family. The nurse who focuses on the family with the individual as context would interview the adult children of a woman with Alzheimer's disease to discover how the family copes with caring for their mother at home.

There are five ways of viewing the family in family nursing (Friedman et al., 2003) (see Figure 16.2):

- The first level is to view the family as context to the client. The CHN focuses nursing care on the individual, with the family as a secondary focus.
- In the second level, the family is viewed as a sum of its individual family members or parts. Healthcare is provided to each individual family member and this is viewed as providing family healthcare. This is not the same as viewing the whole family as the focus of care.
- In the third level of family nursing practice, the focus is on family subsystems. Family dyads, triads, and other family subsystems are the focus of care, for example, a

CHN who focuses on the care of the new mother and her baby during a home visit. Other areas of focus could be caregiving issues and bonding attachment.

- Family as client is the fourth way of viewing the family. The unit of care is the entire family. The nurse does not focus on either the individual or the family, but concentrates on both the individual and the family simultaneously. The interaction that occurs among members of the family is emphasized. In the family-as-client approach to care, the family is in the foreground and individuals are in the background. The nurse would assess each person within the family and provide healthcare for all family members.
- A fifth level of family nursing conceptualizes family as a component of society. The family is seen as one of society's basic institutions. Nursing practice that focuses on the family as client is **family systems nursing**.

Working with families from a systems perspective helps the nurse understand ways in which family members interact, what the family norms and expectations are, how effectively members communicate, how families make decisions, and how families cope with needs and expectations (Rentfro, 2006, p. 154).

Nurses who practise at this level will have extensive knowledge about family dynamics, family systems theory, and family assessment and intervention.

Theoretical Underpinnings of Family Health Nursing

Theories help us to "make sense" of our world; theories that are relevant to families inform and guide nursing practice. Family social science theories, family therapy theories, and nursing models and theories all contribute to the emerging field of family nursing theories. Theories that are oriented to practice are relevant to nurses working with families (Friedman et al., 2003); for example, Neuman's Health System Model (Neuman & Fawcett, 2002) is frequently used by CHNs. The McGill Model (Feeley & Gottlieb, 2000) and the Developmental Model of Health and Nursing (Allen &

FIGURE 16.2 Five Ways of Viewing the Family

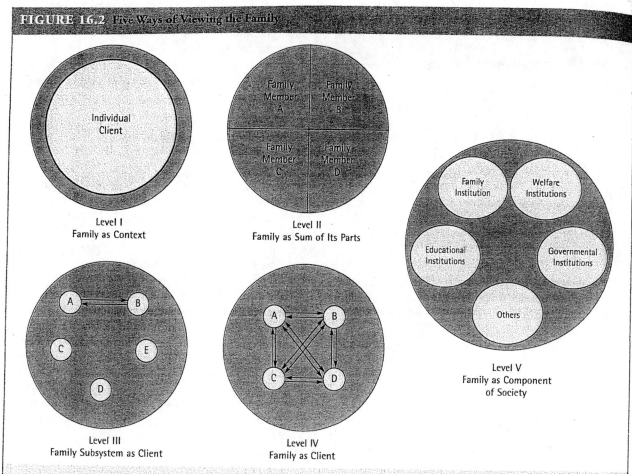

Source: Reproduced with permission from Friedman, M. M., Bowden, V. R., & Jones, E. G. (Eds.). (2003). Family nursing: Research, theory, and practice (5th ed.). Upper Saddle River, NJ: Prentice Hall, p. 37. © Reprinted by permission of Pearson Education, Inc. Upper Saddle River, NJ.

Warner, 2002) are examples of family theories emerging within nursing.

No one theory or conceptual model, however, is sufficient for describing the multifaceted nature of family processes and relationships (Harmon Hanson & Rowe Kaakinen, 2005; Hartrick Doane & Varcoe, 2005; RNAO, 2006). In order to fully understand a variety of perspectives about families and thereby increase the potential for a variety of nursing interventions, CHNs will need to have the knowledge and skill to utilize and integrate multiple theories within the contexts of health promotion and determinants of health. The guiding question becomes: "How do these theories sensitize me to particular families and how will they enhance and/or constrain my ability to responsively attend to particular families at particular times?" (Hartrick Doane & Varcoe, 2005, p. 48).

Although every family is unique, all families share some universal characteristics. Riley-Lawless (2010, p. 477) lists five of the most important characteristics for CHNs to consider:

- Every family is a small social system.
- Every family has its own cultural values and rules.
- Every family has structure.
- Every family has certain basic functions.
- Every family moves through stages in its life cycle.

These universal characteristics reflect the importance of culture as well as structural–functional theory, systems theory, and theories of family development—all theories from the social sciences that have been applied to families. **Structural–functional theory** focuses on how the family structure contributes to and affects family functions. **Systems theory** focuses on the interaction between members of the family system and between the family system and other systems (Artinian, 1999). **Family developmental theory** refers to stages and tasks as presented in Table 16.1. This is a lifecycle approach, which suggests that families move through typical and shared developmental stages, experiencing growth and development in a similar manner to that of individuals (Hitchcock, Schubert, & Thomas, 2003).

The theories, frameworks, and assessment models discussed in this chapter all recognize that the CHN and the family are engaged in a social process of exploration, negotiation, and mutual goal setting, centred within the family–nurse relationship. Interventions are grounded in the contexts of family structure and function, family development, family support and environment, health work and potential health promotion, education and advocacy, determinants of health, and the principles of primary health care.

TABLE 16.1 Family Life Cycle Developmental Stages and Tasks (for North American Middle Class)

Stage	Tasks
Forming partnerships and/or marriage	Commitment to and establishing a new family
Child bearing families	Adjustment to parenthood and new family members
Families with ■ Preschool children ■ School-age children ■ Teenagers	Adjusting to changes in the partner relationship Meeting age-appropriate developmental needs of children
Launching children	Adjustment to needs of young adults leaving and/or re-entering the family
Middle-aged parents	Maintaining supportive relationships with children and across generations
Aging parents	Adjustments to retirement, end of life

FAMILY ASSESSMENT

"A **family assessment** is an exploration between the nurse and family to gain insight into the family's perspective of the event, their strengths and need for support" (RNAO, 2006, p. 23).

During the assessment process, the nurse facilitates the family in discovering and articulating the often unexamined assumptions, context, and expectations underlying its perception of reality. This means that

■ the assessment process takes time, sensitivity, and flexibility.
■ the assessment process starts from the perspective of the family and/or the community.

■ assessments take place in an atmosphere of openness, awareness, mutual collaboration, and relationship-building.
■ assessments are holistic.
■ assessment tools can be adapted and adjusted to identified needs by the client and the nurse, such as time and area of focus.

Regardless of the concepts, models, and tools utilized, a comprehensive family assessment uses open-ended questions, and is detailed and inclusive. Nursing assessments are ongoing, which means they change and develop over time as data are shared with the family and collected by the nurse. An assessment is not "done to" the family, but is rather a process that the nurse facilitates. The act of facilitation sets the tone for building the relationship between the nurse and the family. The assessment process is the first stage of the nursing process, and provides the foundation for planning, interventions, and evaluation of nursing care. It is important, however, for nurses to complete the assessment in an engaging manner since many families may be deterred by a prescribed, impersonal assessment check-list (Hartrick Doane & Varcoe, 2005).

The Friedman Family Assessment Model (Friedman et al., 2003), the Calgary Family Assessment Model (Wright & Leahey, 2009), the McGill Model (Feeley & Gottlieb, 2000; Gottlieb & Rowat, 1987), and the Developmental Model of Health and Nursing (Allen & Warner, 2002) are examples of family assessment models. The latter three were developed in Canada. Essential features of the models are presented in Table 16.2.

Friedman Family Assessment Model

The Friedman Family Assessment Model has six broad categories (see Table 16.2) (Friedman et al., 2003). Identifying data include family composition, cultural background, religious identification, social class status, and recreational activities. The developmental stage is assessed along with the family's history

TABLE 16.2 Components of Family Assessment Models

Friedman Family Assessment	Calgary Family Assessment Model	McGill Model	Developmental Model of Health and Nursing
Identifying data	Developmental stage and history of family	The family as the subsystem	The family as the primary social system
Developmental stage and history of family	Structural	Health as the focus of work	Health work
Environmental data	Developmental	Learning as the process through which health behaviours are acquired	Health potential
Family structure	Functional		Competence in health behaviours
Family functions		Family collaborates with the nurse in the learning process	Health status
Family coping			

Source: Adapted from Registered Nurses' Association of Ontario (2006). Supporting and strengthening families through expected and unexpected life events (rev.suppl.). Toronto, Canada: Registered Nurses' Association of Ontario.

and the history of both parents' family of origin. Environmental data include characteristics of the home, neighbourhood, and community; the family's geographic mobility; associations with the community and use of community resources; and the family's social support system. **Family structure** looks at communication patterns, power structure, role structure, and family values. Affective, socialization, and healthcare functions are assessed in the family functions category. The sixth category, family stress and coping, includes assessment of stressors and strengths along with coping strategies (Friedman et al., 2003). Each category has many subcategories. The nurse and the family decide which areas need in-depth exploration based on the focus for nursing intervention.

Calgary Family Assessment Model

Wright and Leahey (2009) first developed the Calgary Family Assessment Model (CFAM) in 1983 at the University of Calgary. The CFAM has been conceptualized as a branching model with three major categories: structural, developmental, and functional. As in Friedman's model, it has many subcategories. Each nurse decides which subcategories should be explored and assesses each family accordingly. The nurse and the family move back and forth across the branches to build a story of the family and its interactions.

Interventions are conceptualized in the Calgary Family Intervention Model (CFIM), which complements the CFAM and provides a framework for family functions in three domains: cognitive, affective, and behavioural. Interventions focus on promoting, improving, and sustaining effective family functioning. The most effective interventions are congruent with the family's beliefs and values, the articulation of which is facilitated during the assessment (Wright & Leahey, 2009).

McGill Model

The McGill Model has been developed and refined over time by faculty and students at the McGill University School of Nursing (Gottlieb & Rowat, 1987). This model emphasizes family, health, collaboration, and learning. The family is an active participant, with the nurse, in its own healthcare.

One of the goals of nursing, based on the McGill Model, is to help families use the strengths of the individual family members and of the family as unit, as well as resources external to the family system, to cope, achieve their goals, and develop (Feeley & Gottlieb, 2000).

Health consists of processes that are dynamic and multidimensional, especially the processes of coping and development.

FIGURE 16.3 Genogram

Another valuable tool assessment is the genogram, which is used to build a picture of family structure, relationships, and boundaries. This genogram shows the family of Mr. and Mrs. W., who were married in 1990. Mrs. W. is 52 years of age and lives with her 53-year-old husband and their two children, who are nine and 13 years of age. The oldest daughter is in Grade 8 and the younger daughter is in Grade 4 at the local elementary school. Mr. W.'s father died of stomach cancer in 2000 and Mrs. W.'s mother died of pancreatitis in 1962. Mrs. W. did not know her father. Mrs. W. was diagnosed with locally advanced breast cancer in 2008. Mrs. W. works as a researcher and Mr. W. works as an administrator. The W. family is used as a case study later in the chapter.

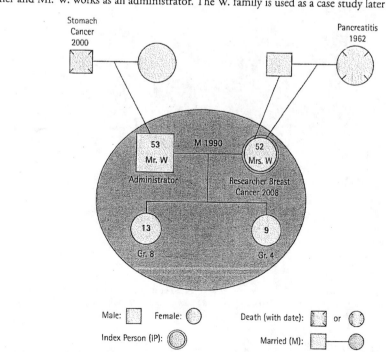

The assessment phase of the McGill Model requires an exploratory approach by the nurse, with the nurse creating a supportive environment so that the family's perceptions and strengths can emerge. Learning needs are identified and the initiative for planning can be with the nurse or the family (Gottlieb & Rowat, 1987). It is during the implementation phase that the family becomes an active learner in collaboration with the nurse. Arising from the McGill Model, the Developmental Model of Health and Nursing emphasizes health as a process, the nurse as an empowering partner, and the potential for families to demonstrate strengths and positive growth.

Many family assessment tools are available (Friedman et al., 2003; RNAO, 2006; Rowe Kaakinen & Harmon Hanson, 2005; Salopek, 2010; Tarko & Reid, 2004). So how does the CHN decide on an assessment tool that will then guide interventions? It is not a case of "one size fits all" or of designing the "perfect" model. Rather, it is having the openness, knowledge, and skill to evaluate existing theories, models, and tools in light of what would be most appropriate and effective for the client, and integrating and adapting as necessary.

Two valuable tools for all assessments are the genogram and ecomap. The **genogram** (see Figure 16.3) is used to build a picture of family structure, relationships, and boundaries. Another tool that is especially useful for CHNs is the **ecomap** (see Figure 16.4), which visually represents a family's connections and the nature of relationships with the larger community and can be used to assess resources and strengths (Tarko & Reed, 2004; Wright & Leahey, 2009).

FIGURE 16.4 Ecomap

The ecomap displays the family members' contact with larger systems; relationships between family members and other community institutions (such as schools, work, etc.)

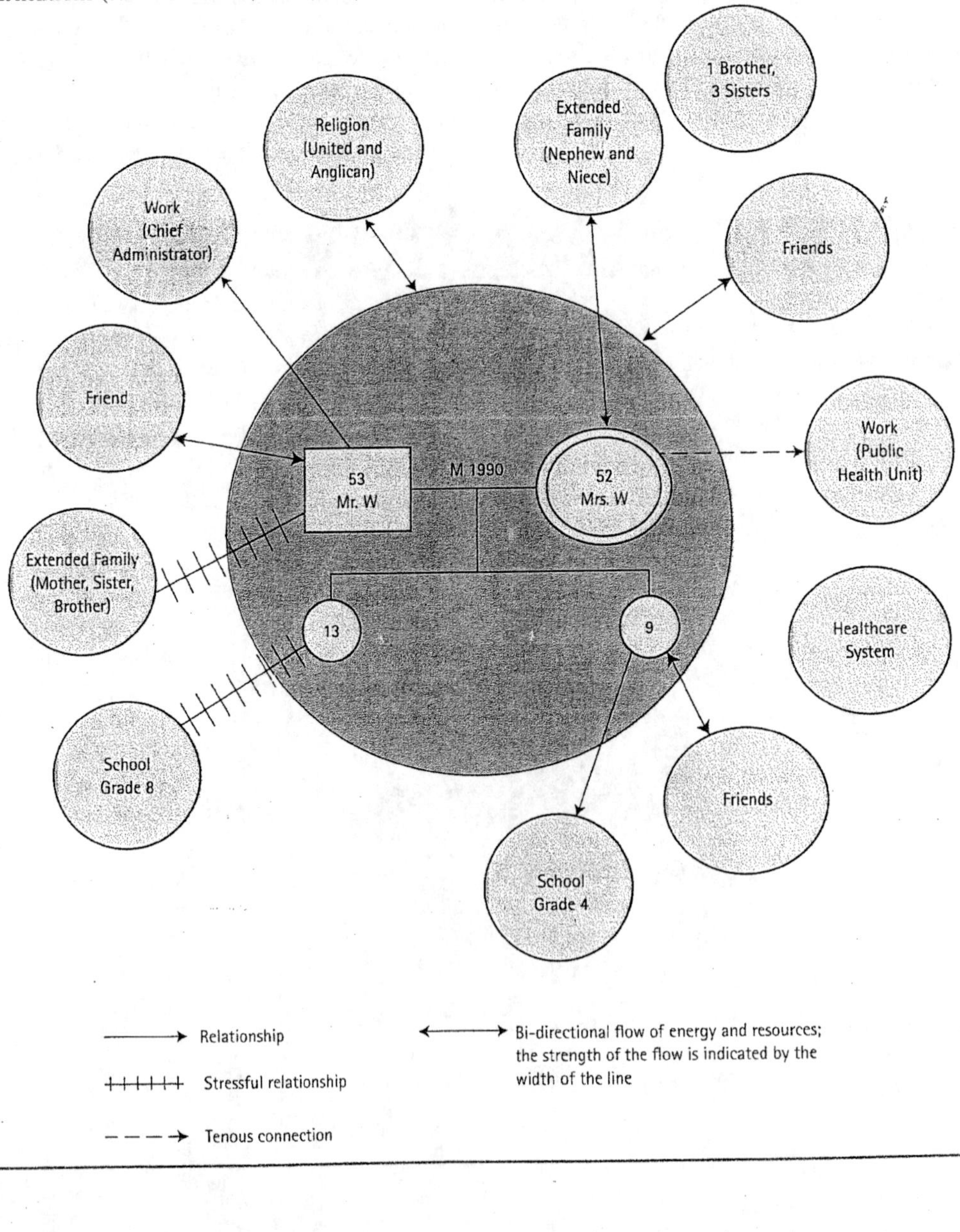

The Family Home Visit

The CCHN Standards and the PHCC are excellent guidelines from which to assess, plan, implement, and evaluate family care. In the context of the family home visit, we begin by focusing on the CCHN Standards of Building Relationships and Professional Responsibility and Accountability, since building a collaborative relationship is the crucial link to the other CCHN Standards of health promotion, building capacity, and facilitating access and equity.

The family home visit represents the "roots" of nursing practice. Historically, nurses visited families in their homes prior to institutionalized medicine. Being invited into the home by a family continues to be one of the privileges of a CHN. The major benefit of the family visit is that it allows the nurse to observe and interact with a family in their natural environment. It also allows nurses to better understand the needs of the collective family in addition to the individual members.

Families have the right to decide the level at which they wish to participate in the nurse–client relationship (RNAO, 2006). Thus, the goals for service are tailored according to the desires and needs of the family. Goals can be preventative, for example, reviewing healthy infant and child development, and/or building capacity to cope with an acute or chronic illness.

CCHN STANDARDS: BUILDING RELATIONSHIPS AND PROFESSIONAL RESPONSIBILITY AND ACCOUNTABILITY

The first stage of a family home visit is building the relationship. Successful family home visits require thought in order to establish mutuality and trust in the nurse–patient relationship. This approach is especially necessary if the family feels vulnerable, or has fears that they will be judged or reported to child-care authorities (Jack, DiCenso, & Lohfeld, 2005). A collaborative relationship facilitates an assessment of family strengths; an understanding of the family fears, issues, and concerns; and identifies opportunities to collaboratively plan, intervene, and evaluate the desired goals.

Past models of nursing care focused on compliance. Nurses would provide advice. Families were then expected to follow this advice (Greenwood, Wright, & Nielsen, 2006). In contrast, Doane and Varcoe (2006) emphasize the need for relational nursing to promote "responsibility instead of blame, understanding instead of defensiveness, connection rather than guilt or anger and effectiveness rather than a sense of powerlessness and frustration" (p. 15). It is crucial that the empowerment in decision making be the foundation of family nursing (Aston, Meagher-Stewart, Sheppard-Lemoine, Vukic, & Chircop, 2006; Benzein, Hagberg, & Saveman, 2008). Nurses need to use their expert position to create empowering situations with the family while they make decisions in order to help build the family's confidence. The nurse and family relationships need to complement each other. The nurse needs to create a dialogue with the family to give and gain information, as well as to identify family strengths and

resources in and outside of the family "to promote health and to prevent or alleviate suffering" (Benzein et al., 2008, p. 106). Each family member's perceptions of an event or a situation need to be validated. Aston et al. advise nurses "to listen, be patient and wait for the right moment" (p. 65). Nurses need to ask questions to elicit the family's current level of knowledge on the health issues, their past history of approaches to resolve issues, and their desired approaches toward change, prior to providing advice.

Doane and Varcoe (2006) argue that

. . . it is not too difficult to care for families who meet our expectations, who behave in ways we consider to be safe and appropriate, who treat each other the way we think they ought to and who align their actions with our nursing goals. (p. 7)

When CHNs experience difficulties in building a trusting relationship with families or when nursing goals don't align with family values or difficulties, CHNs need to be aware of any "hard spots" that can be the basis of connecting across differences to understand the families' strengths and capacity to cope. Hard spots can occur when family members feel invisible and isolated, or when families are struggling with complex health problems that disrupt the regular patterns and rituals of daily life. Families may face emotional and psychological challenges related to suffering or losses that affect their identity, sense of hope, and feeling of security for the future.

A nurse's initial contact with a family is very important in order to build an affinity. First contact often occurs during a phone call when the nurse introduces her/himself, states the purpose of the visit, and schedules a visit. Visits should include multiple family members in order to allow family members to voice their thoughts and concerns. CHNs must also be conscious of their own safety when planning a family visit. They should be cognizant of scheduled visit times and possible safety concerns (e.g., history of family violence, environmental conditions such as weather, etc.).

During the first visit, the CHN should reintroduce her/himself, restate the purpose of the visit, and present identification. The nurse should then engage the family with "small talk" at the beginning of the visit to relax the family. Next, it is important to review confidentiality and duties to report so the family will be aware of the professional responsibilities associated with the role of the family nurse.

CHNs should invite the family to narrate and interpret their story through posing a series of reflective questions. This approach gives the CHN an opportunity to understand the emotional meanings of the families' experiences. For example, if families have perceptions of suffering, they may seek to understand their spiritual needs and find sources of joy. Crying may be an outlet that leads to consoling and healing (Benzein et al., 2008).

The Calgary Family Nursing Unit has spent 25 years advancing the art and science of making a family visit (Bell, 2008). Examples of questions that nurses can use to help familiarize themselves with the hopes and concerns of the family are provided in Table 16.3 (Wright & Leahey, 2009). Benzein et al. (2008) argue that posing reflective questions is powerful in an interview because it can promote healing and

TABLE 16.3 Family Interview Questions

1. How can I be most helpful to you and your family (or friends) during your care? (Clarifies expectations and increases collaboration.)

2. What has been most and least helpful to you and your family in past healthcare experiences? (Identifies past strengths and problems to avoid and successes to repeat.)

3. What is the greatest challenge facing your family right now? (Identifies actual or potential suffering, roles, and beliefs.)

4. With which of your family members or friends would you like us to share information? With which ones would you like us not to share information? (Indicates alliances, resources, and possible conflictual relationships.)

5. What do you need to best prepare you or your family for _____? (Identifies appropriate community resources.)

6. Who do you believe is suffering the most in your family right now? (Identifies the family member who has the greatest need for support and intervention.)

7. What is the one question you would like to have answered during our meeting right now? I may not be able to answer this question at the moment, but I will do my best or will try to find the answer for you. (Identifies most pressing issue or concern.)

8. How have I been most helpful to you today? How could we improve? (Shows a willingness to learn from families and to work collaboratively.)

Source: Adapted from Wright, L. M., & Leahey, M. M. (2009). Nurses and families: A guide to family assessment and intervention (5th ed.). Philadelphia, PA: F. A. Davis. (p. 252).

well-being. For example, "What worries you the most in the family?" (p. 109) can give the family the opportunity to identify their fears and concerns. Other questions will allow the family to name their strengths and reinforce coping mechanisms that assisted them in managing past complex situations. CHNs can purposively use silence while asking questions to allow the family time to reflect on their experiences.

Nurses need to clarify their role and understand the family's expectations with regard to their desired support/services. This can occur by asking "What do you expect of this conversation?" (Benzein et al., 2008, p. 109). Nurses can share their own reflections; however, Limacher and Wright (2006) suggest that **commendations** (affirmations that reflect family strengths and resources over time) should be used carefully, since past traumas can influence the family's perceptions of commendations as unwelcome, superficial, and ego-boosting statements. When used appropriately, "commending a family's competence, resilience, and strengths and offering them a new opinion or view of themselves, a context for change is created that allows families to discover their own solutions to problems and enhance healing" (Wright & Leahey, 2009, p. 151).

When developing the plan of care, nursing goals must be set mutually with the families, and families need to feel emotionally and physically safe to assess the emotional and material resources that are needed to influence their health.

Understanding the families' motivations for change is important since an approach that motivates one member of the family may be a deterrent for another. Clinical notes should be completed after each visit (in a private place) to record the assessment data, the plan of care, the implementation of the interventions, as well as an evaluation of any progress toward the goals. Over the course of the visits, the nurse must ensure that the progress made can be sustained (Benzein et al., 2008).

The decision to end the family visits also should be mutual. At this time, the CHN should review and summarize the family's strengths, and list the strategies used for health promotion, healing, and building capacity at the termination of the visits. Nurses can also include their personal reflections without judgment (Benzein et al., 2008; Wright & Leahey, 2009).

Wright and Leahey (2009) identify three common errors that occur in family visits: (a) failure to establish the context for change, (b) taking sides, and (c) giving too much advice prematurely. Nurses can avoid making these errors by ensuring that they obtain a clear understanding of the family's most pressing concern, while validating each member's perspective. Each family member needs equal time to acknowledge the suffering in the family and the sufferer. Nurses need to remain engaged, not take sides, and seek mutual understanding. A nurse should not offer advice or guidance until a thorough assessment has been completed and after the nurse has established that the advice "fits" with the family's perspective of a possible solution. The nurse should always be aware of personal experiences and biases. Finally, the intervention needs to be evaluated from the family's perspective and adapted according to the family's response.

CHNs should consider rehearsing and videotaping mock interviews to hone their interviewing skills, especially their verbal and non-verbal language. For example, many nurses need to learn to become comfortable with periods of silence, since they can give the impression that time is going very slowly, while in reality little time has passed.

CANADIAN RESEARCH BOX

Are communities aware of postpartum depression?

Sealy, P. A., Fraser, J., Simpson, J. P., Evans, M., & Hartford, A. (2009). Community awareness of postpartum depression. *Journal of Obstetric, Gynecologic & Neonatal Nursing, 38*, 121–133. doi:10.1111/j.1552-6909.2009.01001.x

Postpartum depression (PPD) is one of the most common complications that can occur during the postpartum period and can have serious effects on the mother, infant, and family. A major barrier for postpartum women and their families in becoming aware of PPD is the primary health caregiver's lack of awareness of this disorder. This research used cross-sectional population-based surveillance data from eight communities in southern and eastern Ontario, Canada. A random selection of adults 18 years of age and older with telephones were surveyed to explore awareness of PPD and its symptoms and available community resources for women with PPD. The vast majority of respondents were aware of PPD (90.1% ± 0.6% confidence interval) ($n = 58750$) as compared with the baby blues (62.5% ± 1.1%). Awareness of PPD, the baby blues, their symptoms, and sources of assistance varied according to the demographic profiles of the respondents (family structure, education, and language spoken at home).

Awareness of the term "postpartum depression" does not necessarily imply awareness of its symptoms or sources of assistance. Public education is needed to address this fact in order to provide social support and encourage treatment for symptomatic women and their families. Education should target individuals with lower levels of education and non-English-speaking groups.

Discussion Questions

1. How does a postpartum woman's social support network influence her well-being when feeling symptoms of postpartum depression?
2. What community education is needed?

CCHN STANDARDS: HEALTH PROMOTION AND BUILDING CAPACITY

Bomar (2004) defines **family health promotion** as "the process of achieving family well-being in the biological, emotional, physical, and spiritual realms for individual members and the family unit" (p. 11). Further, Black and Lobo (2008) describe **family resilience** as "the successful coping of family members under adversity that enables them to flourish with warmth, support, and cohesion" (p. 33). Family resilience factors can be developed across the lifespan but they are often enhanced during experiences of problem-solving when stressors are subdued. Nurses must have the conviction to assist the family to identify their strengths, to secure extra-familial resources, and to identify their potential for growth through use of family protective and recovery factors. Family protective and recovery factors may include

- having a positive outlook (optimism, confidence, and humour).
- spirituality (belief system of hope and triumph).
- family member accord (cohesion, nurturance, avoidance of parental conflict).
- flexibility (stable family roles, situational and developmental adjustments).
- family communication (clarity, collaborative problem solving.
- financial management (family warmth despite financial problems).
- family time (togetherness with tasks).

CASE STUDY

A mother touches her right breast and feels a painful lump. Panicked, she tells herself it is probably just another cyst. The feeling of relief is wonderful when the mammogram and ultrasound of the breast are negative. The radiologist says "It's from the mastitis you experienced 13 years ago." However, the lump doesn't go away despite antibiotics and anti-inflammatory drugs. Months pass. The lump seems to be growing. When her breast swells to the size of a cantaloupe, she finds out that she has locally advanced breast cancer. Now what? She wonders if she will live to Christmas and what she is going to tell her girls.

Rose, the younger daughter who is 9 years old, is terrified. Her best friend's mother has just died of a brain tumour; Rose wonders if her mom is next. Rose begins to have stomach and headaches, and is not sleeping. She does not want to go to school and leave her mother. Charlotte, the older daughter who is 13 years old, focuses all of her attention on school and has difficulty talking about what is happening to her mother. John, her husband, must leave for a week-long conference. He wonders if he should leave his family.

Discussion Questions

1. Describe how you would assess the family's ability to cope with the cancer diagnosis and help this family "survive" this unexpected and potentially traumatic event.
2. What family nursing interventions could you employ, and how would you assess the effectiveness of those interventions?

- shared recreation (develop social and cognitive skills, families that play together).
- routines and rituals (embedded activities that bring the family closer).
- support network (individual, family, community to share resources).

CCHN Standard: Facilitating Access and Equity

Spiritual, religious, and cultural considerations must be addressed in order for the CHN to demonstrate the application of the CCHN standard of facilitating access and equity. Access to resources and services should be based on the needs of the family, with an understanding of those needs in a cultural context. Greenwood et al. (2006) suggest that

> Cultural safety recognizes that relationships between nurses and the people they work with are sites of struggle over meaning, the outcomes of which have material and spiritual health effects

on our collective well-being. Cultural safety seeks that nurses work reflexively with people in ways that acknowledge practice always involves the meeting of two cultures and subjectivities that are relationally emergent and contingent on each other and require constant innovation and variation. (p. 206)

Cultural determinants also impact the ability of families to care for members during illness. For example, Ochieng (2003) emphasizes the need to understand the kinship system and involve the extended families in the care of the sick child. In Western society, examples of extended families may include families of African, African-Caribbean, and Asian descent. Nurses need to understand the diversity and functions of the extended family. For example, we need to try to understand and appreciate minority, ethnic child-rearing styles to find useful background information. Ochieng cautions that even though immigrant families may experience stresses related to poverty and discrimination, they may not communicate their hopes and fears to outsiders. Nurses need to be careful to offer care in an approach that does not alienate the family and assists them to buffer experiences of discrimination. CHNs must especially be careful to examine their need to educate minority ethnic families to conform to the socially constructed norms, values, and behaviours of the indigenous population.

CANADIAN RESEARCH BOX

What are the family caregivers' perceptions of, barriers to, and facilitators for relationship-building with in-home healthcare providers?

Gantert, T. W., McWilliam, C. L., Ward-Griffin, C., & Allen, N. (2009). Working it out together: Family caregivers' perceptions of relationship-building with in-home service providers. *Canadian Journal of Nursing Research*, 41(3), 44–63.

This study explored the perceptions of family caregivers of seniors, and barriers and facilitators of relationship-building with their in-home healthcare providers. The method used in this study was interpretive phenomenology. The study sample consisted of 11 family caregivers within one home care program for seniors in southwestern Ontario, Canada. Data were collected using face-to-face semi-structured interviews.

The results of the data analysis revealed that the relationship-building process consisted of a dynamic process with facilitators and barriers at contextual and individual levels. The researchers described the importance of health-care providers' use of empathy to advance relationship-building. Study participants described how healthcare providers tended to focus on task-oriented aspects of care rather than on developing partnerships with family caregivers. In addition, family caregivers identified the lack of time and continuity in assignment of service providers as important barriers that influence relationship-building. The researchers suggest that family caregivers are important partners in care and that healthcare providers ought to attend to relationship-building strategies.

Discussion Questions

1. What are some relationship-building strategies that a nurse could employ in order to develop a more collaborative partnership with family caregivers?

2. How can the nurse address some of the barriers to relationship-building in this context?

Case management is a collaborative approach used by CHNs to coordinate and facilitate the delivery of healthcare services. A CHN case manager works with individuals, families, and other healthcare providers to facilitate all necessary services for care provided in community settings during times of illness and other healthcare conditions requiring nursing intervention. The model was first introduced in 1985 as an outgrowth of primary care nursing and described by Cohen and Cesta (2005) as "an opportunity for the nursing profession to define its role in the changing healthcare industry" (p. 3). Traditional nursing care delivery systems are not able to deal with "the many constraints, economic limitations, and continual changes in today's health care settings" (p. 9). The model also challenges the profession to define nurses' work in terms of its autonomous value to the client. The goal of case management is to arrive at quality, cost-effective client outcomes. The provision of client care using a case manager is becoming a more recognized strategy. Case management is meant to ensure that patients receive needed care and services and that those services are delivered in an efficient manner (Cohen & Cesta, 2005). Nurses in community settings use the case management approach to identify and assess clients, plan care, provide or delegate care, and follow up with an evaluation of care. For nurses working with families, this would mean the best outcomes for individual clients within families and the family as a whole. Canadian nurses have a lengthy history of providing family-centred care to vulnerable individuals and connecting them to services with the purpose of promoting health and preventing disease (Baxter & Markle-Reid, 2009; Sword, Krueger, & Watt, 2006).

In Canada, restructuring during the 1990s resulted in two major mechanisms for managed care to save healthcare dollars. The first was decreasing the length of stay in hospitals (early discharge); the second was decreasing the time spent delivering homecare services. The danger of these was that cost containment, not quality of life, became the main determining factor (Daiski, 2000). The result has been many complaints about deteriorating home care services and the detrimental impact of the changes on patients and their families. Scarce resources have been redirected away from the supportive care required by frail older people (McWilliam, 2008). "Inadequate professional follow-up care often forces families to take over these responsibilities" (Daiski, 2000, p. 75). With the demographic shift toward an aging population, more pressure will be put on informal caregivers with a simultaneous increase in the number of nurses necessary for providing care in community settings (O'Sullivan Burchard, 2005).

Once embraced as a model to increase nursing's influence in the system, case management has come under criticism for its focus on cost containment. Nurses as case managers are "particularly suited for case management roles because of their broad range of assessment and coordination skills related to health" (Fraser & Strang, 2004). This is a very challenging situation for nurses, who must determine the most appropriate services to meet the needs of the client while providing the most benefit at the least cost.

FUTURE RESEARCH DIRECTIONS

Loveland-Cherry (2006) notes that it is timely to review the state of family intervention research. She argues that progress has been made on research on interventions in family, since family nursing is "gaining recognition as a critical environment related to health" and family interventions are "gaining credibility with funding agencies" (p. 5). Family nursing can involve the individual alone; multiple family members, such as a child and parent; or it can involve the whole family system. Domains of family interventions also involve multiple areas, including "behaviour modification or skill development, behavioural therapy, problem solving, or some combination" (p. 4). Loveland-Cherry also emphasizes the need for future research to work on the complex issues of measurement, exploration of new analytical strategies, clarification of the dynamics of interventions, determinations of critical dimensions for tailoring family interventions, and establishment of links between family system characteristics and individual outcomes.

Knafl and Deatrick (2006) are attempting to move family nursing approaches beyond primarily qualitative approaches to quantify and analyze the responses of the family as a unit during a chronic illness. They are testing the functional categories, such as thriving, accommodating, enduring, struggling, and floundering, while recognizing that individual responses of family members may be discrepant. This research broadens the scale of family nursing to test the generalizability of family nursing theory.

McLeod and Wright (2008) are examining the meaning of family spirituality and spiritual care in practice, using a qualitative (hermeneutic) approach through individual and community stories and rituals. These researchers suggest that

> . . . serious illness often creates suffering and precipitates a search for spiritual meaning. . . . Spiritual care requires literacy in reading the spiritual, a willingness to respond to the particular and the unpredictable, and a belief that good care demands a wise and thoughtful response to the suffering other. (p. 118)

It is theorized that nurses can use a spiritual approach to reinterpret memories in order to facilitate healing and find meaning in turmoil. "Many health professionals are caught up in the need to intervene to deliver the powerful word instead of listening to what unanswered questions might have to say" (p. 138). The crux of good spiritual care is understanding the unpredictability of spirituality and suffering, while knowing how to balance the tension of unanswered questions during conversations with families.

Van Riper (2006) examined the role of the family nurse in the era of genomic healthcare. Nurses who take advantage of the family history to trace the prevalence of illness in the family already have an advantage in understanding some of the role of the family nurse, but need to combine this knowledge with that of the technological advances of genetic testing. She discussed the practice competencies and addresses some of the ethical and social issues associated with the pros and cons of families determining whether they will undergo genetic testing.

Finally, there is a debate occurring around whether or not international family nursing needs a professional organization. Curry (2006) argues that a professional organization could

- promote the care of families in health and illness.
- explore cultural and national definitions of family nursing.
- manage resources.
- prepare students.
- provide opportunities for socialization.
- disseminate information, especially research information.

At this time there is no answer as to whether there is a critical mass to support the need for an international professional organization. Nevertheless, Harmon Hanson (2005b) suggests that the need for family nursing as a specialty has never been greater with the movement toward increased levels of community-based care. She fears that family nursing is becoming "anemic if not dying" (p. 336), as the curriculum is being diluted and as nursing faculties become less familiar with the content of this specialty. Evidence of the disturbing dilution of research on family nursing is found with the closure of the Family Nursing Unit at the University of Calgary in 2007 after 25 years of exemplary practice (Bell, 2008; Gottlieb, 2007).

SUMMARY

This chapter is an overview of family care in community settings. It is not all-encompassing, but provides a glimpse into a nursing specialty. The changing composition of the family and the social demographics of the family have been presented so that nurses can understand that families in the future may be smaller and more multicultural. We described the myths of the romanticized and stigmatized families, and that all families have strengths and the capacity to grow through health promotion activities or during times of stress resulting from an illness. We have also discussed the importance of CHNs being self-aware of their own biases and the need to surmount the "hard spots" in family nursing to build productive and satisfying relationships with families. We emphasized the need to use the CCHN Standards and the PHCC to guide the practice of the family nurse especially in evaluating her/his practice. Case management in a family context was also discussed. Finally, areas of future research have been examined.

We support that family nursing should be considered a specialty and that all interactions with clients must take into consideration their families. CHNs need to take a leadership role to advocate for families within the global context of poverty, violence and terrorism, threats of pandemic illness and environmental change, and the lack of access to healthcare (Feetham, 2005). Families benefit when nurses collaboratively assist them to access family and outside resources in order to reduce stress and suffering in the family as they encounter illness and build capacity to promoting health.

The future of family health nursing will be influenced by health policy, health promotion agendas, economics, changes in the nursing profession, family demands, health promotion lifestyle changes, and the growing emphasis by family and healthcare professionals on capacity building with families to transform their health (Bomar, 2004, p. 34).

KEY TERMS

romanticized family, p. 267
stigmatized family, p. 267
family, p. 268
family forms, p. 268
family function, p. 268
family healthcare nursing, p. 268
family systems nursing, p. 269
structural–functional theory, p. 270
systems theory, p. 270
family developmental theory, p. 270
family assessment, p. 271
family structure, p. 272
genogram, p. 273
ecomap, p. 273
commendations, p. 275
family health promotion, p. 276
family resilience, p. 276
case management, p. 277

REVIEW QUESTIONS

Choose the one alternative that best completes the statement or answers the question.

1. Family forms encompass which of the following types?
   a) nuclear families
   b) homosexual families
   c) single parent families
   d) any combination of two or more persons who are bound together over time by ties of mutual consent, birth, and/or adoption or placement

2. Which of the following statements regarding Canadian sociodemographic changes is true?
   a) Married couples are the majority.
   b) The population is getting younger.
   c) Life expectancy is decreasing.
   d) The number of childless couples is greater than those with children.

3. Which of the following nursing actions best describes the CCHN standard of Promoting Health?
   a) upholds the duty to report suspected child abuse
   b) facilitates family access to community resources
   c) reflects on the potential impact of personal values and beliefs on nurse–family interventions
   d) offers family commendations
   e) uses a family assessment framework to assess the family as client

4. Which of the following nursing actions best describes the CCHN standard of Building Family Capacity?
   a) documents family interventions
   b) refers the family to appropriate resources
   c) reflects on the potential impact of personal values and beliefs on nurse–family interventions
   d) assists the family to identify and build upon family strengths

5. Which of the following nursing actions best describes the CCHN standard of Building Relationships?
   a) participates in continuing education activities
   b) refers the family to appropriate resources
   c) identifies the purpose of the family home visit and collaborates with members to establish goals
   d) assists the family to identify and build upon family strengths

6. Which of the following nursing actions best describes the CCHN standard of Facilitating Access and Equity?
   a) participates in continuing education activities
   b) researches the resources available in the community and advocates for families
   c) seeks family feedback regarding goals
   d) uses principles of family systems nursing to assess the family

7. What is the goal of family case management?
   a) to control the provision of services to ensure equitable distribution among all families according to need
   b) to contain costs in accordance with the budget allocated for health services
   c) to provide a structured care plan to ensure the delivery of quality healthcare according to best practice guidelines
   d) to facilitate the provision of appropriate resources and services in an efficient manner to meet the needs of clients and families

STUDY QUESTIONS

1. Define the concept of family and identify some common family functions.

2. Describe the demographic shifts that are changing the composition of Canadian families.

3. What are the levels of conceptualizing the family in family nursing theory?

4. Describe the key differences between a genogram and an ecomap.

5. Identify the components of a family home visit.

6. Define case management and its role in family-centred care.

---

*After working through these questions, go to the MyNursingLab at **www.pearsoned.ca/mynursinglab** to check your answers.*

INDIVIDUAL CRITICAL THINKING EXERCISES

1. Draw your family genogram and ecomap. Describe the roles of family members, the quality of the intra-family relationships, and the strengths of your family.

2. Identify some factors that make a family vulnerable.

3. Describe a crisis experience in your family and the family resilience factors that assisted your family to cope with the crisis.

4. Compare your beliefs about your family with those of a romanticized or stigmatized family.

5. What impact could your values and beliefs about family have on your nurse–family relationships?

GROUP CRITICAL THINKING EXERCISES

1. Differentiate between viewing the family as client and the family as context. Drawing on your experiences, provide an example to illustrate an example of each concept (family as client and family as context).

2. Describe an approach to the assessment of a family for each of the CCHN standards: Promoting Health, Building Capacity, Building Relationships, Facilitating Access & Equity, and Demonstrating Professional Responsibility and Accountability. Provide concrete examples to illustrate the application of each standard in family nursing.

3. Roleplay a family–nurse situation. Practise the family interview questions listed in Table 16.3.

REFERENCES

Allen, F. M., & Warner, M. (2002). A developmental model of health and nursing. *Journal of Family Nursing, 8*(2), 96–135.

Artinian, N. T. (1999). Selecting a model to guide family assessment. In G. D. Wegner & R. J. Alexander (Eds.), *Reading in family nursing* (2nd ed., pp. 447–459). Philadelphia, PA: Lippincott.

Aston, M., Meagher-Stewart, D., Sheppard-Lemoine, D., Vukic, A., & Chircop, A. (2006). Family health nursing and empowering relationships. *Pediatric Nursing, 32*(1), 61–67.

Baxter, P., & Markle-Reid, M. (2009). An interprofessional team approach to fall prevention for older home care clients "at risk" of falling: Healthcare providers share their experiences. *International Journal of Integrated Care, 9,* e15.

Bell, J. M. (2008). The family nursing unit, University of Calgary: Reflections on 25 years of clinical scholarship (1982–2007) and closure announcement. *Journal of Family Nursing, 14*(3), 275–288.

Benzein, E. G., Hagberg, M., & Saveman, B-I. (2008). Being appropriately unusual: A challenge for nurses in health-promoting conversations with families. *Nursing Inquiry, 15*(2), 106–115.

Black, K., & Lobo, M. (2008). A conceptual review of family resilience factors. *Journal of Family Nursing, 14*(1), 33–55.

Bomar, P. J. (2004). Introduction to family health nursing and promoting family health. In P. J. Bomar (Ed.), *Promoting health in families: Applying family research and theory to nursing practice* (3rd ed., pp. 3–37). Philadelphia, PA: Saunders.

Cohen, E. L., & Cesta, T. G. (2005). *Nursing case management: From essentials to advanced practice applications.* St. Louis, MO: Mosby.

Community Health Nurses Association of Canada (CHNAC). (2008). *Canadian community health nursing standards of practice.* Ottawa, ON: Author.

Cooley, M. L. (2009) A family perspective in community/public health nursing. In F. A. Maurer & C. M. Smith (Eds.), *Community/public health nursing practice* (4th ed., pp. 327–344). St. Louis, MO: Saunders.

Curry, D. M. (2006). Does international family nursing need a professional organization? *Journal of Family Nursing, 13*(4), 395–402.

Daiski, I. (2000). The road to professionalism in nursing: Case management or practice based in nursing theory? *Nursing Science Quarterly, 13*(1), 74–79.

Denham, S. A. (2005). Family structure, function, and process. In S. M. Harmon Hanson, V. Gedaly-Duff, & J. Rowe Kaakinen (Eds.), *Family health care nursing theory, practice, and research* (3rd ed.). Philadelphia, PA: F. A. Davis.

Department of Justice Canada. (2009). *Civil Marriage Act.* Retrieved from http://www.canada.justice.gc.ca/eng/news-nouv/nr-cp/2005/doc_31376.html

Doane, G. H., & Varcoe, C. (2006). The "Hard Spots" of family nursing. *Journal of Family Nursing, 12*(1), 7–21.

Feeley, N., & Gottlieb, L. N. (2000). Nursing approaches for working with family strengths and resources. *Journal of Family Nursing, 6*(1), 9–24.

Feetham, S. (2005). Family nursing: Challenges and opportunities: Providing leadership in family nursing from local to global health. *Journal of Family Nursing, 11*(4), 327–331.

Fraser, K. D., & Strang, V. (2004). Decision-making and nurse case management. *Advances in Nursing Science, 27*(1), 32–43.

Friedman, M. M., Bowden, V. R., & Jones, E. G. (Eds.). (2003). *Family nursing: Research, theory, and practice* (5th ed.). Upper Saddle River, NJ: Prentice Hall.

Gottlieb, L., & Rowat, K. (1987). The McGill model of nursing: A practice-derived model. *Advances in Nursing Science, 9*(4), 51–61.

Gottlieb, L. N. (2007). A tribute to the Calgary family nursing unit: Lessons that go beyond family nursing. *Canadian Journal of Nursing Research, 39*(3), 7–11.

Greenwood, S., Wright, T., & Nielsen, H. (2006). Conversations in context: Cultural safety and reflexivity in child and family health nursing. *Journal of Family Nursing, 12*(2), 201–224.

Harmon Hanson, S. M. (2005a). Family health care nursing: An introduction. In S. M. Harmon Hanson, V. Gedaly-Duff, & J. Rowe Kaakinen (Eds.), *Family health care nursing: Theory, practice, and research* (3rd ed., pp. 3–37). Philadelphia, PA: F. A. Davis.

Harmon Hanson, S. M. (2005b). Family nursing: Challenges and opportunities: Whither thou goeth family nursing. *Journal of Family Nursing, 11*(4), 336–339.

Harmon Hanson, S. M., & Rowe Kaakinen, J. (2005). Theoretical foundations for nursing of families. In S. M. Harmon Hanson, V. Gedaly-Duff, & J. Rowe Kaakinen (Eds.), *Family health care nursing: Theory, practice, and research* (3rd ed., pp. 69–95). Philadelphia, PA: F. A. Davis.

Hartrick Doane, G., & Varcoe, C. (2005). *Family nursing as relational inquiry: Developing health-promoting practice.* Philadelphia, PA: Lippincott, Williams & Wilkins.

Hitchcock, J. E., Schubert, P. E., & Thomas, S. A. (Eds.), (2003). *Community health nursing: Caring in action.* Albany, NY: Delmar.

Hunt, R. (2009). Family care. In R. Hunt (Ed.), *Introduction to community-based nursing* (4th ed., pp. 79–117). Philadelphia, PA: Lippincott.

Jack, S. M., DiCenso, A., & Lohfeld, L. (2005). Vulnerable families' participation in home visits: A theory of maternal engagement with public health nurses and family visitors. *Journal of Advanced Nursing, 49*(2), 182–190.

Knafl, K. A., & Deatrick, J. A. (2006). Family management style and the challenge of moving from conceptualization to measurement. *Journal of Pediatric Oncology Nursing, 23*(1), 12–18.

Limacher, L. H., & Wright, L. M. (2006). Exploring the therapeutic family intervention of commendations. *Journal of Family Nursing, 12*(3), 307–331.

Loveland-Cherry, C. J. (2006). Where is the family in family interventions? *Journal of Family Nursing, 12*(1), 4–6.

McLeod, D. L., & Wright, L. M. (2008). Living the as-yet unanswered: Spiritual care practices in family systems nursing. *Journal of Family Nursing, 14*(1), 118–141.

McWilliam, C. L. (2008). Sharpening the focus of research on in-home and community care for older persons. *Canadian Journal of Nursing Research, 40*(1), 5–8.

Neuman, B., & Fawcett, J. (Eds.). (2002). *The Neuman Systems Model* (4th ed.). Upper Saddle River, NJ: Prentice Hall.

Ochieng, B. M. N. (2003). Minority ethnic families and family-centred care. *Journal of Child Health Care, 7*(2), 123–132.

O'Sullivan Burchard, D. J. H. (2005). Family nursing: Challenges and opportunities: What will the challenges for family nursing be over the next few years? *Journal of Family Nursing, 11*(4), 332–335.

Public Health Agency of Canada. (2007). *Core competencies for public health in Canada.* Ottawa, ON: Author.

Rank, J. (2009). *Television and family—The social uses and influence of television on families.* Retrieved from http://family.jrank.org/pages/1681/Television-Family-Social-Uses-Influence-Television-on-Families.html

Registered Nurses' Association of Ontario. (2006). *Supporting and strengthening families through expected and unexpected life events* (Revised). Toronto, ON: Author.

Rentfro, A. R. (2006). Health promotion and the family. In C. L. Edelman & C. L. Mandle (Eds.), *Health promotion throughout the lifespan* (6th ed., pp. 152–177). Philadelphia, PA: Mosby.

Riley-Lawless, K. (2010). Theoretical bases for promoting family health. In J. Allender, C. Rector, & K. Warner (Eds.), *Community health nursing: Promoting and protecting the public's health* (7th ed., pp. 476–493). Philadelphia, PA: Lippincott, Williams & Wilkins.

Rowe Kaakinen, J., & Harmon Hanson, S. (2004). Theoretical foundations for family nursing practice. In P. J. Bomar (Ed.), *Promoting health in families: Applying family research and theory to nursing practice* (3rd ed., pp. 93–116). Philadelphia, PA: Saunders.

Rowe Kaakinen, J. R., Gedaly-Duff, V., Padgett Coehlo, D., & Harmon Hanson, S. M. (Eds.). (2010). *Family health care nursing: Theory, practice, and research* (4th ed.). Philadelphia, PA: F. A. Davis.

Salopek, P. G. (2010). Working with families: Applying the nursing process. In J. Allender, C. Rector, & K. Warner (Eds.), *Community health nursing: Promoting and protecting the public's health* (7th ed., pp. 494–523). Philadelphia, PA: Lippincott, Williams & Wilkins.

Statistics Canada. (2007a, Sept. 12). 2006 Census: Families, marital status, households and dwelling characteristics. *The Daily.* Retrieved from http://www.statcan.gc.ca/daily-quotidien/070912/dq070912-eng.pdf

Statistics Canada. (2007b, July 17). 2006 Census: Age and sex. *The Daily.* Retrieved from http://www.statcan.gc.ca/daily-quotidien/070717/dq070717a-eng.htm

Statistics Canada. (2009). Married-couple families with children aged 24 and under is largest family structure, but declining (97-553-XIE). Retrieved from http://www12.statcan.ca/census-recensement/2006/as-sa/97-553/p3-eng.cfm

Sword, W. A., Krueger, P. D., & Watt, M. S. (2006). Predictors of acceptance of a postpartum public health nurse home visit: Findings of an Ontario survey. *Canadian Journal of Public Health, 97*(3), 191–196.

Tarko, M., & Reed, K. (2004). Family assessment and intervention. In P. J. Bomar (Ed.), *Promoting health in families: Applying family research and theory to nursing practice* (3rd ed., pp. 274–303). Philadelphia, PA: Saunders.

Vanier Institute of the Family. (2010). *Families count: Profiling Canada's families IV.* Ottawa, ON: Author.

Van Riper, M. (2006). Family nursing in the era of genomic health care. *Journal of Family Nursing, 12*(2), 111–118.

Wright, L. M., & Leahey, M. M. (2005). The three most common errors in family nursing: How to avoid or sidestep. *Journal of Family Nursing, 11*(2), 90–101.

Wright, L. M., & Leahey, M. M. (2009). *Nurses and families: A guide to family assessment and intervention* (5th ed.). Philadelphia, PA: F. A. Davis.

ADDITIONAL RESOURCES

Readings

Hudson, P., & Payne, S. (Eds.). (2009). *Family careers in palliative care: A guide for health and social care professionals.* New York, NY: Oxford University Press.

Rowe Kaakinen, J., Gedaly-Duff, V., Padgett Coehlo, D., & Harmon Hanson, S. M. (Eds.). (2010). *Family health care nursing: Theory, practice, and research* (4th ed.). Philadelphia, PA: F. A. Davis.

Wright, L. M., & Bell, J. M. (2009). *Beliefs and illness: A model for healing.* Calgary, AB: 4th Floor Press.

Websites

Canadian Child Care Federation
http://www.cccf-fcsge.ca

Canadian Nurses Association
www.cna-nurses.ca

Public Health Agency of Canada
http://www.phac-aspc.gc.ca/

Statistics Canada
http://www.statcan.gc.ca

The Vanier Institute of the Family
http://www.vifamily.ca

About the Authors

Patricia Sealy, RN, BA, BScN (University of Windsor) MScN (nursing administration), PhD (sociology in health and aging and policy and program evaluation) (University of Western Ontario), is the Nurse Researcher Educator and an Adjunct Assistant Professor with the Labatt Family School of Nursing at the University of Western Ontario. Her research interests are postpartum depression and the application of the CCHN standards and the Public Health Core Competencies in public health nursing practice.

Julia Smith, RN, BSc (University of Guelph), MSc(A) Nursing (McGill), PhD (c) Epidemiology & Biostatistics (University of Western Ontario), has experience in family nursing and community health. She has taught community health nursing courses at the University of Windsor. Her research interests include family structure and children's mental health.

The authors gratefully acknowledge Dr. Linda Patrick (University of Windsor) and Kathryn Edmunds in authorship of earlier editions of this chapter. In addition, the authors acknowledge Dr. Marilyn Evans (University of Western Ontario), Charlene Beynon (Middlesex-London Health Unit), and Ashley Hoogenboom (Middlesex-London Health Unit) for their valuable feedback on this chapter.

School Health

17

Yvette Laforêt-Fliesser, Carol MacDougall, and Irene Buckland

OBJECTIVES

After studying this chapter, you should be able to:

1. Explain the importance of the school as a setting for child and youth health promotion.
2. Discuss the common health concerns encountered in the school-aged population.
3. Describe Canadian and international school-based health promotion models.
4. Understand the history of community health nurses' roles and contributions in Canadian schools.
5. Describe the roles and functions of community health nurses within the comprehensive school health approach.
6. Identify challenges and opportunities for the future development of community health nursing in school settings.

INTRODUCTION

School-aged children and youth need a supportive healthful environment to foster optimal developmental and educational milestones. The academic success and optimal health and well-being of school-aged children and youth will ultimately determine Canada's place in the world (Health Council of Canada, 2006). Today, more than 5.1 million Canadian children and adolescents attend school every day (Brockington, 2010). While many factors influence the physical, social, and emotional well-being of children and youth, research is increasingly viewing the school setting as having a positive impact on most of the health behaviours and outcomes of this population (Boyce, King, & Roche, 2008). Because schools play a key role in child and youth development, they must position themselves prominently as partners in any health promotion effort (Kendall, 2008).

Schools have been an important setting for community health nurses (CHNs) to provide health promotion services and programs. They are settings where children and youth learn, play, and love; where adults work; and where families and neighbourhoods gather to engage in various educational and community activities (Vince Whitman & Aldinger, 2009). In some communities, especially in rural Canada, the school-based CHN may be the only health professional providing service on an ongoing basis (Varpalotai & Leipert, 2006). CHNs work within a primary health care model by offering a broad spectrum of services to promote and protect the health of individuals, families, groups, and aggregates within the school community.

Level of education attained, and, in particular, literacy, are significant determinants of long-term health and quality of life (Ronson & Rootman, 2004). While dropout rates are improving in Canada, more resources for non-involved, at-risk adolescents and teen parents would further decrease the dropout rate and increase return-to-school rates (Ungerleider & Burns, 2004). CHNs can enable students to complete their education by facilitating access to health and social services such as early identification and referral of students with mental health or other health concerns. Initiating school nutrition programs and support programs that help pregnant and parenting teens stay in school are examples of how CHNs can impact the social determinants of health in school settings.

This chapter begins with a brief overview of growth and development in school-aged children and youth, and a discussion of some of the important health and social concerns in this population. Two socioenvironmental frameworks for health promotion will be presented: comprehensive school health (CSH) and the health promoting school (HPS), followed by a brief historical perspective on school health. The diverse roles and functions of CHNs within school communities will then be examined within these frameworks.

THE IMPORTANCE OF THE SCHOOL YEARS

Healthy children and youth are an important predictor of a society's overall health. How children and adolescents negotiate the transitions from early to middle childhood and from adolescence to adulthood are important indicators of how healthy and well they will be as adults. Middle childhood extends from age 6 to the onset of puberty at 10 to 12 years, when children shift from seeing themselves as the centre of the world to realizing that the world is a complex place in which they must find a place (Davies, 2004). The transition to middle childhood is marked by entry into the formal education system, when children begin to move from home and their family into wider social contexts that strongly influence their development. During these years, the child is driven by basic needs to achieve competence, autonomy, and relationships with others. School-aged children seek opportunities to master and demonstrate new skills, make independent decisions, control their own behaviour, and form good relationships with peers and adults outside the family. Nearing the end of this period, children who have successfully mastered these developmental tasks and not yet entered puberty are likely to appear confident, competent, reasonable, and composed. They are capable of reasoning, looking at situations from multiple perspectives, and using many adaptive strategies of self-regulation (Davies).

Just as early life experiences influence a child's readiness for school, success at school is associated with fewer health problems and greater success throughout life. To be happy, healthy, confident, and secure children and youth need "love, nurturing, nutrition, security, stimulation and health care" (Health Council of Canada, 2006, p. 8). In most cases, the child's family will first meet this requirement; however, it is often the school setting where the child will experience nurturing and caring outside the family. A caring family together with an adequate income is the most important health determinant for children.

Adolescence begins with puberty and ends with the beginning of adulthood. The transition to this life stage involves a balance of school, extracurricular activities, and engagement in the workforce. The developmental tasks associated with adolescence include achieving independence, adjusting to sexual maturation, establishing co-operative relationships with peers, preparing for meaningful work or a career, establishing intimate relationships, and developing a core set of values (Canadian Institute for Health Information [CIHI], 2005; Registered Nurses Association of Ontario [RNAO], 2010). Other developmental outcomes related to successful transition to adulthood are "engagement with and participation in the community, empowerment to make healthy and responsible choices, and realistic hope for the future" (CIHI, p. 21).

COMMON HEALTH CONCERNS

Almost one in nine Canadian children and youth under 18 live in poverty, with the plight being even worse for First Nations and off-reserve Aboriginal children—one in four, and two in five, respectively (Campaign 2000, 2008). Child poverty rates are also very high for new immigrants, visible minorities, and children with disabilities. Children and youth living in poverty are disadvantaged in almost every way and the health effects last a lifetime. They are more likely to live in unsafe neighbourhoods where exposure to violent and illegal activity occurs. These same conditions also create fewer opportunities for them to be physically and socially active (Ontario Public Health Association [OPHA], 2004). Approximately one in five Canadian children lives in small or rural areas that have limited access to public transportation, specialist services, and recreation opportunities (Health Council of Canada, 2006).

While most Canadian children and youth are relatively healthy, their health status is often described in terms of risky activities and problem behaviours. Health concerns commonly addressed in school settings include unintentional injuries, communicable diseases, inactivity and unhealthy eating, mental health issues, and **risky behaviours** (Boyce et al., 2008; CIHI, 2005). The following section briefly outlines each of these health concerns in school-aged children and youth.

Unintentional Injuries

Unintentional injuries are "the leading cause of death for children ages one to fourteen . . . [and] . . . account for more deaths in children and youth than all other causes of death combined" (Leitch, 2007, p. 4). The unintentional injury death rate varies for children of different age groups, with the highest rate in male youth. Car crashes are the main cause of injury death for children and youth (Ramage-Morin, 2008). Sports are a major cause of non-fatal injuries among all youth (Pickett, 2004). For children under age 10 in Canada, unintentional injury to the brain/skull resulted in the highest incidence of death or hospitalization (Smartrisk, 2009). Prevention initiatives have made a difference; for example, serious head injuries from bicycle crashes have dropped in regions where bicycle helmet legislation has been implemented (Macpherson, To, Macathur, Chipman, Wright, & Parkin, 2002).

Communicable Diseases

Immunization is often considered one of the most important public health achievements of the 20th century. Just 100 years ago, infectious diseases were the leading cause of death around the world. Today, in Canada, they cause fewer than 5% of all deaths (Canadian Public Health Association [CPHA], 2001). Immunization against vaccine-preventable communicable diseases is one of the most cost-effective public health interventions. Public health units are mandated by provincial health legislation to collect and review immunization information on students relating to measles, mumps, rubella, tetanus, diphtheria, and polio; and, in some jurisdictions, to hepatitis B, human papilloma virus, and meningitis, as well as annual influenza immunization. Free universal vaccinations are available in most provinces and territories. However, not all children and youth have up-to-date immunizations due to barriers such as lack of transportation, transiency, childcare problems, and religious and personal beliefs (Health Council of Canada, 2006).

Inactivity and Unhealthy Eating

Overweight and obesity in Canadian 12- to 17-year-olds has more than doubled in the last 25 years (Shields, 2006) and is becoming a major health concern. "Given the prevalence of childhood obesity, and given its contributions to many diseases, this is the first generation that may not live as long as their parents" (Leitch, 2007, p. 95). A federal government report recently revealed that 26% of Canadian children and youth aged 2 to 17 years are overweight or obese. For aboriginal children, the numbers are of great concern where 55% of on reserve children and 41% of off reserve children are either overweight or obese (Parliament of Canada, 2007). Two major factors contribute to this health problem: a lack of physical activity and poor food choices. Sedentary activity and obesogenic environments have contributed to what many call an obesity epidemic. "Almost half of Grade 6 to Grade 10 students in Canada are physically inactive, the problem being particularly worrisome in girls" (Boyce et al., 2008, p. 43). Fewer than half of Canadian children and youth eat sufficient fruits and vegetables on a daily basis.

Children living in lower socioeconomic situations are at increased risk of being overweight or obese as opposed to children living in higher socioeconomic groups (Health Council of Canada, 2006). Low-income families have much less choice when it comes to food and to opportunities for physical activity. Many rely on food banks for ongoing support. In 2008, 37% of Canadian food bank clients were children less than 18 years of age (Food Banks Canada, 2008). Inadequate nutrition impacts a child's ability to learn, as well as develop physically (Ontario Ministry of Health and Long-Term Care, 2004).

Mental Health

"The mental health of children and youth is as important as physical health. . . .The onset of most mental illnesses occurs during adolescence and young adulthood" (Government of Canada, 2006, p. 6). An estimated 1.2 million—or 15 percent—of young Canadians live with anxiety, attention deficit, depression, addiction, and other disorders (Mental Health Commission of Canada, 2006). According to the Health Council of Canada (2006),

> . . . these mental health conditions affect their lives at home, at school, and in the community. . . . In 2002, more than six per cent of youth and young adults experienced a major depressive episode in the previous year, six per cent reported suicidal thoughts, and five per cent had social anxiety disorder. (p. 20)

Almost 29% of Canadian children 12 and under have developmental or behaviour problems that often persist into

adulthood, thus seriously affecting their ability to lead happy, healthy lives. Suicide rates decreased slightly between 2000 and 2003; however, suicide is still the cause for 9% of early adolescent deaths and 22% of older youth deaths. Boys in Grade 6 (26%) and Grade 10 (22%) reported that they felt low at least weekly in the previous six months; 24% and 38% of girls in Grade 6 and 10, respectively, reported feeling low at least weekly in the previous six months. This gender gap appears to be increasing from previous years (Boyce, et al., 2008).

"In 1998–1999, males aged 15 to 19 years were more likely to complete their suicide attempts; hospitalization rates for suicide attempts were over two times higher among females aged 15 to 19 years" and "hospitalization rates for eating disorders in girls under age 15 increased by 34% from 1987 to 1999" (CIHI, 2005, p. 32). In some Aboriginal communities suicide is a grave concern, with rates for Aboriginal youth being five to six times that of non-Aboriginal youth in Canada (Health Canada, 2005). With early detection and intervention, most children can experience improvement in mental health conditions. Programs and services are more effective when they are part of a comprehensive approach for nurturing all children (Health Council of Canada, 2006).

Risky Behaviours

While risk-taking is a normal part of the growth and development of adolescents, in some cases it can be a symptom of deeper underlying issues. Risky behaviours can include alcohol and drug use, smoking habits, and unprotected sexual activity. The use of cannabis peaked in 2002 but dropped significantly in 2006 with just under 40% of boys and girls reporting having tried the drug. However, in 2006, the rate of weekly alcohol use increased from 1 to 8% between Grades 6 and 10 for girls and from 2 to 18% for boys; 16% of Grade 8 students reported having used alcohol to get drunk at least twice. By Grade 10, the proportion had increased to 39% (Boyce, et al., 2008). In 2004, 62% of 15- to 17-year-olds and 91% of 18- to 19-year-olds drank alcohol (Adlaf, Begin, & Sawka, 2005). Smoking tobacco among youth 15 to 19 years declined to 15% in 2008 from 18% in 2003, with more boys (18%) reporting smoking than girls (13%) thus reversing a trend of a higher prevalence of smoking among girls (Health Canada, 2008).

In 2005, 43% of youth 15 to 19 reported having sexual intercourse at least once, down from the 47% in 1996–1997. Eight percent of boys and girls reported having had sex before age 15, indicating a 4% decline from 1996–1997 (Rotermann, 2008). While these trends are encouraging, 33% of youth reported having multiple partners and 20% of 15- to 17-year-olds and 30% of 18- to 19-year-olds reported having sex without a condom. These patterns of sexual activity have contributed significantly to the number of chlamydia cases among 15- to 19-year-olds, which increased from 1063.7 to 1362 per 100 000 youth between 1998 and 2002 (Public Health Agency of Canada [PHAC], 2005). Between 1997 and 2001, pregnancy rates among 15- to 19-year-old girls declined from 43 to 36 per 1000 girls (CIHI, 2005, p. 32).

Experimentation in the above risky behaviours is mostly responsible for the morbidity and mortality in adolescence. There is strong evidence that teens who engage in one "risky behaviour" tend to engage in several other risk behaviours (CIHI, 2005). Many of the behaviours that begin during this time can continue into adulthood, with negative long-term health consequences. Thus, all known risk factors must be acknowledged and incorporated into a community's plan for health promotion and disease and injury prevention with children and youth. Positive relationships with families, peers in schools, and community members may lessen the potential harm of these high-risk behaviours and encourage more health-enhancing behaviours. Individual capacity and coping skills, such as personal competence and a sense of control over one's life, also play an important role in supporting mental and physical health (Boyce, et al., 2008; CIHI, Government of Canada, 2006). Creating supportive environments and opportunities for connecting with caring, committed adults, engaging in age-appropriate decision-making and problem-solving, and meaningful youth participation can provide both prevention and health promotion benefits (Weare & Markham, 2005).

SCHOOL-BASED HEALTH PROMOTION MODELS

The term **Comprehensive School Health (CSH)** was coined in the 1980s to describe the socioecological approach to school-based health promotion in Canada and in the United States. The American model evolved into the **Coordinated School Health Program (CSHP)**, which includes eight components to effectively address major health risks identified among the school-aged population (Allensworth & Institute of Medicine, 1997; Marx, Wooley, & Northrop, 1998):

- health education
- physical education
- health services
- nutrition services
- health promotion for staff
- counselling, psychological, and social services
- healthy school environment (physical and psychosocial)
- parent and community involvement

The concept of the **Health Promoting School (HPS)** was developed at a special symposium in Scotland in 1986 and provided the World Health Organization (WHO) with an opportunity to test the principles and strategies set out in the Ottawa Charter for Health Promotion. The HPS model had three main elements: (a) formal curriculum time allocated to health-related issues in subjects such as biology, social education, health studies, and physical education; (b) the hidden curriculum, referring to the social and physical environment including staff/student relationships, relationships between the school and community, and school meals; and (c) health and caring services including screening, prevention, and child guidance (Young, 2005). By the

mid-1990s, the Global School Health Initiative began to expand these concepts under WHO's leadership and guidance and created policy documents, international guidelines, and services to support the implementation of HPS (Vince Whitman & Aldinger, 2009). The HPS movement further broadened and refined its ideas through the lens of a settings approach endorsed in the *Jakarta Declaration on Health Promotion into the 21st Century* (WHO, 1997). A **settings approach** promotes a healthy working and living environment, integrates health promotion in daily activities, and works collaboratively with the community (Ontario Ministry of Health Promotion, 2010).

More recently, the International Union for Health Promotion and Education [IUHPE] (2008) has produced protocols and guidelines for HPS based on evidence-based quality practices from around the world. While school-based health promotion programs may be known by names other than Health Promoting Schools, they still integrate the same core elements of policy, skills-based health education, health and social services, and a healthy social and physical environment (Vince Whitman & Aldinger, 2009). Table 17.1 illustrates the commonalities among the models used in different jurisdictions around the world.

In Canada, CSH gained momentum following a national conference in 1990 that produced a consensus statement on CSH subsequently endorsed by more than 20 national organizations (Canadian Association for School Health [CASH], 1991). In 2007, the consensus statement was revised to reflect a unifying vision for educators, health professionals, policy makers, parents, and youth. CSH is now defined as "a multi-faceted approach that includes teaching health knowledge and skills in the classroom, creating health-enabling social and physical environments, and developing linkages with parents and the wider community to support optimal health and learning" (CASH, 2007). The four main components are: (a) teaching and learning; (b) health and other support services; (c) a supportive social environment; and (d) a healthy physical environment. This approach emphasizes the creation of dynamic, collaborative partnerships among children and youth, parents, teachers, principals, school councils, and members of community agencies concerned about the health and learning of children (CASH, 2007). Partnerships and policies are viewed as integral to all four components of CSH.

Health Canada, CASH, the Canadian Council on Learning, and more recently the Public Health Agency of Canada (PHAC) have played important roles in promoting CSH through research, education, project development, and networking activities. An increasing emphasis on school improvement and school effectiveness has resulted in schools linking student health and academic success. In 2005, provincial and territorial deputy ministers of education and health and the PHAC formed the Pan-Canadian Joint Consortium for School Health (JCSH) to support federal–provincial/ territorial co-operation and inter-ministerial co-ordination within jurisdictions. The consortium serves to

- Strengthen cooperation among ministries, agencies, departments, and others in support of healthy schools;

TABLE 17.1   Comparison of HPS-CSH Approaches Around the World

Model/Approach	Elements/Components				
Comprehensive School Health (Canadian Association for School Health)	Teaching and Learning	Healthy Physical Environment	Supportive Social Environment	Health and Other Support Services	Note: Healthy Policies and effective linkages with partners are embedded in each of the four components
International Union for Health Promotion and Education (IUHPE)	Individual Health Skills and Action Competencies	School's Physical Environment	School's Social Environment	Health Services Home and Community Links	Healthy School Policies
Focusing Resources on Effective School Health (FRESH-WHO)	Skills-based health education	Safe water and sanitation	Health-related school policies [school policies promoting good health and a non-discriminatory, safe, and secure physical and psychosocial environment] Pupil awareness and participation	Access to health and nutrition services Partnerships between education and health Community partnerships	Health-related school policies
Comprehensive School Health (Canadian Joint Consortium for School Health)	Teaching and Learning	Social and Physical Environment		Partnerships and Services	Healthy School Policy
Health Promoting School (WHO)	Provides skills-based health education	Strives to provide a safe, healthy environment		Engages health and education officials, teachers and their representative organizations, students, parents, and community leaders in efforts to promote health Provides access to health services Strives to improve the health of the community	Implements health-promoting policies and practices
Health Promoting School (Australia)	Curriculum, Teaching and Learning	School Organization, Ethos, and Environment		Partnerships and Services	Note: Policies contribute to achieving Health Promoting Schools
Coordinated School Health Program (USA)	Health Education; Physical Education	Healthy School Environment (physical and psychosocial; includes Nutrition Services)		Health Services; Nutrition Services; Counselling and Psychological Services; Family/Community Involvement; Health Promotion for Staff	

Souce: Adapted from the Table 1: Commonalities Among Healthy School Approaches, in School Health Guidance *Document, pp. 13–14. Ontario Ministry of Health Promotion. @ Queen's Printer for Ontario, 2010. Reproduced with permission.*

FIGURE 17.1 The Pan-Canadian Joint Consortium for School Health Model for Comprehensive School Health

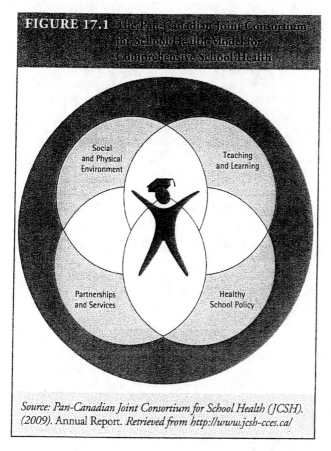

Source: Pan-Canadian Joint Consortium for School Health (JCSH). (2009). Annual Report. Retrieved from http://www.jcsh-cces.ca/

■ Build the capacity of the health and education sectors to work together more effectively and efficiently; and

■ Promote understanding of, and support for, the concept and benefits of comprehensive school health initiatives. (JCSH, 2009, p. 4)

According to the JCSH, comprehensive school health encompasses the **whole school environment** that supports students in becoming healthy and productive members of society through actions illustrated in four distinct but interrelated pillars (see Figure 17.1): social and physical environment; teaching and learning; healthy school policy; and partnerships and services.

In Canada, the terms HPS and CSH are essentially considered synonymous, and some regions use the term Healthy Schools; for clarity, we will use the term CSH in the remainder of this chapter. Table 17.2 outlines the key components of CSH and HPS models. At the end of this chapter, you will find a list of provincial and territorial websites that link you to important resources available in your jurisdiction.

HISTORICAL PERSPECTIVES ON SCHOOL HEALTH NURSING IN CANADA

CHNs in Canada have a long history of working in school communities. With the emergence of public health nursing at the turn of the 20th century, schools became one of the initial settings for the provision of health education and preventive programs (see Chapter 1). Medical inspection programs were initiated in most schools to counteract absenteeism of children due to communicable disease. Public health officials proposed that poor health inhibited a child's academic performance and could potentially have harmful effects on that child's future economic and social well-being. In several Canadian cities, boards of education initially established school health programs in which the CHNs moved between school and home providing preventive health teaching, screening, and counselling in addition to their primary role in communicable disease control (McKay, 2009).

For most of the 20th century, CHNs in school settings primarily focused on individual and family counselling, classroom health teaching, screening, case finding programs, immunization programs, and advising school staff about student health problems. Interventions were based on a biomedical model where the emphasis was on the prevention and control of disease. Schools were one of the settings in a district or neighbourhood that received the services of the generalist CHN. District nursing created opportunities for the nurse to really know the community, where regular communication and collaboration with local family physicians, pharmacists, businesses, and other health professionals occurred. School children and their families were often known to the nurse through home visiting or clinic work in the district. With the emergence of health promotion in the mid-1970s, CHNs addressed lifestyle issues through health education, health communication campaigns, and individual or group counselling in addition to the traditional screening and immunization programs. The 1986 Ottawa Charter introduced a new way of thinking about health promotion, including the important idea that health is created and maintained in the settings of people's lives, the school being an important one for children and youth after the home and family (Whitehead, 2006).

While CHNs across Canada have provided leadership in promoting the benefits of socioenvironmental approaches for school-based health promotion, they have encountered a number of challenges. In 1990s and into the early part of the 21st century, health services restructuring and changing public health mandates at the provincial/territorial level reduced or eliminated CHNs in schools or placed constraints on their practice at a time when CSH was being introduced in many jurisdictions (Falk-Rafael, Fox, & Bewick, 2005). The fragmentation of these programs into a restructured health service has often contributed to the invisibility of CHNs and other staff (Meagher-Stewart & Aston, 2005).

Despite these challenges, CHNs in Canada have played an important role in advocating for school-based comprehensive health promotion. They have made progress in articulating their health promotion and illness prevention roles within schools, in challenging the political forces that shape their practice, and in lobbying for the integration of CSH approaches into mandated public health programs and services (Macleod, Huskisson & Keys, 2009; Ontario Public Health Association, 2005).

TABLE 17.2 Components of a Comprehensive School Health/Health Promoting Schools Approach

Teaching and Learning	K–12 Health and Physical Education **curriculum**	■ emphasize generic skill development (e.g., information seeking, decision making, problem solving, refusal skills, critical thinking, media awareness, coping, personal goal setting, social skills, building relationships, conflict resolution)
	Relevant, high-quality teaching/learning materials	
	Commitment to **teacher preparation**: pre-service and in-service training	
	Empowerment approaches that consider individual and social contexts, promote **action competence**, and:	■ encourage students to participate in local **community** action
	■ use active and cooperative learning techniques	
	■ develop health knowledge, attitudes, and behaviours	Cross-curriculum support for health
Services	Health services (e.g., physical, mental, public health)	Parks and recreation/Boys' and Girls' Clubs/YMCAs and YWCAs
	Guidance and career education	Access to community-based services
	Social work	"Healthy School" coordinators (provincial level, school board level, and local school level)
	Psychology	
	Child protection	Government, school board, and school policies/guidelines and funding facilitating access to services
	Police services	
	Early identification, assessment, referral, treatment, and follow-up	
Supportive Social Environment	Welcoming and positive environment	**Democracy**/involving students in decision-making/active student participation (e.g., in setting classroom rules, on a school health committee, on a student council, in peer leadership)
	Supportive relationships	
	Clear expectations and limits	High degree of staff participation
	Inclusive environment that celebrates diversity and ensures **equity**	Encouragement of staff and student autonomy
		Role-modelling by parents, teachers, peers
	Collaborative, partnership approach with input from students, parents, administration, teachers, and local community agencies	Mentoring programs
		Universal, non-stigmatizing student nutrition/food programs
	Establishment of **sustainable** structures and processes (e.g., school health committees/teams) to identify and address health issues and **measure success**	Media reinforcing healthy behaviours
		Government, school board, and school policies/guidelines supporting health
Healthy Physical Environment	Clean and hygienic **environment**	Smoke-free policy enforcement
	Acceptable air quality and ventilation	Availability of healthy food choices
	Safe water	Safe food-handling practices
	Adequate lighting	Safe and healthy school policies/guidelines (e.g., prohibiting harassment, discrimination, violence, alcohol and drug use, as well as focusing on their prevention)
	Low-allergen environment	
	Safe playground equipment and injury prevention measures in the school	

Note: The words in bold refer to the 10 key principles of the Health Promoting School concept as identified at the First International Conference for Health Promoting Schools in Greece, 1997: 1. Democracy, 2. Equity, 3. Empowerment and Action Competence, 4. School Environment, 5. Curriculum, 6. Teacher Training, 7. Measuring Success, 8. Collaboration, 9. Communities, 10. Sustainability.

ROLES OF THE SCHOOL-BASED NURSE

In Canada, CHN practice in school communities is grounded in the principles and strategies of CSH/HPS and is consistent with the Community Health Nurses of Canada (CHNC) Standards of Practice (CHNC, 2008), the Public Health Nursing Discipline Specific Competencies (CHNC, 2009), and the roles and activities of public health/community health nurses in Canada recently described by CPHA (2010). The roles of the school-based CHN can focus on the health of individuals, groups, or the entire school population. One-on-one work with individuals, whether counselling or providing clinical services, can evolve into identifying a need for small group or psycho-educational interventions. Individually focused or small group focused strategies may also uncover

CASE STUDY

Most provincial and territorial ministries of education have passed special legislation to integrate and accommodate exceptional children and youth in publicly funded schools. In the past, many children with complex medical or developmental needs attended special residential or day schools. These schools were often part of the district PHN's caseload for targeted programs such as immunization and health education. With integration of these students into public schools, many jurisdictions have developed special services within their home care programs or community and social services to address the unique and often complex medical needs of this population. These nursing services include providing information and consultation about health issues relating to the special needs, planning of community care, providing treatments in the school setting or at home, and training of alternate caregivers.

Discussion Questions

1. What role might a PHN or CHN who provides nursing support services to individual students play in broader school-based health promotion activities?

2. Identify any advocacy issues that the visiting CHN and the school's CHN or PHN might address together?

3. Discuss how your jurisdictions currently support children and youth with special needs in schools.

specific health concerns within the school community requiring a whole school intervention using a comprehensive school health approach. The neighbourhood or broader community may also be engaged by the CHN and school partners to address more complex or systemic problems.

Working with Individuals

Today, clinical services provided by CHNs may include immunization, sexual health services, vision and hearing screening, and health counselling and referral. CHNs are also employed by visiting nurse agencies or departments in regional health authorities and provide clinical services to support students with special needs (see Case Study).

The important counselling role of CHNs in school communities, especially high schools, contributes to successful adolescent health programs, along with personal skill training in learning life and social skills and dealing with peer pressure and peer influences (Ardiles, 2009). CHNs have the clinical expertise and knowledge to provide this initial assessment, support, and referral as needed, as they practise from a solution-based approach that optimizes the problem-solving and coping abilities of young people and families. Moreover,

CHNs often work within an anticipatory guidance approach that prepares youth and their families for expected stressful events before they occur (RNAO, 2010). However, individual counselling is rarely included within mandated public health services. Even in jurisdictions supportive of this CHN role, most CHNs are on-site only a few hours per week, so it is important that additional counselling services be provided by other professionals such as social workers, guidance counsellors, and psychologists. Collaborative partnerships among public health, school boards, and community agencies can share responsibility for funding these types of support services in schools.

School boards with a significant rural population may enter into an agreement with the local public health unit for CHNs to offer counselling services to both elementary and secondary school students. Health unit CHNs may work with students for stress or coping-related issues, self-esteem, sexual health, and relationship difficulties with peers and parents. They may also link students and their families to other health and social services in the community. This type of school-based counselling service yields a high degree of satisfaction among staff, students, and parents (Perth District Health Unit, 2007).

The **school-based health clinic** is another model that is gaining acceptance in many jurisdictions. Secondary-school Teen Health Clinics are a model of care in various communities. Rural students often have limited access to community services, and urban students often have to take time out from classes to attend off-site medical appointments. Public health agencies can work with a number of community partners, including school police officers, physicians, and alcohol and drug service workers, to provide school-based comprehensive health services to high school youth. The majority of students often prefer to seek health services at school rather than at an off-site agency (Wellington–Dufferin–Guelph Health Unit, 2001).

In Nova Scotia, the **Youth Health Centre (YHC)** model offers a comprehensive range of services within a population health and youth-centred approach. These centres often operate within high schools, where youth receive accessible, confidential, and non-judgmental programs and services, including health education, health assessment and intervention, referral, and support and follow-up by CHNs and other health providers (Halifax Regional School Board and Capital Health, 2005). Additionally, the YHC coordinators support student action teams, provide health curriculum support through classroom presentations, and coordinate immunization clinics in the school. The Halifax model integrates individual-focused services, as well as opportunities for group work and peer-led student action teams that address whole-school issues.

Working with Small Groups

Group learning or group discussion is an effective approach to actively engage children and youth in creating a circle of **peer support** and formal or informal learning. Topics may include smoking cessation, healthy relationships, sexual health and sexuality, parenting, anger management, self-esteem, decision making, birth control methods, or puberty discussion. It can involve the training of peer leaders to lead a variety of activities during lunch, at recess, or after school. Such group learning is particularly valuable because it enables a peer group as a whole to experience a shift in social norms, and collectively increase its awareness, knowledge, and critical-thinking skills in a caring, supportive, and non-judgmental environment.

Building Structures and Processes for Comprehensive School Health

Some health concerns that arise during individual or small group work may benefit from further school-wide action. The CSH process is, in essence, the community health nursing process applied in collaboration with a school community. Integral to this process is the development of effective working relationships with the community client (CHNC, 2008). The core nursing skills of mutual respect, caring, listening, assessing, enabling, and empowering are critical to the CHN's work with school communities and school boards. A CHN's practice in school can be complex and challenging because relationships with school staff, parents, students, superintendents, or community partners occur within a complex, changing, and often ambiguous environment that may present conflicting circumstances for the CHN. Chapter 3 noted that CHNs practising in schools are often PHNs. They have specialized skills in working with groups and in population health promotion. In addition to meeting the needs of individuals, families, or groups, a PHN uses a macroscopic approach in assessing and planning interventions that address the broader determinants of health within a community. The use of **community development principles** is particularly relevant when building capacity in school communities. (See MyNursingLab, "A Day in the Life of a School-based CHN").

In facilitating CSH, it is important to determine the school community's level of readiness, its strengths or assets, and its areas of interest or concern. Some school communities

may have a health champion who can easily facilitate the school's participation in health promotion activities. Other school communities may be immersed in their academic focus and the CHN has a role in assisting them to see the link between health and learning before any action is possible. Some schools may be operating within a school board that has a strategic priority for promoting student health, while another board's emphasis may be focused on character-building.

The formation of strong partnerships between boards of education and public health agencies at the local level enables sustainable implementation of CSH. Examples of effective partnerships include joint committees for curriculum and policy development, which support the health of students and the school environment (MacDougall & Laforêt-Fliesser, 2009). Joint development of a local comprehensive school health initiative or adoption of a provincial initiative greatly increases the commitment of principals and school staff, as their participation becomes part of expected school improvement efforts and is actively recognized by school board leaders (Ontario Ministry of Health Promotion, 2010). Central planning of professional development and networking and celebration events for school health committee representatives contributes greatly to building and maintaining momentum within schools and school boards. Today's schools are fast-paced, ever-changing environments, and CHNs need to work closely with school board superintendents, consultants, principals, and teachers to adapt the health agenda and their practice to fit with the reality of daily school life.

CSH is a flexible health promotion approach that empowers individuals and school communities to take action for health. A CHN can engage a school in reflecting on the following questions: How effective is the health, physical education, and other curriculum delivery? Is the school aware of and able to access support services from the board and local community to support the health of students, staff, and families in the school community? Does the school have a democratic and supportive social environment with shared decision making? Is the physical environment supportive of the health curriculum being taught in the classroom? (MacDougall, 2004a).

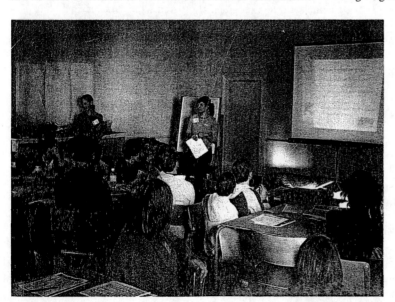

Photo 17.1

A public health nurse and public health promoter leading a Youth Leadership Workshop with Grade 5–7 youth.

Credit: Courtesy of Rebecca Dahle

The JCSH (2010a) provides Healthy School Planner, an online tool that helps Canadian schools assess the state of their environment and surveys students on specific health issues such as healthy eating, physical activity, or tobacco. Several jurisdictions have developed their own assessment tools that foster discussion about the school's strengths and health issues and what it can do about them, including the Healthy School Profile (Middlesex–London Health Unit, 2010), a visioning approach used in British Columbia schools (British Columbia Ministry of Children and Family Development, 2003), and a community development approach used in Calgary schools (Macleod et. al., 2009). Potential activities, services, and programs within the four components of the Comprehensive School Health approach are illustrated in Table 17.2.

CHNs play an important facilitative role in raising awareness among principals, teachers, students, and parents about "the possibility of addressing school health issues in a partnership structure" through **school health committees or action teams** (MacDougall, 2004b, p. 48) (see MyNursingLab "The School Health Committee/Action Team"). It is critical to involve a diverse group of representatives so they can share their concerns about various aspects of school life that need to be improved. Such inclusive participation of students is essential for the success of healthy school initiatives (MacDougall & Laforêt-Fliesser, 2009)). Ideally, the chairperson should come from the school community itself to encourage local ownership of the health committee from the outset.

CANADIAN RESEARCH BOX

What is the impact of the comprehensive school health model on school children?

Coughlin, R., & Juby, B. (2009). *The comprehensive youth pilot project: Applying best practice principles, focussing on changing school resiliency and using the comprehensive school health model as a framework for delivery: An evaluation of the impact on grades six, seven and eight youth in three pilot school communities. Final report.* Toronto, ON: Toronto Public Health.

This study evaluated the impact of a program designed to increase youth involvement and school resiliency. The "Child Resiliency: Assessing Developmental Strengths" questionnaire was administered to Grade 6 to 8 students in three intervention and three comparison schools located in three high priority Toronto neighbourhoods and repeated 18 months later. A key finding in the pre-test was that students felt a lack of connection with their school, parents, and community and desired a mentoring relationship for themselves either as a mentor or mentee. Schools that implemented mentoring programs reported an increase in positive behaviour and self-esteem in mentees. While the average number of developmental strengths typically drops as students move from grades 6 to 8, the intervention schools in this study showed no significant change over the study period, compared to a significant drop in developmental strengths in comparison schools. Students on the school health committees reported that once they were given a voice, and it was heard, they were able to make substantial change in their school. The school PHNs identified a need for ongoing professional development on effectively engaging youth and organizations, and integrating a strength-based approach in their day-to-day practice with schools.

Discussion Questions

1. Review websites or literature on resiliency, developmental assets or strengths, and protective factors, and discuss ways in which a CHN can support a school community to enhance its assets.

2. Discuss the meaning of a "strength-based approach" and how a CHN could operationalize this in working with students and schools.

3. Identify some key principles of effective youth or student engagement and discuss the importance of using these in a CHN's daily practice.

Formulating Action Plans

The School Health Committee or Action Team creates a place to discuss and build upon a school's strengths or assets while addressing health concerns and planning appropriate action. When formulating a plan to address an identified health issue, the action team should identify strategies or activities within each of the four component areas to achieve a degree of comprehensiveness that is more likely to have a meaningful impact on the school community. For example, if student nutrition is the priority concern of the school, then the components of the plan might look like this:

1. Teaching and learning—In-service for teachers so they are better prepared to deliver the nutrition curriculum;

2. Partnerships and services—Consult with a public health nutritionist, dietitian, or nurse to explore the many ways student nutrition could be addressed throughout the school, or to suggest community agencies that could assist students who may have significant nutritional issues, such as eating disorders or unhealthy weights;

3. Healthy school policies—Establish universal student nutrition programs, such as breakfast, snack, or lunch programs; establish healthy school nutrition policies that address foods offered at school events and for fundraising;

4. Supportive physical and social environment—Assist students to run a healthy tuck shop; engage youth in finding solutions for healthier high school cafeteria menus; encourage parents to reinforce healthy eating in the purchases they make for lunches and home meals.

The CHN can be instrumental in the planning process and link the school to a wide range of health-sector and community-based resources, including issue-specific public health resources (MacDougall & Laforêt-Fliesser, 2009).

Aggression between young people, which can take the form of physical, verbal, social, and electronic bullying, sexual

Table 17.3 A Healthy School's Approach to Violence Prevention

Component	
Teaching and learning	■ Whole School Survey conducted to confirm bullying as an issue ■ "ABC" Anti-Bullying Crew raised money for the purchase of Anti-Bullying Integrated Resource Units for students from JK– Grade 8 from (Community Alliance for York Region (CAYR)) ■ Classroom teaching of related curriculum for all grades ■ Grade-specific learning materials created to enhance curriculum ■ Taught students about the Stop, Think, Act, and Reflect (STAR) problem-solving and decision-making model ■ Fridge magnets, personal badges, and bookmarks distributed to all students ■ Newsletter inserts created to keep families informed about the initiative
Healthy school policy	■ Anti-Bullying Pledge designed by students and signed by the entire school was plaqued and hung in the school entrance ■ Increased reporting of harassment/bullying incidents on the playground helped to break the previous "code of silence," which was a barrier to help-seeking and bystander involvement ■ Posters were created by students and hung in the halls
Partners and services	■ Whole school assembly held to present new banner and highlight anti-bullying messages and activities from the CAYRE Program. School Board Director attended and affirmed these activities ■ OPP victim service workers and school social worker supported students as needed following a serious bullying incident at the school ■ Public Health Nurses worked closely with the school community to create and implement an action plan ■ Evaluation of the project completed
Healthy physical and social environment	■ Suggestion box placed in a private but accessible location and used for ongoing feedback from students ■ Large banner with "STAR" message made for the school ■ Health Walls posted relevant violence prevention information ■ Positive problem-solving messages posted throughout the school ■ Staff supervision around and behind portables ■ Time-out room set up to talk with students ■ Media invited to school "kick off" assembly ■ Peer mediators took part in a workshop on defining and dealing with playground bullying

harassment, and racial discrimination, is another prevalent issue in schools today (Craig, 2004). Table 17.3 provides an example of a comprehensive approach to violence prevention in schools.

Addressing Common Health Concerns

Health promotion programs in schools focus on increasing the students' awareness about healthy eating, active living, safety issues, avoiding substance use, healthy sexuality, and developing healthy relationships, including sexual health, sexuality, and violence prevention. Research and government policy are focusing on the need to promote young people's **developmental assets** or strengths that play important roles in protecting youth and promoting healthy choices (CIHI, 2005). Scales (1999) explains that "the more assets young people possess, the fewer risky behaviours they engage in—less violence, less problem alcohol and other drug use, less early sexual intercourse, less delinquency" (p. 113). *Internal assets* include a commitment to learning, a positive value system, social skills, and positive self-identity. *External assets* include support (for example, from family, adults, school, and neighbourhood), empowerment, clear boundaries and expectations, and opportunities for constructive use of time. School-wide programming that focuses on promoting these assets in all the children and youth, rather than just in the high-risk students, is the most recommended approach. Some specific targeted programs will still be needed however, to support those with diagnosed concerns such as depression, substance use, eating disorders, sexually transmitted infections, and so on.

Researchers have identified general characteristics of programs/policies that may contribute to healthy youth development (CIHI, 2005):

1. Interventions that address common factors associated with multiple determinants of health, e.g., policy initiatives, education, youth-focused media and marketing, skills training, peer support, and community activities; address underlying factors such as influences of early childhood, family, school, community, and peers.

2. Approaches that support healthy youth development, e.g., instead of focusing on problem behaviours, focus on positive youth development through programs that promote a sense of belonging; bonding and connections to caring, committed adults; age-appropriate responsibility for decision making and problem solving; and leadership roles and activities that are youth friendly and encourage youth ownership and participation.

3. Approaches that engage youth, e.g., in meaningful structured activities such as sports, music, arts, and community work.

The Health Council of Canada (2006) similarly identifies 10 key ingredients for effective child and youth health programs and these are discussed further in MyNursingLab. Additionally, listen to the MyNursingLab audiovideo presentations that provide perspectives on school connectedness and youth development.

Two health concerns, which are receiving a great deal of attention, are childhood obesity and the mental health of children and youth. According to the Dietitians of Canada (2004), overweight and obesity are complex health factors that are linked to a number of determinants of health and have been proven to be difficult to prevent and manage. Multifaceted interventions across multiple settings such families, schools, and community are more likely to have a more positive effect. Creating a healthy school environment that supports healthy eating requires student, parent, and staff education; food and nutrition policies; positive role modelling by school staff; healthy, reasonably priced, and appropriate food choices; safe food practice; appropriate scheduling of nutrition breaks; and student nutrition programs. CHNs can work in collaboration with dietitians to guide schools and school boards in accessing appropriate resources, in developing school nutrition policies, and in facilitating the planning and implementation of activities in each of the four components of CSH. The Canadian Best Practices Portal for Health Promotion and Chronic Disease Prevention (http://www.cbpp-pcpe.phac-aspc.gc.ca) is an excellent source of information on best practices in relation to nutrition and other health issues.

Promoting mental health through schools provides another opportunity for CHNs to use their clinical knowledge and expertise in prevention and health promotion. The characteristics of effective **mental health promotion programs** in schools include:

1. Providing a backdrop of universal, multi-dimensional, coherent programs and services that promote the mental health of all and then effectively targeting those with special needs.

2. Creating supportive climates that promote warmth, empathy, positive expectations, and clear boundaries.

3. Tackling mental health problems early when they first manifest themselves and then taking a long-term approach that considers the child's development over time.

4. Identifying and targeting vulnerable and at-risk groups and helping people acquire the skills and competencies that underlie mental health.

5. Involving end users and their families in ways that encourage a feeling of ownership and participation, and providing effective training for those who run the programs, including helping them to promote their own mental health (JCSH, 2010b; Weare & Markham, 2005, p. 118). [See MyNursingLab for links to audiovisual resources.]

FUTURE CHALLENGES AND OPPORTUNITIES

Schools are unique settings in which CHNs can work collaboratively to optimize the health of school-aged children and youth, their families, and school personnel. The significant health concerns in this population identified at the beginning of this chapter reinforce the need for an expanded health promotion role of the CHN in schools. While comprehensive school health promotion has gained momentum in this country, CHNs struggle to work within a broad scope of practice that is consistent with socioenvironmental and population health approaches. Wicklander (2005) submits that school nurses have unique insight into the health needs of individual students and the school community. Additionally, they have the clinical expertise and knowledge to support school staff within a whole school approach. In the United Kingdom, the National Healthy Schools Standard has provided an explicit framework for strengthening the public health role of nurses within schools that "encompasses a multi-dimensional and multi-sectoral understanding of the health promotion and health protection needs of the school-aged child" (Brooks, Kendall, Bunn, Bindler, & Bruya, 2007, p. 228).

CANADIAN RESEARCH BOX 17.2

What is the relationship between school-level factors and the health and well-being of students?

Saab, H., & Klinger, D. (2010). School differences in adolescent health and wellbeing: Findings from the Canadian health behaviour in school-aged children study. *Social Science and Medicine, 70*(6), 850–858.

A secondary analysis of the *2006 Canadian Health Behaviour in School-aged Children* (HBSC) study of 9670 Grade 6–10 students and 187 administrators was used to assess the relationship between student and school-level factors and three student health and well-being outcomes: self-rated health, emotional well-being, and subjective health complaints. School-level factors included the school's academic and SES standing, problem behaviours, and student aggression.

The findings identified that both individual and school-level factors are associated with students' reported health. Increased health outcomes are associated with increased family and neighborhood wealth, two-parent families, higher levels of student achievement, and the quality of one's neighbourhood. Girls generally reported lower health outcomes across schools. Schools having increased problem behaviours also had students with lower levels of reported health and life satisfaction. The study suggests that schools may be able to differentially impact those students' background factors that impact their reported health outcomes. These factors need more attention in health promotion efforts that involve neighborhoods and communities.

Discussion Questions

1. Discuss how the findings of this study support a socioecological approach to health promotion.

2. As a CHN, how might you work with a school to develop initiatives aimed at students struggling both emotionally and academically?

In Canada, there is an urgent need to increase the number of CHNs working in school communities. We need to evaluate the work that CHNs are currently doing in schools across the country and to examine different models for providing CHN services in schools. CHNs have the competencies that foster collaboration between the health and education sectors to better promote and protect the health of students, staff, and their families.

SUMMARY

This chapter describes the importance of the school years and the evolution of the role of CHNs in promoting the healthy growth and development of children and youth in the school setting. It describes both international and national movements for healthy schools, including comprehensive school health, health promoting schools, and coordinated school health programs. This chapter illustrates the importance of building committee structures and processes within schools that involve students, parents, teachers, administrators, CHNs, and other community partners. CSH offers CHNs the opportunity to work within a broad scope of practice that incorporates one-on-one, small group, and population health strategies using a socioenvironmental approach.

KEY TERMS

risky behaviours, p. 284
Comprehensive School Health (CSH), p. 286
Coordinated School Health Program (CSHP), p. 286
Health Promoting School (HPS), p. 286
settings approach, p. 286
whole school environment, p. 288
school-based health clinic, p. 290
Youth Health Centre (YHC) model, p. 290
peer support, p. 290
community development principles, p. 291
school heath committee or action team, p. 292
developmental assets, p. 293
mental health promotion programs, p. 294

REVIEW QUESTIONS

Choose the one alternative that best completes the statement or answers the question.

1. A new CHN has been assigned to an inner city secondary school and is beginning to gain an understanding of common health concerns in the adolescent population. Which of the following factors put teens at greatest risk for health concerns and early death?

   a) poverty, aboriginal status, sporting injuries, exposure to infectious disease

   b) Aboriginal status, regular alcohol use, driving to school, poverty

   c) gender, overweight, out-of-date immunization status, attention deficit and hyperactivity disorder (ADHD)

   d) smoking, unprotected sex, attention deficit and hyperactivity disorder

2. The CHN has been asked to develop a healthy lifestyle program for youth. How would the nurse engage youth in the planning process?

   a) Complete a literature review to determine the common needs of youth.

   b) Arrange a youth-led focus group with potential program participants to identify strengths and areas of need.

   c) Arrange for youth to rotate the responsibility for chairing the meetings.

   d) Facilitate a forum to discuss youth needs with parents, teachers, and community partners.

3. An assessment of the school's health confirms that bullying is a prominent issue that needs to be addressed. A number of activities are put in place: (1) Classroom teaching of violence prevention curriculum is offered for all grades; (2) The media are invited to a school kick-off assembly where students will be taught a problem-solving/decision-making model. The assembly invites the school board's consultant on violence prevention, the local police, and a social worker; (3) A large banner promoting the anti-bullying campaign

is unveiled and hung in the hallway. Which of the four components of comprehensive school health are reflected in the above activities?

a) teaching and learning, supportive social environment, health and other support services

b) teaching and learning, supportive social environment, health promotion

c) health promotion, health and other support services, teaching and learning

d) teaching and learning, health and other support services, healthy physical environment

4. Two teachers approach the CHN to discuss their observations of what children are eating at lunch and recess. A large number of students are consuming processed and pre-packaged junk food, minimal fruits and vegetables, and pop; some have no lunch at all. The CHN speaks to other teachers and staff and to a few parents to validate the concern. What sources of information can the CHN access or consult to complete an assessment of the situation?

a) Consult a Community Health Status Report.

b) Conduct a formal assessment using key informant interviews, surveys, or focus groups.

c) Contact a local business that provides age-appropriate lunches to schools.

d) Consult a Public Health Dietitian to provide ideas to improve student nutritional habits.

5. A number of students are reporting incidents of sexual harassment and homophobia in a high school's corridors. The school's Health Action Team discusses several ways to address the issue in an effort to prevent this behaviour. Which of the following actions would be the most effective first step in establishing an effective prevention initiative?

a) Act quickly and involve as many people as possible to consider multiple approaches.

b) Encourage students to use health services and engage the offenders in group counselling.

c) Take considerable time to fully assess those students who are known as homophobic and encourage family and community involvement.

d) Implement a poster contest to encourage positive messaging throughout the school.

STUDY QUESTIONS

1. Compare and contrast health promotion work with individuals versus with school communities.

2. Discuss the challenges for CHNs working in school settings.

3. Explain the school-based health promotion models and their components (i.e., Comprehensive School Health, Health Promoting Schools, Coordinated School Health Program).

4. List the potential partners to form the School Health Committee/Action Team.

5. List the common health concerns or problems found in school settings.

6. List the 10 key ingredients for effective child and youth health programs.

After working through these questions, go to the MyNursingLab at www.pearsoned.ca/mynursinglab to check your answers.

INDIVIDUAL CRITICAL THINKING EXERCISES

1. What are the main assumptions underlying comprehensive school health work, in particular work with school health committees?

2. Think of a school you attended in your past, and identify an issue that you believe would have benefitted from a comprehensive school health approach.

3. How might a CHN in a school promote the health of families who have children in the school?

4. Considering the growth and development of children and youth, what potential health issues are likely to arise and how would you use the Healthy Schools framework to address them?

5. What are the benefits of a Healthy Schools approach for students, teachers, and entire school community?

6. Analyze your level of comfort, knowledge, and skill base in facilitating a Healthy Schools approach. What would increase your comfort, knowledge, and skill with each component?

GROUP CRITICAL THINKING EXERCISES

1. Imagine a high school has a sudden increase in the number of teens becoming pregnant. (Or: Imagine an elementary school is experiencing a high incidence of bullying.) Describe how you would work with the school community to assist it to address this issue.

2. Review current provincial or territorial legislation to determine what health services are provided in schools.

3. What barriers exist for school-aged children and youth with complex medical needs? How would you address these?

4. In developing a health profile for a school community, what assessment questions would you ask for each component of CSH? What methods might you use for various stakeholders: students, parents, teachers, administration, and community members?

5. A high school administration wants to find ways to prevent substance use and abuse among its students. Identify five or six points that you would want to address with school staff, students, and parents.

REFERENCES

Adlaf, E. M., Begin, P., & Sawka, E. (Eds.). (2005). *Canadian addiction survey: A national survey of Canadians' use of alcohol and other drugs: Prevalence of use and related harms.* Ottawa, ON: Canadian Centre on Substance Abuse.

Allensworth, D. D., & Institute of Medicine (U.S.) Committee on Comprehensive School Health Programs. (1997). *Schools and health: Our nation's investment.* Washington, DC: National Academy Press.

Ardiles, P. (2009). *Best practice guidelines for mental health Promotion Programs: Children and Youth.* Retrieved from http://www.camh.net/About_CAMH/Health_Promotion/ Community_Health_Promotion/Best_Practice_MHYouth/ index.html

Boyce, W. F., King, M. A., & Roche, J. (2008). *Healthy settings for young people in Canada.* Ottawa, ON: Public Health Agency of Canada. Retrieved from http://www.phac-aspc .gc.ca/dca-dea/yjc/index-eng.php

British Columbia Ministry of Children and Family Development. (2003). *Healthy schools resource guide.* Retrieved from http://www.mcf.gov.bc.ca/early_childhood/pdf/ healthy_schools_website.pdf

Brockington, R. (2010). *Summary public school indicators for the provinces and territories, 2001–2001 to 2007–2008.* Cat. No. 81-595-M2010083. Ottawa, ON: Statistics Canada.

Brooks, F., Kendall, S., Bunn, F., Bindler, R., & Bruya, M. (2007). The school nurse as navigator of the school health journey: Developing the theory and evidence for policy. *Primary Health Care Research and Development, 8,* 226–234.

Campaign 2000. (2008). *Family security in insecure times: The case for a poverty reduction strategy for Canada.* Retrieved from http://www.campaign2000.ca/reportcards/national/ 2008EngNationalReportCard.pdf

Canadian Association for School Health [CASH]. (1991). *Comprehensive school health: A consensus statement.* Retrieved from http://www.cash-aces.ca/index.asp?Page =consensus

Canadian Association for School Health. (2007). *Comprehensive school health: Canadian consensus statement* (revised). Retrieved from http://www.safehealthyschools .org/CSH_Consensus_Statement2007.pdf

Canadian Institute for Health Information [CIHI]. (2005). *Improving the health of young Canadians.* Ottawa, ON: Author.

Canadian Public Health Association [CPHA]. (2001). The value of immunization in the future of Canada's health system. Retrieved from http://resources.cpha.ca/CCIAP/ data/268e.pdf

Canadian Public Health Association [CPHA]. (2010). *Public health-community health nursing practice in Canada: Roles and Activities.* Ottawa, ON: Author.

Community Health Nurses of Canada. (2008). *The Canadian community health nursing standards of practice* (revised). Toronto, ON: Author.

Community Health Nurses of Canada. (2009). *Public health nursing discipline specific competencies Version 1.0.* Toronto, ON: Author.

Craig, W. (2004). Bullying and fighting. In W. Boyce (Ed.), *Young people in Canada: Their health and well-being* (pp. 87–96). Ottawa, ON: Health Canada.

Davies, D. (2004). *Child development: A practitioner's guide* (2nd ed.). New York, NY: Guilford Press.

Dietitians of Canada. (2004). *Eating, physical activity and body weight trends in Canadian children and youth: Backgrounder for* Eat Well Live Well. Retrieved from http://www .dietitians.ca/child/pdf/backgrounder.pdf

Falk-Rafael, A., Fox, J., & Bewick, D. (2005). Report of a 1999 survey of public health nurses: Is public health restructuring in Ontario, Canada moving toward primary care? *Primary Health Care Research and Development* (6), 172–183.

Food Banks Canada. (2008). *Hunger count.* Retrieved from http://www.cafb-acba.ca/main2.cfm?id=10718648-B6A7- 8AA0

Government of Canada. (2006). *The human face of mental health and mental illness in Canada.* Retrieved from http://www.phac-aspc.g.ca/publicat/human-humain06/ pdf/human_face_e.pdf

Halifax Regional School Board and Capital Health. (2005). *The youth health centre model in Halifax regional municipality.* Unpublished manuscript.

Health Canada. (2005). *Acting on what we know: Preventing youth suicide in First Nations.* Retrieved from http://www .hc-sc.gc.ca/fniah-spnia/pubs/promotion/_suicide/ prev_youth-jeunes/

Health Canada. (2008). *Canadian tobacco use monitoring survey.* Retrieved from http://www.hc-gc.ca/hc-ps/tobac- tabac/research-recherche/stat/_ctums-esutc_2008/wasve- phase-1_summary-sommaire-eng.php

Health Council of Canada. (2006). *Their future is now: Healthy choices for Canada's children and youth.* Retrieved from http://www.healthcouncilcanada.ca/docs/rpts/2006/ HCC_ChildHealth_EN.pdf

International Union for Health Promotion and Education [IUHPE]. (2008). *Achieving health promoting schools: Guidelines for promoting health in schools.* Retrieved from http://www.dashbc.org/upload/HPS_Guidelines_2008.pdf

JCSH Canadian Joint Consortium for School Health. (2009). *annual report.* Retrieved from http://eng.jcsh-cces.ca/upload/ JCSH%20Annual%20Report%202009%20English% 20Sept%2029%2009%20WebReady.pdf

JCSH Canadian Joint Consortium for School Health. (2010a). *The school health planner.* Retrieved from http://www.healthyschoolplanner.uwaterloo.ca/ jcshsite_app/controller/index.cfm

JCSH Canadian Joint Consortium for School Health. (2010b). *Schools as a setting for promoting positive mental health: Better practices and perspectives.* Retrieved from http:// eng.jcsh-cces.ca/upload/JCSH%20Positive% 20Mental% 20Health%20Perspectives%20Better% 20Practices.pdf

Kendall, P. R. W. (2008). An ounce of prevention revisited: A review of health promotion and selected outcomes for children and youth in B.C. schools. *Public Health Officer's annual report 2006.* Victoria, BC: Ministry of Health. Retrieved from http://www.hls.gov.bc.ca/annual.html

Leitch, K. K. (2007). *Reaching for the top: A report by the advisor on healthy children and youth.* Ottawa, ON: Health Canada.

MacDougall, C. A. (2004a). School health committees: Making "healthy schools" happen. *Canadian Association for*

Health Physical Education Recreation and Dance Journal, 70(2), 27–29.

MacDougall, C. A. (2004b). School health committees: Perceptions of public health staff. ProQuest Digital Dissertations database Publication No.AAT MQ91427. Toronto, ON: Ontario Institute for Studies in Education University of Toronto.

MacDougall, C. A., & Laforêt-Fliesser, Y. (2009). Canada: The evolution of healthy schools in Ontario, Canada: Top-down and bottom-up. In C. Vince Whitman & C. Aldinger (Eds.), *Case studies in global school health promotion: From research to practice* (pp. 143–157). New York, NY: Springer.

Macleod, C., Huskisson, R., & Keys, E. (2009). *Advancing health promotion in school nursing practice: Taking the best from the past to shape the future.* Paper presented at the 3rd National Community Health Nurses Conference Blazing our Trail: Tools, tactics & taking charge. Calgary, Alberta.

Macpherson, A. K., To, T. M., Macarthur, C., Chipman, M. L., Wright, J. G., & Parkin, P. C. (2002). Impact of mandatory helmet legislation on bicycle-related head injuries in children: A population-based study. *Pediatrics, 110*(5). Retrieved from http://www.cmaj.ca/cgi/content/abstract/166/5/592

Marx, E., Wooley, S., & Northrop, D. (1998). *Health is academic: A guide to coordinated school health programs.* New York, NY: Teachers College Press.

McKay, M. (2009). Public health nursing in early 20th century Canada. *Canadian Journal of Public Health, 100*(4), 249–250.

Meagher-Stewart, D., & Aston, M. (2005). *Fostering citizen participation and collaborative practice: Tapping the wisdom and voices of public health nurses in Nova Scotia.* Ottawa, ON: Public Health Agency of Canada.

Mental Health Commission of Canada. (2006). *Out of the shadows at last: Transforming mental health, mental illness and addiction services in Canada.* Retrieved from http://www.parl.g.ca/39/1/parbus/commbus/senate/Com-e/SOCI-E/re-e/rep02may06-e.htm

Middlesex-London Health Unit. (2010). *Healthy schools toolkit.* Retrieved from http://www.healthunit.com/articlesPDF/161155.pdf

Ontario Ministry of Health and Long-Term Care. (2004). *Healthy weights, healthy lives. Chief Medical Officer of Health report.* Toronto, ON: Author.

Ontario Ministry of Health Promotion. (2010). *School health guidance document.* Retrieved from http://www.mhp.gov.on.ca/en/healthy-communities/public-health/guidance-docs/SchoolHealth.pdf

Ontario Public Health Association. (2004). *Public health responds to the challenge to reduce poverty and enhance resiliency in children and youth.* Toronto, ON: Author.

Ontario Public Health Association. (2005). *Child and youth health: Strengthening interministerial integration.* Toronto, ON: Author.

Parliament of Canada. (2007). *Healthy weights for healthy kids: Report of the Standing Committee on Health.* Retrieved from http://www.ccfn.ca/pdfs/healthyweightsforhealthykids.pdf

Perth District Health Unit & Huron-Perth Catholic District School Board. (2007). *Evaluation of a collaborative pilot program for school-based public health nurse services in Perth County Catholic elementary schools.* Retrieved from http://www.pdhu.on.ca/pdf/pilot.pdf

Pickett, W. (2004). Injuries. In W. Boyce (Ed.), *Young people in Canada: Their health and well-being.* Ottawa, ON: Health Canada.

Public Health Agency of Canada [PHAC]. (2005). *Canada communicable disease report,* Volume 31S2. Ottawa, ON: Author.

Ramage-Morin, P. L. (2008). *Motor vehicle accident deaths. 1979–2004.* Ottawa, ON: Statistics Canada.

Registered Nurses Association of Ontario [RNAO]. (2010). *Nursing best practice guideline: Enhancing healthy adolescent development.* Toronto, ON: Author.

Ronson, B., & Rootman, I. (2004). Literacy: One of the most important determinants of health today. In D. Raphael (Ed.), *Social determinants of health: Canadian perspectives* (pp. 155–169). Toronto, ON: Canadian Scholars' Press.

Rotermann, M. (2008). Trends in teen sexual behaviour and condom use. *Health Reports, 19*, 1–5.

Saab, H., & Klinger, D. (2010). School differences in adolescent health and wellbeing: Findings from the Canadian health behaviour in school-aged children study. *Social Science and Medicine, 70*(6), 850–858.

Scales, P. C. (1999). Reducing risks and building developmental assets: Essential actions for promoting adolescent health. *Journal of School Health, 69*(3), 113–119.

Shields, M. (2006). Overweight and obesity among children and youth. *Health Reports* (Statistics Canada, Catalogue no. 82-003-XIE), *17*(3), 27–42.

Smartrisk. (2009). *The economic burden of unintentional injury in Canada.* Retrieved from http://www.smartrisk.ca/downloads/research/publications/burden/EBI-Eng-Final.pdf

Ungerleider, C., & Burns, T. (2004). The state and quality of Canadian public education. In D. Raphael (Ed.), *Social determinants of health: Canadian perspectives* (pp. 139–153). Toronto, ON: Canadian Scholars' Press.

Varpalotai, A., & Leipert, B. D. (2006). Rural schools/rural communities: Partnerships between physical and health educators and public health nurses. In E. Singleton & A. Varpalotai (Eds.), *Stones in the sneaker: Active theory for secondary school physical and health educators* (pp. 203–222). London, ON: The Althouse Press.

Vince Whitman, C., & Aldinger, C. (2009). Introduction and Background. In C. Vince Whitman & C. Aldinger (Eds.), *Case studies in global school health promotion: From research to practice* (pp. 3–17). New York, NY: Springer.

Weare, K., & Markham, W. (2005). What do we know about promoting mental health through schools? *Promotion and Education, 12*(3/4), 118–122.

Wellington-Dufferin-Guelph Health Unit. (2001). *Student health services study: Final report.* Unpublished manuscript.

Whitehead, D. (2006). The health-promoting school: What role for nursing? *Journal of Clinical Nursing, 15*, 264–271.

Wicklander, M. K. (2005). The United Kingdom National Healthy School Standard: A framework for strengthening the school nurse role. *Journal of School Nursing, 21*(3), 132–138.

World Health Organization. (1997). *Jakarta declaration on leading health promotion into the 21st century.* Retrieved from http://www.who.int/hpr/NPH/docs/jakarta_declaration_en.pdf

Young, I. (2005). Health Promotion in schools—A historical perspective. *Promotion and Education, 12*(3/4), 112–117.

ADDITIONAL RESOURCES

Readings

Adelman, H. S., & Taylor, L. (2006). Mental health in schools and public health. *Public Health Reports, 121*(3), 294–298.

CSH Canadian Joint Consortium for School Health. (2010). *Schools as a setting for promoting positive mental health: Better practices and perspectives.* Retrieved from http://eng.jcsh-cces.ca/upload/JCSH%20Positive%20Mental%20Health%20Perspectives%20Better%20Practices.PDF

Ontario Ministry of Health Promotion. (2010). *School health guidance document.* Toronto, ON: Queens Printer. Retrieved from http://www.mhp.gov.on.ca/en/healthy-communities/public-health/guidance-docs/SchoolHealth.pdf

Websites

A National Assessment of Effects of School Experiences on Health Outcomes and Behaviours of Children
http://www.phac-aspc.gc.ca/hp-ps/dca-dea/publications/schobc-esrcscj/pdf/schobc-esrcscj-eng.pdf

Canadian Joint Consortium on School Health
http://www.jcsh-cces.ca

Canadian School Health Community
http://www.canadianschoolhealth.ca

Centre for Addictions and Mental Health
http://www.camh.net/About_CAMH/Health_Promotion/Community_Health_Promotion/Best_Practice_MHYouth/index.html

Communities and Schools Promoting Health
http://www.safehealthyschools.org

Healthy School Planner
http://www.healthyschoolplanner.uwaterloo.ca/jcshsite_app/controller/index.cfm

Public Health Agency of Canada/Health Canada: "Voices and Choices" Planning for School Health Assessment Tool
http://www.phac-aspc.gc.ca/hp-ps/dca-dea/prog-ini/school-scolaire/vc-ss/index-eng.php

About the Authors

Yvette Laforêt-Fliesser, RN, BScN, MScN (University of Western Ontario), CCHN(C), is an independent consultant in community and public health with over 35 years of progressive experience in public health and community nursing, academia, management, training, and research. An Adjunct Associate Professor at the University of Western Ontario, her practice and research interests include family and community health, school-based nursing practice, and mental health promotion. Yvette is an active member of the Ontario Healthy Schools Coalition and is a member of the Board of Directors of the Community Health Nurses of Canada. She is currently serving on the CNA Certification in Community Health Nursing Examination Committee.

Carol MacDougall, RN, BScN (McGill University), MA (Ontario Institute for Studies in Education, Department of Curriculum, Teaching and Learning, University of Toronto), has worked for 12 years as a Public Health Nurse in Toronto schools, five years as the School Health Consultant in Planning and Policy with Toronto Public Health, and is currently the Public Health Manager, School and Sexual Health, at the Perth District Health Unit in Stratford, Ontario. She has been involved in provincial advocacy for Comprehensive School Health since 1990, and is Co-Chair of the Ontario Healthy Schools Coalition.

Irene Buckland, RN, BScN, MScN (University of Western Ontario), has worked in public health as a program manager and a PHN for over 12 years. She has also worked for several years as a professor and clinical instructor in both college and university nursing programs. Irene participated in the School Health Benchmarking Project sponsored through the Ontario Teaching Health Units and is a member of the Ontario Healthy Schools Coalition.

The authors would like to thank Middlesex-London and Perth District Health Units PHNs for their contributions to the case studies and for their ongoing commitment to advancing Healthy Schools in Ontario.

chapter

18

Gender and Community Health

Joy L. Johnson and John L. Oliffe

OBJECTIVES

After studying this chapter, you should be able to:

1. Distinguish between the concepts of sex and gender.
2. Apply a gender lens to community health nursing practice.
3. Describe how the community health needs of men and women may differ.
4. Develop community nursing strategies to meet the health needs of men and women living in the community.

INTRODUCTION

Gender is often taken for granted in community health nursing. We design programs and interventions without asking whether the programs are equally suited to the needs of women and men. Before reading further, think about the ways your own gender influences your life. Consider the ways it influences how you dress, what you talk about, who you are friends with, when and where you may feel unsafe, and to whom you go for help. While we often think about gender as something that is "natural," it is something that we as individuals cultivate and develop and society reinforces through social relations and institutions. Societies are organized along the fault lines of gender, which means that in our society men and women are thought of, live their lives, and are treated as different kinds of people with different bodies and different roles, responsibilities, and opportunities (Jackson, Pederson, & Boscoe, 2009). When we really begin to think about gender, we realize that it influences many aspects of our lives. Indeed, it has been recognized as a key social determinant of health.

The **social determinants of health** are the conditions in which people are born, grow, live, work and age. These circumstances are shaped by the distribution of money, power, and resources at global, national and local levels. The social determinants of health are mostly responsible for health inequities—the unfair and avoidable differences in health status seen within and between countries. The World Health Organization's [WHO] Commission on Social Determinants of Health [CSDH] (2008) report and the Public Health Agency of Canada's *Report on the State of Public Health in Canada 2008* (Public Health Agency of Canada, 2008) both stress the importance of considering how different social determinants impact health. Social determinants of health

such as gender, socioeconomic status, education level, age, geographic location, race/ethnicity, Aboriginal identity, and immigrant status play intersecting roles in shaping Canadians' health and access to health services.

Responding to increasing concern about these persisting and widening inequities, the WHO established the Commission on Social Determinants of Health (CSDH) in 2005 to provide advice on how to reduce them (CSDH, 2008). One of the chapters in this report focuses on gender equity and health. The authors of the report argue that gender inequities damage the health of women and girls throughout the world, particularly in low and middle income countries. This is because girls and women have less power, privilege, and access to resources than do men. In some countries girls are valued less, receive less education, are fed less, and are restricted in what they can do. This inevitably influences their health outcomes. Is the same true in Canada where it is often assumed that women and men have equal opportunity?

HEALTH OUTCOMES OF CANADIAN MEN AND WOMEN: STATISTICS AND TRENDS

Life expectancy is one indicator of the health of a population, while sex differences in life expectancy tell a story about the health of men and women in that population. Mortality figures show that as of 2005, Canadian women had an average life expectancy at birth of 82.7 years while Canadian men live to an average of 78 years. Women continue to outlive men, although men have recently made greater gains in life expectancy. The past 10 years have seen women's life expectancy increase by 1.6 years and men's by 2.9 years (Statistics Canada, 2008). See Table 18.1.

TABLE 18.1	Life Expectancy at Birth, by Sex; Canada, 1995–2005		
	Both Sexes	Men	Women
1995	78.2	75.1	81.1
1996	78.4	75.7	81.2
1997	78.6	75.7	81.3
1998	78.8	76.0	81.5
1999	79.0	76.2	81.7
2000	79.4	76.7	81.9
2001	79.6	77.0	82.1
2002	79.7	77.2	82.1
2003	79.9	77.4	82.4
2004	80.2	77.8	82.6
2005	80.4	78.0	82.7

Data sources: Vital Statistics Birth and Death Databases, estimates of population by age and sex for Canada, the provinces, and the territories. Statistics Canada. (www.statcan.gc.ca) CANSIM, Table 102-0511 and Catalogue no. 84-537-XIE. Last modified: 2010-01-05.

These subtle shifts in life expectancy reflect behaviours such as the increased tobacco use rate among women starting in the 1960s, as well as scientific advances that have improved clinical outcomes for cancer and cardiac disease, and improved overall nutritional status. There is speculation that the life expectancy gap will continue to narrow, and we may also begin to see a decline in life expectancy over the next decade due in part to rising rates of obesity and diabetes.

It is important to recognize that men and women are not monolithic categories but groups of individuals with multiple and intersecting identities connected to socioeconomic status, race, age, and sexual identity. Even as Canadians enjoy a publically-funded healthcare system and generally good health, access to and utilization of healthcare services is not equal across the board. Socioeconomic status, sexual orientation, and Aboriginality impact the social resources Canadian men and women have that allow them to access care. Poor, Aboriginal, and gay and lesbian Canadians continue to be vulnerable to discrimination and social and political disempowerment; a reality that impacts negatively on health.

Although Canada ranks well internationally in terms of life expectancy and quality of life for its citizens, not every Canadian's health reflects this and differing social locations impact Canadians' health in important ways. Assessing differences and disparities in health status, health behaviours, and utilization of healthcare services based on sex and gender is one step in ensuring that all Canadians benefit equally from Canada's public health system.

CONCEPTUAL DEFINITIONS

The concepts of sex and gender are often used interchangeably. While highly related, these terms are not equivalent. As a CHN, it is important that you think about the implications of both "sex" and "gender" as you plan and deliver programs and interventions.

Sex refers to the biological makeup of and differences between females and males. It is a concept that encompasses anatomy, physiology, genes, and hormones that all influence how we function and see ourselves. Although conceptualizing sex usually relies on the female/male binary, in reality, individuals' sex characteristics exist on a continuum. Thus, using a binary understanding of male/female cannot account for all the variety in human sex characteristics. Still, the majority of people today, researchers included, tend to think of both animals and humans as being comprised of two sexes. As our understanding of the complexities of sex increases, we will be better able to address—in both everyday life and in research—the nuances of the continuum of sex (Johnson, Greaves, & Repta, 2007).

Sex plays an important role in health because individuals may experience various processes differently based on their biology. For example, male and female bodies respond differently to alcohol, drugs, and therapeutics due to differences in hormones, body composition, and metabolism. In fact, the constitution of the female body is inherently different from the male body—from cellular metabolism to blood chemistry. Indeed, some researchers claim that "every organ in the body—not just those related to reproduction—has the capability to respond differently on the basis of sex" (Gesensway, 2001, p. 935).

There are important sex-based differences at the cellular level arising from chromosomal dissimilarity. While we know that a male liver cell is not the same as a female liver cell, we do not know enough about the exact nature of these differences or whether these differences affect the development of disease or responses to treatment. We do know that male and female cells exist in different environments and respond accordingly. It is increasingly clear, therefore, that cellular differences can create dissimilar patterns in the progression of disease in men and women to impact their health status in diverse ways.

There are also sex-specific differences in many diseases and conditions that might arise from the influence of sex hormones (Gesensway, 2001). For example, men have heart attacks at a younger age than women do, largely because premenopausal women benefit from the hormonal protection of estrogens. Scientists are also currently examining whether disease conditions such as stroke and schizophrenia are influenced by hormones.

These emergent findings emphasize the need to include both female and male animals and women and men in biomedical and clinical research because results from one group cannot necessarily be applied to the other. Ignoring the influence of sex compromises the validity and generalizability of the study findings and can be detrimental not just to the research enterprise but also to the health of individuals.

Gender refers to the array of socially constructed roles and relationships, personality traits, attitudes, behaviours, values, relative power, and influence that society ascribes men and women on a differential basis. Gender is culturally based, historically specific, and constantly changing. For example, what it means to be a man in Canada may be different from what it means to be a man in Greece or China. Gender refers to the socially prescribed and experienced dimensions of "femaleness" or "maleness" in a society, and is manifested at many levels (Johnson, Greaves, & Repta, 2007).

Gender roles are the behavioural norms applied to males and females in societies that influence their everyday actions, expectations, and experiences. Gender roles are expressed and enacted in a range of ways, from how we dress or talk, to what we may aspire to do, to what we feel are valuable contributions to make as a woman or a man. In some cultures, these roles are sharply defined and differentiated, allowing and disallowing women (and men) from certain tasks, jobs, opportunities, and/or spaces. In some cultures, there is more gender equity and the lines between gender roles can blur. Either way, gender roles often categorize and control individuals within institutions such as the family, labour force, and education systems. For example, in some cultures men are ascribed the "breadwinner" role in the family, while women are expected to fulfill more nurturing and caretaking roles that include domestic chores, child care, and the emotional work of relationships. We still talk about women in "non-traditional jobs," thereby giving recognition to the fact that there is a pattern in which certain forms of paid employment are seen as "men's" jobs and others as "women's." These differences in gender roles are associated with social status: in almost every society, higher power and prestige is conferred on individuals occupying masculine gender roles. It is also important to acknowledge how governments often enforce these roles and power differentials by providing higher rates of pay to men for performing similar jobs to those of women (Connell et al., 1999).

Gender identity describes how we see ourselves as women and men and affects our feelings and behaviours. Both women and men develop their gender identity in the face of strong societal messages about the "correct" gendered role for their presenting sex. Gender identities are malleable and actively constructed over time and culture, underpinning "an ongoing process of becoming" (Knaak, 2004, p. 302). Gender identity evolves and can change depending on the context. For example, a man may feel that his masculine identity is threatened when he experiences illness (Charmaz, 1995). Socially, a woman working in a typically masculine environment might see herself, act, and dress in a different way than she does at home. Closely tied to gender identity are the concepts of masculinity and femininity. **Masculinity theories** suggest that men's performances, perceptions, and practices around health and illness are informed and influenced by gender norms. For example, many men are reluctant to seek professional help for depression because the illness and their actions in seeking help suggest weakness and are both decidedly unmasculine. As a result masculine ideals including self-reliance, stoicism, and emotional control can be lost and negatively impact many men's self-perceptions about their masculinity (Oliffe & Phillips, 2008). Likewise **femininity** can be thought of as the gender norms that are ascribed to women. In the context of health, women often ascribe to feminine ideals about being competent in self-care as well as being the primary health provider to the men and children in their lives (Lee & Owen, 2002).

Gender relations refer to how we interact with or are treated by people in the world around us, based on our ascribed gender. They affect us at all levels of society and can restrict or make available various opportunities. Gender relations interact with our race, ethnicity, class, and other identities. In most societies, gender relations reflect differential power between women and men and often disadvantage women. Gender affects not only our personal relationships with others, but also guides our interactions within larger social units, including family and the workplace. For example, the gendered relationships between men and women have been found to influence the interpersonal dynamics related to tobacco reduction in pregnant and postpartum women (Bottorff, Kalaw, Johnson, Stewart, Greaves, & Carey, 2006). Likewise, prostate cancer is often referred to as a couples' disease because the illness and many treatments directly impact gender relations (Bottorff, Oliffe, Halpin, Phillips, McLean, & Mroz, 2008).

Institutionalized gender reflects the distribution of power between the genders in the political, educational, religious, media, medical, and social institutions in any society. These powerful institutions shape the social norms that define, reproduce, and often justify different expectations and opportunities for women and men and girls and boys, such as social and family roles, job segregation, job limitations, dress codes, health practices, and differential access to resources such as money, food, or political power. These institutions often impose social controls through the ways that they organize, regulate, and uphold differential values for sexes and genders and women and men. These restrictions reinforce each other, creating cultural practices and traditions that are difficult to change and often come to be taken for granted. For example, some have argued that many family and general practice clinics are feminized environments that men do not feel welcome in. From the colour of the walls to the types of magazines available, all can suggest that the environment favours women.

GENDER, SEX, AND HEALTH OUTCOMES

Sex and gender are powerful determinants that influence the health of the community. This is because *every cell in our body is sexed and every person is gendered.* This means that biologically men and women differ in terms of the diseases they develop, the symptoms they experience, and the ways they respond to medicines and other treatments. Likewise, women and men's varying alignments to gender ideals mediate their experiences and expressions about health and illness.

The effects of sex and gender sometimes combine and lead to particular health outcomes. For example, research has found that women are more likely to experience depression because of both their sex characteristics and gender roles. Hormones, the activity of the hypothalamic–pituitary–adrenal (HPA) axis in response to stress, and reduced thyroid function have all been posited as important biological factors that make women more likely than men to suffer from depression (Kuehner, 2003). But gender is also associated

TABLE 18.2 The Ten Leading Causes of Death among Canadian Men and Women, 2004

Males		Females	
Rank Order of Causes of Death	Number of Deaths	Rank Order of Causes of Death	Number of Deaths
Malignant Neoplasms	35 156	Malignant Neoplasms	31 791
Heart Disease	27 076	Heart Disease	24 924
Cerebrovascular Disease	5 959	Cerebrovascular Disease	8 667
Accidents	5 416	Chronic Lower Respiratory Diseases	4 717
Chronic Lower Respiratory Diseases	5 324	Alzheimer's Disease	3 940
Diabetes	4 020	Diabetes	3 803
Intentional Self-Harm	2 734	Accidents	3 570
Influenza Pneumonia	2 557	Influenza Pneumonia	3 172
Kidney Disease	1 816	Kidney Disease	1 725
Alzheimer's Disease	1 596	Intentional Self-Harm	879

*Source: Statistics Canada. (2008). Sex ratio, ranking, number, and percentage of male and female deaths for the 10 leading causes,
Canada, 2004. Retrieved from http://www.statcan.gc.ca/daily-quotidien/081204/t081204c2-eng.htm*

with different rates of depression among men and women. Factors such as poverty, low level of education, social isolation, and lack of power can increase the risk for depression, and are often unequally distributed among the genders. Additionally, women's multiple roles within work and family settings can result in work overload, and can affect women's mental health (Kuehner).

As another example, both sex and gender relations influence the risk of contracting infectious diseases and their outcomes. For example, women face specific sex- and gender-based inequities when it comes to contracting HIV and seeking medical care for HIV infection. This is in part because the vagina is anatomically and physiologically more susceptible to contracting sexually transmitted infections (STIs) than is the penis (Darroch & Frost, 1999). Also, gender relations lead to women having less power in and control over sexual relationships, putting them at greater risk of contracting HIV (Amaro & Raj, 2000). Finally, due to gender roles, women may delay seeking treatment for HIV/AIDS because of family and childcare obligations.

While men and women develop and experience disease differently, they share the 10 leading causes of death. All of these causes can be targeted by CHNs for primary or secondary prevention.

Gender and Equity

The valuation of men and masculine ideals over women and feminine ideals is one way that "gender is a part of all human interactions" and "is a 'stable' form of structured inequality" (Ettorre, 2004, p. 329). These experiences and cultural values can foster inequity for both men and women. Gender can constrain our everyday life decisions and thereby affect our health. For example, gender has been demonstrated to affect decisions about income, employment, housing, and child care. Men's and women's opportunities are constrained by

gender, and this in turn creates inequities and affects their health. **Gender inequity** occurs when men and women are not provided the same opportunities in society. **Gender bias** is the root of gender inequities and generally arises from three problems:

1. Overgeneralization—when it is assumed that what is good for men is good for women
2. Gender and sex insensitivity—ignoring gender and sex as important variables
3. Double standards—assessing the same situation differently on the basis of gender

To combat gender inequity in our practices as CHNs we need to adopt an approach that will help sensitize us to sex and gender issues.

THE GENDER LENS AND COMMUNITY HEALTH NURSING PRACTICE

The use of a **gender lens** is one way to ensure that nursing programs and interventions are appropriate for women and men, and girls and boys. You can liken the use of a gender lens to putting on a pair of eyeglasses. Through one lens of the glasses, you see the participation, needs, and realities of women. Through the other lens, you see the participation, needs, and realities of men. Your sight or vision is the combination of what each eye sees. Increasingly, gender-based analyses are being used by governments and agencies to ensure that the programs and interventions they develop are equitable. For example, Health Canada's (2000) *Gender Based Analysis Policy* is an important driver in encouraging policy makers to account for gender in their work (Tudiver, 2009).

A *gender lens* helps us to assess the differential impact that a proposed or existing policy, program, or intervention might have on men and women. It is applied by considering a series of questions in relation to a program or an intervention. Ideally, you might want to modify these questions depending on the program or intervention you are considering. To start thinking about a gender lens, one needs to thoughtfully consider a number of questions highlighted in the box below.

Applying a Gender Lens to Depression

A CHN has been asked to develop a depression awareness campaign for college students. The nurse researches evidence about how best to engage college students and raise awareness about depression. During the development of the program, a gender lens is applied in the following ways:

1. How is the problem/issue you are addressing different for men and women?

   - Depression is experienced and expressed in different ways by men and women. Women typically become sad and may cry in talking about how they feel. Men's depression may manifest as anger and irritability, claiming intolerable stress as the underpinning problem.
   - While women are more likely to be diagnosed and treated for depression, men are more likely to commit suicide. This may inadvertently position depression as a women's illness and suicide as the action of men.

2. How are the different contexts in the lives of men and women, boys and girls addressed?
   - This program focuses on college students, but these students come from a variety of contexts. Young women and men living away from home amid diverse pressures around finances, academic performance, and transitions from school to career may render this group particularly vulnerable.

3. How is diversity within subgroups of women and men, girls and boys identified and taken into account?
   - Certain groups such as gay, lesbian, and transgendered college students may be socially isolated and particularly vulnerable to depression. These groups may also be difficult to reach because of their desire to be somewhat anonymous to ensure their safety.
   - International students may also be particularly vulnerable and ethnicity may affect the ways that people understand and acknowledge depression. For example, some individuals of Asian ancestry might talk about feeling "sad" but deny depression as a face-saving strategy.

4. What intended and unintended outcomes for men and women can be identified?
   - The broad aim of the program is to foster dialogue about depression among college students in signalling how it may "look" different among men and women.
   - To detail strategies that might encourage people to prevent or recognize and seek help for depression.
   - A screening program that does not specially address both genders and marginalized groups may ultimately further disadvantage particular groups.

5. What other social, political, and economic realities are taken into account?
   - Mental illness can at times be a stigmatizing condition. Efforts are required to not further stigmatize those who might seek assistance for depression.
   - Depression and some downstream indicators of depression including absenteeism, substance overuse and violence result in significant disease burden. Therefore, prevention and awareness-raising efforts make sound economic and social sense.
   - There may be particular times including mental health awareness week that could aid the momentum for launching a "new" community health depression campaign targeted to men and women who attend college.

Based on the analysis, the nurse develops campaigns that target college men and women in discretely different ways. The nurse is especially careful to use a variety of images that represent a diversity of men and women and engages the campus health services department to ensure they have recent information about gender differences and depression.

CANADIAN RESEARCH BOX 18-1

What speaks to fathers who smoke tobacco?

Johnson, J. L., Oliffe, J. L., Kelly, M. T., Bottorff, J. L., & Le Beau, K. (2009). The readings of smoking fathers: A reception analysis of tobacco cessation images. *Health Communication, 24*(6), 1–16.

For decades, pregnant women and mothers were targeted with messages about the dangers of tobacco use, but the National Health Service (NHS) in the United Kingdom wanted to directly engage dads in family health and tobacco cessation. An image of flowers arranged to read "Dad" on a freshly covered grave was developed as part of the NHS's pregnancy and smoking campaign, titled Emotional Consequences, and was disseminated via billboards and posters throughout the U.K. A team of Canadian researchers in British Columbia decided to show this and four other images to 20 new dads who continued to smoke and to conduct qualitative interviews in which they solicited their responses to the images. They were interested in understanding how these dads read and received the smoking cessation messages.

Many of the men expressed feelings of sadness or distress as they looked at the image and read the accompanying caption. Men focused on the mound of dirt at the centre point of the photograph, indicating that this unpleasant, sensory aspect of the composition held meaning around their own mortality and the consequences of a smoking-induced death on their family. The overarching message "smoking kills" prompted a 28-year-old tradesman to comment, "Wow . . . it's pretty surreal . . . pretty in your face . . . it really hits home." Most of the men's responses related to their identity as a provider and protector for their family. In these ways, the men's alignment with dominant ideals about good fathering practices created dissatisfaction about being a dad who smokes. A 40-year-old Canadian man of South Asian ancestry explained, "I'm thinking about my babies, my family, they are losing, they'll be frustrated for sure, they will have a problem. . . ." In these ways we begin to see how gender—and in this example masculine ideals—can be used to message men about the far-reaching impact of their smoking. That said, it is also important to note that a few men continued to position smoking as a central signifier of their masculinity. For example, a 27-year-old man who began to smoke heavily while serving a prison sentence in the past defended his smoking:

Well, I like to think that I'm invincible so I don't contemplate death much and if I do die then, you know, I'm a Christian so I believe it's meant to be and there's a reason for it so if the Higher Being decides to take me off the planet, well there's a lesson to be learned by someone, maybe, you know, it will be for the good in the end.

This research study illustrates the complexity of gender and diversity in men's masculine identities, while also providing direction for how we might develop gender-savvy community health messages to support fathers committed to tobacco reduction or smoking cessation.

Discussion Questions

1. In your view, what types of images would be most effective to encourage fathers to quit smoking?
2. If you were to design a smoking cessation campaign, what steps might you take to ensure the images have the intended impact?
3. How might the partner's and child's reaction to the NHS DAD image influence a dad who smokes?

WOMEN'S HEALTH

Often when we think of women's health, we focus only on reproductive health issues (e.g., birth control, conception, birth, breastfeeding), or diseases that affect the reproductive system (e.g., breast cancer, ovarian cancer). While these issues and conditions are important, we need to recognize that a woman's health perspective embraces everything that impacts women both directly and indirectly as a product of the practices and interactions with those around them.

In Canada, women's health has been a particular concern of policy makers for over 40 years. The *Report of the Royal Commission on the Status of Women* (Minister of Supply and Services Canada, 1970) was released in 1970. While the report did not explicitly address women's health, the release of this report and its 167 recommendations played a key role in improving services for women. The women's health movement was developed in response to the need to improve health services for women. Of particular concern were the health system's tendency to medicalize natural processes such as menstruation and birth, and its tendency to show a paternalistic attitude toward women and reproductive rights, and violence against women. In 1993, the Canadian Women's Health Network was established whose mandate was to help share information and resources and act as a "watchdog" on emerging issues. In order to foster knowledge development in the field of women's health, in 1996 the Government of Canada funded five Centres of Excellence for Women's Health, whose mandate was to conduct community-based and policy-relevant research that would improve the lives of Canadian women and their families. This was followed in 1999 by the establishment of a Women's Health Strategy (Greaves, 2009).

Over the past decade, women's health has expanded to include a consideration of all of the health issues affecting the lives of women. As we made headway on a number of women's health issues, there was a conceptual shift to examine how the health system could be more responsive to women, and attention was turned to issues of woman-centred care and how health reform might be affecting healthcare for women. Most recently, many of the women's health issues have become embedded in broader concerns about gender and health. At times, the term "gender" is conflated with women's concerns. While concerns about gender and health helped to raise the issue about how both men and women are at times inequitably treated in the health system, there is a need to continue to exclusively focus on the specific community health needs of women and men.

Women living in the community have specific needs and issues that require nurses' attention. The aging of the Canadian population means that many women will experience chronic illness and disability. As the primary caregivers in our society, women will continue to experience the stress associated with multiple roles. Particular groups of women, such as Aboriginals and immigrants, are particularly disenfranchised and require special attention from community health providers. Women continue to remind us that health professionals are often not sensitive to their needs and tend to overprescribe medications, and that the health system is not responsive to their concerns (Hendrikson, 2009). Of particular concern is the fact that women continue to lack the resources they require for good health.

CASE STUDY

The research evidence suggests that while many women quit smoking during pregnancy, many relapse in the postpartum period. One of the major factors associated with relapse is having a partner who smokes. Women smoke for a variety of reasons; in addition to struggling with addiction, they may smoke to manage difficult emotions or to get a much needed time out from their hectic schedules.

Discussion Questions

1. In what ways is tobacco use a women's health issue?
2. How might gender relations affect women's tobacco use?
3. What might a women-centred approach to smoking cessation programming involve?

CASE STUDY

Support groups are commonly used in the context of community health as a vehicle to share knowledge and resources and offer support to individuals faced with common afflictions. These groups have been used to support men facing illnesses such as prostate cancer. Prostate cancer support groups (PCSGs) play a variety of functions and, on occasion, men's partners attend.

Discussion Questions

1. In what ways are PCSGs typically masculine?
2. What similarities and differences might we expect in breast cancer support groups?
3. How might CHNs guide the efforts of PCSGs?

MEN'S HEALTH

Targeted men's health initiatives and dedicated policy are often leveraged by the population data discussed earlier in this chapter. That is, men die earlier than women, and oftentimes from seemingly preventable causes (e.g., suicide, motor vehicle accidents). Typically, the ensuing logic positions men as needing focused attention and services, or, less proactively, a competing victim discourse emerges to lobby for men's health *rather* than women's health (e.g., research and screening in prostate versus breast cancer). Less often discussed is the interconnectedness of men's health and women's health. For example, there are many examples whereby men's health and illness practices impact others, most often their partner(s) and family. Although men's health is often discussed, to date there is no Canadian network, or single point of contact, for gathering research evidence, collating examples of good practice, or examining policy in order to explore how to best promote the health of men in ways that work with (rather than compete against) advances in promoting women's health (Robertson, Galdas, McCreary, Oliffe, & Tremblay, 2009).

Although the history of men's health in Canada is modest, strong evidence linking men's health and illness practices to dominant ideals of masculinity have emerged over the last decade. For example, men typically deny illness and attempt to self-manage for long periods before reluctantly consulting a healthcare professional. Following these masculine scripts enables many men to affirm their masculinity in doing what men typically do (i.e., self-reliance and stoicism) and aligning with what society expects of them. A less often discussed artefact of men's practices dedicated to avoiding "being seen" as weak (a label assigned to men who give in and/or waste the time of busy healthcare professionals with benign issues) is that the vast majority of men are seen in Canadian emergency rooms rather than family or general practice.

In turning our attention to community health nursing, similar challenges prevail. Men's health promotion has grappled with how as well as where to best engage their target audiences (Lee & Owens, 2002; Robertson, 2007). Social marketing has been put forward as a means to taking health information and services to the places that men ordinarily inhabit, including the pub and sporting events (Courtenay, 2004). It can be reasonably argued that effective community nursing practices might lead the way to engaging men more fully with their health because they operate within many locales in which men ordinarily reside. Although masculine ideals guide the health and illness practices of men, the ways in which men interpret, align, and produce masculinity reveals significant diversity within and across men's lives.

CANADIAN RESEARCH BOX 18.2

Why are teenage boys more likely to smoke marijuana?

Haines, R. J., Johnson, J. L., Carter, C. I., & Arora, K. (2009). "I couldn't say, I'm not a girl"—adolescents talk about gender and marijuana use. *Social Science and Medicine, 69,* 2029–2036.

Recent studies suggest that in comparison to girls, adolescent boys in Canada smoke marijuana more frequently, and are more likely to report problematic use. While patterns of use differ for girls and boys, there is limited research that investigates why this difference exists. This qualitative study was based on in-depth interviews with 26 teen boys and 19 teen girls who used marijuana. When asked about their marijuana use in relation to their social activities and relationships, adolescents referenced masculine and feminine ways and reasons for using marijuana, as well as gendered social dynamics present when girls and boys smoked together. The majority said that they knew more boys who smoked, that boys smoked greater amounts of marijuana, and smoked more frequently. Frequent users were referred to as "stoners," an identity positioned as the domain of boys. Girls' habitual use was typically described as inappropriate or inauthentic. While boys smoking marijuana were cast as cool and macho, girls who smoked were described as "annoying," "giggly," or too "immature" to handle being high. Girls who smoked marijuana were often labelled as "heaty," a slang term referring to obvious or uncool behaviour. The findings have practical implications for adolescent substance use prevention strategies. One possibility is to draw from the identities of the "stoner guy" and "heaty girl" to encourage adolescents to think critically about the gendering of marijuana use, and to interrogate norms of masculinity and femininity within the context of adolescence. Prevention programming that ignores the gendered dynamics of smoking marijuana may have limited resonance for young people.

Discussion Questions

1. What would a gender-sensitive drug prevention program look like?
2. How might other risk behaviours that adolescents engage in be gendered?
3. How can we be gender sensitive in our public health programming without reinforcing gendered stereotypes?

TOWARD GENDER APPROPRIATE COMMUNITY HEALTH NURSING PRACTICE

Gender considerations are relevant to *all* community health nursing programming and practice. By applying a gender lens, we can start to consider the ways programs and practices can better meet the needs of men and women. However, caution must be exercised when planning gender appropriate community health interventions. We do not want to inadvertently enforce gendered stereotypes or gender dominance. For example, youth-directed anti-tobacco campaigns seeking to counter the "gendered cool" of smoking present in tobacco advertising can also run the risk of reinforcing gender biases by focusing on smoking as diminishing physical attractiveness and female beauty and emphasizing connections between smoking, erectile dysfunction, and a loss of male sexual virility (Haines, Poland, & Johnson, 2009; Lacroix & Auger, 2007). While tending to structures that design and deliver community health policy and programs it is important to consider their potential for reinforcing or disrupting gender ideals. By delivering and evaluating gender-appropriate community nursing programs, we will better engage end users to advance the well-being of all Canadians. In addition, we will develop our collective expertise for how gender can most effectively be integrated to future community health programs.

SUMMARY

It is clear that "one size does not fit all" when it comes to community health. Nursing strategies in community health need to be gender sensitive. We cannot assume that the approaches commonly used with women will be effective with men (nor the reverse). **Gender appropriate public health interventions** are tailored approaches that ensure than the unique needs of men and women are met. Assessing differences and disparities in health status, health behaviours, and utilization of healthcare services based on sex and gender is an important step in ensuring that all Canadians benefit equally from Canada's health system.

In this chapter, we have highlighted the differences between the concepts of sex and gender and have demonstrated how these concepts are relevant to community health practice. Applying a gender lens to one's practice can help to shed light on the unique health needs that men and women have, and can help us to appropriately tailor our approaches.

KEY TERMS

social determinants of health, p. 300
sex, p. 301
gender, p. 301
gender roles, p. 302
gender identity, p. 302
masculinity theories, p. 302
femininity, p. 302
gender relations, p. 302
institutionalized gender, p. 302
gender inequity, p. 303
gender bias, p. 303
gender lens, p. 303
gender appropriate public health intervention, p. 307

REVIEW QUESTIONS

Choose the one alternative that best completes the statement or answers the question.

1. A nurse learns that the teenage boys in her community are reluctant to attend the clinic for STI testing. The nurse should
   a) teach the young men the importance of safe sex.
   b) explore ways to make the clinic more welcoming to young men.
   c) teach the importance of STI testing at the high school.
   d) focus on providing STI testing services for girls.

2. Which of the following statements is false?
   a) One's sex affects one's gender.
   b) Gender and sex are the same.
   c) Gender is social, sex is biological.
   d) Gender and sex are made up of many dimensions.

3. In developing an obesity prevention program for young men, a nurse should

   a) understand that body image is a women's issue.

   b) consider how the issue of obesity may be different for men and women.

   c) encourage lots of exercise because this is what men like.

   d) make sure a man leads the program.

4. Men may use the health system less than women because

   a) they tend to be less ill than women.

   b) they are more resilient and require less healthcare than women.

   c) they are more likely to engage in preventive practice.

   d) they are influenced by societal norms that view help-seeking as a sign of weakness.

5. In delivering quality care to men and women, a nurse should

   a) always assume that because men and women are different they need different healthcare.

   b) offer separate programs for men and women.

   c) never assume that men and women are different.

   d) consider the ways that programs need to be tailored to meet the needs of men and women.

STUDY QUESTIONS

1. What distinguishes sex from gender?

2. What is a gender lens and how is it used?

3. How do Canadian men's and women's life expectancy and causes of death differ?

4. How do sex and gender affect health outcomes?

5. When should gender considerations be made in community health nursing?

*After working through these questions, go to the MyNursingLab at **www.pearsoned.ca/mynursinglab** to check your answers.*

INDIVIDUAL CRITICAL THINKING EXERCISES

1. Consider the table of contents in this textbook. In what ways are gender considerations relevant to topics covered in this text?

2. Imagine a world without gender—what would the world be like?

3. How do I as a community nurse influence the gender performances of men and women clients within my practice?

4. In what ways are my expectations different for men and women in my practice?

5. In your practice experiences, who is more likely to engage in health promoting behaviour—men or women?

GROUP CRITICAL THINKING EXERCISES

1. Stand up and position yourself on a continuum from one side of the room to another. On one side of the room is the most feminine; on the other is the most masculine. After placing yourself on the continuum look around and see where everyone else is. Discuss why you placed yourself where you did? How do your observations inform our understanding of gender?

2. Now place ourself on a continuum for how men and women typically do health (most similar to atypical). What specific gendered aspects of health informed your positioning?

3. *Picturing smoking dads*—In small groups, discuss your interpretations and critique of the DAD image (see Canadian Research Box 18.1) in addressing the following questions:

   ■ How might we more effectively message the 27-year-old father about his continued smoking?

   ■ What masculine roles, identities, and relations were operating for the fathers who were prompted to reduce or cease smoking by this image?

   ■ What would the equivalent message "look" like and "say" to moms who smoke?

REFERENCES

Amaro, H., & Raj, A. (2000). On the margin: Power and women's HIV risk reduction strategies. *Sex Roles, 42*(7), 723–749.

Bottorff, J. L., Kalaw, C., Johnson, J. L., Stewart, M., Greaves, L., & Carey, J. (2006). Couple dynamics during women's tobacco reduction in pregnancy and postpartum. *Nicotine and Tobacco Research, 8*, 499–509.

Bottorff, J. L., Oliffe, J. L., Halpin, M., Phillips, M., McLean, G., & Mroz, L. (2008). Women and prostate cancer support groups: The gender connect? *Social Science and Medicine, 66*, 1217–1227.

Charmaz, K. (1995). Identity, dilemmas of chronically ill men. In D. Sabo & D. F. Gordon (Eds.), *Men's health and illness: Gender, power and the body* (pp. 266–291). Thousand Oaks, CA: Sage.

Commission on the Social Determinants of Health. (2008). *Closing the gap in a generation: Health equity through action on the social determinants of health. Final report of the Commission on Social Determinants of Health.* Geneva, Switzerland: World Health Organization.

Connell, R., Schofield, T., Walker, L., Wood, J., Butland, D. L., Fisher, J., & Bower, J. (1999). *Men's health: A research agenda and background report.* Canberra, Australia: Department of Health and Aged Care.

Courtenay, W. (2004). Making health manly: Social marketing and men's health. *The Journal of Men's Health and Gender, 1*(2–3), 275–276.

Darroch, J. E., & Frost, J. J. (1999). Women's interest in vaginal microbicides. *Family Planning Perspectives, 31*(1), 16–23.

Ettorre, E. (2004). Revisioning women and drug use: Gender sensitivity, embodiment and reducing harm. *International Journal of Drug Policy, 15*(5–6), 327–335.

Gesensway, D. (2001). Reasons for sex-specific and gender-specific study of health topics. *Annals of Internal Medicine, 135*(10), 935–938.

Greaves, L. (2009). Women, gender and health research. In P. Armstrong & J. Deadman (Eds.), *Women's health: Intersections of policy research and practice* (pp. 3–20). Toronto, ON: Women's Press.

Haines, R. J., Poland, B. D., & Johnson, J. L. (2009). Becoming a "real" smoker—cultural capital in young women's accounts of substance use, *Sociology of Health and Illness, 31*(1), 66–80.

Haines, R. J., Johnson, J. L., Carter, C. I., & Arora, K. (2009). "I couldn't say, I'm not a girl"—adolescents talk about gender and marijuana use. *Social Science and Medicine, 69*, 2029–2036.

Health Canada. (2000). *Health Canada's gender-based analysis policy.* Ottawa, ON: Author.

Hendickson, T. (2009). Marginalized women's voices: Crucial for research, policy and practice. In P. Armstrong & J. Deadman (Eds.), *Women's health: Intersections of policy research and practice* (pp. 251–262). Toronto, ON: Women's Press.

Jackson, B. E., Pederson, A., & Boscoe, M. (2009). Waiting to wait: Improving wait times evidence through gender-based analysis. In P. Armstrong & J. Deadman (Eds.), *Women's health: Intersections of policy research and practice* (pp. 35–52). Toronto, ON: Women's Press.

Johnson, J., Greaves, L., & Repta, R. (2007). *Better science with sex and gender: A primer for health research.* Vancouver, BC: Women's Health Research Network.

Johnson, J. L., Oliffe, J. L., Kelly, M. T., Bottorff, J. L., & Le Beau, K. (2009). The readings of smoking fathers: A reception analysis of tobacco cessation images. *Health Communication, 24*(6), 1–16.

Knaak, S. (2004). On the reconceptualizing of gender: Implications for research design. *Sociological Inquiry, 74*(3), 302–317.

Kuehner, C. (2003). Gender differences in unipolar depression: An update of epidemiological findings and possible explanations. *Acta Psychiatrica Scandinavica, 108*(3), 163–174.

Lacroix, C., & Auger, N. (2007). Beauté et tabagisme: L'utilisation des données probantes dans la prévention du tabagisme chez les jeunes. *Revue Canadienne de Santé Publique, 98*(5), 400–401.

Lee, C., & Owens, R. (2002). The psychology of men's health series. Philadelphia, PA: Open University Press.

Minister of Supply and Service Canada. (1970). *Report of the Royal Commission on the Status of Women.* Ottawa, ON: Supply and Services Canada.

Oliffe, J. L., & Phillips, M. (2008). Depression, men and masculinities: A review and recommendations. *Journal of Men's Health, 5*(3), 194–202.

Public Health Agency of Canada. (2008). *The chief public health officers' report on the state of public health in Canada.* Ottawa, ON: Author.

Robertson, S. (2007). *Understanding men and health: Masculinities, identity and well-being.* Berkshire, England: Open University Press.

Robertson, S., Galdas, P., McCreary, D., Oliffe, J. L., & Tremblay, G. (2009). Men's health promotion in Canada: The current state of play. *Health Education Journal, 68*, 266–272.

Statistics Canada. (2008). Life expectancy, abridged life table, at birth and at age 65, by sex, Canada, provinces and territories, annual (years). Table 102-051. CANSIM (database).

Tudiver, S. (2009). Integrating women's health and gender analysis in a government context: Reflections on a work in progress. In P. Armstrong & J. Deadman (Eds.), *Women's health: Intersections of policy research and practice* (pp. 21–34). Toronto, ON: Women's Press.

ADDITIONAL RESOURCES

Readings

Armstrong, P., & Deadman, J. (Eds.). (2008). *Women's health: Intersections of policy, research and practice.* Toronto, ON: Women's Press.

Institute of Medicine. (2001). *Exploring the biological contributions to human health: Does sex matter?* Washington, DC: National Academy Press.

Johnson, J. L., Greaves, L., & Repta, R. (2008). *Better science with sex and gender.* Vancouver, BC: Women's Health Research Network. (Available at http://www.whrn.ca/resources.html)

Mechakra-Tahiri, S. D., Zunzunegui, M. V., Préville, M., & Dubé, M. (2010). Gender, social relationships and depressive disorders in adults aged 65 and over in Quebec. *Chronic Diseases in Canada, 30*(2). (Available at http://www.phac-aspc.gc.ca/publicat/cdic-mcc/30-2/ar_03-eng.php)

Robertson, S. (2007). *Understanding men and health: Masculinities, identity and well-being.* Maidenhead, UK: Open University Press.

Films/Videos

100% Woman—A documentary film by Karen Duthie
http://www.100percentwoman.com/XXY http://www.imdb.com/title/tt0995829/

The Disappearing Male
http://www.cbc.ca/documentaries/doczone/2008/disappearingmale/

Websites

WHO Gender, Women, Health
http://www.who.int/gender/en/
Gender & Health Collaborative Curriculum
http://genderandhealth.ca/
Health Canada Gender Based Analysis Policy
http://www.hc-sc.gc.ca/hl-vs/pubs/women-femmes/sgba-policy-politique-ags-eng.php
European Men's Health Forum
http://www.emhf.org/

About the Authors

Joy Johnson, PhD, RN, FCAHS, is a Professor in the School of Nursing at the University of British Columbia and the Scientific Director of the Canadian Institutes of Health Research, Institute of Gender and Health. She has conducted research focused on a variety of community health issues, including tobacco use, marijuana use, harm reduction for crack cocaine use, sexual health, and mental health. Her research focuses on the ways that gender, diversity, and place shape the health of individuals and communities.

John Oliffe, PhD, M.Ed, RN, is an Associate Professor in the School of Nursing at the University of British Columbia and a Canadian Institutes of Health Research New Investigator and Michael Smith Foundation for Health Research Scholar. His program of research in men's health and masculinity focuses on smoking and fathering, immigrant men's health, prostate cancer, and men's depression. He has published empirical and methods articles to illustrate and guide policy, nursing practice, and the "doing" of gender and health research.

Older Adult Health

Lori Schindel Martin

OBJECTIVES

After studying this chapter, you should be able to:

1. Discuss population trends of older adults in Canada within a global context.

2. Examine societal myths related to aging.

3. Describe the philosophical underpinnings of, the population health context of, and the Age-Friendly Community Program for aged care.

4. Understand the range of healthcare needs and services for older adults.

5. Identify the resources necessary for holistic care of older adults living at home or transitioning into long-term care environments.

6. Discuss community health nursing roles and challenges in maintaining and promoting the health and well-being of older adults.

INTRODUCTION

Within the last decade, the study of the aging process and its impact on individuals, families, and communities has expanded to give us a growing body of knowledge about the experiences of older adults and their corresponding healthcare needs. While many older adults in Canada desire to live as independently as possible in their own homes, co-ordinated resources must be available to maintain their needs (Cranswick & Dosman, 2008; Statistics Canada, 2008; Turcotte & Schellenberg, 2007). This chapter will explore the factors related to the assessment, maintenance, and promotion of the health of older adults. CHNs must acquire competent knowledge and skills to care for older persons so that they can experience life and living with vitality and strength; chronic illness and dying with comfort, dignity, and connectedness.

POPULATION TRENDS

In this chapter, the terms **older adults, older persons,** and **aged persons** will be used interchangeably, and will refer to Canadians aged 65 and older. Age 65 is considered the standard marker for an older adult, although there is debate about whether 65 years reflects the age at which someone becomes "old" (Turcotte & Schellenberg, 2007). The term "aged care" will be used to refer to the services and resources delivered to older adults.

Canadian and global statistics support that the world population is rapidly aging and this trend will continue at an even faster rate into the future (Statistics Canada, 2008) (see Figure 19.1). It is predicted that over 20% of the world's population will be comprised of older people by 2050, meaning 2 billion older people in both developed and under-developed countries (World Health Organization, 2003).

From a Canadian demographic context, the number of older adults over 65 years living in Canada increased from 2.4 to 4.2 million between 1981 and 2005. It is expected that the number of older persons in Canada will increase to 9.8 million between 2005 and 2036. This will represent an increase in older adults from 13.2% to 24.5% of the total Canadian population (Statistics Canada, 2006). By 2056 it is projected that the proportion of Canadians age 65 and older will be 1 in 4. For Canadians age 80 and older the proportion will be 1 in 10, which is triple that of 2005 (Cranswick & Dosman, 2008). (See Figure 19.2 and MyNursingLab.)

SOCIETAL MYTHS ABOUT AGING

The negative attitudes in society that marginalize and discriminate against older adults subject them to having unmet healthcare needs. Older adults are often stereotyped as dependent, frail, disabled, intellectually incapable, and inactive. This results in a societal belief that older adults are an expensive drain on healthcare resources, rather than contributors

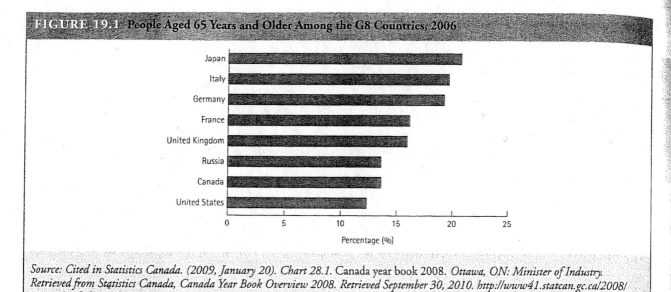

FIGURE 19.1 People Aged 65 Years and Older Among the G8 Countries, 2006

Source: Cited in Statistics Canada. (2009, January 20). Chart 28.1. Canada year book 2008. Ottawa, ON: Minister of Industry. Retrieved from Statistics Canada, Canada Year Book Overview 2008. Retrieved September 30, 2010. http://www41.statcan.gc.ca/2008/70000/grafx/htm/ceb70000_000_1-eng.htm h

to society (Canadian Network for the Prevention of Elder Abuse, 2010). In fact, more older adults are continuing to participate in the labour force past retirement age, with the numbers of those actively employed expected to increase as more baby boomers (those between the age of 45 and 60) reach 65 (Cranswick & Dosman, 2008; Statistics Canada, 2008). Older persons consider themselves to be in much better overall health compared with their predecessors of 25 years ago. The proportion of older adults with low income after taxes fell by 5% and the overall average income of married elderly couples rose by 18% between 1996 and 2006.

FIGURE 19.2 Percentage of Canadian Population Composed of Persons Aged 65 or Older, 1921 to 2005 and Projections to 2056

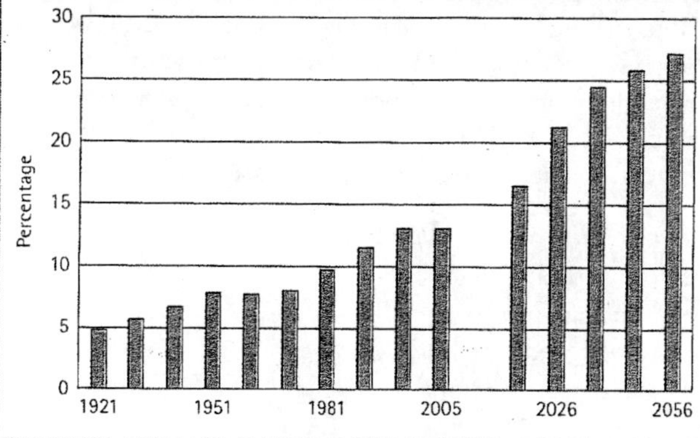

Source: Cited in Turcotte, M., & Schellenberg, G. (2006). A portrait of seniors in Canada (Catalogue No. 89-519, p. 11). Ottawa, ON: Minister of Industry. Retrieved from http://www.statcan.gc.ca/pub/89-519-x/89-519-x2006001-eng.pdf

Thus, the economic status of older adults is considered to be more stable than that of previous generations (Statistics Canada).

In addition, only a small proportion of older adults rely on the healthcare system for any care as many live independently in their homes. According to Cranswick and Dosman (2008), 83% of men and 75% of women over the age of 65 years are living at home, in comparison with 17% and 25% respectively, who live in facility-based care. Interestingly, both groups are living with a range of chronic illnesses that must involve professional services on a daily basis (Statistics Canada, 2006). However, those older adults who require help to remain at home are often supported by a large community of social networks, compared with past generations who were cared for by their children. This is thought to be because many older adults have had fewer children who have then moved away from their hometowns for employment. (See MyNursingLab.) These trends indicate that it is imperative that we cease thinking of aging as a pathology. It is not enough that the social environment becomes elder friendly. Rather, we must advance our thinking from elder friendly to becoming "elder essential" (Gueldner, 2009).

PHILOSOPHICAL UNDERPINNINGS OF AGED CARE

One of the primary philosophical tenets of **aged care** or **elder care** embraces respect for the older individuals experiencing a life transition or chronic illness. It is imperative that CHNs seek to understand each "unique individual's life story" within the context of the aging process. While an appreciation of ethical principles such as "autonomy" is necessary for compassionate practice, no single concept is more important than the recognition and honouring of the "personhood" of the individual. By uncovering the individual's life history, hopes, fears, frustrations, pleasures, strengths, beliefs, and personal values, CHNs will be able to develop a relationship of trust based on *unconditional positive regard* for that person. With this understanding, CHNs can assist the individual in living life as fully as possible within the constraints of any chronic health condition, disability, or loss.

A complementary philosophical tenet is *maximization of remaining strengths*, whereby the physical and emotional abilities of the older adult are continually encouraged and incorporated into daily activities (Brooker, 2007; Clarke, Hanson, & Ross, 2003). It is imperative that the CHN identify and maximize the remaining strengths of the individual, rather than focusing on the inherent disabilities associated with any chronic conditions. CHNs can assist their clients to live within the parameters of maximum wellness that are possible within the limitations of their illness and the available resources.

An additional complementary philosophical tenet is *partnership*. Older people should and want to be involved in their care as active partners rather than as passive recipients of care. Therefore, CHNs act as facilitators of services to empower older adults and their family members to navigate the system, and to engage them in decision-making and self-management strategies wherever possible (Pringle Specht, Taylor, & Bossen, 2009).

POPULATION HEALTH AND OLDER ADULTS

In order to facilitate healthcare and influence health policy for broad communities of older adults, CHNs can assess service needs using a population health framework. **Population health approach** is a lens through which CHNs consider the macro-level health issues of communities and larger groups, moving beyond the micro level of the health of individual persons. This approach focuses on the analysis of how factors such as lifestyles and living conditions affect the health of certain groups. This analysis can result in the identification of disease prevention and health promotion strategies that reduce health inequities (Raphael, 2009; Thompson, 2010). The concept of population health as it relates to the healthcare of older adults refers to a systematic, scientific approach to the maintenance and improvement of the overall health of those Canadians over 65 years of age. While determinants of health are similar across populations, there are unique features of each when considered within the context of older adults. For example, one determinant of health is social support networks. As the number of friends and family resources dwindle, older adults may increasingly rely on the healthcare system and their immediate neighbourhoods for opportunities to interact with other people. Thus, neighbourhoods become a determinant of health that must be assessed for quality of support. One example of a population health framework that has been implemented in

Canada is the Age-Friendly Community Program initiative described below.

AGE-FRIENDLY COMMUNITY PROGRAMS

Traditionally, planning and delivery of healthcare for older adults was through a biomedical lens. This biomedical framework focused on the treatment of illnesses associated with aging, rather than health promotion. Over the past two decades there has been a movement toward providing community-based services that accommodate the unique needs of the older population. This movement is based on the belief that older adults should be partners in planning their healthcare, and should be supported in their familiar community setting as long as possible. It is reported that older adults view the ideal community-based services available as those that provide a continuum of service in the home setting and in the community to improve health status and level of independence. Older adults also want services that enable participation in community life, prevent prolonged stays in healthcare institutions, and relieve excess stress on family members or other caregivers (Turcotte & Schellenberg, 2007). (See MyNursingLab.)

Various community-based programs have been developed using the above principles in one form or another over the years. The World Health Organization [WHO] (2007) recently recommended the **Age-Friendly Communities program**, which is based on communities adapting their services and environments to meet the needs of a wide range of older adults. The aged persons actively engage as participants in the planning of health and social service delivery and evaluation of these services with respect to inclusiveness and promotion of health and security. This notion of "active ageing" depends on determinants such as gender, culture, social factors, physical environment, and behavioural conditions that interact to influence how well individuals age. (See Figure 19.3.) WHO developed a guide for age-friendly communities based on a participatory action research study. Halifax, NS, Saanich, BC, Portage la Prairie, MB, and Sherbrooke, QC, were the four Canadian communities that were engaged with other international sites to develop the guide. The Age-Friendly Communities movement has implications for the role of the CHN with respect to community assessment. A checklist of age-friendly community features includes

- outdoor spaces and buildings;
- transportation;
- housing;
- respect and social inclusion;
- social participation;
- communication and information;
- civic participation and employment; and
- community support and health services. (WHO, 2007)

Reviewing these determinants of health and involvement in the community can assist the CHN to identify those older

FIGURE 19.3 Determinants of Active Aging

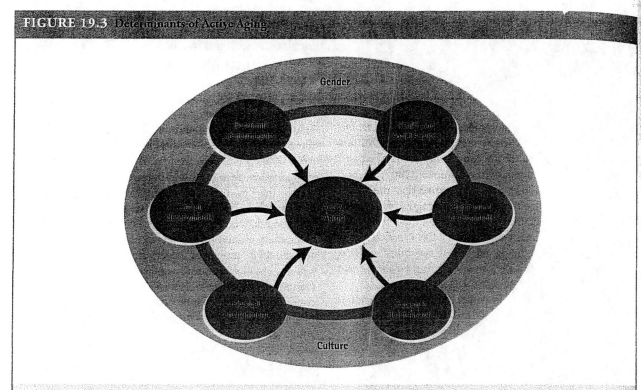

adults at risk for poor health and requiring assistance to access resources to remain in the community.

ASSESSMENTS AND RESOURCES NEEDED FOR AGED-CARE SUPPORT

The evidence-based conceptual knowledge of the CHN working with older adults is extensive. Given the movement toward caring for older adults with complex care requirements while they continue to live at home, it will be essential that the CHN have an awareness of a variety of screening and disease prevention tools. These include, but are not limited to, such clinical issues as physical activity and fall prevention; continence; mental health disorders such as anxiety, delirium, and depression; substance abuse; medication misuse and polypharmacy; pain management; social isolation; sexual relationships; housing; poverty; food security; elder abuse and neglect; and end-of-life care. In addition, the CHN must understand the principles of advanced care planning; ethics and legalities; competency and cognitive impairment; adherence/compliance; culture, ethnicity, and diversity; family systems; local, provincial/territorial government standards; leadership and advocacy. Some of these areas of assessment are discussed in more detail in resources associated with this chapter. (See MyNursingLab.)

Physical Activity and Fall Prevention

It is estimated that between 28–79% of older adults are physically inactive. This is a concern considering that physical activity reduces the risk of chronic illness and contributes to the overall strength, flexibility, mobility, and cognitive function that will maintain autonomy and independence (Health Canada, 2002a). Thus, it is critical that CHNs assess the physical activity levels of their clients. In addition, CHNs must be aware of community resources and programs available to enhance physical activity. Isolated and rural communities may not have access to such programs, and, therefore, creative adaptations can be developed and encouraged.

It is insufficient for the CHN to provide information to older adults about why they *should* exercise. While exercise does reduce risk associated with stroke, cardiac disease, and diabetes, it is clearly not enough to provide this information and then expect older adults to change their health behaviours. In the instance of the individual who enjoys watching television and reading novels, the CHN would need to take into account the physical activities the older adult prefers and previously enjoyed. A conversation about these activities is important to engage the person in creating, planning, and building an exercise program that fits his or her unique personality, preferences, and needs. The CHN can also identify new activities in the older person's community that would strengthen social networks. A possible intervention here, therefore, is mobilizing a community organization to offer a book club for older adults that includes a walk or swimming event just

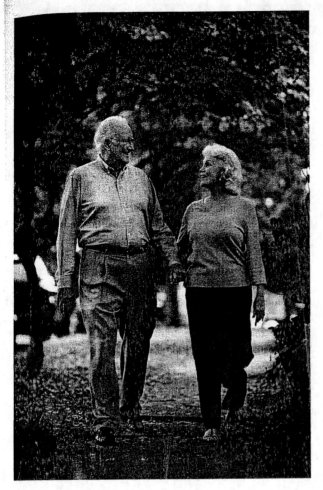

Photo 19.1

Physical activity is important for older adults.

Credit: Steve Cole / iStockphoto.com

CANADIAN RESEARCH BOX

What factors influence older adults' participation in exercise?

Weeks, L. E., Profit, S., Campbell, B., Graham, H., Chircop, A., & Sheppard-LeMoine, D. (2008). Participation in physical activity: Influences reported by seniors in the community and in long-term care facilities. *Journal of Gerontological Nursing, 34*(7), 36–43.

This qualitative study identified factors influencing the likelihood that seniors will exercise. The study built on previous research indicating that higher fitness levels associated with exercise will improve mobility, reduce falls, improve the management of chronic illness, improve mental health, and enhance independence. Of the 24 participants, 17 were community-dwelling seniors and 7 lived in a nursing home. Participants completed socio-demographic and physical activity profiles and engaged in 45-minute personal interviews about the perceptions, barriers, and facilitators to exercise. Interviews were audiotaped and transcribed. The findings revealed that past experiences, life transitions, and future concerns influence seniors' participation in exercise. Other influencing factors are inter-generational influences, establishment of early physical activity patterns, family transitions, changing health status, and future health concerns.

Understanding of an individual's life history is paramount so that CHNs provide encouragements that foster exercise based on the individual's preferences and previous activity patterns. This study is important because adequate physical activity in the later years of life is central to overall health and well-being.

Discussion Questions

1. What implications do the results of this study have for the health promotion education that a CHN would give an older adult living at home whose main activity is watching television programs and reading novels?

2. What additional health history and physical assessments would the CHN perform in order to collect data to create a fitness program for this older adult?

prior to every meeting. The key point here is that the older adult must be directly involved in building opportunities for exercise into everyday events that have meaning and purpose.

Falls are a common health problem associated with older persons. It is estimated that 30% of older people living in the community experience one or more falls each year (Liu-Ambrose, Ashe, Graf, Beattie, & Khan, 2008). Of those older adults who have fallen, 50% will fall repeatedly; it is estimated that falls result in 87% of hospitalizations from unintentional injuries and are the etiology of 75% of the deaths resulting from such injuries (Health Canada, 2002b).

Falls are preventable occurrences, unlike other accidental events. Therefore, CHNs can play a critical role in fall prevention. Falls are the result of a series of inter-related determinants that can be classified under biological, behavioural, environmental, and socioeconomic factors, many of which are modifiable (Health Canada, 2002b; Rose, 2008). When these risk factors occur in combination, they increase the likelihood of fall incidents. Evidence suggests that older adults prefer information about falls presented in the context of health promotion and independence, rather than focusing on fall prevention strategies alone (Hughes et al., 2008).

Mental Health

Older persons are at risk for mental health difficulties including depression, delirium, dementia, anxiety disorders, medication misuse, and substance abuse. The changes associated with aging, such as physiological impact from chronic illnesses, diminishing social networks, financial instability, and life transitions all contribute to mental illness. According to the Centre for Addiction and Mental Health [CAMH] (2008), the number of older Canadians with mental health concerns is predicted to increase as the population ages. The signs and symptoms of mental illness include sleep disturbance, concentration difficulties, psychomotor slowing or agitation, depressed mood, loss of interest, personality changes, decreased self-care capabilities, memory changes, disorganized thinking, social withdrawal, and excessive worry. Since CHNs often are the first contact for older adults experiencing mental illness, they must have the knowledge and skill to identify older adults for referral to appropriate diagnostic and treatment centres. CHNs also need to know the variety of mental health services available to their clients that can assist with diagnosis and the development and monitoring of treatment plans. The client should be assisted to identify resources that are based on the recovery model, wherein older adults identify their own strengths, gain control of their lives, reclaim their sense of self, set their own goals, and form supportive networks with others. CHNs will need to be aware of the types of treatments that an older adult is receiving in order to assist with outcome monitoring. (See Chapter 21.)

Medication Misuse and Polypharmacy

Ramage-Morin (2009) reported that over a half million older persons in both facility-based and home environments often are taking multiple medications inaccurately. CHNs must assess the number and types of medications used by older adults. Medications include, but are not limited to, antihypertensives, calcium channel blockers, diabetes medications such as insulin and hypoglycemics, laxatives, and antacids. Older adults often use neuroleptic medications such as antipsychotics, anxiolytics, hypnotics, and sedatives. These medications are associated with elevated risk of adverse events such as falls, delirium, and cognitive dysfunction.

Food Security and Nutrition

Access to preferred safe, nutritious, and affordable food is a concern for many older adults, in particular those who are functionally dependent. It is estimated that as many as 60% of older adults with health conditions that warrant hospitalization or admission to nursing homes experience malnutrition. This is a concern because malnutrition is associated with decreased body weight, muscle mass, autonomy, and quality of life, and increased likelihood of bone fracture, immuno-suppression, early institutionalization, and mortality. Thus, CHNs must engage in promotion of optimal nutrition and screening of those older people who are at risk for undernourishment. Providing at-risk, frail older adults who are community-dwellers with nutritional supplementation will increase overall quality of life and well-being (Health Canada, 2002b).

Social Isolation

Isolation and loneliness are feelings that are often experienced by older adults. The extent of their social networks, including kinship and friendship, forms part of the nursing assessment. Poor social support is a risk factor for mental health issues, self-neglect, and high rates of morbidity and mortality (Lucie, Gavin, Gosselin, & Laforest, 2009). Older adults over the age of 75, women in particular, are less likely to have connections with friends or neighbours (Lindsay, 2008). (See Chapter 18.) CHNs who are knowledgeable about the community resources, programs, and activities can enhance the social networks for their older clients. For example, senior centres and adult daycare programs are a potential resource providing group activities that can be enjoyed by older adults with a variety of interests.

Sexual Expression, Sexuality, and Intimate Relationships

Sexual relationships are thought to contribute significantly to the positive quality of life of older adults. Older adults do not often share their experiences with sexuality because of perceived social stigma. Late life sexuality among older adults, particularly among older women, is therefore infrequently explored (Penhollow, Young, & Denny, 2009). Older adults prefer their healthcare providers to bring up the subject of sexual health with them, even if the older person seems reluctant to initiate a discussion themselves (Smith & Christakis, 2009). Therefore, CHNs should discuss sexual health with their clients in order to provide them with health education that will increase overall quality of life and reduce the risk of sexually transmitted infection. Addressing older adults' sexuality can serve to enhance their self-esteem, contribute to healing from depression, improve the quality of intimate relationships, and enhance energy (Rheaume & Mitty, 2008; Wallace, 2008). (See Chapter 29.)

Elder Abuse

While there is no single accepted definition, **elder abuse** is considered to include single or repeated acts or the lack of appropriate action on the part of family, friends, neighbours, or professional caregivers where there is an expectation of trust. It is estimated that 4–10% of older people living in Canada experience abuse (Health Canada, 2008). In their systematic review of the literature, Cooper, Selwood, and Livingstone (2008) found that only a small proportion of instances of elder abuse are detected; therefore, currently published prevalence data is thought to be unreliable. Any abuse or neglect results in harm or distress to an older person. The abuse can be physical, psychological, sexual, financial, or mental. The signs and symptoms of elder abuse include unexplained injury, unusual financial transactions, depression, fear, anxiety, and social withdrawal (Advocacy Centre for the Elderly, 2009; Phelan, 2008; The Ontario Network for the Prevention of Elder Abuse, 2009; World Health Organization, 2002).

Opening up this topic for discussion will give older people the necessary strength to talk about something they may consider taboo or shameful. In addition, it will empower older people who might initially deny abuse, but then reconsider reporting it as trust with the CHN develops (Mackay, 2008). CHNs can intervene by providing empathy and information about community support agencies. Provision of caring and resources instills a sense of hope in the older adult.

CASE STUDY

Mrs. Singh lives alone in an apartment. She has lived in Canada for 30 years. Her husband died six months ago and she has no family in Canada. A neighbour has assumed responsibility for Mrs. Singh, paying bills and accompanying her to the bank. Recently, her family doctor noted that Mrs. Singh lost 20 pounds over the past four months and her blood pressure is elevated. Blood work indicates she is malnourished. When a referral is made to conduct a home assessment, the CHN notes that Mrs. Singh's apartment is crowded with furniture and stacks of newspaper that block her access to the bedroom. She has been sleeping on a chair in front of her television. Her refrigerator contains a half-empty container of yogurt. The cupboard contains a bag of rice, some raisins, and an over-ripe banana. There is no other food in the apartment. Mrs. Singh's medications are in a bowl on the kitchen table. Mrs. Singh says she takes "one pill of each color every morning". She does not know what they are for. The neighbour is present during the visit and often answers the CHN's questions, speaking sharply to Mrs. Singh in her native language. Mrs. Singh defers to the neighbour and seems afraid. Both women appear anxious for the CHN to leave.

Discussion Questions

1. What key issues come to mind in this case?

2. What assessments should the CHN complete? How would this be used to formulate a care plan?

End-of-Life Care

The focus of **end-of-life care** is on achieving comfort and ensuring respect for a person nearing death due to a life-threatening illness. End-of-life care promotes the maximization of quality of life for the person, his or her family, and loved ones (Health Canada, 2009). It may extend over many months or years, and be experienced by those older adults who are living with advanced Alzheimer disease or neurological diseases such as multiple sclerosis (MS) or Parkinson's disease, cancer, complications of long-standing Type 2 diabetes, cardiovascular disease, and stroke. While it is very possible that older persons will experience a sudden acute illness that will result in a sharp decline in health ending in death, it is as likely that CHNs will provide end-of-life care within the context of prolonged chronic illness. Regardless of the etiology behind the need for end-of-life care, the principles are the same: quality of life, management of symptoms; psychological, functional, emotional and spiritual support; caregiver and bereavement support, and the centrality of the client's beliefs, values, and experiences as the basis for the goals of end-of-life care (Health Canada, 2007; Matzo, 2008).

End-of-life care occurs in many modalities across the healthcare continuum, ranging from the home to hospice and hospitals. As many Canadians would prefer to be cared for and to die at home (Quality End-of-Life Care Coalition of Canada, 2008), CHNs need to be knowledgeable about pain and symptom assessment and management strategies, spiritual needs and supports, and the community resources to support the clients and their families, including adjuvant therapies and techniques such as music, massage, and aromatherapy (Meraviglia, Sutter, & Gaskamp, 2008). Through effective counselling and communication skills, CHNs assist older adults in life review, reminiscence, and advanced care planning, and to express their grief, sorrow, fears, and concerns (National Initiative for the Care of the Elderly, 2009).

LONG-TERM CARE FOR OLDER ADULTS

Long-term care (LTC) services are those necessary over an extended period of time to maintain the health integrity of older adults. These services range from residential LTC to home- and community-care services designed and integrated to meet the growing needs of older adults. While many aged persons are high functioning and independent, with no need of support services, a proportion of older persons will require access to healthcare services either in their own home, in the community, or in LTC facilities. If the requirements for care extend to include many hours, care attendants, or an interdisciplinary team, the services may be provided in a residential care setting such as a supportive housing complex, a retirement home, a nursing home facility, or a chronic care facility/hospital. LTC services are not publicly insured under the Canada Health Act. In addition, the federal government endorses provincial autonomy in the implementation and regulation of LTC services. Consequently, there is a variation in governance, legislation, services, and associated funding across the country (Health Canada, 2005). (See Chapter 2.) In most Canadian communities, access to LTC is overseen by a Regional Health Authority or a Community Care Access Centre (CCAC). Although provinces and territories of Canada differ in their focus, most have legislation that ensures services are equitably available to people in their own homes as an alternative to facility-based care by applying consistent and uniform assessment criteria.

The following section describes the two main components of LTC services: home and community support services and residential care. It is important to note here that each territory and province in Canada uses terminology that is unique to their own region; however, the main focus of each component is the same.

Home and Community Support Services

A number of home and community support services are available to assist older adults to manage their own care while living at home. Most regions of Canada have the following main categories of home and community support services available:

Professional Services Professional services include nursing care, occupational therapy, and physiotherapy assessment and treatment, social work services, speech–language pathology services, and nutritional assessment and education. Visits are made to the home of the older adult by registered healthcare professionals to assess healthcare needs, to plan care requirements, and to tender out provision of care to a contracted service provider. For example, a visiting registered care provider may be contracted to provide consultation and care related to wound management, falls, continence, personal care, pain management, or palliation. Supplies for service requirements may be provided although, depending on funding, costs may be absorbed by the client or reimbursed through private insurance.

Personal Care Support Personal care services are available in many regions of Canada through a contracted service provider. **Personal care attendants** assist the older adult with a variety of daily living activities such as bathing, dressing, toileting, and eating. These attendants are typically non-regulated and supervised by a registered nurse. In some regions of Canada, these attendants also assume the duties described under the homemaking section.

Homemaking Homemaking services assist the older person with light housekeeping, menu planning, grocery shopping, meal preparation, laundry, banking, paying bills, and the making of and accompaniment to healthcare appointments.

Community Support Services Community support services vary among communities, and can include delivery of prepared meals, subsidized adapted transportation, adult day programs, day attendance respite services, social and recreational services, and security and emergency response services. Many communities include such out-patient specialty clinics as wheelchair and seating assessment, fall prevention, wound management, swallowing assessment, palliative care, and chronic pain consultation, diabetic management, foot care services, and continence assessment. In addition, there are community support groups available that offer education and information around particular chronic disease experiences.

Private Home Care Services Private pay services are increasingly utilized by older adults living in their own homes. These include the hiring of paid companions and paid home shopping services that are not regulated or funded by local communities or government bodies.

Long-Term Facility-Based Care

Long-term facilities provide accommodation and 24-hour supervised care. The services include professional assessment, personal care, meals, laundry, and housekeeping. The care is governed by provincial and territorial legislation (Health Canada, 2005).

Long-term facility-based care services offer older adults an environment that provides accommodations with the corresponding level of professional and healthcare support needed to maximize quality of life. The type and funding of services will vary among communities across the country but can be summarized in the following main categories of residential care. Any of these services may be available on a temporary or "respite" basis for families needing a break from care-giving in the home. CHNs can help support families through the decision-making process as they consider care options. The older adult should be part of the decision-making process when selecting accommodations. This process matches service requirements with the cognitive and functional capacity of the older person.

Supportive Housing and Group Homes Supportive housing and group homes are selected by older adults who require minimal to moderate levels of support. Widowed persons who no longer wish to remain in the matrimonial home may move to a supportive apartment complex or group home. The services offered may include meal preparation, housekeeping, planned group activities, and on-site staff who can respond to emergencies. The goal is to strengthen supportive community networks. Many communities have subsidies available that allow rent to be geared to income.

Retirement Homes Retirement homes or "assisted living residences" are for older adults who require minimal to moderate levels of support including meals, social and recreational programs, emergency response, supervision of medications, and some assistance with bathing, grooming, toileting, and ambulation. Nursing services are not necessarily provided unless there is a tenant agreement that specifies this. Retirement homes are either privately or publicly owned facilities often not subsidized by governmental funding. It is typical that the resident and/or family pay a fee to live in the home. In some regions of Canada rent increases are controlled through legislation.

Nursing Homes Nursing homes are designed for older persons or individuals requiring high-level 24-hour care, including skilled nursing staff. Typically, a person must meet a minimum threshold of care needs to be eligible for admission. Nursing homes are sometimes referred to as "intermediate care" or "extended care" homes. These homes are typically inspected and regulated by government. They may be charitable or operated by regional government (not-for-profit) or privately owned (for-profit). Older persons in such facilities typically have chronic illnesses. In addition, some nursing homes specialize in hospice/end-of-life care, dialysis treatments, dementia care, or convalescence/ rehabilitation. Residents pay for a percentage of the costs associated with accommodation and care delivery, but in many regions of Canada care is subsidized by government. The majority of persons living in nursing homes will remain there through their final journey with chronic illness until the end of their lives.

Chronic Care Facilities Some regions of Canada have higher levels of care in **chronic care facilities** funded by government. Those living in chronic care have concomitant chronic illnesses requiring services from an advanced-practice, interdisciplinary team where the nurse-to-client ratio is higher than in nursing homes. They may require ventilation, artificial feeding, dialysis, and other intensive treatment to maximize quality of life.

Hospice While many community-based agencies and nursing homes offer hospice or palliative care to older adults through home health nurses, the hospice setting is a facility that specializes in delivery of end-of-life care. **Hospice** organizations offer physical, emotional, psychological, and spiritual support to older persons and their families who are experiencing such life-threatening illnesses as cancer. Services include pain and symptom management in addition to other concerns related to death, dying, and grief.

ROLE OF THE COMMUNITY HEALTH NURSE

CHNs play a vital role in providing continuity in assessment, promotion of optimal physical and mental functioning, and follow-up for older adults who are striving to enhance their overall health while remaining at home (Grove, Loeb, & Penrod, 2009). Regardless of location, community size, or concomitant chronic illnesses, CHNs aim to promote optimal overall health for the older adults and ensure that their life is vibrant and meaningful. CHNs, therefore, collaborate with the multidisciplinary healthcare team to identify service gaps and needs arising that have medical, social, or spiritual implications. This section discusses some of the key activities of CHNs.

Integrating Specialized Knowledge

The evidence-based knowledge of the CHN providing consultation for older adults is extensive. Some of the essential knowledge includes the following: advanced care planning; ethics and legalities; competency and cognitive impairment; risk (e.g., falls, fire, elder abuse, restraint use, neglect, poverty); delirium; depression, and other chronic mental health disorders; behavioural disorders; addiction and substance abuse; pain and symptom management; end-of-life care; culture, ethnicity, and diversity; nutrition; polypharmacy; infection control; wound management; family systems; local or provincial/territorial government LTC standards; leadership; advocacy; and completing related assessments. These skills enable the CHN to identify the potential exacerbation of symptoms and plan for comprehensive, interdisciplinary care. For example, the CHN's identification of a swallowing difficulty may indicate the need to work in interdisciplinary partnership with a speech–language pathologist and a nutritionist in order to plan for the nutritional and eating requirements of an individual who has experienced a stroke.

Providing Education and Support

CHNs working with older adults must develop effective listening skills to provide emotional and educational support. CHNs can reinforce interventions prescribed by other members of the healthcare team through ongoing education and followup. They support clients and their families who are considering transition to facility-based care. CHNs often assist family caregivers to recognize the need for respite care when an older adult's care needs go beyond what they can provide. **Respite care** is temporary residential or day care for clients in order to provide relief for the caregivers. Female caregivers are less likely to receive assistance from other family members, and are therefore more likely to experience burnout (Brazil, Thabane, Foster, & Bedard, 2009). CHNs also facilitate advanced care planning for older persons experiencing progressive and debilitating illness. Their involvement minimizes the strain of repeated exacerbations of illness, hospital admissions and discharges, inevitable fluctuations in health status, and the emotional trauma often associated with admission to a long-term care facility (Graham, Ivey, & Neuhausen, 2009).

Providing Educational and Clinical Support to the Broader Community

CHNs are in a unique position to assist with the professional development of other care providers working with older people. For example, CHNs may act in the role of a clinical supervisor to non-regulated staff. In such a supervisory role, the CHN will provide guidance and feedback to the front-line caregiver. It is very important for CHNs to use various approaches to coach and mentor colleagues working with older adults within the context of strong, trust-based interpersonal relationships.

CANADIAN RESEARCH BOX 19.2

How is practice knowledge about aged care shared in LTC settings?

Janes, N., Fox, M., Lowe, M., McGilton, K., & Schindel Martin, L. (2009). Facilitating best practice in aged care: Exploring influential factors through critical incident technique. *International Journal of Older People Nursing, 4*, 166–176.

This qualitative study explored the perspective of facilitators of evidence-based practice for older adults living in long-term care homes across regions of the province of Ontario.

Thirty-four participants provided examples of their experiences promoting best aged-care practices. The participants shared 123 stories through interviews or an online narrative, open-ended questionnaire. The stories were analyzed by a team of researchers using a thematic analysis approach. The findings revealed that nurses approach knowledge-transfer activities in long-term care settings with care. They consider individual and contextual factors that impact on knowledge sharing. On an individual level they reflect on the unique traits of the staff, for example, their emotional strengths and learning styles. On a contextual level, facilitators of best aged-care practices are attuned to the leadership, culture, and workload requirements that impact on the total environment of practice. Facilitators of best aged-care practice reported that their greatest successes came from acknowledging the skills and strengths of their target group and placing educational interventions within the context of interpersonal relationships based on trust and competence.

This study supports the conclusion that CHNs must be aware of the strengths and learning needs of the staff they supervise. Mentorship and peer support should take place within the context of positive work relationships.

Discussion Questions

1. What implications do the results of this study have for the way a CHN would create a positive relationship with a non-regulated worker such as a Personal Care Attendant (PCA)?

2. Discuss specific strategies that the CHN would use to involve a PCA in planning for the care of an older adult living in their own home who is at high risk for falling. How would you educate the PCA on the assessment of fall risk and the implementation of prevention strategies?

Making Referrals and Establishing Community Provider Partnerships

CHNs must have extensive knowledge of the resources available in the immediate community. Based on client assessment, CHNs may refer older adults to community partners for services that are beyond their scope of practice, e.g., homemakers, recreational therapists, pastoral care workers, social workers, occupational therapists, physiotherapists, speech–language pathologists, pharmacists, and other complementary therapists providing massage, reflexology, Reiki, therapeutic touch, and music therapy. CHNs can advocate for those clients who may be at risk for abuse or exploitation. Therefore, CHNs will need to establish positive relationships with law enforcement providers such as community police and protection services.

Participating in Research

CHNs can actively participate in the development of evidence-based practice for aged care, including dissemination of research in the practice setting. For example, a CHN with a specialty in pain management may conduct a systematic review to develop best practice guidelines for older adults living in nursing homes.

ISSUES, TRENDS, AND CHALLENGES IN AGED CARE

The multifaceted nature of care for older adults requires commitment, energy, compassion, and creativity. In many provinces and territories, the care of older adults is not well funded. Thus, many healthcare services are not readily available in sufficient quantity to effectively manage chronic illness and disability (Wilson & Truman, 2005). Despite recent trends to shift the direction of care to community-friendly services, there will continue to be uncertainty with respect to sustainable public funding for services designed for older adults. Many myths are associated with the level of expertise required to practice gerontological nursing, possibly because the complexity of care and the capacity for autonomous practice are not well understood by practicing nurses. The acute care sector is represented as "exciting" in the media, contributing to nursing shortages in aged care. The many care levels available for older adults can lead to confusion about appropriate resources; therefore, it is necessary to develop a seamless and integrated service system between and across the sectors.

Of continued deep concern is the lack of public and political will to ensure that older adults have access to support and care (Chapman, Keating, & Eales, 2003). Health policy will need to reflect an aging population; therefore, it will become necessary to revisit ethical and moral obligations to care for society's more vulnerable members. It is estimated that older adults with chronic illnesses such as heart disease, diabetes, depression, obesity, and cancer account for 46% of the global burden of disease (WHO, 2006). Therefore, CHNs will be responsible for piecing together comprehensive care programs for a growing number of older individuals living with chronic illness. CHNs must participate in public education about the needs of an aging society, and how these needs translate into healthy public policy. A major advocacy role of CHNs, therefore, is educating stakeholders, policy makers, and the public to ensure that dollars are made available for high quality care for vulnerable older adults.

Additional issues that represent challenges and opportunities for improvement within aged care include

- ineffective use of professional skills.
- high client-to-staff ratios.
- inadequate servicing of rural communities.
- poorly integrated services with limited access.
- limited research-based literature that supports the development and implementation of best practice initiatives.

Encouraging trends have arisen suggesting that these issues will be addressed. Provincial governing bodies are legislating to ensure investment in the development, implementation, and evaluation of care models specific to older adults. Many acute care facilities have developed elder-friendly hospitals designed to reduce de-conditioning so that elder clients can be discharged home. These initiatives provide supports so that older persons function independently at home. Traditionally, health prevention programs have focused on younger adults. Funding dollars are now being invested to develop health promotion and maintenance programs designed for older adults (Wilson & Palha, 2007). In addition, Canadian scholars, clinicians, and researchers are forming collaborative teams to build knowledge that improves health outcomes, application of clinical practice guidelines, and cost effective expenditures specific to aged care (National Initiative for the Care of the Elderly [NICE]. Best practice guidelines and initiatives are being launched by the Registered Nurses Association of Ontario [RNAO], Canadian Gerontological Nursing Association [CGNA], Seniors Health Research Transfer Network [SHRTN], and Translating Research in Elder Care [TREC]). In order to support an evidence-based approach to long-term care, many communities are in the process of building virtual library resources that allow CHNs and other members of the interdisciplinary team who practise in the field to access research literature, thereby enhancing quality practice (Brazil et al., 2004).

SUMMARY

This chapter presented the healthcare needs, services, and resources available for older adults living in Canada. The main challenge to CHNs working with aged persons is to further develop services and interventions despite economic constraints and political/social deterrents. While the federal government is sponsoring activity to move these services forward, and provincial governments and health policy analysts are recognizing an urgent need for quality improvements, there are many competing health priorities that limit success. CHNs are challenged to harness public and political interest to encourage forward momentum for a growing population demographic of older persons. They must work in collaborative fashion with the recipients of care, broader communities, and other practice disciplines, using evidence-based data sources to steer healthcare policy and service delivery in the area of aged care toward a positive, equitable, and integrated whole. The healthcare of older persons will be a primary concern for considerable time to come; consequently, it will be essential that committed, articulate, passionate, research-informed CHNs with political savvy help their clients plot a course through the future.

KEY TERMS

older adults, older persons, and aged persons, p. 311
aged care or elder care, p. 312
population health approach, p. 312
Age-Friendly Communities Program, p. 313
elder abuse, p. 316
end-of-life care, p. 317
long-term care, p. 317
professional services, p. 318
personal care attendants, p. 318
homemaking services, p. 318
community support services, p. 318

long-term facilities, p. 318
long-term facility-based care service, p. 318
supportive housing and group homes, p. 318
retirement homes, p. 318
nursing homes, p. 318
chronic care facilities, p. 319
hospice, p. 319
respite care, p. 319

REVIEW QUESTIONS

Choose the one alternative that best completes the statement or answers the question.

1. Mr. Dennis Ho is a 79-year-old Chinese-speaking gentleman who is being cared for by his 76-year-old wife. Mr. Ho has been diagnosed with dementia of the Alzheimer's Disease type (AD). Mr. Ho's daughter Janis has requested a referral for assessment for community care through the family doctor because she believes her mother is experiencing caregiver burn-out.

    As the CHN assigned to carry out a home assessment visit, you would give Mrs. Ho

    a) memory testing to determine if she is able to understand AD.

    b) a pamphlet that explains in detail how the brain is affected by AD.

    c) the phone number of a support group for people with spouses with AD.

    d) the phone number of a counselor who specializes in AD.

2. During the visit Mr. Ho becomes quite angry with the CHN and says that he thinks her many questions are rude. In response to his anger, the CHN should:

    a) use a firm tone of voice to establish his or her authority.

    b) listen and explain why the CHN has come to visit.

    c) listen and try to identify and summarize his concerns.

    d) smile, nod, and leave right away after making a follow-up appointment.

3. After completing the assessment, the CHN determines that the Ho family is eligible for a care attendant to assist Mr. Ho with bathing and dressing, and provide Mrs. Ho with some assistance with grocery shopping, meal preparation, and housekeeping. To facilitate acceptance of services, the CHN should:

    a) tell the Ho family they need the services to prevent admission to a long-term care facility.

    b) instruct the Ho family how to schedule the care attendant to increase their autonomy.

    c) telephone Janis to have her schedule the care attendant so she can stay involved.

    d) collaborate with the Ho family, including Janis, so they are all involved in the decision-making process.

4. Mr. Ho begins to experience problems with falling in the bathroom. The CHN should focus her fall risk assessment on:

a) biological factors because the natural aging process and a low body mass are the main reasons for falls in older adults.

b) behavioural factors because the CHN should ensure that Mr. Ho eliminates all alcohol and starts using a cane.

c) environmental factors because there may be some adaptations to the bathroom such as installation of grab bars that might decrease risk of falls.

d) socioeconomic factors because Mr. Ho is most likely falling because his financial situation is unstable.

5. Mr. Ho begins to experience wakefulness during the night. Mrs. Ho is worried about this because the wakefulness is accompanied by weight loss and increased irritability during the day. The CHN should:

a) reassure Mrs. Ho that these are the expected signs and symptoms associated with AD as it progresses.

b) ask Mrs. Ho to keep careful records of the number of hours that Mr. Ho sleeps each night.

c) tell Mrs. Ho to admit her husband to a nursing home because the sleeplessness will decrease her quality of life.

d) assess Mr. Ho for signs and symptoms of depression such as psychomotor slowing, depressed mood, and social withdrawal.

STUDY QUESTIONS

1. Describe recent demographic trends with respect to older adults living in Canada.

2. List four societal myths about older adults and explain how these contribute to stigma and ageism.

3. Explain the philosophical tenets that underpin aged care.

4. Describe the features of an age-friendly community.

5. Name and describe four of the assessment/resource areas needed for aged-care support.

6. Describe the role of the CHN in providing healthcare for older adults.

7. Outline the similarities and differences between the typical long-term care services available for older adults.

*After working through these questions, go to the MyNursingLab at **www.pearsoned.ca/mynursinglab** to check your answers.*

INDIVIDUAL CRITICAL THINKING EXERCISES

1. Arrange a home visit with a client you have cared for in an acute care setting who has recently been discharged. Have a conversation about the following:

a) What changes have you seen in the delivery of healthcare in your region of Canada over the last decade? The last five years? How have these impacted your overall health and quality of life?

b) Think back on your interactions with the healthcare system in the last two years. Can you describe a positive experience? An experience that was not positive? Can you provide any suggestions for how CHNs might play a positive role in overall health of older adults?

c) What is the single most important piece of advice you would give to CHNs working with older adults?

d) After the conversation is over, write a short reflection on how the information shared by the older adult has impacted on your opinions, ideas, or beliefs about the role of the CHN working with older adults.

2. Select two to three of the websites listed under Additional Resources. Write a short description of each website. How are they the same? Different? Identify something about best aged-care practices that you found particularly surprising and explain why.

3. Visit a pharmacy in your neighbourhood. Look for any pamphlets or brochures that deal with the education needs of older adults with respect to their medication. What are the strengths/weaknesses of this educational material? What thoughts do you have about how CHNs could participate in an educational program designed to help older adults understand their medication?

4. You are a CHN in a large Canadian city (for example, Vancouver, Calgary, Winnipeg, Montreal, Halifax, St. John's, or Toronto). Identify a neighbourhood where the highest concentration of residents is over the age of 65. Investigate the cost for transportation (by taxi or by bus) to the closest grocery store and hospital. Estimate the monthly cost for an older adult to visit these locations twice a week. What implications does this cost have for the overall health of older adults in this neighbourhood? How would this compare to a rural area of Canada?

5. Access the website for the Canadian Mental Health Association (http://www.cmha.ca). Identify the programs and services for older adults that are available in your province. What are the strengths and weaknesses of the services and programs available? How do you think these services could be improved?

GROUP CRITICAL THINKING EXERCISES

1. Cinemeducation is the use of film to promote discussion that will enhance the knowledge and sensitivity of healthcare professionals working with older adults (DiBartolo & Seldomridge, 2009). Select one of three Canadian films, *Away from Her* (loss of self and relationships in the face of Alzheimer's Disease, transition to long-term care, family support); *The Company of Strangers* (aging, older women, grief, reminiscence, support networks); or *Housecalls* (independence/dependence and transition from community to long-term care). Each of these films portrays older adults as

they seek to overcome health issues. Watch the selected film as a group, or assign a different film to each group. Discuss the following issues:

a) Identify the stages of grief displayed by each of the older adult characters in the film selected. How are their grief experiences the same and/or different?

b) Describe how what you learned from this film could be used in your work with older clients.

c) Identify an ethical principle displayed in the film and discuss ways to advocate for clients in a similar situation.

2. Ageism is pervasive in Canadian society. It is important to recognize myths, labels, and stereotypes that reinforce healthcare providers' negative attitudes about older adults. These myths and labels should be challenged. Select a news program, commercial, film, or television show. After viewing the selected media clip or article, discuss the following issues:

a) Identify common myths, labels, and stereotypes.

b) Discuss how these serve to reinforce negative viewpoints about older people.

c) Write a letter to the editor, TV sponsor, or journalist explaining your position and requesting a change.

3. One of the social determinants of health is access to preferred affordable, nutritious food. Visit a local food bank and determine how many older adults use its services on a monthly basis.

a) Note the kinds and quality of available food and discuss how this relates to the common chronic health conditions experienced by many older adults (diabetes and heart disease).

b) Create a menu for three meals (one day) out of these foods, estimating the cost and nutritional value.

c) Write a short letter to the editor of the local newspaper describing your findings.

REFERENCES

Advocacy Centre for the Elderly. (2009). *Elder abuse.* Retrieved from http://www.advocacycentreelderly.org/elder/index.htm

Brazil, K., Thabane, L., Foster, G., & Bedard, M. (2009). Gender differences among Canadian spousal caregivers at the end of life. *Health and Social Care in the Community, 17*(2), 159–166.

Brooker, D. (2007). *Person-centred dementia care: Making services better.* Philadelphia, PA: Jessica Kingsley.

Canadian Network for the Prevention of Elder Abuse. (2010). *Ageism.* Retrieved from http://www.cnpea.ca/ageism.htm

Centre for Addition and Mental Health. (2008). *Improving our response to older adults with substance abuse, mental health and gambling problems: A guide for supervisors, managers and clinical staff.* Ottawa, ON: Author.

Chapman, S., Keating, N., & Eales, J. (2003). Client-centred, community-based care for frail seniors. *Health and Social Care in the Community, 11*(3), 253–261.

Clarke, A., Hanson, E. J., & Ross, H. (2003). Seeing the person behind the patient: Enhancing the care of older people using a biographical approach. *Journal of Clinical Nursing, 12*(5), 697–706.

Cooper, C., Selwood, A., & Livingston, G. (2008). The prevalence of elder abuse and neglect: A systematic review. *Age and Ageing, 37,* 151–160.

Cranswick, K., & Dosman, D. (2008). *Canadian social trends: Eldercare: What we know today.* Publication 11-008-X, No. 86 2008002. Ottawa, ON: Statistics Canada. Retrieved from http://www.statcan.gc.ca/pub/11-008-x/2008002/article/10689-eng.htm

DiBartolo, M., & Seldomridge, L. A. (2009). Cinemeducation: Teaching end-of-life issues using feature films. *Journal of Obstetric, Gynecologic, and Neonatal Nursing, 35*(8), 30–36.

Graham, C., Ivey, S., & Neuhausen, L. (2009). From hospital to home: Assessing the transitional care needs of vulnerable seniors. *Gerontologist, 49*(1), 23–33.

Grove, L., Loeb, S., & Penrod, J. (2008). Selective optimization with compensation: A model for elder health programming. *Clinical Nurse Specialist, 23*(1), 25–32.

Gueldner, S. (2009). Moving from elder friendly to elder essential: A global mandate. *The Gerontologist, 49*(1), 131–135.

Health Canada. (2002a). *Healthy aging: Physical activity and older adults.* Cat. no. H39-612/2002-4E. Ottawa, ON: Minister of Public Works and Government Services. Retrieved from http://www.phac-aspc.gc.ca/seniors-aines/alt-formats/pdf/publications/pro /healthy-sante/workshop-atelier/phys-eng.pdf

Health Canada. (2002b). *Healthy aging: Prevention of unintentional injuries among seniors.* Cat. no. H39-612/2002-6E. Ottawa, ON: Minister of Public Works and Government Services. Retrieved from http://www.phac-aspc.gc.ca/seniors-aines/alt-formats/pdf/publications/pro/healthy-sante/workshop-atelier/prevention-eng.pdf

Health Canada. (2005). *Health care system: Long-term facilities-based care.* Retrieved from http://www.hc-sc.gc.ca/hcs-sss/home-domicile/longdur/index_e.html

Health Canada. (2007). *Canadian strategy on palliative and end-of-life care.* Cat. no. H21-244/2007. Retrieved from http://www.hc-sc.gc.ca/hcs-sss/alt_formats/hpb-dgps/pdf/pubs/2007-soin_fin-end_life/2007-soin-fin-end_life-eng.pdf

Health Canada. (2008). *Elder abuse: It's time to face the reality.* Retrieved from www.seniors.gc.ca/quick-facts_eaa_canada.09

Health Canada. (2009). *Palliative and end-of-life care.* Retrieved from http://www.hc-sc.gc.ca/hcs-sss/palliat/index-eng.php

Hughes, K., van Beurden, E., Eakin, E., Barnett, L., Patterson, E., Backhouse, J. . . . Newman, B. (2008). Older persons' perception of risk of falling: Implications for fall-prevention campaigns. *American Journal of Public Health, 98*(2), 351–357.

Lindsay, C. (2008). Do older Canadians have more friends now than in 1990? *The General Social Survey.* Cat. no. 89-630-X. Ottawa, ON: Statistics Canada. Retrieved from http://www.statcan.gc.ca/pub/89-630-x/2008001/article/10652-eng.pdf

Liu-Ambrose, T., Ashe, M., Graf, P., Beattie, L., & Khan, K. (2008). Increased risk of falling in older community-dwelling women with mild cognitive impairment. *Physical Therapy, 88*(12), 1482–1491.

Lucie, R., Gavin, L., Gosselin, C., & Laforest, S. (2009). Staying connected: Neighbourhood correlates of social participation among older adults living in an urban environment in Montreal, Quebec. *Health Promotion International, 24*(1), 46–57.

Mackay, K. (2008). To screen or not to screen: Identification of domestic violence in Canadian emergency departments. *Canadian Journal of Emergency Medicine, 10*(4), 329–330.

Matzo, M. (2008). The universal nursing obligation: All gerontological care is palliative care. *Journal of Gerontological Nursing, 34*(7), 3–4.

Meraviglia, M., Sutter, R., & Gaskamp, C. (2008). Providing spiritual care to terminally ill older adults. *Journal of Obstetric, Gynecologic, and Neonatal Nursing, 34*(7), 8–14.

National Initiative for the Care of the Elderly. (2009). *When someone close to you is dying.* Toronto, ON: Author. Retrieved from http://www.nicenet.ca/files/EOL-_Booklet_%28v.11%29.pdf

The Ontario Network for the Prevention of Elder Abuse. (2009). *What you need to know about elder abuse.* Retrieved from http://www.onpea.org/english/pdfs/InfoSheetWhatYouNeedToKnow.pdf

Penhollow, T., Young, M., & Denny, G. (2009). Predictors of life, sexual intercourse, and sexual satisfaction among active older adults. *American Journal of Health Education, 40*(1), 14–22.

Phelan, A. (2008). Elder abuse, ageism, human rights and citizenship: Implications for nursing discourse. *Nursing Inquiry, 15*(4), 320–329.

Pringle Specht, J., Taylor, R., & Bossen, A. (2009). Partnering for care: The evidence and the expert. *Journal of Obstetric, Gynecologic, and Neonatal Nursing, 35*(3), 16–21.

Ramage-Morin, P. (2009). Medication use among senior Canadians. *Health Reports, 20*(1). Cat. no. 82-003-XPE. Ottawa, ON: Statistics Canada. Retrieved from http://www.statcan.gc.ca/pub/82-003-x/2009001/article/10801-eng.pdf

Raphael, D. (Ed.). (2009). *Social determinants of health* (2nd ed.). Toronto, ON: Canadian Scholars' Press.

Rheaume, C., & Mitty, E. (2008). Sexuality and intimacy in older adults. *Geriatric Nursing, 29*(5), 324–349.

Rose, D. (2008). Preventing falls among older adults: No "one size suits all" intervention strategy. *Journal of Rehabilitation Research and Development, 45*(8), 1153–1166.

Smith, K., & Christakis, N. (2009). Association between widowhood and risk of diagnosis with a sexually transmitted infection in older adults. *American Journal of Public Health, 99*(11), 2055–2062.

Statistics Canada. (2006). Unpaid work, age groups, and sex for the population 15 years and over of Canada, Provinces, Territories, Census Divisions and Census Subdivisions. *2006 Census of population.* Retrieved from http://www12.statcan.ca/english/census06/data/topics/RetrieveProductTable.cfm

Statistics Canada. (2008). *Canada year book 2008.* Cat. no. 11-402-X. Retrieved from http://www.statcan.gc.ca/pub/11-402-x/2008000/pdf/seniors-aines-eng.pdf

Thompson, V. (2010). *Health and health care delivery in Canada.* Toronto, ON: Mosby.

Turcotte, M., & Schellenberg, G. (2007). *A portrait of seniors in Canada.* Cat. no. 89-519-XIE. Ottawa, ON: Statistics Canada. Retrieved from http://www.statcan.gc.ca/pub/89-519-x/89-519-x2006001-eng.pdf

Wallace, M. (2008). Assessment of sexual health in older adults. *American Journal of Nursing, 108*(7), 52–60.

Wilson, D., & Palha, P. (2007). A systematic review of published research articles on health promotion at retirement. *Journal of Nursing Scholarship, 39*(4), 330–337.

Wilson, D., & Truman, C. (2005). Comparing the health services utilization of long-term care residents, home-care recipients and the well elderly. *Canadian Journal of Nursing Research, 37*(4), 138–154.

World Health Organization. (2002). *Missing voices: Views of older persons on elder abuse.* Geneva, Switzerland: Author. Retrieved from http://www.who.int/ageing/projects/elder_abuse/missing_voices/en/

World Health Organization. (2003). *Gender, health and aging.* Retrieved from http://www.who.int/gender/documents/en/Gender_Ageing.pdf

World Health Organization. (2006). *Global strategy on diet, physical activity and health. Facts related to chronic disease.* Retrieved from http://www.who.int/dietphysicalactivity/publications/facts/chronic/en

World Health Organization. (2007). *Global age-friendly cities: A guide.* Geneva, Switzerland: Author. Retrieved from http://www.who.int / ageing/age_friendly_cities_guide/en/

ADDITIONAL RESOURCES

Readings

Alzheimer Society of Canada. (2010). *Rising tide: The impact of dementia on Canadian society.* Toronto, ON: Author. Retrieved from http://www.alzheimer.ca/docs/RisingTide/Rising%20Tide_Full%20Report_Eng_FINAL_Secured%20version.pdf

National Initiative for the Care of the Elderly. (2009). *When someone close to you is dying.* Toronto, ON: Author. Retrieved from http://www.nicenet.ca/files/EOL-_Booklet_%28v.11%29.pdf

The Ontario Network for the Prevention of Elder Abuse. (2009). *Safety planning for older persons.* Retrieved from http://www.onpea.org/english/pdfs/InfoSheetSafetyPlanning.pdf

Waddel, C. (2010). *Advancing population health in Canada: What we can learn from children's mental health.* SFU Canada Research Chairs Seminar Series. Retrieved from http://www.youtube.com/watch?v=LHR8rK8l9Dg

Films

National Film Board of Canada, & Scott, C. (1990). *The company of strangers* (a/k/a *Strangers in good company*).

Canada: NFB. 100 minutes. See http://www.onf-nfb.gc.ca/eng/collection/film/

National Film Board of Canada, & McLeod, I. (2005). *House calls*. Canada: NFB. 55 minutes. See http://www.onf-nfb.gc.ca/eng/collection/film

Polley, S. (2006). *Away from her*. Canada: Mongrel Media. 100 minutes. See http://www.mongrelmedia.com

Websites

The Canadian Network for the Prevention of Elder Abuse (CNPEA)
http://www.cnpea.ca

The Canadian Gerontological Nursing Association (CGNA)
http://www.cgna.net

National Initiative for the Care of the Elderly (NICE)
http://www.nicenet.ca

Seniors Health Research Transfer Netork (SHRTN)
https://www.ehealthontario.ca/portal/server.pt/community/home/204

About the Author

Dr. Lori Schindel Martin, RN, PhD, Associate Professor, has held several advanced nursing practice positions in gerontological nursing over the past 20 years. Her program of research focuses on the healthcare needs of seniors living with cognitive impairments. Current research studies include evaluating professional development programs developed to enhance the management of responsive behaviours exhibited by residents with dementia in long-term care facilities, and an exploration into the mealtime experiences of older adults with cognitive impairments. Lori currently teaches in the undergraduate and graduate programs at Ryerson University. She is the Chair of the Gentle Persuasive Approaches (GPA) Steering Committee, a national initiative focusing on the development and evaluation of educational objects designed to enhance the practice of front-line staff working with frail older adults in long-term care facilities. She is also actively involved in the Ontario Gerontological Nursing Association, an interest group of the Registered Nurses Association of Ontario (RNAO).

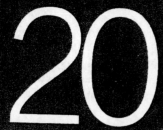

chapter 20

Gay, Lesbian, Bisexual, and Transgender Clients

Anne Katz

OBJECTIVES

After studying this chapter, you should be able to:

1. Understand the societal attitudes and healthcare risks confronting gay, lesbian, bisexual, and transgender clients in communities and healthcare settings.
2. Relate the meaning of disclosing homophobia and heterosexism.
3. Identify strategies that community health nurses can employ to make the healthcare system more gay-positive and to reduce challenges of access for gay, lesbian, bisexual, and transgender clients.
4. Understand the challenges of disclosing sexual orientation to healthcare providers.

INTRODUCTION

Conservative estimates suggest that 2% to 3% of the North American population self-identify as gay (homosexual) or lesbian (Blank, 2005), and less commonly as bisexual or transgender. **Homosexuality** refers to people whose sexual and emotional attraction is to persons of the same sex. While **homosexual** refers to both men and women, most women prefer to be called **lesbians** and many men prefer to be called **gay**; this removes the word "sexual" from the descriptor and is thought to be more politically correct. Aboriginal or First Nations people may prefer the term "two-spirited," which refers to the duality of the male and female in one person. A **bisexual** person is one who is attracted to both men and women. **Transgenders** are men or women who believe that their physical body and sexual characteristics do not match their self-concept (a man's mind in a woman's body or vice versa). These individuals will often dress and act the way they feel rather than according to their sexual characteristics and may choose to undergo sexual reassignment surgery where their physical sex organs are surgically altered. Acknowledging one's sexual orientation to the self and others is termed **coming out**. There are various theories about the nature of homosexuality and bisexuality; some claim this is genetically determined and cannot be altered, while others maintain this is a lifestyle choice that can be controlled, denied, or accepted.

Most nurses can expect to encounter at least some gay, lesbian, bisexual, and, less commonly, transgender clients, in all age groups from adolescents to older adults. These numbers will reflect regional variation, with large metropolitan cities having more gay/lesbian/bisexual/transgender residents than smaller cities or rural towns. The purpose of this chapter is to describe the factors in Canadian society that contribute to ill health in gays, lesbians, and bisexual individuals, and to identify strategies that CHNs can use to mitigate these influences.

SOCIETAL ATTITUDES

Some gay/lesbian/bisexual clients choose to not disclose their sexual orientation, or limit disclosure to a limited group that they trust. This reluctance to disclose or fear of the consequences of disclosure relates to two essential concepts: homophobia and heterosexism. **Homophobia** describes a fear, often irrational, of gay men and lesbian women on the part of heterosexuals. This fear is not usually based on experience or knowledge of gays and lesbians but rather on myths and assumptions. It is often manifested in derogatory language, jokes, and discriminatory treatment of those individuals perceived or known to be gay or lesbian. At its very worst, it may involve extreme violence (gay bashing) toward those perceived to be homosexual. More often it is manifested as bullying in schools and social situations when young persons are seen to be "different" from their peers or identify themselves as lesbian, gay, or bisexual.

Some gay/lesbian individuals may have subconsciously accepted a negative view of homosexuals as abnormal and even deviant and thus experience self-loathing and lack of self-acceptance; this is termed **internalized homophobia**. It is often manifested as low self-esteem and self-loathing resulting in high-risk activities such as substance abuse and high-risk sexual activity.

Heterosexism, on the other hand, refers to viewing the world through the lens of heterosexuality as the norm and a lack of realization or acknowledgement that alternatives to this exist. This is acted out constantly in everyday society by the assumption that everyone is heterosexual and that anything else is not "normal." Examples of heterosexism in healthcare systems abound. Asking clients about their marital status is itself a heterosexist assumption, as most gays or lesbians cannot be or are not married. This situation is changing in Canada, however, with legislation protecting the rights of same-sex couples to marry having been enacted in the recent past. The usual choices for partner status include married, separated/divorced, widowed, or single. How does a lesbian woman who is in a long-term relationship answer this question? Heterosexism serves to alienate gays and lesbians, and while it is not as overtly threatening as homophobia, the social and psychological effects are far reaching and are known to delay entry into the healthcare system. In contrast, individuals who are gay-positive recognize the diversity of human sexual and emotional attraction and are open to gay, lesbian, and bisexual individuals and couples.

Many healthcare providers describe themselves as being neutral in their practice related to the sexual orientation of their clients. This is based on the belief that healthcare should be accessible to all and not based on the particular needs of any one group or population (Brotman et al., 2002). This may result in healthcare providers not asking about sexual orientation when meeting a new client or ignoring disclosure in an attempt to appear accepting. It is more appropriate to acknowledge this disclosure and reflect acceptance and caring, which will further encourage the client to share sensitive information that may influence care (Williams-Barnard et al., 2001). Acting in neutral manner may in fact be seen as a negative response (Boehmer & Case, 2004).

HEALTHCARE RISKS RELATED TO HOMOSEXUALITY

Because of the invisibility of sexual minorities in our society, the reality of their healthcare needs and health risks are not readily apparent. Up until the mid-1970s, homosexuality was classified as a mental illness, and much attention was focused on "curing" homosexuals (Brotman et al., 2002). This usually involved intensive psychiatric therapy, including classical aversion therapy using electric shocks. In the 1980s, the HIV/AIDS epidemic appeared and attention was primarily focused on gay men as vectors and victims of this disease. Lesbians in the healthcare system are often even more invisible and unless they identify as such may be regarded as single women. Because many lesbians do not have children, they are at increased risk of cancers such as breast and ovarian cancer, which are both associated with childlessness. Smoking and other substance abuse rates are also higher among lesbians

than the general population, and this may be related to the stress of living as a sexual minority, internalized homophobia, or social factors such as peer group acceptance of these behaviours (Lehmann et al., 1998).

Many healthcare providers equate sexual orientation with sexual behaviour and focus exclusively on the apparent link between the two. They thus see gays and lesbians only in the context of their sexual activities and perceived risks associated with these and ignore other healthcare risks that are not associated with gender. Healthcare providers frequently make assumptions about both the healthcare status and risks for disease of their gay/lesbian/bisexual clients, and these assumptions are often erroneous (Bonvicini & Perlin, 2003). Examples of these assumptions include the belief that all gay men have anal intercourse and are at high risk for HIV and other STIs, and that lesbians never have penetrative sex. While gay men have been disproportionately affected by the HIV/AIDS epidemic since the 1980s, many gay men do not have anal intercourse, preferring other acts of sexual expression that do not place them at higher risk for HIV infection, and some lesbians do have penetrative sex with men occasionally and yet continue to identify as lesbian. Even participating in anal sex can be safe if condoms are used consistently. Homosexual youth are often assumed to be HIV infected regardless of their risk activities (Ginsburg et al., 2002).

The most significant health risk for gays and lesbians is thought to be the avoidance of routine healthcare due to a variety of concerns (Harrison & Silenzio, 1996); many of these concerns are related to the actual or perceived reactions of the healthcare providers to the client's homosexuality. Lesbians do not have mammograms and Pap tests as often as heterosexual women, and gay men are less likely to seek out preventive healthcare for themselves. Mental health issues such as depression are also major concerns for this population; however, how this is viewed is vitally important. As lesbians and gay men age, these issues persist and may be compounded by lack of social support, difficulties finding assisted housing where the individual or couple may feel comfortable, and lack of knowledge about financial planning (McMahon, 2003).

Homosexuality is not a mental health problem, but society's traditional view of homosexuality as deviant has contributed to gay and lesbian people having conflicting feelings about their sexual orientation. This results in high levels of depression in this population and an increased risk of suicidal ideation and attempts (Igartua et al., 2003). In the past, medical textbooks have described homosexuality as a deviation from the norm, further cementing negative attitudes. Internalized homophobia is seen to be central to this phenomenon; if individuals find it difficult to accept who they are because of negative societal messages that have been absorbed, this causes a significant amount of self-doubt and self-loathing, resulting in destructive behaviours and high-risk activities. The stresses that many in this population are exposed to have been termed "minority stress," referring to the negative effects on mental health of stigma, prejudice, and discrimination (Meyer, 2003). Encompassed in this concept is the expectation of rejection, the need to hide and conceal, internalized homophobia, and coping mechanisms used to adapt to the hostile environment that is created.

Gay youth are more likely to be targets of hate crimes and violence in schools and may experience abuse in their intimate partner relationships, often associated with substance and alcohol abuse (Bonvicini & Perlin, 2003). The consequences of bullying are far reaching and may continue into adulthood, where the occurrence of post-traumatic stress disorder has been associated with bullying at school (Rivers, 2004). Gay youth are also more likely to become homeless; they are either evicted from their family home due to conflict about their sexual orientation or flee for their safety when emotional, sexual, and/or physical abuse becomes untenable (Rew et al., 2005). (See Chapter 26.)Gay youth are more likely to be self-destructive in their behaviours; this is theorized to occur because of psychological distress and shame (Mcdermott, Roen, & Scourfield, 2008).

Gay men, lesbians, and bisexuals of colour and/or with visible or invisible disabilities face additional challenges, both within larger society and within the gay/lesbian community (Parks et al., 2004). They have to confront the norms of both the majority and minority communities and cultures in which they live. Aboriginal or First Nations people who are gay or lesbian face additional challenges based on historical and familial patterns of abuse and trauma with high levels of psychological distress and increased use of mental health services (Balsam et al., 2004).

DISCLOSURE OF SAME-SEX ATTRACTION OR RELATIONSHIP

Coming Out

Disclosure of sexual orientation is recognized as being difficult no matter when it occurs in the lifespan. The amount of difficulty relates to the nature of the relationship (telling a parent), the age of the individual (adolescent versus adult), and the value placed on the relationship (friend or relative versus stranger). Hiding one's sexual orientation is thought to lead to poor health outcomes (Cole et al., 1996), as well as risk-taking behaviour such as smoking and alcohol and substance abuse (Case et al., 2004). Gay/lesbian adolescents are at increased risk for suicide, and as many as 30% to 40% of homosexual teens have attempted or seriously contemplated harming themselves. Risk of suicide has been noted to be highest around the time when disclosure to parents is being planned or has occurred (Igartua et al., 2003). Youth who are in the process of coming out experience health risks dependent on where in the process they are. Those who do not have connections in the gay and lesbian community appear to suffer significant psychological distress as they struggle to accept their sexual orientation. Later in the process, when they are connected to a social group, their risk for alcohol and substance abuse increases, as does high-risk sexual activity. This may reflect the reality of where young gay and lesbian people meet their peers; interactions frequently occur at bars and other places where this population is able to meet and may centre around activities that are not always healthy (Wright & Perry, 2006).

Transgender youth are especially vulnerable as society is particularly blind to the existence of individuals who do not fit into the traditional male or female mould. Gender-atypical behaviour is less acceptable in boys than in girls, and these youth experience significant adversity in school and the family. They often run away, become involved in street activities, and suffer the consequences of survival sex (exchanging sex for food, shelter, or money) and all that this entails (Grossman & D'Augelli, 2006). These youth often dress as the sex they feel like and are open to ridicule, harassment, and sometimes violence. Fear of the consequences of disclosing their transgender status is a major factor in mental health and contributes to fear of personal safety in many social as well as family situations.

Disclosing to Healthcare Providers

Communication is seen to be a central part of the problems that gays and lesbians face in their healthcare interactions. Coming out or disclosing sexual orientation is an essential element of good health for gays, lesbians, and two-spirited people; however, in the healthcare arena, it is a constant process, as with each new care provider encountered the process must be repeated and the same fears and concerns about the reaction are experienced over and over again (Brotman et al., 2002). Not disclosing (being "closeted") is associated with shame and hiding, and leads to ill health both physically and mentally. Lesbians have been noted to find it more difficult to disclose to healthcare providers (Klitzman & Greenberg, 2002), which may reflect the lack of power many women experience in society and in the healthcare system. However, other evidence suggests that women are more likely than men to disclose to their healthcare providers (Neville & Henrickson, 2006). The difference may lie in the gender of the healthcare provider, as many women prefer a female care provider and may feel more comfortable disclosing than a male homosexual to a male healthcare provider.

CANADIAN RESEARCH BOX 20.1

How do gays, lesbians, and bisexual individuals use the Canadian healthcare system?

Tjepkema, M. (2008). Healthcare use among gay, lesbian, and bisexual Canadians. *Health Reports, 19*(1), 53–64.

This study used data from the 2003–2005 Canadian Community Health Survey to provide a snapshot of healthcare usage of Canadians aged 18 to 59 who self-identified as gay, bisexual, or lesbian in a large, population-based survey. Two years of data were used in the analysis because of the relatively small numbers of respondents who identified as either gay, lesbian, or bisexual in any one year.

An estimated 346 000 identified as gay, lesbian, or bisexual, representing 1.9% of Canadians. Gays and lesbians were older (ages 35–44), while those who identified as bisexual were below 35 years of age. Gays, lesbians, and bisexuals were more likely to consult mental health services than their heterosexual counterparts. Lesbians were less likely to have Pap tests or to consult family doctors than straight women. Bisexuals generally had more unmet healthcare needs compared to heterosexuals.

This is important information for health policy makers; attempts should be made to facilitate access by these individuals to primary and preventive health services. It is also important that recognition be given to the fact that gays, lesbians, and bisexuals should not be regarded as homogenous and care should be taken to address the specific health needs of each group.

Discussion Questions

1. Why are bisexual individuals less likely to access healthcare?

2. Why do these individuals in the study access mental health services more than do heterosexual individuals?

SOCIAL INCLUSION

So what can nurses do to be inclusive with gay/lesbian/bisexual clients? The first step is to address our own assumptions, beliefs, and attitudes about homosexuality (see the *Gay Affirmative Practice Scale* in this chapter's Appendix). These are likely to be reflective of the attitudes we absorbed growing up in our own families. Many of us may not ever have explored our attitudes to homosexuality and may not be aware of how heterosexist we are. Think about what you believe about homosexuality and where those beliefs came from. Have they changed over the years, or are they the same as they were when you were growing up? Do you know anyone who is lesbian, gay, bisexual, or transgender? Can you recall caring for a self-identified homosexual client and what that was like? What did you have to do to overcome assumptions or attitudes that got in the way of providing non-judgmental care? Perhaps this has never presented a challenge to you, or perhaps you cannot remember taking care of a gay/lesbian client. This may be because you have never asked the right questions or have appeared to be non-accepting and so a gay/lesbian client has never disclosed to you. It is highly unlikely that you have *never* come across a gay/lesbian client; you just did not know at the time that the client was gay or lesbian!

Reflect whether you regularly use inclusive language when taking a history from a new client. Do you ask if the client has a partner and if that partner is a man or woman? Most heterosexual clients will readily tell you that their partner is a man (or woman), and even if gay/lesbian clients do not disclose to you at that point, or state that they are not partnered at the present time, you have indicated by your choice of language that you are aware something other than heterosexual relationships exist. This may allow the gay/lesbian client to be more open at this or a future appointment. If the client does identify as being gay/lesbian or bisexual, do not ignore the comment but rather acknowledge this fact and inform the client that openness will allow for a better therapeutic relationship. Another way of asking this question is to ask whether the client is sexually active, and if so, whether sex is with men, women, or both. This removes the assumption that sex is only something that happens in the context of a relationship and may allow disclosure of bisexuality that occurs outside of an established relationship. Directly asking if the client is gay or lesbian can itself raise a barrier, as the client may not self-identify as such but may in fact be having sexual relations with someone of the same or the opposite sex.

Consider the forms that we ask clients to complete. Is the language contained in these forms inclusive or exclusive? Think about advocating for a change in the section usually marked as "marital status." This can be changed to "relationship or partner status" and include the option of same-sex relationship (gay, lesbian, or bisexual) along with the usual single, married, separated/divorced, or widowed. However, for clients who are in same-sex marriages, the term "married" does apply and should be used.

It is also important to be truthful about the level of confidentiality that is possible related to the clients and their health history. Many gay/lesbian/bisexual clients, especially teens, are very concerned about this (Ginsburg et al., 2002). Though complete confidentiality is a goal to aim toward, it is not always possible, and the clients need to know what information about them may be accessible to others and to tailor their disclosure and health-related information accordingly.

Think about the educational material that is given to clients and look to see if there are any images of same-sex couples used as illustration. The same goes for posters that are displayed on the walls of clinics and hospitals. These seemingly minor details can speak volumes to the gay/lesbian clients who attend the clinic/hospital about their safety in disclosing sexual orientation. Familiarize yourself with resources in the community that are gay/lesbian friendly; know the names and contact information of gay-positive or gay-identified counsellors and other healthcare providers. Have information on hand to give out to clients, including websites and other resources that target gay/lesbian/bisexual individuals.

The U.S Gay and Lesbian Medical Association suggest the following to promote open and honest relationships between healthcare providers and gay patients/clients: the creation of a welcoming environment (brochures and posters showing same-sex couples); use of inclusive forms, languages, and discussions; the development of a written confidentiality policy that outlines what information is collected and how it is shared; and training and evaluation of staff to maintain standards of respect and confidentiality (Dunn, Scout, & Taylor, 2005).

CANADIAN RESEARCH BOX 20.2

How do Quebec youth who are not heterosexual identify themselves?

Igartua, K., Thombs, B. D., Burgos, G., & Montoro, R. (2009). Concordance and discrepancy in sexual identity, attraction, and behavior among adolescents. *Journal of Adolescent Health, 45*(6), 602–608.

This study described the agreement and discrepancy between sexual identification, attraction, and behaviour in Quebec adolescents aged 14 years and older. The participants surveyed were 1951 students from 14 high schools in Montreal, Quebec, who anonymously completed the Quebec Youth Risk Behaviour Survey related to assessing sexual orientation (sexual identity, sexual attraction, and sexual behaviour). Of those surveyed, 3.4% reported gay/lesbian or bisexual (GLB) identity, while an additional 3.4% were unsure of their sexual identity, 9.0% reported same-gender attraction, and 4% reported same-sex sexual behaviour. The study concluded that non-heterosexual youth are not a homogenous group and that in assessing sexual orientation, it is important to assess multiple dimensions including identity, attraction, and behaviour. Furthermore, non-heterosexual youth are potentially at risk for the negative effects of direct and indirect discrimination.

Discussion Questions

1. What is the difference among identity, attraction, and behaviour?
2. Why is it important to discriminate among these concepts?

ROLE OF THE COMMUNITY HEALTH NURSE

Community health nurses have a vital role to play in both modelling and encouraging respect and tolerance in all aspects of daily life and especially in the various arenas where they work with members of the community. Nurses who work in schools have a particularly important role to play in affecting the health and physical and mental safety of gay, lesbian, bisexual, or transgender youth. It is vitally important that the needs of this vulnerable and invisible population are identified and addressed both on an individual and a school-based level. There is much work to be done in sensitizing teachers, coaches, aides, and other youth to the challenges facing these youth every day in our schools and playgrounds. This needs to occur within the context of the client's cultural and religious affiliations; communities where homosexuality is strictly forbidden present a challenge for the individual who wants to come out but also wants to maintain ties with family and members of the community.

CHNs can also advocate for social inclusion and equity in health in our diverse nation by influencing the attitudes and knowledge of community members. This may start at the level of the family, where nurses can help a young gay person come out to their family and support the family in accepting this. This work can then extend to the school, the community centre, and perhaps even to the level of civic and provincial politics. As advocates for our clients and communities, we can both support their best interests and encourage change when inequity and disparity are identified. Creating a society based on tolerance and respect is the responsibility of each of us as citizens, and nurses, by virtue of the trust granted us by the people we work with, and we are ideally suited to encourage this.

CASE STUDY

You are a CHN in an inner-city clinic and you are contacted by the guidance counsellor at a local high school. She wants you to take part in some educational sessions she is organizing at the high school for World AIDS Day. She tells you that she is concerned that the gay students in the school are not practising safe sex, so she wants you to make sure they know about condoms.

Discussion Questions

1. What additional questions would you need to ask this counsellor before agreeing to participate in any activity at the school?
2. How do you identify gay students in a high school and specifically target them for education?
3. How would you approach this topic in a high school population?

Though it is important to consider our own attitudes, beliefs, and practices, it is also important to challenge these same attitudes and actions among fellow students, co-workers, and colleagues. While you may be gay-positive, other people you encounter in class and in clinics and hospitals may not be, and they will have equal opportunities to interact with gay/lesbian/bisexual clients and potentially cause harm through their words and actions. Including fellow students in an exploration of attitudes, knowledge, and beliefs will give you a good idea of how easy or difficult it may be to change homophobic or heterosexist attitudes and practices.

SUMMARY

This chapter has described some of the challenges that lesbians, gay men, bisexuals, and transgenders face in our society as a whole and our healthcare systems in particular. It has also presented strategies for nurses to confront their own attitudes to gay, lesbian, bisexual, and transgender clients and to help in the development of greater accessibility for this population to our healthcare system.

KEY TERMS

homosexuality, p. 326
homosexual, p. 326
lesbians, p. 326
gay, p. 326
bisexual, p. 326
transgender, p. 326
coming out, p. 326
homophobia, p. 326
internalized homophobia, p. 327
heterosexism, p. 327

REVIEW QUESTIONS

Choose the one alternative that best completes the statement or answers the question.

1. Lesbians are less likely to have which of the following:
   a) mammograms
   b) Pap tests
   c) depression screening
   d) STI screening

2. Gay youth are more likely to become homeless because of which of the following:
   a) eviction from home
   b) they flee for their safety because of abusive home situations
   c) arguments with siblings
   d) they are the victims of emotional abuse

3. Delaying coming out may lead to which of the following:
   a) increased risk of poor health outcomes
   b) better relationships with peers
   c) lower self-esteem
   d) less risk of bullying

4. Lesbians are at greater risk of the following diseases:
   a) heart disease
   b) breast and ovarian cancer
   c) STIs
   d) suicidal ideation

5. Which of the following may increase satisfaction with care for lesbians, gays, bisexuals, and transgendered individuals?
   a) screening for mental health issues
   b) use of inclusive forms and language
   c) a "don't ask, don't tell" policy
   d) routine and universal STI and HIV testing

STUDY QUESTIONS

1. How is homophobia usually enacted?

2. What are some of the risks of being neutral about homosexuality as a nurse or other healthcare provider?

3. Why is internalized homophobia a threat to general well being?

4. What are some of the special issues related to gay youth?

5. When is the time of highest risk of suicide for gay youth?

6. How can we make healthcare settings more accepting of gay, lesbian, and transgender clients?

7. How can nurses work within their communities to support gay, lesbian, bisexual, and transgender youth?

8. What can you as a school nurse contribute to the health and well-being of these youth?

9. What is the time of the highest risk for suicide among gay, lesbian, bisexual, and transgender youth?

10. What are the special issues for gay, lesbian, and transgender youth of colour or of minority social groups?

> *After working through these questions, go to the MyNursingLab at* **www.pearsoned.ca/mynursinglab** *to check your answers.*

INDIVIDUAL CRITICAL THINKING EXERCISES

1. What is your belief about homosexuality? Do you think it is genetic or a learned phenomenon (i.e., nature or nurture)? What factors in your life may have influenced your thinking?

2. A client comes to you and discloses that she is a lesbian. Do you enter this into her chart or tell other members of the health team about this? Why or why not?

3. How would you address a transgender client who has male genitalia but dresses as a woman?

4. What are your feelings regarding caring for a patient with HIV/AIDS? What are your ethical responsibilities regarding caring for such a patient? You may find it helpful to draw upon the CAN Code of Ethics when thinking about these questions.

5. What, if any, ethical issues can arise from refusing to care for a patient with HIV/AIDS?

6. Do you think that gays and lesbians should have access to specialized clinics for their healthcare? Why or why not?

GROUP CRITICAL THINKING EXERCISES

1. Identify homophobic or heterosexist attitudes that you have witnessed as a student at the university and during clinical experiences. How did you deal with these?

2. Do you think that a gay nurse should be "out" in the workplace? Why or why not?

3. Would you be comfortable working with another nurse who is gay, lesbian, or bisexual? What, if any, concerns do you have and why?

REFERENCES

Balsam, K., Huang, B., Fieland, K., Simoni, J., & Walters, K. (2004). Culture, trauma, and wellness: A comparison of heterosexual and lesbian, gay, bisexual, and two-spirit native Americans. *Cultural Diversity and Ethnic Minority Psychology, 10*(3), 287–301.

Blank, T. O. (2005). Gay men and prostate cancer: Invisible diversity. *Journal of Clinical Oncology, 23*(12), 2593–2596.

Boehmer, U., & Case, P. (2004). Physicians don't ask, sometimes patients tell: Disclosure of sexual orientation among women with breast carcinoma. *Cancer, 101*(8), 1882–1889.

Bonvicini, K., & Perlin, M. (2003). The same but different: Clinician–patient communication with gay and lesbian patients. *Patient Education and Counseling, 51,* 115–122.

Brotman, S., Ryan, B., Jalbert, Y., & Rowe, B. (2002). The impact of coming out on health and health care access: The experiences of gay, lesbian, bisexual and two-spirit people. *Journal of Health and Social Policy, 15*(1), 1–29.

Case, P., Austin, S. B., Hunter, D. J., Manson, J. E., Malspeis, S., Willett, W. C., et al. (2004). Sexual orientation, health risk factors, and physical functioning in the Nurses' Health Study II. *Journal of Women's Health, 13*(9), 1033–1047.

Cole, S. W., Kemeny, M. E., Taylor, S. E., & Visscher, B. R. (1996). Elevated physical health risk among gay men who conceal their homosexual identity. *Health Psychology, 15*(4), 243–251.

Dunn, P., Scout, M. A., & Taylor J. S. (Eds.). (2005). *Guidelines for care of lesbian, gay, bisexual and transgender patients.* San Francisco, CA: Gay and Lesbian Medical Association.

Ginsburg, K., Winn, R., Rudy, B., Crawford, J., Zhao, H., & Schwarz, D. (2002). How to reach sexual minority youth in the health care setting: The teens offer guidance. *Journal of Adolescent Health, 31,* 407–416.

Grossman, A., & D'Augelli, A. (2006). Transgender youth: Invisible and vulnerable. *Journal of Homosexuality, 51*(1), 111–128.

Harrison, A., & Silenzio, V. (1996). Comprehensive care of lesbian and gay patients and families. *Primary Care, 23*(1), 31–47.

Igartua, K., Gill, K., & Montoro, R. (2003). Internalized homophobia: A factor in depression, anxiety, and suicide in the gay and lesbian population. *Canadian Journal of Community Mental Health, 22*(2), 15–30.

Klitzman, R., & Greenberg, J. (2002). Patterns of communication between gay and lesbian patients and their health care providers. *Journal of Homosexuality, 42*(4), 65–75.

Lehmann, J., Lehmann, C., & Kelly, P. (1998). Development and health care needs of lesbians. *Journal of Women's Health, 7*(3), 379–387.

Mcdermott, E., Roen, K., & Scourfield, J. (2008). Avoiding shame: Young LGBT people, homophobia and self-destructive behaviours. *Culture, Health and Sexuality, 10*(8), 815–828.

McMahon, E. (2003). The older homosexual: Current concepts of lesbian, gay, bisexual, and transgender older Americans. *Clinics in Geriatric Medicine, 19,* 587–593.

Meyer, I. (2003). Prejudice, social stress, and mental health in lesbian, gay, and bisexual populations: Conceptual issues and research evidence. *Psychological Bulletin, 129*(5), 674–697.

Neville, S., & Henrickson, M. (2006). Perceptions of lesbian, gay and bisexual people of primary healthcare services. *Journal of Advanced Nursing, 55*(4), 407–415.

Parks, C., Hughes, T., & Matthews, A. (2004). Race/ethnicity and sexual orientation: Intersecting identities. *Cultural Diversity and Ethnic Minority Psychology, 10*(3), 241–254.

Rew, L., Whittaker, T., Taylor-Seehafer, M., & Smith, L. (2005). Sexual health risks and protective resources in gay, lesbian, bisexual and heterosexual homeless youth. *Journal for Specialists in Pediatric Nursing, 10*(1), 11–19.

Rivers, I. (2004). Recollections of bullying at school and their long-term implications for lesbians, gay men, and bisexuals. *Crisis, 25*(4), 169–175.

Wright, E., & Perry, B. (2006). Sexual identity distress, social support, and the health of gay, lesbian, and bisexual youth. *Journal of Homosexuality, 51*(1), 81–110.

Williams-Barnard, C., Mendoza, D., & Shippee-Rice, R. (2001). The lived experience of college student lesbians' encounters with health care providers. *Journal of Holistic Nursing, 19*(2), 127–142.

ADDITIONAL RESOURCES

Clipsham, J., Hampson, E., Powell, L., Roeddling, D., & Stewart, K. (2007). *A positive space is a healthy place: Making your community health centre, public health unit or community agency inclusive to those of all sexual orientations and gender identities.* Toronto, ON: OPHA.

MacDonnell, J. A. (2009). Fostering nurses' political knowledges and practices: Education and political activation in relation to lesbian health. *Advances in Nursing Science, 32*(2), 158–172.

Public Health Agency of Canada. (2010). *Questions and answers: Sexual Orientation at schools.* Retrieved from http://www.phac-spc.gc.ca/publicat/qasos-qose/qasos-qose-eng.php

Websites

Alberta Teachers' Association—List of Resources (books, videos, etc.)
http://www.teachers.ab.ca/For%20Members/Professional%20Development/Diversity%20and%20Human%20Rights/Resources/Pages/Resources.aspx

Egale Canada, a national organization that advances equality and justice for lesbian, gay, bisexual, and trans-identified people and their families across Canada
http://www.egale.ca

PFLAG Canada, a registered charitable organization that provides support, education, and resources to parents, families, and individuals who have questions or concerns about sexual orientation or gender identity
http://www.pflagcanada.ca

About the Author

Anne Katz, RN, PhD, was born and raised in South Africa. She emigrated to Canada after completing her basic nursing training with a specialty in midwifery. Her nursing experience in Winnipeg includes caring for HIV/AIDS-infected individuals at the Village Clinic, a centre of excellence for the care of individuals with HIV/AIDS. She is an adjunct professor at the University of Manitoba and is currently the clinical nurse specialist and sexuality counsellor at the Manitoba Prostate Centre.

Appendix 20A
Gay Affirmative Practice Scale

This questionnaire is designed to measure clinicians' beliefs about treatment with gay and lesbian clients and their behaviours in clinical settings with these clients. There are no right or wrong answers. Please answer every question as honestly as possible.

For items 1 to 15, please rate how strongly you agree or disagree with each statement about treatment with gay and lesbian clients on the basis of the following scale:

SA = Strongly agree
A = Agree
N = Neither agree nor disagree
D = Disagree
SD = Strongly disagree

1. In their practice with gay/lesbian clients, practitioners should support the diverse makeup of their families. _____
2. Practitioners should verbalize respect for the lifestyles of gay/lesbian clients. _____
3. Practitioners should make an effort to learn about diversity within the gay/lesbian community. _____
4. Practitioners should be knowledgeable about gay/lesbian resources. _____
5. Practitioners should educate themselves about gay/lesbian lifestyles. _____
6. Practitioners should help gay/lesbian clients develop positive identities as gay/lesbian individuals. _____
7. Practitioners should challenge misinformation about gay/lesbian clients. _____
8. Practitioners should use professional development opportunities to improve their practice with gay/lesbian clients. _____
9. Practitioners should encourage gay/lesbian clients to create networks that support them as gay/lesbian individuals. _____
10. Practitioners should be knowledgeable about issues unique to gay/lesbian couples. _____
11. Practitioners should acquire knowledge necessary for effective practice with gay/lesbian clients. _____
12. Practitioners should work to develop skills necessary for effective practice with gay/lesbian clients. _____
13. Practitioners should work to develop attitudes necessary for effective practice with gay/lesbian clients. _____
14. Practitioners should help clients reduce shame about homosexual feelings. _____
15. Discrimination creates problems that gay/lesbian clients may need to address in treatment. _____

For items 16 to 30, please rate how frequently you engage in each of the behaviours with gay and lesbian clients on the basis of the following scale:

A = Always   R = Rarely
U = Usually   N = Never
S = Sometimes

16. I help clients reduce shame about homosexual feelings. _____
17. I help gay/lesbian clients address problems created by societal prejudice. _____
18. I inform clients about gay affirmative resources in the community. _____
19. I acknowledge to clients the impact of living in a homophobic society. _____
20. I respond to a client's sexual orientation when it is relevant to treatment. _____
21. I help gay/lesbian clients overcome religious oppression they have experienced based on their sexual orientation. _____
22. I provide interventions that facilitate the safety of gay/lesbian clients. _____
23. I verbalize that a gay/lesbian orientation is as healthy as a heterosexual orientation. _____
24. I demonstrate comfort about gay/lesbian issues to gay/lesbian clients. _____
25. I help clients identify their internalized homophobia. _____
26. I educate myself about gay/lesbian concerns. _____
27. I am open-minded when tailoring treatment for gay/lesbian clients. _____
28. I create a climate that allows for voluntary self-identification by gay/lesbian clients. _____
29. I discuss sexual orientation in a non-threatening manner with clients. _____
30. I facilitate appropriate expression of anger by gay/lesbian clients about oppression they have experienced. _____

Scoring Instructions

Using the chart below, please give each answer the indicated number of points. After all questions have been answered, add up the total number points. Higher scores reflect more affirmative practice with gay and lesbian clients.

Items 1–15	Items 16–30	Points
Strongly agree	Always	5
Agree	Usually	4
Neither agree nor disagree	Sometimes	3
Disagree	Rarely	2
Strongly disagree	Never	1

Source: Copyright © 2002 Catherine Lau Crisp, PhD Illegal to photocopy or otherwise reproduce without expressed permission of author. In addition, please do not change any of the wording on the version at http://ccrisp.googlepages.com/GAP.doc

21

Mental Health

Elaine Mordoch

OBJECTIVES

After studying this chapter, you should be able to:

1. Understand the historical context and current challenges surrounding mental health and illness in Canadian society.

2. Discuss the effects, impact, and risk factors for mental illness and how they affect the vulnerable populations.

3. Examine the causes of suicide, the "at risk" groups, and related assessment, intervention, and prevention strategies.

4. Explain mental health legislation that dictates the provision of services for people with mental illness.

5. Analyze the organization of services in the mental health system and selected models of care.

6. Consider nursing's current role in community mental health and future directions for practice.

INTRODUCTION

Mental illness (MI) affects the life trajectory of individuals, disrupts family processes, and impacts communities and society with lost productivity and costly treatment. Stigma and discrimination influence the identification and treatment of people with MI and their families. Services are often neither timely nor adequate to facilitate recovery from MI. Realizing that community services must incorporate rehabilitation, treatment, prevention, and mental health promotion, community mental health nurses (CMHNs) have the potential to establish best practices with this population. Mental health can impact the ability of all people, with or without MI, to enjoy life and deal with its challenges. This chapter discusses challenges facing persons with MI, available services, and strategies to promote mental health within Canadian society.

HISTORICAL CONTEXT AND CHALLENGES

Historically, mental healthcare in Canada has taken place within a context of culture, gender, and social–political attitudes. Formal management of people with MI (PMI) began in poor houses and jails that provided little but containment. In the mid-19th century, large institutional hospitals or

asylums were built to provide more humane care. Hospitals were first built in Quebec, New Brunswick, Nova Scotia, Manitoba, British Columbia, and Prince Edward Island, followed by Saskatchewan and Alberta. Although physically isolated from their homes and families, PMI were believed to be in safe healing environments where they followed structured therapeutic routines (Sussman, 1998).

Efforts to define psychiatry (which was introduced in 1846) and to find a cure for mental illnesses prevailed. When expectations that patients would return to the community proved unrealistic, the asylums became overcrowded and understaffed, deteriorating to warehouses for PMI (Nolan, 1993). The resultant inhumane care evoked public outcry, demanding humane treatment and educated caregivers.

In the 1960s, a philosophical shift proposed that humane treatment would be best achieved in the community. Concurrently, the discovery of the psychotropic medications chlorpromazine and lithium, and cost containment measures associated with large institutions, contributed to deinstitutionalization, wherein long-stay institutions were depopulated and people with major mental illnesses were placed in community hospitals and other community facilities. Deinstitutionalization resulted in a decrease in bed capacity in provincial mental hospitals from 47 633 beds in 1960 to 15 011 beds in 1976, and a rise in general hospital psychiatric beds from 844 to 5836 (Goering, Wasylenki, &

Durbin, 2000). The resources that former residents needed to live in the community were underestimated. People discharged from the institutions were now marginalized and vulnerable, with families lacking adequate resources to assist them (Davis, 2006).

CURRENT DEVELOPMENTS IN CANADA

Today, several important trends influence psychiatric/mental health services: the consumer and family movements, the rehabilitative recovery model, and the Mental Health Commission of Canada. Through effective lobbying, consumer and family movements advanced health promotion strategies and rehabilitative resources for patients (Davis, 2006). Concurrently, the **recovery model of rehabilitation** identified life beyond symptom management. It is based upon a collaborative, consumer-driven process that challenges previous conceptions of intervention goals (Anthony, 2000). Consumers expect active collaboration with care providers rather than passive participation in dictated treatment. These trends are influencing changes within the Mental Health Act, service delivery, research, policy development, and the relationship between service providers, PMI, and their families. Despite these significant advances, Canada remains the only G8 country without a national mental health strategy. *Out of the Shadows at Last: Transforming Mental Health, Mental Illness and Addictions Services in Canada* (Kirby & Keon, 2006) was Canada's first national report on mental health services as compared to 300 reports on the physical healthcare system (Kirby, 2008).

In 2007, the federal government initiated The Mental Health Commission of Canada (MHCC). Its mandate is to reform mental health policies and improve service delivery, facilitate a national approach to mental health issues, diminish stigma and discrimination, and disseminate evidence-based research to governments, stakeholders, and the public. The Commission is developing five strategic initiatives: (1) a 10-year anti-stigma campaign to change public attitudes toward mental illness; (2) development of a national strategy to address mental illness in collaboration with all members of the mental health community; (3) the homelessness research demonstration projects; (4) the Partners for Mental Health Program; and (5) the development of a Knowledge Exchange Center to facilitate access to evidence-based information and encourage collaboration across Canada (Kirby, 2008).

While most PMI receive services within their communities, poor integration of services, alienation of psychiatric hospitals, community mental health programs, and private practitioners continue to fragment service delivery. Rural and remote areas lack access to appropriate and timely mental health services (Ryan-Nicholls & Haggarty, 2007). Comprehensive services that address socioeconomic factors such as housing, income, and supportive resources to facilitate living in the community are needed to assist PMI and their families in their daily lives (Kirby & Keon, 2006). Recognition of the impact of social health determinants, the need for consumer involvement within policy development, the value of self-help groups and peer consultations, and the importance of policy based on a recovery model will assist PMI to live more satisfying, hopeful, and productive lives.

STIGMA AND DISCRIMINATION

The 10-year anti-stigma campaign *Opening Minds*, initiated by the MHCC, recognizes that stigma and discrimination are a reality facing PMI (Corrigan & Wassel, 2008). Cultural beliefs, superstitions, and poor understanding of MI contribute to fear, stereotyping, and avoidance of PMI. Stigma causes people to conceal their illness and delay or refuse treatment and follow-up care (Corrigan & Wassel; Harper, Stalker, Palmer, & Gadbois, 2008). Stigma affects health determinants such as housing, where discrimination limits consumers' ability to secure safe and affordable housing. People with co-morbid MI and physical disabilities are doubly jeopardized by stigma from society and healthcare professionals (Bahm & Forchuk, 2008).

Language is embedded with underlying biases and requires careful consideration in its use. Debate exists regarding terms describing PMI. The terms "consumer" and "survivor" are currently used. **Consumer** describes people with MI who are choosing care from a critical stance of the available treatment. **Survivor** describes people who resist care and labels that they find unhelpful in their recovery process. Survivors actively challenge status quo treatments and advocate for alternative treatments and social changes (Speed, 2006). Nurses must be cognizant of terminology and respect the language that PMI prefer.

CANADIAN MENTAL HEALTH ORGANIZATIONS

Providing community mental health services in Canada is the responsibility of provincial health ministries. In most provinces, mental health services are governed by regional health authorities without an overriding national strategy (Kirby, 2008). Many community organizations exist that have arisen from the consumer, recovery, and family movements.

Community mental health programs such as the Canadian Mental Health Association operate under the provincial mental health division. The **Canadian Mental Health Association (CMHA)** is an umbrella organization founded in 1918 to fight and prevent MI, and promote the mental health of people living in their own communities. The CMHA has a national office, provincial divisions, and local community-based branches. Local branches provide resources, mental health programs, and other human services to individuals, families, and groups. This is accomplished through self-help, community resources, and the support of family, friends, and neighbours. Services such as housing, income, education, leisure opportunities, employment, peer and social supports, and self-esteem are based on factors that determine health and wellness. See MyNursingLab for other organizations.

TABLE 21.1 Twelve-Month Prevalence of Mental Disorders and Substance Dependence Measured in the 2002 Mental Health and Well-Being Survey (CCHS 1.2)

Mental Disorder or Substance Dependence	Total**		Men		Women	
	Number	%	Number	%	Number	%
Any measured mood disorder, anxiety disorder, or substance dependence*	**2 660 000**	**11.0**	**1 220 000**	**10.2**	**1 440 000**	**11.7**
Any mood	1 310 000	5.3	510 000	4.2	800 000	6.3
▪ Major depressioin	1 200 000	4.8	450 000	3.7	740 000	5.9
▪ Bipolar disorder	240 000	1.0	120 000	1.0	120 000	1.0
Any anxiety	1 160 000	4.8	430 000	3.6	730 000	5.9
▪ Panic disorder	380 000	1.5	130 000	1.0	250 000	2.0
▪ Agoraphobia	180 000	0.7	40 000	0.4	140 000	1.1
▪ Social anxiety disorder (Social phobia)	750 000	3.0	310 000	2.6	430 000	3.4
Any substance dependence	760 000	3.1	550 000	4.5	210 000	1.7
▪ Alcohol dependence	640 000	2.6	470 000	3.9	170 000	1.3
▪ Illicit drug dependence	190 000	0.8	130 000	1.1	60 000	0.5
Eating Attitude Problems	**430 000**	**1.7**	**60 000**	**0.5**	**360 000**	**2.9**
Moderate Risk for/or Problem Gambling	**490 000**	**2.0**	**320 000**	**2.6**	**170 000**	**0.5**
▪ Problem Gambling	120 000	0.5	70 000	0.6	50 000	0.4
▪ Moderate Risk for Problem Gambling	370 000	1.5	250 000	2.0	130 000	0.1

* Respondents could have reported symptoms that met the criteria for more than one condition.
** Numbers have been rounded to the nearest 10 000.

Source: Adapted from Statistics Canada, Canadian Community Health Survey, 2002, Mental Health and Well-being, *Cycle 1.2 (accessed September 30, 2010).*

MENTAL ILLNESS AND ITS EFFECTS

Mental illness (MI) refers to a group of diagnosable diseases or disabilities of the mind described as some combination of altered thinking, mood, behaviour, or will that can be linked with distress or impaired functioning (Mental Health Act, 1990, amended 2010). **Mental health** is the capacity to think, feel, and act in ways that enhance the enjoyment of life and ability to face life's challenges. "It is a positive sense of emotional and spiritual well-being that respects the importance of culture, equity, social justice interconnections, and personal dignity" (Government of Canada, 2006, p. 2). Having an MI does not negate the importance of nurturing mental health.

Each year, 3% of the Canadian population experience serious MI (SMI) and 18% experience mild to moderate MI (Kirby & Keon, 2006). One in five Canadian adults will require mental health services at some point in their lifetime (Statistics Canada, 2003). In Canada, the *Diagnostic and Statistical Manual,* 4th edition, with text revisions (DSM-IV TR) is used to diagnose MI. It has been criticized for gender bias, cultural insensitivity, and reliance on non-empirical evidence. Efforts to address these biases are ongoing (Davis, 2006). For example, chronic trauma experiences, such as childhood sexual abuse, have not been adequately explained by post-traumatic stress disorder. The terms "complex post-traumatic stress disorder," and "disorders of extreme stress" have been suggested to capture the experience of chronic traumatization (Harper et al., 2008). For a description of specific MIs, see MyNursingLab and Table 21.1.

Children and the elderly suffer from particular mental illnesses, with estimates of 14 to 15% of Canadian children experiencing clinically significant problems (depression, behavioural disorder, substance abuse, anxiety, eating disorders, attention deficit disorder), and 15 to 30% of the elderly suffering with dementia and Alzheimer's disease (Southern Alberta Geriatric Mental Health Working Group, 2003; Waddell, Hua, Garland, Dev Peters, & McEwan, 2007). (See Table 21.2.)

TABLE 21.2 Mental Health and Mental Illness

Who is affected?
- ▪ Mental illness affects all Canadians at some time through a family member, friend, or colleague.
- ▪ 20% of Canadians will personally experience a mental illness in their lifetime.
- ▪ Mental illness affects people of all ages, education and income levels, and cultures.
- ▪ Approximately 8% of adults will experience major depression at some time in their lives.
- ▪ About 1% of Canadians will experience bipolar disorder (or "manic depression").

How common is it?
- ▪ Schizophrenia affects 1% of the Canadian population.
- ▪ Anxiety disorders affect 5% of the household population, causing mild to severe impairment.
- ▪ Suicide accounts for 24% of all deaths among 15- to 24-year-olds and 16% among 25- to 44-year-olds.
- ▪ Suicide is one of the leading causes of death in both men and women from adolescence to middle age.
- ▪ The mortality rate due to suicide among men is four times the rate among women.

Source: From Canadian Mental Health Association, "Fast Facts: Mental Health/Mental Illness" adapted from "The Report on Mental Illness in Canada," October 2002. EBIC 1998 (Health Canada 2002), Stephens et al., 2001.

THE IMPACT OF MENTAL ILLNESS

The World Health Organization (WHO) states that five of the 10 leading causes of disability are related to mental disorders, and that within 20 years depression will be the second leading cause of worldwide disability, and the first in developed countries (World Health Organization, 2001). Disability increases the risk for poverty due to underemployment and unemployment. People cannot maintain adequate employment and are forced to live in unsafe and demoralizing conditions that perpetuate stigma (Bahm & Forchuk, 2008; National Council of Welfare, 2006). PMI are disproportionately represented in the homeless and prison populations. These disproportionate numbers suggest that social systems and treatment options are inadequate (Olley, Nicholls, & Brink, 2009).

PMI are at risk for accidents, suicide, and premature deaths from treatable medical conditions. PMI experience increased diabetes, HIV, chronic obstructive pulmonary disease, gastrointestinal disorders, and cardiovascular disorders, some of which are related to side effects of medications. Other factors such as heavy smoking and co-occurring disorders (e.g., the co-existence of a diagnosable MI and an addiction) increase the risk of health problems (Jones, Macias, Barrieres, Fisher, Hargreaves, & Harding, 2004).

RISK FACTORS

The etiology of MI is not fully understood, with links between specific brain dysfunction and disorders remaining unclear. Psychiatric illness is best explained as a combination of complex interactions between genetics, environment, biology, and personality. *The Human Face of MI in Canada* (Government of Canada, 2006) discusses the etiology of MI under three categories: genetics and heredity, poverty, and violence.

Genetic and hereditary influences on schizophrenia, autism, and bipolar illness were supported by considerable research due to the push for biological evidence in the 1990s, the Decade of the Brain (Rutter, Pickles, Murray, & Eaves, 2001). Neuro-imaging techniques identifying minute neurological and anatomical abnormalities have generated new biomedical explanations of MI.

Conversely, *poverty*, when combined with a genetic predisposition, can cause MI due to the accompanying ongoing stress, despair, and anger. The effects of MI may cause the individual to "drift" downward into poverty. A significant number of people with disabilities and substance abuse problems are on welfare as they face multiple barriers to compete successfully in the job market (National Council of Welfare, 2005). (See Chapter 27.)

Research demonstrates a favourable relationship between neighbourhood factors and positive mental health. This perspective reinforces the inclusion of strategies affecting the broad determinants of health in service models and prevention efforts. Canadian research connecting mental well-being and neighbourhood influences highlights the importance of key neighbourhood characteristics. These influences are grouped into clusters that study participants viewed as influential toward mental well-being. (See Figure 21.1.)

Violence, such as childhood sexual abuse (CSA), with a global prevalence of 6 to 11% for girls and 2% for boys, increases the risk of adult mental disorders. Studies report that 83% of women in a psychiatric hospital had experienced CSA,

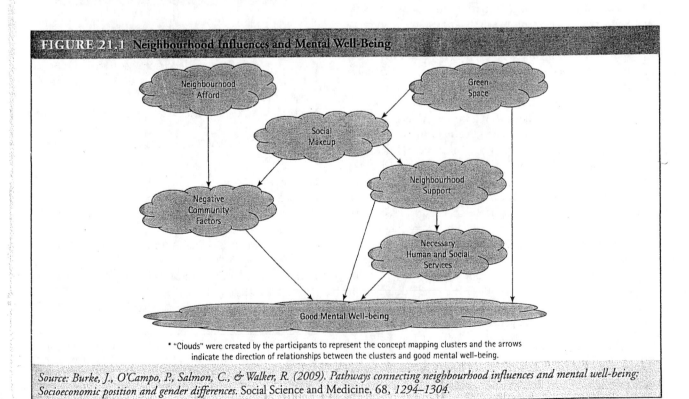

FIGURE 21.1 Neighbourhood Influences and Mental Well-Being

* "Clouds" were created by the participants to represent the concept mapping clusters and the arrows indicate the direction of relationships between the clusters and good mental well-being.

Source: Burke, J., O'Campo, P., Salmon, C., & Walker, R. (2009). *Pathways connecting neighbourhood influences and mental well-being: Socioeconomic position and gender differences.* Social Science and Medicine, 68, 1294–1304.

while 80% of young adults who experienced CSA met the criteria for a DSM-IV disorder (Government of Canada, 2006). Victims of CSA are at increased risk for depression, panic disorder, alcohol and drug abuse, post-traumatic stress disorder, and suicide. Complex trauma reactions, resulting from multiple and ongoing episodes of violence, have been identified in children exposed to chronic maltreatment and traumatic experiences (Cook et al., 2005). For women who are socially marginalized, poor, and have SMI, the effects of violence are compounded (Government of Canada). Violence in the form of teasing and bullying often takes place in school settings. Abada, Hou, and Ram (2008) identified girls, immigrant children, and children living in single-parent households as frequent victims of harassment leading to depression and poor health outcomes. (See Chapter 26 and Table 21.3.)

Children

The prevalence of MI causing significant distress and impairment in children is estimated at 15% of the Canadian population, with only one in six children receiving care (Cloutier, Cappelli, Glennie, & Keresztes, 2008). Accessing treatment is problematic in conjunction with a Canadian health policy that does not emphasize prevention (Waddell et al., 2007). Services for diagnosis and treatment are critical to prevent deterioration that increases the likelihood of adult disorders. For example, 90% of people diagnosed with co-occurring substance abuse and mental disorders developed their first symptoms at the average age of 11 years (Ministry of Children and Family Development, British Columbia, 2003). Children suffer from anxiety, mood disorders leading to suicidal thoughts

TABLE 21.3 Risk Factors Potentially Influencing the Development of Mental Health Problems and Mental Disorders in Individuals

Individual Factors	Family/Social Factors	School Context	Life Events and Situations	Community and Cultural Factors
▪ prenatal brain damage ▪ prematurity ▪ birth injury ▪ low birth weight, birth complications ▪ physical and intellectual disability ▪ poor health in infancy ▪ insecure attachment in infant/child ▪ low intelligence ▪ difficult temperament ▪ chronic illness ▪ poor social skills ▪ low self-esteem ▪ alienation ▪ impulsivity	▪ having a teenage mother ▪ having a single parent ▪ absence of father in childhood ▪ large family size ▪ antisocial role models (in childhood) ▪ family violence and disharmony ▪ marital discord in parents ▪ poor supervision and monitoring of child ▪ low parental involvement in child's activities ▪ neglect in childhood ▪ long-term parent unemployment ▪ criminality in parent ▪ parent substance misuse ▪ parental mental disorder ▪ harsh or inconsistent discipline style ▪ social isolation ▪ experiencing rejection ▪ lack of warmth and affection	▪ bullying ▪ peer rejection ▪ poor attachment to school ▪ inadequate behaviour management ▪ deviant peer group ▪ school failure	▪ physical, sexual and emotional abuse ▪ school transitions ▪ divorce and family breakup ▪ death of family member ▪ physical illness/impairment ▪ unemployment, homelessness ▪ incarceration ▪ poverty/economic insecurity ▪ job insecurity ▪ unsatisfactory workplace relationships ▪ workplace accident/injury ▪ caring for someone with an illness/disability ▪ living in a nursing home or aged care hostel ▪ war or natural disasters	▪ socioeconomic disadvantage ▪ social or cultural discrimination ▪ isolation ▪ neighbourhood violence and crime ▪ population density and housing conditions ▪ lack of support services including transport, shopping, recreational facilities

* Many of these factors are specific to particular stages of the lifespan, particularly childhood; others have an impact across the lifespan, for example socioeconomic disadvantage.

Source: Commonwealth Department of Health and Aged Care 2000, Promotion, Prevention and Early Intervention for Mental Health—A Monograph, Mental Health and Special Programs Branch, Commonwealth Department of Health and Aged Care, Canberra. @ Commonwealth of Australia reproduced by permission.

and actions, conduct disorder, attention deficit disorder, developmental delays, substance abuse, and eating disorders. Causative factors for MI in children may include genetic and hereditary influences, traumatic and abusive experiences, social pressures, and low self-esteem. Youth suicide is concerning, with high incidents in some First Nations communities (Niezen, 2009). Although identified as at-risk for psychopathology, behavioural and emotional problems, and physical illness, services for children whose parents have an MI are not well integrated into the mental health system (Mordoch & Hall, 2008). Current estimates suggest that a significant number (15.6%) of Canadian children are exposed to parental MI (Bassani, Padoin, & Veldhuzein, 2008).

The lack of professionals specializing in children's mental health, the stigma related to MI, and the difficulty of diagnosing children's behaviour over their growth and developmental life

---

Signs of Mental Illness in Children and Youth

Changes in behaviour: an active child becomes quiet and withdrawn; a good student starts getting poor grades, avoiding places

Changes in feelings: feeling unhappy, worried, guilty, angry, fearful, hopeless, or rejected

Physical symptoms: frequent headaches, stomach or back aches, problems eating or sleeping, decreased energy

Changes in thoughts: saying things that indicate low self-esteem, self-blame, or **suicidal thoughts**

Abuse of alcohol and/or drugs

Difficulty coping with regular activities and everyday problems

Little regard for the rights of others: thefts, vandalism

Odd or repetitive movements beyond regular play such as spinning, hand-flapping, or head banging

Deliberate self-harm

Source: Adapted from HereToHelp. (2009). Could my child have a mental disorder? Children, youth and mental disorders fact sheet. Retrieved from http://www.heretohelp.bc.ca/publications/factsheets/child-youth-md

---

CANADIAN RESEARCH BOX

How do children living with parents with mental illness understand mental illness?

Mordoch, E. (2010). How children understand parental mental illness: "You don't get life insurance, What's life insurance?" *Journal of the Academy of Child and Adolescent Psychiatry, 19*(1), 19–25.

The objectives of this study were to understand how children living with parental mental illness (PMI) understand mental illness (MI) and what they want to tell other children. The study design was a secondary analysis of a grounded theory study exploring Canadian children's perceptions of living with PMI. Interviews with 22 children ages 6 to 16 years, living with a parent with depression, bipolar disorder, or schizophrenia and receiving treatment for the MI were reread, coded, and analyzed along with data categories, their properties, field notes, and memos from the original data. The findings revealed that children had limited understanding of MI and received few factual explanations of what was happening. Limited information on MI caused undue hardship. Younger children worried about their parent dying, while older children were concerned about developing mental illness. Children offered suggestions to help other children living in these circumstances. This study identified the importance of raising awareness of children living with PMI and identifies them as a population requiring services. It incorporates children's perceptions of what they know and what they need to know. Mental health and primary health care clinicians have opportunities to assist children within collaborative care models.

Discussion Questions

1. Why do you think children often do not have adequate information about mental illness?

2. How could intervention services be changed to inform children in a supportive and sensitive manner?

---

spans, contribute to inadequate treatment. Canada urgently requires a multifaceted approach to children's mental health concerns inclusive of assessment, treatment, and universal mental health promotion for all children. Telemental health services may enhance services in rural and remote areas (Cloutier et al., 2008). Prevention programs remain a low priority in Canadian health policy. Researchers are working toward informing policy makers about evidence-based programs that may be replicated in Canada (Waddell et al., 2007). (See the box "Signs of Mental Illness in Children and Youth" and Figure 21.2.)

Refugees and Immigrants

Eighteen percent of people living in Canada are immigrants. During their first 10 years in Canada, 30% live in poverty, which may predispose them to developing mental health problems. Refugees are at increased risk for post-traumatic stress disorder related to their past experiences (Government of Canada, 2006). There is need for language- and culturally sensitive services and an enhanced understanding of the social context in which immigrants and refugees live (Chow, Law, & Andermann, 2009; Simich, Malter, Moortag, & Ochocka, 2009) (see Chapter 8). Immigrant women are vulnerable to MI due to their multiple social roles and limited autonomy (Reitmanova & Gustafson, 2009). Accessing mental health services is often problematic. Resources outside of formal medical services, such as social and health workers who practise in the communities, may be better able to offer services (Crooks, Hynie, Killan, Giesbrecht, & Castleden, 2009).

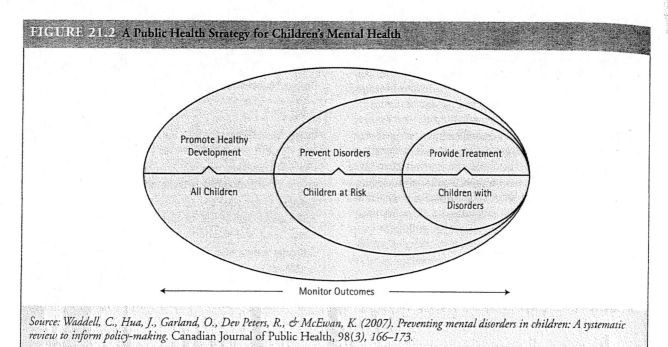

FIGURE 21.2 A Public Health Strategy for Children's Mental Health

Source: Waddell, C., Hua, J., Garland, O., Dev Peters, R., & McEwan, K. (2007). Preventing mental disorders in children: A systematic review to inform policy-making. Canadian Journal of Public Health, 98(3), 166–173.

Prison Inmates

Prison inmates have elevated rates of mental disorders and substance abuse, with 1 to 2% having an intellectual disability and 7% of inmates being estimated to have SMI (Olley et al., 2009). In the maximum-security settings, up to 78.3% of women and 51% of men have alcohol and drug addictions. In addition, 43% of inmates have a diagnosable mental disorder. Most inmates are male (97%) and under the age of 50 years (Government of Canada, 2006). Mental health services are too often inadequate and inaccessible. MI is under-diagnosed in prison populations. (See Chapter 25.)

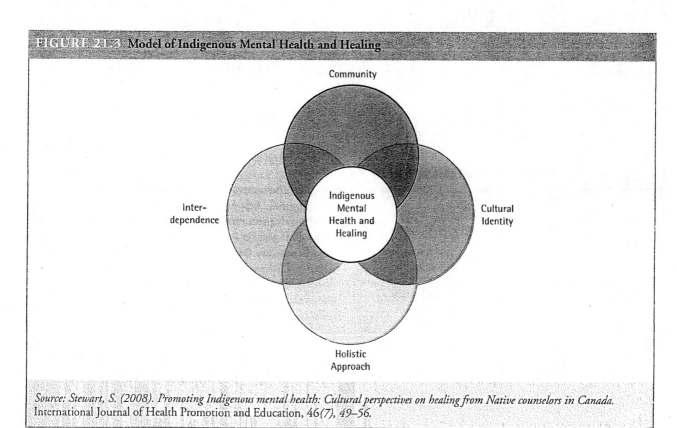

FIGURE 21.3 Model of Indigenous Mental Health and Healing

Source: Stewart, S. (2008). Promoting Indigenous mental health: Cultural perspectives on healing from Native counselors in Canada. International Journal of Health Promotion and Education, 46(7), 49–56.

Aboriginal People

Risk factors influencing Aboriginal people are historical oppression, post-colonization, and the lack of appropriate mental health therapies honouring Aboriginal perspectives. The legacy of colonization contributes to elevated rates of alcoholism, suicide, domestic violence, and community demoralization in addition to the social structural problems experienced in many communities (Kirmayer, Tait, & Simpson, 2009). For example, the Inuit people of Nunavut face tremendous social problems with high incidences of suicide, domestic violence, and substance abuse as well as overcrowding, unemployment, and legal difficulties. Societal changes, socioeconomic conditions, and interpersonal problems contribute to high mental health needs (Law & Hutton, 2007). Despite a high proportion of mental health problems, services are underused by Aboriginal people. In all individual mental health problems and treatment, consideration of the impact of the collective identity and political situations of Aboriginal people is crucial for healing (McCormick, 2009). Most mental health services do not incorporate an Aboriginal understanding of mental health, illness, and healing (Stewart, 2009). (See Chapter 22 and Figure 21.3.)

Serious Mental Illness

SMI and homelessness signify social justice issues in nursing practice. Mental illness is a risk factor for unstable housing and becoming homeless. People with SMI are disproportionately represented in the Canadian homeless population, with estimates that 1/3 of homeless people have an SMI (Forchuk et al., 2008). People without MI who become homeless may develop MI as a result of their circumstances. Poverty, lack of affordable housing, and inadequate discharge planning from hospitals to shelters or the street exacerbate this societal problem. For people with SMI, debates ensue over a Treatment First or Housing First approach to the problem (Kirkpatrick & Byrne, 2009). Policy changes related to housing and discharge planning are needed to alleviate hardship for people with SMI.

CANADIAN RESEARCH BOX 21.2

What is the experience of individuals with major mental illness after they have been homeless and received housing and support?

Kirkpatrick, H., & Byrne, C. (2009). A narrative inquiry: Moving on from homelessness for individuals with a major mental illness. *Journal of Psychiatric and Mental Health Nursing, 16*, 68–75.

This narrative study examined the experience of people with major mental illness who had previously been homeless and "moved on" to receive housing with supports as part of the Ontario's strategy to reduce homelessness. The sample was composed of 12 participants who were interviewed three times over a period of six months. Various situations had led to their homelessness. All described homelessness as being "on the move," going from shelter to shelter or street. Place and a series of places were central to this experience. Permanent housing and supports helped the participants to "move on" and reconnect with family, jobs, and hope for their futures. Their stories send messages of hope, courage, and survival. The study highlights the need for nurses to be aware of the importance of the concept of 'place' in recovery from mental illness.

Discussion Questions

1. Why do you think the authors have stressed the importance of nurses understanding the "concept of place" in recovery from mental illness?
2. How do you think CMHNs can influence policies for affordable safe housing and adequate supports to assist homeless people with mental disorders in their recovery?

SUICIDE IN CANADA

Suicide is a public health concern affecting all ages and socioeconomic classes. The Canadian prevalence of suicide is at the mid to high range, with 18.7% of men and 5.2% of women completing suicide. Suicide is the fifth leading cause of death in Canada, the leading cause of death for men aged 25 to 29 years and 40 to 49 years, and the second leading cause of death in youth 10 to 24 years of age (Health Canada, 2003). Deaths by suicide are likely underestimated, as deaths may be labelled as undetermined or accidental. Stigma surrounding suicide prevents populations at risk and their families from seeking help and discussing suicide. Survivors of suicide often feel isolated and experience complex emotions. Survivors of suicide need encouragement to attend self-help groups, where they may benefit from discussion with other group members who have experienced suicide deaths (Government of Canada, 2006).

Contributing Factors to Suicide

Suicidal behaviours are classified as suicidal ideation, suicide attempt, and completed suicide (Statistics Canada, 2003). **Suicidal ideation** refers to thoughts about suicide; 13.4% of people had seriously thought about suicide during their lifetime. As suicide attempts are not always reported, their incidence is likely under reported. Statistics indicate that 3.1% of the population over 5 years of age has attempted suicide, with women attempting more than men. Hospitalization rates are higher for women, peaking between the ages of 15 and 19 years and again in mid-life. Mortality due to completed suicides is four times higher among men. Men have historically chosen more fatal methods and been reluctant to seek help. This trend is changing with some women choosing more lethal suicide methods. A significant proportion of people with suicidal ideation and attempts do not perceive a need for or do not access mental healthcare prior to the event. Outreach and

TABLE 21.4 Contributing Factors to Suicidal Behaviour among Canadians

Predisposing Factors	Precipitating Factors	Protective Factors
MI (depression, bipolar, schizophrenia)	Physical illness	Tolerance for frustration
Substance abuse	Substance abuse	Adaptive coping skills
Previous suicide attempt	Isolation, rejection	Positive expectations for the future
Male	Suicide of a friend	One healthy relationship with a confidante
Aboriginal	Early loss	Sense of humour
Losses: divorce, job, relationships, stature in society	Sexual identity issues Difficulty with peers, social supports, unstable family, family history of suicide Risk taking, self-destructive behaviour, legal problems	Strong family and social support

Source: Adapted from Government of Canada. (2006). The human face of mental health and mental illness in Canada: Suicide assessment, intervention and prevention. *Ottawa, ON; Author. Retrieved from http://www.phac-aspc.gc.ca/publicat/human-humain06/index-eng.php*

educational programs may decrease this trend (Pagura, Fotti, Katz, & Sareen, 2009).

Developmental crisis, impulsivity, and lack of life experiences make youth particularly vulnerable to suicidal thoughts and attempts. Aboriginal youth aged 15 to 24 years are at increased risk, with boys having five times greater risk and girls having seven times greater risk compared to the general Canadian population. Seniors also face multiple losses of friends and family, health problems, and diminished capacity, and in facing their own mortality may choose to end life (Government of Canada, 2006). Due to the stigma associated with their sexual identity, gay, lesbian, bisexual, and transgender (GLBT) youth are at increased risk for suicide. People who "come out" may face increased harassment, while not "coming out" may lead to extreme isolation. GLBT youth require sensitive assessment to determine their suicide risk (King et al., 2008).

Aboriginal People

Aboriginal people have a suicide rate twice the national average. Although the suicide rate varies among communities, it has shown little change since 1979. Inuit people in Nunavut have one of the highest suicide rates in the world, with a suicide rate 6.8 times higher than the national Canadian average. This rate continues to rise, particularly among youth. The high incidence of youth suicide in First Nations communities represents a significant loss of potential years of life. Addictions and depression, both factors in increasing the risk of suicide, are disproportionately represented in the First Nations population (Government of Canada, 2006; Law & Hutton, 2007. (See Table 21.4.)

Prompt and accurate assessment of suicide lethality is crucial to ensure the safety of the individual. Nurses must be comfortable asking directly about suicidal ideation, the suicide plan, the means, and if the person has access to the means.

Ropes, firearms, and medications should be removed until the person has received treatment and is safe. Acutely suicidal people require suicide observation in a safe environment. Survivors of suicide often feel isolated and emotionally overwhelmed. They require specific resources to manage their grief and to restore their mental health. Suicide prevention efforts at the provincial, territorial, and national levels must both be population-wide and target at-risk populations. Efforts to reduce stigma, increase pubic awareness of suicidal behaviours, restrict access to lethal means (guns, access to bridges, quantities of over-the-counter medications), and incorporate universal and culturally sensitive mental health promotion in public policy are needed to address the problem of suicide in Canada (Government of Canada, 2006).

CARING FOR MENTAL HEALTH CLIENTS IN THE COMMUNITY

CMHNs work with individuals, families, aggregates, and populations affected by the major mental illnesses, personality, eating, and trauma-related disorders and mental health issues across the life span. CMHNs implement specific target-group intervention and contribute to population-wide interventions that have the potential to influence population incidence. Nurses have a unique opportunity to advocate on issues that impact the mental well-being of Canadians and mental healthcare for people with MI.

Community Mental Health Service Delivery

The **Mental Health Act** (2010) is a legal document that provides humane and just care to people with MI, while protecting society and individuals with MI from harm. It is evoked when acute treatment services are needed on an involuntarily basis. PMI and family members often have diverse opinions when an involuntary admission is enacted, with PMIs feeling that their rights are violated and family members expressing concerns that their loved ones require treatment. While the mental health act covers multiple details on the rights of PMI, this discussion focuses on two central issues: committal and compulsory treatment orders.

Committal Mental health acts across Canada vary in their wording and focus on the criteria for curtailing an individual's freedom. There is general consensus that harm to others or self-harm is a key deciding factor, with some provinces adding the criteria of potential physical and mental deterioration. Manitoba, Alberta, and British Columbia include potential physical and mental deterioration, while Ontario has specified this may be a criterion only when there is evidence of past successful psychiatric treatment (Davis, 2006). CMHNs need to be familiar with the Mental Health Act in their province and issues related to the diverse perspectives of PMI, their families, and the public.

Compulsory Treatment Orders Compulsory treatment orders (CTOs) decree that PMIs be compliant with treatment or they must return to the hospital. The laws on CTOs vary among provinces, with Saskatchewan, Ontario, and British Columbia having statutes for CTOs. There is a trend toward this type of legislation (Davis, 2006).

SERVICE ORIENTATION

Discussion regarding resource allocation for an adequate balance of mental health services in the institutional and community sectors continues. Service reorganization has not yet provided comprehensive supports to enable recovery from MI nor implemented a national, population-based, mental health promotion strategy. Practising CMHNs will be aware of the need for improvement in mental health services.

Three main problems affect service orientation. First, while the move from institutions to intersectoral community services is expected to ultimately reduce costs, currently both systems must be operated with continued community services investment. An institutional bias requiring public funding of physician and hospital services disadvantages people with limited incomes when trying to obtain alternative services. In remote and rural regions, adequate mental health services are lacking. Second, comprehensive services must be intersectoral and address the basic determinants of health to enable recovery. Housing is a major problem, with 27% of people with MI unable to find and afford adequate housing (Kirby & Keon, 2006). Third, stigma and discrimination are formidable barriers preventing people from accessing services. The principles of recovery, which challenge society's assumptions regarding MI, are beginning to be implemented into policy and services.

Mental health resources are organized around primary, secondary, and tertiary services. Primary intervention's goal is to prevent new cases and the rate of development of mental disorder in the community. It occurs through case finding of at-risk individuals and mental health promotion. Key strategies promote healthy growth and development of individuals and resourcefulness of the family and the community. Secondary intervention focuses on the early screening and diagnosis of PMI, healing strategies, and the health promotion of individuals, families, and communities. The goal is to reduce episodes of acute distress and the prevalence of MI in the community. Tertiary intervention focuses on treatment and case management of people with MI with emphasis on rehabilitation and recovery through tangible resources, psychoeducation, and rehabilitative strategies. The goal of tertiary intervention is to reduce the severity of the illness and associated disability and to assist people in recovery from MI.

Organization of Services in the Mental Health System

Emergency Services Emergency services, consisting of admissions to hospital and crisis stabilization units, are initiated through general hospitals' emergency wards, where services are organized for medical emergencies, not psychiatric emergencies. General or psychiatric hospitals provide services for serious acute illness, while **crisis stabilization units** provide services to less-acutely ill people, generally judged by indicators of self-harm or homicide. Additional services include 24-hour mobile crisis response teams and professional and peer support telephone crisis lines.

Outpatient clinics and specialized programs, for example, eating disorder programs and child and adolescent treatment clinics, may be offered as follow-up services in the form of day hospitals, day treatment, and daycare settings. Community mental health workers follow people with MI in the community but often carry large caseloads that leave little time for consistent intervention.

Case Management Case management is a best-practice model providing assistance to PMIs and families to negotiate the mental health system. Case managers co-ordinate long-term care, providing and negotiating services for holistic needs related to physical health, leisure, education, and housing. Case management fosters continuity and coordination of care.

Assertive Community Treatment Assertive community treatment (ACT) is a comprehensive, long-term, intensive case management approach to treating persons who have an SMI, a functional impairment, and are "intensive users of the health care system" (British Columbia Minister of Health, 2003). **Functional impairment** refers to an inability to look after hygiene, nutritional needs, and finances and to develop or sustain support systems. Outreach services decrease hospitalizations by addressing compliance issues and improving the quality of community life. Programs exist in many areas of Canada and are noted in best practice documents as vital to co-ordination of services for this difficult-to-serve population.

Primary Health Care Services Primary health care services include a wide range of services, and the first contact is often a general practitioner with little time and limited expertise in mental illness. This can result in over prescribing medications and fewer people being assessed by mental health specialists. Integrating mental health practitioners with primary health care providers is a goal of the collaborative care movement. This shared care could involve telephone access to psychiatrists or on-site psychiatrists at clinics (Davis, 2006).

Early Intervention Programs Early intervention programs arose in response to treatment delays. These programs attempt to intervene prior to a full-blown episode of MI to mitigate the illness's effects. The Early Psychosis Intervention (EPI) program addresses the stigma and demoralization associated with MI, supports family, and actively seeks timely treatment and follow-up (Thomas & Nandrha, 2009).

Co-occurring Disorder Programs Co-occurring disorders refer to the existence of a psychiatric diagnosis and an additional diagnosis of substance abuse. Currently, programs exist that address both MI and addiction. People with anxiety disorders and depression have higher rates of substance dependence than the general population. Acceptance of both addictions and MIs as conditions requiring treatment that may be long term, inclusive of relapse, is crucial (Davis, 2006).

Self-Help and Peer Support These programs are an integral part of services for PMI and their families and allow them to share their lived experiences with one another. Recommendations to fund these programs from public funding attest to their value. Current discussion suggests increasing the number of paid peer support helpers and peer counsellors. Research in this area is new but shows promise for innovation (Kirby & Keon, 2006).

Mental Health Promotion Mental health promotion emphasizes positive mental health and recognizes the personal, social, economic, and environmental factors that contribute to mental health. Mental health promotion is becoming increasingly prominent in the mental health and public health systems (Kates, 2008). Recommendations to include mental health promotion in a Pan-Canadian Healthy Living Strategy and the development of a *Canadian Mental Health Guide* demonstrate the growing trend to incorporate mental health promotion at a policy level. Suicide prevention efforts inclusive of a national policy to decrease suicidal behaviour and completed suicides in Canada are under discussion.

Mental Health Service Delivery Models

The Recovery Model The recovery model arose from the writings of PMIs who were in the mental health system. These writings challenged professional attitudes, suggesting that MI irrevocably led to deterioration and diminished lives (Anthony, 2000). In consultation with the Boston University Center for

TABLE 21.5   Assumptions about Recovery

Factors	Reasons
Can occur without professionals.	Consumers hold the key to recovery.
Consumers must have people to believe in them and stand by them.	Someone must be there in time of need.
Recovery is not based on a theory of causation of MI.	There is hope for the future
Recovery can occur even though symptoms reoccur.	Recovery occurs within MI.
Recovery is unique.	There is no one path.
Recovery means choices.	That one has options is important.
Recovery from the consequences of the illness is difficult.	Consequences include stigma, discrimination, segregation, effects of treatment.

Adapted from Anthony, W. (2000). A recovery oriented service system: Setting some service level standards. Psychiatric Rehabilitation Journal, 24(2), 159–168.

Psychiatric Rehabilitation, the recovery model has been implemented in parts of the mental health system. The assumptions of recovery challenge the status quo to reexamine psychiatric mental health service delivery. Essential services are crisis intervention, case management, rehabilitation, enrichment, rights protection, basic support, self-help, wellness, and prevention. Current interest and a growing body of evidence posit that service and policy recommendations incorporate recovery principles (Kirby & Keon, 2006). (See Table 21.5.)

Collaborative Care Model The Canadian Collaborative Mental Health Initiative has created a body of evidence-based research papers and toolkits available from www.ccmhi.ca. The initiative has proposed collaboration among primary health care services, consumers and families, and interdisciplinary healthcare providers to provide optimal mental healthcare for all Canadians. A collaborative mental healthcare model consists of consumers, family and caregivers, and multidisciplinary healthcare providers from mental health and primary care services to provide more coordinated and effective service. This model delivers mental health promotion, prevention, detection, and treatment of mental illness, rehabilitation, and recovery support.

Nursing Role in Case Finding and Referral

Early identification and treatment of MI reduces its severity and promotes quicker recovery. For example, timely referral can decrease secondary problems of substance abuse and depression commonly associated with anxiety disorders.

CMHNs providing mental health promotion programs will have opportunities to assess people at risk or who are not receiving appropriate services. CMHNs play an important role in screening for physical health problems and adherence to medical treatment in the SMI population who are at risk for physical disorders and non-adherence to treatment plans (Jones et al., 2004). Within family nursing, CMHNs can assess children living with a parent with MI and ensure that the children's needs are met. CMHNs may also refer parents to parenting programs to assist them with parenting skills.

Advocacy is needed to negotiate the mental health system (Kirby & Keon, 2006). Finding services when one is stressed is difficult. CMHNs ease this tension for PMI and their families, ensuring their concerns are represented and their rights are protected, and accessing appropriate services. CMHNs advocate for funding for new community programs based on needs and best practice evidence, serve on advisory boards, and lobby to influence healthy public policy. They play a significant role in advocating to reduce social inequities that impede mental health and recovery from MI.

Nursing Role in Education and Counselling

CMHNs provide education to the general public, to targeted groups, and to individuals and families. The Recovery and Collaborative Care models provide a framework for developing therapeutic relationships with consumers, families, and communities. Within therapeutic relationships, CMHNs promote self-care, develop coping abilities, and foster social support networks. In crisis, nurses work with PMI and families to find appropriate resources. Individual and group educational counselling promotes discussion of the signs of MI, medication, treatment options, and the recovery model. CMHNs support peer and self-help recovery-based programs; facilitate cognitive behavioural therapy groups; and organize educational programs for the general public to promote mental health and reduce risk factors associated with mental illness. Programs that inform schools and children of ways to protect children from CSA help to reduce the risk of abuse, a precursor to mental health problems. Programs can offer information on specific illnesses, stigma, and suicide prevention. CMHNs can create educational programs to increase public awareness of the issues surrounding MI and mental health.

FUTURE DIRECTIONS AND IMPLICATIONS FOR NURSING

Reports on mental health services in Canada demonstrate the need for continued support for PMI and their families and have called for integrated comprehensive services from diverse sectors, such as income and housing (Davis, 2006). Increased recognition of peer support programs, family contributions to care, self-help, and the principles of recovery are beginning to change service delivery. Nurses will face challenges to address the needs of specific populations at risk for mental health problems, contribute to innovative programs for mental health promotion targeted at the Canadian population, and support policy changes at the national level and commit to the anti–mental health stigma campaign

Changes in the community mental health system call for comprehensive funding to address societal barriers that impede PMI. Vulnerable target populations such as children, adolescents, First Nations people, inmates, people with co-occurring disorders, and SMI will require specific nursing intervention and health promotion strategies. Nurses have the opportunity to be part of the changes that are occurring. They can prepare themselves to address gaps in mental health services. Nurses play a key role in facilitating peer programs, self-help groups, and family advocacy and support groups. The Recovery Model outlines approaches to working with people with MI while acknowledging the support structures that people require to live successfully in the community. Future directions require focused nursing efforts to affect policy and health determinants and to work collaboratively in new ways and relationships

CMHNs have the capacity to encourage and support clients and families to become actively involved in the work of the Commission. CMHNs' grounding in the realities that clients, families, and communities face, propels them to advocate for services and to work collaboratively with their families and community partners. CMHNs will provide valuable input in knowledge exchange and translation by engaging in pertinent research, and facilitating dissemination of research findings (Mental Health Commission of Canada, 2009).

CASE STUDY

Gloria is a 27-year-old Cree woman recently admitted to the hospital from a remote reserve. She is admitted for depression with suicidal thoughts. Recently, Gloria lost her infant daughter as the result of sudden infant death syndrome. Since then she has had continual thoughts of harming herself and difficulty sleeping. She describes her husband as a good man who sometimes drinks and beats her. Gloria has experienced both physical and sexual abuse as a child. She states that she has forgiven the people who hurt her. Gloria has been unable to look after her older daughter (age 4). Her daughter is now living with her grandparents in Gloria's home community several hundred kilometres away from Gloria's present community. Gloria feels isolated in her new community and has no confidantes. When asked about her life, she states she lives in a shack and everything is wrong. She is unkempt and requires dental care. Gloria is put on a trial of antidepressant medication. The plan is to return her to the reserve when she is stable. There are limited mental health resources on the reserve.

You are the primary nurse who will be looking after Gloria while she is in the hospital. You will be responsible for discharge planning upon her return to the reserve.

1. What do you assess as the personal issues in Gloria's situation that contribute to her depression?

2. How can you implement care with Gloria around these issues?

3. What are the systemic issues that impact on Gloria's situation?

4. How will you plan for discharge in order to help Gloria remain safe?

SUMMARY

When working with PMI, their families, and their communities, nurses are practising in a system that is undergoing change. New models propose reconfigurations of care that honour personal narratives of PMI and families, and change the nurse–person relationship. These changes will challenge nursing to examine practice and nursing's openness to innovations. Population data sets will assist nurses to identify vulnerable groups and direct healthcare and promotion efforts toward them. As colonialism's effects on mental health are recognized and traditional Aboriginal wisdom is incorporated into therapies for First Nations communities, nurses are challenged to learn different ways to promote healing. As cultural diversity increases within Canadian society, nurses will consider alternative ways of understanding MI. Perhaps, most importantly, the Recovery Model and the integration of a Collaborative Model of mental healthcare will help nurses to focus on consumers' abilities to build meaningful lives and strengthen nurses' resolve to change the inequities that influence the mental well-being of people living with MI.

KEY TERMS

recovery model of rehabilitation, p. 335
consumer, p. 335
survivor, p. 335
Canadian Mental Health Association (CMHA), p. 335
mental illness (MI), p. 336
mental health, p. 336
suicidal ideation, p. 341
Mental Health Act, p. 342
emergency services, p. 343
crisis stabilization units, p. 343
case management, p. 343
emergency services, p. 343
case management, p. 343
assertive community treatment (ACT), p. 343
functional impairment, p. 343
early intervention programs, p. 344
co-occurring disorders, p. 344
mental health promotion, p. 344
recovery model, p. 344

REVIEW QUESTIONS

Jake is a 35-year-old man who has a co-occurring disorder of schizophrenia and alcohol abuse. He lives in a rooming house in the center of the city. He has been on long acting medication for the past three years. His symptoms are reasonably controlled. During the day he wanders around the neighbourhood, with no apparent destination.

1. Using a recovery model approach, what intervention would you suggest?
   a) Encourage Jake to attend AA.
   b) Develop a multidisciplinary team to support Jake in rehabilitation efforts.
   c) Leave Jake to wander as he pleases.
   d) Consult with psychiatry to change his medication.

2. Jake has been abusing alcohol since he was 20 years old. He says alcohol helps him to "drown out the voices." How can you assist Jake with his alcohol abuse behaviours?
   a) Tell him he must abstain from alcohol for health reasons.
   b) Suggest he try meditation.
   c) Link him to a Co-Occurring Disorder Intervention (CODI) resource.
   d) Refer him to an AA group.

3. Jake is having difficulty at his residence. The landlord has issued a warning that if there are further complaints about Jake from the other tenants, Jake will be evicted. Jake is concerned and agitated. How can you initially help Jake with this problem?
   a) Inform Jake there is a housing shortage and he must behave.
   b) Ask Jake if he has any relatives in the city.
   c) Inform Jake of the city shelter mission.
   d) Ensure Jake's rights are not being violated due to stigma and discrimination.

4. Jake is standing outside the library talking to himself, muttering, and making bizarre facial grimaces. As the CMHN for Jake, you are most concerned Jake is
   a) blocking pedestrian traffic.
   b) embarrassing himself in public.
   c) decompensating and becoming psychotic.
   d) requiring removal from the street.

5. Jake requires a brief hospitalization, is stabilized on medication, and is discharged back to his rooming house. His neighbours and landlord are worried he will not stay on his medication and will become violent. They also feel he is vulnerable, wandering around the neighbourhood. How can the nurse assist Jake to remain well?
   a) Inform him that he will be back in the hospital if he does not stay on his meds.
   b) Tell him that people in his building are afraid of him.
   c) Suggest an alternative activity for wandering.
   d) Request a para professional helper to assist him and find a community meal program for him to attend

STUDY QUESTIONS

1. Knowing the history of the mental health system in Canada can help nurses understand current issues. From what you have read about the process of deinstitutionalization, how do you think this may have impacted the current problems in the mental health system?

2. Suicide continues to be a troubling problem in Canadian society. Identify groups who are at risk for suicide. Explain four strategies you might use in your community nursing practice to decrease suicide in these groups.

3. Define mental health promotion and consider how you would implement strategies to promote mental health in the frail elderly living in the community, new immigrant mothers, and suburban high school students.

4. Consider the risk factors for mental illness. How can community mental health nurse reduce risk factors within their practice communities?

5. Recently there has been a national report on the state of mental health services in Canada. Identify and discuss four recommendations from the national report.

After working through these questions, go to the MyNursingLab at **www.pearsoned.ca/mynursinglab** *to check your answers.*

INDIVIDUAL CRITICAL THINKING QUESTIONS

1. What strategies might a community mental health nurse use to promote the mental health of elementary school age children?

2. How would a community mental health nurse implement the Recovery Model with a depressed client and their family?

3. Why do you think "people first" language (i.e., a person with schizophrenia rather than schizophrenic) is important?

4. What issues are important to consider in designing mental health services for diverse cultural groups?

5. What are the unique challenges that face First Nations people in restoring mental health and healing to their communities?

GROUP CRITICAL THINKING QUESTIONS

1. How might CMHNs ensure that the physical and mental health needs of people with MI are met within a primary health care clinic?

2. How might CMHNs influence and develop a national suicide prevention strategy?

3. How can the principles of recovery be implemented and researched within the mental health system?

REFERENCES

Abada, T., Hou, F., & Ram, B. (2008). The effects of harassment and victimization on self-rated mental health among Canadian adolescents. *Social Science and Medicine, 67,* 557–567.

Anthony, W. A. (2000). A recovery service system: Setting some systems level standards. *Psychiatric Rehabilitation Journal, 24*(2), 160–166.

Bahm, A., & Forchuk, C. (2008). Interlocking oppressions: The effect of a co-morbid physical disability on perceived stigma and discrimination among mental health consumers in Canada. *Health and Social Care in the Community, 17*(1), 63–70.

Bassani, D. G., Padoin, C. V., Phillip, D., & Veldhuzein, S. (2008). Estimating the number of children exposed to parental psychiatric disorders through a national health survey. *Child and Adolescent Psychiatry and Mental Health, 3*(1), (6). doi:10.1186/1753-2000-3-6

British Columbia Ministry of Health Services. (2003). *Historical perspective: Mental health resource utilization in British Columbia (1997/98 to 1999/00). Prior to health authority restructuring in 2001.* Victoria, BC: Ministry of Health Services.

Chow, W., Law, S., & Andermann, L. (2009). ACT tailored for ethnocultural communities of metropolitan Toronto. *Psychiatric Services, 60*(6), 847.

Cloutier, P., Cappelli, M., Glennie, E., & Keresztes, C. (2008). Mental health services for children and youth: A survey of physicians' knowledge, attitudes and use of telehealth services. *Journal of Telemedicine and Telecare, 14,* 98–101.

Cook, A., Spinazzola, J., Ford, J., Lanktree, C., Blaustein, M., Cloitre, M. et al. (2005). Complex trauma in children and adolescents. *Psychiatric Annals, 35*(6), 390–396.

Corrigan, P. W., & Wassel, A. (2008). Understanding and influencing the stigma of mental illness. *Journal of Psychosocial Nursing and Mental Health Services, 48*(1), 42–48.

Crooks, V. A., Hynie, M., Killan, K., Giesbrecht, M., & Castleden, H. (2009). Female newcomers' adjustments to life in Toronto, Canada: Sources of mental stress and their implications for delivering primary mental health care. *Springer Science+Business Media, Geo Journal.* doi:10.1007/s107/s10708-009-9287-4

Davis, S. (2006). *Community mental health in Canada: Policy, theory, practice.* Vancouver, BC: UBC Press.

Forchuk, C., MacClure, S. K., Van Beers, M., Smith, C., Csternik, R., Hoch, J., & Jensen, E. (2008). Developing and testing an intervention to prevent homelessness among individuals discharged from psychiatric wards to shelters and "no fixed address." *Journal of Psychiatric and Mental Health Nursing, 15,* 569–575.

Goering, P., Wasylenki, D., & Durbin, J. (2000). Canada's mental health system. *International Journal of Law and Psychiatry, 23*(3–4), 345–359.

Government of Canada. (2006). *The human face of mental health and mental illness in Canada 2006* (Cat. no. HP5-19/2006E). Ottawa, ON: Minister of Public Works and Government Services. Retrieved from http://www.phac-aspc.gc.ca/publicat/human-humain06/index-eng.php

Harper, K., Stalker, C. A., Palmer, S., & Gadbois, S. (2008). Adults traumatized by child abuse: What survivors need from community-based mental health professionals. *Journal of Mental Health, 17*(4), 361–374.

Health Canada. (2003). *Acting on what we know: Preventing youth suicide in First Nations.* Retrieved from http://www.hc-sc.gc.ca/fniah-spnia/pubs/promotion/_suicide/prev_youth-jeunes/section1-eng.php

Jones, D. R., Macias, C., Barriers, P. J., Fisher, W. H., Hargreaves, W. A., & Harding, C. M. (2004). Prevalence, severity, and co-occurrence of chronic physical health problems of persons with serious mental illness. *Psychiatric Services, 55*(11), 1250–1257.

Kates, N. (2008). Promoting collaborative care in Canada: The Canadian collaborative mental health initiative. *Families, Systems and Health, 26*(4), 466–473.

King, M., Semlyen, J., Tai, S., Kilaspy, H., Osborne, D., Popelyk, D., & Nazereth, I. (2008). A systematic review of mental disorder, suicide and deliberate self harm in lesbian, gay and bisexual people. *BMC Psychiatry, 8*(70). doi:10.1186/1471-244X-8-70

Kirby, M. J. (2008). Mental health in Canada: Out of the shadows forever. *Canadian Medical Association Journal, 178*(10), 1320–1322.

Kirby, M. J., & Keon, W. J. (2006). *Out of the shadows at last: Transforming mental health, mental illness and addictions services in Canada.* Ottawa, ON: Standing Senate Committee on Social Affairs, Science and Technology.

Kirkmayers, L. J., Tait, C., & Simpson, C. (2009). The mental health of Aboriginal peoples in Canada: Transformations of identity and community. In L. J. Kirkmayer & G. Valaskakis (Eds.), *Healing traditions. The mental health of Aboriginal peoples in Canada* (pp. 3–35). Vancouver, BC: UBC Press.

Kirkpatrick, H., & Byrne, C. (2009). A narrative inquiry: Moving on from homelessness for individuals with a major mental illness. *Journal of Psychiatric and Mental Health Nursing, 16*, 68–75.

Law, S., & Hutton, E. (2007). Community psychiatry in the Canadian Arctic: Reflections from a 1 year continuous consultation series in Iqaluit, Nunavut. *Canadian Journal of Community Mental Health, 26*(2), 123–140.

McCormick, R. (2009). Aboriginal approaches to counseling. In L. J. Kirkmayer & G. Valaskakis (Eds.), *Healing traditions: The mental health of Aboriginal peoples in Canada* (pp. 337–353). Vancouver, BC: UBC Press.

Mental Health Act. (2010). *RSO 1990 Chapter M7.* Retrieved from http://www.e-laws.gov.on.ca/html/statutesenglish/elaws_statutes_90m07_e.htm

Health Commission. (2009). *Mental health strategy for Canada.* Retrieved from http://www.mentalhealthcommission.ca/Pages/index.htm

Ministry of Children and Family Development British Columbia. (2003). *New children's mental health plan first in Canada.* Vancouver, BC: Author.

Mordoch, E., & Hall, W. (2008). Children's perceptions of living with a parent with a mental illness: Finding the rhythm and maintaining the frame. *Qualitative Health Research, 18*(8), 1127–1144.

National Council of Welfare. (2006). *Welfare incomes 2006–2007.* Retrieved from http://www.ncwcnbes.net/en/research/welfare-bienetre.html

Niezen, R. (2009). Suicide as a way of belonging: Causes and consequences of cluster suicides in Aboriginal communities. In L. J. Kirmayer & G. Guthrie Valaskakis (Eds.), *Healing traditions: The mental health of Aboriginal peoples in Canada* (pp. 178–194). Vancouver, BC: UBC Press.

Nolan, P. W. (1993). A history of the training of asylum nurses. *Journal of Advanced Nursing, 18*(8), 1193–1201.

Olley, M., Nicolls, T., & Brink, M. (2009). Mentally ill individuals in limbo: Obstacles and opportunities for providing psychiatric services to corrections inmates with mental illness. *Behavioural Sciences and the Law, 27*, 811–831.

Pagura, J., Fotti, S., Katz, L., & Sareen, J. (2009). Help seeking and perceived need for mental health care among individuals in Canada with suicidal behaviours. *Psychiatric Services, 60*(7), 943–949.

Reitmanova, S., & Gustafson, D. J. (2009). Mental health needs of visible minority immigrants in a small urban center: Recommendations for policy makers and service providers. *Journal of Immigrant Minority Health, 11*, 46–56.

Rutter, M., Pickles, A., Murray, R., & Eaves, L. (2001). Testing hypotheses on specific environmental causal effects on behavior. *Psychological Bulletin, 127*, 291–324.

Ryan-Nicholls, K. D., & Haggarty, J. M. (2007). Colloborative mental health care in rural and isolated Canada: Stakeholder feedback. *Journal of Psychosocial Nursing, 45*(12), 37–45.

Simach, L., Malter, S., Moortag, S., & Ochoka, J. (2009). Taking culture seriously: Ethnolinguistic community perspectives on mental health. *Psychiatric Rehabilitation Journal, 30*(3), 208–214.

Southern Alberta Geriatric Mental Health Working Group. (2003). *Summary report of the Southern Alberta Geriatric Mental Health Working Group.* Calgary, Alberta, 1–12.

Speed, E. (2006). Patients, consumers and survivors: A case study of mental health service user discourses. *Social Science and Medicine, 62*, 28–38.

Statistics Canada. (2003, updated 2004, 2007). *Canadian community health survey: Mental health and well-being.* Retrieved from http://www.statcan.ca/bsolc/english/bsolc?catno=82-617-X&CHROPG=1

Stewart, S. (2008). Promoting Indigenous mental health: Cultural perspectives on healing from Native counselors in Canada. *International Journal of Health Promotion and Education, 46*(7), 49–56.

Sussman, S. (1998). The first asylums in Canada: A response to neglectful community care and current trends. *Canadian Journal of Psychiatry, 43*, 260–264.

Thomas, S. P., & Nandrha, H. S. (2009). Early intervention in psychosis: A retrospective analysis of clinical and social factors influencing duration of untreated psychosis. *Primary Care Companion Journal of Clinical Psychiatry, 11*(5), 212–214.

Waddell, C., Hua, J., Garland, O., Dev Peters, R., & McEwan, K. (2007). Preventing mental disorders in children: A systemactic review to inform policy-making. *Canadian Journal of Public Health, 98*(3), 166–173.

World Health Organization. (2001). *The world health report 2001. Mental health: New understanding, new hope.* Retrieved from http://www.who.int/whr/2001/en/index.html

World Health Organization. (2002). *The world health report 2002. Reducing risks, promoting health life.* Retrieved from http://www.who.int/whr/2002/en/index.html

ADDITIONAL RESOURCES

Readings

Mordoch, E., & Hall, W. (2008). Children's perceptions of living with a parent with a mental illness: Finding the rhythm and maintaining the frame. *Qualitative Health Research, 18*(8), 1127–1144.

Stewart, S. (2008). Promoting Indigenous mental health: Cultural perspectives on healing from Native counselors in Canada. *International Journal of Health Promotion and Education, 46*(7), 49–56.

Videos

The Interventionist: Chronicles of a mental health crisis team. National Film Board of Canada, 2006.

Flight from Darkness [DVD]. Trevoor Grant, 2007.

Waddel, C. (2010). *Advancing population health in Canada: What we can learn from children's mental health.* SFU Canada Research Chairs Seminar Series. Retrieved from http://www.youtube.com/watch?v=LHR8rK8l9Dg

Websites

Anxiety Disorders Association of Canada
http://www.anxietycanada.ca

Canadian Association for the Mentally Ill
http://www.cami.org

Canadian Federation of Mental Health Nurses
http://www.cfmhn.ca/about_us.html

Canadian Mental Health Association
http://www.cmha.ca

Canadian Network for Anxiety and Mood Treatments
http://www.canmat.org/

Canadian Psychiatric Research Foundation
http://www.cprf.ca

Health Canada, Mental Health
http://www.hc-sc.gc.ca/hl-vs/mental/index-eng.php

Mood Disorders Society of Canada
http://www.mooddisorderscanada.ca

National Network for Mental Health
http://www.nnmh.ca

Schizophrenia Society of Canada
http://www.schizophrenia.ca

Mental Health Commission of Canada
http://www.mentalhealthcommission.ca/Pages/index.html

University of Pennsylvania, Authentic Happiness
http://www.authentichappiness.sas.upenn.edu/Default.aspx

About the Author

Elaine Mordoch, RN, PhD (University of Manitoba) has been passionate about psychiatric/mental health nursing throughout her nursing career. She has practised as a primary nurse in acute psychiatry, and facilitated groups for the well elderly living with depression and for women identifying abuse in their relationships. She has developed and managed COPE (Care of Psychiatric Emergencies) for a tertiary hospital general emergency unit with a focus on family care and intermediate follow-up services. Her research interest focuses on children and families living with parental mental illness. She is particularly interested in children's perceptions of their lives and ways to strengthen families. She is also interested in the long-term effects of childhood sexual abuse on adult survivors. Currently she teaches psychiatric/mental health nursing and counselling skills in the Faculty of Nursing and in the Aboriginal Focus Programs at the University of Manitoba.

22

Aboriginal Health

Rose Alene Roberts

OBJECTIVES

After studying this chapter, you should be able to:

1. Identify culturally appropriate nursing practice for Aboriginal communities.
2. Describe historical impacts that relate to the current health status of Aboriginal peoples in Canada.
3. Describe Aboriginal peoples' healthcare delivery systems including funding implications.
4. Identify healthcare issues that are important in Aboriginal communities.
5. Describe how culture and policy can impact on the health of Aboriginal communities.

INTRODUCTION

This chapter is a broad overview of community health nursing in Canadian Aboriginal communities. Waldram et al. (2006) state, "Currently, the Indian, Inuit, and Métis peoples are recognized as 'Aboriginal peoples' under Section 35 of the Constitution, and their 'existing Aboriginal and treaty rights [are] recognized and affirmed.' While the courts and politicians continue to wrangle about the legal implication of this section, clearly the Constitution establishes the Aboriginal peoples as unique, with special status within Canada" (p. 12). As part of the decolonizing process, Indian organizations are more commonly referring to themselves as **First Nations**; the Inuit and Métis have already decolonized their names. First Nations, Métis, and Inuit peoples are often recognized as being **vulnerable populations**, meaning they are more likely than other populations to have adverse health outcomes (Flaskerud & Winslow, 1998). This has occurred not only through colonization, but also by the overwhelming poverty found within many of the communities. Community health nurses (CHNs) need to adapt knowledge and skills to provide meaningful community health nursing care in Aboriginal communities. Nurses who choose to practise in Aboriginal communities must come prepared to deal with complex issues in health and nursing.

In this chapter, the history of Aboriginal people is outlined from **pre-European contact** (prior to exploration and settlement by Europeans) to contemporary times. The historical context is important in order to provide culturally appropriate community healthcare to Aboriginal populations. Healthcare services are delivered to First Nations and Inuit by a distinctly different system, whereas healthcare is delivered to the Métis in typically the same method as to non-Aboriginals. Included is the description of the funding of First Nations and Inuit healthcare systems. Finally, cultural, policy, and health issues important to the Aboriginal people of Canada in the modern context are discussed. The CHN can influence changes to improve the health of the descendants of Canada's First Peoples.

FIRST NATIONS HISTORY

Pre-European Contact

North America's Aboriginal peoples have maintained that they are the original inhabitants of the Americas. That fact is not questioned; however, the date and path of the arrival of humans to this continent are still being debated (Dickason, 2002a). Most tribes have a version of a creation story of being the original inhabitants of North America. Unearthed artifacts prove that humans arrived and resided in the Americas during the later Ice Ages. The first inhabitants of the Americas arrived with the necessary skills to survive in harsh environments (Ricciuti, 1990). Despite the hardships, cultures developed and adapted to the locale (Ballantine & Ballantine, 1993). However, the lives of Aboriginal people were profoundly altered by colonization. Mann (2005) presents somewhat controversial theories, based on research, of the possibility that the Americas may have been more densely populated as many as twenty or thirty thousand years earlier than history accepts.

Before the arrival of the Europeans on this continent, an estimated 18 million inhabitants and more than 2200 languages flourished. First Nations peoples of Canada had an oral history (Dickason, 2002a). Aboriginal languages evolved into dialects spoken in different areas of a region, leading to the following linguistic and cultural groupings: Arctic, Western Subarctic, Eastern Subarctic, Northeastern Woodlands, Plains, Plateau, and Northwest Coast (Waldram et al., 2006). These cultures were based on the resources of the area that the people inhabited. For example, the Plains people were hunter-gatherers who provisioned their **bands** or **tribes** by hunting and harvesting the fauna and flora of the prairies, including following the bison herds (Schultz, 1962). The Haudenosaunee (Six Nations) in the Ontario regions grew up to 80% of their food requirements, while the tribes along the Northwest Coast met their needs from the abundance in the oceans (Dickason, 2002a). Thus, cultural and historical diversity of Aboriginal peoples in Canada clearly existed before the arrival of the colonizers.

Childcare and education were the responsibility of the extended family (Sherman, 1996). The adults provided for themselves and the community. Methods of food preservation were devised to store food for less plentiful seasons. Housing materials included animal hides or the trees of the woodlands. Any less fortunate members of the band were provided sustenance by the whole group. Sharing of resources among the group was expected and ensured the survival of the community; for example, among the Northwest Coast tribes, the potlatch was a method of redistributing resources. Transgression by anyone was dealt with according to custom law. The culture of the group included spirituality; one facet involved connection with all living and non-living things—this was a belief shared by most Aboriginal people. Life, if not ideal, was valued, and individuals knew their roles and purpose (Fleet, 1997).

Aboriginal communities had traditional beliefs about health. Shamans and herbalists held the knowledge of curing illness. Mothers or grandmothers practised folk medicine to care for their families, using medicines that were common to their geographical area. The medicine wheel philosophy, which encompassed all nature, was extensively used by numerous tribes, with regional variability.

European Contact

Initial contact with Europeans was on Canada's east coast and extended into the Hudson Bay area over a significant period of time. Explorers and fur traders from England and France began to explore and to harvest the plentiful animals for the fur trade. Missionaries made their way westward to bring Christian doctrine. The newcomers brought diseases such as smallpox, tuberculosis, and measles, which decimated the population by the thousands. For example, Mann (2005) cites research that the initial Aboriginal population's small homogeneous gene pool made them more susceptible to European diseases. Biochemistry research of measles vaccine responses of an Aboriginal group concluded that "virgin-soil Indians" were more susceptible to European diseases, while "virgin-soil Europeans" had acquired immunity. The result was the devastation and fragmenting of Aboriginal cultures. Furthermore, resources that had supplied Aboriginal livelihoods, such as the buffalo and the beaver, became scarce; thus adding to the susceptibility to depopulating epidemics.

The establishment of Canada as a country brought settlers from Europe into virtually all areas of the country. The process of establishing colonies and settlements in Canada required treaty negotiations with the original inhabitants and the subsequent establishment of reserves, which created further problems, including malnutrition, starvation, and death. At the time of European contact, Canada was estimated to have 50 to 60 languages. Many of those languages became extinct, and the rest continued to dwindle over time (Waldram et al., 2006), further contributing to the decimation of Aboriginal culture (Chrisjohn et al., 1994).

Post-European Contact

Even though there were about 500 distinct tribes in the early 1600s, the land was legally considered empty and therefore claimable (Fleet, 1997). Britain developed the **treaty** method with the Indians to claim land that the Aboriginal people occupied. The **British North America (BNA) Act** of 1867 gave Canada its birth as a country, but The Royal Proclamation specified that only the British government could buy Indian lands or negotiate treaties. Private individuals or other nations (including Canada) could not go into Indian communities to buy land directly (Dickason, 2002b). The **Indian Act** of 1876 was passed to ensure that the terms of the treaties were observed.

As a result of the treaties, First Nations peoples were relegated to living on **reserves**. Those who came from agrarian cultures had lived their entire lives in villages; however, hunter-gatherers were a nomadic society whose territories were reduced to small plots of land, some as small as a few acres, and in many cases the land was of no economic value. The Indian reserves were governed by the federal government under the Indian Act (Venne, 2002). Individuals called **Indian agents** were assigned to carry out the terms of the treaty. Once accustomed to having freedom, First Nations people found that they now required written permission from the Indian agents to leave the reserve and became dependent on them for all aspects of their sustenance (Canada, Department of Indian & Northern Affairs, 1997). First Nations reserves are located in all of Canada's provinces, but not in the territories. Some reserves are adjacent to or located within urban centres. The reserves located in the south are easily accessible. Farther north, most reserves are remote and isolated unless they are located near an urban centre. Most reserves are governed by an elected chief and council for two- to four-year terms of office. **The Department of Indian Affairs and Northern Development** was and continues to be the government department responsible for managing the reserves and the treaty Indians.

The Residential School Legacy

Residential schools were first established by the missionaries in the late 1800s in various locations of Canada. The federal government took over the administration of some residential schools as a response to the treaty right to education. Leaders of First Nations communities wanted schools built on the reserves. However, the federal government decided that residential schools would be cheaper; furthermore, a similar system in the United States was showing promise in assimilating the American Indian children into the white society. Approximately 135 residential schools were operated through an agreement between the federal government and the Roman Catholic Church, the Church of England, the Methodist Church, and the Presbyterian Church between 1892 and 1969 (Aboriginal Healing Foundation, 1999). After the withdrawal of the federal government, some residential schools continued to operate into the 1970s, 1980s, and 1990s. The vast majority of residential schools were in the western provinces. The number of children sent to residential schools has been estimated to be more than 150 000, and in 1991 the Assembly of First Nations estimated that approximately 105 000 to 107 000 survivors were still alive; that figure has dropped to about 86 000 today (Aboriginal Healing Foundation, 2007).

The premise of the residential schools was to assimilate the children through a process of education, religious and otherwise, as well as cultural degradation—teaching the children to be ashamed of their heritage in order to facilitate the assimilation process. Parents were legally required to send their children; failure to do so meant incarceration, at which point the children were wards of the state and would be sent to residential schools anyway. Physical, emotional, and sexual abuse was rampant in the schools, and little was done to stop it or to punish the abusers. Living conditions were often far below acceptable levels in modern society's terms. Children often went hungry; children report their parents bringing them food on their weekend visits to supplement their substandard diet (Aboriginal Healing Foundation, 1999). Some children report being forced to steal food from the kitchens. The education they received was also substandard. As late as the 1950s, more than 40% of the teaching staff at the schools had no professional training (Aboriginal Healing Foundation, 1999). Cultural degradation practices included physical and emotional abuse for speaking a traditional language, cutting of hair (hair has strong cultural and spiritual implications), imposing foreign religious practices, and intentional separation from visiting parents. The residential school experiences of Aboriginal peoples continue to have a detrimental impact on Aboriginal communities. Generational and intergenerational issues such as high rates of suicide, addictions, violence, and abuse plague Aboriginal communities. The intergenerational impact of loss of parenting skills has now been felt by two generations and is starting to be felt by a third generation.

The Aboriginal Healing Foundation (AHF) was established in 1998 as a response to the findings of the 1996 Royal Commission on Aboriginal Peoples regarding residential school survivors (Aboriginal Healing Foundation, 2007). The AHF was provided with a $350 million one-time fund to assist communities in healing from the residential school trauma (Aboriginal Healing Foundation, 2007). Furthermore, the federal government signed the Indian Residential Schools Settlement Agreement in 2005 which was intended to acknowledge every survivor's experience. There are three sections of the Agreement: lump sum payments for every survivor—$10,000 for ever having attended and $3,000 for each year of attendance; an Independent Assessment Process for students who suffered physical/sexual/psychological abuse; and a commemorative section including more funding for the AHF (Indian and Northern Affairs, 2009). Aboriginal communities are striving to reweave the strands of their social, cultural, and spiritual worlds. Community-based healing initiatives funded through the Aboriginal Healing Foundation have helped the healing process in some communities. Compensation for survivors has been ongoing since the Agreement was ratified through the court systems on September 17, 2007 (Indian and Northern Affairs, 2009).

Treaty Status

An understanding of how treaty status is acquired and defined is indispensable to understanding the healthcare of Aboriginal people. The status of being a treaty Indian in Canada is not only acquired by birth but also legislated by the Indian Act. A **registered** or **status Indian** is recognized under the Indian Act and has a unique registration number called a treaty number. Non-status Indians are culturally Indians, but because their tribe did not sign a treaty or their treaty status was lost through the Indian Act policies, they are not recognized as Status Indians by the federal government. One of the main goals of the Indian Act was assimilation. There were several ways one could lose treaty status, otherwise known as enfranchisement, such as entering the armed forces, obtaining a university education, becoming a Christian minister, gaining access to vote, or, for a woman, marrying a non-status man.

Prior to 1985, the definition of an Indian was any male person of Indian blood belonging to a recognized band, any child of such a person, and any woman legally married to such a person (Furi & Wherrett, 1996). There was an amendment to the Indian Act in 1985; many of the issues relating to loss of treaty status were intended to be resolved through the passing of **Bill C-31**. For example, a status woman who marries a non-status man no longer loses her treaty status, and neither do her children. Furthermore, individuals who had lost their status could apply for its return. However, the assimilative intent of the Indian Act remains in Bill C-31, because there are limitations on how far treaty status can be passed on generationally. In two generations of intermarriage, whether the non-status spouse is male or female, the children lose their treaty status. There have been several court challenges to this aspect of Bill C-31; however, no definitive changes or decisions have been made since it was enacted in 1985 (Furi & Wherrett, 1996). The **Inuit** are in a separate category, because no treaties were signed in the far north, but they are treated in the same manner as registered Indians by the federal government (Waldram et al., 2006). The isolation, cold, and inhospitable environment are the likeliest reasons treaties were not signed in the far north; that is, settlers were unlikely to have wanted the land. The Métis, who were the mixed-blood children born of Aboriginal and non-Aboriginal parents, are legally considered the same as non-status Indians. The Métis are considered Aboriginal peoples of Canada under the Constitution and are acquiring rights, such as hunting. Métis acquire services through the Office of the Interlocutor at the federal government level.

CONTEMPORARY ABORIGINALS

A White Paper was written in 1969 (Health Canada, 2005a) for the purpose of abolishing the treaties and the Indian Act and disassembling the government departments responsible for reserves and treaty Indians. Generally, a White Paper is a government report on an investigation into a given topic. Often, a White Paper offers recommendations that become policy or law. However, this White Paper never became policy or legislation (Canada, Department of Indian & Northern Affairs, 1997), because of an unprecedented show of force and unity among Aboriginal communities. Though the White Paper did not succeed in terminating the First Nations and Inuit relationship with the federal government, its very attempt appears to have created a resurgence in the culture of Canada's Aboriginal people (Schouls, 2002). Today, there is increasing interest in speaking the languages of the remaining 11 language families: Algonquian, Athapaskan, Eskimo–Aleut, Haida, Tlingit, Siouan, Tsimshian, Wakashan, Salishan, Kutenai, and Iroquoian.

Canada's Aboriginal peoples' rights were given recognition in the Canadian Constitution. Several attempts have been made to define the treaty rights. The federal government attempted to clarify governance issues through its First Nations Governance Act (FNGA), The FNGA would allow effective self-governance for Aboriginal people (Canada, Department of Indian & Northern Affairs, 2002). However, once again, Aboriginal communities, political bodies, and community groups acted in unity to prevent this act being passed by parliament into law. Another federal initiative spearheaded by Prime Minister Paul Martin was intended to improve the lives of Aboriginal people, with a $5 million dollar budget over a 10-year period (Patterson, 2006). This agreement was signed by the federal government, all provincial and territorial governments, as well as Aboriginal organizations in November 2005. However, due to the change in government, the principles of the agreement were never formally adopted at the federal government level (Patterson, 2006).

First Nations, Métis, and Inuit Health Status

The deplorable health status of First Nations, Métis, and Inuit populations has been a controversial issue within Canadian society for decades. Applying the health determinants to the Aboriginal population shows disparities in virtually all areas. It is often easier to access statistical data on First Nations due to the unique identifying number on their health cards; Métis and Inuit populations are more difficult. Information presented here is as current and comprehensive as possible; however, the reader is encouraged to keep in mind the limitations inherent in missing/unavailable data.

In addition to the cultural disorganization caused by colonization are the issues borne from the culture of poverty (Bartlett, 2003). Because reserves effectively excluded First Nations people from mainstream Canadian society, poverty became permanent (Allender & Spradley, 2001). There are also Métis settlements. Most are found in the western prairie provinces; however, the majority (69%) of the Métis population can be found interspersed within the general rural and urban populations (Women of the Métis Nation, 2007), while the Inuit live in settlements throughout the far north. Low socioeconomic status can be found in all Aboriginal populations, regardless of rural, urban, or remote location and more than 50% of Aboriginal children live in poverty (Chansonneuve, 2005).

The effects of the residential school legacy on education levels are still being felt, with 26% of the population having a less than grade 9 education. This figure jumps to 44% for older adults (50–64 years old) (Chansonneuve, 2005). The Métis population was living in very similar conditions to the First Nations at the turn of the century and, despite the federal government's initial resistance, Métis students attended the residential schools. Exact figures are difficult to obtain; however, Métis students comprised up to 9% of the residential school populations in Canada and currently 17% of those over the age of 15 have a less than grade 9 educational level (Chansonneuve, 2005). First Nations communities have been addressing this issue by reclaiming their own educational institutions, including curriculum and the training of Aboriginal teachers. Aboriginal individuals graduating from postsecondary institutions increased from 33% in 1996 to 38% in 2001 (Statistics Canada, 2003).

Employment indicators are closely related to education levels and socioeconomic status; therefore, it is not surprising that employment rates are low among Aboriginal peoples. On reserve unemployment rates are four times that of the general population (27.7% versus 7.3%) (Health Canada, 2009). The Inuit unemployment rate is 22% and 20% among the Métis Chansonneuve, 2005; NAHO, 2007). Even of those who are employed, a significant portion earn less than $10 000 per year. There is improvement in the labour participation rates and the employment rates of First Nations peoples (Health Canada, 2009), so the expectation is that there is similar improvement among the Inuit and Métis.

Health determinants cite physical environment as one of the factors that determine the health of individuals in a community. On-reserve housing is often substandard by Canadian standards (Health Canada, 2009), and smoke alarms are not mandatory in such homes. Utilities that are considered essential in urban homes, such as electricity, heating, and indoor plumbing, are not always available to all First Nations community homes. Furthermore, urban dwelling Aboriginal peoples are often found in the poorer areas of town such as the inner city, which is often rampant with substandard rental housing. Risk factors inherent with unsafe physical environments affect health; this is demonstrated in the high rates of mortality and morbidity from injury and trauma, chronic illness, depression, and family violence (Sebastian, 2000). Illnesses such as TB and respiratory diseases, transmission of which is exacerbated by crowded housing, continue to be a health threat. For example, the rates of TB in the Inuit population are 70 times that of the general population (NAHO, 2007a). Respiratory diseases among Aboriginal children are one of the leading causes of hospitalization and death. (Smylie & Adomako, 2009). Burns caused by fires are another area of concern. Health Canada (2007) reports that nearly half of the Aboriginal communities under its jurisdiction lack adequate fire protection services. The nurse must be an advocate for clients and community to improve housing standards and safety for Aboriginal communities.

Trauma and injury, whether accidental or intentional, are also related to physical environments and are high on the list of health issues besetting Aboriginal populations. Communities that practise a hunting and gathering culture may be prone to injuries related to their particular lifestyle, such as from firearms, boats, ATVs, snowmobiles, or other hunting equipment. Alcohol is often a contributing factor to injuries and death caused by injuries, both accidental and intentional.

In the area of personal health practices and coping skills, lifestyle illnesses caused by drug and alcohol abuse, such as organ damage and FASD, continue to be over represented among Aboriginal populations. Smoking rates continue to be very high—58.8% versus 24.2% in the general population (Health Canada, 2007). According to the 2002–2003 First Nations Regional Longitudinal Survey, the majority (73%) of First Nations adults are overweight or obese (Health Canada, 2007). Therefore, it is not surprising that diabetes, of which being overweight is a common risk factor, has reached epidemic proportions in Aboriginal communities. Mortality rates from diabetes for Aboriginal women living in First Nations communities are five times higher than the national average. Diabetes is also being diagnosed at a younger age. Rates of amputation, blindness, and kidney failure are higher among Aboriginal populations. Nurses must understand the health promotion and health education needed to change the lifestyle of those affected by diabetes (McMurray, 1999). Cancer, which has been relatively uncommon in Aboriginal populations, has steadily been increasing and there are certain issues that are common in relation to cancer screening, diagnosis, and treatment. Screening programs have generally received a low uptake, diagnosis is often at advanced stages, and remote locations hamper cancer treatment, which typically takes place in larger urban centres (Shahid & Thompson, 2009).

Healthy child development is an important health indicator for Aboriginal populations, because the birth rate is almost twice that of the general Canadian population. Furthermore, the overall Aboriginal population is younger, with 25% of Métis, 35% of Inuit and 32% of First Nations populations being 15 years or younger (Smylie & Adomako, 2009). Lack of childcare, lack of food security, and low immunization rates for children are serious concerns for Aboriginal communities, both on and off reserve.

Health and social indicators of Aboriginal peoples highlight the grim statistics relative to health, the justice system, education, and the social and child welfare system. But the resilience of individuals, families, and communities is resulting in their being educated and participating as members of mainstream Canadian society (Mercredi & Turpel, 1993).

Aboriginal peoples are moving to urban communities in increasing numbers, often to seek a better life for their children. However, the same problems that plague reserve and remote communities can also be apparent for urban dwellers. Those problems present themselves as unemployment, inadequate housing, social exclusion, lack of childcare, food insecurity, lack of transportation, and intermittent access to healthcare.

The picture is not all bleak. Aboriginal people are adapting to Western society and are represented in all occupations, including education, health, justice, business, and the trades. Some individuals receive a Western-based education and return to work and live in their communities, while others elect to remain in urban settings. The National Aboriginal Achievement Awards showcase the talent in the Canadian Aboriginal community. It is important to become aware of the positive aspects of being Aboriginal. It counteracts the negative stereotyping of Aboriginal people.

The national profile of First Nations communities and their health status highlights the dire need for change. The relatively new health determinants have emphasized the health needs of the Canadian Aboriginal people. The change has to be made to the social determinants of health, such as income, physical environments, and employment, to overcome the poverty and third-world conditions present in too many First Nations communities.

HEALTH STATUS OF ABORIGINAL WOMEN

Several reports have stated that Aboriginal women continue to be overrepresented in statistics relating to poverty, violence, abuse, and overall health status (Dion-Stout et al., 2001; Royal Commission on Aboriginal Peoples [RCAP], 1996; Saskatchewan Women's Secretariat, 1999). While it is important to present epidemiological evidence in order to provide an overview of health and illness within a population, the author wishes to offer the following cautionary note to the reader. Aboriginal communities and peoples have repeatedly stated that they have been over-researched, and the research has consistently portrayed primarily negative health status; this runs the risk of creating institutional and health professional biases and perpetuating the negative stereotypes. This concept is no different when it comes to Aboriginal women.

It is difficult to obtain population-level health indicators for Métis populations, as has previously been stated. One source that provides inclusive information is the Census. According to the Canadian 2001 Census, Aboriginal women comprise 1.7% of the Canadian population (n = 499 605) (Statistics Canada, 2002). When compared with Aboriginal males, females are more likely to be married, separated, divorced, or widowed. Women are more likely to have attained higher education levels, including high school, trades, and postsecondary education. However, they earn less overall income, work more part-time jobs, and depend on government sources more than men do (Statistics Canada, 2002).

The 2002/2003 First Nations Regional Longitudinal Health Survey (RHS) reports similar findings. This is not surprising considering that the RHS is run concurrently with the Census, but the RHS does provide data on a wider array of health indicators. In regard to First Nations women living on reserves, 56% live in smoke-free homes, which is positive as women are more likely to live with children under the age of 15 (National Aboriginal Health Organization [NAHO], 2006). Women reported less use of alcohol and marijuana as well as receiving fewer alcohol- and drug-treatment programs than men. In terms of preventive and screening services, women were more likely to have accessed such services. Coincidentally, women also reported more barriers and problems accessing healthcare services. First Nations women are being diagnosed earlier with diabetes (20–34 age group) and they also are more likely to be obese or morbidly obese. They also report higher rates of arthritis, allergies, hypertension, asthma, stomach/intestinal problems, rheumatism, and osteoporosis. First Nations women were also more likely to report feeling blue, sad, or depressed for two weeks or more in the previous year, as well as to having ever attempted suicide. Furthermore, 20% reported they had attended residential school and they believed this affected their health negatively. However, women also reported they had support systems in place when they needed to talk to someone. An interesting finding is that 70% of respondents stated they talked to family and friends, compared to only 29% who talked to their family physician (NAHO, 2006).

Healthcare practitioners need to be aware of the pre-Confederation history of Canada and Aboriginal peoples, and the effect this has on health-seeking behaviours. A study of Mi'kmaq patients reported favourable encounters with the health system when there was compassion and a non-discriminatory attitude among healthcare workers (Baker & Daigle, 2000). The avoidance of health systems that are not culturally safe does little to acknowledge patterns of individual or institutional discrimination (Browne & Fiske, 2001). Examples of negative encounters included dismissal by healthcare providers, and negative stereotypes including lack of parenting skills, marginalization, situations of vulnerability, and disregard for personal circumstances. Positive or affirming encounters were situations where the women were active participants in healthcare decisions, received exceptional care, received affirmation of personal and cultural identity, and developed a long-term relationship with healthcare providers (Browne & Fiske, 2001).

This brief synopsis of the health status of Aboriginal women is not intended to be the complete picture. Health determinants are intended to be guidelines to assess equality among communities and populations; the reader must remain aware that these guidelines have been drawn up by the dominant society. Community initiatives such as Naspici Miyomahcihowin (Continuous Good Health): A Community-Based Research Project Examining the Health Needs of Aboriginal Women in Saskatoon encourages Aboriginal women to determine their own health requirements, incorporating their cultural values and beliefs throughout the process (Saskatoon Aboriginal Women's Health Research Committee, 2004). Aboriginal communities are continuing to strive for improvement in health outcomes, and more often than not the leaders are women.

FIRST NATIONS HEALTHCARE

A component of working with First Nations communities is knowing the larger healthcare system that enacts policy to establish the practice and standards for First Nations healthcare systems. Healthcare provision is considered a treaty right by First Nations and Inuit; however, government policy states that healthcare provided to First Nations is benevolence by the federal government. Deagle (1999) contends that Canada's healthcare system operates under a three-tier system, with the Aboriginal populations in the lowest position. The federal government, through its Health Minister and department and the **First Nations and Inuit Health Branch (FNIHB)** (formerly Medical Services Branch of Health Canada), provides the health services and support for First Nations and Inuit living on reserves. First Nations are increasingly assuming local control through the transfer of health services (see Appendix 2A at the end of Chapter 2). Health services for the Métis are provided by the provincial healthcare systems. Furthermore, First Nations and Inuit living off reserve get their healthcare services provided within the provincial healthcare system, and then the province asks for reimbursement from the federal government. The territories assume responsibility for their Aboriginal populations through their agreements with Ottawa. The FNIHB is based in Ottawa, where policy is planned. The First Nations and Inuit health policy is administered by the regional branches in each province, headed by a regional director.

Part of the politics of First Nations, Métis, and Inuit are the national organizations that represent their interests in Ottawa. For example, the Assembly of First Nations elects a Grand Chief, who negotiates with federal officials for program funding of First Nations healthcare. The Inuit Tapiriit Kanatami represents the Inuit, and the Métis National Council represents the Métis.

Why do CHNs need to know about government and its functions? The answer is that it affects how healthcare is delivered to First Nations on a daily basis. It is advantageous to know and understand policies, thereby increasing the effectiveness of healthcare practitioners. When the governing party changes, often the agreements that have been in place are altered, deleted, or replaced by new legislation.

For acute care services, First Nations healthcare systems interface with the greater Canadian healthcare system, primarily because hospitals are a provincial responsibility. The degree of interfacing required with the surrounding communities depends on the type and scope of health services that exist on the reserves. The more remote and isolated the reserve, the more likely it is that the healthcare services include comprehensive care, including short-term acute care services. The federal government operated Indian hospitals but has been divesting itself of this responsibility.

The process for community-based health services is different. The governance for health services is derived from the chief and council, the governing authority for First Nations. Once the band council resolution is signed, a health committee or health board can be formed to begin the process of exploring community-based health services for its membership. First Nations health authorities were established to prepare for the transfer of control of health services to First Nations. Various types of funding arrangements are available to First Nations groups seeking to administer their own health programs (see Appendix 2A).

CANADIAN RESEARCH BOX 22.1

How is health knowledge used in Aboriginal communities?

Smylie, J., Kaplan-Myrth, N., McShane, K., Metis Nation of Ontario–Ottawa Council, Pikwakanagan First Nation, & Tungasuvvingat Inuit Family Resource Centre. (2009). Indigenous knowledge translation: Baseline findings in a qualitative study of the pathways of health knowledge in three Indigenous communities in Canada. *Health Promotion Practice, 10*, 436–446.

The premise for this study, which was to assess whether public health programs are ineffective in Indigenous communities, is related to failing to take into consideration local understandings of health and illness as well as local mechanisms of knowledge sharing. Three communities in Ontario—urban Métis, urban Inuit, and semi-rural First Nations—participated in focus groups and key informant interviews.

Each community identified specific themes that were distinct for each, however, five common themes were also identified, namely:

1. Valuing experiential knowledge—health information is evaluated based on personal experience.
2. Influence of community structure on health information dissemination—for a cohesive community, word-of-mouth is a very effective method; dispersed population groups or social fragmentation makes for difficult dissemination.
3. Preference for "within the community" messages—incorporation of culturally appropriate icons, symbols, and language in messages was preferred.
4. Dissemination through family and community networks—this was the most important mode of information sharing.

5. Local effects of colonization—different levels of tension exist between traditional knowledge systems and Western knowledge systems.

Implications for policy and practice indicate that local knowledge systems need to be incorporated in health promotion materials. The one-size-fits-all approach of FNIHB is not an appropriate policy.

Discussion Questions

1. As a CHN, how might you use the findings in your program planning?
2. In the Western education system, experiential learning is not always a prerequisite for uptake of information—taking the first theme into consideration, how would you facilitate a new treatment procedure into the community?

Cultural Issues in Community Health Nursing in Aboriginal Communities

First Nations' healthcare systems are varied in scope and practice. The nurse may practise in a large healthcare system that utilizes nursing skills in a limited scope. In contrast, the nurse may arrive in a remote northern community where the expectation is that all nursing roles will be met by one individual (Cradduck, 1995). Giger and Davidhizar's (1998) conceptual framework states that there are six key cultural phenomena in all cultures: communication, space, time, social organization, environmental control, and biological variations. The Giger and Davidhizar transcultural assessment model is one tool that can be utilized in assessing Aboriginal populations to develop culturally appropriate community health nursing care.

Development of competent, culturally appropriate nursing care (Andrews & Boyle, 1999) for Aboriginal clients requires the CHN to keep in mind the historical, cultural, and changing clinical healthcare delivery system. As noted earlier, the traditional lifestyles of Canada's Aboriginal peoples profoundly changed because of colonization. Reserves effectively excluded First Nations from participation in mainstream Canadian society (McMurray, 1999).

Aboriginal populations continue to remain a distinct cultural segment of Canadian society. Traditional holistic health beliefs, traditional medicine, and herbal medicine are deemed acceptable alternatives to Western medicine by some Aboriginals. First Nations communities are societies in themselves. Based on a culture continuum, the society may have different members who are traditionalists, traditionalists/modernists, or modernists. Each group's strengths and challenges present for interesting nurse practice. The CHN must learn protocol for communicating with the traditionalists, who may possess cultural manners, diet, and health beliefs contrary to nursing knowledge and skills (Holland & Hogg, 2001). For example, some individuals believe that bear grease is the best treatment for abrasions and wounds. The CHN must respect the client's health beliefs, yet attempt to maintain sterile wound care. The outcome is establishing sufficient trust with the client so that the wound heals without infection and the client continues to seek the required healthcare.

Rumbold (1999) states that ethics provides a framework for dealing with issues, problems, and dilemmas. An understanding of ethical or moral theories helps a person decide on an appropriate line of action, although it may not necessarily provide the answer. Nurses need to study ethics because they often have to deal with moral or ethical problems. Nurses need to examine their own beliefs and values. Rumbold makes the case that nurses who move from one culture to another need to be informed of the values and norms of the society to which they are moving. It does not mean that they should abandon their own ethical values (Rumbold, 1999). Aboriginal communities can present dilemmas in which it is crucial that CHNs make wise choices. Dilemmas may be related to childcare, family violence, or geriatric abuse (Dumont-Smith, 2001). Aboriginal nurses working with First Nations communities may find different challenges, such as a personal tension between cultural practices and their knowledge of health science. Clients may assume a belief system (e.g., traditional medicine) that is not included in the nurse's practice. The Aboriginal Nurses Association of Canada (ANAC), formed in 1975, provides support to Aboriginal and non-Aboriginal nurses practising in First Nations communities and can be accessed on their website (http://www.anac.on.ca).

Nurses contemplating employment with FNIHB or a First Nations health authority should prepare by doing prior research on the tribe's culture, language, geographic location, education, economy, and healthcare system. CHNs require excellent skills for assessment, planning, implementing, and evaluating community health programs (see Chapters 13 and 14). Knowing your client, whether it is the individual, family, or community, facilitates evidence-based decision making. The nurses should be genuinely interested in the health of the Aboriginal clients requiring community health nursing. Required skill sets include the ability to remain objective and to resist stereotyping the community and its residents despite frequent negative media attention. The person who wishes to become familiar with the health status of the First Nations populations could begin by reviewing the First Nations Regional Longitudinal Health Survey (RHS). The RHS describes Canada's first peoples' health, using the cultural framework. Adult, youth, and children's results are available as national and regional reports. Data on the Métis and Inuit are still relatively difficult to obtain, however, the National Aboriginal Health Organization has both Métis and Inuit sectors.

Health personnel must continually be recruited, and nurses often must relocate to remote or isolated First Nations communities (Tarlier et al., 2003). Retention of health personnel for only short lengths of time can result in some communities becoming distrustful of new nurses. This can provide another challenge to the nurse's communication skills (Sundeen et al., 1998).

CANADIAN RESEARCH BOX

How might end-of-life care differ for Aboriginal clients?

Hampton, M., Baydala, A., Bourassa, C., McKay-McNabb, K., Placsko, C., Goodwill, K., . . . Boekelder, R. (2010). Completing the circle: Elders speak about end-of-life care with Aboriginal families in Canada. *Journal of Palliative Care, 26*(1), 6–14.

In this study, the researchers asked the question, "What would you like non-Aboriginal healthcare providers to know when providing end-of-life care for Aboriginal families?" (p. 6). Using community action research methodology, and following OCAP (ownership, control, access, and possession) principles for research with Aboriginal people, the researchers were assisted by two elders throughout the research process. Five additional elders (key informants) from various Aboriginal communities in southern Saskatchewan participated in open-ended interviews. While there was diversity in the traditions, several common themes did emerge from the analyses. These were completing the circle; gathering of community; care and comfort; moments after death; and grief, wake, funeral. Additional outcomes of the study included two videos—one for Aboriginal families and one for non-Aboriginal healthcare providers. The authors note that this research reinforces the notion that cultural values and beliefs lead to end-of-life needs that are important to clients and their families.

Discussion Questions

1. Given cultural diversity among Aboriginal peoples in Canada, how could this research be valuable to CHNs anywhere in the country?

2. How might the new CHN approach this topic when settling in to a new Aboriginal practice setting?

Formal and informal leadership in First Nations communities can be difficult to grasp. CHNs require the skills to assess the community and outline the health priorities and health issues of the population. They have to decide on the course of action in consultation with the community. Historically, First Nations people made decisions on a consensus basis; some communities continue to make decisions in this way (Cookfair, 1991). CHNs have to find roles that can be filled by a non-member health professional, perhaps as a consultant who provides information the community can use to make its best decision. Alternatively, the nurse may be seen as the individual who makes the decisions. The nurse must rely on community-development knowledge and allow the community to make its own decisions over time. It is easy to assume control of the decision making if you are seen as the individual with the best health knowledge. However, it is important to consult and work with the community in all phases of health program development (Smylie, 2000). Elders are traditionally seen as the knowledge keepers of communities, and as such they can be important allies and sources of knowledge.

Policy Issues Affecting Community Health Nursing in Aboriginal Communities

Unlike public health nursing in urban communities, First Nations and Inuit healthcare systems vary in size and services offered. Nurses who seek employment in an Aboriginal community must establish a network of colleagues who can assist with information when required. Health professionals establish liaisons with other service agencies or professional organizations such as the ANAC to promote the population health approach.

CHNs must also be aware of competing policies. For instance, the federal government is responsible for the healthcare of Aboriginal people; thus, nursing services are provided for home care clients by FNIHB. However, the Department of Indian Affairs is responsible for funding personal care and home support services. The nurse must be innovative in coordinating the home care services for clients from two service agencies. In addition, the CHN may be requested to supervise staff responsible for personal care, homemaking, and transportation.

Health education and promotion are part of the everyday contact with communities and groups. CHNs need to make the effort to make these activities culturally appropriate. The medicine wheel framework is an excellent teaching tool and, because of its diversity, can be adapted to virtually any health issue. Medicine wheels are found in the United States and southern Canada, mostly in Alberta and Saskatchewan; they are made of stone and small boulders set in various circular patterns. However, their origins and meaning have been lost in time. Some say they are for navigation using the stars or to mark events such as the solstice. Whatever significance they had for the original inhabitants of North America, they still influence the thinking and lives of Canadian Aboriginal people today. Not unlike other aboriginal cultures in the world, Canadian Aboriginals have a holistic belief about life.

Traditional world views of Aboriginal peoples emphasize the interconnectedness of all things, and this concept is the basis of the medicine wheel framework. Most First Nations in Canada have holistic beliefs, yet not all believe in the medicine wheel philosophy. The present significance of the medicine wheel is that it provides a framework for the holistic beliefs of the descendents of those original inhabitants of Canada.

The medicine wheel usually represents four quadrants of the emotional, physical, mental, and spiritual aspects of health and wellness (see Figure 22.1).

It is said that a balance has to be maintained in the four aspects for an individual to maintain optimal health. On first glance, the medicine wheel model can be simple; however, the concepts it represents are complex. The four directions are represented, just as the races of humankind are represented. The different teachings of how one can lead a purposeful life are also represented. The four life stages of infancy, childhood, adulthood, and the elder are also represented. The four components of our humanness are the physical, the intellectual,

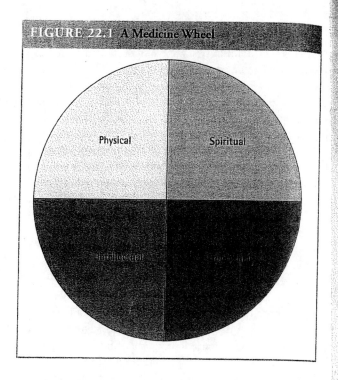

FIGURE 22.1 A Medicine Wheel

the spiritual, and the emotional. Colours, animals, and characteristics such as strength, humility, and illumination are also assigned to their respective quadrants. Today, the medicine wheel philosophy is being taught by elders to the youth in Aboriginal populations across North America. Examples can be found online where communities have adapted the medicine wheel to issues including HIV/AIDS, diabetes, family violence, and addictions.

An alternative framework can be found in the First Nations cultural framework of the national First Nations and Inuit Regional Longitudinal Health Survey (NAHO 2005). The two are similar but cannot be deemed to be the same.

Part of the community health nursing practice in Aboriginal communities is the evaluation component of health programs. Nurses should recognize that nursing standards of practice can be maintained through continuous quality improvement. First Nations health systems are becoming members of the Canadian Council on Health Services Accreditation.

CASE STUDY

A First Nations community has a total population of 3200. Two thousand members live on the reserve and 1200 members live off-reserve. The community is located near a mid-size city. The unemployment level is consistently at 70%. Most families rely on social services for their subsistence. Sixty percent of the population is 18 years of age or less. The education level is at the junior- to high-school range. The community is governed by an elected Chief and eight Councillors.

Most homes are 25 to 35 years old and have indoor plumbing, central heating, and electricity. However, potable water is delivered by water trucks. Sewage disposal is the community sewage system, but rural homes have a septic tank sewage disposal system. The climate is temperate, with cold winters and dry summers.

The community-controlled school system goes from Kindergarten to Grade 6, and six of the 10 teachers are Aboriginal. The community no longer practises its Aboriginal beliefs, and fewer than 5% of the school children speak their language. High school students are bused for an hour each way to attend school in the nearby city. Most families end up being single-parent households.

The economy is based on school transportation, employment with the band administration, the band-controlled school, and two privately owned gas stations/convenience stores. The school principal has initiated a good recreation program for the students, and Aboriginal teacher assistants keep the students interested in being physically active. Parents participate in the school activities. However, once the students are bused to attend school in the city, parents do not display much interest in school activities. Most of the adults attended the residential school at the neighbouring First Nations community, and most of them completed middle school.

The Health Centre is readily accessed by the population for all community health programs. The Chief and Council transferred control of the health programs five years ago to a health administrator hired from another First Nations community. Immunization levels are at 55% for all ages. Chronic disease rates for diabetes, arthritis, and circulatory diseases have not been assessed since prior to the health program transfer. The First Nations and Inuit Health Branch continue to provide support for the CHN. During your orientation at the Regional FNIHB office, the zone nurse manager informs you that one of the priorities is the immunization program because the Canada Disease Weekly has reported pertussis in the area. On weekends, parents leave the community to shop in the nearby city. They frequent the bars to drink alcohol and gamble on the video lottery terminals. Children are often left in the care of elderly grandparents or alone at home to fend for themselves until their parents return.

There have been disturbing developments in the community in the last five years. Family violence, child neglect, and an increased number of motor vehicle accidents and house fires are causing concern for the various community agencies. The frequency of fetal alcohol spectrum disorder is not known. In the last five months, five teenagers have attempted suicide.

You are the new nurse. When you arrive, a lone community health representative is there to welcome you to the Health Centre. She seems to know the community very well, as people greet her warmly on the way to the Health Centre. The people that you meet appear very

glad that you have arrived at the community. They greet you heartily and make you feel welcome.

Discussion Questions

1. How would you, as the CHN, use the nursing process to begin planning to improve the population health?
2. Whom would you ask to help you familiarize yourself with the community?
3. List the resiliency factors of the community.
4. What factors make this First Nations community a vulnerable community?
5. Describe how you will begin to work on the immunization program.

SUMMARY

The chapter outlined the historical and current health issues affecting Aboriginal populations in Canada. Nurses working in Aboriginal communities must understand the distinction between First Nations status and non-status, Métis, and Inuit because it affects nursing services delivery. The employers of nurses working in Aboriginal communities can be the federal, provincial, or local health authorities, each with its own organizational complexities.

Aboriginal populations have immense health challenges that nurses must assess in order to plan health services. Nurses may be responsible for the implementation of health services and programs, and should have the skills to evaluate the efficacy of health programs for Aboriginal communities. In addition, nurses must have the communication skills to allow effective interaction with Aboriginal leadership and other service agency personnel. Advance preparation for working with First Nations and Inuit should be a priority for nurses contemplating employment in First Nations and Inuit communities to lessen the possible effects of culture shock. Nurses working with Canadian Aboriginals face complex challenges in a rewarding practice setting.

KEY TERMS

Aboriginal, p. 350
First Nations, p. 350
vulnerable populations, p. 350
pre-European contact, p. 350
bands, p. 351
tribes, p. 351
treaty, p. 351
British North America (BNA) Act, p. 351
Indian Act, p. 351
reserves, p. 351
Indian agents, p. 351

REVIEW QUESTIONS

1. Which of the following is the legal term used to describe ANY descendants of the people who inhabited Canada prior to the arrival of Europeans?

   a) First Nations person

   b) Registered Indian

   c) Aboriginal person

   d) Status Indian

2. The Indian Act was originally designed to

   a) assimilate the First Nations population.

   b) uphold the treaty obligations of the government.

   c) create a dependent segment of society.

   d) protect the land base reserved to status Indians.

3. Residential schools were initially established by

   a) missionaries.

   b) the federal government.

   c) the Roman Catholic Church.

   d) the Church of England.

4. One of the intergenerational impacts of the residential school legacy is lack of parenting skills. Creating parenting programs in the community should follow this principle:

   a) Do a literature review and apply the most recent research findings.

   b) Establish partnerships with respected Elders in the community.

   c) Create the program and offer it once to test it out.

   d) Create a poster display outlining the effects on children who lack appropriate parenting.

5. The medicine wheel health belief model encompasses the following human concepts:

   a) environment, physical, spiritual, intellectual.

   b) mind, body, spirit.

   c) spiritual, physical, emotional, mental.

   d) nature, stars, animals, humans.

STUDY QUESTIONS

1. What is the difference between a Status and a non-Status Indian?

2. Why are Aboriginal women more likely to be diagnosed with diabetes at a younger age?

3. Is healthcare a treaty right for First Nations people in Canada?

4. What did the 1969 White Paper unintentionally create?

5. Describe five effects of the residential school legacy that can still be seen in Aboriginal communities today.

6. Bill C-31 created a spike among which sectors of the First Nations population in Canada?

After working through these questions, go to the MyNursingLab at **www.pearsoned.ca/mynursinglab** *to check your answers.*

INDIVIDUAL CRITICAL THINKING EXERCISES

1. The Chief of the First Nations community that employs you has just asked to see the chart of one of the clients in your care. How would you handle the situation? How do you maintain security for client records?

2. An Elder in the community believes cancer is spread through personal contact. How would you go about ameliorating this knowledge deficit?

3. A mother brings in her child for immunization and you notice the mother has several large bruises on her face and arms. What course of action do you take?

4. There is an increase in dental caries among the school age children, which corresponds with the installation of a pop machine in school. The proceeds from the pop machine are to be used to build a skating rink. What are your options?

5. An intoxicated female client comes into the clinic with lacerations on her arms and face. During your treatment of her, she starts swearing at you and attempting to hit you. What are your professional and personal responsibilities in this situation?

GROUP CRITICAL THINKING EXERCISES

1. The routine water sample of the First Nations community indicates heavy growth of E. coli. As the nurse manager, how would you deal with this threat to public health? Whom would you contact?

2. There is an unexpected increase in the school age children's responses to the yearly tuberculin Mantoux test. As the community health nurse, what would you do, in addition to instituting a preventive medication regime for the children? Who could you contact for assistance?

3. The community you work in believes that children are a gift from the Creator; therefore, there doesn't seem to be

any incentive to prevent teen pregnancy. You know the health risks to teen moms and their babies. What are some ways you could approach this issue from a community health promotion perspective?

REFERENCES

Aboriginal Healing Foundation. (1999). *Annual report 1999*. Retrieved from http://www.ahf.ca/about-us/annual-reports

Aboriginal Healing Foundation. (2007). *Lump sum compensation payments research project: The circle rechecks itself*. Ottawa, ON: Aboriginal Healing Foundation.

Allender, J. A., & Spradley, B. W. (2001). *Community health nursing: Concepts and practice* (5th ed.). Toronto, ON: Lippincott.

Andrews, M. M., & Boyle, J. S. (1999). *Transcultural concepts in nursing* (3rd ed.). Philadelphia, PA: Lippincott.

Baker, C., & Daigle, M. C. (2000). Cross-cultural hospital care as experienced by Mi'kmaq clients. *Western Journal of Nursing Research, 22*(1), 8–28.

Ballantine, B., & Ballantine, I. (Eds.). (1993). *Native Americans: An illustrated history*. Atlanta, GA: Time.

Bartlett, J. G. (2003). Involuntary cultural change, stress phenomenon and Aboriginal health status. *Canadian Journal of Public Health, 94*, 165–167.

Browne, A. J., & Fiske, J. (2001). First Nations women's encounters with mainstream health care services. *Western Journal of Nursing Research, 23*(2), 126–147.

Canada, Department of Indian and Northern Affairs. (1997). *First Nations in Canada*. Ottawa, ON: Author.

Canada, Department of Indian and Northern Affairs. (2002). *A summary of the First Nations Governance Act*. Ottawa, ON: Author.

Chansonneuve, D. (2005). *Reclaiming connections: Understanding residential school trauma among Aboriginal People*. Ottawa, ON: Aboriginal Healing Foundation.

Chrisjohn, R. D., Young, S. L., & Maraun, M. (1994). *The circle game: Shadows and substance in the residential school experience in Canada: A report to the Royal Commission on Aboriginal Peoples*. Penticton, BC: Theytus.

Cookfair, J. M. (1991). *Nursing process and practice in the community*. Toronto, ON: Mosby.

Cradduck, G. R. (1995). Primary practice. In M. J. Stewart (Ed.), *Community nursing: Promoting Canadians' health* (pp. 454–471). Toronto, ON: Saunders.

Deagle, G. (1999). The three-tier system. [Editorial]. *Canadian Family Physician, 45*, 247–249.

Dickason, O. P. (2002a). Reclaiming stolen land. In J. Bird, L. Land, & M. Macadam (Eds.), *Nation to nation: Aboriginal sovereignty and the future of Canada* (pp. 34–42). Toronto, ON: Irwin.

Dickason, O. P. (2002b). *Canada's First Nations: A history of founding peoples from earliest times* (3rd ed.). Don Mills, ON: Oxford.

Dion-Stout, M., Kipling, G. D., & Stout, R. (2001). *Aboriginal women's health research synthesis project*. Ottawa, ON: Women's Health Bureau.

Dumont-Smith, C. (2001). *Exposure to violence in the home: Effects on Aboriginal children*. Ottawa, ON: Aboriginal Nurses Association of Canada.

Flaskerud, J. H., & Winslow, B. J. (1998). Conceptualizing vulnerable populations health-related research. *Nursing Research, 51*(2), 69–78.

Fleet, C. (1997). Introduction. In C. Fleet (Ed.), *First Nations firsthand: A history of five hundred years of encounter, war, and peace inspired by the eyewitnesses* (pp. 7–9). Edison, NJ: Chartwell.

Furi, M., & Wherrett, J. (1996). *Indian status and band membership issues*. Retrieved from http://www.parl.gc.ca/information/library/PRBpubs/bp410-e.htm

Giger, J. N., & Davidhizar, R. E. (1998). *Canadian transcultural nursing assessment and intervention*. Toronto, ON: Mosby.

Grace, L. S. (2003). Hepatitis A among residents of First Nations reserves in British Columbia, 1991–1996. *Canadian Journal of Public Health, 94*, 173–175.

Health Canada-FNIAH. (2009). *A statistical profile on the health of First Nations in Canada: Determinants of health, 1999–2003*. Retrieved from http://www.hc-sc.gc.ca/fniah-spnia/pubs/aborig-autoch/2009-stats-profil/index-eng.php#tab-cont-mat

Health Canada-FNIHB. (2005a). *Indian health policy 1979*. Retrieved from http://www.hc-sc.gc.ca/ahc-asc/branch-dirgen/fnihb-dgspni/poli_1979-eng.php

Health Canada-FNIHB. (2005b). *Ten years of health transfer First Nations and Inuit control*. Retrieved from http://www.hc-sc.gc.ca/fniah-spnia/pubs/finance/_agree-accord/10_years_ans_trans/index-eng.php

Holland, K., & Hogg, C. (2001). *Cultural awareness in nursing and health care: An introductory text*. New York, NY: Oxford University Press.

Indian and Northern Affairs. (2009). *Indian residential schools*. Retrieved from http://www.ainc-inac.gc.ca/ai/rqpi/index-eng.asp

Lalonde, M. (1974). *A new perspective on the health of Canadians: A working document*. Ottawa, ON: Canada, National Health and Welfare.

Mann, Charles C. (2005). *1491: New revelations of the Americas before Columbus*. New York, NY: Vintage Books.

McMurray, A. (1999). *Community health and wellness: A sociological approach*. Toronto, ON: Mosby.

Mercredi, O., & Turpel, M. E. (1993). *In the rapids: Navigating the future of First Nations*. New York, NY: Penguin.

National Aboriginal Health Organization (NAHO) First Nations Centre. (2006). *First Nations Regional Longitudinal Health Survey (RHS) 2002/03: Report on selected indicators by gender*. Retrieved from www.rhs-ers.ca/english/pdf/rhs2002-03reports/rhs2002-03-report_on_selected_indicators_by_gender.pdf

National Aboriginal Health Organization (NAHO) Inuit Tattarvingat. (2007). *Overview of Inuit health*. Retrieved from http://www.naho.ca/inuit/e/overview/

Patterson, L. L. (2006). *Aboriginal roundtable to Kelowna Accord: Aboriginal policy negotiations, 2004–2005*. Retrieved from http://www.parl.gc.ca/information/library/prbpubs/prb0604-e.htm

Ricciuti, E. (1990). *The natural history of North America.* New York, NY: Gallery.

Royal Commission on Aboriginal Peoples (RCAP). (1996). *Report of the Royal Commission on Aboriginal Peoples: Perspectives and realities.* Vol. 4. Ottawa, ON: Author.

Rumbold, G. (1999). *Ethics in nursing practice* (3rd ed.). Toronto, ON: Bailliere Tindall.

Saskatchewan Women's Secretariat. (1999). *Profile of Aboriginal women in Saskatchewan.* Regina, SK: Author.

Saskatoon Aboriginal Women's Health Research Committee. (2004). *Naspici miyomahcihowin (continuous good health): A community-based research project examining the health needs of Aboriginal women in Saskatoon.* Winnipeg, MB: The Prairie Women's Health Centre of Excellence.

Schouls, T. (2002). The basic dilemma: Sovereignty or assimilation. In J. Bird, L. Land, & M. Macadam (Eds.), *Nation to nation: Aboriginal sovereignty and the future of Canada* (pp. 34–42). Toronto, ON: Irwin.

Schultz, J. W. (1962). *Blackfeet and buffalo: Memories of life among the Indians.* Norman, OK: University of Oklahoma Press.

Sebastian, J. G. (2000). Vulnerability and vulnerable populations: An overview. In M. Stanhope & J. Lancaster (Eds.), *Community and public health nursing* (5th ed., pp. 638–661). Toronto, ON: Mosby.

Shahid, S., & Thompson, S. C. (2009). An overview of cancer and beliefs about the disease in Indigenous people of Australia, Canada, New Zealand and the US. *Australian and New Zealand Journal of Public Health, 33,* 109–118.

Sherman, J. (1996). *Indian tribes of North America.* New York, NY: Todri Productions.

Smylie, J. (2000). A guide for health professionals working with Aboriginal people. *Journal of the Society of Obstetricians and Gynecologists of Canada, 22*(12), 1056–1061.

Smylie, J., & Adomako, P. (2009). *Indigenous children's health report: Health assessment in action.* Retrieved from http://www.stmichaelshospital.com/pdf/crich/ichr_report.pdf

Statistics Canada. (2002). *2001 Census Aboriginal population profiles.* Retrieved from http://www12.statcan.gc.ca/english/Profil01/AP01/Index.cfm?Lang=E

Statistics Canada. (2003). *Education in Canada: Raising the standard.* Retrieved from www12.statcan.ca/english/census01/Products/Analytic/companion/educ/canada.cfm#aboriginal

Sundeen, S. J., Stuart, G. W., Rankin, A. D., & Cohen, S. A. (1998). *Nurse–client interaction: Implementing the nursing process* (6th ed.). Toronto, ON: Mosby.

Tarlier, D. S., Johnson, J. L., & Whyte, N. B. (2003). Voices from the wilderness: An interpretive study describing the role and practice of outpost nurses. *Canadian Journal of Public Health, 94,* 180–184.

Venne, S. (2002). Treaty-making with the Crown. In J. Bird, L. Land, & M. Macadam (Eds.), *Nation to nation: Aboriginal sovereignty and the future of Canada* (pp. 45–52). Toronto, ON: Irwin.

Waldram, J. B., Herring, D. A., & Young, T. K. (2006). *Aboriginal health in Canada: Historical, cultural and epidemiological perspectives.* Toronto, ON: University of Toronto Press.

Women of the Métis Nation. (2007). *Health policy paper.* Retrieved from http://www.laa.gov.nl.ca/laa/naws/pdf/WMNHealthPaper.pdf

ADDITIONAL RESOURCES

Websites

Aboriginal AIDS Network
http://www.caan.ca

Aboriginal Nurses Association of Canada (ANAC)
http://www.anac.on.ca

First Nations and Inuit Health Branch
http://www.hc-sc.gc.ca/ahc-asc/branch-dirgen/fnihb-dgspni/index-eng.php

National Aboriginal Health Organization (NAHO)
http://www.naho.ca

Population Health Approach
http://www.phac-aspc.gc.ca/ph-sp/index-eng.php

About the Author

Dr. Rose Alene Roberts is a member of the Lac La Ronge Indian Band and is originally from the community of Stanley Mission, Saskatchewan. She has an undergraduate degree in nursing, and master's and doctoral degrees in Community Health and Epidemiology, all from the University of Saskatchewan. Dr. Roberts currently holds a faculty position of Assistant Professor at the College of Nursing, University of Saskatchewan. Her research interests include cancer in Aboriginal populations, alternative healing modalities, residential school survivorship, and autoimmune diseases.

Rural Health

Judith Kulig, Martha MacLeod, Norma Stewart, and Roger Pitblado

OBJECTIVES

After studying this chapter, you should be able to:

1. Define and describe the meaning of rural in a Canadian context.
2. Investigate the impact of the rural context on the health status and access to care experienced by rural residents.
3. Identify the challenges associated with being a community resident in rural Canada.
4. Understand the context of rural nursing practice and its interrelationship with the care of clients in rural areas.

INTRODUCTION

This chapter introduces concepts relevant to caring for clients in rural areas. The character of rural and remote Canada is delineated, with an emphasis on diversity. The discussion provides a contextual understanding of clients who live in these areas and some of the practice characteristics of rural nurses.

The rewards and challenges of rural nursing, including the key features of this practice, are identified and explained in depth. Sample questions enable opportunities for discussion and application of the materials presented.

THE CHARACTER OF RURAL/REMOTE CANADA

Definitions

Approximately 95% of Canada's land mass, or 9.5 million square kilometres, consists of rural and remote areas (Public Health Agency of Canada, 2002). However, longstanding debate exists about the definitions of key terms including rural, remote, northern, and isolated. Pitblado (2005) has noted two main ways to define rural: technical and social.

Technical approaches to the definition of rural include locators or geographic regions, like the location of hospitals, roads, or specific political areas (i.e., provinces, counties). Statistics Canada (du Plessis, Beshiri, & Bollman, 2001) has examined six possible ways to define rural, with each emphasizing different criteria such as population size, population density, and settlement or labour market contexts. One example is the definition of "census rural," which refers to "individuals living in the countryside outside centres of 1000 or more population" (du Plessis et al., 2001, p. 6). Another example, from the Organisation of Economic Co-operation and Development (OECD), is the definition of "rural communities" that include "individuals in communities with less than 150 persons per square kilometre" (du Plessis et al., p. 6). Other technical definitions focus on distances and interrelated features to define rural. In practice disciplines such as nursing and medicine, a common application of this approach is to use degrees of rurality for the purposes of financial reimbursement for working in isolated locations. For example, the First Nations and Inuit Health Branch (FNIHB) within Health Canada (2005) uses the following designations for that purpose:

1. *Non-isolated community* includes communities with road access less than 90 kilometres to physician services;
2. *Semi-isolated community* includes communities with road access greater than 90 kilometres to physician services;
3. *Isolated community* refers to communities with good telephone service, scheduled air transportation flights but no roads; and
4. *Remote, isolated community* means the communities have no scheduled air flights, minimal telephone or radio access, and no roads.

Examination of the FNIHB designations highlights the importance of access to services and the types of locally available health services. Transportation and communication

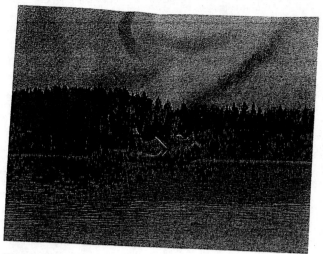

Photo 23.1

Float plane landing on Lac La Ronge, adjacent to La Ronge, Saskatchewan

Credit: Courtesy of Dr. Judith C. Kulig / University of Lethbridge

limitations are important factors in their differentiation. A wide variety of indices of rurality exist, such as the Canadian General Practice Rurality Index (Leduc, 1997) or the Rurality Index of Ontario (Kralj, 2001). Many of these indices are based on point systems that give various weights to characteristics such as the number of family physicians in a community, availability of physician specialists, presence and characteristics of the nearest hospital, availability of ambulance services, and so on. Many of these indices of rurality are only of theoretical value as they have never been put into operation. And almost all of them have been designed with physicians in mind—not nurses. A recent article on the perceptions of rurality by rural RNs (Kulig, et al, 2008) concluded that there was no benefit in developing a national numerical index of rurality based on distance to services because of the variability of absolute distance (ranging from 20 to 1000 km). In addition, most rurality models focus on deficits rather than the strengths of rural communities.

Social approaches to define rural refer to the nature of the rural community, with such features as specific services that are normally associated with larger population sizes (e.g., specific types of stores or restaurants) (Pitblado, 2005). Although this social nature of place in defining rural is relevant to healthcare service delivery, particularly the recruitment and retention of health professionals including registered nurses (RNs), there has been limited work done on examination of its specific meaning. The rural RNs who discussed perceptions of rural and remote focused on the larger responsibilities held by RNs who work in such settings and having a dual role of professional and friend with their clients (Kulig et al., 2007). The population that Statistics Canada designates as "rural and small town" refers to those "individuals in towns or municipalities outside the commuting zone of larger urban centres" (du Plessis et al., 2001, p. 6). Using this definition, 20% of Canadians are rural and live in communities with populations of less than

10 000 people. This is the definition of rural employed in this chapter. It was selected because of its growing use in studies of a wide variety of rural issues in Canada, including the determinants of health and the delivery of healthcare.

Diversity of Rural

Rural economies vary by the specific geographic features of the land itself. Hence, rural communities may be dependent upon natural resources that permit oil exploration, forestry, fishing, or farming activities. Of late, some rural communities are becoming increasingly dependent upon alternative economic ventures such as tourism because of changes in the local economy and the inability to financially survive solely on natural resources, the prices of which are highly influenced by global markets. Rural Canada is not homogenous. Therefore, this chapter provides examples from a variety of natural-resource rural communities rather than generalizing to one type of rural community. It is incumbent on nurses to determine the socioeconomic context of the rural community within which they work.

The geographic **diversity of rural** communities influences the types of services available (i.e., ability to access roads, telephones, satellite transmission), while the economy of the rural community has an impact on the cycle of activities within the community. Thus, during seeding and harvest within an agricultural community, there is less opportunity for RNs to work with groups or the entire community on health promotion activities. The type of natural resource base of the community will also influence health status. For example, in 2006 there were 327 060 farm operators across Canada (Statistics Canada, 2008b). The most common reported injuries were sprains or strains (43.9%), followed by fractures (27%) and nerve or open wounds (23.4%) (Statistics Canada, 2006). Operators on medium-sized farms had the highest incidence of injury because they worked the longest hours without reliance on hired help in comparison to those on the largest farms (Maltais, 2010). Farm operators are also aging, possibly contributing to the higher incidences of injury in an industry that continues to have one of the highest fatality rates (Maltais, 2007).

Being Rural

Although there has been some discussion about whether there is a "type" of rural person, emphasizing such notions can lead to generalizations and inaccurate descriptions of the variety of people who live in rural settings. It is more useful for nursing practice to discuss the intersection between living rural and the meanings of health and health status.

Rural residents have been the focus of studies examining the meaning of health. Research that focused on the health beliefs of rural Canadians in two western provinces found that being healthy was defined as having a holistic relationship among mental, social, physical, and spiritual aspects (Thomlinson, McDonagh, Baird, Crooks, & Lees, 2004). The participants differentiated sickness as a curable and short-term condition, whereas illness was chronic and life-threatening.

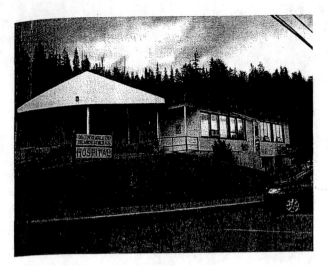

Photo 23.2

Queen Charlotte Islands General Hospital, Queen Charlotte City, British Columbia

Credit: Martha MacLeod / University of Northern British Columbia

Practitioners were encouraged to build a trusting relationship with rural residents and examine their health complaints in a holistic manner.

Other research with rural residents focuses specifically on their health status, examining differences in disease patterns and occurrences. For example, one study found a lower proportion of those living in small-town regions, rural regions, and northern regions who rate their health as excellent. Specific conditions such as arthritis are higher than the national average among rural regions and those in northern regions had a higher prevalence of hypertension (Mitura & Bollman, 2003). Another study (DesMeules et al., 2006) that examined health status and health determinants among the rural population found that

- rural areas reported higher proportions of people with low income and less than secondary education level. On the other hand, a strong sense of community belonging was reported by rural residents in greater proportions than by their urban counterparts.
- health-related factors, such as the prevalence of smoking and obesity, were elevated in rural Canada, while analyses of other health influences, such as dietary practices and leisure-time physical activity, indicated lower practice levels in rural areas.
- life expectancy at birth was significantly higher in urban areas.
- higher overall mortality risks among rural communities appear to be driven by higher death rates from such causes as circulatory diseases, injuries, and suicide; residents of the most rural areas are often at highest risk.
- incidence rates of most cause-specific cancers were lower in rural areas.
- respiratory disease mortality risks were for the most part significantly higher among rural residents.
- women living in the most rural areas had higher risks of dying from diabetes.

the importance of disease prevention and health promotion is well recognized in public health and clinical settings. What is less clear is whether conventional strategies, mostly developed by urban program planners for urban residents, are equally effective in rural settings.

Beyond the above health conditions, rural residents also experience other issues common in urban settings but not well understood in rural areas. A case in point is rural elder abuse and domestic violence in general. Rural communities often lack the resources to address these issues from legal and social standpoints (Spencer, 2000). One study found that service delivery for those who experience elder abuse in rural communities is under threat by centralization of such services including the removal of clergy, police, and care providers (Harbison, Coughlan, Karabanow & VanderPlaat, 2005).

Unique Groups of People in Rural Areas

In addition to unique geographic features that affect the livelihood and everyday life cycle of rural residents, a number of **unique groups** of people live in rural areas. For many of these groups, challenges are inherent in being diverse and living in a rural environment. Thus, some may feel excluded, whereas others want to live separate from larger society and prefer rural living where they can co-exist with other groups but not be expected to interact with others. It is part of the role for nurses to assess the rural community within which they live to determine its diversity and the strengths or needs that arise from such diversity. Many groups could be included for further discussion in this chapter; however, the emphasis is on Aboriginal people and unique religious groups, including the Amish, Hutterites, Mennonites, and Conservative Dutch. Discussing these groups in some detail provides the opportunity to examine the intersection between diversity and living rural with implications for nursing practice, while also providing examples of how to work with other diverse groups. General principles in relation to assessing and caring for multicultural clients are identified in Chapter 8 and for those with alternative sexual orientations are discussed in Chapter 18. The complexity of such individual situations is beyond the scope of this chapter but needs to be considered by rural nurses who may encounter such individuals in their practice.

Identifying unique groups in rural areas is important for the development and implementation of appropriate nursing care. However, accurate statistics regarding the number of these groups living in rural areas are usually not available. In general, few databases exist that provide community-specific demographic profiles of rural populations. Thus, an accurate picture of rural residents, including their health status, is often not readily available. Although precise statistics may be lacking, it is essential for rural nurses to be aware of the diversity of the rural population and the implications it has for health status and provision of health services.

Aboriginal People Aboriginal people includes First Nations, Métis, and Inuit groups. (See Chapter 22.) In 2006, there were

1 172 790 Aboriginal people in Canada (Statistics Canada, 2006). Aboriginal people are increasingly becoming urban dwellers, with 623 470 currently living in urban settings (Statistics Canada, 2008a). Many will continue to live in rural settings on or off-reserve. For example, there are now 308 490 Aboriginal individuals living on reserve and 240 825 living in rural areas (Statistics Canada, 2008a). Consequently, in order to provide appropriate care, nurses working in such settings need to understand the historical context of Aboriginal people; their healthcare issues; the policy context of healthcare delivery, including the transfer of health services to local control (Kulig et al., 2003; Kulig, MacLeod & Lavoie, 2005); and the challenges and rewards of working with Aboriginal people. Community nursing practice increasingly acknowledges the social determinants of health experienced by rural Aboriginal peoples (i.e., inadequate housing and water; lack of infrastructure supports on reserve; and inadequate social supports within family units).

Unique Religious Groups Unique religious populations who live predominantly in rural communities include the Anabaptist groups, specifically the Amish, Hutterites, and Mennonites. Each of these three groups has its own particular lifestyle based upon the desire to have the freedom to live according to religious principles with no interference by government intervention. All three live by the principles of adult baptism, pacifism, and separation from the physical world. In addition, they also emphasize a literal interpretation of the Bible. Most of the members of these groups work in the agricultural sector. Hutterites in Canada number 30 665 (Statistics Canada, 2008c), with the majority residing in Alberta, Manitoba, and Saskatchewan. The Hutterites live a communal lifestyle with each member contributing through specific duties such as cooking or animal husbandry. Conservative Mennonites in Canada more often referred to as the Low-German-Speaking Mennonites. This group is made up of individuals and families whose ancestors lived in Canada but moved to Mexico and other Central and South American countries in the 1920s (Bensen, 1998; DeLuca & Krahn, 1998; Sawatzky, 1971). For religious and economic reasons they are now returning to Canada, mainly to Alberta, Manitoba, and Ontario, where many of them live according to a strict interpretation of the Bible (dictating that, for example, they cannot use devices such as radios). Their religious beliefs impact their health knowledge and behaviours, including the silence surrounding childbearing that prohibits the sharing of information about this important life transition (Kulig, Wall, Hill, & Babcock, 2008). Another unique religious group is the Conservative Dutch, who are also predominantly agricultural-based and live according to a traditional interpretation of the Bible. Variations within all of these groups exist and thus it would not be appropriate to generalize from one Hutterite, Mennonite, or Conservative Dutch family to another. However, generally speaking, literacy levels can be low among these groups and hence specifically targeted health teaching approaches need to be developed to ensure concepts are understood and can be applied. There are also specific health issues that are more common in each of these groups. Among Hutterites heart disease is common due to their high-fat and -caloric diet; genetic disorders are also not uncommon among them because of the

close relationship between spouses (Brunt, 1998). Such diseases as diabetes, autoimmune disorders (i.e., rheumatoid arthritis), and congenital malformations (i.e., inborn errors of metabolism) have been found as disease clusters among Conservative Mennonites because of their close genetic relationships (Jaworski et al., 1998). Immunization is not accepted among many Conservative Dutch families because they believe that immunizations challenge the will of God, who is ultimately responsible for a child's life (Kulig, Meyer, Hill, Handley, Lichtenberger, & Myck, 2002).

The Challenges Experienced by Rural Communities

Several challenges are faced by rural communities and their residents in Canada. It is commonly acknowledged that the population of rural Canada is increasing only in predominantly rural regions that are within commuting distance of large urban areas (du Plessis et al., 2001). Thus, many more distant rural areas are experiencing an out-migration of all age groups (Rothwell, Bollman, Tremblay, & Marshall, 2002). Generally speaking, there are fewer individuals to contribute to the functioning of the community. Youth migration out of rural communities has escalated, thus further decreasing the community's future workers and residents (Tremblay, 2001). There is less infrastructure in rural communities, thus resources such as retail businesses and healthcare delivery services are more limited. Rural communities are more often dependent upon a limited range of economic opportunities; boom and bust cycles play into this, leading to an overall decreased availability of employment for individuals. Finally, there is a perception of a loss of political voice within the rural regions of Canada, decreasing the sense of independence and autonomy for which rural residents are often known (Government of Canada, 1998) and a call for implementing recommendations that can build sustainable rural communities (Alberta Association of Municipal Districts & Counties, 2009). Rural poverty has recently been recognized despite being "invisible" by the urban sector of the country. The rural poor are also disadvantaged because they have to travel longer distances for services and pay more for services and resources in their home communities (Fairbairn & Gustafson, 2006). Rural poverty is exacerbated by the declining population and the subsequent declining resources in rural communities.

All of these challenges have impacts on health status in general and on healthcare delivery in particular. For example, the loss of youth and economic opportunities in rural communities leads to fewer individuals available to provide care to elderly parents and other relatives. In communities that are dependent on oil and gas extraction, there may be many single men or young families with few supports. Therefore, nursing practice needs to be designed to specifically address the particular situation in each rural community. For example, in some rural communities, there is access to technologies such as telehealth; this virtual environment would allow for health education such as prenatal teaching or on-line support programs for individuals with chronic illnesses. Rural-based CHNs need to become familiar with e-health initiatives and their use to positively impact their clients' health (Wathen & Harris, 2007).

THE REALITIES OF RURAL NURSING PRACTICE

Although all graduates of nursing programs in Canada are prepared for a generalist role, working with clients in rural communities as a nurse stretches the meaning of being a generalist. Primarily, this is due to the wide range of practice demands on nurses in small communities. It is compounded by the statistical profile of rural RNs discussed below. However, it is also due to several key issues that are particularly at play for rural RNs. These issues include **leadership, quality work environments, education for rural settings,** and **policy issues for rural environments.** Each of these is subsequently discussed in depth.

Statistics

Analyses (Canadian Institute for Health Information [CIHI], 2002; MacLeod, Kulig, Stewart, Pitblado, & Knock, 2004; Pitblado, 2005) of the Registered Nurses Database (RNDB) reveal that there were 41 500 RNs working in rural Canada in 2000. The majority were female (95.6%), with 50.3% working full time. Rural RNs have an average age of 42.9 years. Rural RNs have achieved lower levels of education at entry to practice and throughout their nursing careers; 18.5% of rural RNs have achieved a baccalaureate degree as their highest level of education. Lower education is associated with limited access to nursing education (i.e., access to degree education for rural RNs came much later than for RNs in urban settings) as well as an historical lack of emphasis on needing a degree within many rural settings.

Nurse-to-client ratios vary by rural region, but on average there were 62 nurses per 10 000 in rural Canada compared to 78 per 10 000 in urban Canada. There is also an east to west trend, with higher nurse-to-population ratios in Eastern Canada.

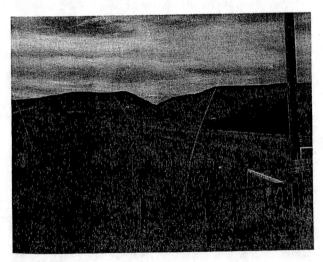

Photo 23.3

Ranch Country, near Nanton, Alberta

Credit: Courtesy of Dr. Judith C. Kulig / University of Lethbridge

Key Features of Rural Nursing

Regardless of practice setting, all rural nurses are faced with addressing issues in clinical practice, leadership, the work environment, and education. Rural nursing practice is shaped by the context of rural communities, with their limited transportation, communications, and other resources. Within small communities, rural nurses provide care to clients, who also may be friends and neighbours, with a wide range of conditions. Rural nurses experience practice as being multi-faceted and complex, with considerable decision-making challenges, few resources, and little backup. (MacLeod, Martin-Misener, Banks, Morton, Vogt, & Bentham, 2008). It demands considerable knowledge and skills to be responsive to community needs (CARRN, 2008). For example, CHNs in northern British Columbia found they could be more responsive to high-risk and vulnerable families when they focused on creating working relationships with families instead of focusing on 'home visiting' protocols, because their services to families happened in many locations in the community, including the grocery store (Moules, MacLeod, Hanlon, & Thirsk, 2009).

Leadership In the narrative component of the study "The Nature of Nursing Practice in Rural and Remote Canada," almost all nurses talked about issues related to nursing leadership (Ulrich & MacLeod, 2005). Issues included finding ways of working through conflicting priorities, coping with having leaders at a distance, and creating support networks. Leadership was more effective when leaders set up possibilities for quality practice, even in situations of few resources. When leaders planned for the realities of rural practice, nurses felt supported. For nursing leaders, providing the appropriate support at a distance was a challenge; for nurses, seeking and accepting that support was equally challenging. Both nursing managers and nurses needed to work creatively within organizations that did not always understand the realities of their practice.

Quality Work Environments Creating quality work environments in rural practice settings is particularly challenging. A central challenge is that many nurses in rural settings work alone all the time (Andrews, Stewart, Pitblado, Morgan Forbes, & D'Arcy, 2005) or with few colleagues during much of their everyday work. Orientations that include discussion about working alone and safety issues when entering homes or travelling on isolated roads can help. A strategy for developing a quality work environment in rural or remote practice includes developing consistent expectations and approaches among managers and nurses to address practice issues at the site level. This includes relevant rural practice standards; policies and practices that support rural nurses' scope of practice; practice-driven, rural-focused nursing education programs; rural reality-based preceptorship and mentorship programs; and the development of sustained processes for direct rural nursing involvement in local and regional planning (Ulrich & MacLeod, 2005).

Nursing Education for Nursing Practice A few nursing programs in Canada are rural-focused due to their geographic location. Examples include the University of Lethbridge, the University of Northern British Columbia, and the University of

Saskatchewan, which include rural placements and theoretical content related to rural nursing. Other programs include Aurora College in the Northwest Territories and the Nunavut Arctic College, which partners with Dalhousie University to offer a four-year collaborative degree program. All of these nursing programs are locally available, addressing the geographic barriers for those who wish to pursue an education experience. However, these programs also incorporate information that is specifically pertinent to providing care in their locale.

Research with rural nurses has provided some direction about the specific needs for nurses who want to work in rural communities (MacLeod et al., 2004). Two themes exist: (1) creating a relevant curriculum, including using reality-based cases and offering at least part of the curriculum in rural settings, and (2) providing infrastructure supports, including incorporating telehealth education and mentoring programs in the workplace that help with the transition of new graduates in rural and remote communities (MacLeod et al., 2004). Rural and remote nurses report that specialty continuing education for rural and remote practice is difficult to attain and nurses would like programs that prepare them for the realities of practice, keep them up to date with changes in practice, and are flexible and accessible (MacLeod et al., 2008; MacLeod, Ulrich, Lindsey, Fulton, & John, 2008; Martin Misener et al., 2008). Other studies among rural healthcare professionals in Canada (Curran, Fleet, & Kirby, 2006; Penz, D'Arcy, Stewart, Kosteniuk, Morgan, & Smith, 2007) and New Zealand (Janes, Arrol, Buetow, Coster, McCormick, & Hague, 2005) acknowledge workplace issues, including lack of access to computers, as a barrier to continuing education and learning.

Although the Internet is commonly thought of as a solution for continuing education for individuals who live in rural communities, one recent Canadian study has shown that Internet use is not common among rural nurses as an avenue to locate information (Kosteniuk, D'Arcy, Stewart, & Smith, 2006). Rural and remote RNs were more likely to use information sources central to their own work environment (e.g., colleagues, in-service) than peripheral sources such as the Internet or library. This study also found, however, that nurses who had more recently graduated and were in positions of authority or in multiple positions that required ongoing research use, and who had been employed fewer than five years, had significantly greater odds of using the Internet (Kosteniuk et al.). We can therefore anticipate that more recent graduates of nursing programs who are employed by workplaces that emphasize the need for evidence-based practice and provide infrastructure support for technology would be more amenable to accessing continuing education over the Internet.

CANADIAN RESEARCH BOX 28.1

Why do rural and remote nurses leave their nursing positions?

Stewart, N., D'Arcy, C., Kosteniuk, J., Andrews, M. E., Morgan, D., Forbes, D., . . . Pitblado, R. (2010, July). Moving on? Predictors of intent to leave among rural and remote RNs in Canada, *Journal of Rural Health.* doi:10.1111/j.1748-0361.2010.00308.x

Health human resources remain a challenge in many rural and remote settings. This paper explores the predictors of intent to leave (ITL) for all nursing positions in rural and remote practice settings in Canada. We hypothesized that both job and community satisfaction would have an impact on ITL. A national cross-sectional mail survey of RNs in rural and remote Canada comprised the data set ($n = 3051$), which was from The Nature of Nursing in Rural and Remote Canada national study (Stewart et al, 2005). In this sample, the majority were female (94.8%) with an average age of 43 years, and with a diploma (69.6%) as their highest level of education. One in five planned to leave their position in the next 12 months and 64% had five years or more of experience as an RN. ITL (dependent variable) was assessed according to 41 potential predictors (independent variables in three categories [the individual RN, the workplace, and the community context]). Logistic regression was used to analyze the data. The findings revealed that RNs were more likely to intend to leave their nursing positions if they were male, had higher perceived stress, had higher education, and had no dependent children or relatives. In addition, RNs were more likely to be planning to move on if they were working in advanced practice, remote settings, and had lower community satisfaction, lower satisfaction with autonomy and scheduling in their jobs, and the requirement to be on call. The importance of the community context in predicting the RN intent to leave is a unique feature of rural settings and can be used to develop policies and guidelines to offset turnover.

Discussion Questions

1. What initiatives could communities take to enhance the individual RN's satisfaction with the community context?

2. What is the responsibility of healthcare agencies in assisting RNs seeking further education and preparation? What is the individual RN's responsibility in this regard?

3. What could CHNs do to help recruit and retain RNs in rural communities?

CANADIAN RESEARCH BOX 28.2

What contributes to resiliency in rural communities?

Kulig, J., Edge, D., Reimer, W., Townshend, I., & Lightfoot, N. (2009). Levels of risk: Perspectives of the Lost Creek Fire. *Australian Journal of Emergency Management, 24*(2), 33–39.

The purpose of this pilot study was to identify how resiliency is manifested in rural communities that have experienced disasters. Community resiliency is defined as the ability of a community to deal with adversity and ultimately become stronger. Several studies have contributed to its theoretical development (see, for example, Kulig, Edge, & Joyce, 2008). The interactions that are created at the community level lead to an expression of a sense of community and to community action. Community resiliency has much potential for rural nursing because it focuses on the strengths and assets of communities while identifying ways in which community members and nurses can work together.

The study examined the Crowsnest Pass in southern Alberta, which experienced the Lost Creek Fire in 2003. The Crowsnest Pass is a single municipality comprised of the amalgamation of the towns of Coleman and Blairmore, the villages of Bellevue and Frank, several improvement districts, and 13 hamlets (the largest being Hillcrest Mines). The community had experienced several other major disasters in its history (e.g., the Frank Slide and the Hillcrest Mine Disaster), thereby demonstrating its resiliency. However, the Lost Creek Fire was the worst wildfire in the community's history. It resulted in a 31-day state of emergency which included the evacuation of Hillcrest Mines and the southeast area of Blairmore. In total, 21 000 hectares burned and the total cost for controlling the fire was $40 million. Fortunately, no structures or loss of life occurred but the natural environment was dramatically changed and the realization that all rural communities are vulnerable to wildfires was reinforced to the community members.

Thirty qualitative interviews were conducted with individuals who experienced evacuations, assisted in dealing with the evacuation and overall management of the fire within the community, and those within government who were involved with controlling the fire. The interviews were analyzed while data collection was being conducted and examined within the larger context of the theoretical frameworks of community resiliency and the history of the community in experiencing and dealing with disasters.

The major findings from the study include (1) the historical context of dealing with disaster helped the community to cope with and work through the Lost Creek Fire experience and (2) both individuals and the community were identified as vulnerable but in different ways. Individual vulnerability included being-at-risk and feeling-at-risk. Being-at-risk was associated with internal (age; dependence on others) and external (having no house insurance) individual circumstances. Those people feeling-at-risk included the wives and families of the fire fighters. Community vulnerability included being-at-risk for issues such as economic concerns (loss of business or employment due to the wildfire). The experience of risk can impact both individual and community resiliency. Those at risk may reside in communities that are relatively resilient, just as the levels of individual resiliency may impact resiliency at the community level. Studies that address community vulnerability and resiliency in relation to disasters are increasingly important given the heightened vulnerability of rural communities and their members due to climate change and inter-related changes in the environment (e.g., loss of forests due to pine beetle infestation).

Currently, a three-year mixed method study is being conducted to further examine community resiliency in communities that have undergone wildfires. LaRonge, Saskatchewan and Barriere, British Columbia are the focus of this study, which includes compilation of a community profile based upon existing local and regional data, qualitative interviews, and household surveys in each community plus one comparative community (www.ruralwildfire.ca).

Discussion Questions

1. As a rural nurse, identify what your role is within disaster mitigation and management. In addition, provide specific examples how you would assist families to prepare for evacuation and return to their community.

2. Discuss the links between community resiliency and your practice as a rural community health nurse. How can you work with rural community members to enhance resiliency?

CASE STUDY

The Gibbons family lives on their family farm 90 km east of a small city (population 68 000). After completing high school at the local community school, Nancy and John were married in the Anglican Church. Nancy is now 45 and John is 46. Nancy has been an active mother, raising their three sons while also volunteering in the community. John and his son Peter work on the farm together, which has been in the family for two generations. The older two sons, Jack and Ian, live and work in cities that are three hours and five hours, respectively, from the family farm. Both Jack and Ian are married and have children. Their jobs, family life, and other responsibilities mean that they are not able to visit on the farm very often.

Nancy has had an uneventful health history; she had regular physical examinations and three normal pregnancies. A few years ago she had a hysterectomy, and from a health perspective was expecting to enjoy retirement with her husband and their sons, daughters-in-law, and grandchildren. About a year ago, Nancy began to feel "unwell." She was tired, shaky, and having difficulties sleeping. Four months ago, tests revealed that she had amyotrophic lateral sclerosis (ALS), a terminal condition for which there is no cure.

She was referred to home care for assessment, but John refused to have them in the home and instead has provided all care to Nancy. The ALS Society was notified by home care about Nancy's diagnosis and has called and offered to visit and assist in any way possible. John would agree only after Peter convinced his mother and father that it could be helpful. While the ALS Society was at the home, John expressed his frustration at his wife's deteriorating condition and related he was unsure if he could continue providing care by himself. Nancy is now dependent upon John to bathe her, assist her with feeding, and transfer her to the toilet. She is also frequently in pain, and due to the muscle weakness is at risk for falls. Depression has set in and Nancy has said that "life is not worth living." At the same time, she wants to die peacefully at the farm and does not want to be moved into the city hospital. John is increasingly upset about his wife's condition and appears overwhelmed and bewildered; he realizes he needs support to continue to care for Nancy in their home.

It takes some time but John finally agrees to have a home care nurse return, do another assessment, and set up equipment resources such as oxygen and personal care aides on a routine basis. The home care nurse also refers the family to the palliative care nurse. Peter calls his brothers and asks that they come home to visit their mother as soon as possible.

Discussion Questions

1. Describe the roles and responsibilities of a home care and palliative care nurse in this case study.

2. Identify three factors related to living in a rural setting that provide challenges in the delivery of nursing care for Nancy Gibbons. Identify how a home care nurse could address these factors.

3. Identify three rural community factors that could provide assistance to the Gibbons family. Identify how a home care nurse could incorporate these factors into a care plan for Nancy.

Source: This case study is a modified version from the Nursing Education in Southern Alberta (NESA) problem-based curriculum used by the collaborative partners The University of Lethbridge and Lethbridge College.

Policy Issues in Rural/Remote Environments Most policies in Canada, with health policies being no exception, are based upon an urban perspective with little consideration of their applicability in rural environments. In order for this situation to be changed, the following key issues need to be addressed.

- Having a specific individual champion in Canada that focuses on the importance of addressing the unique situation experienced by rural residents would be beneficial.
- Few RNs are educationally prepared for work in the policy arena (Kulig, Nahachewsky, Thomlinson, MacLeod, & Curran, 2004), and although nurse educators have been encouraged to include information about the policy cycle and its application in their curriculum (Murphy, 1999) it will be some time before any change is realized.
- Relevant information about the nature of rural communities, including the number and location of rural residents

and their health issues, is not readily available. Some organizations have lobbied to have this altered (e.g., Canadian Rural Health Research Society, 2008).
- The perspectives of rural residents and their involvement in setting the policy agenda, even at their local level, needs to be acknowledged and respected as a key component of rural development (Morton, Glasgow, & Johnson, 2004). Rural RNs have a key role in helping this to transpire (Kulig et al., 2004).

SUMMARY

This chapter has focused on the unique nature of caring for clients in rural areas. Precise definitions of rural are lacking and need to include both technical and social characteristics. Rural residents experience challenges including depopulation, distance to services, and the need to develop local initiatives. Nurses who practise in rural areas would benefit from educational supports including continuing education by distance delivery methods and the development of appropriate work expectations given the rural settings. Many diverse groups within rural Canada offer opportunities for a rewarding nursing practice.

KEY TERMS

technical approaches, p. 363
social approaches, p. 364
diversity of rural, p. 364
unique groups, p. 365
leadership, p. 367
quality work environments, p. 367
education for rural settings, p. 367
policy issues for rural environments, p. 367

REVIEW QUESTIONS

1. Heather is a rural home care nurse who has been caring for Tom, a 67-year-old man diagnosed with terminal cancer. At one visit, Tom's wife, Charlene, asks if they can call Heather at her home when she is not on call because they prefer her as their nurse. If Heather agrees to this situation, she would be compromising

   a) ethical standards.

   b) professional boundaries.

   c) union standards.

   d) regional health policies.

2. Mr. Field, a farmer with valvular disease, has just come on to Jane's caseload. Jane has noticed that many of her home care clients have circulatory conditions. Jane's experience illustrates that in rural communities

   a) circulatory disease mortality rates are the norm in rural areas and cannot be altered.

   b) circulatory disease mortality rates are higher in rural areas compared to urban areas.

c) circulatory disease mortality rates are equally common in rural and urban areas.

d) circulatory disease mortality rates are not common in rural areas and Mr. Field is an exception.

3. Safety concerns for home care RNs working on-call and driving at night on deserted roads have increased. To address these concerns, the RNs have requested a meeting with the nurse manager and the area administrator. The meeting would be most productive if the discussion reflected:

a) professional practice standards.

b) professional boundaries.

c) principles of teaching and learning.

d) community capacity.

4. Anita has been working in the local rural home care unit for a number of years and her family is originally from the community. There isn't anywhere that Anita goes where someone does not know her. One day she is in the grocery store and is approached by Mrs. Hewett enquiring if it is true that Mrs. Nyl is gravely ill and has been sent home to die. The most appropriate way for Anita to handle this situation is to

a) remind Mrs. Hewett what time visiting hours are at the hospital.

b) tell Mrs. Hewett that it is not up to her to provide a patient update.

c) tell Mrs. Hewett that to stop bothering her when she is doing her personal errands.

d) politely explain to Mrs. Hewett that she is not able to disclose the information and encourage her to contact Mrs. Nyl since they have been close friends for years.

5. Rural community members have

a) higher life expectancies, lower respiratory disease mortality rates

b) higher life expectancies, higher respiratory disease mortality rates

c) lower life expectancies, higher respiratory disease mortality rates

d) lower life expectancies, lower respiratory disease mortality rates

STUDY QUESTIONS

1. Maria is a 35-year-old Low German–speaking Mennonite woman who has just had her fifth child. She was diagnosed with gestational diabetes and requires follow-up to more closely monitor her health. What actions could the PHN take to assist Maria?

2. Timothy has been working as a public health nurse in a transferred Aboriginal community for the past four years. Two months ago the community experienced a wildfire that required evacuation; several homes were lost due to the fire, and much of the landscape was permanently altered. What are three things Timothy can do

to help the community rebuild and prepare for future natural disasters?

3. Identify what public health nurses can do in order to generate information about the communities they work within.

4. A group of undergraduate nursing students are developing a health promotion project for a farming community. In order to be successful, what do they need to take into consideration?

5. Identify four concepts that would be discussed in a rural nursing course for nursing students.

6. Identify four challenges to working as a rural nurse in the community.

After working through these questions, go to the MyNursingLab at www.pearsoned.ca/mynursinglab to check your answers.

INDIVIDUAL CRITICAL THINKING EXERCISES

1. Examine the provincial or territorial nursing standards related to professional boundaries and identify three challenges in the provision of care within rural communities. As a professional registered nurse, how would you address the challenges without jeopardizing ethical standards and professional boundaries?

2. Jacob Hofer is a 56-year-old Hutterite colony boss who is experiencing chest pains and fatigue. Consider his unique religious background and lifestyle as well as his rural agricultural setting and outline three nursing strategies that can be implemented in his care plan.

3. The community care office you work within as a home care nurse will be moving to a primary care model in the next year. Identify how you can describe this change to your home care clients and what it means to the care that they will receive. What does it mean for you as a nurse? How might it affect your practice?

4. Your rural community shares a border with a non-community-based health services Aboriginal community. Both locations have experienced RN shortages. Consider ways in which the two communities and two health services can work together for the benefit of the clients. What barriers would need to be addressed? What actions might facilitate collaboration? Where would you need to seek support?

5. You work in a long-term care facility that has just developed a support group for rural families caring for a relative with dementia, which is most commonly caused by Alzheimer disease. After the first six months of the service, only three family members have attended the group, even though you are sure that many others could benefit from the support. What issues could make families reluctant to participate in this service?

GROUP CRITICAL THINKING EXERCISES

1. You work part time as a CHN in a two-nurse office in a rural community. The other nurse works full time. You are both responsible for implementing the full range of public health programs. Because of the difficulty in finding casual replacements over the last two months, you deferred your vacation and have worked more than full time. You have just received a call that the full-time nurse has gone on sick leave. As your manager, who works 200 km away, tells you this, she adds that the Medical Health Officer has identified two TB cases in your community. Your manager asks you to work overtime again. You are debating what your answer should be. As a group,

   a) identify the personal and professional concerns you would face in this situation.

   b) identify the dilemmas being faced by the public health administration.

   c) identify the potential impacts on client and community safety.

   d) identify strategies, including ones that reflect interprofessional practice, to address the above concerns.

2. You are the new community nurse in an outpost setting on a community-based Aboriginal reserve. Two other nurses are stationed at the centre but they are from the community and live with their spouses away from the station. You are the only nurse who works at the outpost accommodation. This particular community (population of 545) is fly-in only with interruptions of flight service due to inclement weather. As a group,

   a) identify the priorities you would engage in as the new nurse.

   b) identify the process you would use to assess the community.

   c) identify how you would develop a relationship with the other nurses and community residents.

3. You are part of a group of CHNs who receive the latest statistics that discuss the health status of Canadian residents. The report lacks sufficient details about rural Canadians and their health status. In order to address this scenario, discuss the following:

   a) Identify the shortfalls of using inappropriate data in your work as CHNs.

   b) Identify agencies that collect information about rural residents and their health status.

   c) Identify a process to work with your program managers to address the limitations of the data.

   d) Identify a process to work with your program managers to contact the relevant agencies about the limitations of the data.

4. You are a CHN in a logging/ranching community of 1500 residents. There is only one physician in town and a limited health centre facility. In the community, when the logging and ranching slows down over winter, some individuals are able to go south for a vacation. This year when one couple returns, the husband develops symptoms indicative of a new flu strain. A few days later it is confirmed that the man has the new flu strain. Within a week, several other people have similar symptoms and are also confirmed to have the new flu strain.

   a) Identify the key individuals you would need to work with in this circumstance; include a list of their roles in addressing the situation.

   b) Identify the main elements of a pandemic plan to curtail the spread of the new flu strain.

   c) Identify the process that you would use to work with community members in implementing a pandemic strategy.

   d) Discuss the ramifications to your regular workload and the impact on your personal life.

5. You have been a home care nurse working in several eastern coastal communities for the last 5 years. It is a job that you love mostly because of the people you care for and the diversity within your everyday work. You are currently mentoring an undergraduate nursing student from an urban-based university nursing program. The student has made it clear that it was not her choice to come to a rural area or to do home care. As a group, identify how you will address the student's issues in a productive manner. Identify ways in which you can encourage the student to see the benefits of her education experience in a rural area.

REFERENCES

Alberta Association of Municipal Districts and Counties. (2009). *One vision, many voices: How to build a sustainable rural Canada.* Edmonton, AB: Author.

Andrews, M. E., Stewart, N. J., Pitblado, J. R., Morgan, D. G., Forbes, D., & D'Arcy, C. (2005). Registered nurses working alone in rural and remote Canada. *Canadian Journal of Nursing Research, 37*(1), 14–33.

Bensen, J. (1998). Protective retreat: Mexico's Mennonites consider a new migration. *World and I, 13*(8), 1–6.

Brunt, H. (1998). Canadian Hutterites. In R. E. Davidhizar & J. N. Giger (Eds.), *Canadian transcultural nursing* (pp. 230–245). Toronto, ON: Mosby.

Canadian Institute of Health Information. (2002). *Supply and distribution of registered nurses in rural and small town Canada, 2000.* Ottawa, ON: Author.

Canadian Rural Health Research Society. *About us.* Retrieved from http://crhrs-scrsr.usask.ca/

Curran, V., Fleet, L., & Kirby, F. (2006). Factors influencing rural health care professionals' access to continuing professional education. *Australian Journal of Rural Health, 14*(2), 51–55.

DeLuca, S. A., & Krahn, M. A. (1998). Old Colony Mexican–Canadian Mennonites. In R. E. Davidhizar & J. N. Giger (Eds.), *Canadian transcultural nursing* (pp. 343–358). Toronto, ON: Mosby.

DesMeules, M., Pong, R., Lagacé, C., Heng, D., Manuel, D., Pitblado, R. J., . . . Koren, I. (2006). *How healthy are rural Canadians? An assessment of their health status and health determinants.* Ottawa, ON: Canadian Population Initiative, Canadian Institute for Health Information.

du Plessis, V., Beshiri, R., & Bollman, R. (2001). Definitions of rural. *Rural and Small Town Analysis Bulletin, 3*(3) 1–17. #21-006-XIE. Ottawa, ON: Statistics Canada. Available at statcan.gc.ca

Fairbain, D., & Gustafson, L. J. (2006). *Understanding freefall: The challenge of the rural poor.* Interim Report of the Standing Senate Committee on Agriculture and Forestry. Retrieved from http://www.parl.gc.ca/39/1/parlbus/commbus/senate/com-e/agri-e/rep-e/repintdec06-e.pdfS

Government of Canada. (1998). *Rural solutions to rural concerns.* National Rural Workshop Final Report. Retrieved from http://www.rural.gc.ca/ nrw/final_e.html

Harbison, J., Coughlan, S., Karabanow, J., & VanderPlaat, M. (2005). A clash of cultures: Rural values and service delivery to mistreated and neglected older people in Eastern Canada. *Practice: Social Work in Action, 17*(4), 229–246.

Health Canada. (2005). *Ten years of health transfer First Nation and Inuit control.* First Nations and Inuit Health Branch. Retrieved from http://www.hc-sc.gc.ca/fnihspni/pubs/agree-accord/10_years_ans_trans/5_agreement-entente_e.html

Janes, R., Arroll, B., Buetow, S., Coster, G., McCormick, R., & Hague, I. (2005). Rural New Zealand health professionals' perceived barriers to greater use of the internet for learning. *Rural and Remote Health, 5*(4). Online. 11 pages.

Jaworski, M. A., Slater, J. D., Severini, A., Hennig, K. R., Mansour, G., Mehta, J. G., . . . Yoon, J.-W. (1998). Unusual clustering of diseases in a Canadian Old Colony (Chortitza) Mennonite kindred and community. *Canadian Medical Association Journal, 138,* 1017–1025.

Kosteniuk, J., D'Arcy, C., Stewart, N., & Smith, B. (2006). Central and peripheral information source use among rural and remote Registered Nurses. *Journal of Advanced Nursing, 55*(1), 100–114.

Kralj, B. (2001). Measuring "rurality" for purposes of healthcare planning: An empirical measure for Ontario. *Ontario Medical Review,* October, 33–52.

Kulig, J., Andrews, M. E., Stewart, N., Pitblado, R., MacLeod, M., Bentham, D., . . . Smith, B. (2008). How do Registered Nurses define rurality? *Australian Journal of Rural Health, 16*(1), 28–32.

Kulig, J., Edge, D., & Joyce, B. (2008). Understanding community resiliency in rural communities through multimethod research. *Journal of Rural and Community Development, 3*(3) (online).

Kulig, J., Macleod, M., & Lavoie, J. (2007, February). Nurses and First Nations and Inuit community-managed primary health services. *The Nature of Rural and Remote Nursing, 5.* Retrieved from http://www.ruralnursing.unbc.ca/factsheets/factsheet5.pdf

Kulig, J., Meyer, C., Hill, S., Handley, C., Lichtenberger, S., & Myck, S. (2002). Refusals and delay of immunization within southwest Alberta. *Canadian Journal of Public Health, 93*(2), 109–112.

Kulig, J., Nahachewsky, D., Thomlinson, E., MacLeod, M., & Curran, F. (2004). Maximizing the involvement of rural nurses in policy. *Nursing Leadership, 17*(1), 88–96.

Kulig, J., Thomlinson, E., Curran, F., Nahachewsky, D., MacLeod, M., Stewart, N., & Pitblado, R. (2003). *Rural and remote nursing practice: An analysis of policy documents.* Lethbridge, AB: University of Lethbridge. R03-2003.

Kulig, J., Wall, M., Hill, S., & Babcock, R. (2008). Childbearing beliefs among Low-German-speaking Mennonite women. *International Nursing Review, 55*(4), 420–426.

Leduc, E. (1997). Defining rurality: A general practice rurality index for Canada. *Canadian Journal of Rural Medicine, 2*(2), 125–134.

MacLeod, M., Kulig, J., Stewart, N., & Pitblado, R. (2004). *Nursing practice in rural and remote Canada.* Canadian Health Services Research Foundation. http://www.chsrf.ca

MacLeod, M., Kulig, J., Stewart, N., Pitblado, R., & Knock, M. (2004). The nature of nursing practice in rural and remote Canada. *The Canadian Nurse, 100*(6), 27–31.

MacLeod, M., & Ulrich, C. (2005). *Nursing leadership at a distance: Addressing the experience of rural and remote nurses.* Proceedings of the National Nursing Leadership Conference, Ottawa, ON, February 13–15, 2005.

MacLeod, M. L. P., Martin-Misener, R., Banks, C., Morton, M., Vogt, C., & Bentham, D. (2008). "I'm a different kind of nurse": Advice from nurses in rural and remote Canada. *Canadian Journal of Nursing Leadership, 21*(3), 24–37.

MacLeod, M. L. P., Ulrich, C. H., Lindsey, L., Fulton, T., & John, N. (2008). The development of a practice-driven, reality-based program for rural acute care registered nurses. *Journal of Continuing Education in Nursing, 39*(7), 298–304.

Maltais, V. (2007). *Risk factors associated with farm injuries in Canada.* Ottawa, ON: Statistics Canada.

Maltais, V. (2010). *Risk factors associated with farm injuries in Canada.* 2010 catalogue # 21-601-MWE From the Agriculture and Rural Working Paper Series. Retrieved from http://www.statcan.gc.ca/bsolc/olc-cel/olc-cel?catno=21-601-MWE&lang=eng

Martin Misener, R., MacLeod, M. L. P., Banks, K., Morton, M., Vogt, C., & Bentham, D. (2008). "There's rural, and then there's rural": Advice from nurses providing primary healthcare in northern remote communities. *Canadian Journal of Nursing Leadership, 21*(3), 54–63.

Mitura, V., & Bollman, R. (2003). The health of rural Canadians: A rural–urban comparison of health indicators. *Rural and Small Town Analysis Bulletin, 4*(6), 1–23. #21-006-XIE. Ottawa: Statistics Canada. Retrieved from http://www.statcan.gc.ca

Morton, L., Glasgow, N., & Johnson, N. (2004). Reaching the goal: Less disparity, better rural health. In N. Glasgow, L. Morton, & N. Johnson (Eds.), *Critical issues in rural health* (pp. 283–291). Ames, IA: Blackwell.

Moules, N. J., MacLeod, M. L. P., Hanlon, N., & Thirsk, L. (2009). "And then you'll see her in the grocery store": The working relationships of community health nurses and high priority families in rural and northern Canadian communities. *Journal of Pediatric Nursing, 25*(5), 327–334.

Murphy, N. (1999). A survey of health policy content in Canadian graduate programs in nursing. *Journal of Nursing Education, 38*(2), 88–91.

Penz, K., D'Arcy, C., Stewart, N., Kosteniuk, J., Morgan, D., & Smith, B. (2007). Barriers to participation in continuing education among rural and remote nurses: Results from a national survey. *The Journal of Continuing Education in Nursing, 38*(2), 58–68.

Pitblado, J. R. (2005). So, what do we mean by "rural," "remote," and "northern"? *Canadian Journal of Nursing Research, 37*(1), 163–168.

Pitblado, J. R., Medves, J., & Stewart, N. J. (2005). For work and for school: Internal migration of Canada's rural nurses. *Canadian Journal of Nursing Research, 37*(1), 102–121.

Public Health Agency of Canada. (2002). *Rural health in rural hands: Strategic directions for rural, remote, northern and Aboriginal communities.* Retrieved from http://www.phac-aspc.gc.ca/rh-sr/pdf/rural_hands.pdf

Rothwell, N., Bollman, R., Tremblay, J., & Marshall, J. (2002). Migration to and from rural and small town Canada. *Rural and Small Town Analysis Bulletin, 3*(6), 2–22. #21-006-XIE. Ottawa, ON: Statistics Canada. Retrieved from http://www.statcan.gc.ca

Sawatzky, H. L. (1971). *They sought a country: Mennonite colonization in Mexico.* Berkeley, CA: University of California Press.

Spencer, C. (2000). Abuse and neglect of older adults in rural communities. *Gerontology Research News, 19*(1), 7–10.

Statistics Canada. (2006). *Snapshot of Canadian agriculture.* Retrieved from http://www.statcan.gc.ca/ca-ra2006/articles/snapshot-portrait-eng.htm#5

Statistics Canada. (2008a). *First Nations peoples: Selected findings of the 2006 Census.* Retrieved from http://www12.statcan.gc.ca/english/census06/data/topics/

Statistics Canada.(2008b). *Labour force, farm operators by country of birth, by province (2006 Censuses of Agriculture and Population).* Retrieved from http://www.statcan.gc.ca/pub/95-629-x/8/4182944-eng.htm

Statistics Canada. (2008c). *Population in collective dwellings, by province and territory (2006 Census).* Retrieved from http://www40.statcan.gc.ca/l01/cst01/famil62b-eng.htm

Stewart, N., D'Arcy, C., Pitblado, R., Morgan, D., Forbes, D., Remus, G., . . . MacLeod, M. (2005). A profile of registered nurses in rural and remote Canada. *Canadian Journal of Nursing Research, 37*(1), 122–145.

Thomlinson, E., McDonagh, M., Baird Crooks, K., & Lees, M. (2004). Health beliefs of rural Canadians: Implications for rural practice. *Australian Journal of Rural Health, 12,* 258–263.

Tremblay, J. (2001). Rural youth migration between 1971 and 1996. *Rural and Small Town Analysis Bulletin, 2*(3), 1–10. #21-006-XIE. Ottawa, ON: Statistics Canada. Retrieved from http://www.statcan.gc.ca

Ulrich, C., & MacLeod, M. (2005). *Overcoming distance and accommodating diversity: Creating a practical northern nursing strategy.* Proceedings of the National Nursing Leadership Conference, Ottawa, ON, February 13–15, 2005.

Wathen, C. N., & Harris, R. (2007). "I try to take care of myself: How rural women search for health information. *Qualitative Health Research, 17,* 639–651.

ADDITIONAL RESOURCES

Readings

Hegney, D., Pearson, A., & McCarthy, A. (1997). *The role and function of the rural nurse in Australia.* Adelaide, SA: University of Adelaide.

Ross, J. (Ed.). (2008). *Rural nursing: Aspects of practice.* Dunedin, New Zealand: Rural Health Opportunities.

Stewart, N., Kulig, J., Penz, K., Andrews, M. E., Houshmand, S., Morgan, D., . . . D'Arcy, C. (2006). *Aboriginal registered nurses in rural and remote Canada: Results from a national survey.* Saskatoon, SK: University of Saskatchewan. R06-2006.

Stewart, N., & MacLeod, M. (2005, August). RNs in nurse practitioner positions in rural and remote Canada. *The Nature of Rural and Remote Nursing, 3.* Retrieved from http://www.ruralnursing.unbc.ca/factsheets/factsheet3.pdf

Websites

British Columbia Rural & Remote Health Research Network
http://www.bcrrhrn.ca

Canadian Association for Rural & Remote Nursing
http://www.carrn.com

Canadian Centre for Health and Safety in Agriculture
http://www.cchsa-ccssma.usask.ca/

Canadian Rural Health Research Society
http://crhrs-scrsr.usask.ca

Canadian Rural Revitalization Foundation
http://www.crrf.ca

Centre for Rural and Northern Health Research
http://www.cranhr.ca

Rural Policy Research Institute
http://rupri.org

About the Authors

All four authors were co-principal investigators for the study "The Nature of Nursing Practice in Rural and Remote Canada."

Judith C. Kulig, RN, DNSc (University of California San Francisco), is a Professor in the Nursing Program in the Faculty of Health Sciences at the University of Lethbridge. She conducts a research program related to rural health that focuses on community resiliency of rural communities, unique populations in rural communities, and nursing practice in rural communities.

Martha L. P. MacLeod, RN, PhD (University of Edinburgh), is Professor and Chair, School of Nursing at the University of Northern British Columbia. Her research program is on rural and northern practice and its development.

Norma J. Stewart, RN, PhD (University of British Columbia), is a Professor in the College of Nursing at the University of Saskatchewan. Her research program has focused on dementia care and rural health services.

Roger Pitblado, PhD (University of Toronto), Professor Emeritus & Senior Research Fellow in the Centre for Rural and Northern Health Research at Laurentian University. His research deals with geographical variations in health status and the relative locations of health human resources, with a particular emphasis on rural Canada.

chapter 24

Environmental and Occupational Health

Shelley Kirychuk and Niels Koehncke

CHAPTER OBJECTIVES

After studying this chapter, the student should be able to:

1. Explain how the environment influences health.
2. Identify elements common to environmental factors, including frameworks for defining environmental factors.
3. Outline the environmental health assessment.
4. Be knowledgeable about legislation and regulations that relate to environmental health.
5. Apply the nursing process to the practice of environmental health.

INTRODUCTION

"The environment is everything that isn't me."
(Einstein)

Einstein defined the environment in the broadest of terms. In the context of this chapter, this definition implies that environmental health encompasses all parameters that impact health and that are not the person. The influence of environmental factors on health is receiving increased public, political, scientific, and media attention. Globally, the diseases with the largest absolute burden attributable to modifiable environmental factors include diarrhoea, lower respiratory tract infections, unintentional injuries (i.e., workplace injuries, industrial accidents, pedestrian and cycling accidents, and radiation), and malaria (see Figure 24.1) (Prüss-Üstün, 2006). Compared to other countries, Canada is considered healthy in terms of the environmental burden of disease (see Table 24.1), although vulnerable and disparate groups would differ from the national average. The World Health Organization (WHO) has estimated that 23% of all deaths can be attributed to environmental factors (Prüss-Üstün, 2006). This significant statistic highlights the importance of understanding how the environment influences health. This chapter will provide an overview of environmental health, including the environmental health assessment and environmental legislation, with emphasis on the role of the nursing profession.

DEFINING ENVIRONMENTAL HEALTH

The WHO defines **environmental health** as all aspects of human health, disease, and injury that are determined by factors in the environment (Prüss-Üstün, 2006). These **environmental factors** include the effects of *chemical, physical, and biological agents* as well as impacts related to the broad physical and social environment (i.e., housing, urban development, land use and transportation, industry, and agriculture) (Prüss-Üstün, 2006).

Health and environmental factors are often inextricably linked. Environmental health is a relatively new area in health; *A New Perspective on the Health of Canadians* was the first documented acknowledgement by a Canadian federal agency that health included environment, genetics, and lifestyle (Lalonde, 1981). Environmental factors have the potential to impact health at the *individual, family, community, and population levels,* and the ability to initiate, promote, sustain, or stimulate disease and/or disease conditions. At the individual level, environmental exposures can occur at home, at work, and during social and recreational activities. The environmental factors an individual is exposed to, alone or in combination, can produce no, minimal, or substantial health effects.

The complexity of environmental health factors requires a multidisciplinary approach. The role of the multidisciplinary team is to anticipate, recognize, evaluate, and control for environmental factors that arise and have the potential to cause impaired well-being at the individual, community, or population level. The team identifies *modifiable environmental factors* that are realistically amenable to change using available technology, policy, prevention, and public health measures. Community health nurses (CHNs) form part of the multidisciplinary team that may also include physicians, industrial hygienists, toxicologists, engineers, safety professionals, scientists, provincial health and safety officials, workplace safety officials, urban planners, lobbyists, or others. As members of this multidisciplinary team, CHNs must be

FIGURE 24.1 Diseases with the Largest Environmental Contribution

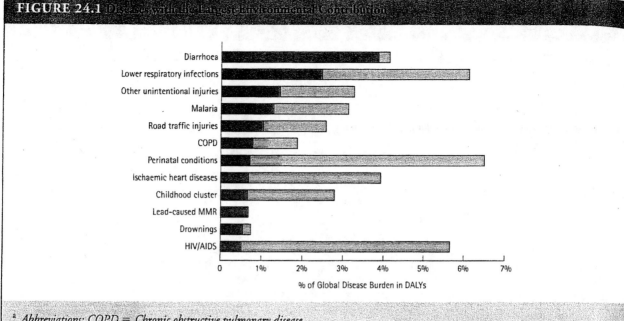

% of Global Disease Burden in DALYs

^a *Abbreviations: COPD = Chronic obstructive pulmonary disease*
^b *Lead-caused mental retardation is defined in the WHO list of diseases.*
^c *DALYs represent a weighted measure of death, illness, and disability.*
^d *For each disease the fraction attributable to environmental risks is shown in dark orange. Light orange plus dark orange represents the total burden of disease.*

Source: Prüss-Üstün, A. (2006). In Corvalán, C., World Health Organization. (Eds.), *Preventing disease through healthy environments: Towards an estimate of the environmental burden of disease.* Geneva: World Health Organization, p. 11.

knowledgeable about how specific factors in the environment (including chemical, physical, and biological hazards) can impact human health. CHNs have the training and background to identify potential health impacts from environmental factors, including the disparate influences on vulnerable and disadvantaged populations, and have the opportunity to lead interventions at the individual, community, and population level to reduce the burden of environmental disease.

DPSEEA Framework

Defining environmental health requires understanding what constitutes an environmental factor. For this purpose, the WHO uses a very broad framework called the **DPSEEA framework** (Driving forces, Pressures, State, Exposures, Effects, and Actions). This framework categorizes environmental health factors into driving forces (D), pressures (P), the state of the environment (S), exposure (E1) defined as the interaction between people and the environment, and resulting health effects (E2) related to the amount of exposure (Briggs, 1999).

- **Driving forces (D):** Driving forces are factors that create pressures, which can influence the state of the environment. Examples include poverty, population density, population growth, age structure, urbanization, and technology.

- **Pressures (P):** The environment can be altered by pressures. Such pressures could include production and consumption of resources as well as waste management. Pressures may be modifiable environmental factors. For example, public health policy could minimize the extent to which driving forces generate pressures.

- **State of the Environment (S):** The state of the environment can be altered in response to pressures (i.e., resource availability, air pollution). However, the environmental state can impact health only following human exposure. **Risk assessment** determines the environmental hazards important in human health.

- **Exposure and Effects (EE):** Exposures occur through inhalation, ingestion, and absorption of hazards (i.e., indoor air pollution, animal and or human waste and by-products, water quality and supply, lead, radiation, communicable diseases, occupational exposures). The health effects relate to the exposures that occur. Vulnerable, hypersensitive, and disadvantaged populations may have differential health outcomes to similar exposure levels.

- The "**A**" in the model represents the **Actions** undertaken to affect the environmental factor, including policy changes, pollution monitoring, environmental improvements, and education/awareness programs (adapted from Briggs, 1999).

TABLE 24.1 Canadian Profile of Environmental Burden of Disease

Population	32.3 million
Under age 5 mortality rate (2006)	6/1000 live births
Life expectancy (2006)	80 years

Environmental burden of disease for selected risk factors, per year

Estimates based on national exposure and WHO country health statistics 2004

Risk Factor	Exposure	Deaths/ Year	DALYs/1000 capita/year
Water, sanitation, and hygiene (diarrhoea only)	Improve water: 100%	—	0.2
Outdoor air	Mean urban PM_{10}: 21 μg/m³	2700	0.4
Main malaria vectors	No transmission		

Yearly burden attributable to the risk factors

Environmental burden of disease (preliminary), per year

Estimates based on Comparative Risk Assessment, evidence synthesis, and expert evaluation for regional exposure and WHO country health statistics 2004

DALYs/1000 capita	(World – lowest: 14, highest: 316)	15
Deaths		36 800
% of total burden		13%

Indicates how much is preventable through healthier environments (could be used for intercountry comparison)

Environmental burden by disease category [DALYs/1000 capita], per year

Disease Group	World's Lowest Country Rate	Country Rate	World's Highest Country Rate
Diarrhoea	0.2	0.3	107.0
Respiratory infections	0.1	0.1	71.0
Malaria	0.0	—	34.0
Other vector-borne diseases	0.0	0.0	4.9
Lung cancer	0.0	1.2	2.6
Other cancers	0.3	2.3	4.1
Neuropsychiatric disorders	1.4	2.4	3.0
Cardiovascular disease	1.4	2.4	14.0
Chronic Obstructive Pulmonary Disease	0.0	0.4	4.6
Asthma	0.3	1.0	2.8
Musculoskeletal diseases	0.5	0.9	1.5
Road traffic injuries	0.3	0.4	15.0
Other unintentional injuries	0.6	1.2	30.0
Intentional injuries	0.0	0.7	7.5

Indicates how the preventable environmental burden of disease is spread across disease groups in Canada (for intracountry comparison)

Note: DALYs (disability-adjusted life years) represent a weighted measure of death, illness, and disability.

Source: World Health Organization. (2009). Country profiles of environmental burden of disease. Retrieved from http://www.who.int/quantifying_ehimpacts/national/countryprofile/en/index.html

FIGURE 24.2 Environmental Influences on Health

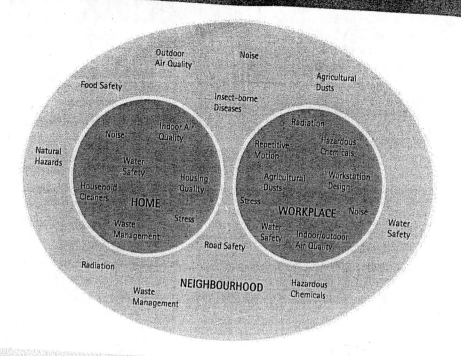

Source: Modified from WHO: Environmental Burden of Disease Series, No. 1 Introduction and methods: Assessing the environmental burden of disease at national and local levels. Figure 2.1 Environmental hazards and risk factors; and Myres, A. W., & Betke, K. (2002). Healthy environments = healthy people. Health Policy Research Bulletin, Issue 4. Ottawa, ON: Minister of Health: Her Majesty the Queen in Right of Canada, p. 6.

CHNs would most typically be actively involved in environmental health at the exposure and effects (EE) and action (A) levels. Knowledge of all factors in the framework is important to appreciate the complexities related to environmental exposures and health outcomes. The DPSEEA framework can explain how environmental factors of concern will differ locally, regionally, and nationally. For example, driving forces, such as poverty, create pressures, such as poor sanitation and hygiene, which create an environmental state with high risk of diarrhoea (Prüss-Üstün, 2006).

Environmental Factors

An estimated 24% of the global disease burden and 23% of all deaths can be attributed to environmental factors.

(WHO)

Modelling Environmental Influences on Health Exposure to individual environmental factors will primarily occur at home, at work, or during recreational activities. These factors have the potential to impact health individually or in combination. For example, indoor and outdoor air quality are two main environmental factors related to acute lower respiratory infections in various parts of the world, with contributing environmental factors including tobacco smoke, solid fuel use, housing conditions, and possibly hygiene. The major risk factors worldwide for diarrhoea are attributed to water, sanitation, and hygiene (Prüss-Üstün, 2006). Figure 24.2 outlines some common hazards in the home, workplace, and recreational environments that have the potential to impact health.

CANADIAN RESEARCH BOX 24.1

Can differing manure systems influence bioaerosols in buildings housing swine?

Létourneau, V., Nehmé, B., Mériaux, A., Massé, D., & Duchaine, C. (2010). Impact of production systems on swine confinement buildings bioaerosols. *Journal of Occupational and Environmental Hygiene, 7*(2), 94–102.

This study compared the levels of environmental contaminants between bioaerosols from swine confinement buildings using three types of manure systems: conventional, source separation, and litter. Swine workers suffer from a high prevalence of respiratory symptoms and these symptoms are associated with the number of hours working in a swine confinement building. Long-term effects of working in a swine confinement building include reduced respiratory function, wheezing, chronic bronchitis, and asthma. Bioaerosols from swine confinement buildings are composed of animal proteins, bedding material, feed, waste, soil, and micro-organisms. Micro-organisms in swine bioaerosols include bacteria, fungi, and viruses, as well as their metabolites and fragments, such as endotoxin.

RESULTS: There was no statistically significant difference between total dust and endotoxin in bioaerosols from the three types of swine confinement buildings. Culturable bacteria and fungi were significantly higher in swine confinement buildings using sawdust litter than those using conventional and source separation manure systems.

PRACTICAL IMPLICATIONS: Better understanding of swine bioaerosols could help to improve indoor air quality in swine confinement buildings and lower respiratory symptoms in swine workers.

Discussion Questions

1. From an environmental health perspective, what are some of the factors that were included in this study?
2. From the results of this study, what types of information could a nurse provide to a swine worker suffering from respiratory symptoms?

CANADIAN RESEARCH BOX

Can safety practices prevent machinery-related farm injuries?

Narasimhan, G., Peng, Y., Crowe, T., Hagel, L., Dosman, J., & Pickett, W. (2010). Operational safety practices as determinants of machinery-related injury on Saskatchewan farms. *Accident Analysis and Prevention, 42*, 1226–1231.

This study examined the association between safety practices and machinery-related farm injury. In North America, agriculture is one of the most hazardous occupations. On average, 177 hospitalizations per 100 000 Canadians are reported annually due to machinery-related farm injury. Existing theory suggests that use of safety devices on machinery can attenuate exposure of workers to physical safety risks.

RESULTS: From the Saskatchewan Farm Injury Cohort Study (SFIC), 159 machinery-related injuries on 2390 farms were reported in 2006. It was found that tractors, combines, and augers were the largest single types of machinery related to farm injury. Farm residents of age 45–64 years reported the highest number of machinery-related injuries, at 62%; residents of the 20–44 year age group reported 25% of injuries, residents 65 years of age and older reported 13%, and residents under 20 years of age reported 1% of injuries. The majority of machinery-related injuries occurred on grain farms (90%), which was the most common type of farm studied. Farms that used safety devices less frequently were 1.94 times more likely to report machinery-related injuries. Therefore, there is an association between an increased risk of machinery-related injury and less frequent use of safety devices on machines.

PRACTICAL IMPLICATIONS: Injury prevention programs that focus on the use of safety devices could help to lower the rate of machinery-related farm injury.

Discussion Questions

1. What is unique about the agricultural setting in terms of health and health risks?
2. From the above data, is there a particular age group(s) of farm residents that appear at risk for machinery-related injuries? Explain.
3. What are some methods for reducing risk in this group?

Categorization of Environmental Factors Individual environmental factors are typically categorized as chemical, physical, biological, psychological, and ergonomic.

- **Chemical factors** are in the form of vapours, gases, dusts, fumes, and mists. Chemicals may be raw materials in original form or by-products of the chemical breakdown or production process.
- **Physical factors** include ionizing and non-ionizing radiation, noise, vibration, and extremes in temperature and pressure.
- **Biological factors** are any living organisms or their components or properties that can cause an adverse health effect, such as micro-organisms (bacteria, viruses, fungi), pests and insects, and animals.
- **Psychological factors** are individual stress or distress events that have the ability to impact health, such as illness, death, birth, job promotion, finances, and interpersonal conflict.
- **Ergonomic factors** include factors that influence the compatibility or "fit" between the person and his or her immediate environment, task, job, or activity. Examples of problematic ergonomic factors that could lead to illness or injury include improperly designed or utilized tools or work areas, as well as poor work procedures, such as improper lifting or reaching, poor visual conditions, or repetitive motion activities.

Routes of Entry The four common routes of entry for individual environmental factors (chemical, physical, or biological) are inhalation, absorption, injection, and ingestion.

- **Inhalation** involves inhaling agents directly into the respiratory tract and lungs.
- **Absorption** refers to entrance through the skin, regardless of whether the skin is intact or damaged. Some substances may be absorbed by way of openings or through hair follicles, while others may dissolve in fats and oils of the skin (i.e., organic lead compounds and organic phosphate pesticides and solvents such as toluene and xylene). Some compounds can produce systemic poisoning through direct contact with the skin (cyanides, aromatic amines, amides, and phenols).
- **Injection** can involve accidental or intentional injection of agents from either a high velocity source (i.e., an agent released under high pressure) or a point source (i.e., needle puncture).

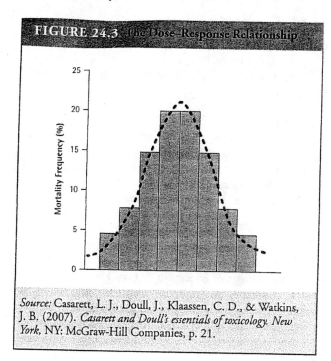

FIGURE 24.3 The Dose-Response Relationship

Source: Casarett, L. J., Doull, J., Klaassen, C. D., & Watkins, J. B. (2007). *Casarett and Doull's essentials of toxicology.* New York, NY: McGraw-Hill Companies, p. 21.

■ **Ingestion** includes knowingly or unknowingly eating or drinking a harmful agent and subsequently having a toxic compound absorbed from the gastrointestinal tract into the bloodstream.

Degree of Hazard The relationship between the dose of an agent and the response it elicits is a fundamental concept in toxicology (Figure 24.3). The level of harm depends on the level of exposure. The **degree of hazard** from exposure to environmental factors depends on (1) the nature of the agent involved, (2) the intensity of the exposure, and (3) the duration of the exposure. Key elements to consider include how much of the agent is required to produce an effect, the probability of the agent entering the body at levels required to produce an effect, the rate at which the agent is generated or emitted, the total contact time, and the use of any measures that might reduce the level of exposure (e.g., ventilation or personal protective equipment).

Hazard Control When an environmental factor is recognized, three strategies are typically employed to control for exposure. The appropriate types of controls will depend on the exposure in question.

Engineering controls are the first line of defense by providing or creating a design, structure, enclosure, or system to engineer the exposure away. Examples of engineering controls include substitution (i.e., replacing a substance of concern with something associated with less or no effects), changing the design of a process so that exposures do not or are less likely to occur (i.e., building enclosures, isolating the hazard from the public), and adding ventilation to dilute or to remove the agent.

Administrative controls are utilized when engineering controls are not feasible, or are insufficient, or in the case of sensitive individuals. An example of an administrative control

is removing the individual from the source of exposure or limiting their contact time with the exposure. In the case of an occupational exposure, this could include changing the job functions of the individual to prevent the exposure from occurring. A classic example of administrative control is limiting time spent performing a repetitive task in order to prevent musculoskeletal injury.

The third form of control is personal protective equipment (PPE). PPE is worn to protect an individual from a known exposure (i.e., respirators to prevent inhalation exposures, gloves to prevent absorption). Although PPE is effective in reducing exposures, individual actions can dictate the effectiveness of the PPE. For example, PPE must be worn properly and fit appropriately to be effective. Due to these limitations, PPE should always be considered a last line of defense; engineering and administrative controls are preferable when feasible.

"All things are poisons; there is none which is not a poison. The right dose differentiates a poison and a remedy." (Paracelsus 1493–1541)

Dose–Response Exposures to an agent may result in a dose–response that has no effect, a minimal effect, or an acute and/or a chronic health outcome. **Dose–response** histograms, such as Figure 24.3, are often utilized as a means to portray the relationship between the dose of an agent and the elicited responses in a population. The dose–response histogram indicates the frequency of health events associated with varying doses of an agent and forms a bell-shaped curve known as a *normal frequency distribution.* The curve indicates the differences in susceptibility among individuals. In a normally distributed population, the mean ±1 standard deviation (SD) represents 68.3% of the population. The left end of the curve represents hyper-susceptible members of the population, and the right end of the curve represents the resistant population. In other words, those at the left end of the curve experience an effect at lower doses, while those at the right end experience an effect only at high doses. A population will always contain individuals that fall at either end of the curve and at points in between. Individuals at the hyper-susceptible end of the curve may require additional resources to control for exposures, while individuals at the resistant end of the curve might not appear to suffer from above average levels of exposure, though falling in the latter group should not preclude use of appropriate exposure control measures outlined above.

ENVIRONMENTAL HEALTH ASSESSMENT

An **environmental health assessment** is performed to examine possible links between environmental exposures and health outcomes. Some individuals may have a specific environmental exposure concern, such as arsenic in well water. Others may have more generalized concerns about environmental exposures or are looking to environmental exposures as the cause of unexplained symptoms. In these cases, a more detailed inventory of possible environmental exposures must be taken. It is not uncommon for the individual to present with concerns about a potential exposure in the absence of any notable symptoms or health effects. Certain populations might also be considered vulnerable to environmental factors, including children, elderly, pregnant, and immune-compromised individuals.

Personal Exposure History

An important part of assessing the influence of environmental exposures is the individual interview. The **individual interview** involves asking the individual about the nature of his or her environmental exposures, when and where they occur, the circumstances of how they occur, and whether or not he or she feels any ill effects from those exposures. The impacts of biology (genetics), sociology (habits), occupation, the home environment, and past exposure history must all be considered in the assessment. Specifically, the individual interview includes occupational, residential, and recreational information.

Occupational information would include present and past jobs and work exposures, as well as any protective measures related to work exposures. The workplace may be a significant source of chemical, physical, biological, psychological, or ergonomic factors. Duration of exposure, including number of hours a day, days a week, and number of years of exposure are important aspects in the assessment. Source agents of exposure as well as by-products should be included in an assessment.

When working as an occupational health nurse, the assessment of the work environment is an essential component in health and safety programming in order to recognize and control for hazards (chemical, physical, biologic, ergonomic, or psychological). An occupational health nurse would be involved in assessing the work site, providing healthcare, doing medical assessments, and providing emergency response among other things. A work-site assessment identifies actual or potential worker exposures from the work processes and materials (raw materials, by-products, and end-products).

Residential information includes water sources (i.e., well water, city water), dampness and mould issues (i.e., history of floods, water damage), and indoor air quality issues. Residential information can provide additional insights into potential exposures. For example, different exposures, such as biologic, zoonotic, injury, and water quality factors exist between rural and urban residences. Rural and remote populations may not only be differentially exposed to certain environmental factors, but other factors within the framework assessment may also impact health in comparison to urban counterparts. For example, persons in rural and remote areas may have less access to healthcare. Some of the issues of importance are described in Chapter 22, "Aboriginal Health" and Chapter 23, "Rural Health."

Recreational information would include social activities and community exposures. Environmental factors associated with industries and processes within the community would be documented during a community assessment, as described in Chapter 13, "Community Assessment."

Determining whether an individual or a group has experienced an effect from an environmental exposure can be difficult for a variety of reasons. First, environmental exposures may be associated with latent health conditions, highlighting the importance of collecting information from as far back as the individual can provide. Second, the combined effect of one or more exposures from home, work, and social activities can make it difficult to attribute one particular exposure to a particular effect. Third, many environmentally related conditions and illnesses are characterized by signs and symptoms that are very similar to those of more typical "non-environmental" illnesses (for instance, mild respiratory infections can present with symptoms that are sometimes confused with allergy to an environmental agent). Fourth, in cases of low-level environmental exposures and mild or uncertain health effects, attempts to attribute cause to a particular exposure may be extremely difficult. Finally, considerable "background noise" in the form of co-existing health conditions, other exposures (i.e., workplaces, smoking) and inherited factors may be present. The challenge lies in recognizing all potential sources of exposures and factors of influence, then attempting to attribute the cause of illness or symptoms to an exposure.

Environmental Epidemiology

Environmental epidemiology is utilized to clarify relationships between environmental factors and human health effects. Epidemiological studies might (1) characterize health effects from known exposures, (2) characterize exposures and effects in populations and attempt to determine dose–response relationships, or (3) report on a disease pattern for which there is no causal explanation and where attempts were made to identify potential agents. Cross-sectional, cohort, ecological, case-control, and community intervention study designs, including adaptations to these designs, are utilized in environmental epidemiology studies. Although environmental health is a relatively new field, researchers have been performing environmental epidemiology studies for centuries. In the 1800s, John Snow published his epidemiological work on the transmission of cholera in an essay, "On the Mode of Communication of Cholera." Contrary to common belief at that time, Snow suggested that cholera entered the body via ingestion rather than inhalation (Snow, 1860). Chapter 9 introduces epidemiology and relationships to community health nursing.

Environmental Indicators

For some environmental factors, **environmental indicators** are monitored to assist in recognizing community and population exposures that have the potential to impact health. Indicators provide a simple way to convey complex environmental information. Through the Canadian Environmental Sustainability Indicators (CESI) initiative, the Canadian federal

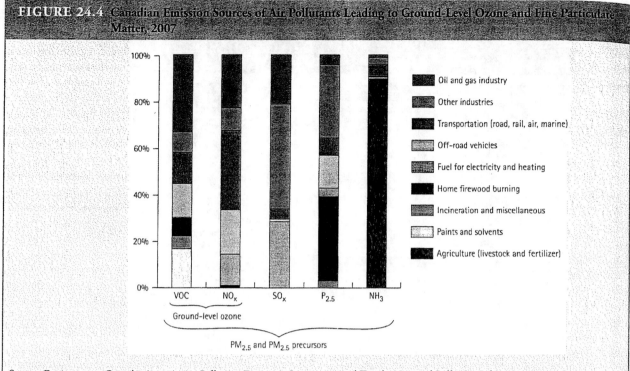

FIGURE 24.4 Canadian Emission Sources of Air Pollutants Leading to Ground-Level Ozone and Fine Particulate Matter, 2007

Source: Environment Canada. (2007). *Air Pollutant Emissions Summaries and Trends, National Pollutant Release Inventory,* Ottawa, ON. Retrieved from http://www.ec.gc.ca/indicateurs-indicators/default.asp?lang=En&n=ADF1A74C-1www.phac-aspc.gc.ca/ph-sp/pdf/perspect-eng.pdf

government reports on three environmental indicators: (1) air quality, (2) water quality, and (3) greenhouse gas emissions.

Air quality indicators track ground-level ozone and fine particulate matter (PM$_{2.5}$) (see Figure 24.4). Ground-level ozone has the ability to impact plant, animal, and human health. Fine particulate matter (PM$_{2.5}$) can be inhaled deep into the lungs and can be the cause of chronic and/or **acute health effects.** Long-term high-level exposures may be associated with chronic cardiovascular and respiratory health outcomes whereas short-term high-level exposures can impact vulnerable populations (i.e., individuals with pre-existing heart or lung disease, infants, or the elderly).

Water quality indicators measure the extent and severity of water pollution by tracking a wide range of substances in water across Canada. Water quality is considered a broad reflection of ecosystem health. Health outcomes related to water quality include waterborne illnesses (*E. coli, Giardia* and *Cryptosporidium*) from untreated or undertreated water supplies, infant methemoglobinemia from nitrate exposure in drinking water systems, or mercury poisoning from consuming high amounts of contaminated fish.

Greenhouse gas indicators track Canada's greenhouse gas emissions and identify sources. Typical greenhouse gases are carbon dioxide, methane, nitrous oxide, and ozone. Greenhouse gas emissions can be considered a pressure using the DPSEEA model. Greenhouse gases can potentially impact climate, which could influence ecosystems with resultant health outcomes (i.e., changes in disease patterns caused by insects, bacteria, or pathogens).

Risk Assessment, Risk Management, and Risk Communication

Risk assessment, risk management, and **risk communication** are tools utilized in environmental health for assessing, managing, and communicating risks associated with environmental factors (see Figure 24.5).

Risk assessment is the systematic process for describing and quantifying the level of exposure to particular substances that will result in increased risks to health (Covello & Merkhofer, 1993). Risk assessment typically involves an estimation of risk either through direct association, based on assumptions utilizing the best available information (dose–response curves), or generalizations based on animal models.

Risk management options include minimal intervention (i.e., enhancing public awareness) to maximum intervention (i.e., legislation).

Risk communication is the process of making risk assessment and risk management information comprehensible and taking the necessary steps to distribute and present that information accordingly. CHNs are typically involved in risk communication at the prevention level. Anticipating and recognizing potential environmental factors of concern are important first steps in preventing exposures, while education is a primary preventive strategy in environmental health. Applying the basic principles of disease prevention, including primary, secondary, and tertiary levels of prevention, is important when planning strategies for environmental health.

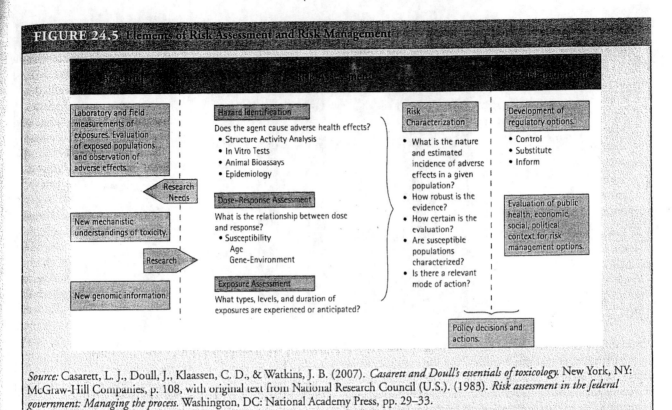

FIGURE 24.5 Elements of Risk Assessment and Risk Management

Source: Casarett, L. J., Doull, J., Klaassen, C. D., & Watkins, J. B. (2007). *Casarett and Doull's essentials of toxicology.* New York, NY: McGraw-Hill Companies, p. 108, with original text from National Research Council (U.S.). (1983). *Risk assessment in the federal government: Managing the process.* Washington, DC: National Academy Press, pp. 29–33.

Primary prevention involves promoting activities that prevent the actual occurrence of a specific environmentally related illness or disease. Such activities might include immunization, counselling about reducing exposures, supporting development of policy and standards related to environmental health, educating about healthy lifestyles related to environmental health (i.e., teaching parents about minimizing exposure to lead during home renovations and in consumer products), as well as supporting and practising positive activities, such as washing fruit and vegetables under running water before eating them.

Secondary prevention involves promoting early detection or screening of environmentally related disease and limiting disability. Secondary prevention activities include assessing for blood lead levels in at-risk young children, assessing urine for arsenic in individuals with arsenic content in their water supply, and recommending x-rays for individuals occupationally exposed to asbestos.

Tertiary prevention involves recovery or rehabilitation of an environmentally related disease or condition after the disease has developed. Tertiary prevention activities include assisting in distribution of information as well as taking action (treatment, medical management) in the event of an acute environmental health-related incidence (i.e., *E. coli* in a water source). See the following Case Study.

CASE STUDY

In May 2000, drinking water contaminated with *E. coli* and *Campylobacter* bacteria killed seven people and made over 2300 ill in Walkerton, Ontario. Reporters from around North America descended on the area, trying to get to the bottom of Canada's worst outbreak of *E. coli* contamination. After the tragedy, the Ontario government established a Public Inquiry led by the Honourable Dennis O'Connor. Commissioner O'Connor's findings were released in two volumes. *The Report of the Walkerton Inquiry, Part One: The Events of May 2000 and Related Issues* (O'Connor, 2002a) reported on the events in Walkerton and the causes of the tragedy. It was released in January 2002 and contained 28 recommendations. The inquiry found contributing factors to the incident that included lack of monitoring of chlorine levels in the drinking water, deregulation of water testing, and cuts to the Environment Ministry by the Ontario government. *Part Two: A Strategy for Safe Drinking Water* (O'Connor, 2002b) was released in May 2002 and contained 93 recommendations. This latter report stated:

> While it is not possible to utterly remove all risk from a water system, the recommendations' overall goal is to ensure that Ontario's drinking water systems deliver water with a level of risk so negligible that a reasonable and informed person would feel safe drinking the water. (p. 5)

The Ontario government introduced numerous new pieces of legislation and regulations in response to the inquiry findings. These include the *Safe Drinking Water Act (SWDA)*, the *Sustainable Water* and *Sewage Systems Act*, the *Nutrient Management Act,* and the *Drinking Water Systems Regulation.* A companion study on the

Walkerton incident conservatively estimated the economic impact of the Walkerton water incident at more than $64.5 million (Livernois, 2002).

Discussion Questions

1. Imagine that you were a community health nurse in May 2000 when people first began to fall ill. Who should be members of the multidisciplinary team necessary to address the initial illnesses and determine the source of the illnesses? Once the initial acute incident passed, what would be some roles that you as a community health nurse could be involved in?

2. Using the DPSEEA model, what may have been some of the important environmental factors related to this event?

ENVIRONMENTAL LEGISLATION

Legislating controls for environmental factors (policy development) is a maximal intervention, as it sets and administrates safe levels of exposure. Due to the complexity of environmental factors, numerous provincial and national government agencies have responsibilities with respect to legislation. The examples that follow are legislation and policies that have been developed in relation to environmental health.

Health Canada

Hazardous Products Act (HPA) prohibits the advertising, sale, and importation of hazardous products. *Food and Drugs Act (FDA)* ensures the safety of food, drugs, cosmetics, and therapeutic devices. *Pest Control Products Act (PCPA)* governs the importation, manufacture, sale, and use of pesticides.

Environment Canada

Canadian Environmental Assessment Act (CEAA) ensures all new projects with federal involvement include an environmental impact assessment, including an assessment of human health impact. *Canadian Environmental Protection Act (CEPA)* governs pollution prevention and protection of the environment and human health. *Fisheries Act* is administered by the Department of Fisheries and Oceans to control pollutants released to water frequented by fish.

Provincial Responsibility

Workplaces *Workplace Exposure Limits:* Provincial labour departments and ministries of labour in Canada are responsible for occupational health and safety legislation and for setting occupational standards for exposure, which are often referred to as **occupational exposure limits** (OELs). However, certain industries in Canada fall under federal jurisdiction with respect to health and safety, such as air transportation, including airports, aerodromes, and airlines; grain elevators; feed and seed mills; banks; and most federal Crown corporations. The provinces are also responsible for enforcing workplace health and safety legislation and exposure limits for employers within their boundaries who do not fall under federal jurisdiction. The American Conference of Governmental Industrial Hygienists (ACGIH) researches and publishes suggested exposure limits for contaminants based on available current scientific knowledge. Many provincial jurisdictions in Canada rely on the suggested exposure limits published by the ACGIH and adopt them as legal OELs.

Environment Provincial ministries of the environment and health legislate policies for air quality, water quality, and health. For example, provincial legislation often regulates air emissions originating in a given province (i.e., the Clean Air Act in Saskatchewan) and protects provincial air, land, and water resources by regulating and controlling potentially harmful activities and substances (i.e., the Ontario Environmental Protection Act).

ROLE FOR NURSES IN ENVIRONMENTAL HEALTH

The mission of health professionals in environmental health is to prevent, anticipate, recognize, evaluate, and control for those environmental exposures that could bring harm to a population. In terms of toxicology of environmental factors, the most attention has focused on occupational settings and, in particular, manufacturing settings. However, over the past two decades greater emphasis has been placed on other settings, including communities, homes, schools, hospitals, offices, and daycares. Nurses are practising in all these settings with designations as community nurses, public health nurses, school nurses, or occupational health nurses, and, as such, many are actively involved in addressing exposures to environmental factors.

The environments we live, work, and play in have the potential to impact health; nurses have a role in preventing exposures to and reducing health risks from environmental factors. The nursing curriculum provides the foundation for considering environmental factors as contributors to impaired health. The Canadian Nurses Association has developed tools to support nurses in addressing environmental health issues in areas ranging from clinical practice, administration, research, and education through to policy (Canadian Nurses Association, 2009). The influence of environment on community health and well-being is an important component of community health nursing practice.

Occupational Health Nursing

Occupational health nursing is a branch of nursing dealing with health, safety, treatment, care, and prevention of illness or injury in a workplace setting. Whereas CHNs apply the practice of nursing in a wide variety of community settings, occupational health nurses (OHNs) apply the practice of nursing to the workplace setting and to specific populations of workers. CHNs and OHNs share common competencies in the practice of nursing.

They are registered nurses with additional training, skills, and education in health and safety and are often hired by industry to provide services on site. The Canadian Nurses Association (CNA) offers certification in Occupational Health Nursing. The Canadian Occupational Health Nurses Association (COHNA/ACIIST) is the national association for OHNs in Canada, and provides a national voice to influence health and safety regulations across the country (http://www. cohna-aciist.ca/).

OHNs often work as part of a larger team of occupational health professionals at a workplace or for a workforce. That team might also include industrial hygienists, safety professionals, engineers, management, and physicians. However, on-site physicians are much less common in the workplace than they used to be; it is not unusual for the OHN to be the front-line healthcare provider and emergency response coordinator for a workplace. The experience and scope of practice for an OHN at a workplace can be very broad, encompassing everything from emergency response and first aid to policy planning and prevention initiatives. The CNA outlines the key competencies for the occupational health nursing certification exam (http://www.cna-nurses.ca/CNA/nursing/certification/specialties/biblio/default_e.aspx).

OHN Certification Competencies

1.0 Provision of Occupational Health, Safety and Environmental Nursing

The occupational health nurse

1.1 Practices in accordance with occupational health, safety and environmental nursing standards of practice, codes of ethics, and applicable professional legislation.
1.2 Practices in compliance with legislation, codes, regulations, and standards (e.g., communicating, interpreting and utilizing jurisdictional occupational health and safety legislation and regulations, workers' compensation, human rights, labour laws, relevant collective agreements, organizational policies).
1.3 Complies with legislative requirements for due diligence regarding record keeping.

2.0 Recognition, Evaluation and Control of Workplace/Environmental Health and Safety Hazards

2.1 Identifies potential and existing workplace/environmental health and safety hazards (physical, chemical, biological, ergonomic, psychosocial, and safety).
2.2 Assesses the level of risk (immediate, long-term, and continuous) and severity of hazards based on probability that harm may occur in a specific situation.
2.3 Applies principles of hazard control.

3.0 Health Assessment, Planning, Implementation, Monitoring, and Evaluation

3.1 Assess, plans, implements, recommends, and monitors interventions to promote employee health and wellness
3.2 Develops, implements, and evaluates programs and procedures for health surveillance
3.3 Collects, analyses, uses, and communicates aggregate data for prevention, identification of trends, and statistical or research purposes.

4.0 Assessment, Care, and Case Management of Injuries and Illnesses

4.1 Applies the nursing process to implement appropriate interventions to minimize effects of illness and injury.
4.2 Uses a combination of ongoing data-gathering activities to evaluate ill or injured employees
4.3 Identifies the implications for fitness to work for disorders.
4.4 Identifies occupational or non-occupational injuries and illnesses, assesses limitations, and recommends workplace accommodation as required.
4.5 Provides and coordinates ability/case management.
4.6 Counsels employees in the prevention and management of both occupational and non-occupational illnesses and injuries.

5.0 Environmental, Health, Safety, Wellness Promotion and Education

5.1 Provides leadership to empower employees and management to adopt strategies directed towards both organizational and individual health, safety, and wellness.

6.0 Environment, Health, Safety, and Wellness Management

6.1 Manages environment, health and safety, and wellness services

CASE STUDY

A member of the community presents with hearing loss. The following information is ascertained during the health assessment:

- Present work: welder
- Past work: grain elevator agent for five years; underground potash mine worker for 25 years
- Residence/living: acreage with three horses, 25 head of cattle, one dog, and one indoor cat.
- Activities: rifle expert (spends about 100 hours a year at the shooting range).

Discussion Questions

1. Describe the categorized environmental factors that may have influenced the person's hearing.

2. Is it possible to determine the effect from each of these exposures on his current health condition?

3. What information may assist in counselling this individual?

SUMMARY

The health of individuals and communities is often closely linked to their environment and to exposures in that environment. Assessing the impact of environmental exposures requires a multidisciplinary approach and a thorough understanding of the factors that influence those exposures and potential health outcomes.

Frameworks for categorizing environmental health factors, such as the World Health Organization's DPSEEA framework, are useful for creating a system of factors in a decision-making context. Environmental factors can include chemical, physical, biological, psychological, and ergonomic factors. Typically, personal exposure to such factors occurs through inhalation, absorption, ingestion, or injection. Determining the potential extent of exposure to such factors and possible effects requires careful individual assessment and, where applicable, understanding of dose–response effects and toxicology of the factors in question. Risk assessment, risk management, and risk communication are important tools utilized in environmental health to (1) describe, characterize, and quantify the exposure, (2) intervene as needed for control and prevention, and (3) make the information available to and comprehensible by the general public. Controlling for hazards can occur through engineering, administration (including legislation), and personal protective equipment.

The nursing profession plays a very important role in preventing exposures to and reducing effects from environmental exposures. As front-line healthcare professionals in both rural and urban settings, nurses may often be the first to encounter those with ill effects from environmental exposures, whether from home, work, or community.

KEY TERMS

REVIEW QUESTIONS

1. The World Health Organization has developed a framework for categorizing environmental factors. This framework categorizes environmental factors under the headings:

   a) Dormancy, Public Health, Sentinel Events, Ecosystem, Environment and Air Quality

   b) Driving Forces, Pressures, State, Exposure, Effects, Action

   c) Driving Forces, Population Health, Structure, Elements, Ecosystem, Actions

   d) Dormancy, Pressures, Status, External, Effects, Actions

2. Which of the following diseases is considered to have a large burden of attributable environmental factors?

   a) multiple sclerosis

   b) radiation sickness

   c) diarrhoea

   d) cancer

3. The World Health Organization (WHO) defines environmental health as

   a) healthy rivers, soil, and ecosystems.

   b) all aspects of human health, disease, and injury that are determined by factors in the environment.

c) all aspects of animal health, disease, and injury that are determined by factors in the environment.

d) low levels of harmful agents in the environment.

4. An example of a Driving Force in the DPSEEA framework would be

a) indoor air pollution.

b) water quality.

c) occupational exposures.

d) population growth.

5. Excessive noise exposure in the environment would be an example of exposure to what type of environmental factor?

a) chemical factor

b) physical factor

c) biological factor

d) psychological factor

e) ergonomic factor

6. Which of the following is considered a common route of entry for environmental factors into the body?

a) radiation

b) diffusion

c) inhalation

d) convection

7. The process of making risk assessment and risk management information comprehensible and taking steps to distribute that information is known as

a) a press conference.

b) an editorial.

c) risk communication.

d) knowledge dissemination.

8. Examples of strategies to control exposure to environmental factors include:

a) Look, Listen, Feel.

b) Engineering, Administrative, and Personal Protective Equipment.

c) Driving Forces, Pressures, State, Action.

d) Internal, External, Combined.

9. The branch of nursing dealing with health, safety, treatment, care, and prevention of illness and injury in the workplace setting is known as

a) Environmental Health Nursing.

b) Community Nursing.

c) Occupational Health Nursing.

d) Clinical Nursing.

STUDY QUESTIONS

1. Using the DPSEEA framework, choose a particular driving force and describe the pressures generated, how these pressures alter the state of environment, what types of hazards may be present, possible routes of exposure, and actions that could improve environmental health issues.

2. What are the five categories of environmental factors? Categorize the environmental influences listed in Figure 24.2 into types of environmental factors.

3. What are the four routes of entry for environmental factors?

4. List the three hazard control strategies for environmental factors in order of preferred use.

5. Describe the three types of information gathered during an individual interview.

6. What are five challenges to environmental health assessments?

7. Describe the three environmental indicators measured by the federal government.

8. Provide examples of primary, secondary, and tertiary prevention in terms of environmental health.

*After working through these questions, go to the MyNursingLab at **www.pearsoned.ca/mynursinglab** to check your answers.*

INDIVIDUAL CRITICAL THINKING EXERCISES

1. Name three issues in your local news that relate environment to health. Is there a role for nursing in these issues?

2. What are some of the roles of a community health nurse in the field of environmental health?

3. What are some of the roles of a community health nurse in the field of occupational health?

4. Think of an example of how a community health nurse might be involved in risk communication and prevention.

5. A person living on an acreage presents with general concerns about exposure to pesticides and related chemicals from a neighbouring agricultural (grain) operation. He has been experiencing some unexplained symptoms, including "frequent colds" and headaches, more often than usual. The neighbouring operation has been applying fertilizers and pest control products by both tractor and aircraft. Describe how you might go about investigating the concern and gathering more information.

GROUP CRITICAL THINKING EXERCISES

1. Propose ways of incorporating environmental health principles into nursing practice, education, research, and policy.

2. Identify policies (including legislation) at the community level (municipal and/or urban level), provincial/territorial level, and national level that have an influence on the health outcomes of clients in your community.

3. Think of an industry in your community. Identify five potential hazards in this industry. For each of the potential hazards, identify at least one control method to reduce or eliminate the hazard.

REFERENCES

American Conference of Governmental Industrial Hygienists (ACGIH). (2008). *Threshold limit values for chemical substances and physical agents and biological exposure indices.* Cincinnati, OH: ACGIH.

Briggs, D. (1999). *Environmental health indicators: Framework and methodologies for the protection of the human environment occupational and environmental health* (series No. 99.10). Geneva, CH: World Health Organization.

Canadian Nurses Association. (2009). *Nursing and environmental health.* Retrieved from http://www.cna-nurses.ca/CNA/issues/environment/default_e.aspx

Casarett, L. J., Doull, J., Klaassen, C. D., & Watkins, J. B. (2007). *Casarett and Doull's essentials of toxicology.* New York, NY: McGraw-Hill.

Covello, V. T., & Merkhofer, M. W. (1993). *Risk assessment methods: Approaches for assessing health and environmental risks.* New York, NY: Plenum Press.

Environment Canada. (2007). *Air pollutant emissions summaries and trends, National Pollutant Release Inventory.* Ottawa, ON: Author. Retrieved from http://www.ec.gc.ca/indicateurs-indicators/default.asp?lang=En&n=ADF1A74C-1 www.phac-aspc.gc.ca/ph-sp/pdf/perspect-eng.pdf

Livernois, J. (2002). *The Walkerton Inquiry Commissioned Paper 14: The economic costs of the Walkerton water crisis.* Ottawa, ON: Ontario Ministry of the Attorney General, Queen's Printer for Ontario. Retrieved from http://www.uoguelph.ca/~live/WICP-14-Livernois1.pdf

Myres, A. W., & Betke, K. (2002). Healthy environments = healthy people. *Health Policy Research Bulletin,* Issue 4. Ottawa, ON: Minister of Health: Her Majesty the Queen in Right of Canada.

National Research Council (U.S.). (1983). *Risk assessment in the federal government: Managing the process.* Washington, DC: National Academy Press.

O'Connor, D. R. (2002a). *The report of the Walkerton Inquiry, part one: The events of May 2000 and related* issues. Ottawa, ON: Queen's Printer for Ontario. Retrieved from http://www.attorneygeneral.jus.gov.on.ca/english/about/pubs/walkerton/

O'Connor, D. R. (2002b). *The report of the Walkerton Inquiry, part two: A strategy for safe drinking water.* Ottawa, ON:

Queen's Printer for Ontario. Retrieved from http://www.attorneygeneral.jus.gov.on.ca/english/about/pubs/walkerton/

Pope, A. M., Snyder, M. A., & Mood, L. H. (Eds.). (1995). *Nursing, health and the environment: Strengthening the relationship to improve the public's health.* Washington, DC: National Academy Press.

Prüss-Üstün, A. (2006). In C. Corvalán & World Health Organization. (Eds.), *Preventing disease through healthy environments: Towards an estimate of the environmental burden of disease.* Geneva, Switzerland: World Health Organization.

Snow, J. (1860). *On the mode of communication of cholera* (2nd ed.). London, UK: John Churchill.

World Health Organization. (2009). *Country profiles of environmental burden of disease.* Retrieved from http://www.who.int/quantifying_ehimpacts/national/countryprofile/en/index.html

ADDITIONAL RESOURCES

Websites

Canadian Association of Physicians for the Environment
http://www.cape.ca/

Canadian Environmental Sustainability Indicators. 2008.
http://www.ec.gc.ca/indicateurs-indicators/default.asp?lang=en

Community Based Environmental Monitoring Network. Offers assistance to individuals, community groups and organizations in the initiation of environmental monitoring.
http://www.envnetwork.smu.ca/

Creating a Healthy Environment for Kids.
http://www.healthyenvironmentforkids.ca/english/

Health Canada regulations
http://www.hc-sc.gc.ca/english/about/acts_regulations.html

Health Canada: Environment and Workplace Health
http://www.hc-sc.gc.ca/ewh-semt/index-eng.php

Inventory of Federal, Provincial and Territorial Environmental and Occupational Health Data Sources and Surveillance Activities.
http://www.hc-sc.gc.ca/ewh-semt/pubs/eval/inventory-repertoire/index-eng.php

Public Health Agency of Canada: Environment and Public Health
http://www.phac-aspc.gc.ca/chn-rcs/eh-es-eng.php?rd=environ_eng

United Nations Economic Commission for Europe. Globally Harmonized System of Classification and Labelling of Chemicals (GHS).
http://www.unece.org/trans/danger/publi/ghs/ghs_welcome_e.html

About the Authors

Shelley Kirychuk, BSN, MSc, MBA, PhD, is an Assistant Professor at the University of Saskatchewan. She is a nurse and holds a Master's Degree in Preventive Medicine and Environmental Health and a PhD in Interdisciplinary studies with focus on occupational health and hygiene. Her research, teaching, and extension activities have focused on respiratory and occupational exposures as well as health and hygiene of agricultural and rural populations.

Niels Koehncke, MD, MSc, FRCPC, is an Assistant Professor at the University of Saskatchewan and Director of the Occupational Medicine Clinic at Royal University Hospital. He is a specialist in Occupational Medicine, providing clinical consultation to patients with concerns about occupational and environmental exposures. He is an active instructor, teaching occupational and environmental health to medical, undergraduate, and graduate students. His research areas of interest include agricultural health and safety, noise exposure, and respiratory exposures in mining.

The authors would like to acknowledge the contributions of Natasha Just and Gillian Binsted in reviewing and rewriting for this chapter.

25

Correctional Health

Cindy Peternelj-Taylor and Phil Woods

OBJECTIVES

After studying this chapter, you should be able to:

1. Understand the role of the nurse in correctional health.
2. Describe the Canadian offender population.
3. Examine common health challenges seen in correctional settings.
4. Analyze professional challenges and ethical responsibilities experienced by nurses in correctional environments.
5. Reflect on ongoing education, research, and practice developments relative to nursing in correctional settings.

INTRODUCTION

Correctional nursing is simply defined as "the practice of nursing and the delivery of [client] care within the unique and distinct environment of the criminal justice system" (American Nurses Association, 2007, p. 1). Nurses practising in the criminal justice system primarily work in correctional settings, including jails, detention centres, prisons, healing lodges, correctional centres, youth custody facilities, and halfway houses. They are primarily responsible for providing healthcare services to a large and diverse population. Through their use of clinical assessment and triage skills, they engage in primary, secondary, and tertiary intervention strategies including early case finding, infection control, treatment and medication administration, health promotion, illness prevention, as well as rehabilitative services and end-of-life care (see the box "Levels of Prevention in Correctional Health"). As per the Corrections and Conditional Release Act (CCRA), and various provincial and territorial corrections acts, clients incarcerated in correctional facilities are entitled to physical and mental healthcare in accordance with professional and community standards (Canadian Public Health Association [CPHA], 2004). Nurses represent the largest group of healthcare professionals working with incarcerated individuals, and as such they have a significant role to play. Timely identification, treatment, and management of healthcare concerns not only contributes to the health of the individual client, but also further contributes to the health and safety of other offenders, facility staff, and the community at large.

Levels of Prevention in Correctional Health

Primary Prevention

Illness prevention (control of communicable diseases, immunization, suicide prevention, violence prevention)
Health promotion
Provision of education and information
Classification of stressors
Political involvement
Appropriate referrals
Advocacy

Secondary Prevention

Assessment, evaluation, diagnosis
Community consultation
Crisis intervention
Program planning and implementation
Substance abuse treatment
Sex offender treatment
Aggressive behaviour control
Life and social skills training
Acute inpatient psychiatric nursing
Suicide risk assessment and management
Creation and maintenance of a therapeutic milieu
Short-term therapy
Counselling, psychotherapy
Medication administration and management
Emergency and trauma care

Tertiary Intervention

Case management
After-care services/community reintegration
Rehabilitation
Vocational training
Relapse prevention
End-of-life/palliative care
Compassionate release
Spiritual care

Correctional facilities are not generally considered part of the traditional healthcare system; by default they are responsible for the provision of healthcare services to a diverse group of individuals who have come into conflict with the law, including those who are remanded in custody while awaiting trial (charged but not yet sentenced), and those found guilty and sentenced by the courts to various periods of time in custody. Federal, provincial, and territorial governments share the administration of correctional services in Canada. Generally, individuals receiving a sentence of two years less a day are the responsibility of either provincial or territorial correctional centres, while those sentenced to two years or greater serve their sentences within federal correctional institutions operated by the Correctional Service of Canada (CSC). Those on remand tend to have greater and more complex healthcare needs than sentenced inmates, who may have had these issues addressed during the remand period.

On an average day in 2004–2005, approximately 152 600 adults were under custodial or community supervision; approximately 32 100 adults were in provincial/territorial or federal custody in Canada; approximately 120 500 were under community supervision; while an additional 9600 (approximately) adults were held on remand (Beattie, 2006). Figures for the average daily count were not provided in the 2005–2006 report, but a 3% increase in admission was reported, 232 810 to custody and 109 539 to community supervision. While the majority of those in custody are male, females accounted for 11% of provincial and 6% of federal admissions sentenced to custody, and 12% of all remand admissions, representing an upward trend in all admissions for females (Landry, Sinha, & Beattie, 2008). On any given day in 2008–2009, there were seven youth in custody for every 10 000 youth in the general population. This number represents a decline of 4% from the previous year and a 15% decline from 2004–2005 (Calverley, Cotter, & Halla, 2010). The health and psychosocial issues experienced by this large captive group are extremely complex and contribute to treatment challenges during incarceration and upon release from custody.

HEALTHCARE OF THE CORRECTIONAL POPULATION

Historically, those who are incarcerated have experienced limited and inconsistent exposure to our healthcare system. They may experience many of the same age- and gender-specific healthcare concerns common to the general population; morbidity and mortality data suggest higher rates of disease and disability when compared to non-incarcerated populations (CPHA, 2004). For many individuals, healthcare received while incarcerated may be the first real opportunity that they have had to address their healthcare needs. Numerous opportunities exist for correctional nurses to provide leadership in the provision of health promotion and illness prevention, especially if individuals are motivated to make lifestyle changes that would improve their overall health status.

The correctional system provides care for offenders with all types of acute and chronic illnesses (CPHA, 2004). The lifestyle of many offenders includes substance abuse, which gives rise to various drug and alcohol withdrawal syndromes, diverse infectious diseases, and the need for long-term treatment interventions. Crowded living conditions can result in higher exposure to infectious diseases, a concern of public health officials worldwide, as most clients eventually return to the community (Thomas, 2005). Furthermore, the "deinstitutionalization movement" that began in Canada in the 1960s and continues today has frequently been blamed for the criminalization of the mentally ill. Peternelj-Taylor (2008), in a recent editorial, affirms that prisons were never designed to meet the needs of individuals requiring treatment for mental illness, and much controversy exists around how they can meet these needs. Finally, it is not uncommon for nurses to care for clients who have experienced multiple traumas such as sexual assaults, stabbings, and/or beatings.

Provincial correctional facilities (and to a lesser extent territorial facilities) admit extremely large numbers of offenders on a daily basis. Clearly, the volume, turnover, and lengths of stay, which can range from a few hours to years, definitely impact on the professional nursing role. Daily admissions to federal correctional facilities are minimal compared to provincial correctional facilities, so the care they are able to provide is different. Clients presenting with acute healthcare problems are assessed and triaged by nurses, and those requiring acute emergency care are normally transferred to a local community general hospital for further assessment and treatment. Nursing staff, in collaboration with the facilities' physicians, manage other less urgent issues. Nurses frequently assist the clients to bring chronic conditions under better control by attending to treatment protocols, assessing for complications, preventing recurrence of health problems, attending to health promotion needs, and preparing for eventual discharge to the community.

Special Populations in Correctional Settings

It could be argued that all individuals who are incarcerated have special needs requiring the attention of correctional nurses. However, the unique needs of offenders who experience mental illness, those who are elderly, women, youth, and those from culturally diverse backgrounds are highlighted here to draw attention to the healthcare concerns and the overall disparities experienced by offender populations.

Offenders with Mental Illness Deinstitutionalization has resulted in an influx to correctional facilities of individuals with serious mental illness. Prior to this, police would transport individuals exhibiting bizarre behaviours in public to a mental health facility; now they have few choices but to remand the individual in custody in a local jail or remand centre.

In *Out of the Shadows at Last: Transforming Mental Health, Mental Illness, and Addiction Services in Canada*, the final report of the Standing Senate Committee on Social Affairs, Science and Technology (2006), a mother whose son has bipolar disorder poignantly shared her concerns regarding the lack of mental health beds within the healthcare system:

> [I]ncarcerating mentally ill people in jails and prisons is cruel, unjust and ineffective. Prisons do not have adequate or appropriate facility resources or medical care to deal with the mentally ill. Poorly trained staff is unable to handle the difficulties of mental illness. The mentally ill suffer from illogical thinking, delusions, auditory hallucinations, paranoia, and severe mood swings. They do not always comprehend the rules of jails and prisons. They are highly vulnerable and prone to bizarre behaviour that prison staff must deal with and inmates must tolerate. (p. 300)

The CPHA (2004) reports that epidemiological studies in the CSC have found high prevalence of mental disorder in inmates, often with two or more coexisting disorders, and higher rates of psychosis, depression, anxiety, and personality disorder when compared to the Canadian population. Over the past 10 years, the number of those with significant mental health problems has doubled in federal correctional institutions. According to the CSC (2008), one of the major challenges they currently have with the changing offender profile is that more than one out of 10 male offenders, and one out of five female offenders, are identified at admission as presenting with mental health problems. Since 1997 they have seen a growth rate of 71% in men, and 61% in women. In a prevalence study of mental illness in inmates in the Ontario correctional facilities, the prevalence of schizophrenia was 4.5%, depression 5.6%, bipolar 5.2%, antisocial personality disorder 4.1%, adjustment disorder 3.4%, anxiety 1.9%, and attention deficit hyperactive disorder 1.5% (total 26.2%) (Brown, Girard, & Mathias, 2006). Although these figures are somewhat lower than those identified by the CSC, the discrepancy is most likely due to how mentally ill inmates are assessed and labelled in Ontario facilities. Similar high prevalence rates are reported in other countries. In a survey of psychiatric morbidity among prisoners in England and Wales, Singleton et al. (1998) report a high prevalence of mental illness and personality disorder in both remanded and sentenced males and females. A more recent study by the U.S. Department of Justice reported that 64% of local jail inmates, 56% of state prisoners, and 45% of federal prisoners have symptoms of serious mental illness (James & Glaze, 2006).

Generally, correctional facilities are not in a position to provide mental healthcare at the same standard as that found within community mental health systems. Indeed, the Office of the Correctional Investigator [OCI] (2006) emphasized that treatment within federal facilities was often non-existent, or unsatisfactory, when compared to the community standard. Subsequently, the OCI has reported that improvements have been made; however, the most recent report (OCI, 2009) highlights that "mental healthcare delivery and related services and supports in federal corrections are perhaps the most serious and pressing issues facing the Service today" (p. 7). Furthermore, the CPHA (2004) highlights the need for more proactive standardized mental health intake assessments rather than reactive, crisis-oriented services. However, the CPHA (2004) also notes that promoting mental health in a correctional setting is challenging at best, as the environment is coercive by definition.

Correctional nurses must conduct mental health assessments on all new admissions, and, moreover, be astute to assessing those who may become mentally ill while incarcerated. Often, those with a mental illness are withdrawn, non-communicative, and suicidal. The nurse requires highly developed assessment and communication skills to elicit data necessary to identify those with mental illness (or mental health problems) and to ensure their safety. It is very important that those with psychosis, or those who have decompensated, are housed in an area where they can be protected from predatory inmates, as those with mental illness can be victimized and/or physically bullied for their medications. Individuals with mental illness are especially vulnerable within correctional systems, due to the pecking order that exists within the prison subculture.

Although policies vary across the country and across jurisdictions, individuals presenting as mentally ill at the time of remand require an advocate to ensure that they move through the justice system as quickly as possible and that appropriate transitional discharge plans are in place; the role of the advocate often falls to the correctional nurse. There is a great opportunity for nurses to work with external community-based organizations in order to meet the treatment and release needs of this vulnerable group. By collaborating with various community agencies, correctional nurses can gain their assistance with the provision of mental health services while the client is in custody and these same agencies can provide the link to their home community upon release. Increasingly, through the administration of community-based treatment and support services, **diversion programs** and policies have been implemented as a way of redirecting individuals with mental illness who come into conflict with the law from the criminal justice system to appropriate mental health services. In general, there are three types of diversion in Canada: pre-arrest and pre-booking diversion; court diversion; and mental health courts (Canadian Population Health Initiative, 2008). Such schemes hold promise for humane treatment and reduced recidivism among this population.

All inmates are assessed for suicidal thoughts and plans on admission, and reassessed throughout their incarceration as necessary. Suicide may be viewed by inmates as the only way to cope with their charges (and/or their sentence), family responsibilities that cannot be met, fear of the actions of fellow inmates, and the living conditions within the correctional facility. For the mentally ill, severity of current psychotic symptoms is related to current risk of suicide (Tandon &

Jibson, 2003). Offenders may be placed on a suicide watch if assessment indicates, and referred to a psychiatrist for further assessment, medication, other treatments, and admission to hospital as necessary.

In most settings, mentally ill inmates are generally supervised 24 hours per day by correctional staff; training and experience varies among this group, and minimal training in mental health theory and practice is often the norm. Even though it is recognized that they are primarily responsible for containment and security, the OCI (2006) has recommended that suitable educational programs should be an integral part of the training of all front-line correctional staff. It is important that correctional staff have the necessary skills to identify those with mental health problems, to provide appropriate supervision, and to make referrals to healthcare accordingly (Appelbaum, 2010). In turn, correctional nurses should be advocating for mental healthcare that is consistent with the community standard. Correctional officers cannot, and should not, be replacing nurses.

The Aging Offender Unfortunately, for an increasing number of Canadians, growing old in prison is a harsh reality; this is a trend also experienced in other Western countries. Individuals over the age of 50 years are among the fastest-growing subgroup found within correctional environments. On average, correctional clients are thought to be 10 to 12 years older physiologically when compared to their chronological age (Beckett, Peternelj-Taylor & Johnson, 2003).

Common physical healthcare needs experienced by this population include cardiovascular disease, pulmonary disorders, diabetes, arthritis, cancer, and Alzheimer's disease and other dementias. The mental health issues most evident in this group include stress, social isolation, depression, and suicide (CPHA, 2004).

Prisons and correctional facilities were never designed for an aging population; subsequently, the increased "greying population" in many facilities has resulted in the need for significant improvements in relation to accommodation planning, program development, palliative care, and reintegration options (OCI, 2006). For many elderly and infirm correctional clients, the fear of dying while imprisoned is a terse reality.

Although the CCRA and various pieces of provincial and territorial legislation provide for *parole or release by exception*, also known as *compassionate release* (often to community-based long-term care facilities), it is rarely utilized, as ongoing fears about community safety, acute bed shortages in long-term care, and the stigma associated with incarceration are factors impacting on placement. The public in general is not interested in having convicted criminals residing in long-term care facilities (regardless of their health status). Encinares (2007) has reported that offenders with dementia are particularly difficult to place in the community. As a result, correctional nurses are responsible for developing and providing services geared specifically to the elderly, including palliative care services (Beckett et al., 2003; Duggleby, 2005).

Women's Issues Women most likely to be incarcerated have grown up in poor communities, have limited education and job skills, are victims as well as perpetrators of crime, and are the primary caregivers for dependent children (Blanchette & Brown, 2006; Fisher & Hatton, 2009; Lewis, 2006). And, like "free" women, they are likely to experience multiple roles such as mother, daughter, wife, sister, and friend (Harner, 2004) and to be responsible for the emotional maintenance of the family unit, even when they are not with their families. The fear of losing custody of their children is an ever-present reality (Canadian Centre on Substance Abuse [CCSA], 2006).

Studies indicate that 50 to 70% of female inmates report physical and/or sexual abuse (Heney & Kristiansen, 2002). Common health concerns experienced by incarcerated women include substance abuse and related sequelae; infectious diseases including HIV, AIDS, and hepatitis B (HBV) and C (HCV); pregnancy-related concerns; gynecological problems; urinary incontinence (especially within the aging population); obesity; and chronic health disorders such as asthma, hypertension, heart disease, and diabetes (Fisher & Hatton, 2009; Maeve, 2003). Blanchette and Brown (2006) report that the mental health needs of women are quantitatively and qualitatively different from their male counterparts. In particular, female offenders experience higher levels of anxiety disorders (including post-traumatic stress disorder), depression, psychopathy, and borderline personality disorder (including self-injurious behaviour), serious mental illness (e.g., schizophrenia and depression), and chronic health disorders. Cloyes, Wong, Latimer, and Abarca (2010) in a recent study addressing recidivism, community tenure, and illness severity for people with serious mental illness (SMI) released from a state prison found that women with SMI were at greater risk for repeated incarceration due to factors related to the intersection of gender and mental disorder.

Reproductive issues require considerable attention for women who are pregnant and incarcerated, and nurses are often thrust into a counselling role regarding the woman's choice and decision making surrounding pregnancy. Nurse-to-nurse collaboration with local hospitals is critical, as hospital nurses are often unaware of the extra security precautions that are required during medical transfers. For example, labour and delivery nurses are not generally accustomed to working with women who are in shackles and accompanied by correctional officers. Following delivery, special provisions must be made so the woman has contact with her child in order to facilitate normal mother–child bonding (Ferszt & Erickson-Owens, 2008; Fogel & Belyea, 2001; Hufft & Peternelj-Taylor, 2008). The mother may require help with parenting skills, and community agencies are often called upon to assist with these skills while the mother is in custody, and again upon her release. If there is a prior history of child abuse, the newborn may be taken into care as per the authority of provincial or territorial child protection services. In such cases, women may need additional support in relation to the grieving process over the loss of their children. Pregnant women who are addicted to opiates and/or are involved in a methadone maintenance program will need to have this program either initiated or continued to prevent damage to the fetus from opiate withdrawal.

Women who are incarcerated are often interested in learning more about their health, including family-planning services. It is not uncommon for nurses in correctional centres to work with community partners in developing programs that focus on the needs of women related to prenatal, birth, and postpartum needs. Furthermore, nurses have been actively involved in the development and implementation of a number of programs including those related to self-harming behaviours (Roth & Pressé, 2003); gender-specific substance abuse treatment (Fortin, 2010); the use of storytelling to enhance health promotion among Aboriginal women (Rowan et al., 2004); and a weight and body image program ("Caring in Corrections," 2010).

Overall, providing safe nursing care to women who are incarcerated requires gender-sensitive strategies and consideration of their vulnerability. Clearly good correctional health-care is good public health. As such, strengthening partnerships with community such as re-entry programs, which include healthcare, housing, parenting, education, and employment are critical (Fisher & Hatton, 2009).

Youth Youth ages 12 to 17 residing in youth centres and youth and adult shared facilities are sentenced under the authority of the Youth Criminal Justice Act (YCJA). More often than not, youth in custody present with significant psychiatric morbidity, and partake in risky behaviours that increase their chances of contacting HIV, hepatitis, and other STIs. These higher rates are often attributed to inadequate coping skills that are common among incarcerated youth (Griel & Loeb, 2009).

Youth in custody frequently present with a variety of symptoms consistent with schizophrenia, anxiety disorders, depression, and behavioural disorders, although they may never have had a formal diagnosis as such (Shelton, 2004). The first episode of schizophrenia may be seen in this age group and needs to be considered by nurses when conducting mental health assessments. Symptom presentation is often more subtle in this age group. For example, the youth may be withdrawn, display an abnormal affect, and demonstrate a minor thought disorder. A suicide assessment of every youth is also necessary since studies have found that 11% of non-incarcerated people with a first episode of psychosis have attempted suicide (Tandon & Jibson, 2003). In addition, youth in custody often experience higher rates of fetal alcohol spectrum disorder, significant substance abuse issues, self-harm, suicidal ideation, and high rates of physical, sexual, and emotional abuse, and many are involved with a child protection agency at the time of their arrest (Latimer & Fosse, 2004).

Canada has had the reputation of incarcerating more youth per capita than any other Western country, even though the YCJA mandates that alternatives to incarceration be considered. However, as noted in the most recent report *Youth Custody and Community Services in Canada, 2008/2009* (Calverley et al., 2010) a reduction in incarceration rates is being realized. Aboriginal youth however, continue to be highly represented in corrections when compared to their non-Aboriginal counterparts. According to the 2006 Census, Aboriginal youth represented approximately 6% of all youth in the Canadian

population, yet 27% of youth remanded in custody, 36% the youth sentenced in custody, and 24% of youth admitt to probation (Calverley, et al., 2010).

Youth require life skills and substance abuse progran plus education in prevention of sexually transmitted disease family planning, and parenting skills. A recent study on th prevalence of HIV and HCV in youth in secure custod found 0% prevalence of HIV and 0.4% of HCV. Howeve many youth reported engaging in risky behaviours: 33.3% injected drugs with a used needle, and 78% engaged in vagi nal or anal intercourse without a condom (Calzavara et al. 2006).

Nurses have to be aware of treatment boundaries and the power inherent within their professional roles (Bunner & Yonge, 2006). A participant in Shelton's (2003) study lamented that "the big problem is when patients get attached to staff. For some kids, this is as good as it gets. In many ways you're the parent this kid wished he had" (p. 49).

Culturally Diverse Offenders The cultural diversity of Canada as a whole is reflected in the demographic profile of Canadian correctional facilities. As in other Western societies, people of colour are over represented within correctional systems. Historically, Aboriginal people have been disproportionately represented in provincial, territorial, and federal correctional systems when compared to their representation in the overall population. In 2007–2008, Aboriginal adults accounted for 22% of those sentenced to custody, even though they represented only 3% of Canada's adult population. Throughout Canada, the number of Aboriginal adults incarcerated exceeds their representation in the general population. For example, in Quebec, Aboriginal offenders are two times more likely than the general population to be incarcerated, while in Saskatchewan, their representation is seven times greater (Perreault, 2009).

The overrepresentation of Aboriginal people within the criminal justice system has been attributed to the commingling of a number of complex factors including rapid culture change, cultural oppression, marginalization, and the long-term effects of the residential schools (Kirmayer et al., 2000), which together have contributed to high rates of poverty, substance abuse, and victimization within families and communities of origin (CSC, 2010). Perreault (2009) further suggests that a lack of a high school diploma and employment contributes to overall incarceration rates particularly in the 20 to 34 age group. The OCI (2009) continues to be critical of the federal government's response to Aboriginal offenders, citing the need for a greater range and variety of Aboriginal-specific programming.

There has been a growing awareness in recent years of the need to provide culturally competent care in all areas of healthcare (Srivastava, 2007); the same can be said for correctional systems. Charles (2010), in a recent article, cautions that "despite the nature of the commitment, nurses must provide culturally competent care" (p. 432). Increasingly, specific cultural practices are incorporated into programming offered within correctional facilities. For example, in collaboration with First Nations, Inuit, and Métis communities, as part of the rehabilitation process, elders, healers, and community leaders often lead traditional activities, including sweet grass ceremonies, smudging, and sweat lodges. Mason (2010) notes that it is important to continue to engage Aboriginal peoples in collaborative dialogue around Aboriginal correctional programming.

COMMON HEALTH CHALLENGES

For many individuals, healthcare received while incarcerated may be the first real opportunity that they have had to address their healthcare needs. Numerous opportunities exist for correctional nurses to provide leadership in the provision of health promotion and illness prevention, especially if individuals are motivated to make lifestyle changes that would improve their overall health status.

Substance Abuse

Substance abuse, including alcohol, nicotine, cocaine, opiates, benzodiazepines, cannabis products, and hallucinogens, is a major problem within correctional systems worldwide, and this problem is no different in Canada, although different levels of the problem are reported. The CPHA (2004) has reported that the majority of federally incarcerated inmates meet criteria for substance or alcohol abuse disorders. Likewise, the CSC (2010) reports that there continues to be a high prevalence of substance abuse within its correctional facilities (80% overall, 95% Aboriginal men, 77% women). The Ontario correctional system has reported that 7.1% of inmates have a definite substance abuse diagnosis (Brown et al., 2006). However, 85% have a substance abuse note on their correctional files, and the severity of withdrawal syndromes varies, requiring nurses to be astute in their assessments and observations regarding how withdrawal is manifested. Furthermore, nurses have to be alert for drug-seeking attempts and differentiate those who are simply trying to manipulate the system from those who legitimately require medications for health-related problems.

Harm reduction, including methadone maintenance treatment (MMT) and prison needle and syringe programs (PNSP), is the most widely accepted approach for dealing with substance abuse in many correctional institutions worldwide (Canadian HIV/AIDS Legal Network, 2008, 2010; Thomas, 2005). These strategies are not only controversial, they are also generally misunderstood by correctional administrators and healthcare professionals alike. From a public health perspective, such programs are both morally and fiscally responsible, and contribute to the protection of the community at large (Canadian HIV/AIDS Legal Network, 2008). To date, no correctional facility in Canada has adopted a PNSP, despite pleas from advocacy groups such as the Canadian HIV/AIDS Legal Network and the Prisoner' HIV/AIDS Support Action Network. Instead, bleach kits, for the purposes of decontaminating injection equipment, are available in some jurisdictions. However, bleach is at best considered a

second-line strategy in the absence of clean needles and syringes, as disinfection alone does not kill all viruses such as HBV and HCV (Canadian HIV/AIDS Legal Network, 2010; National Collaborating Centre for Infectious Diseases [NCCID], 2008; Thomas, 2005).

As of 2002, most Canadian correctional facilities had adopted policies that allowed for the continuation of MMT for those placed in custody while in treatment. And although full access to MMT programs (including initiation and maintenance) has been recommended by both professional and advocacy groups (Registered Nurses Association of Ontario [RNAO], 2009; Canadian HIV/AIDS Legal Network, 2008), to date, many jurisdictions do not allow for the initiation of MMT for those already in custody (Canadian HIV/AIDS Legal Network, 2008; Thomas, 2005). MMT, like other harm-reduction strategies, is controversial. Unfortunately, the lack of understanding among many correctional staff members (including nurses) contributes to the belief that methadone administration simply gives offenders a drug that replaces the illicit drug they were taking prior to arrest. Correctional officers' concerns often stem from the fact that methadone is a highly valued commodity within correctional systems, which can lead to inmate attempts to divert the drug and to bully/muscle other inmates for it. Consequently, the procedure for administration of methadone is tightly supervised, and can be time consuming. Concerns regarding violence and diversion are typically successfully addressed once the MMT program has been established (Canadian HIV/AIDS Legal Network, 2008).

The RNAO (2009) outlines common MMT-related issues that are specific to correctional environments in its recently published clinical best practice guideline *Supporting Clients on Methadone Maintenance Treatment*. Correctional nurses are often challenged with balancing the goals of harm reduction and MMT with the goals of custody, and as such, this best practice guideline is particularly noteworthy as it offers information related to the perceptions of methadone, administration of methadone, discharge/release planning, and related issues specific to correctional environments.

Infectious Diseases

The prevalence of blood borne and sexually transmitted infections and tuberculosis among offender populations is a real concern for correctional authorities. The prevalence of blood borne infections such as HIV, HBV, and HCV are higher in the incarcerated population, primarily as a result of the high-risk behaviours demonstrated by offenders before and during incarceration such as tattooing, ear and body piercing, intravenous drug use, and risky sexual activity.

A CSC study found that in 2000 and 2001 the number of reported infections of hepatitis B in the federal facilities was 13 and 43, respectively. This corresponded to a 0.1% prevalence rate in 2000 and a 0.3% prevalence rate in 2001. The rate in the general population was estimated to be between 0.5% and 1.0% in 2000 (De, 2002). The prevalence of HCV in an Ontario study during 2003 to 2004 was

17.6%. HCV prevalence was 15.9% in adult males and 30.2% in adult females, while HIV prevalence was reported to be 2% (Calzavara et al., 2006). In Ontario, HIV antibody prevalence in provincially held adult female inmates was 1.8%, and 2% in males held provincially. The study concluded that, based on 52 876 admissions per year, one could expect a projected 1097 HIV-positive inmates and 9208 HCV-positive inmates.

The HIV infection rate in federal facilities is 1.7% for males and 4.7% for females (CSC, 2003). However, as in the Canadian population, true prevalence rates are unknown because screening for HIV and other blood borne infections is voluntary. It is estimated that up to 70% of federal inmates remain unscreened. Across the country, incarcerated women have a rate of infection 2.5 times that of men, which raises the question whether this difference is due to an actual higher infection rate, or women request testing more often than men (NCCID, 2008).

The Saskatchewan Ministry of Corrections, Public Safety and Policing will be piloting a one-year opt-out project, whereby female offenders will be informed that an HIV test will be performed as part of their routine medical intake examination unless they decline and choose to opt out of the testing. Modelled after the Centers for Disease Control (2009) HIV testing implementation guidance for correctional settings, this pilot project will be the first of its kind in a Canadian correctional facility, and will bring together the collaborative efforts of community-based organizations and corrections. Nursing will have an integral role in the successful implementation and evaluation of this novel pilot project (S. Bolt, personal communication, June 4, 2010).

In 2004, 53 (0.40%) federal offenders had genital chlamydia, 11 (0.08%) had gonorrhoea, and 10 (0.08%) had syphilis (CSC, 2004). Preliminary unpublished data suggest that in 2008, 131 (1.01%) federal offenders had chlamydia, 9 (0.07%) had gonorrhoea, while 21 (0.16%) cases of syphilis were reported (J. Smith, personal communication, June 10, 2010). The highest rates for reported chlamydia and gonorrhoea infection for both men and women were found in the Prairie Region; the majority of cases of reported syphilis however were found among offenders in Quebec (PHAC & CSC, 2008).

Harm-reduction strategies such as condoms, dental dams, and water-based lubricants are available to offenders who request such products. However, sexual activity between offenders can result in a citation for misconduct. Consequently, they are ambivalent about requesting these products. On one hand, they are being responsible by using a coping mechanism to prevent spread of disease; on the other hand, by merely requesting these products they are risking misconduct. Prisoners HIV/AIDS Support Action Network (PASAN) and other advocacy groups such as the Canadian HIV/AIDS Legal Network further recommend that bleach be freely available and that correctional centres introduce PNSPs (Canadian HIV/AIDS Legal Network, 2010). However, many offenders have charges of drug possession and/or trafficking, and governments are loath to be seen as condoning criminal behaviour. Such harm-reduction programs, although endorsed by the

healthcare community and advocacy groups alike, continue to be deemed controversial and subject to the political whim of governments, as was illustrated in the cancellation of the safe tattooing project that had been piloted in six federal correctional facilities (Canadian Broadcast Corporation, 2006). This is another example where correctional policies (e.g., custody) and healthcare interventions (e.g., caring) often collide.

The prevalence of tuberculosis (TB) infections in previously TB skin test naive or negative inmates in Ontario was 7.5% for the 12 months ending March 2006. Of these, one inmate was diagnosed with active TB (Ferris, personal communication, 2006). The estimated active TB rate among federal offenders is five times higher than in the general population in Canada. In 2004, four cases of incident TB were reported among offenders under the supervision of the CSC (PHAC & CSC, 2008). TB in crowded correctional settings represents a public health challenge worldwide (CPHA, 2004; Centers for Disease Control and Prevention, 2006), and concerns regarding tuberculin skin test conversion among offenders and staff alike are a real concern for provincial, territorial, and federal correctional authorities (PHAC & CSC, 2008).

Nurses are often the first healthcare providers to assess inmates for infectious disease. This assessment is important in case finding and subsequent medical treatment. Nurses also implement infection-control precautions to prevent subsequent infection of staff and other inmates. Health education for inmates and staff on the prevention of infection transmission is a good example of a primary prevention strategy.

In 2003, the Ontario government declared a provincial emergency because of severe acute respiratory syndrome (SARS). At that time, not much was known about the disease and its control or treatment. The strategy from the beginning was to prevent offenders or staff with symptoms of SARS from entering the facilities. As a precaution, restrictions were placed on visits to facilities in the greater Toronto area where SARS cases had been reported. A screening tool was also developed by a group of senior nurse leaders, and correctional nurses in Ontario identified several inmates who required voluntary quarantine as directed by the local public health unit. These inmates were isolated in the province's correctional facilities. Several other inmates, identified with SARS-like symptoms, were sent to hospital and returned to the facility once SARS had been ruled out. As well, several staff members were advised to leave work and consult with public health, Telehealth Ontario, or their family physicians. Approximately 6000 inmates were screened using this tool.

Similarly, in 2009, the pandemic HINI flu virus saw correctional nurses directly involved in the development of policies related to infection prevention and control measures, clinical assessment and management, laboratory testing, antiviral treatment, and outbreak control measures in closed facilities (Public Health Branch, Health Services Sector, 2009). Correctional systems followed Health Canada's guidelines regarding immunization; however, controversies did arise in some jurisdictions when it was discovered that inmates with pre-existing health conditions were immunized before healthy "law-abiding" citizens and correctional staff (Canadian Broadcast Corporation, 2009; Matas, 2009). In total, 56% (8120) of offenders under the jurisdiction of the CSC received the H1N1 vaccine; a total of 51 laboratory-confirmed cases were reported across the CSC between November 2009 and April 2010. Further detailed analysis of data is in progress (J. Smith, personal communication, June 10, 2010).

Correctional Staff and Infectious Diseases Nurses function within a very narrow margin when addressing staff members' "need to know" and inmates' confidentiality. Nurses cannot provide confidential information regarding diagnoses; however, they must educate and inform correctional staff of infection control and other healthcare procedures. The pressure from staff for confidential healthcare information will continue, as will the need for nurses to protect that confidentiality. Most nurses do find a way to provide health education to correctional staff and alleviate some of their work-related stress. For example, nurses can instruct correctional officers regarding the principles of harm reduction; the use of universal precautions, standard practices; airborne, droplet, and direct-contact isolation procedures; and the need for confidentiality in health-related matters.

PRACTICE SETTING

The effects of the correctional environment can be particularly severe, given the interpersonal climate, organizational culture, and social context. The incarceration experience represents a significant, stressful life event, as separation from family and friends, limitations on privacy, overcrowding, and the fear of assault can severely impact the offender's health status and quality of life. Furthermore, power, control, and implicit authority are manifested in the physical and interpersonal environments of correctional systems and can be incompatible with the achievement of health-related treatment goals (Peternelj-Taylor, 2010).

Access to clients can be difficult depending on the mandate of the institution and the clients' specific healthcare needs. For instance, in many correctional facilities, offenders are housed in units with two-person cells and a common day area. Depending on the institution, they may be allowed out of their cells for up to 12 hours per day, and healthcare must be provided within this time frame. In some settings, assessment of health concerns and provision of minor interventions is provided in the living unit, and more complex care is provided in a centralized ambulatory healthcare clinic. In many facilities a correctional officer accompanies the nurse or supervises the nurse for every offender contact, and this officer must maintain visual contact of the offender at all times. And although the nurse respects the officer's security responsibilities, the nurse must maintain client confidentiality while providing health care and eliciting health-related information.

The priorities of the correctional system focus on confinement and security, and matters of security will often take precedence over nursing care. It is not uncommon for nurses to have to wait while the officer completes security-related tasks. And although nurses, as employees of correctional facilities, must abide by the correctional policies that govern all correc-

tional employees, correctional nurses often find themselves in a "catch 22" position as they face the competing tensions enmeshed in their collective responsibilities. Not only are they responsible to the offender, who is their client, they are also responsible to their profession, to the correctional system which is their employer, and to the community at large (Storch & Peternelj-Taylor, 2009). In order to develop therapeutic relationships and provide professional and ethical care, correctional nurses often are faced with confronting their own reactions to offenders' alleged offences, or the crimes for which they have been sentenced. It is also important that they not get caught up in the sensationalism that surrounds a particular offender, or the setting in which nursing practice takes place.

While professional autonomy in practice has often been described as a factor related to job satisfaction in correctional nursing in general ("Caring in Corrections," 2010; Smith, 2005), in practice this often means working alone, and professional isolation is a concern for correctional nursing (Greifinger, 2007; LaMarre, 2006; Shelton, 2009). In some instances, there may only be one registered nurse for as many as 200 offenders, on the day and evening shifts. This large caseload results in nurses having to set priorities based on assessment of individual client needs. In other settings, nursing practice may reflect a more traditional approach to healthcare, for instance in secure treatment facilities operated by provincial, territorial, and federal correctional agencies.

Regardless of the setting, the therapeutic treatment needs of clients must always be considered within the context of maintaining security. For instance, nurses need to be ever vigilant regarding security awareness. This includes **static security**, the structural environmental features common to correctional facilities (e.g., video monitoring, internal barriers, perimeter fences or walls, personal protection alarms, staffing patterns, policies related to counting offenders, and counting equipment), and **dynamic security**, which addresses such things as institutional policies and procedures related to interpersonal security (e.g., developing professional relationships, "knowing" the client in one's care, managing professional boundaries, and methods of operation). Nurses must be attentive to the materials left with clients, as many could be fashioned into weapons; likewise, in some settings, dental floss may be used (and disposed after use) only in the healthcare clinic, rather than being allowed in the client's living area. Nurses working in other community settings certainly understand the need for innovation; nurses working in a correctional setting require similar "thinking outside the box."

COMMUNITY CONNECTION

Increasingly, correctional facilities are being identified as a "public health opportunity" (CSC, 2003). From a public health perspective, the health of the incarcerated population is a reflection of the state of the health of the community at large. Offenders come to prison from the community, and they will return to the community upon their release; in short, correctional health affects public health (NCCID, 2008). Harm-reduction strategies as discussed are recommended for disease prevention and control within correctional facilities, and have direct implications for the community at large, as the majority of those in custody will eventually reintegrate into the community. Attending to the comprehensive needs of this population requires interdisciplinary and intersectoral collaboration between healthcare, criminal justice, education, social services, non-governmental organizations, and the voluntary sector. Such partnerships need to be established, nurtured, and evaluated (Peternelj-Taylor, 2010).

In 2001, Freudenberg challenged practitioners, researchers, and policy makers to ask new research questions, develop new policies, and implement new programs that improve health and social services, emphasize community reintegration efforts, and support alternatives to incarceration. This agenda is still relevant today and continues to address contemporary concerns. Correctional nurses are in key positions to collaborate with the staff in community-based residential facilities, to ensure a safe release for offenders transitioning to the community. Organizations such as the St. Leonard's Society of Canada (and its affiliate members), and other not-for-profit charitable organizations, are excellent resources for correctional nurses as they work with offenders, preparing them for release into the community.

POLICY DEVELOPMENT

Nurses are especially well situated to influence, develop, and change correctional healthcare policies. For example, nurses have played a huge role in initiating and implementing non-smoking policies in many correctional facilities across the country. Through the implementation of this public health initiative, healthier living and work environments have been created for all concerned. Nurses have also been staunch advocates for the development of policies related to infection control courses for delivery in local and regional facilities; prenatal and postnatal program development in women's institutions; resource management (including staffing and scheduling patterns); the introduction of telemedicine and automated external defibrillators; mental healthcare delivery in secure mental health treatment units, and policies regarding palliative care and end-of-life care.

Since the SARS outbreak of 2003, and the emergence of pandemic H1N1 flu virus in North America in 2009, correctional nurses are now at the forefront of policy development in relation to pandemic planning.

PROFESSIONAL DEVELOPMENT AND RESEARCH IN CORRECTIONAL NURSING

Recognition of correctional nursing as a specialized area of nursing practice is critical to the ongoing growth and development of this specialty area. In 2005, the RNAO Correctional

Nurses Interest Group was established by correctional nurses, the first such group in Canada. In 2007, the Forensic Nurses Society of Canada was approved as an emerging special interest group of the Canadian Nurses Association, and represents all forensic nursing specialties, including correctional nursing. However, unlike the American Nurses Association (2007), who publish *Corrections Nursing: Scope and Standards of Practice*, and the Royal College of Nursing (2009), who publish *Health and Nursing Care in the Criminal Justice Service*, comparable formal professional nursing documents that provide guidance and direction to nurses working in Canadian correctional facilities are non-existent.

The ongoing evolution of correctional nursing as a specialty is further dependent on the establishment of a nursing culture that supports and nurtures the development of nursing research. And although correctional nursing has undergone significant transformations in professional role development in recent years, the professional literature remains largely anecdotal as correctional environments have attracted very few nurse researchers (Peternelj-Taylor, 2005). This has resulted in a severe scarcity of research in correctional nursing in Canada and elsewhere, even though a goldmine of research opportunities exists within correctional environments. Freudenberg (2007), in discussing a research agenda for correctional health, has declared that "correctional research has to be considered a branch of population health research and therefore address the broadest questions that affect the health of the public" (Freundenberg, 2007, p. 429).

Nursing has a pivotal research role to play in the correctional milieu, both in the translation and interpretation of research relevant to incarcerated populations and in the identification of important nursing research questions that emerge from practice. There are unique issues with this population, for example ensuring that consent is free, informed, and given without expectation of special favours. Therefore, guidelines are in place that clearly prevent the offer of privileges, early release, or favourable parole assessments in return for participation in a research study during incarceration (Peternelj-Taylor, 2005).

Since 1989, the College of Nursing, University of Saskatchewan, in collaboration with the Regional Psychiatric Centre (Prairies), Correctional Service of Canada, has sponsored a biennial nursing conference that showcases the unique contributions nurses make to healthcare within the criminal justice system. This international forum provides opportunities for clinical practitioners, educators, administrators, researchers, and policy makers to learn about matters of interest to correctional nurses. Additionally, correctional environments are being selected more frequently as community and mental health placements for senior nursing students.

Embracing a research agenda with incarcerated populations will provide new insights into nursing practice in this domain. Canadian Research Boxes 25.1 and 25.2 highlight two recent Canadian projects.

CANADIAN RESEARCH BOX

What health promotion and literacy needs are identified for women in conflict with the law?

Hall, J., & Donelle, L. (2009). Research with women serving court-mandated probation of parole orders. *Canadian Journal of Nursing Research, 41*(2), 36–53.

The authors reported the results of a pilot study exploring the health promotion and health literacy needs of women in conflict with the law. They also discuss the challenges that occurred as a result of the research. Twelve women, ranging in age from 25 to 45, agreed to participate. They completed a demographic survey, two health literacy assessments, and were interviewed on health promotion and literacy issues. The researchers note that three themes emerged from the data:

- perception that the participants' health was influenced by others (such as people being judgmental);
- participant access to health information (such as community clinic or specialized health services for vulnerable populations); and
- recommended changes to the healthcare system (such as outreach to ask them questions and to see what their needs are).

Unfortunately, these were not discussed for the reader. Rather, this research article focuses on the challenges experienced by the researchers that affected and influenced the research process during this pilot study.

Four challenges are summarized and discussed:

- participant recruitment, which required shifting strategies due to some resistance experienced by community workers;
- methods of data collection and how they tackled issues to do with time, space, and place (as related to the transient nature of the study population);
- the physical and emotional safety of the research team and the participants; and
- professional and personal tensions, particularly in relation to research team members witnessing activities or disclosures that had the potential to cause legal, ethical, or moral tensions, while at the same time.

From the issues they encountered, recommendations for future research with women offenders are made in relation to the careful consideration to the research setting that is selected (e.g., selecting closed custody vs. open custody in the community); the method of data collection (with body mapping and photo voice being proposed as additional data collection strategies); and how community collaborators are engaged (e.g., working with a community advisory committee).

Discussion Questions

1. Offenders are considered a vulnerable population. Are there other vulnerable populations to which this research may apply?
2. How might a nurse use the information gleaned from this study to address future research projects with women offenders?

CANADIAN RESEARCH BOX

What are the STI issues identified by inmates?

Zakaria, D., Thompson, J. M., Jarvis, A., & Borgatta, F. (2010, March). *Summary of emerging findings from the 2007 national inmate infectious diseases and risk-behaviours survey.* Ottawa, ON: Correctional Service of Canada.

The results of the 2007 National Inmate Infectious Diseases and Risk Behaviours Survey (NIIDRBS), a 50-page self-administered questionnaire, completed by a large sample of federal offenders ($n = 3370$) serving time under the jurisdiction of the Correctional Service of Canada (CSC), are reported. The study was designed to gain information from offenders on issues relevant to blood-borne sexually transmitted infections (BBSTIs), particularly HIV and HCV, based upon the past six months in prison. The major findings of the study illustrate that:

- The proportion of offenders reporting high-risk drug- and sex-related risk behaviours significantly declined in prison compared to the community. However, 34% of men and 25% of women continued to use non-injection drugs, 17% of men and 14% of women injected drugs, and 17% of men and 31% of women had oral, vaginal, or anal sex. Men were more likely to report risky injection practices, while women reported risky sexual behaviour.
- Offenders' awareness of how to access harm-reduction items was high, and those reporting risky sexual and injecting behaviour were associated with an increased demand for harm reduction items, suggesting that harm reduction items are being utilized as intended. Sexually active offenders (57%) reported an attempt to get condoms, lubricant, and/or dental dams; 87% reported awareness of available bleach, and the majority of offenders who reported injection drug use, being tattooed, and/or being pierced reported using bleach to clean the equipment.
- Opportunities were identified to improve the care of HIV-positive offenders, particularly in relation to (1) transmission pathways and CSC's policies regarding privacy, confidentiality, and discrimination; and (2) treatment interruptions. Overall, 67% worried about discrimination, while of those who started treatment, 60% reported past treatment interruptions.

- Inmate knowledge of HIV and HCV in regard to modes of transmission, prevention, testing, and treatment revealed some deficiencies: 21% of respondents were unaware that there is no cure for HIV. Overall, offenders were more knowledgeable about HIV compared to their knowledge of HCV.
- A substantial proportion of inmates were tested for HIV (71% men, 85% women) and HCV (74% men, 83% women) during their most recent incarceration with CSC. Of those ever tested, 4.6% (4.5% men, 7.9% women) reported being HIV-positive, while 31% (30.8% men, 37% women) reported being HCV-positive. Aboriginal women were identified as a particularly high-risk group, as they reported the highest rates of HIV (11.7%) and HCV (49.1%). Of those not tested, the most frequently reported reason was not being offered the test.
- Although not possible to attribute reported infections since admission to risk behaviours in the correctional environment, rates of self-reported infections since admission to CSC institutions were explored. The number of self-reported HIV cases was too few to examine (< 5). The HCV infection rate among men was 16 per 1000 (or 1.6%). Women were 4.5 times more likely to report an STI since admission.

While the authors identify some limitations to the study, such as the complexity and length of the questionnaire, measurement error, and social desirability bias, they conclude that greater knowledge has been associated with behaviours that could ultimately reduce the transmission of HIV and HCV, and efforts to increase offender knowledge should continue. Risky sexual behaviour and injecting practices are modifiable; therefore, continued education and awareness campaigns emphasizing use of harm reduction items are key prevention strategies. Examination of the findings suggest many implications for clinical practice including increasing awareness of health education programs; promoting screening and testing throughout incarceration; and ensuring culturally sensitive and appropriate interventions designed to decrease risk behaviours and increase harm-reducing behaviours.

Finally, the authors report that future analyses will address factors associated with in-prison drug use, sexual activity, and testing for HIV/HCV. However, the question of why inmates continue to engage in risky behaviours despite adequate knowledge and availability of harm-reduction items remains unanswered in this study and requires additional research.

Discussion Questions

1. How might a correctional nurse or community health nurse use the information gleaned in this study when implementing health promotion programs for incarcerated persons?
2. Despite their availability, many offenders choose not to use harm-reduction items. How might this information be utilized in practice? What are the policy implications?

CASE STUDY

An 18-year-old male is admitted to a local detention centre, charged with the sexual assault of a child. On assessment, you find that he is quiet, has difficulty establishing eye contact, and simply answers "yes" or "no" to most questions asked. His affect is incongruent with the topic under discussion. He tells you he has been smoking three joints per day for the last year. The police call and want to know his HIV, HBV, and HCV status, as the victim's family wants their child treated if such a risk is present.

Discussion Questions

1. What are your thoughts and feelings about this young man? The child? The child's family?
2. What might you do to work through your feelings in order to provide care for your client?
3. What might your working nursing diagnosis be? What other data would you need to collect?
4. How would you respond to the request for information regarding the inmate's HIV, HBV, and HCV status?

SUMMARY

Correctional nursing, as a specialty area of practice, has undergone significant transformations in role development in recent years. Accepting the challenge to provide nursing care in environments where healthcare delivery is not the primary goal can lead to a myriad of personal and professional issues for nurses. Correctional nursing is collaborative and interdisciplinary by its very nature; the most successful healthcare outcomes are achieved when nurses and correctional officers share a common vision, one of professionalism in the provision of security and quality nursing care to those in custody (Hufft & Kite, 2003).

KEY TERMS

correctional nursing, p. 390
criminalization of the mentally ill, p. 391
diversion programs, p. 392
static security, p. 397
dynamic security, p. 397

REVIEW QUESTIONS

1. Responsibility for health services for individuals who have come into conflict with the law in Canada fall under the jurisdiction of the
   a) Canada Health Act.
   b) Corrections and Conditional Release Act.

c) Provincial or Territorial Mental Health Act.

d) Canadian Public Health Act.

2. In the Canadian correctional population the precise prevalence of infectious diseases such as HIV, HVB, and HVC is not known because

a) authorities do not have the resources to screen upon admission.

b) testing for infectious diseases is on a voluntary basis only.

c) authorities do not want individuals to be stigmatized as a result of testing.

d) harm reduction strategies are not in place in all institutions.

3. Safety and security are major concerns in controlled environments, and security awareness training prepares nurses to work with both the static and dynamic security systems. Dynamic security systems are best described as

a) policies, staffing patterns, and methods of operation.

b) video monitoring, locked units, security personnel.

c) security orientation, key control, personal portable alarms.

d) monitoring contraband, perimeter fences, locked doors.

4. Maggie, an RN who works on a sex offender treatment unit views prevention as integral to her correctional nursing role. An example of her role in primary prevention is

a) conducting a relapse prevention group for the clients in the sexual offender treatment program.

b) developing a medication management program for the clients also diagnosed with a mental disorder.

c) applying principles of crisis intervention following any suicide attempts made during treatment.

d) participating in a community-based committee whose focus is interpersonal violence.

5. Mr. Martino, 65 years of age, is found guilty of committing manslaughter and sentenced to 10 years in a federal penitentiary. Shortly after his transfer to Saskatchewan Penitentiary, he is diagnosed with cancer of the liver. His physical health deteriorates very quickly, and the treatment team recommends that he be transferred to a long-term care facility. In Canada application would be made for

a) probation. c) clemency.

b) medical leave. d) parole by exception.

STUDY QUESTIONS

1. What are the nursing implications associated with the implementation of a methadone maintenance (MMT) program within a correctional facility?

2. Discuss the reasons why correctional nurses often find themselves in a "catch 22" position when working with offenders in correctional settings.

3. Identify and briefly discuss the common healthcare challenges encountered by incarcerated women.

4. What knowledge, skills, and abilities do nurses need to possess to be successful in their work in secure environments?

5. Increasingly, correctional facilities are being identified as a "public health opportunity." Discuss.

6. What issues need to be considered when implementing harm-reduction strategies in correctional facilities, such as the distribution of condoms, dental dams, water-based lubricants, and having bleach accessible?

After working through these questions, go to the MyNursingLab at www.pearsoned.ca/mynursinglab to check your answers.

INDIVIDUAL CRITICAL THINKING EXERCISES

1. What types of assessment tools would you need to assess inmates for their most prevalent health problems?

2. What information would you give to a correctional officer when asked what an inmate's positive TB skin test means?

3. Define "vulnerability" within the context of nursing research. How is this definition relevant to individuals who are incarcerated? What guidelines exist to protect correctional clients as research participants?

4. What would be the advantage of having standards for practice for Canadian nurses who work in correctional facilities?

5. If you were a correctional nurse in your community, what community-based organizations and resources would you collaborate with in meeting the needs of offenders in your care?

GROUP CRITICAL THINKING EXERCISES

1. What is the role of the nurse in advocating for individuals with mental illness who find themselves in conflict with the justice system?

2. In comparison to other Western countries, Canadian statistics regarding youth incarceration, especially youth of Aboriginal ancestry, are particularly alarming. What factors contribute to this phenomenon in Canada?

3. Nurses who chose to work in correctional environments are often asked the following questions: "Why would you want to work there?" "How can you stand working with those criminals?" "Aren't you afraid of getting hurt?" What are your initial thoughts about these questions? What do you think is behind such questions?

REFERENCES

American Nurses Association. (2007). *Corrections nursing: Scope and standards of practice.* Silver Spring, MD: Author.

Appelbaum, K. L. (2010). The mental health professional in a correctional culture. In C. L. Scott (Ed.), *Handbook of correctional mental health* (2nd ed.). Washington, DC: American Psychiatric Publishing.

Beattie, K. (2006). Adult correctional services in Canada, 2004/2005. *Juristat, 26*(5) (Catalogue No: 85-002 XIE). Ottawa, ON: Canadian Centre for Justice Statistics.

Beckett, J., Peternelj-Taylor, C., & Johnson, R. (2003). Growing old in the correctional system. *Journal of Psychosocial Nursing and Mental Health Services, 41*(9), 12–18.

Blanchette, K., & Brown, S. L. (2006). *The assessment and treatment of women offenders: An integrative perspective.* Chichester, UK: John Wiley & Sons.

Brown, G., Girard, L., & Mathias, K. (2006, June). *Identifying the psychiatric care needs of adult offenders in the Ontario correctional system.* Paper presented at the 20th Annual Mental Health Centre, Penetanguishene Forensic Conference: Mentally disordered offenders: What have we learned in 20 years? Penetanguishene, ON.

Bunner, K., & Yonge, O. (2006). Boundaries and adolescents in residential treatment settings: What clinicians need to know. *Journal of Psychosocial Nursing and Mental Health Services, 44*(9), 38–44.

Calverley, D., Cotter, A., & Halla, E. (2010). Youth custody and community services in Canada, 2008/2009. *Juristat, 30*(1) (Statistics Canada Catalogue No. 85-002-X). Ottawa, ON: Canadian Centre for Justice Statistics.

Calzavara, L., Burchell, A., Meyers, T., Swantee, C., Feron, M., Ford, P., et al. (2006). *Prevalence and risk factors for HIV and hepatitis C in Ontario's jails and detention centres (2003–2004).* Toronto, ON: University of Toronto Press.

Canadian Broadcast Corporation. (2006, December 4). *Prison tattoo parlours get the axe.* Retrieved from http://www.cbc.ca/canada/story/2006/12/04/tattooprogram.html

Canadian Broadcast Corporation. (2009, November 5). Inmates should get priority H1N1 shots: Advocates. *The Canadian Press.* Retrieved from http://www.cbc.ca/canada/montreal/story/2009/11/05/que-prisoners-h1n1-shot.html

Canadian Centre on Substance Abuse. (2006). *Fact sheet: Self harm among criminalized women.* Retrieved from http://www.ccsa.ca/NR/rdonlyres/6EC2EA26-D953-4E82-AC09-A1B9BEF7DAC1/0/ccsa0113382006e.pdf

Canadian HIV/AIDS Legal Network. (2008). *Opioid substitution therapy in prisons: Reviewing the evidence.* Canadian HIV/AIDS Legal Network. Retrieved from http://www.aidslaw.ca/publications/publicationsdocEN.php?ref=163

Canadian HIV/AIDS Legal Network. (2010). *Under the skin: A people's case for prison needle and syringe programs.* Retrieved from http://www.aidslaw.ca/publications/publicationsdocEN.php?ref=1014

Canadian Institute for Health Information. (2008). *Improving the health of Canadians: Mental health, delinquency and criminal activity.* Ottawa, ON: Author.

Canadian Population Health Initiative. (2008). *Improving the health of Canadians: Mental health, delinquency and criminal activity.* Ottawa, ON: Author. Retrieved from http://secure.cihi.ca/cihiweb/dispPage.jsp?cw_page=PG_1250_E&cw_topic=1250&cw_rel=AR_1730_E

Canadian Public Health Association. (2004). A health care needs assessment of federal inmates. *Canadian Journal of Public Health, 95*(supplement 1), S1–S63.

Centers for Disease Control and Prevention. (2006, July). Prevention and control of tuberculosis in correctional and detention facilities: Recommendations from CDC. *Morbidity and Mortality Weekly Report, 55*(RR-9), 1–64.

Centers for Disease Control and Prevention. (2009, January). *HIV testing implementation guidance for correctional settings.* Retrieved from http://www.cdc.gov/hiv/topics /testing/resources/guidelines/correctional-settings/

Charles, C. E. (2010). Providing culturally competent care for the criminally insane inmate. *Issues in Mental Health Nursing, 31,* 432–434.

Cloyes, K., Wong, B., Latimer, S., & Abarca, J. (2010). Women, serious mental illness and recidivism: A gender-based analysis of recidivism risk for women with SME released from prison. *Journal of Forensic Nursing, 6,* 3–14.

Correctional Service Canada. (2003). *Infectious diseases prevention and control in Canadian federal penitentiaries 2000–01* (Cat. No. 0-662-67144-9). Ottawa, ON: Author.

Correctional Service Canada. (2008). *2008–2009 Report on plan and priorities.* Ottawa, ON: Minister of Public Works and Government Services.

Correctional Service Canada. (2010, March). *Issues and challenges facing CSC.* Retrieved from http://www.csc-scc.gc.ca/text/pblct/sb-go/pdf/7-eng.pdf

De, P. (2002). Infectious diseases in Canadian federal penitentiaries. *Forum on Corrections Research, 14*(2), 15–19.

Duggleby, W. (2005). Fostering hope in incarcerated older adults. *Journal of Psychosocial Nursing and Mental Health Services, 43*(9), 15–20.

Encinares, M. (2007). Community care of elderly offenders with dementia. *Journal of Chinese Clinical Medicine, 21*(1), 34–41.

Ferszt, G. G., & Erickson-Owens, D. A. (2008). Development of an educational support group for pregnant women in prison. *Journal of Forensic Nursing, 4,* 55–60.

Fisher, A. A., & Hatton, D. C. (2009). Women prisoners: Health issues and nursing implications. *Nursing Clinics of North America, 44*(3), 365–373.

Fogel, C. I., & Belyea, M. (2001). Psychosocial risk factors in pregnant inmates: A challenge for nursing. *American Journal of Maternal Child Nursing, 26*(1), 10–16.

Fortin, D. (2010, March). Correctional programs for women offenders. *Let's Talk, 34*(2), 11.

Freudenberg, N. (2001). Jails, prisons, and the health of urban populations: A review of the impact of the correctional system on community health. *Journal of Urban Health: Bulletin of the New York Academy of Medicine, 78*(2), 214–235.

Freudenberg, N. (2007). Health research behind bars: A brief guide to research in jails and prisons. In R. Greifinger (Ed.), *Public health behind bars: From prisons to communities.* New York, NY: Springer.

Greifinger, R. B. (2007). Thirty years since *Estelle v Gamble*: Looking forward, not wayward. In R. B. Greifinger (Ed.), *Public health behind bars: From prisons to communities.* New York, NY: Springer.

Griel, L. C., & Loeb, S. J. (2009). Health issues faced by adolescents incarcerated in the juvenile justice system. *Journal of Forensic Nursing, 5,* 162–179.

Harner, H. M. (2004). Relationships between incarcerated women: Moving beyond stereotypes. *Journal of Psychosocial Nursing, 42*(1), 38–46.

Heney, J., & Kristiansen, C. (2002). *Working with women in conflict with the law: A trainers' guide.* Toronto, ON: Ministry of Public Safety and Security.

Hufft, A., & Kite, M. M. (2003). Vulnerable and cultural perspectives for nursing care in correctional systems. *The Journal of Multicultural Nursing and Health, 9*(1), 18–26.

Hufft, A., & Peternelj-Taylor, C. (2008). Ethical care of pregnant adolescents in correctional settings. *Journal of Forensic Nursing, 4,* 94–96.

Hume, L. (2004). A gender specific substance abuse program for federally sentenced women. *Forum on Corrections Research, 16*(1), 40–41.

James, D. J., & Glaze, L. E. (2006, September). Mental health problems of prison and jail inmates. *Bureau of Justice Statistics Special Report.* U.S. Department of Justice, Office of Justice Programs. Retrieved from http://www.ojp.usdoj.gov/bjs/pub/pdf/mhppji.pdf

Kirmayer, L. J., Brass, G. M., & Tait, C. L. (2000). The mental health of Aboriginal peoples: Transformations of identity and community. *Canadian Journal of Psychiatry, 45*(7), 607–616.

LaMarre, M. (2006). Nursing role and practice in correctional facilities. In M. Puisis (Ed.), *Clinical practice in correctional medicine* (2nd ed., pp. 417–418). Philadelphia, PA: Mosby Elsevier.

Landry, L., Sinha, M., & Beattie, K. (2008). Adult correctional services in Canada, 2005/2006. *Juristat, 28*(6) (Catalogue No. 85-002-X). Ottawa, ON: Canadian Centre for Justice Statistics.

Latimer, J., & Fosse, L. C. (2004, February). *A one-day snapshot of aboriginal youth in custody across Canada: Phase II.* Department of Justice Canada. Retrieved from http://www.justice.gc.ca/en/ps/rs/rep/2004/snap2/index.html

Lewis, C. (2006). Treating incarcerated women: Gender matters. *Psychiatric Clinics of North America, 29,* 773–789.

Maeve, K. M. (2003). Nursing care partnerships with women leaving jail: Effects on health and crime. *Journal of Psychosocial Nursing and Mental Health Services, 41*(9), 30–40.

Magnall, J., & Yurkovich, E. (2010). A grounded theory exploration of deliberate self-harm in incarcerated women. *Journal of Forensic Nursing, 6,* 88–95.

Mason, R. (2020, March). Aboriginal correctional programs. *Let's Talk, 34*(2), 10.

Matas, R. (2009, October 26). B.C. Inmates to receive flu vaccine before prison staff. *The Globe and Mail.* Retrieved from http://www.theglobeandmail.com/news/national/british-columbia/bc-inmates-to-receive-flu-vaccine-before-prison-staff/article1339295/

Milligan, S. (2008). Youth custody and community services in Canada, 2005/06. *Juristat, 28*(8) (Statistics Canada Catalogue No. 85-002 X). Ottawa, ON: Canadian Centre for Justice Statistics.

National Collaborating Centre for Infectious Diseases. (2008, April). *Primary HIV prevention interventions in prisons and upon release.* Retrieved from http://www.nccid.ca/en/files/Evidence_reviews/HIV_Prevention_in_Prison_Eng_2008_04_18.pdf

Office of the Correctional Investigator. (2006). *Annual report of the Office of the Correctional Investigator 2005–2006* (No. PS100-2006). Ottawa, ON: Minister of Public Works and Government Services Canada. Retrieved from http://www.oci-bec.gc.ca/rpt/pdf/annrpt/annrpt20052006-eng.pdf

Office of the Correctional Investigator. (2009). *Annual report of the Office of the Correctional Investigator 2008–2009* (No. PS100-2009). Ottawa, ON: Her Majesty the Queen in Right of Canada. Retrieved from http://www.ocibec.gc.ca/rpt/pdf/annrpt/annrpt20082009-eng.pdf

Perreault, S. (2009, July). The incarceration of Aboriginal people in adult correctional services. *Juristat, 29*(3) (Catalogue no. 85-002-x). Ottawa, ON: Canadian Centre for Justice Studies.

Peternelj-Taylor, C. (2005). Conceptualizing nursing research with offenders: Another look at vulnerability. *International Journal of Law and Psychiatry, 28,* 348–359.

Peternelj-Taylor, C. (2008). Criminalization of the mentally ill. *Journal of Forensic Nursing, 4*(4), 185–187.

Peternelj-Taylor, C. (2010). Forensic psychiatric and mental health nursing. In W. Austin & M. A. Boyd (Eds.), *Psychiatric nursing for Canadian practice* (2nd ed., pp. 835–849). Philadelphia, PA: Lippincott, Williams & Wilkins.

Public Health Agency of Canada & the Correctional Service of Canada. (2008*). Infectious Disease Surveillance in Canadian Federal Penitentiaries 2002–2004.* Retrieved from http://www.csc-scc.gc.ca/text/pblct/infectiousdiseases02-04/index-eng.shtml#tphp

Public Health Branch, Health Services Sector. (2009). *CSC interim guidance for managing seasonal influenza and novel influenza viruses including Pandemic (H1N1) 2009* (Version 3).

Registered Nurses Association of Ontario. (2009). *Supporting clients on methadone maintenance treatment.* Toronto, ON: Author. Retrieved from http://www.rnao.org/Storage/58/5254_BPG_Managing_Methadone_Treatment.pdf

Roth, B., & Pressé, L. (2003). Nursing interventions for parasuicidal behaviors in female offenders. *Journal of Psychosocial Nursing and Mental Health Services, 41*(9), 20–29.

Rowan, J., Auger, S., Toto, H., Simpson, S., & McNab, C. (2004). The use of stories for healing interventions with women. *Forum on Corrections Research, 16*(1), 42–44.

Royal College of Nursing. (2009). *Health and nursing care in the criminal justice service.* London, UK: Author. Retrieved from http://www.rcn.org.uk/__data/assets/pdf_file/0010/248725/003307.pdf

Shelton, D. (2003). The clinical practice of juvenile forensic psychiatric nurses. *Journal of Psychosocial Nursing and Mental Health Services, 41*(9), 43–53.

Shelton, D. (2004). Experiences of detained young offenders in need of mental health care. *Journal of Nursing Scholarship, 36*(2), 129–133.

Shelton, D. (2009). Forensic nursing in secure environments. *Journal of Forensic Nursing, 5,* 131–142.

Singleton, N., Meltzer, H., Gatward, R., Coid, J., & Deasy, D. (1998). *Psychiatric morbidity among prisoners in England and Wales*. London, UK: The Stationery Office.

Smith, S. (2005, February). Stepping through the looking glass: Professional autonomy in correctional nursing. *Corrections Today, 54–56*, 70.

Srivastava, R. H. (2007). Understanding cultural competence in health care. In R. H. Srivastava (Ed.), *The healthcare professional's guide to clinical cultural competence* (pp. 3–27). Toronto, ON: Mosby Elsevier.

Standing Senate Committee on Social Affairs, Science and Technology. (2006, May). *Out of the shadows at last: Transforming mental health, mental illness and addiction services in Canada*. Retrieved from http://www.parl.gc.ca/39/1/parlbus/commbus/senate/com-e/soci-e/rep-e/rep02may06-e.htm

Storch, J., & Peternelj-Taylor, C. (2009). Ethics for health care providers: Codes as guidance for practice in prisons. In D. Hatton & A. Fisher (Eds.), *Women prisoners and health justice* (pp. 109–116). Oxford, UK: Radcliffe.

Tandon, R., & Jibson, M. D. (2003). Suicidal behavior in schizophrenia: Diagnosis, neurobiology and treatment implications. *Current Opinion in Psychiatry, 16*(2), 193–197.

Thomas, G. (2005). Harm reduction policies and programs for persons involved in the criminal justice system. *Harm reduction for special populations in Canada*. Canadian Centre on Substance Abuse. Retrieved from http://www.ccsa.ca/NR/rdonlyres/B092A5D6-C627-4503-8F21-8A1AB8923B3A/0/ccsa0039002005.pdf

Williams, N. H. (2007). Prison health and the health of the public: Ties that bind. *Journal of Correctional Health Care, 13*(2), 80–92.

ADDITIONAL RESOURCES

Websites

Canadian Association of Elizabeth Fry Societies
http://www.elizabethfry.ca

Canadian HIV/AIDS Legal Network
http://www.aidslaw.ca

Children and Youth: Crime Prevention through Social Development
http://www.ccsd.ca/cpsd/ccsd/index.htm

Correctional Service Canada
http://www.csc-scc.gc.ca

Corrections and Conditional Release Act
http://www.laws.justice.gc.ca/eng/acts/C-44.6/index.html

Custody and Caring: International Conference on the Nurse's Role in the Criminal Justice System
http://www.usask.ca/nursing/custodycaring/index.php

Forensic Nurses Society of Canada
http://www.forensicnurse.ca/

Human Rights Watch
http://www.hrw.org

John Howard Society of Canada
http://www.johnhoward.ca

Ministry of Community Safety and Correctional Services (Ontario)
http://www.mcscs.jus.gov.on.ca/English/english_default.html

National Commission on Correctional Health Care
http://www.ncchc.org

Office of the Correctional Investigator
http://www.oci-bec.gc.ca/index-eng.aspx

Prisoners' HIV/AIDS Support Action Network
http://www.pasan.org

Registered Nurses' Association of Ontario Correctional Nurses Interest Group
http://www.rnao.org/Page.asp?PageID=122&ContentID=1452&SiteNodeID=113&BL_ExpandID=

Royal College of Nurses Nursing in Criminal Justice Forum
http://www.rcn.org.uk/development/communities/rcn_forum_communities/prison_nurses

St Leonard's Society of Canada
http://www.stleonards.ca/?s=announcements&p=currentannouncements

Youth Criminal Justice Act
http://www.laws.justice.gc.ca/en/Y-1.5/

About the Authors

Cindy Peternelj-Taylor, RN, MSc, DF-IAFN (University of Saskatchewan), is a Professor with the College of Nursing, University of Saskatchewan, and a Distinguished Fellow—International Association of Forensic Nurses. She is a graduate of Lakehead University and the University of Saskatchewan and is currently completing doctoral studies with the University of Alberta. Much of Cindy's career has focused on professional role development for nurses who work with vulnerable populations in forensic psychiatric and correctional settings. She is a member of the Editorial Board of the *Journal of Psychiatric and Mental Health Nursing* and is the Editor-in-Chief, *Journal of Forensic Nursing*. Her current research explores the lived experience of engagement with forensic patients in secure environments.

Phil Woods, RPN, PhD (Anglia Polytechnic University), is a Professor and Associate Dean Research, Innovation and Global Initiatives, with the College of Nursing, University of Saskatchewan. He trained as a mental health nurse in the United Kingdom and is a registered psychiatric nurse in Saskatchewan. Phil has a PhD in Nursing Studies. He has an extensive personal portfolio of forensic-related research and is a well-known author of mental health and forensic nursing articles and books. His specific research interests are risk assessment and management, violence prediction, and developing mental health and forensic mental health practice. Phil is currently undertaking research projects involving Saskatchewan psychiatric acute units, forensic units, and correctional institutions in relation to violence prediction and risk assessment and management.

chapter

Violence in Societies

Margaret M. Malone

26

OBJECTIVES

After studying this chapter, you should be able to:

1. Analyze critically the concepts of violence and societal violence and their implications for women, children, youth, and seniors.

2. Examine the health and social costs of violence, especially for marginalized and/or at-risk populations.

3. Explore critical social theories and approaches to societal violence.

4. Scrutinize current debates about 'universal screening' and 'case finding' for intimate partner violence within the context of community health nursing.

5. Develop ethical and culturally safe health-promoting strategies to address violence for individuals, families, groups, communities, and societies.

6. Discuss the role of the community health nurses in eliminating violence in society locally, nationally, and globally.

INTRODUCTION

Violence is a major public health and social justice problem of epidemic proportion in Canada and globally. Moreover, violence is a multi-faceted problem with biological, psychological, emotional, social, economic, political, cultural, and environmental roots. The World Health Organization (WHO) (2002a) states, "Violence is a universal scourge that tears at the fabric of communities and threatens the life, health, and happiness of all of us" (p. 1).

WHO (2002b) defines **violence** as:

> The intentional use of physical force or power, threatened or actual, against oneself, another person, or against a group or community, that either results in or has a high likelihood of resulting in injury, death, psychological harm, maldevelopment or deprivation. (p. 5)

Importantly, WHO (2002b) definition includes the word "power" in addition to the phrase "use of physical force." The inclusion of power helps to expand the dominant societal understanding of violence to "include acts that result from a power relationship, including threats and intimidation" (p. 5). Including power also draws attention to less visible forms of violence, such as "neglect" and "omission."

However, as can be seen in its Declaration on the Elimination of Violence Against Women, the United Nations General Assembly (UN) (1993) clearly moves beyond individual victim blaming to focus on underlying root causal factors within social, political, economic, and cultural contexts.

The term **"violence against women"** means any act of gender-based violence that results in, or is likely to result in, physical, sexual, or psychological harm or suffering to women, including threats of such acts, coercion, or arbitrary deprivation of liberty, whether occurring in public or in private life (UN, p. 2).

Moreover, the UN Declaration states that violence against women encompasses, but is not limited to, physical, sexual, and psychological violence within the family and the community, and by states. These include

- spousal battering.
- sexual abuse of female adults and children.
- dowry-related violence.
- rape, including marital rape.
- female genital mutilation and other traditional practices harmful to women.
- non-spousal violence.
- violence through exploitation.
- sexual harassment and intimidation in workplaces, educational institutions, and elsewhere.
- forced prostitution and trafficking.
- violence perpetrated or condoned by states, e.g., rape in war.

Community health nurses (CHNs) are frequently the first members of health-care teams to encounter individuals experiencing violence and abuse. Moreover, CHNs are strategically located within communities where assessment, intervention, prevention, and health promoting initiatives can be developed, researched, implemented, and evaluated. However, while there are significant "expectations for an active and consistent response by healthcare professionals to women experiencing the effects of violence," these expectations "may not match the realities of professional preparation" (Wathen et al. (2009, p. 1). Furthermore, given the prevalence of violence, especially violence directed at women, female children, and youth, some professional nursing organizations in Canada and the United States "recommend that health-care support staff routinely ask all female patients" (Jack, Jamieson, Wathen, & MacMillah, 2008, p. 152) who enter the health-care system about their exposure to intimate partner violence (IPV)—"a procedure referred to as universal screening" (p. 152).

However, the context of CHNs' home visits, e.g., postpartum, is very different from clinical and other institutional settings (Jack et al., 2008). It is important to differentiate between 'screening' and 'case-finding,' the latter being part of an in-depth nursing assessment often conducted over multiple visits. In this instance, "questions about IPV are posed in any assessment of clients who show signs or symptoms of abuse" (p. 165).

This chapter outlines some of the statistics regarding the ongoing violence in our societies; analyzes critically who is often missing and/or less visible in statistics, drawing attention to people who are marginalized, socially excluded, and/or at risk; and considers the detrimental physical, mental, cultural, and social health effects of violence. It also describes theoretical frameworks rooted in equity and social justice: critical social theories that focus on the intersections of gender, race, age, socioeconomic status, education, sexuality, ability, ethnicity, culture, religion or spirituality, nationality, and geographic location, with attention throughout to cultural safety and cultural humility. It illustrates how these frameworks can help CHNs identify violence in individuals' lives, families, groups, communities, and societies; raise critical awareness of violence's health impacts; and guide prevention, health promoting, and empowering strategies to eliminate violence in society.

CRITICAL ANALYSIS OF VIOLENCE IN SOCIETIES AND HEALTH IMPLICATIONS

Central to understanding violence within families, communities, and societies are some of the underlying beliefs and pervasive 'common' knowledge that can mask the incidence and prevalence of violence in our everyday lives. For example, many cling to a family ideal that assumes love between members, shared norms and values, happiness, caring, nurturing and, above all, *safety*. Moreover, we often assume that violence occurs between strangers, not to newborn infants, children, adolescents, pregnant women, Aboriginal women, immigrant and refugee women, disabled people, same-sex partners, or seniors. Violence happens in our families and communities, among our neighbours, friends, co-workers, and clients.

Violence also cuts across genders, social classes, races, abilities, education levels, sexualities, age brackets, ethnicities, cultures, religions and spiritualities, and nationalities. Therefore, reading statistics critically is essential. For example, while sexual assault against men and boys is often underreported and largely neglected in research (WHO, 2002b), women are "more likely than men to be the victims of the most severe forms of spousal assault, as well as spousal homicide, sexual assault, and criminal harassment (stalking)" (Statistics Canada, 2006, p. 13). Indeed, 83% of spousal-assault victims are female (Statistics Canada, 2009).

Some women are particularly vulnerable: immigrants, refugees, children, and disabled women, women in military contexts, women who are pre-natal or post-natal, separating or divorcing, in institutions, poor, elderly, or Aboriginal. For example, spousal violence rates for Aboriginal women "remain more than three times higher than for non-Aboriginal women or men" as do severe and "potentially life-threatening forms of violence" (Statistics Canada, 2006, p. 65). Furthermore, "poverty and economic dependence, combined with racism and indifference from legal authorities" increases their vulnerability to violence (Canadian Feminist Alliance for International Action [CFAIA], 2010, p. 5). In developed and developing countries, women with HIV and AIDS are vulnerable to violence (Lewis, 2006; Nolan, 2007).

WHO (2004) argues for "prevention of interpersonal violence as a whole rather than focusing on individual subtypes" (p. 3). However, when nurses conduct assessments and develop prevention and health promotion strategies, it is equally important to attend to marginalized and socially excluded populations, while focusing on common risk factors. The following sections draw attention to marginalized and at-risk populations and combine individual and community-based assessment, prevention, and health promotion strategies needed to eliminate violence in societies.

Violence, Women, Health, and Social Costs

Violence against women occurs in every society. Similar to most countries, violence against women is a pervasive problem of epidemic proportions in Canada. The most comprehensive Canada-wide study, the National Violence against Women Survey (Statistics Canada, 1994) reported that 25% of the 12,300 women surveyed (16 and over) stated they had been abused by an intimate partner, and 10% had been assaulted at least once during the previous 12 months. Females were the victims in 85% of reported cases of spousal violence. However, it is important to note that the 2004 General Social Survey found that only 28% of spousal-violence victims reported abuse to the police (36% of females victims and 17% of male) (Statistics Canada, 2009, p. 24). The number of women killed by their male spouses (current or estranged) was three times the number of men killed by their spouses, and spousal homicide for Aboriginal women was eight times the rate for non-Aboriginal women (Statistics Canada, 2006).

"Ignoring violence as a factor in women's health and well-being not only leads to misdiagnosis and inadequate treatment, it also disregards the full extent of the personal and social consequences of violence" (Health Canada, 1999a, p. 2). These include "death, injury, chronic pain, poor gynaecologic and general health outcomes, posttraumatic stress disorder, depression, anxiety and substance abuse" (Wathen et al., 2009, p. 2). Furthermore, "women who experience violence use more healthcare services yet are at risk for marginalization in the healthcare system due to the complexity of their physical and mental health needs" (Health Canada, p. 2).

In 1995, the combined health and social costs of violence against women were estimated at $4.2 billion annually (Statistics Canada, 2006). In the United States, direct medical and health services are estimated at $4.1 billion (United Nation Development Fund for Women [UNDFW], 2007) while in England and Wales the estimated total costs are 10.2 billion US dollars (WHO, 2004, p. 2). Although research is required to capture more specific data within countries and between countries, clearly, the health and social cost of violence in societies is staggering. "Violence against women impoverishes individuals, families, and communities, reducing the economic development of each nation" (UNDFW, p. 1). Therefore, violence against women impacts us all.

Violence, Children, Youth, and Health

According to the United Nations, up to 275 million children witness and/or are exposed to violence at home annually (UN, 2006). Violence against children also occurs in schools and streets, in places of work and entertainment, and in care and detention centres. Pinheiro (2006) noted that perpetrators include "parents, family members, guardians, teachers, caregivers, law enforcement authorities, and other children. And no country is immune, whether rich or poor." Violence has devastating consequences for children's health and well-being; it "places at risk not only their health, but also their ability to learn and grow into adults who can create sound families and communities" (p. xi).

Violence against children and youth takes many forms. For example, **child maltreatment** is "harm, or risk of harm, that a child or youth may experience while in the care of a person they trust or depend on" (Jack, Munn, Cheng, & MacMillan, 2006, p. 1). Harm may occur through direct actions or neglecting to provide basic human needs: "human nurturance, food, clothing, shelter, necessary healthcare, and provisions for safety" (McAllister, 2000, p. 8). Moreover, "relative to physically abused children, neglected children have more severe cognitive and academic deficits, social withdrawal, and limited peer interaction, and internalizing (as opposed to externalizing) problems" (Hildyard & Wolfe, 2002, p. 679).

We still do not know how many children and youth experience abuse and neglect. However, Trocme et al. (2005) found that among the 103 297 "substantiated" reports of child maltreatment by Canadian child welfare services in 2003 (excluding Quebec), neglect was the most common form of child abuse (30%), followed by exposure to domestic violence

(28%), physical abuse (24%), emotional maltreatment (15%), and sexual abuse (3%). Girls were more often sexually abused (63%) and emotionally maltreated (54%) than boys, and boys were more often physically abused (54%) than girls.

Moreover, "the rate of sexual assault against children and youth committed by family members was 4 times higher for girls than for boys" (Statistics Canada, 2008, p. 26). In 2003, the cost of child abuse to child victims and adults was estimated at $15 billion (Statistics Canada, 2006).

According to the Native Women's Association of Canada [NWAC], 2007), within Aboriginal communities in Canada, three-quarters of sexual-assault survivors are under 18 and female. Of these, 50% are under 14 and almost 25% under 7. It states: "This is a shameful demonstration of Canada's failure to protect the basic human rights of Aboriginal women and girls" (p. 5).

UNDFW (2007) reports that young women and some young men are particularly vulnerable to coerced sex and are increasingly infected with HIV/AIDS. Harmful traditional practices in some African, Asian, and Middle Eastern countries, as well as within some immigrant communities in Europe, North American, and Australia, put approximately two million girls a year at risk of mutilation, and they are killed in dowry murders and "honour killings" (predominantly in South Asia, with instances reported in Canada and other western countries). Early marriage, especially in Africa and some Asian countries, leaves young girls vulnerable to sexual violence, jeopardizing their health, risking exposure to HIV/AIDS, and limiting their chances of attending school. Child prostitution and trafficking across the globe ensnares girls and boys in sexual exploitation.

Policy makers tend to focus on immediate problems rather than on the "roots" of the problems, and on interventions rather than actions to prevent the roots taking hold (McMurtry & Curling, 2008). Violence is preventable if its underlying causes are identified and addressed (UN, 2006).

Violence, Older Adults, and Health

Elder abuse and neglect is a significant and growing problem. A systematic review found that 6% of older people reported significant abuse the previous month, "probably an underestimate because some people are reluctant to report abuse" (Ploeg, Fear, Hutchinson, MacMillian, & Bolam, 2009, p. 188). This is troubling "in view of the expected doubling of the number of older adults world-wide from 1995 to 2025" (Ploeg et al., p. 188).

Difficulties in defining elder abuse persist. In the Toronto Declaration on the Global Prevention of Elder Abuse (WHO, 2002b), **elder abuse** is described as "a single or repeated act, or lack of appropriate action, occurring within a relationship where there is an expectation of trust which causes harm or distress to a older person. It can be of various forms: physical, psychological/emotional, sexual, financial, or simply reflect intentional or unintentional neglect" (p. 2).

Elder neglect involves "the failure of a caregiver to meet the needs of an older adult who is unable to meet those needs alone" (Health Canada, 1999a, p. 2). Behaviours such as denial of food, water, medication, medical treatment, therapy, nursing services, health aids, clothing, and visitors are included. Caution has been expressed about subsuming elder abuse under family violence, lest we miss the vulnerability arising from age, gender, and health status (Killick & Taylor, 2009) combined with cultural contexts (WHO, 2002b).

Only a small proportion of elder abuse comes to the attention of the health, social service, and justice systems. Abuse and maltreatment of older adults is 14 times less likely to be reported than abuse of 18- to 24-year-olds because of emotional, physical, or financial dependence on abusers, embarrassment (especially if abusers are adult children), or fear of institutionalization (Statistics Canada, 2004). In healthcare focus groups with older people in eight countries (Argentina, Austria, Brazil, Canada, India, Kenya, Lebanon, and Sweden), seniors often mentioned "lack of knowledge on the part of health professionals about ageing and older people, and also about elder abuse" (WHO/INPEA, 2002, p. 19). The extent of the costs of elder abuse has yet to be determined.

Violence, Aboriginal Peoples, and Health

The Aboriginal Healing Foundation (Bopp, Bopp, & Lane, 2006) defines **Aboriginal family violence and abuse** as a multidimensional social syndrome, not simply undesirable behaviour; systemic; intergenerational; involving community breakdown; linked to need for healing from trauma; and linked to historical experience. Violent crime is increasing in many Nunavut communities (Pauktuutit Inuit Women of Canada, 2006). Family violence and its effects on Aboriginal peoples has led to high health disparities related to social, economic, cultural, and political inequities (Adelson, 2005). Examples include much higher infant mortality and lower life expectancy than the Canadian average, and higher rates of chronic disease, injury, suicide, and obesity. Violence puts Aboriginal women (children and youth) at significant risk for poverty, drug and/or alcohol use; increased exposure to HIV and other sexually transmitted infections (Varcoe & Dick, 2008); persistent higher rates in morbidity and mortality, chronic diseases, suicides, and injuries relative to other Canadians (Kurtz et al., 2008).

Attitudinal change is vital in removing barriers faced by Aboriginal peoples; however, health issues must be addressed in culturally safe and appropriate ways (McMurray, 2007). "Understanding how the intersecting dynamics of gender, rural living, poverty, racism, and colonialism create risk for Aboriginal women provides a basis for developing policies that aim to strengthen the well-being of women, particularly their economic well being" (Varcoe & Dick, 2008, p. 42).

Violence, Immigrants, and Health

Canada is one of the most culturally diverse countries in the world, yet there is a dearth of research addressing differential experiences of violence by race, ethnicity, class, and culture.

Fong's (2000) research with Chinese Canadian women showed that immigrant women "experienced a great deal of pain and hardship due to their isolation, burden of childcare responsibilities, lack of English skills, unfamiliarity with the new environment and new culture, lack of an adequately paid job, and/or financial dependence on their husbands" (p. iv), in addition to abusive relationships. Yet these same women "employed a wide range of strategies to resist the abuse and protect themselves from different dangerous situations" (p. iv). Agnew (1998) captured similar experiences for immigrant women from Asia, Africa, and the Caribbean who suffered wife abuse.

Immigration and resettlement greatly influence the health of immigrants and refugees (Beiser, 2005; Guruge, 2010; Guruge & Khanlou, 2004) and can be compounded by violence. Cultural, linguistic, and systemic barriers to health and healthy behaviours unique to diverse immigrant populations must be taken into account when developing strategies to prevent violence in immigrant and refugee families. Furthermore, "instead of looking at limitations and weaknesses, our society needs to focus more on these women's strengths when examining how they deal with abuse in intimate relationships" (Fong, 2010, p. 212) and recognize their "resilience and ability to change even with limited resources" (p. 212). However, as "helping professionals, we should not expect abused women to take steps before they are ready or that go beyond their boundaries" (p. 214).

Knowing more about the ways in which violence is experienced and perceived by immigrant and refugee women and their children will help enhance the capacities of communities and society at large to respond to violence and "to develop culturally, linguistically, and contextually appropriate interventions and programs" (Guruge, 2010, p. 283), together with culturally safe prevention and health promoting strategies.

CANADIAN RESEARCH BOX 26.1

What are the perceptions of older immigrant women and their responses to abuse and neglect?

Guruge, S., & Kanthasamy, P. (2010, March). *Older women's perceptions of and responses to abuse and neglect in the post-migration context.* Toronto, ON: Wellesley Institute. Retrieved from http://www.wellesleyinstitute.com

As health research on violence against older immigrant women is limited, this qualitative study explored the experiences of and responses to abuse/violence and neglect among a group of older immigrant women. In-depth individual interviews ($n = 18$) and focus group discussions ($n = 25$) were conducted with a group of older women from the Sri Lankan Tamil community in Ontario. Thematic analysis revealed that women experiencing abuse/violence spoke of financial, physical, emotional, and sexual abuse along with threats, control, and neglect that they or others in their community experienced. The abusers included husbands, children, and children-in-law. Power and control exerted by the community and society were also addressed.

It is important for CHNs to address family and community expectations of older immigrant women that may lead to abusive situations. Other recommendations include language training and further education and employment opportunities for older women; linguistically and culturally appropriate services, supports, and care; and removal of immigration sponsorship criteria.

Discussion Questions

As a CHN, you are asked to join the School of Nursing curriculum committee to address the societal need for nursing education on violence.

1. What would your contributions be?

2. What approaches would you bring to this initiative?

3. What outcomes would you anticipate from this committee?

Sexual Orientation, Gender Identity, Violence, and Health

The health of lesbian, gay, bisexual, transsexual, transgendered, two-spirit, intersex, queer, or questioning (LGBTTTIQQ) people "is compromised by direct assaults such as hate crimes, physical violence and verbal assaults as well as chronic stress caused by stigmatization" (RNAO, 2007b, p. 1). However, LGBTTTIQQ people are as diverse as the general population (Brotman & Ryan, 2001); therefore, sexism and heterosexism interact with racism, classism, and ableism, together with ethnicity, culture, religion, and nationality complicate obtaining knowledge of the prevalence of violence against LBGTTTIQQs.

Although violence occurs in all types of relationships, non-prototypical relationships, e.g., lesbian and gay couples (with or without children), are often overlooked (Seelau & Seelau, 2005). Therefore, prevalence of violence has been more difficult to assess. However, "experts estimate rates comparable to heterosexual couples" (Seelau & Seelau, p. 363).

"There is overwhelming evidence that LGBTTTIQQ people in Ontario and Canada experience barriers to inclusive and appropriate care" (RNAO, 2007a, p. 3) because of "practices by healthcare institutions and health professionals that are heterosexist and discriminatory" (p. 1). Therefore, the Society of Obstetricians and Gynaecologists of Canada alerted healthcare workers regarding the need to assess for partner abuse in lesbian relationships while being sensitive to difficulties in disclosing sexual orientation compounded by revealing experiences of partner abuse (Davis, 2000).

RNAO (2007a) also reported that in educational environments, homophobia and heterosexism contribute to LBGTTTIQQ adolescents dropping out of school; "becoming street-involved and homeless; high suicide and attempted suicide rates; and internalized shame and low self-esteem" (p. 3). Gochros and Bidwell (1996) challenge healthcare workers to develop innovative early intervention programs for lesbian and gay youth while acknowledging the formidable barriers to providing these services.

STRATEGIES TO ELIMINATE VIOLENCE IN SOCIETIES

Brown (1991) asserted that "violence in any society persists because there is a role for it, because it serves a purpose. Violence persists . . . because people opposed to it have been addressing its manifestations rather than its **root causes**" (p. 104). Most researchers and people working with individuals, families, groups, communities, and populations agree that violence is rooted in power and control. Moreover, abuse of women, children, youth, and the elderly often "occur[s] within familial relationships because these are sites of power" (Neysmith, 1995, p. 48). Definitional problems about what constitutes violence and abuse persist, but this should not preclude acting now to prevent violence and promote health.

Violence is an insidious, pervasive, and frequently deadly social problem. Eradicating violence must address multiple levels in multiple sectors of society—simultaneously locally, nationally, and globally. Guided by the Canadian Community Health Nursing Standards of Practice (Community Health Nurses Association of Canada, 2008) and the Public Health Nursing Discipline Specific Competencies (Community Health Nurses of Canada, 2009), we propose the following theoretical frameworks, approaches, and culturally safe and empowering strategies.

THEORETICAL FRAMEWORKS AND APPROACHES

Critical Social Theories

Critical social theories include liberation work against poverty and illiteracy; feminist scholarship on oppression of women; lesbian and gay studies; and critical perspectives on race and ethnic relations, gender inequalities, and health promotion (Stevens & Hall, 1992). These include theories of violence. In defining violent societies, critical theorists (1) analyze the social, economic, political, cultural, and environmental ways individuals and groups are harmed by social institutions and states and (2) act on these health-damaging effects at the community level for structural change.

"The interwoven process of critical reflection and action is a theoretical key to effective community health nursing practice" (Stevens & Hall, 1992, p. 81). Through theory, research, and evidence-informed practice, critical questions could be raised to examine social justice, equity, and social change (Schim, Benkert, Bell, Walkerm, & Danford, 2007).

Intersectionality

Understanding the intersections of race, ethnicity, class, genders, abilities, sexualities, culture, age, and religious beliefs (Andersen & Collins, 2004; Varcoe, Hankivsky, & Morrow, 2007) expands our capacity to work effectively against violence (Hankivsky & Varcoe, 2007). As CHNs, we must shift our thinking and put front and centre those who have been devalued, marginalized, and socially excluded. Andersen and Collins (2004) argue that, "This shift is central to thinking about race, class, and gender in ways that transform, rather than buttress existing social formations" (p. 61). **Intersectionality** shifts the focus, blame, responsibility, and explanations of violence against women from the individual to the social context, including the culture of violence that "encompasses the violence of racism, poverty, heterosexism, and other forms of inequity" (Hankivsky & Varcoe, p. 482).

We must really hear and understand the experiences and concerns of marginalized, socially excluded, and at-risk populations and provide culturally safe and sensitive services to those who have experienced violence within their communities. When developing health promotion programs related to violence, e.g., for immigrant women, CHNs must be respectful of culture and tradition while working for change. Changing our thinking requires examining our own biases, beliefs, and feelings about these issues.

Central to working effectively in cultures different from one's own are the concepts of cultural competence, cultural safety, and cultural humility. "**Cultural competence** is the application of knowledge, skill, attitudes and personal attributes required by nurses to provide appropriate care and services in relation to the characteristics of their clients" (Canadian Nurses Association [CNA], 2004, p. 1). However, **cultural safety** shifts the focus from nurses' competencies to giving "power to community members to say whether or not they feel safe, and professionals need to enable the community members to express the extent to which they feel risk or safety, resulting in changes in behaviours in health professionals as appropriate" (Israel, Eng, Schulz, & Parker, 2005, p. 11). **Cultural humility** is a process that requires humility and commitment to ongoing self-reflection and self-critique, including identifying and examining one's own patterns of unintentional and intentional racism and classism, addressing existing power imbalances, and establishing and maintaining "mutually beneficial and non-paternalistic partnerships with communities" (Israel et al., 2005, p. 11). The capacity to reflect on our own experiences is a major principle in CHN practice (CHNC, 2008). (See Chapter 8.)

Empowerment and Community Participation Approaches

Empowerment is a dynamic, action-oriented process that focuses on power relations and intervention strategies in creating relationships with greater equity in resources, status, authority, and health. The process of community empowerment can begin at any point along a continuum that includes personal, small group, community organization, partnerships, and social and political action (Laverack, 2004). CHNs can engage community participants in problem identification, planning, development, implementation, and evaluation processes. In this process, "power over" becomes "power with" in the personal and collective work

to eliminate violence and its associated health disparities in individuals, families, communities, and societies (see Chapters 6, 7, 10, and 13).

ROLE AND FUNCTION OF THE COMMUNITY HEALTH NURSE

Assessment at the individual level can facilitate critical awareness of the extent of violence in communities and societies. Assessment includes addressing the safety of the person, including cultural safety, in addition to being critically aware of violence, indicators of abuse and neglect, the importance of asking about abuse, how to ask about abuse, individual risk factors, case finding, routine universal comprehensive screening, community resources, prevention and health promoting strategies, and connecting individual harm with the social, political, economic, environmental, and cultural context in which it occurs to make political action possible. As individual CHNs and as a collective, we are all part of the multi-sectoral prevention and health promotion initiatives required to meet the goal of eradicating violence.

Assessment, Prevention, and Health Promoting Strategies

First, *safety of the person* is key. Poorly designed and implemented assessment strategies put women, children, and elders in violent, abusive, or neglectful relationships at substantial risk. Within the context of cultural safety and cultural humility, the environment must *be safe* and individuals must *feel safe* before they can discuss their experiences. A short-form ABCD-ER Mnemonic Tool can guide this process.

Short-Form ABCD-ER Mnemonic Tool:
Guiding Principles for Screening

A: *Attitude* and *Approachability* of healthcare professionals
B: *Belief* in the woman's account of her own experience of abuse
C: *Confidentiality* is essential for disclosure
D: *Documentation* that is consistent and legible
E: *Education* about serious health effects of abuse
R: *Respect* for the integrity and authority of each woman's life choices and *Recognition* that the process of dealing with identified abuse must proceed at her pace, directed by her decisions.

Source: Reproduced with permission from the Middlesex-London Health Unit, London, Ontario, Canada. (2000). Task force on the health effects of women abuse: Final report (p. 34). London, ON: Author. While the information contained in the materials is believed to be accurate and true, no responsibility is assumed by MLHU for its use.

FIGURE 26.1 Battering in Intimate Relationships: "The Power and Control Wheel"

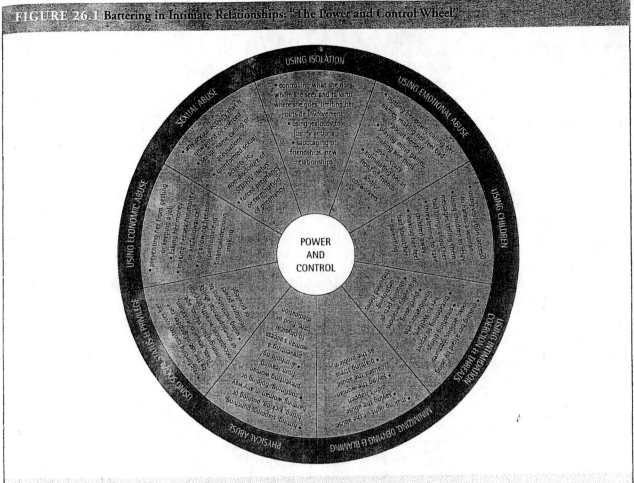

Source: Reproduced with permission from the Middlesex-London Health Unit, London, Ontario, Canada. Originally developed by The Domestic Abuse Intervention Project, Duluth, USA. Further adapted by The London Battered Women's Advocacy Centre.

Second, CHNs must become *critically aware* of violence and abuse, understanding that it cuts across all ages, races, genders, sexualities, cultures, religions, abilities, classes, nationalities, etc. The Power and Control Wheel (Figure 26.1) outlines some of the tactics used by abusers.

Third, CHNs need to know *indicators* of emotional abuse and neglect for children, youth, adults, and elders. Indicators for all groups include depression, withdrawal, low self-esteem, severe anxiety, fearfulness, being overly passive or compliant, sleep disturbances, suicide attempts, and physical abuse, present or suspected. For children, indicators include failure to thrive in infancy, emotional instability, physical complaints with no medical basis, over- or underachievement, and inability to trust. For adults, indicators include feelings of shame and guilt, substance abuse, discomfort or nervousness around caregivers or relatives, social isolation (Health Canada, 1996), somatic complaints in women, post-traumatic stress, unemployment or underemployment of male partners, common-law relationships, or recently separated. Note that "it has not yet been determined which indicators precede or succeed abuse" (Jack et al., 2008, p. 153).

Fourth, CHNs must understand the importance of *asking about abuse.* An important signal of support, asking can

prevent further abuse. Asking lets a woman know that violence is an important health issue and that she will be believed, respected, supported, and heard. Moreover, naming the problem raises awareness and makes it public and political. Cultural safety, cultural humility, sensitivity, and language must be considered in CHNs' practice.

CANADIAN RESEARCH BOX 26.2

Does an interactive curriculum that integrates dating violence prevention reduce physical dating violence (PDV)?

Wolfe, D. A., Crooks, C., Jaffe, P., Chido, D., Hughes, R., Ellis, W., Stitt, L., & Donner, A. (2009). A school-based program to prevent adolescent dating violence: A cluster randomized trial. *Archives of Pediatrics and Adolescent Medicine, 163*(8), 692–699.

Adolescent dating violence was found to be one of the strongest precursors to intimate partner violence in adulthood. For adolescents, dating violence is defined as acts ranging from threats of harm, to punching or hitting with an object, emerging during critical, stressful transition periods that involve new pressures and responsibilities for handling conflict and emotions in unfamiliar contexts. Given the importance of reducing the cycle of violence, this study evaluated efforts to educate high school students about healthy dating behaviours and ways to avoid or reduce PDV and associated risks.

This study used a randomized trial with 2.5 year follow-up with a pre-specified subgroup analysis by sex. Grade 9 student participants were enrolled in required health classes (1722 students, ages 14–15, in 20 public schools). They received a 21-month curriculum delivered by teachers, enhanced by additional training in the dynamics of dating violence and healthy relationships. Relationship skills to promote safer decision making with peers and dating partners were emphasized. Control schools targeted similar objectives without training manuals.

The results indicated that the primary outcome at 2.5 years was self-reported PDV during the previous year and that PDV was greater in the control versus intervention students. It was concluded that the teaching of youths about healthy relationships as part of their required health curriculum reduced PDV and increased condom use 2.5 years later at a low per-student cost.

Discussion Questions

1. As CHNs, how would you develop a health promotion program to raise awareness and reduce bullying and harassment in schools? What theoretical frameworks would guide your program? On what would you take action? How would you take action? With whom would you take action?

2. What ethical and cultural safety issues would you consider?

3. With whom and how would you evaluate your program?

Fifth, CHNs need to learn *how* to ask about abuse. Privacy is key (Jack et al., 2008). Direct, specific questions are best and should be non-threatening, non-blaming, open-ended, and always preceded by genuinely supportive statements of concern (see the box "Screening for Woman Abuse"). When CHNs do post-partum home visits, discussions of intimate partner violence (IPV) are "best held when there is a bond of trust between the provider and the client and when the client does not feel rushed" (Jack et al., p. 164).

Sixth, CHNs need to understand *individual risk factors* to intervene in the cycle of violence. Social determinants of health (income, social status, employment, working conditions, personal health, food security, early childhood development, coping skills, gender, race, ethnicity, age, sexuality, religion, culture, abilities, and social environment) should be considered when assessing risk.

Seventh, through *case finding* and/or *routine universal comprehensive* screening, CHNs can demonstrate connections between individual harm and social contexts. **Case**

finding is conducted within in-depth nursing assessments, possibly over multiple home visits, where CHNs ask any clients who show signs of abuse about IPV (Jack et al., 2008). "Screening means imbedding questions about abuse in a health history or incorporating validated screening instruments into the history and assessment process" (RNAO, 2005, p. 15), regardless of the woman's reasons for seeking healthcare (Jack et al., 2008).

- **Universal screening** occurs when nurses ask every woman over a specified age about her experience of abuse.
- **Routine screening** is performed on a regular basis regardless of whether or not signs of abuse are present.
- **Indicator-based screening** refers to screening after nurses observe one or more indicators that suggest a woman may have been abused (RNAO, 2005).

Screening for Woman Abuse: Developing a Personal Style

Screening protocols should be flexible so that they can change to fit each situation. The process may vary depending on healthcare or community settings, the relationship of CHNs to women, presenting problems, the women's histories, and role of each CHN in meeting women's health needs. A few suggestions:

- Ask simple, direct questions.
- Maintain a matter-of-fact tone of voice and relaxed demeanour.
- Ensure your body language, facial expressions, and words all convey the same thing: that you are willing to hear what the woman has to say and willing to help.
- Emphasize that all women are screened routinely for abuse as part of healthcare interactions.
- Use screening as an opportunity to educate women about the prevalence, dynamics, and health effects of abuse.
- Use neutral terms in asking about abuse. (Someone of the same sex may have abused the woman.)

Ways to Ask About Abuse: Some Sample Questions

- We know that abuse and violence in the home affect the health of many women. I wonder if you ever experience abuse or violence at home?
- Have you ever felt unsafe or threatened in your own home?

Physical Abuse

- The injuries you have suggest to me that someone may have hit you. Did anyone hit you?

Emotional Abuse

- Does anyone close to you call you names, criticize your friends or family, or try to control what you do?

Sexual Abuse

- Have you ever been forced to have sex with your partner when you did not want to?

Sources: Adapted from Health Canada. (1999). A handbook for health and social services professionals responding to abuse during pregnancy (p. 24). Ottawa, ON: Health Canada, Health Promotion and Services Branch. (Cat. No. H72-21/165-1998E); and Middlesex-London Health Unit. (2000). Task force on the health effects of women abuse: Final report (pp. 33–34). London, ON: Author.

The most comprehensive approach is one that combines routine and universal screening for all females 12 and older (RNAO, 2005, p. 23). The choice of approach taken must consider the individual needs of the client and the social and cultural circumstances in which they live.

Eighth, CHNs must *make appropriate referrals* for abused women, children, seniors, and men; for example, to

shelters; sexual assault supports; women's centres; child advocacy centres; children's aid services; crisis telephone lines (e.g., kids-help lines, distress lines); medical services, health care centres; counselling services for women, children, Aboriginals, immigrants, and seniors; legal aid, lawyer referral services; Aboriginal services; immigrant and refugee services; ethno cultural organizations addressing abuse; police; victim assistance services (police based, court based); programs for men who abuse women and men who have been abused; self-help clearinghouses and networks; community resources centres. (Health Canada, 1999b, p. 41)

Ninth, CHNs must work collaboratively to *develop broad-based, comprehensive health promoting strategies* that include primary, secondary, and tertiary prevention approaches to family violence. These should include ethical, research, and evaluative components. CHNs should also address the diversity and cultural context of their community by attending to gender, race, class, age, ethnicity, ability, sexuality, language, literacy, and culture in an effort to highlight "missing voices" and bring an end to their absence in statistics, research, literature, prevention, and health promoting strategies.

Tenth, when CHNs *connect individual harm with social, economic, cultural, environmental, and political contexts,* it makes violence public and political. CHNs can initiate political actions supported by critical theoretical frameworks (Stevens & Hall, 1992). This means

- *taking a stand.* CHNs have a responsibility to diverse communities vulnerable to the oppressive, health-damaging conditions of violence.
- *asking critical questions* to expose oppressive situations. For example, why has a unified effort to eradicate violence not occurred? Whose interests does violence serve? Whose interests are suppressed or ignored?
- *working with communities* to name violence and solve its related health problems. Targeting problems people identify, such as violence and abuse, situates CHNs' efforts in communities' struggles.

- *forming alliances* with community members and groups concerned with violence in families to create solidarity and use collective strength to work for healthy social change. Sustaining alliances requires ongoing commitment supported by sufficient funding.

Eleventh, *develop and ensure cultural safety.* This involves (i) developing cultural awareness: recognizing that, e.g., health relationships are unique, power-laden, and culturally dyadic; (ii) developing cultural awareness and sensitivity, e.g., recognizing inherent cultural difference; (iii) exploring one's own experience and realities and the impact these may have on others; (iv) committing to preserving and protecting others' cultures; and (v) analyzing power imbalances, institutional discrimination, colonization, and colonial relationships related to violence and health (National Aboriginal Health Organization, 2008).

Twelfth, use the *Ottawa Charter for Health Promotion's five areas for action* (WHO & Canadian Public Health Association, 1986) while ensuring cultural safety to guide your practice (see Chapter 6). Develop personal skills, e.g., cultural awareness related to violence; create supportive environments, e.g., culturally safe violence-free environments; strengthen community action, e.g., partnerships, participation, and protection from violence; build healthy public policies, e.g., culturally safe violence free policies and practices; and reorient health (and social) services, e.g., culturally safe theories, policies, curricula, and practices aiming to prevent violence in societies while promoting health.

Thirteenth, *take action guided by the Bangkok Charter for Health Promotion in a Globalized World* (WHO, 2005). Advocate for health and freedom from violence based on human rights and solidarity; invest in sustainable policies, actions, and infrastructure to address determinants of health; build capacities for leadership, health promoting practice, research and knowledge sharing, and health literacy; regulate and legislate to ensure high levels of protection from harm and enable equal and equitable opportunities for health and well-being for all people; and build partnerships and alliances with public, private, and international organizations, non-governmental organizations, and civil society to create culturally safe and sustainable actions.

Fourteenth, *build in measurable evaluation strategies from the start* that address the following questions: (1) To what extent does the community organize effort to prevent violence and promote health improve the lives of community members, and if so, which members and how many? (2) Does participating give community members a sense of power, strength, and imagination as a group and help build structures for future healthy social change? (3) Does the struggle to politically educate community members enhance their capacities for critiquing and challenging systems that enable and permit so much violence in societies (Minkler & Pies, 2002)?

Learning how to do this work takes time, care, and commitment. Because there are many complex intersecting issues, this work requires dynamic alliances with individuals, families, groups, and communities concerned with violence in societies, while remaining critically conscious of cultural

CASE STUDY

Serena, a 30-year-old Mexican Canadian woman, recently gave birth to her first child, a small, healthy girl. During her short hospital stay, Serena attended postnatal classes, including one on breastfeeding. She appeared to be confident in caring for her baby. However, in the presence of her husband during the discharge planning meeting, the nurse noted Serena appeared quite nervous.

You do a follow-up home visit as part of the "Healthy Mother, Healthy Baby" program co-sponsored by the Community Health Department and the hospital. Serena welcomes you and informs you that her husband is out buying groceries. You assess the health of mother and baby and offer support and advice about breastfeeding. You invite Serena to the local "Mothers and Babies Group," but Serena, who seems quite interested, does not think her husband will let her go. She mentions that when the baby cried for a while last evening her husband became angry, telling her to keep the baby quiet because he needed his sleep. Serena appears anxious about her husband's impending return.

Discussion Questions

1. Given Serena's concerns about her husband, what is your first response?

2. How will you initiate assessment of her situation?

3. What are your priorities?

safety, power imbalances, institutional discrimination, colonization, and relationships with colonizers related to violence and health. See Additional Resources at the end of this chapter. Other resources may be obtained at women's centres, clinics, shelters, and health and social service agencies.

SUMMARY

Violence in societies is a social act that involves a serious abuse of power and control. Violence is endemic in our individual lives and in our families, communities, and societies, cutting across class, race, age, ethnicity, sexualities, abilities, religions, and national boundaries.

Violence is located within historical, economic, cultural, social, environmental, and political contexts. There are connections between what happens in our individual lives and in our families, communities, and societies, and between what happens in our societies, communities, families, and in our individual lives. In our work to address and eradicate violence, CHNs and our allies must make these connections visible. Simultaneously, CHNs can work collaboratively to facilitate social changes at the level of individual, family, group, community, and society.

CHNs who guide their practice with critical social theories and intersectional frameworks, while working with people where they live, affirm those who are dealing with experiences of violence in their lives as active, engaged subjects in their own struggle. Culturally safe participatory empowering strategies can facilitate this process. "Empowerment influences people's ability to act through collective participation by strengthening their personal and organizational capacities, challenging power inequities, and achieving outcomes on many reciprocal levels in different domains" (Wallerstein, 2006, p. 19), while working collaboratively to eliminate violence in our lives, families, communities, and societies.

KEY TERMS

violence, p. 405
violence against women, p. 405
child maltreatment, p. 407
elder abuse, p. 407
elder neglect. p. 407
Aboriginal family violence and abuse, p. 408
root causes, p. 409
critical social theories, p. 410
intersectionality, p. 410
cultural competence, p. 410
cultural safety, p. 410
cultural humility, p. 410
empowerment, p. 410
screening, p. 412
case finding, p. 412
universal screening, p. 412
routine screening, p. 412
indicator-based screening, p. 412

REVIEW QUESTIONS

Choose the one alternative that best completes the statement or answers the question.

1. For prevention of violence strategies to be possible, community health nurses need to learn about violence in societies and work to decrease barriers to effective healthcare for those who are socially isolated, marginalized, and/or at risk to violence in their lives. Which one of the following is a significant barrier for community health nurses?

   a) Professional healthcare preparation

   b) Cultural and language barriers

   c) Lack of institutional support for healthcare care providers in assessing for violence.

   d) Awareness of pervasiveness of violence locally, nationally, and globally

2. Canada is one of the most culturally diverse countries in the world, yet there is a lack of specific data addressing differing experiences of violence. One of the major implications of this lack of specific data about violence is

a) specific healthcare needs are overlooked.

b) cultural safety is not built into assessment, intervention, and prevention of violence strategies.

c) difficulties in defining violence.

d) frequency of reporting violence may be reduced.

3. When CHNs connect individual experiences of violence with the social, cultural, economic, environmental, and political contexts, it makes violence public and political. Therefore, it is important to include which one of the following in political action strategies:

a) Aim strategies at the individual level rather than the collective level.

b) Build connections with your local members of parliament.

c) Work primarily with healthcare professionals to name and solve violence.

d) Take a stand with diverse, socially isolated, marginalized, and at-risk populations.

4. When CHNs assess for violence, which of the following is essential?

a) attitude of the CHN

b) respect for the individual the nurse is assessing

c) the safety of the individual being assessed

d) confidentiality

5. CHNs are encouraged to use theory to inform their practice. Which one of the following theoretical frameworks would be best to guide nurses' practice in relation to violence?

a) empowerment

b) critical social theory

c) cultural safety

d) intersectional theory

5. Analyze critically ongoing debates about universal screening and case finding as they relate to CHN practice. What factors would you consider when deciding how best to proceed in assessing for violence?

6. How can CHNs work collaboratively to

a) raise awareness of violence in societies?

b) appropriately and ethically assess for violence and abuse?

c) prevent violence in societies?

d) promote health while working to eliminate violence locally, nationally, and internationally?

> *After working through these questions, go to the MyNursingLab at* **www.pearsoned.ca/mynursinglab** *to check your answers.*

INDIVIDUAL CRITICAL THINKING EXERCISES

1. Examine critically your perspectives, assumptions, and biases about people who have experienced violence or abuse. Think about where, when, from whom, and/or how you developed these ideas.

2. How is violence represented in the media? Give two examples. Drawing on the material in this chapter, compare critically your examples, addressing the strengths and limitations of each.

3. Critically analyze the implications these media representations have for the community's understanding of violence, for health and healthcare, and for CHN theory and practice.

4. Youth who regularly access the Internet are confronted with images of violence and human degradation, especially depictions of women and children as sexual objects and not fully functioning human beings.

a) Analyze critically how you respond to these images.

b) Address how you, as a CHN, might assist in creating public awareness about the potential for personal sexual exploitation of youth via the Internet.

5. Violence is endemic. This can lead one to feeling overwhelmed with the immensity of the problem and unsure how, when, where, and with whom to act. At the personal level, consider how you might relate across differences when assessing, intervening, and/or preventing violence while promoting health.

STUDY QUESTIONS

1. Analyze critically the following concepts: violence; violence against women; violence in societies; root causes.

2. Cultural competence, cultural safety, and cultural humility are similar concepts yet offer differing understandings and directions for CHNs working on violence in societies. Compare and contrast these concepts, addressing their strengths and limitations together with their directional focus for CHN practice.

3. Drawing on two different marginalized and/or at-risk populations addressed in this chapter, analyze critically the health and social costs of violence.

4. Examine critically the relevance of critical social theory, intersectionality, cultural safety, and empowerment as theoretical frameworks to guide CHNs working on violence in societies.

GROUP CRITICAL THINKING EXERCISES

1. You are a nurse in an urban community health centre serving a mixed-income, ethnically and racially diverse community. A number of women recently disclosed that they are "victims" of violence. After reading on this topic and talking with other healthcare providers, you realize that

violence is much more pervasive than you imagined. You and your colleagues begin to think about strategies to address violence in the community. Using critical theories and other CHN frameworks and approaches, while attending to the critical analysis of current statistics, develop a health promotion program to address this problem.

2. Your local school board recently launched a Gender-Based Violence Policy. Your Community Health Department was asked to assist in implementing this policy at one of the local high-schools. You and some of your nursing colleagues were asked to be part of the pilot project team.

   a) As CHNs, what would you have to consider before embarking on this endeavour? Where would you begin? What would you need to know? Who would you need to connect with? As CHNs, how might you begin to tease apart your own agendas from that of the school board and the high school?

   b) If active involvement of people, beginning with what they define as their needs, is required to facilitate true community participation, as CHNs, on what would you take action? How would you take action? With whom would you take action?

   c) If ethical and culturally safe practices have not been considered in development of this Gender-Based Violence Policy, as CHNs, how would you ensure their inclusion to enable healthy social change?

   d) As members of this pilot project team, what ethical and evaluative questions should be included? At what point in the pilot project should these be integrated?

3. Representatives from the CHNs' staff made a presentation to the local Board of Health about prevalence estimates of elder abuse together with a systematic review of the literature revealing extremely low reporting of elder abuse. The Board of Health asked the CHNs to develop and implement a broad-based community awareness campaign about elder abuse. Drawing upon the material presented in this chapter, answer the following questions.

   a) As CHNs, where would you begin? What do you need to do? What do you need to know? Where would you get this information? Who would you involve in this effort? At what point would you involve them—why, where, and how? What health promoting and empowering communication approaches and strategies will you use for this campaign? What would be your primary goals and objectives for your communication strategies?

   b) What resources will you need? How will you access these resources? What health literacy and linguistic factors would you need to consider? What strategies will you use in this campaign? Who will you involve in these strategies and/or campaign? Who will be the target group(s)? What ethical considerations will you address?

   c) How will you implement your health promoting campaign—where, when, how, and with whom?

How will you assess the results of your program? How and to whom will you communicate the results of this campaign?

REFERENCES

Adelson, N. (2005). The embodiment of inequity: Health disparities in Aboriginal Canada. *Canadian Journal of Public Health, 96*(S2), S45–S61.

Agnew, V. (1998). *In search of a safe place: Abused women and culturally sensitive services.* Toronto, ON: University of Toronto Press.

Andersen, M. L., & Collins, P. H. (2004). Shifting the center. In M. L. Andersen & P. H. Collins, *Race class and gender: An anthology* (5th ed., pp. 15–22). Toronto, ON: Thomson/Wadsworth.

Beiser, M. (2005). The health of immigrants and refugees in Canada. *Canadian Journal of Public Health, 96*(S2), S30–S44.

Bopp, J., Bopp, M., & Lane, P. Jr. (2006). *Aboriginal domestic violence in Canada.* Ottawa, ON: The Aboriginal Healing Foundation. Retrieved from http://www.ahf.ca

Brotman, S., & Ryan, B. (2001, March). *Critical issues in practice with gay, lesbian, bisexual, and two-spirited people: Educational module for professionals in the fields of health and allied health.* Montreal, PQ: McGill School of Social Work.

Brown, R. (1991). Attack violence at its roots. *Canadian Woman Studies/Les Cahiers de la Femme, 12*(1), 12–15.

Canadian Feminist Alliance for International Action (CFAIA). (2010, February). *No action: No progress: Canadian Feminist Alliance for International Action report on Canada's progress in implementing priorities made by the United Nations Committee on the Elimination of Discrimination against women in 2008.* Ottawa, ON: Author.

Canadian Nurses Association. (2004, March). *Position statement: Promoting culturally competent care.* Ottawa, ON: Author.

Canadian Nurses Association. (2008). *Code of ethics for registered nurses: 2008 centennial edition.* Ottawa, ON: Author. Retrieved from http://www.cna-nurses.ca/CNA/documents/pdf/publications/Code _of_Ethics_2008_e.pdf

Community Health Nurses Association of Canada. (2008). *Canadian community health nursing standards of practice.* Ottawa, ON: Author.

Community Health Nurses Association of Canada. (2009). *Public health nursing discipline specific competencies.* Toronto, ON: Author.

Davis, V. (2000). Lesbian health guidelines. SOGC clinical practice guidelines. *Journal of the Society of Obstetricians and Gynecologists of Canada, 2*(3), 202–205.

Fong, J. (2010). Chinese immigrant women confronting male violence in their lives. In J. Fong (Ed.), *Out of the shadows: Women abuse in ethnic, immigrant, and Aboriginal communities* (pp. 186–214). Toronto, ON: Women's Press.

Fong, J. S. (2000). *Silent no more: How women experienced wife abuse in the local Chinese community.* Unpublished doctoral dissertation, York University, Toronto, ON.

Gochros, H., & Bidwell, R. (1996). Lesbian and gay youth in a straight world: Implications for health care workers. *Journal of Gay and Lesbian Social Services, 5*(1), 1–17.

Guruge, S. (2010). Perceptions of intimate male partner violence and determinants of women's responses to it: Findings from a study in the Sri Lankan Tamil Community in Toronto. In J. Fong (Ed.), *Out of the shadows: Women abuse in ethnic, immigrant, and Aboriginal communities* (pp. 264–283). Toronto, ON: Women's Press.

Guruge, S., & Khanlou, N. (2004). Intersectionalities of influence: Researching the health of immigrant and refugee women. *Canadian Journal of Nursing Research, 36*(3), 32–47.

Hansivsky, O., & Varcoe, C. (2007). From global to local and over the rainbow: Violence against women. In M. Morrow, O. Hanskivsky, & C. Varcoe (Eds.), *Women's health in Canada: Critical perspectives on theory and policy* (pp. 477–506). Toronto, ON: University of Toronto Press.

Health Canada. (1996). *Emotional abuse: Information from the National Clearinghouse on Family Violence.* Ottawa, ON: Public Health Agency of Canada. (Cat. No. 72-22/18-1996E).

Health Canada. (1999a). *Abuse and neglect of older adults: Information from the National Clearinghouse on Family Violence.* Ottawa, ON: Public Health Agency of Canada. (Cat. No. H72-22/6-1998E).

Health Canada. (1999b). *A handbook for health and social services professional responding to abuse during pregnancy.* Ottawa, ON: Health Canada, The National Clearinghouse on Family Violence. (Cat. No. H72-21/165-1998E).

Hildyard, K. L., & Wolfe, D. A. (2002). Child neglect: Developmental issues and outcomes. *Child Abuse and Neglect, 26,* 679–695.

Israel, B. A., Eng, E., Schulz, A. J., & Parker, E. A. (Eds.) (2005). *Methods in community-based participatory research for health.* San Francisco, CA: Jossey-Bass.

Jack, S., Munn, C., Cheng, C., & MacMillan, H. (2006). *Child maltreatment in Canada: Overview paper.* National Clearinghouse on Family Violence. Ottawa, ON: Government of Canada.

Jack, S. M., Jamieson, E., Wathen, C. N., & MacMillan, H. L. (2008). The feasibility of screening for intimate partner violence during postpartum home visits. *Canadian Journal of Nursing Research, 40*(2), 150–170.

Killick, C., & Taylor, B. J. (2009). Professional decision making on elder abuse: Systematic narrative review. *Journal of Elder Abuse and Neglect, 21,* 211–238.

Kurtz, D. L. M., Nyberg, J. C., Van Den Tillart, S., Mills, B., & The Okanagan Urban Aboriginal Health Research Collective (QUAHRC). (2008). Silencing of voice: An act of structural violence. *Journal of Aboriginal Health, 4*(1), 53–63.

Laverack, G. (2004). *Health promotion practice: Power and empowerment.* Thousand Oaks, CA: Sage.

Lewis, S. (2006). *Race against time: Searching for hope in AIDS-ravaged Africa* (2nd ed.). Toronto, ON: House of Anansi Press.

McAllister, M. (2000). Domestic violence: A life-span approach to assessment and intervention. *Lippincott's Primary Care Practice, 4*(2), 174–189. PMID: 11143628

McMurray, A. (2007). *Community health and wellness: A socio-ecological approach* (3rd ed.). Marrickville, Australia: Elsevier Australia.

McMurtry, R., & Curling, A. (2008, November). *The review of the roots of youth violence: Volume 2 Executive summary.* Retrieved from http://www.rootsofyouthviolence.on.ca/english/reports/volume2.pdf

Minkler, M., & Pies, C. (2002). Ethical issues in community organization and community participation. In M. Minkler (Ed.), *Community organizing and community building for health* (pp. 120–136). New Brunswick, NJ: Rutgers University Press.

National Aboriginal Health Organization. (2008, July). *Cultural competency and safety: A guide for health care administrators, providers, and educators.* Retrieved from http://www.naho.ca/publicaions/culturalCompetency.pdf

Native Women's Association of Canada. (2007). *Violence against Aboriginal women and girls: An issue paper.* Ottawa, ON: Author.

Neysmith, S. M. (1995). Power in relationships of trust: A feminist analysis of elder abuse. In M. J. MacLean (Ed.), *Abuse and neglect of older Canadians: Strategies for change* (pp. 43–54). Toronto, ON: Thompson Educational.

Nolan, S. (2007). *28 stories in Africa.* Toronto, ON: Alfred A. Knopf Canada.

Onyskiw, J. E. (2002). Health and the use of health services of children exposed to violence in their families. *Canadian Journal of Public Health, 93*(6), 416–420. Retrieved from http://www.ncbi.nlm.nih.gov/pubmed/12448862

Pauktuutit Inuit Women of Canada. (2006). *National strategy to prevent abuse in Inuit communities and sharing knowledge, sharing wisdom: A guide to the national strategy.* Ottawa, ON: Author.

Pinheiro, P. S. (2006). *World report on violence against children.* Geneva, Switzerland: United Nations, Secretary-Generals Study on Violence against Children. Retrieved from http://www.unicef.org/violencestudy/1.%20World%20Report%20on%20Violence%20against%20Children.pdf

Ploeg, J., Fear, J., Hutchinson, B., MacMillian, H., & Bolam, G. (2009). A systematic review of interventions for elder abuse. *Journal of Elder Abuse and Neglect, 21*(3), 187–210.

Registered Nurses' Association of Ontario (RNAO). (2005). *Woman abuse: Screening, identification and initial response.* Toronto, ON: Author.

Registered Nurses' Association of Ontario. (2007a). *Embracing cultural diversity in health care: Developing cultural competence.* Toronto, ON: Author.

Registered Nurses' Association of Ontario. (2007b, June). *Position statement: Respecting sexual orientation and gender identity.* Toronto, ON: Author.

Schim, S. M., Benkert, R., Bell, S. E., Walker, D. S., & Danford, C. A. (2007). Social justice: Added metaparadigm concept for urban heath nursing. *Public Health Nursing, 24*(1), 73–80.

Seelau, S. M., & Seelau, E. P. (2005). Gender-role stereotypes and perceptions of heterosexual, gay and lesbian domestic violence. *Journal of Family Violence, 20*(6), 363–371.

Statistics Canada. (1994). *Violence against women survey.* Ottawa, ON: Author. (Cat. No. 11-001E).

Statistics Canada. (2004). *Family violence in Canada: A statistical profile, 2004.* Ottawa, ON: Canadian Centre for Justice Statistics.

Statistics Canada. (2006, October). *Measuring violence against women: Statistical trends, 2006.* Ottawa, ON: Author. (Cat. No. 85-570-X1E).

Statistics Canada. (2008, October). *Family violence in Canada: A statistical profile 2008.* Ottawa, ON: Statistics Canada, Canadian Centre for Justice Statistics. (Cat. No. 85-224-XIE).

Statistics Canada. (2009, October). *Family violence in Canada: A statistical profile, 2009.* Ottawa, ON: Author. (Cat. No. 85-224-X).

Stevens, P., & Hall, J. (1992). Applying critical theories to nursing in communities. *Public Health Nursing, 9*(1), 2–9.

Trocme, N., Fallon, B., MacLaurin, B., Daciuk, J., Felstiner, C., Black, T., et al. (2005). *Canadian incidence study of reported child abuse and neglect—2003: Major findings.* Ottawa, ON: Minister of Public Works and Government Services Canada. (Cat. No. HP5-1/2005E).

United Nations General Assembly. (1993). *Declaration on the elimination of violence against women.* A/RES/48/104. adopted by the UN General Assembly, 20 December 1993. Retrieved from http://www.un.org/documents/ga/res/48/a48r104.htm

United Nations. (2006, August). *Report of the independent export for the United Nations study on violence against children.* Geneva, Switzerland: United Nations, UNICEF. Retrieved from http://www.unicef.org/violencestudy/reports/SG _violencestudy_en.pdf

United Nations Development Fund for Women. (2007, November). *Violence against women and children: Facts and figures.* Geneva, Switzerland: UNIFEM. Retrieved from http://www.unifem.org

Varcoe, C., & Dick, S. (2008). The intersecting risks of violence and HIV for rural Aboriginal women in a neo-colonial Canadian context. *Journal of Aboriginal Health, 4*(1), 42–52.

Varcoe, C., Hankivsky, O., & Morrow, M. (2007). Introduction: Beyond gender matters. In M. Morrow, O. Hankivsky, & C. Varcoe (Eds.), *Women's health in Canada: Critical perspectives on theory and policy* (pp. 3–30). Toronto, ON: University of Toronto Press.

Wallerstein, N. (2006). *What is the evidence of empowerment to improve health?* Copenhagen, Denmark: WHO Regional Office for Europe (Health Evidence Network Report).

Wathen, C. N., Tanaka, M., Catallo, C., Lebner, A. C., Friedman, M. K., Hanson, M. D., & MacMillian, H. L. (2009). Are clinicians being prepared to care for abused women? A survey of health professional education in Ontario, Canada. *BMC Medical Education, 9*(34). doi:10.1186/1472-6920-9-34

World Health Organization. (Health & Welfare Canada & the Canadian Public Health Association). (1986). *Ottawa Charter for Health Promotion.* Geneva, Switzerland: WHO.

World Health Organization. (2001). *Putting women first: Ethical and safety recommendations for research on domestic violence against women.* Geneva, Switzerland: WHO, Department of Gender and Women's Health, Family and Community Health.

World Health Organization. (2002a). *World report on violence and health: Summary.* Geneva, Switzerland: Author.

World Health Organization. (2002b). *World report on violence and health.* Geneva, Switzerland: Author.

World Health Organization. (2002c). *The Toronto Declaration on the global prevention of elder abuse.* Geneva: Switzerland: Author. http://www.who.int/hpr/aging

World Health Organization. (2004). *Preventing violence: A guide to implementing the recommendation of the world report on violence and health.* Geneva, Switzerland: Author.

World Health Organization. (2005). *The Bangkok Charter for health promotion in a globalized world.* Geneva, Switzerland: Author.

World Health Organization (WHO) & The International Network for the Prevention of Elder Abuse (INPEA). (2002). *Missing voices: Views of older persons on elder abuse.* Geneva, Switzerland: Authors.

ADDITIONAL RESOURCES

Readings

Aboriginal Nurses Association of Canada. (2009). *Cultural competence and cultural safety in nursing education: A framework for First Nations, Inuit, and Metis nursing.* Ottawa, ON: Aboriginal Nurses Association of Canada. http://www.anac.on.ca

Currier, D. M., & Carlson, J. H. (2009). Creating attitudinal change through teaching: How a course on "Women and violence" changes students' attitudes about violence against women. *Journal of Interpersonal Violence, 24*(10), 1735. doi:10.1177/0886260509335239

Fong, J. (Ed.). (2010). *Out of the shadows: Woman abuse in ethnic, immigrant, and Aboriginal communities.* Toronto, ON: Women's Press.

Humphreys, J., & Campbell, J. (Eds.). (2011). *Family violence and nursing practice* (2nd ed.). New York, NY: Springer.

Martin, S. L., Coyne-Beasley, T., Hoehn, M., Mathew, M., Runyan, C. W., Orton, S., & Royster, L-A. (2009). Primary prevention of violence against women: Training needs of violence practitioners. *Violence Against Women, 15*(1), 44–56.

World Health Organization and the International Society for the Prevention of Child Abuse and Neglect. (2006). *Preventing child maltreatment: A guide to taking action and generating evidence.* Geneva, Switzerland: WHO.

Video

Sunnybrook Hospital and Women's College. "Responding to domestic violence in clinical settings"—An e-learning program. Available at http://www.dveducation.ca

Websites

Assaulted Women's Help Line
http://www.awhl.org
Boost for Kids: Child Abuse Prevention & Intervention
http://www.boostforkids.org/
Canadian Women's Health Network
http://www.cwhn.ca
Connect 2 End Violence:
http://www.connect2endviolence.ca/
National Clearinghouse on Family Violence
http://www.phac-aspc.gc.ca/ncfv-cnivf/index-eng.php
Punjabi Community Health Services: Serving Diverse
Communities
http://www.punjabiservices.com/
United Nations: UN Study on Violence against Children,
2006.
http://www.unviolencestudy.org/

About the Author

Margaret M. Malone, RN, PhD, Associate Professor, Daphne Cockwell School of Nursing, Ryerson University. A feminist nurse sociologist, Margaret's community nursing experience informs her research, teaching, and community work. Teaching includes community, urban, population, and global health, with an emphasis on diversity and health promotion. Current program of research addresses violence against women and children with special attention to diverse at-risk populations and theoretical work on the development of a social theory of gender, knowledge, and emotion. Margaret co-leads the Nursing Centre for Research and Education on Violence Against Women and Children, Ryerson University, and is a member of a Canadian Public Health initiative, *Prevention of Violence Canada*.

chapter

27

Poverty and Homelessness

Lynnette Leeseberg Stamler and Aaron Gabriel

OBJECTIVES

After studying this chapter, you should be able to:

1. Describe the multiple definitions of poverty and homelessness and discuss the origins of those definitions.
2. Use the determinants of health framework to assess the influence of poverty and/or homelessness on an individual's or family's health.
3. Describe the community health nurse (CHN) role in advocating for groups and populations affected by poverty and homelessness.

INTRODUCTION

Many factors contribute to homelessness, poverty being significant. In fact, poverty is considered a threat to human development, health, and quality of life (Raphael, 2007); and some authors consider poverty to be the primary contributing factor in homelessness. While there is ongoing interest in poverty and homelessness in the media, it is disheartening to realize that few firm statistics are available that demonstrate the scope of the issue. There seems to be little interest in gathering national homelessness statistics since the 2001 census, and many of the statistics available today are relative and do not provide the "whole picture." For example, the data collection methods for homelessness are most often done using snowball sampling, point in time "guesstimates," and indirect estimations; and while poverty statistics are a bit more fulsome, the varying definitions of poverty contribute to a lack of clarity. Despite the absence of definitive statistics, it is clear from the data available that poverty and homelessness are continuing problems in Canada.

- It is estimated that 150 000 to 300 000 people are homeless in Canada in shelters or on the streets, and that 40 000 people stay in homeless shelters on any given night (Human Resources and Skills Development Canada, 2010).
- "Approximately one in nine Canadian adults, or close to 3 million people, reported that they have either experienced or come close to experiencing homelessness. Respondents in Manitoba and Saskatchewan reported the highest rate, with one in five (20%) respondents voicing concern about homelessness. Rates were also highest (16%) among respondents 45 to 55 years of age, and not surprisingly, among those with income levels less than $40 000 a year (20%)" (The Salvation Army, 2010, p. 3).

- Homeless Aboriginal people are over-represented in terms of the Canadian population. Aboriginals make up 3% of the Canadian population, but they account for 10% of the country's entire homeless population (Regroupement des centres d'amitié autochtones du Québec, 2008).
- In Toronto in 2005, 726 street homeless people had been housed through a "street to homes initiative" (Toronto Shelter, Support & Housing Administration, 2006).
- In the downtown core of Toronto, Canada, it has been estimated that between 900 and 1100 visible individuals are homeless on the street (Berry, 2007).
- In Ontario, there are nearly 130 000 households on waiting lists for social housing (Ontario Non-Profit Housing Association, 2009).
- In Vancouver in 2008, the preliminary homeless count, done in a single 24-hour period, suggested that there were approximately 2592 homeless persons (1547 street/service homeless and 1045 sheltered homeless) and that the total number of homeless persons had increased by 19% from 2005 to 2008 (Greater Vancouver Steering Committee on Homelessness, 2008).
- BC Housing reported that between 2008 and 2009 shelters were at full occupancy 40% of the nights they were open, which met their goals of 50% of the nights or less that they had to turn people away They also report serving 8075 homeless households, 6115 special needs households, 48 234 senior's households, and 28 199 low-income households (BC Housing, 2009).
- From a 2008 point-in-time census, Calgary reported that there were 4060 homeless persons in the city, and that this indicated an 18.2% increase since 2006 (The City of Calgary, 2008).

TABLE 27.1 Low-Income Cut-Offs (LICOs), After Tax, 2008

Size of Family Unit	Rural Areas	Urban Areas Size of Communities			
		Less than 30 000	30 000 – 99 999	100 000 – 499 999	500 000 and over
1 person	$12 019	$13 754	$15 344	$15 538	$18 373
2 persons	$14 628	$16 741	$18 676	$18 911	$22 361
3 persons	$18 215	$20 845	$23 255	$23 548	$27 844
4 persons	$22 724	$26 007	$29 013	$29 378	$34 738
5 persons	$25 876	$29 614	$33 037	$33 453	$39 556
6 persons	$28 698	$32 843	$36 640	$37 100	$43 869
7 or more persons	$31 519	$36 072	$40 241	$40 747	$48 181

Source: Statistics Canada. (2009). Income research paper series: Low income cut-offs for 2008 and low income measures for 2007. *Retrieved from http://www.statcan.gc.ca/pub/75f0002m/75f0002m2009002-eng.pdf. Table found on page 19.*

In this chapter, we will consider the scope of poverty and homelessness in Canada, and the demographic composition of these populations. Using the Health Canada determinants of health as a framework, we will examine the effects of poverty and homelessness on the health of Canadians and the role of CHNs who work with these populations.

POVERTY

One difficulty inherent in discussing poverty is the fact that we have no universally accepted definition of poverty. The measurement of a societal condition (such as poverty) is an essential precondition to taking corrective policy action. It seems that in modern societies, unless a societal condition has some statistical visibility, it is deemed not to exist. For example, even the census does not represent the most deprived citizens in Canada, thereby overlooking the growing income inequity among Canadians (Osberg, 2007). Four common definitions of poverty are used by policy makers; three are government developed.

The **"basic needs"** approach defines **poverty** as lacking food, clothing, and shelter plus other necessities "required to maintain long-term physical well being" (Sarlo, 1996, p. 25). The author of a basic needs measure arbitrarily determines the basic necessities and costs them out. Those who cannot afford these items are, by definition, poor. The **market basket measure (MBM)**, created by Human Resources Development Canada, is similar except that the contents of measure include a non-defined category of essentials in addition to food, clothing, and shelter. Thus the MBM looks at needs beyond purely physical needs. In both measures, the reference family includes two adults and two children. Inferences for other family configurations must be drawn by the users of the measure.

The low-income cut-off measure (LICO) and low-income measure (LIM) are based on family income rather than family costs. The better known of these two measures, the **LICO**, is based on the premise that the average Canadian family spends half its income on food, clothing, and shelter.

Researchers at Statistics Canada therefore concluded that any family that had to spend more than 70% of its income on those three items would have little disposable income to spend on other things such as transportation. The LICO is divided into family sizes ranging from one to seven and more, and is also referenced against the number of people in that family's place of residence. As such the LICO is able to capture how the family rates economically in relation to changing geography and a corresponding change in cost of living (Statistics Canada, 2009). The LICO measure identifies those persons in Canada who make considerably less than the average (see Table 27.1). Although Statistics Canada denies that this is a measure of poverty, it is a commonly used measure to describe that segment of our population that is worst off in economic terms, which some policymakers believe to be synonymous with poverty.

The **LIM** is an alternative measure also developed by Statistics Canada. It is based directly on income and is calculated based on what a single person requires, with the assumption that food, clothing, and shelter should account for 50% of the median income for one person. Other family configurations are considered, and the LIM stratifies between adult and child members of a family. Table 27.2 illustrates the LIM rates which were last calculated by Statistics Canada in 2007 (Statistics Canada, 2009).

One of the advantages of the LICO is that it reflects the community of residence and the composition of the family. This measure assumes that it takes more income to live in a larger centre and to support a larger family. Families with lower incomes than those in Table 27.1 are considered to be living in poverty.

The LICO provides a unique view of poverty in Canada by looking at the issue from the local level and then comparing the incomes with those in other centres. Economic growth is not equally divided among the constituents of a country. As the economy grows and communities prosper, the numbers living in poverty also grow, although at different rates. For example, between 1990 and 1995, metropolitan areas grew by 6.9% overall, while there was a 33.8% increase in the poor population (Lee, 2000). Further, using the LICO and LIM

TABLE 27.2   Low-Income Measures (LIMs), Before Tax, 2007

	Number of Children					
	0	1	2	3	4	5
1 Adult	$18 178	$25 449	$30 903	$36 356	$41 809	$47 263
2 Adults	$25 449	$30 903	$36 356	$41 809	$47 263	$52 716
3 Adults	$32 720	$38 174	$43 627	$49 081	$54 534	$59 987
4 Adults	$39 992	$45 445	$50 898	$56 352	$61 805	$67 259

Source: Statistics Canada. (2009). Income research paper series: Low income cut-offs for 2008 and low income measures for 2007. Retrieved from http://www.statcan.gc.ca/pub/75f0002m/75f0002m2009002-eng.pdf. Table found on page 28.

measures, the Organization for Economic Co-operation and Development (OECD) has been able to show that Canada's poverty rate has been on the rise, even compared to other countries (Hay, 2009).

People can have working income and still be considered poor. A working poor person has been defined as "someone who works the equivalent of full-time for at least half of the year but whose family income is below a low-income threshold" (Human Resources and Skills Development Canada, 2007, p. 6). Several factors contribute to a perception of working poor moving into middle class:

- Recent tax policies have shifted the burden of federal and provincial income taxes onto lower income workers.
- A second tax is the consumption tax, such as the sales tax. The required outlay for basic necessities takes a larger percentage of the poor family's income, thus, they bear a higher burden from consumption taxes.
- Wages, including low-income wages, have only been increasing at or below the rate of inflation. Thus, relative income is stagnant across all but the higher incomes.

Many factors can place persons at risk for living in poverty. Human Resources and Skills Development Canada (2008) completed a report on low income between the years of 2000 and 2006. This report identifies five "high-risk" groups for low income:

- lone parents with at least one child under 18 years of age,
- unattached individuals between the ages of 45 and 64,
- people with physical or mental disabilities that impede working,
- recent (within the past 10 years) immigrants to Canada, and
- Aboriginal Canadians living off reserve.

It is important to note that the above list did not focus on children or the elderly, who are often represented in the low-income ranges. This was potentially because the family/ household income status predicts these groups' income status as both children and elderly often live in shared accommodations. To this end, it is important to note that if the main income earner of a family fell under any of the above categories, the family would also fall under "high risk" for low income, would

have three times the risk of being low income compared to families whose main earner did not fall into the risk categories, and experience persistent low income more often (Human Resources and Skills Development Canada, 2008).

Lee (2000) examined regional differences in the urban poor in Canada. He found that poverty rates were higher in metropolitan areas as compared to smaller urban or rural areas in 1995. This finding was also shared in that Human Resources and Skills Development Canada (2008) found regional differences in the urban poor in Canada, indicating that poverty rates were higher in metropolitan areas. Using 1995 census statistics for cities of over 500 000 people, Lee found Montreal to have the most persons living in poverty, as well as the highest poverty rate. Vancouver and Winnipeg had the next highest rates of poverty, while Toronto had the second highest number of poor people. In relation to centres under 500 000 people, communities in Atlantic Canada and Quebec were more likely to have higher poverty rates than other parts of the country. Cape Breton had the highest incidence of poor persons.

Interestingly, the incidence of low income has decreased throughout all the risk categories except for Aboriginal Canadians living off reserve and recent immigrants (Human Resources and Skills Development Canada, 2008). This suggests that Canada is making some headway into eliminating poverty through programs such as old age security pensions, income supplements, and refundable child tax benefits. But, it seems clear that Canada has much work to do before it wins the war on poverty.

HOMELESSNESS

As with poverty, the definitions of homelessness are many and varied. Murphy (2000) chose to define **homelessness** in its narrowest and most limiting terms, which is, "those using emergency shelters and those sleeping in the street"-(p. 12). In contrast, the Niagara District Health Council (1997, pp. i–ii) identified four categories of homelessness:

- episodic (moves often, has periods of no housing),
- situational (absence of housing due to significant life event such as violence, illness, fire),

- seasonal (able to find housing during winter or other inclement weather), and
- absolute (lives on the street or in shelters for the majority of any given time).

Stearman (1999, p. 5) chose four other categories to describe this population:

- inadequate or inferior housing (lack of basic facilities),
- insecure housing (squatters in buildings or refugee camps),
- houselessness (people who use shelters, institutions, or other short-term accommodation like hotels), and
- rooflessness (living and sleeping outdoors).

While these categories were coined more than a decade ago, they still provide a framework for the CHN to consider poverty in the community of practice.

Once a definition of homelessness has been chosen, the next step is to ascertain how many people fall into that category. However, this presents significant difficulties. The data are incomplete because most population descriptions are a snapshot of time, and many survey methodologies are based on the ability to contact the population in order to count them. In other words, telephone surveys and census surveys assume a fixed address and/or telephone number. Thus the episodic, situational, and seasonal homeless may well be absent in any given counting and the absolute homeless, unless they happen to be in a shelter during census time, may be completely missed. Given these difficulties, it is not surprising that agencies like Statistics Canada are unable or unwilling to publish complete statistics on Canada's homeless population. At best, they can suggest inferences from other data. For example, B.C. Housing (2009) states that approximately 64 900 households in B.C. were unable to find adequate housing without spending 50% or more of their income. Moreover, 28% of off-reserve Aboriginal households lived in core housing, and were disproportionately represented among the homeless. Further, government assisted housing in 2009–2010 is estimated to account for 6% of the province's total house stock from dependent to independent support services. While these numbers are disturbing, they do not include people who have not applied, indicating that a portion of the population is underserved.

Murphy (2000) contends that this inability to be precise is a grave difficulty because "overestimating (the number of homeless) invites public cynicism, [and] underestimating incurs the wrath of service agencies that rely on public funding" (p. 11). She acknowledges that counting people in shelters misses "Canadians whose incomes force them to live in substandard housing with constant fear of eviction if their meager incomes should temporarily disappear. Nor does it address the growing number of poor who must spend up to 70% of their incomes on rent, leaving very little for food, nor those doubling up in accommodations" (pp. 12–13). She notes that some studies have estimated that for every person in a shelter on a given night, there are 1–2 persons living on the street on the same night. As noted earlier, in a single night count, Vancouver had 1045 persons in shelters and 1547 found homeless on the street (Greater Vancouver Steering Committee on Homelessness, 2008). It is evident that Murphy's estimates still hold true today.

A relatively new technology available to community stakeholders is the "Homeless Individuals and Families Information System" (HIFIS) initiative, which collects information related to the population using shelter services. This initiative has been implemented in nearly half of the known shelters in Canada, and was created with the purpose of providing a national understanding of homeless in Canada that can help communities plan for their local challenges. The HIFIS provides software and training to shelter staff that enables the staff to collect a comprehensive set of data on those individuals using the services (Human Resources and Skills Development Canada, 2009).

But what does being homeless really mean? Is it more than not having a roof over one's head? Murray (1990) used Tognoli's (1987) framework to examine the concept of homefullness in light of the homeless population. Tognoli (pp. 657–665) suggested that the following aspects are missing in the life of the homeless person:

- centrality, rootedness, and place attachments;
- continuity, unity, and order;
- privacy, refuge, security, and ownership;
- self-identity and gender differences;
- home as a context of social and family relations; and
- home as a sociocultural context.

It is clear that the homeless are missing much more than a roof. Rather, many of the connections in their life that link them to mainstream society are decreased or absent.

Golden, Currie, Greaves, and Latimer (1999, p. v) summarized the causes of homelessness, including

- increased poverty,
- lack of affordable housing,
- deinstitutionalization and lack of discharge planning, and
- social factors.

Morrell-Bellai, Goering, and Boydell (2000) used qualitative methodology to examine how and why persons become and/or remain homeless. They found that both macro (poverty, unemployment, or poor employment) as well as individual (mental health issues, childhood abuse, and/or substance abuse) vulnerabilities contributed to homelessness. Persons who were chronically homeless frequently indicated severe childhood traumas. Goering, Tolomiczenko, Sheldon, Boydell and Wasylenki (2002) interviewed 300 unaccompanied adult users of homeless shelters. They found fewer differences than similarities between those homeless for the first time and those who had been homeless previous to the study. While they found some indications of childhood homelessness issues as a characteristic of adult homelessness, they concluded that both groups had multiple problem indicators that required immediate intervention. In most of the reports, poverty was listed as a significant factor in homelessness. The issue of homelessness is not confined to large urban centres. The box below illustrates the large number of Canadian settings where homelessness is a challenge.

There are 61 communities in Canada that have significant problems with homelessness and receive funding from the Homelessness Partnering Strategy (HPS) to address their local issues (Human Resources and Skills Development Canada, 2010). These communities are

British Columbia/Yukon

- Kelowna, Kamloops, Nanaimo, Nelson, Prince George, Vancouver, Victoria, Whitehorse

Alberta/NWT/Nunavut

- Calgary, Edmonton, Grande Prairie, Iqaluit, Lethbridge, Medicine Hat, Red Deer, Wood Buffalo, Yellowknife

Saskatchewan

- Prince Albert, Regina, Saskatoon

Manitoba

- Brandon, Thompson, Winnipeg

Ontario

- Barrie, Belleville, Brantford, Dufferin, Guelph, Halton, Hamilton, Kingston, Kitchener, London, North Bay, Ottawa, Peel Region, Peterborough, Region of Durham, Sault Ste. Marie, St. Catharines-Niagara, Sudbury, Thunder Bay, Toronto, Windsor, York Region

Quebec

- Drummondville, Gatineau, Montreal, Quebec City, Saguenay, Sherbrooke, Trois-Rivières

New Brunswick

- Bathurst, Fredericton, Moncton, Saint John

Prince Edward Island

- Charlottetown, Summerside

Nova Scotia

- Halifax, Sydney (Cape Breton)

Newfoundland and Labrador

- St. John's

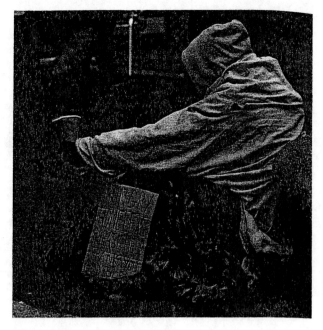

Photo 27.1

It is estimated that 150 000 to 300 000 people are homeless in Canada.

Credit: jon le-bon / Shutterstock

POVERTY, HOMELESSNESS, AND THE DETERMINANTS OF HEALTH

In 2003, Health Canada, based on evidence, identified 12 key determinants of health, sometimes known as the *social determinants of health*. The World Health Organization (WHO) (2009a) described the social determinants of health as "the conditions in which people are born, grow, live, work and age, including the health system. These circumstances are shaped by the distribution of money, power, and resources at global, national and local levels, which are themselves influenced by policy choices. The social determinants of health are mostly responsible for health inequities—the unfair and avoidable differences in health status seen within and between countries." From 2005 to 2008 the WHO established a commission to study health inequities on a global scale and report on

the best way to reduce the inequities. The Commission reported that "closing the health gap" would require "concerted actions across sectors" and presented three recommendations: (1) improving daily living conditions, (2) tackling inequitable distribution of power, money and other resources, and (3) measuring and understanding the problem and assessing the impact of action (WHO, 2009b). Raphael, Curry-Stevens, and Bryant argue that "Despite Canada's reputation as a leader in health promotion and population health, implementation of public policies in support of the social determinants of health has been woefully inadequate" (2009, p. 222). Recently, videos have been produced that discuss determinants of health; they are referenced under Additional Resources at the end of the chapter. In this chapter, we do not reiterate the data that produced these determinants; rather, we discuss how poverty and homelessness affect each one and mention a few of the programs in place to mitigate the effects of poverty and homelessness.

Income and Social Status Our income often dictates where we can afford to live, what we can afford to eat, and the activities we enjoy. The 2006 census indicates that 80% of the Canadian population lives in urban areas (Martel & Caron-Malenfant, 2007). A research group studied the results of the 2001 Census to determine links between health outcomes and living in five urban centres in Canada (Canadian Population Health Initiative, 2006). Findings included that more people living in high-income neighbourhoods tended to rate their health as excellent or very good, report more leisure time activity, and be non-smokers. The

Chief Public Health Officer's Report on the state of public health in Canada 2008 reports that if all the population had the same income levels and mortality rates as our highest income neighbourhoods, the potential for years lost to urban populations would decrease by almost 20% (Minister of Health, 2008) Some provincial governments have put programs in place to assist low-income families in such areas as early kindergarten, subsidized housing, and child benefits; however, families with no fixed address may still have difficulty accessing these programs. Persons who perceive their health as poor may be less likely or able to overcome barriers to seeking healthcare. While LICO recognizes the need for smaller incomes in rural areas, transportation costs are higher and healthcare services may be sparser, due to consolidation of services.

Social Support Networks Historically, Canadians have looked out for each other. This is evident in the way our healthcare and social support systems have evolved. However, the poor and the homeless are less able to meet this determinant of health in several ways.

■ Many of these networks are not available to them. A poor family's circle of friends and relatives may have exhausted the assistance they are able to give, putting strain on the relationships. This absence may come just at a time when the family needs the support desperately.

■ Obtaining money for travel or long-distance communication to continue the relationships may be problematic. Not having a fixed address makes it very difficult to receive mail or other communication from family and friends.

■ Establishing new and meaningful relationships in shelters or when frequently moving is difficult.

■ Poor persons may perceive they have nothing to offer in a relationship and begin to withdraw, increasing a sense of low self-esteem. Children who live in poverty may not learn to access and build social support networks.

Education and Literacy People who are poorly educated are less likely to qualify for high-paying jobs. As our use of technology increases, literacy requirements for many jobs are increasing. Persons with undiagnosed or untreated learning disabilities are more likely to drop out of school, again decreasing the opportunities available. Even if upgrading classes are subsidized and can be reached with affordable transportation, these people may not be able to afford the simplest of supplies to go to school or the childcare required in order to attend.

Employment/Working Conditions Persons with no fixed address and little or no income have difficulty getting identification papers, applying for jobs, or maintaining employment. The jobs they do get are often transitory, hourly-wage jobs with few benefits, forcing them to choose, for instance, between going to a health professional for a personal or family health problem and going to work. Further, persons working in low-paying jobs may be more susceptible to workplace injury, thus further limiting opportunities. While Canada enjoyed a relatively low unemployment rate as late as 2008, the global financial events in 2008 and onwards have increased the numbers of families affected by unemployment.

Social Environments Poverty can be viewed as a social exclusionary factor (see Research Box 27.1). Many persons who are poor and/or homeless are victims of violence or have been deinstitutionalized. Thus, social supports previously available may not be in place. Further, the social definition of poverty can be internalized, contributing to a sense of stigma, feelings of shame and inferiority, and low self esteem (Reutter, Stewart, Veenstra, Love, Raphael, & Makwarimba, 2009).

CANADIAN RESEARCH BOX

How do experiences of social isolation and perceptions of belonging differ between lower-income persons and higher-income persons?

Stewart, M. J., Makwarimba, E., Reutter, L. I., Veenstra, G., Raphael, D., & Love, R. (2009). Poverty, sense of belonging and experiences of social isolation. *Journal of Poverty, 13,* 173–195.

This interprofessional study team interviewed 60 individuals with higher incomes and 59 individuals with lower incomes (using LICO) in Toronto and Edmonton. Six group interviews with low-income participants were also conducted. Further, a telephone survey of both lower- and higher-income individuals was completed. The interviews focused on a sense of belonging, what factors contribute to this sense of belonging, and the effect of income on both the sense of belonging and a feeling of isolation. The telephone surveys consisted of a 110-item investigator-constructed instrument, based on previously validated measures and data from the interviews. While religious organizations were identified as strong places for a sense of belonging, lower-income participants felt precluded from full participation, while higher-income participants did not. In contrast, lower-income participants identified with community or social agencies. Poverty also seemed to isolate lower-income participants from full participation in family events. In fact, lower-income participants described less reciprocal involvement with all sources of belonging or community than higher-income participants, contributing to a sense of isolation. Quantitative results supported the qualitative data—"respondents above the LICO had an odds of reporting a sense of belonging that was 2.31 times as high as for those below the LICO" (pg. 190). This research illustrates the importance of income to a positive social environment.

Discussion Questions

1. What are all the communities you consider yourself a part of? How many of them would be more difficult if poverty was an issue?

2. What activities could the CHN engage in to foster a sense of belonging in neighbourhoods that are lower-income?

Physical Environments Some cities and neighbourhoods are in high pollution geographic areas, exposing the whole population to additional health risks. However, within specific geographic locations, housing that is affordable to the poor family and is not subsidized is frequently substandard, may be unsafe, and is often crowded. Overcrowding, combined with poor hygiene, can contribute to the spread of contagious diseases, including tuberculosis. Further, low-income housing is more likely to be in an unsafe neighbourhood, exposing the inhabitants to increased violence and fewer supports, such as law enforcement. Over the last several years national and local organizations such as Habitat for Humanity have worked to ensure affordable and safe housing for low-income families. While poverty can be less visible in rural communities, inability to maintain or enhance the physical environment (e.g., house, outbuildings) can lead to increased accidents and disease.

Personal Health and Coping Skills The facilities and opportunities available for basic personal hygiene, much less optimal health practices, are more difficult for the poor and the homeless populations. Votta and Manion (2003) found that homeless male youths reported more substance abuse, families that were dysfunctional, difficulties in school, legal problems, and suicide attempts than non-homeless youths. Further, these youth reported less parental support, greater depressive episodes, and increased use of disengagement as a coping style.

Healthy Child Development One of the greatest concerns with poverty and homelessness is their effect on children. One of the most obvious issues is food insecurity, or the lack of access to sufficient nutritious food. This can result in children experiencing difficulties with memory, concentration, energy, problem-solving skills, and creativity (Minister of Health, 2008). Food banks, before-school breakfast programs, and other social activities to encourage healthy eating, where available, are making some inroads to better food security in Canada. Other issues to consider are poor hygiene and increased exposure to hazards and violence, resulting in lower life expectancy for persons who grow up in poverty. One of the less obvious results of poverty is that families with little or no disposable income have difficulty ensuring their children have access to activities that would enhance their development. Even reading to a child at night becomes problematic when one cannot afford books and cannot access a library card due to the lack of fixed address. Constant moving can also interfere with normal progress through public education. Further, poor children who do not dress like other children or have the same type of school supplies may feel more ostracized and victimized by peer bullying.

Biology and Genetic Endowment While biology and genetics may account for vision, hearing, and dental problems, poverty may ensure those problems remain untreated. Poor people may delay seeking help due to their inability to pay for medication or other treatment not covered by the healthcare system. Mortality rates in poorer neighbourhoods are higher than in the general population.

Health Services While geography is frequently a barrier to health services for all Canadians, the poor family faces additional barriers. Despite a strong universal healthcare system, income is required for services such as dental care and pharmaceuticals. Unemployment makes access that much more difficult. The lack of a fixed address can wreak havoc with making healthcare appointments or registering for services. The family seeking care may be faced with health professionals who do not provide culturally safe care, thus encouraging the family to avoid returning for follow up care. When a poor or homeless person is hospitalized, assumptions may be made about the care that can be delivered after discharge—a challenge even for families with adequate income. Mobile health units and the use of technology such as telehealth has increased access for many persons, but still does not always meet the needs of the poor and homeless.

Gender Women generally live longer than men and experience greater incidences of depression, stress overload, and some chronic conditions. When rates of physical activity (often part of leisure time) are included in the equation, risk for chronic illnesses among women increases. Women are more likely to be the victims of family violence. As well, they are more likely to be in the lower employment categories. Lone-parent families continue to experience the lowest levels of family income in Canada, with the greater majority of these headed by women (Statistics Canada. 2008). Further, women who become lone-parent heads of households under the age of 40 tend to remain in poverty (Gadalla, 2008). All these factors contribute to inclusion within the populations of poverty and homelessness.

Culture Each person belongs to several different cultures, including ethnic, neighbourhood, work, club (e.g., the Legion), and religious. Part of belonging to any given culture is the desire to meet that culture's expectations. Poverty and homelessness for many of the reasons already stated may increase the barriers to meeting one's cultural tasks, contributing to decreases in self-worth, and failure to engage in healthy behaviours that are possible.

This limited discussion on the effects of poverty and homelessness on the determinants of health demonstrates that both poverty and homelessness increase the barriers to meeting the determinants and reinforces their interrelatedness. A barrier is anything that prevents the person or family from accomplishing a health task. Barriers may be actual (lack of address or identification, resulting in refusal of services) or perceived (belief that as a poor or homeless person I have nothing to offer a relationship). In the case of poverty and homelessness, the above discussion has identified multiple barriers to each of the determinants of health. When there is a barrier to one determinant of health, that barrier influences several other determinants as well. In the next section, we will consider specific health issues for these populations.

SPECIFIC HEALTH ISSUES OF THE HOMELESS AND POOR

Health issues of the homeless do not differ from those of the general population. Disease severity is related to a number of factors: poverty, cognitive impairment, delays in seeking treatment, non-adherence to therapy, and the adverse health effects of homelessness itself (Hwang, 2001). Adverse health effects of homelessness include, but are not limited to, skin and foot disorders, poor oral hygiene, respiratory tract infections, and hypertension (Hwang). Foot disorders, for example, can be related to improperly fitted footwear or wearing the same footwear for prolonged periods of time. Shoes are sometimes used as pillows to allow the foot to breathe. Socks also may be worn for extended periods of time. All of these factors can impact the treatment of specific foot disorders such as fungal infections, plantar warts, ulcers, and large calluses.

Diseases and conditions often seen by clinicians whose practice includes homeless individuals reflect environmental factors, lifestyle choices, and the impact of poverty on health. Hypertension, cardiovascular disease, diabetes, asthma, renal disease, mental illness, cancer, HIV infection, AIDS, sexually transmitted diseases, infant mortality, trauma caused by violence, and substance abuse are some of the conditions experienced by people who are homeless. An obvious correlation can be found between some of the diagnoses and life on the street. For example, a person sleeping on heating grates may be burned.

To find the relationships between an adverse health effect and a homeless person, the healthcare provider needs to assess the lifestyle of the client. Assessment should include sleeping patterns and where sleep is obtained, food, smoking, substance use, support networks, and income. A thorough assessment of the daily routine of the client is important because it may reveal the relationships. A good understanding of the determinants of health and their application is important when doing the assessment. Other relationships or the weight these relationships place on the health of the person may not be so obvious to the novice clinician.

CASE STUDY

It is 2013 and there has been a new swine flu (H1N1) outbreak in Toronto. You are a CHN working with the homeless population. So far no homeless persons have contracted H1N1, but you need to prepare a plan of action to ensure this at-risk population is aware and protected. You meet a 22-year-old male reporting symptoms of fever, productive coughs, and increasing difficulty breathing. He tells you that he has been living on the street with his girlfriend for two years and reports an unremarkable medical history. He was born in Toronto and works part-time at a nearby grocery store.

You auscultate his lungs and note decreased air entry and slight atelectasis. You recommend a trip to the hospital, but he does not appear concerned and does not want to see a doctor. He promises to come back to the clinic if he feels worse. Four days later, you run into him and his girlfriend at a local shelter. She is displaying his initial symptoms but he appears unchanged.

Discussion Questions

1. Identify the determinants of health and explain their effect on attainment of optimum health for this young man.

2. How would you share relevant information on H1N1 and health maintenance?

3. What might you recommend to the local shelter to prevent further spread?

Case study inspired by Leung, C., Ho, M., Kiss, A., Gundlapalli, A., & Hwang, S. (2008). Homelessness and the response to emerging infectious disease outbreaks: Lessons from SARS. Journal of Urban Health, 85(3), 402–410.

Chronic conditions or the exacerbation of symptoms caused by acute onset in clients who are poor or homeless can also be influenced by both internal and external barriers to health. External barriers can include fragmented healthcare and misconceptions, prejudice, and frustration from the healthcare providers (Plumb, 2000). Poor perception of health issues, competing priorities (shelter, food, safety versus accessing healthcare), and feelings of prejudice are some of the internal barriers (Plumb). Other barriers can also make the delivery of healthcare difficult for this population. Once healthcare is accessed, it can be fragmented if the care is gained at an ER or walk-in clinic. Care in either the ER or a walk-in clinic may be for symptom management with little opportunity to develop a long-term plan of care. If specialist care is needed, access becomes difficult without a valid health card, return phone number to confirm the appointment, and physician to consult with or develop a plan of care.

Researchers working with young mothers who were street involved noted that while the pregnancy and/or birth positively changed many of the perceptions of the women, long-term poverty and health implications were not as strongly considered (King, Ross, Bruno & Erickson, 2009). The challenge in the delivery of healthcare to these populations revolves around clinicians' ability to reduce their own feelings of frustration and comprehend the impact that environment and lifestyle have on a person's health. Also, it is important to be aware that health conditions normally seen in housed 60-year-old people may appear in 40-year-old homeless persons due to the harsher living conditions for the homeless.

CANADIAN RESEARCH BOX

What are mortality rates among residents of shelters, rooming houses and hotels?

Hwang, S. W., Wilkins, R., Tjepkema, M., O'Campo, P. J., & Dunn, J. R. (2009). Mortality among residents of shelters, rooming houses, and hotels in Canada: 11 year follow-up study. *British Medical Journal, 339,* 4036

Housing is an indicator of socioeconomic standing and is a social determinant of health, as such it is understood that homeless persons will experience a lower level of health when compared to the general Canadian population. Most homeless persons live in shelters, hostels, and missions, and persons who are marginally housed may live in low-cost collective dwellings such as the YMCA, rooming houses, and single-room hotels.

Hwang et al. utilized a follow-up method to look at mortality rates in the homeless and marginally housed. Their research was done in an attempt to determine the age- and sex-specific causes of death and the probability of survival to various ages through a nationwide sample of homeless and marginally housed persons. Further, this research looked at the mortality rates among variously categorized homeless and marginally housed individuals in order to determine if there was a difference in mortality rates when compared by income.

To do this, the researchers utilized the 1991 Canadian census, which was distributed to one in five private households and to all persons living in non-institutional collective dwellings serving the homeless or marginally housed. Tax filter data were also used to collect names of individuals so that the researchers could determine mortality using the Canadian Mortality database. Finally, the researchers determined the total pre-tax income of all census sources (for each household or unattached individual), and calculated the ratio of total incomes using the 1991 LICO from Statistics Canada in order to rank the population into fifths. The results of this study indicated that compared to the entire Canadian cohort, the life expectancy was significantly shorter for people living in shelters (by 13 years for men and 8 years for women), rooming houses (11 years for men and 9 years for women), and hotels (8 years for men and 5 years for women). This research also indicated that the premature mortality of the homeless or marginally housed individuals was predominantly caused by alcohol, smoking, violence, injuries, mental disorders, and suicides. Incredibly, it was estimated that the probability of a 25 year old (living in a shelter, rooming house, or hotel) reaching the age of 75 was 32% for men and 60% for women; which is interesting when compared to 51% for men and 72% for women who were a part of the lowest fifth of income. These results suggest that where a homeless or marginally housed person lives is a factor in mortality no matter the level of income.

Discussion Questions

1. You are asked to coordinate the development of a health program for the homeless in your city. Would this research paper be useful in that development? What are its limitations?

2. Using the determinants of health, what ways might specifically targeting housing positively affect the general and emotional health of a homeless or marginally housed individual?

3. Why do you think there is a significantly higher rate of mortality for homeless individuals or marginally housed individuals living in shelters, rooming houses, or hotels, even when compared to individuals in the lowest fifth of income distribution?

ACCESS TO HEALTHCARE

Challenging economic, social, and environmental conditions often result in poor health. Unfortunately, some populations in urban, rural, remote, and northern environments have difficulty accessing mainstream healthcare services. Canadians living in urban and non-urban areas face different difficulties in accessing the care they require, as such community-based front-line health services need to be able to provide necessary care while addressing the local determinants of health. Individuals living in non-urban areas often experience more challenges when accessing healthcare services compared to those living in cities. Rural, remote, and northern areas often struggle with attracting healthcare professionals, leading to a decreased selection in healthcare services. For example, many rural hospitals are staffed by family doctors and there are few specialists. Further, patients seeking health services outside of their community often must travel great distances and usually incur further costs such as taking time off work, having decreased social support from family/friends, and expenses for travel, lodging, and food (Hay, Verga-Toth, & Hines, 2006).

The most common access points for healthcare in rural areas are family doctors, small rural hospitals, community health centres or clinics, nursing stations, and mobile health units. However, the use of telehealth is an option explored in these areas to allow specialists to consult with the local healthcare providers, as well as an avenue for training. Essentially, telehealth involves use of a telephone, written materials, and a video or web-based program. For example, Dr. Patrick McGrath, a professor of psychology and psychiatry at Dalhousie University, and colleagues are providing mental health services to rural persons being treated for post-partum depression and for parents of children with behavioural challenges (Hay, Varga-Toth, & Hines, 2006, p.18).

Travelling healthcare providers, particularly those who are specialized, may stop in underserved communities and rural hospitals to provide services. However, the services may be few and far between due to time constraints, waiting list times, lack of medical resources/supplies, and distances of travel for the healthcare provider. For this reason a proactive form of healthcare services was created wherein the service is brought to those who need it. For example, in Saskatoon, Saskatchewan, a mobile health bus has been staffed with a nurse practitioner and a paramedic in order to provide primary healthcare services closer to home for members of the core community. The services provided on the bus are health checks, blood pressure and sugar checks, chronic disease management, disease prevention, health education, wound care, and follow-up care. The staff also link clients to youth/addiction/mental health services, and community-based organizations and programs (Saskatoon Health Region, 2008).

COMMUNITY HEALTH NURSES' ROLE

CHNs act to provide community empowerment through their public health functions with the goal of providing services to the population, community, families, and individuals in terms of outcomes such as protection, promotion, prevention, and access. By increasing their clinical acumen within their population, CHNs learn or rather take on new roles. One role is that of an advocate through political action (e.g., Cathy Crowe). Another is enabling clients to empower themselves.

Cathy Crowe is an example of a CHN who is committed to this high-risk population. It is fitting that she works in the Canadian city with one of the highest populations of poor, although there are CHNs in most major cities working with this population. Ms Crowe advocates through strong political action for the rights of the homeless. She is noted for legal action she has brought against the Province of Ontario to increase affordable housing, to reduce the number of deaths related to homelessness, and to be accountable for its policies. The Toronto Disaster Relief Committee made these accomplishments possible through strong lobbying of the municipal, provincial, and federal governments. Ms Crowe and others formed the Toronto Disaster Relief Committee in the mid-1990s. She works closely with this Committee and a community health centre. Her strong commitment to this population has lead to the formation of the federal ministry devoted to homelessness (Keung, 2002). Ms Crowe can also be found delivering care to the homeless, carrying the essentials in her backpack. Tent City, a homeless ad hoc city on the shore of Lake Ontario, was part of her practice. Ms Crowe received the first-ever Woodsworth Award for Social Advocacy in recognition of her commitment to social advocacy. The award was named after Jean Woodsworth, a social advocate who fought for the universality of old-age pensions (Keung). Further, in 2004 she received an Atkinson Fellowship award that was extended in both 2007 and 2009 to help fight homelessness during the economic recession. In 2009, she published a book called *Dying for a Home*, and has continued to travel to other Canadian cities to offer support while advocating for the homeless (Crowe, 2009).

Toronto Public Health developed a project for supporting at-risk homeless pregnant and parenting women. Two nurses worked on this project. One nurse worked in the downtown area of Toronto and the other worked in the suburbs where there were hotels serving homeless families. These nurses received referrals from shelters, drop-in health centres, and street hangouts. The nurses coordinated care involving several community services, provided home visits, and made telephone follow-ups. The nurses also accompanied clients to prenatal visits until they were comfortable going alone (Little, Gorman, Dzendoletas & Moravac, 2007).

TECHNOLOGY AND HOMELESSNESS

Technology is a part of everyday living in Canada, and it has been suggested that technology has the capacity to improve the quality of life that people enjoy. However, most people do not reflect on how the technology in their environments affects their lives, or how the lack of that technology may put them at a disadvantage. Although the development of technology is not to blame for poverty or homelessness, it does play an integral role in how everyone interacts with society as a whole.

Le Dantec and Edwards (2008) suggested that "the factors that disadvantage developing nations are also present among the homeless population in industrialized nations and affect the relationship of this population with technology; lower levels of education and literacy restrict access to information, a lack of economic independence restricts access to computers and Internet resources, and limited access to training hinders the uptake of digital technology when it is made available" (p. 628). A qualitative study by Le Dantec and Edwards (2008) used one-on-one interviews from which several themes were developed about the relationship homeless persons have with technology. They suggested that homeless persons use technology regularly especially if there is a perceived benefit. This research indicated that homeless persons place great value in being able to stay connected with family, friends, and important contacts or resources whether by phone, Internet, or in person. This research also indicated that homeless persons utilize computers and the Internet to find resources (such as where they can go for a shower, meals, and job postings), to access information or give tips on how to survive on the streets, and to do social networking on sites without feeling the stigma associated with homelessness. However, several difficulties were reported including finding an affordable and/or available telephone/computer, being able to receive or answer messages on the telephone, the availability of electricity to recharge batteries, literacy and understanding how to use technology, and the time involved in finding sources of technology (i.e.. waiting in line for a public phone or computer, taking public transit).

Le Dantec and Edwards' research suggests that thoughtful technologies, that are socially relevant, could be used as an intervention to reduce homelessness while helping those already at risk. This is a belief shared by several networking sites, such as "Homeless Nation," which describes itself as a website for and by the street community. This website was developed in 2003 by a Montreal-based documentary filmmaker and friends who were interested in the stories of the homeless. This site was created as an access point for online media, a place to share stories and information, a social networking site, a place to locate friends who have gone missing, and most importantly to create social awareness and positive change. Nearly 4500 people have joined the site and it has received several awards; most recently this site was recognized by receiving the UN-based 2009 World Summit Award (Pinchin, 2009).

Recently, in Vancouver, BC, the Lu'ma Native Housing Society began a program to provide free phone numbers and voice-mail to the homeless. This voice mail acts as a means to contact the homeless individual, whether that person is a landlord, prospective employer, healthcare provider, or loved one (Paulsen, 2010). This service provides persons in crisis or transition a reliable way to maintain contact. The telephone numbers are given to the homeless clients through their case-workers. A password and personal greeting are created, and then the clients can manage their own appointments by dialing into the system. This program will also alert the clients to waiting voice mail via their e-mail account, so that the clients receive notice of the mail while it is relevant. Further, the voice-mail program allows organizations to broadcast blanket messages to all clients in the system, whether the message is about possible employment or a safety warning for the area (Foster, 2010).

RESEARCH

Research in the area of homelessness can be difficult for a number of reasons. Not knowing who the homeless people are or where to find them is the most obvious. Other reasons may include, but are not limited to, competing priorities of the client (finding food may take precedence over participation in research), the perception that the endpoint of the research does not make a difference in the daily life of the homeless, and the inability of the researcher to find a funding agency. To overcome some of these barriers, researchers have begun to use the community participation approach to their research. Community participatory research is characterized by using community leaders in partnership with the researchers through the entire research process. That is, the community is involved from the inception, when the gap is identified, to the endpoint of writing the report and disseminating the information. Through this process the community has the opportunity to see a difference in their daily lives as a result of the research process.

Research contributing to the understanding of these populations is limited. It is interesting to note that in a recent search of professional literature, nursing literature was sparse in the areas of homelessness and poverty, and other Canadian researchers appear more likely to study these topics elsewhere in the world rather than at home.

SUMMARY

In this chapter we have explored the definitions and scope of poverty and homelessness in Canada. Recognition of the difficulty in defining and describing these populations separately or together has informed the process. Using the determinants of health as a framework, we have explored the effect of poverty and homelessness on the determinants. Specific health issues for these populations and the CHN's role were explored.

The CHN is the healthcare provider who may have first access to poor or homeless persons through community outreach activities. By initiating communication and making a determined effort to understand their world, the CHN may be able to establish a trusting relationship that enables the nurse and the client to co-create a higher level of health.

KEY TERMS

basic needs, p. 421
poverty, p. 421
market basket measure (MBM), p. 421
low-income cut-off measure (LICO), p. 421
low-income measure (LIM), p. 421
homelessness, p. 422

REVIEW QUESTIONS

1. Poverty is a social condition often considered as predetermining for homelessness. As a CHN, you would like to compile statistics on the homeless population you work with so that you can compare your population to that of Canada as a whole. What measure would you use in order to achieve the most impact for people who create policy related to affordable housing?

   a) market basket beasure (MBM)

   b) low-income cut-offs (LICO)

   c) low-income measures (LIM)

   d) use an independent measure because the others are not accurate

2. Mrs. Bennett, 35-year-old mother of two, brings her youngest child in for complaints of ringing ears and a headache that has gotten worse over two days. The children appear thin for their age and Mrs. Bennett is thin and very pale. A full assessment is done for child and mother. You find out that Mrs. Bennett is a single, working mother who earns minimum wage and often has difficulty paying for rent and groceries. What services might you, as a CHN, suggest to best assist this family?

   a) Suggest they seek placement on an affordable housing list.

   b) Suggest they apply for government support.

   c) Suggest that the children be placed in a school with a breakfast and lunch program.

   d) Give the family information on how to access the community food bank.

Charlie, 27 years old, has been homeless for five years. Two weeks ago Charlie visited a walk-in health clinic where you work as a CHN, and consented to complete a comprehensive nursing assessment.

3. Charlie informs you that he has not had a physical examination in over 5 years, and that he rarely visits a healthcare provider. What should you do to provide Charlie with optimum care?

   a) Call Charlie's family and ask that they let him stay with them.

   b) Assess Charlie for any immediate health concerns and give him pamphlets including Canada's food guide, Participaction recommendations, and "how to dispose of prescriptions safely" when he leaves as a way to prevent future health troubles.

   c) Encourage Charlie to return to the walk-in clinic every six months for a check-up, and any time he does not feel well.

   d) Perform a head-to-toe assessment and refer Charlie to a physician at a hospital emergency department five blocks away.

4. Charlie tells you that during the winter he tries to sleep in shelters or churches, and that during warmer nights he sleeps in parks or bus stop shelters. What category of homelessness does Charlie fit into?

   a) episodic

   b) situational

   c) seasonal

   d) absolute

5. Charlie confides in you that he has had multiple sexual partners, and uses a condom occasionally. Your priority goal in meeting his needs at this time would include ensuring that he

   a) understands the risks of multiple partners.

   b) knows how to access free condoms.

   c) gets regular testing for HIV.

   d) understands his own sexual preferences

STUDY QUESTIONS

1. List three different ways that homelessness can be defined.

2. What is the difference between the LICO and LIM measures of poverty?

3. What is the difference between a family in poverty and the working poor?

4. Identify three ways that a CHN can contribute to ensuring food security in a given community.

5. Discuss the assumption that it is less expensive to live in rural areas.

6. What factors contribute to the statistic that female-headed lone parent families are more likely to live in poverty than those headed by males? Consider all the determinants of health.

After working through these questions, go to the MyNursingLab at www.pearsoned.ca/mynursinglab to check your answers.

INDIVIDUAL CRITICAL THINKING EXERCISES

1. In 1990, the Canadian Public Health Association described the advocacy role of public health nursing as one of helping the socially disadvantaged to become aware of issues relevant to their health and promoting the development of resources that will result in "equal access to health and health-related services." As a nurse working in the community, how would you develop a plan of care for a person living in a shelter? Use the above statement as a guide, paying close attention to accessing healthcare services.

2. Consider how many times a day you are asked for some form of identification. What activities would you be unable to perform if you did not have this identification? How might this affect your health and healthcare?

3. List 10 personal everyday activities that require money for participation and add up the total. What activities would you need to delete if your income was below the LICO level? Would the removal of any of these activities affect your health status? How?

4. "There is evidence that homeless children have more health problems, more hospitalizations, and more developmental problems than poor children who have never been homeless" (Egan, 2002). Using the determinants of health as your guide in the discussion, comment on this quotation and discuss its validity.

5. Consider how a CHN might need to reframe his or her perceptions of healthcare service delivery when working with the homeless populations.

GROUP CRITICAL THINKING EXERCISES

1. Recent extreme heat waves in the summer months have led to growing public health concern regarding the elderly, people with chronic and debilitating health conditions, and people living in poverty and inadequate housing such as rooming houses. Existing public health measures seem to rely on public service announcements that encourage the public to drink lots of fluid and go to the air-conditioned spaces such as libraries. Provide a critique of these measures and consider possible solutions and advocacy measures.

2. "The working poor live on a precipice that can tumble them into homelessness at any time. An illness or an unexpected layoff brings missed paycheques, which lead to skipped utility or rent payments, which snowball into penalties, which end in shutoffs or evictions" (Plumb,

2000). Discuss how a CHN would interact with a person in this situation. Consider advocacy measures and possible research questions that would assist this high-risk clientele.

3. Read about the Calgary 24-hour homeless count. Consider the city or area you live in and make a list of all the agencies in your community that you would include to replicate this in your area.

REFERENCES

BC Housing. (2009). *Annual report 2008/09*. Retrieved from http://www.bchousing.org/resources/About%20BC%20Housing/Annual%20Reports/2009/BCH_Annual_Report_2009.pdf

Berry, B. (2007). A repeated observation approach for estimating the street homeless population. *Evaluation Review, 31*(2), 166–199.

Canadian Population Health Initiative. (2006). *Improving the health of Canadians: An introduction to health in urban places*. Ottawa, ON: The Canadian Institute of Health Information.

Crowe, C. (2009). *Cathy Crowe newsletter #57-summer 2009*. Retrieved from http://tdrc.net/uploads/file/Cathy/newsletter/ccnews_summer09.pdf

Egan, J. (2002, March 24). To be young and homeless. *The New York Times*. Retrieved from http://www.nytimes.com/2002/03/24/magazine/to-be-young-and-homeless.html?pagewanted=9

Foster, J. (2010). *Phonelines are lifelines*. Retrieved from http://www.tenants.bc.ca/ckfinder/userfiles/files/CVM%20-%20Phonelines%20are%20Lifelines.pdf

Gadalla, T. M. (2008). Gender differences in poverty rates after marital dissolution: A longitudinal study. *Journal of Divorce and Remarriage, 49*(3–4), 225–238.

Goering, P., Tolomiczenko, G., Sheldon, T., Boydell, K., & Wasylenki, D. (2002). Characteristics of persons who are homeless for the first time. *Psychiatric Services, 53*(11), 1472–1474.

Golden, A., Currie, W. H., Greaves, E., & Latimer, E. J. (1999). *Taking responsibility for homelessness: An action plan for Toronto*. Toronto, ON: Toronto, Mayor's Homelessness Action Task Force.

Greater Vancouver Steering Committee on Homelessness. (2008). *Metro Vancouver homeless count figures 2008: Preliminary numbers April 8, 2008*. Retrieved from http://www.metrovancouver.org/planning/homelessness/ResourcesPage/2008HomelessCountPreliminaryFS-April.pdf

Hay, D. (2009). *Poverty reduction policies and programs*. Retrieved from http://www.ccsd.ca/SDR2009/Reports/Canada_Report_FINAL.pdf

Hay, D., Varga-Toth, J., & Hines, E. (2006). *Frontline health care in Canada: Innovations in delivering services to vulnerable populations*. Canadian Policy Research Networkers INC. Retrieved from http://www.cprn.org/documents/45652_en.pdf

Human Resources and Skills Development Canada. (2007). *When working is not enough to escape poverty: An analysis of Canada's working poor August 2006*. Retrieved from http://www.hrsdc.gc.ca/eng/cs/sp/sdc/pkrf/publications/research/SP-630-06-06/page00.shtml

Human Resources and Skills Development Canada. (2008). *Low income in Canada: 2000–2006 using the market basket measure*. Retrieved from http://www.servicecanada.gc.ca/eng/cs/sp/sdc/pkrf/publications/research/SP-630-06-06/page06.shtml

Human Resources and Skills Development Canada. (2009). *HPS Success: Enhancing access to and use of good practices, information, data and measures*. Retrieved from http://www.hrsdc.gc.ca/eng/publications_resources/evaluation/2009/ehps/page11.shtml

Human Resources and Skills Development Canada. (2010). *The homelessness partnering strategy*. Retrieved from http://www.hrsdc.gc.ca/eng/homelessness/index.shtml

Hwang, S. W. (2001). Homelessness and health. *Canadian Medical Association Journal, 164*(2), 229–233.

Keung, N. (2002). *Cathy Crowe: Toronto's street nurse*. Retrieved from http://www.ottawainnercityministries.ca/newsArticlesStats/Cathy_Crowe.htm

King, K., Ross, L., Bruno, T., & Erickson, P. (2009). Identity work among street-involved young mothers. *Journal of Youth Studies, 12*(2), 139–149.

Le Dantec, C., & Edwards, K. (2008). Designs on dignity: Perceptions of technology among the homeless. *Conference on Human Factors in Computing Systems—Proceedings*, 627–636. Retrieved from http://www.cc.gatech.edu/~keith/pubs/chi2008-homeless.pdf

Lee, K. (2000). *Urban poverty in Canada: A statistical profile*. Ottawa, ON: Canadian Council on Social Development.

Little, M., Gorman, A., Dzendoletas, D., & Moravac, C. (2007). *Caring for the most vulnerable: A collaborative approach to supporting pregnant homeless youth*. Retrieved from http://www3.interscience.wiley.com/cgi-bin/fulltext/117983044/PDFSTART

Martel, L., & Caron-Malenfant, E. (2007). *Portrait of the Canadian population in 2006, findings*. Retrieved from http://www12.statcan.gc.ca/census-recensement/2006/as-sa/97-550/index-eng.cfm

Minister of Health. (2008). *The chief public health officer's report on the state of public health in Canada 2008*. Retrieved from http://www.phac-aspc.gc.ca/publicat/2008/cpho-aspc/pdf/cpho-report-eng.pdf

Morrell-Bellai, T., Goering, P. N., & Boydell, K. M. (2000). Becoming and remaining homeless: A qualitative investigation. *Issues in Mental Health Nursing, 21*(6), 581–604.

Murphy, B. (2000). *On the street: How we created homelessness*. Winnipeg, MB: J. G. Shillingford.

Murray, A. (1990). Homelessness: The people. In G. Fallis & A. Murray (Eds.), *Housing the homeless and poor: New partnerships among the private, public and third sectors*. Toronto, ON: University of Toronto Press.

Niagara District Health Council. (1997). *Report on homelessness in Niagara*. Fonthill, ON: Author.

Ontario Non-Profit Housing Association. (2009). *ONPHA's 2009 report on waiting list statistics for Ontario: June 2009*. Retrieved from http://www.onpha.on.ca/AM/Template.cfm?Section=Waiting_Lists_2009

Osberg, L. (2007). *A quarter century of economic inequity in Canada: 1981–2006.* Retrieved from http://www.onpha .on.ca/AM/Template.cfm?Section=Waiting_Lists_ 2009&Template=/CM/ContentDisplay.cfm& ContentID=5496

Paulsen, M. (2010, April). *Giving voice(mail) to the homeless.* Retrieved from http://thetyee.ca/Blogs/TheHook/Housing/ 2010/04/30/Giving-voicemail-to-the-homeless/

Pinchin, K. (2009, September). Technology for tomorrow: Homeless find hope through technology, Internet. *The Globe and Mail.* Retrieved from http://www .theglobeandmail.com/news/technology/homeless-find- hope-through-technology-internet/article1296491/

Plumb, J. D. (2000). Homelessness: Reducing health disparities. *Canadian Medical Association Journal, 163*(2), 172.

Raphael, D. (2007). *Poverty and policy in Canada: Implication for health and quality of life.* Toronto, ON: Canadian Scholars' Press.

Raphael, D., Curry-Stevens, A., & Bryant, T. (2009). Barriers to addressing the social determinants of health: Insights from the Canadian experience. *Health Policy, 88*(2–3), 222–235.

Reading, C., & Wien, F. (2009). *Health inequalities and social determinants of Aboriginal peoples' health.* Retrieved from http://www.nccah-ccnsa.ca/docs/nccah%20reports/ LoppieWien-2.pdf

Regroupement des centres d'amitié autochtones du Québec. (2008). *Brief concerning urban Aboriginal homelessness in Quebec.* Retrieved from http://www.reseaudialog.qc.ca/ DocsPDF/URBANABORIGINALHOMELESSNESS.pdf

Reutter, L., Stewart, M. J., Veenstra, G., Love, R., Raphael, D., & Makwarimba, E. (2009). Who do they think they are, anyway? Perceptions of and responses to poverty stigma. *Qualitative Health Research, 19*(3), 297–311.

Saskatoon Health Region. (2008). *"Health bus" services in demand.* Retrieved from http://www.saskatoonhealthregion .ca/news_you_need/media_centre/telling_our_stories/ 2008/econnect_090808.pdf

Sarlo, C. (1996). *Poverty in Canada* (2nd ed.). Vancouver, BC: Fraser Institute.

Statistics Canada. (2008). *Earnings and incomes of Canadians over the past quarter century, 2006 census: Findings.* Retrieved from http://www12.statcan.gc.ca/english/ census06/analysis/income/index.cfm

Statistics Canada. (2009). *Low income cut-offs for 2008 and low income measures for 2007.* Retrieved from http://www .statcan.gc.ca/pub/75f0002m/75f0002m2009002-eng.pdf

Stearman, K. (1999). *Homelessness.* Austin, TX: Raintree Steck-Vaughn.

The City of Calgary. (2008). *Biennial count of homeless persons in Calgary: 2008 May 14.* Retrieved from http://www .calgary.ca/docgallery/bu/cns/homelessness/ 2008_count_executive_summary.pdf

The Salvation Army. (2010). *Poverty shouldn't be a life sentence: A report on the perceptions of homelessness and poverty in Canada.* Retrieved from http://salvationarmy.ca/ documents/PovertyReport2010.pdf

Tognoli, J. (1987). Residential environments. In D. Stokols & I. Altman (Eds.), *Handbook of environmental psychology.* New York, NY: Wiley Interscience.

Toronto Shelter, Support & Housing Administration. (2006). *Quick facts.* Retrieved from http://intraspec.ca/quickfacts .pdf

Votta, E., & Manion, I. G. (2003). Factors in the psychological adjustment of homeless adolescent males: The role of coping style. *Journal of the American Academy of Child and Adolescent Psychiatry, 42*(7), 778–785.

World Health Organization. (2009a). *The social determinants of health.* Retrieved from http://www.who.int/ social_determinants/en/

World Health Organization. (2009b). *Closing the gap in a generation – how?* Retrieved from http://www.who.int/ social_determinants/thecommission/finalreport/ closethegap_how/en/print.html

ADDITIONAL RESOURCES

Beavis, M. A., Klos, N., Carter, T., & Douchant, C. (1997). *Literature review: Aboriginal peoples and homelessness.* Ottawa, ON: Canada Mortgage and Housing Corporation.

Hwang, S., Wilkins, R., Tjepkema, M., O'Campo, P., & Dunn, J. (2009). Mortality among residents of shelters, rooming houses, and hotels in Canada: 11 year follow-up study. *British Medical Journal, 339*(b4036).

Shapcott, M. (2009). Canada needs a national housing strategy that engages key partners from the community up: A submission from the Wellesley Institute to the Commons HUMA Committee for its review of Bill C-304.

Videos

This website has several videos. View the ones relating to poverty and homelessness.

http://www.onf-nfb.gc.ca/eng/collection/film/?id=55345

About the Authors

Lynnette Leeseberg Stamler is a Full Professor and Assistant Dean, College of Nursing, University of Saskatchewan. She has degrees from Olaf College, Minnesota (BSN), the University of Manitoba (MEd – Health Education), and the University of Cincinnati (PhD – Nursing). Her research interests include patient/health education, breast health, diabetes education, nursing education, and, most recently, quality care. She was a VON nurse for four years prior to her career in nursing education. She has been active in research and professional nursing organizations including Sigma Theta Tau International, the Nursing Honor Society. She was President of the Canadian Association of Schools of Nursing from 20082010.

Aaron Gabriel, RN, B.A., B.SN, is a master's student with the College of Nursing at the University of Saskatchewan. She completed a B.A. in psychology prior to her BSN in nursing. Now she is employed as a medical-surgical nurse and is working on her thesis.

28

Substance Use

Hélène Philbin Wilkinson

OBJECTIVES

After studying this chapter, you should be able to:

1. Consider the reasons why people use psychoactive substances.
2. Recognize the differences between substance use, abuse, and dependency.
3. Discuss the scope of substance use and abuse in Canada.
4. Identify the harms associated with substance use and abuse.
5. Describe the relationship between substance abuse and the social determinants of health.
6. Discuss the components of Canada's Federal Drug Strategy and other substance abuse frameworks and models.
7. Develop strategies to address substance abuse problems in communities.
8. Reflect upon your own values and beliefs about substance use and abuse and how the community health nurse can help to address and reduce the harms associated with substance use and abuse.

INTRODUCTION

Substance abuse is a complex public health issue that spans the life cycle and can have severe and permanent consequences for individuals, families, and communities. The overall cost of substance abuse (including alcohol, tobacco, and illicit drugs) is estimated to cost Canadians approximately $40 billion, with tobacco and alcohol accounting for almost 80% of the total cost (Rehm et al., 2006). Substance abuse is also associated with high rates of diseases and other lifestyle-related causes of death and injury. For example, in our country, substance abuse accounts for 21% of all deaths (cancer, cardiac and pulmonary disease, overdoses, motor vehicle accidents, and death by fire), 25% of years of potential life lost, and 19.4% of hospitalizations (Rehm et al., 2006). Considerable non-monetary costs to Canadian society also exist, such as the pain, suffering, and bereavement experienced by families, friends, and victims, which can have profound and lasting effects that cannot be measured in dollars.

Evidence from various fields of inquiry strongly suggests that substance use and abuse is multifactorial—that genetic, psychological, and socioeconomic factors are all determinants of substance use. Just as substance abuse causes poor health, poor health and other socioeconomic disadvantages can contribute to substance abuse (Single, 1999). This socioenvironmental perspective has guided the development of holistic substance abuse strategies that recognize the interrelationships between the person, the substance, and the environment.

Traditionally, nurses have often been described as sentinels on the riverbanks, responding to a problem occurring upstream (Butterfield, 1997). The impact of substance abuse on the individual or the collective is often seen first-hand by the community health nurse (CHN). As such, this chapter is intended to introduce you to the practice of developing comprehensive responses and challenge you to make those critical connections to what is happening upstream in your community.

WHY DO PEOPLE USE DRUGS?

People use different drugs for different reasons, and the reasons vary from drug to drug, from person to person, and from circumstance to circumstance. While certain psychoactive drugs may be prescribed to relieve anxiety, tension, stress, or insomnia, some people may self-medicate to improve performance or to resolve physical or emotional discomfort. The mere availability of a drug may cause individuals to be curious enough to experiment. The danger, however, is that experimental use may lead to other reasons for using, which may in turn result in abuse and/or dependence.

Other people may take drugs to boost their self-confidence or to forget about or cope with traumatic life events or situations.

Immediate gratification from drugs may make people feel good and/or can quickly reduce or eliminate uncomfortable emotions, albeit temporarily. Social pressures to use drugs can be very strong for both young people and adults. However, children are especially vulnerable as they may imitate and interpret their parents' use as a necessary part of having fun or relaxing. Young people may use drugs to rebel against unhappy situations or because they feel alienated, have an identity crisis, or need to be accepted by their peers. The media are also considered a powerful source of influence. Ads often promote drinking or smoking as a social activity or as a factor in the achievement of success.

TERMINOLOGY

The term **drug** refers to a **psychoactive substance** that affects a person's physiological or psychological state or behaviour. In this chapter, *drugs* will be referred to as substances consumed for medicinal and non-medicinal purposes, legally or illegally, and the term will be used interchangeably with the term *psychoactive substances.*

Most people don't think of **alcohol** as a drug, but it is. Ethyl alcohol (made from grain) is present in beer, wine, spirits, and liqueurs, and methyl alcohol (made from wood) is found in solvents, paint removers, antifreeze, and other household and industrial products. The distinction between the two types is important to make when referring to or defining the term and its consumption. At low doses, alcohol acts as a central nervous system depressant, producing relaxation and a release of inhibitions. At higher doses, it can produce intoxication, impaired judgment and co-ordination, even coma and death. Methyl alcohol, when ingested, can cause blindness and other permanent damage to the nervous system.

Tobacco leaves, which are shredded and dried, can be smoked in cigarettes, cigars, or pipes, or be chewed or inhaled. More than 4000 chemicals are found in tobacco, including nicotine, the main psychoactive component that stimulates the central nervous system.

Illicit drugs (illegal drugs) include cannabis (marijuana and hashish), phencyclidines (PCP, ketamine), hallucinogens (LSD, mescaline, psilocybin, MDA), stimulants other than caffeine and nicotine (amphetamines, cocaine, crack), depressants (barbiturates, methaqualone, benzodiazepine), and opiates (heroin, morphine, methadone, codeine). **Inhalants**, also known as volatile solvents, are depressant drugs that produce feelings of euphoria, exhilaration, and vivid fantasies. Their use can cause irreversible brain damage, asphyxiation, and death. Using inhalants such as gasoline or certain illicit drugs such as PCP can cause immediate and serious problems regardless of how or how much is taken or ingested.

Licit drugs (legal drugs) that are used for medicinal purposes are legally available by prescription or sold over the counter and include drugs to relieve pain, control anxiety, or combat insomnia. Some of these drugs are controlled as they have practical licit uses, but they may be used unlawfully and therefore have illicit uses. Licit drugs used for non-medicinal purposes include alcohol and tobacco, either of which can be legally purchased and used by those who are of legal age. In order to clarify which substances are licit and which are illicit, laws in Canada, such as the Controlled Drugs and Substances Act, specifically name those substances which are to be controlled and how they are to be controlled.

Substance use refers to any consumption of psychoactive drugs, which can result in benefits or harm. **Substance abuse** or misuse refers to drug use that leads to adverse physical or psychological consequences, which may or may not involve **dependence**. Drug dependency is progressive in nature and affects the physiological, cognitive, behavioural, and psychological dimensions of a person's health. It is manifested by continuous use despite the presence of problems that are caused by the pattern of repeated self-administration that results in tolerance, withdrawal, and compulsive substance-taking behaviour (American Psychiatric Association, 1994). Dependence can be physical and/or psychological. **Physical dependence** occurs when an individual's body reacts to the absence of a drug, and **psychological dependence** occurs when drug use becomes central to a person's thoughts and emotions. Other forms of dependence such as gambling, Internet social networking, sex, and binge eating are becoming increasingly prevalent and have implications for community health nursing. Should you wish to further explore these impulse control disorders and the concept of dependence, you are encouraged to consult your psychiatric nursing text.

THE SCOPE OF SUBSTANCE USE AND ABUSE IN CANADA

Prevalence patterns of substance use and abuse are influenced by both individual and sociodemographic factors such as age, gender, education, geography, lifestyle, attitudes, and beliefs. The following section is a brief overview of the most common substance use and abuse patterns in Canada. Tobacco, alcohol, and cannabis are the most widely used in this country. The information below gives you a general overview of how many Canadians are affected by the use and abuse of substances. Having access to current data helps to solidify the evidence base you need as a CHN to make informed decisions to help individuals and communities maintain and improve their health. The data presented in the following paragraphs are by no means comprehensive; however, should you wish to further explore prevalence patterns, you are encouraged to consult the federal and provincial websites listed at the end of this chapter. Some of them contain additional documents that highlight age, gender, and regional differences in consumption patterns across Canada.

Tobacco

It is a well-known fact that smoking is the most important cause of preventable illness, disability, and premature death in our country. The evidence suggests that smoking kills more Canadians than suicide, AIDS, vehicle collision and murders combined with alcohol, car accidents, suicides, and murders combined. However, over the past ten years, smoking prevalence patterns have changed considerably. Overall smoking rates in Canada have declined by approximately 28% among people aged 15 years and older. Although there are now fewer adolescent boys and girls who smoke, young adult Canadians (aged 20 to 24 years), males, and people who live in rural areas have the highest prevalence of smoking (Health Canada, 2008b).

CANADIAN RESEARCH BOX 28.1

How do health professionals from different disciplines approach smoking cessation counselling?

Tremblay, M., Cournoyer, D., & O'Loughlin, J. (2009). Do the correlates of smoking cessation counselling differ across health professional groups? *Nicotine and Tobacco Research, 11*(11), 1330–1338.

The *Framework Convention on Tobacco Control*, negotiated by the World Health Organization, proposes that healthcare professionals provide treatment for nicotine dependence. Numerous studies have shown that tobacco cessation counselling by healthcare professionals is effective in increasing cessation rates among smokers.

In Quebec, several measures to promote smoking cessation have been implemented. Some of these have included media campaigns, reimbursement of nicotine replacement therapy through public and private drug insurance plans, and the establishment of 160 smoking cessation centres across the province offering free individual and group counselling. In addition, the Quebec National Public Health Institute collaborated with six of the province's health professional associations to improve cessation counselling among their active licensed members. This study was carried out to guide the development of training and educational interventions for these groups of healthcare professionals, and enable the tracking of their cessation counselling practices over time.

Self-administered questionnaires were mailed to 500 individuals who were randomly selected from the membership lists of active licensed professionals. These included general practitioners (GPs), pharmacists, dentists, dental hygienists, nurses, and respiratory therapists.

The U.S. Public Health Service's Guidelines for the treatment of tobacco use and dependence recommend that healthcare professionals follow a series of five steps when counselling clients in smoking cessation. These are commonly known as the "5As" and include (a) ask patients about their smoking status; (b) advise them to quit; (c) assess their readiness to quit; (d) assist them in their quit attempts or promote motivation to quit; and (e) arrange follow-up appointments. Respondents were asked to rate their counselling practices as they relate specifically to these five steps. In addition, the survey measured their beliefs about their role in cessation counselling; perceptions

about their level of skills/competency or self-efficacy; their knowledge of available community resources; perceptions of barriers to cessation counselling; and their interest in updating their counselling skills.

There was substantial variability in counselling practices across the different groups; however, three factors emerged as being positively associated with smoking cessation practice. These include the belief that counselling is the role of the healthcare professional; the professional's perceived self-efficacy or competency to engage patients in effective counselling; and their knowledge of available community cessation resources. The fact that these factors were consistent among the respondents is notable given the diversity of the professional groups and their roles, patient populations, work settings, and remuneration structures.

Overall, with the possible exception of general practitioners (GPs), the study found that there is room for improvement in the provision of the "5As" of smoking cessation counselling. In terms of specific practices, all groups including nurses were more likely to perform only the first two steps. It appears that asking and advising are relatively simple tasks that can be completed quickly and are therefore usually more common. In contrast, assessing, assisting, referring, and arranging require more time and increased levels of knowledge and skill, as well as awareness of community cessation resources.

Compared with other groups, GPs and pharmacists undertook more counselling with patients who were deemed ready to quit, with GPs performing the most counselling than any other group. This is not surprising, given that GPs in Quebec have been intensively targeted over the last decade with interventions to optimize cessation counselling. GPs and respiratory therapists performed more counselling with patients who were not ready to quit. Dentists and dental hygienists saw the fewest patients per day. Nurses scored fourth in terms of providing counselling sessions.

While nurses were among the groups scoring the highest for the belief that cessation counselling is part of their role and that they perceive to have the skills to engage patients in cessation, their scores were not significant for the other factors, including knowledge of community resources, training, and interest in updating their knowledge. This suggests the need for interventions to improve these areas for nurses. Scores for receiving smoking cessation training during their academic studies were highest among pharmacists, respiratory therapists, and dentists. This finding also suggests that other healthcare professional groups including nurses may benefit from formal training in smoking cessation as part of their academic preparation.

Overall, the study found that the level of perceived competency in counselling practices can be improved. Despite widespread advertising in this province, less than half of the respondents were aware of cessation services available in their communities. If, as the data suggest, knowledge of community resources is associated with the provision of counselling, developing interventions to further increase awareness of local community cessation resources should be a priority among healthcare professionals. The fact that approximately 20% of the respondents do not believe that cessation counselling is part of their role suggests the need for further integration of cessation training into the basic training courses and daily practice of healthcare professionals.

Although research on smoking cessation counselling has focused on physicians, this study confirms that other health professionals including nurses are well situated to engage in this practice. Increased counselling by diverse health professionals may contribute to broader community-based efforts to improve cessation rates. The authors confirm that healthcare professionals, including nurses, are ideally positioned to provide a leadership role in smoking cessation.

Discussion Questions

1. Explore the 5As of smoking cessation counselling (ask patients about their smoking status; advise them to quit; assess their readiness to quit; assist them in their attempts to quit or promote motivation for them to quit; and arrange for follow-up) in the context of the Canadian community health nursing standards of practice. Choose a standard and discuss the indicators or activities that show how a CHN who is providing smoking cessation counselling is meeting the standard.

2. How might a CHN assess a client's readiness to quit?

Alcohol

Most Canadians drink alcohol but do so in moderation. Overall, men tend to drink more than women, and men along with young people between the ages of 15 and 24 years appear to have higher rates of heavy infrequent and frequent drinking. They are also more likely to experience alcohol-related harms (Health Canada, 2008a) than women and other age groups.

Illicit Drugs

Cannabis is the most widely used illicit drug in Canada. Although the overall consumption of illicit drugs is relatively low compared with that of alcohol and tobacco, research reports indicate that the use of some illicit drugs such as hallucinogens is on the rise (Health Canada, 2008a). Illicit drug use is more common among males and young people.

The next most widely used illicit drug in Canada is hallucinogens, followed closely by cocaine, ecstasy, speed, and methamphetamines (Health Canada, 2008a). Anecdotal evidence from substance abuse treatment centres suggests, however, that the use of illicit drugs such as methamphetamines is much more prevalent than is reported in surveys. Anecdotal evidence from communities with high usage rates of methamphetamine or "crystal meth" suggest that use appears to be cutting across socioeconomic and geographic lines.

Over the last 10 to 15 years, the use of **injectable drugs** among Canadians has increased by approximately 53% (Adlaf, Begin, & Sawka, 2005). Additionally, researchers are finding that approximately half of injection drug users, who inject heroin on a regular basis, also inject cocaine or smoke crack/cocaine.

Although overall use of steroids is low in Canada, lifetime use of steroids is most prevalent among males. As for inhalant use, such as glue, it is the highest among children and youth. Some studies involving inmates of detention centres reveal that inhalants were the first drugs ever used by young people. Other studies report inhalant use as high as 60%—an epidemic among certain impoverished populations, such as children living in isolated Inuit and Aboriginal communities. While heavy use of inhalants can be a response to poor life conditions, in some remote communities inhalant abuse is practically non-existent (Canadian Paediatric Society, 2005). Consult Chapter 22 to further understand the health status of the Aboriginal people.

Licit Drugs

In recent years, the abuse of **prescription drugs**, normally prescribed for therapeutic purposes, has received considerable attention in the media. Canada is one of the top 10 countries that have the highest rates for opioid prescriptions, stimulants, and benzodiazepines (Haydon, Rehm, Fischer, Monga, & Adlaf, 2005). The abuse of prescription opiates is a growing global issue and experts are predicting that prescription drug abuse is expected to exceed the abuse of illicit street drugs as many of these prescription drugs are making their way into the illicit drug market with the use of Internet pharmacies and other clandestine non-regulated laboratories.

In Canada, opioid pain relievers, stimulants, sedatives, and tranquilizers are the most commonly used prescription drugs. Of these, opioids and stimulants are the most frequently abused, with rates of abuse being the highest among adolescents between the ages of 15 and 24 years (Health Canada, 2008a). Prescription opioid use is surpassing the use of heroin in our country. The evidence suggests that contributing factors include increases in opioid prescribing practices and the ease of acquiring these pharmaceuticals on the street.

Other licit drugs that are known to be abused for their psychoactive effects include "over-the-counter" medications such as cough medicines, sleep aids, antihistamines, and diet pills. The use of "over the counter" and prescription drugs by older persons is also important to pay attention to since the aging process is frequently accompanied by an increase in chronic and acute illness, and in the total number of prescribed drugs.

Concurrent Disorders

Although previously discussed in Chapter 21, this chapter would be incomplete if we failed to present information about **concurrent disorders**. A concurrent disorder is the term used when referring to people who have co-occurring mental health and substance use problems. In diagnostic terms, a concurrent disorder refers to any combination of mental health and substance use disorders, as defined on either Axis I or Axis II of the DSM-IV.

Having a mental health problem increases the risk of having a substance use problem, just as having a substance use problem increases the risk of having a mental health problem (Health Canada, 2002a). As well, the use of substances can cause behaviours that mimic symptoms of mental health problems. These substance-induced problems may improve as substance use is decreased or stopped; however, almost three of every 10 people who have a mental illness will be dependent on alcohol or drugs, about four of every 10 people who use alcohol in a harmful way, and over half of people who use other substances in a harmful way, will have a mental illness at some time in their lives (Skinner, O'Grady, Bartha, et al., 2004).

HARMFUL CONSEQUENCES OF SUBSTANCE ABUSE

All drugs have adverse and undesirable effects. For example, the long-term use of tobacco can cause lung damage; exposure to second-hand smoke among neonates, infants, children, and adults is associated with an increased risk of a number of acute and chronic conditions; alcohol abuse can cause liver damage; sniffing cocaine can damage nasal passages; and people who inject drugs intravenously can become infected with blood borne pathogens such as HIV and hepatitis B and C.

Every year in Canada, approximately 45 000 people die of tobacco-related disorders; evidence suggests that tobacco surpasses alcohol and illicit drugs as the leading cause of death, hospitalization, and lost years of life. Nicotine dependence or tobacco addiction is the most lethal of all addictions; it is a chronic and relapsing disorder with at least half of smokers dying of tobacco-related illnesses.

Significant social problems caused by the misuse of alcohol in our country include driving under the influence of alcohol, and domestic and interpersonal violence. Although impaired driving rates have dropped over the last couple of decades, the largest number of alcohol-related deaths stem from impaired driving accidents, many of which involve young people. Approximately 40% of young drivers killed in motor vehicle accident have been drinking (Traffic Injury Research Foundation [TIRF], 2009).

Although alcohol remains the primary cause of motor vehicle fatalities in Canada, other drugs such as cannabis, benzodiazepines, and cocaine are also being detected among drivers. In particular, driving after the use of cannabis appears to be increasing in Canada, especially among young drivers (Canadian Centre on Substance Abuse [CCSA], 2009). Alcohol is also frequently involved in snowmobiling and boating accidents in this country. Almost 40% of boating deaths have alcohol involvement, and at least half of all fatally injured snowmobilers in Canada have been drinking (TIRF, 2009).

Other associated harms can include an increase in crime and violent acts; strained relationships; workplace and school absenteeism; and health problems such as ulcers, liver and kidney damage, pancreatic diseases, heart disease, cancer, sexual and reproductive issues, and pre- and postnatal complications.

Although as little as one drink of alcohol every other day can help adults gain some protection against heart disease, heavy drinking does raise blood pressure and can also increase the risk of stroke and heart failure.

The consumption of alcohol during pregnancy can result in **fetal alcohol spectrum disorder** (FASD), which is manifested by developmental, neurological, and behavioural delays in infants and young children. Though the major cause of these conditions is the frequency and volume of an expectant mother's alcohol intake, other contributing factors to consider include genetic predisposition, poor nutrition, age, the lack of prenatal care, and the use of other drugs. Since a safe level of alcohol consumption during pregnancy or while breastfeeding has not been established, public health professionals advise expectant and breastfeeding mothers not to drink alcohol, even in moderation. Consult your maternity and pediatric nursing texts for additional information about the incidence and clinical symptoms of FASD.

People who use drugs that have been obtained illegally can never really know what they are taking. For example, "ecstasy" and "crystal meth," both of which belong to the amphetamine family, can be easily manufactured in clandestine or unregulated illegal labs. As a result, the chemicals and processes vary affecting the strength, purity, and effect of the final product. The consequences can be devastating, including severe dependency and drug reactions, and fatal overdoses. This is evidenced by the sharp increase of mortality rates due to opioids in our country (Dhalla, Mamdani, Sivilotti, Kopp, Qureshi, & Juurlink, 2009).

Several studies have documented a rise in the prevalence of HIV among injection drug users in Canada. Many injection drug users share needles and drug injection equipment, and engage in unprotected commercial sex (CCSA, 2009). Please refer to Chapter 29 for more information on this topic.

Substance abuse affects children's safety, education, and well-being. Children living with parents who use substances, children and youth who have friends who use substances, and children who themselves use substances suffer negative physical, cognitive, emotional, and social consequences. The harmful consequences extend far beyond individuals using substances, their families, and friends. Substance abuse affects community health, safety, and quality of life. Because it impacts the whole community, it requires a total community effort to ensure collective health and well-being.

THE RESPONSE TO SUBSTANCE ABUSE

Given the wide range of individual, social, and cultural factors that can influence patterns of drug use, strategies have shifted from the view that substance abuse is not merely caused by individual psychological or moral factors. Substance abuse is a chronic, multifaceted social problem that requires a range of responses.

Canada's Federal Drug Strategy

Recognizing that a wide range of tools and solutions are needed, Canada developed a framework combining elements of health promotion together with prevention, treatment, harm reduction, and enforcement. These elements have been coined the "pillars" of Canada's Federal Drug Strategy, which represents the need for a balanced approach to address these problems. The "four-pillar" approach is considered a best practice model for ensuring that any substance abuse strategy is comprehensive and co-ordinated.

During the past decade, the Government of Canada renewed and broadened its commitment to the Strategy by making multi-year investments in new areas such as leadership, research and monitoring, partnerships and intervention, and modernized legislation and policy. Additional funding for the Strategy received mixed reviews. Although it has ensured the expansion of prevention and enforcement activities, it has been criticized for its overemphasis on illicit drugs and support of conventional enforcement strategies, while poorly supporting proven, effective harm reduction programs and more costly substances, such as alcohol and pharmaceuticals. Some critics claim that our country has an Americanized strategy, or a Canadianized version of the U.S. "war on drugs." Although progress has been made in the area of treatment and research, many researchers and clinicians in Canada are requesting that we turn our attention to the successful non-conventional harm reduction programs that have been developed by European countries.

Prevention and Health Promotion Prevention and health promotion consist of interventions that seek to prevent or delay the onset of substance use as well as to avoid problems before they occur. Prevention and health promotion is more than education. It also includes strengthening the health, social, and economic factors that can reduce the risk of substance use such as creating alternative activities for youth groups. The main focus is to help people avoid the use of harmful substances and in the case of those who do use, enhance their ability to control their use and prevent the development of substance abuse problems. Awareness campaigns and other education initiatives help people make healthy decisions and participate in health-related activities by increasing knowledge and motivation, changing attitudes, and increasing the skills that are required to avoid or reduce risk. These activities typically consist of programs and services that impart knowledge about substances and help develop refusal skills. They can be developed to target the whole community and/or specific at-risk or high-risk populations. Examples of activities that can be implemented in a couple of these sectors are provided in Table 28.1.

Prevention and health promotion activities may also include policies, health warning labels, and even elements of harm reduction. In fact, it is best practice to combine education and harm reduction with policy changes and other environmental supports, as they are mutually complementary and strengthen the overall impact of prevention activities. Policies such as tobacco by-laws or alcohol and drug legislation can create healthy social and physical environments. Environmental support and controls help to ensure healthy conditions, practices, and policies that make it easier for people to achieve and maintain their health. For example, the presence of recreational activities and self-help groups can provide important

TABLE 28.1 Examples of Substance Abuse Prevention Activities by Sector, Stakeholders, and Target Group

Sector	Stakeholders	Target Group	Activities
Home	Parents, children, local media, mass media, public health, community organizations and groups, health agencies	▪ Children ▪ Youth ▪ Parents	▪ Discuss substance use/abuse issues with children and youth. ▪ Provide skill development programs for parents. ▪ Promote educational materials. ▪ Encourage the development of a home drinking policy. ▪ Encourage alternative healthy activities/behaviours.
Elementary and secondary schools	School administration, public health, students, parents, teachers, guidance counsellors, physical education and health consultants, parent–teacher group, community alcohol and drug consultants	▪ Students (K–12) ▪ Staff ▪ Parents ▪ Teachers ▪ Peer leaders	▪ Develop school policies on alcohol and drugs. ▪ Encourage an integrated drug education curriculum that spans the school years. ▪ Provide ongoing training for those delivering the drug education curriculum. ▪ Hold special events to supplement drug education curriculum. ▪ Organize student interest groups (e.g., students against drunk driving). ▪ Provide early identification and intervention programs in the schools.

Source: Ontario, Ministry of Health, Health Promotion Branch. Community Mobilization Manual [vol. 4] Ideas for Action on Alcohol. 1991. ISBN 0772968616. p. 9. Adapted with permission.

environmental supports for a community. Policy changes are intended to create an environment that is conducive to healthy practices by making it easier to adopt healthy behaviours and more difficult to adopt unhealthy practices. Environmental supports are also present in the workplace. While some workplaces in Canada have instituted drug testing programs in both public and private sectors, many have put in place comprehensive alcohol and drug human resource policies that include strategies for the prevention and management of problems that arise among employees.

Health Recovery Screening, early identification, and treatment and rehabilitation programs are components of health recovery strategies for people who have started to experience problems related to their substance use. The emphasis of screening and early identification is on the detection of signs and symptoms to intervene and reduce consumption levels and effectively manage the problems that have started to develop. **Treatment** and **rehabilitation** are intended to assist people with substance abuse problems as their consumption is considered to be "high risk." These individuals should be provided with a range of options in order to match their recovery needs and personal circumstances with appropriate treatment services. Overall, the purpose in health recovery is to prevent further deterioration and reduce the harms that have resulted from a problematic consumption pattern. The CHN should also be aware that the stigma associated with substance dependence is often a strong deterrent for a person to get help. Later in this chapter, you will be encouraged to pay attention to your own attitudes, which may reflect some of society's misconceptions about people who have substance use problems.

Community treatment services typically include detoxification services, screening, assessment, inpatient and outpatient treatment, and aftercare and follow-up. Additionally, special programs have been designed to address the unique needs of certain population groups such as women, youth, Aboriginal people, inmates of correctional institutions, and impaired driving and drug offenders. Diversion programs such as **drug treatment courts** (DTCs) offer alternatives to incarceration of repeat drug-involved offenders. These programs facilitate access to treatment and help reduce the harms and risk of ongoing dependence and criminal recidivism (Mulgrew, 2003). Currently, there are six DTCs operating in Canada: Edmonton, Ottawa, Regina, Toronto, Vancouver, and Winnipeg. These special courts are working to reduce the number of crimes committed to support drug dependence by providing judicial supervision, comprehensive substance abuse treatment, random and frequent drug testing, incentives and sanctions, clinical case management, and social support services (Harrell, 1998).

The treatment and rehabilitation system in many communities is often structured as a set of individual services, rather than as a continuum. This can create barriers to access appropriate and timely treatment. A **treatment service continuum** should be co-ordinated, provide services that are based on best practices, have medically appropriate care, and meet the diverse needs of individuals including those with concurrent disorders. Research has demonstrated that treatment

services and programs are far more effective and efficient when integrated within various sectors including health, mental health social services, education, and the criminal justice system. For example, screening, when conducted in various points of entry or agencies across multiple sectors, is a good example of integrating access to services throughout the system.

CHNs practising in health centres, homes, schools, and other community-based settings should be aware of the available treatment options in their communities and become familiar with screening and care planning to appropriately refer individuals who need additional support, counselling, and/or treatment. They should have the skills to recognize the signs and symptoms of substance abuse and dependence, and be comfortable raising the topic with clients. Screening can be conducted in a variety of settings, by a variety of individuals, under a variety of conditions. In fact, allied professionals in primary care such as the CHN are significantly more likely to be involved in screening than substance abuse specialists. Additionally, the CHN, in collaboration with professionals from other disciplines, should strive to develop treatment options that acknowledge and integrate concurrent disorders; thus "making every door the right door" along the service continuum in their community.

For this reason, it is important that CHNs understand that they can play a key role as primary screening agents in the community. Training to administer these tools is recommended and CHNs are encouraged to consult local substance abuse specialists in their community, and/or visit the website of the Canadian Network of Substance Abuse and Allied Professionals which is provided in the Additional Resources section of this chapter.

Enforcement The goal of **enforcement** is to strengthen community health and safety by responding to the crimes and community disorder issues associated with the supply (importation, manufacturing, cultivation), distribution, possession, and use of legal and illegal substances.

Enforcement interventions must be linked to the other "pillars" of Canada's Federal Drug Strategy to ensure the social, economic, and emotional complexities of substance abuse are recognized and addressed. As such, effective enforcement also means being visible in communities, understanding local issues, being aware of existing community resources, and participating in improving social conditions and attitudes while upholding public safety.

Although the failure of some law enforcement efforts to counteract illicit drugs has led to recent debates over the decriminalization and/or the legalization of illicit substances, it has also led to the introduction of innovative harm reduction strategies such as drug treatment courts that focus on treating, rather than charging, the substance abuser (Collin, 2006).

Harm Reduction It is important to understand that abstinence is the best goal for drug treatment. Although ideal, it may not always be achievable. Harm reduction is a powerful tool to minimize the harms associated with substance abuse. It offers a wide spectrum of opportunities for the CHN to help strengthen the capacity of individuals and communities experiencing the adverse effects of substance abuse.

Harm reduction is a public health philosophy that has gained popularity in the last two decades; however, some claim that it is a new name for an old concept. It is described as a program or policy designed to reduce drug-related harms without requiring the cessation of drug use (Beirness, Jesseman, Notarandrea & Perron, 2008). Examples include the availability of "light" alcoholic beverages, alcohol server training programs, and impaired driving countermeasures. In the treatment field, the most pre-eminent harm reduction strategies are supervised injection sites, street outreach, needle exchange, and **methadone maintenance treatment** (MMT) programs, all of which allow the individual to live with a certain level of dependency while minimizing risks and other disruptive effects to the person and community.

Street outreach programs tend to target marginalized populations such as street-involved youth, homeless people, sex trade workers, Aboriginal people, and injection drug users who receive information about services that are available in the community as well as counselling and health services. Needle exchange programs provide injection drug users with clean needles and syringes and other health and social support and services. Medically supervised injection sites have health professionals on site to prevent harmful consequences such as overdose, and provide users with information about health, treatment and rehabilitation programs. MMT programs have been introduced across Canada in response to the increasing use of opioids and the extensive cycle of this devastating drug dependency. Methadone alleviates the symptoms of opioid withdrawal by creating stable and sufficient blood levels of methadone. It was developed in Germany as a substitute analgesic for morphine during the Second World War. Researchers in the early 1960s demonstrated its efficacy for opioid dependence, and in 1963, a Canadian researcher established an MMT program in British Columbia, the first of its kind in the world (Health Canada, 2002b). MMT has been demonstrated to improve physical and mental health status; reduce illicit drug use, infectious disease risks, and crime involvement among those involved in treatment; and offers a significant cost benefit to the community given the costs associated with untreated opioid dependency. It is available in some correctional facilities, which is further discussed in Chapter 25.

Some may argue that harm reduction cannot be applied to tobacco since even small quantities of tobacco can be harmful. But consider the recent harm reduction measures that have been put in place and that have created protection for non-smokers in public places in various provinces across Canada. It is often said that harm reduction is not "what's nice, it's what works." The focus is therefore not on the use or the extent of use, but on the harms that are associated with the use. While becoming drug free may be the ultimate goal, it is not required from the outset. The goal is to reduce more immediate and tangible harms.

Harm reduction emerged as a public health strategy that initially involved socially marginal populations such as injection drug users and inmates of correctional facilities. It may therefore provoke debate and controversy as an appropriate strategy for some communities or organizations. Consider the progress that has been made, however, since the introduction of clean needle and syringe exchange and MMT programs. Strong community stakeholder endorsement is essential when considering and planning this approach in order to prevent or minimize an unnecessary public outcry on its appropriateness, which would inadvertently polarize the community, shift the focus from its intended purpose to a debate about other peripheral social issues. On the other hand, such a dialogue may be crucial given its potential to produce a shift in knowledge, attitudes, and values.

A harm reduction message to the public is somewhat different from other types of prevention messages. A harm reduction message might be "avoid problems when you drink" compared to a prevention message such as "drinking less is better." As you work through the case study in this chapter, you will learn that many policies, such as the promotion of low-alcohol beverages, are based on harm reduction principles. Consequently, harm reduction stands in contrast to other models and philosophies such as zero tolerance, abstinence-based health promotion initiatives, and population-based measures like alcohol tax policies and restrictions on availability. Harm reduction focuses on lowering the risk and severity of adverse consequences without necessarily reducing use or consumption. Although different, these approaches are complementary and all have an important role in addressing substance abuse problems in our communities.

CANADIAN RESEARCH BOX

What are the clients' feelings about supervised methadone consumption?

Anstice, S., Strike, C. J., & Brands, B. (2009). Supervised methadone consumption: Client issues and stigma. *Substance Use and Misuse, 44*(6), 794–808.

Pharmacists and other dispensing staff such as nurses play a key role in methadone maintenance treatment (MMT) by preparing, storing, dispensing, and often supervising clients consuming the methadone they have been prescribed. Typically, MMT clients receive between one and seven supervised (daily) doses a week. When clients require supervision with the consumption of their methadone, they are observed by staff to ensure that the dose is swallowed, and are provided with any necessary and immediate assistance and counselling.

The extent to which supervised methadone consumption may influence clients' experiences of MMT is not well understood. Previous studies have found that clients have mixed feelings about supervised methadone consumption. Some clients view it as intrusive, embarrassing, and demeaning, while others believe that supervision is important for compliance and to deter diversion.

There are many factors that can influence client participation and retention in MMT. Such factors include wait lists, cost, dose, program philosophy, and access to counselling. Relationships with providers can also positively or negatively influence treatment outcomes. While the supervision of methadone consumption is an integral part of MMT, it may contribute to stigmatization. Stigma can create barriers to participation and retention in MMT. Although MMT clients have made an important step toward treatment, the stigmatized identity or label of "drug user" often remains, linking them to negative stereotypes and a lower social status, which sets them apart from others. A power imbalance can ensue between the client and the staff dispensing, controlling access to, and supervising the methadone consumption.

This paper explores the role that dispensing staff have in managing stigma in the context of supervised methadone consumption. The authors examine the negative and stigmatizing aspects of supervised methadone consumption from a client's perspective at onsite dispensaries that are connected to MMT programs and community pharmacies. They discuss how stigma is conferred and managed, and examine the challenges of providing non-stigmatizing dispensing services to MMT clients.

Using a convenience sampling method, the authors analyzed the experiences of 64 MMT clients participating in supervised methadone consumption at four methadone programs in Ontario, Canada. Two programs were hosted by public health units and two by AIDS service organizations. All programs were staffed by a coordinator, counsellor/outreach workers, and physicians, with one employing a nurse practitioner. Two programs dispensed methadone at their onsite dispensaries, while the other two dispensed and supervised the methadone consumption at community pharmacies.

Using open-ended questions, participants were asked to discuss their experiences about a number of topics related to the methadone dispensing programs they frequented. Data from these interviews were analyzed using thematic analytic methods.

Three themes dominated clients' accounts of supervised consumption: convenient access to services; relationships with staff, and attributes of the dispensing location/space. These were interwoven with their experiences of feeling stigmatized as an MMT client. In some situations, clients felt that the dispensing context helped them manage or conceal their identity, passing as normal customers in public in discreet locations. In other situations, the dispensing context made them visible as MMT clients, making them feel embarrassed to be taking methadone in public among other customers or using separate entrances and being segregated to be given their dose. Some complained that the connection of some MMT programs to needle exchange services created potential triggers for them by having to encounter former peers and others selling or using drugs. Negative accounts of interactions with dispensing staff tended to focus on feelings of discrimination, with clients complaining they felt patronized, treated with suspicion, and made to wait unnecessarily. This was particularly evident among pharmacy dispensing locations. Although program dispensing locations were less stigmatizing, some

clients reported they also felt demeaned in those locations. Some preferred a business-like transaction, while others preferred dealing with staff who took a personal interest in their lives.

The study found a number of conflicting findings, which suggests that preferences may need to be resolved on an individual basis. Knowing that clients may feel stigmatized as a result of receiving supervised methadone is an important issue for dispensing staff to understand. This means that staff must understand more about the social context of their MMT clients and structure their supervised consumption services to better support individual choice. Addressing specific barriers and stigmatizing experiences may improve MMT outcomes. The findings in this study resonate with those of other previous research on this topic and suggest that they may be generalizable to other MMT clients.

Discussion Questions

1. What strategies would you employ as a CHN working with MMT clients to minimize their feelings of stigma and optimize personal choice and individualized supervised consumption of methadone in either a pharmacy or an agency-sponsored location?

2. What would you include in an orientation/training guide for methadone dispensing staff to help them address and prevent stigmatizing conditions or situations?

3. You are a CHN dispensing methadone in a clinic and a female client discloses she may be three months pregnant. What is your first thought? How do you feel about providing care to this client? What actions will you take to ensure barrier-free access to services and minimize stigma for her and her unborn child?

4. What actions would you take personally and professionally to help reduce the stigma toward people with substance use problems in your community?

Developing Community Interventions

Communities should have a combination of **complementary interventions** such as education, policy, enforcement, screening, early intervention, and various types of treatment and rehabilitation options, all of which are consistent with the various practice expectations of community health nursing. Although some of the frameworks and models presented in this section come from the substance abuse field, they are grounded in the same principles of the population health promotion models presented in Chapter 6.

Developing interventions should be informed by prevalence data, research, best practices, existing community knowledge, and the insight and experience of those affected by the issue. For example, research shows that preventing adolescents from consuming alcohol and tobacco is difficult and that the impact is usually short term. Delaying the onset of substance use and preventing or minimizing harm is much more feasible.

Responding to substance abuse-related problems cannot be done in isolation of the social determinants of health. Taking stock of the community, and its unique strengths and challenges, is essential to understand the context of any problematic substance use and abuse pattern. Social and economic conditions such as limited income, living in unsafe neighbourhoods, and lack of leisure, recreation, job and training opportunities are known to increase the risk of substance abuse and addiction. For example, the sale and distribution of tax-free tobacco accounts for a significant proportion of First Nations' income. As such, smoking cessation among some Aboriginal communities may be more difficult than in others.

Strategies based on sensationalism and shock value should be avoided. Research has shown that while they may produce some deterrence, it is short lived and cannot be sustained over time. Taking the time to assess the community's condition is the first step the CHN should take before defining, supporting, or moving ahead with any intervention. The application of the resiliency theory is particularly valuable because it identifies a community's predominant risk and protective factors. This can help develop interventions that correspond to the root causes of substance use and abuse in the community. **Resiliency** is described as the capability of individuals, families, groups, and communities to cope successfully in the face of significant adversity or risk (Mangham, McGrath, Reid, & Stewart, 1995). The theory of resiliency consists of two fundamental concepts—risk and protective factors—both of which contribute to one's sense of resistance or resiliency. **Risk factors** are considered stresses that challenge individuals, including their own personal and environmental characteristics. When stresses such as substance abuse are greater than one's protective factors, even those who have been resilient in the past may become overwhelmed. **Protective factors** are skills, personality factors, and environmental supports that act as buffers when people are faced with stressful events. Individual protective factors may include literacy and interpersonal skills. Community-based protective factors may consist of a strong economic base, shared values, and good volunteer participation. Assessing factors such as age or social isolation, which may lead to compulsive patterns of drug use, can help the CHN understand why some individuals and communities respond differently to adversity and have different patterns of substance use and abuse. In essence, the theory helps pinpoint predominant risk factors that need to be addressed and the protective factors that need to be optimized (Figure 28.1). The framework is especially important because it supports the integration of health determinants such as employment, and considers the linkages between the person and the community's sociocultural and economic environment. You may want to consult Chapter 13 for further details on this important first step in community development.

As you explore the application of developing substance abuse interventions, you are encouraged to consult Chapter 14 for more detailed information about the process of health planning. Whether CHNs are implementing activities as part of their agency's mandate, leading an intervention with a project team, or collaborating with a community-wide substance abuse committee or task force, their work should reflect the following **guiding principles**, which are embedded in several local, provincial, and national strategic planning documents.

1. **Person Centered**: Creating programs or activities should reflect the needs of the affected population group. Avoid fitting people to programs; work to fit the programs to the people.

2. **Inclusiveness**: Community solutions should be inclusive of all people regardless of societal limitations and perceptions. Their individual insights and experiences are a valued component of the planning process and can be used to generate program ideas, maintain a focus on the person-centered approach, and draw upon the lived experiences of the community.

3. **Non-Stigmatizing**: Interventions should reflect a respect for the dignity of individuals affected by the use or abuse of substances. This means paying attention to stigma ensuring that the social, biochemical, and physiological components to substance abuse are understood and respected. While solutions should respond to the needs of affected individuals, they should also respect their assets, potential, and abilities.

4. **Knowledge and Best Practices**: Local, provincial, and national research provides a good understanding of the extent and consequences of substance abuse. Initiatives and research in other communities and countries can provide a strong knowledge base for moving forward with ideas. There is a wealth of information in Canada and abroad that can help communities with data, best practices, and models that can ensure that decisions are based on evidence. While opinions and anecdotes are helpful, applying validated research and outcomes from other community initiatives improves results. You may want to consult best practice guidelines in smoking cessation and methadone maintenance treatment developed by the Registered Nurses' Association of Ontario (RNAO), as these have achieved a national presence in Canadian nursing (RNAO, 2007; 2009).

5. **Total Community**: Substance abuse is a community-wide problem requiring involvement and action of the total community. Substance abuse affects everyone, not just individual users and their families and friends. It affects neighbourhoods, schools, families, health and community resources, employers, the economy, and many other aspects of the community. Community members must work together to maintain and improve the well-being of the community.

6. **Collaboration**: The complex nature of substance abuse requires innovative approaches that promote partnerships among community members. This maximizes knowledge exchange, a community's assets, and its leverage to acquire additional resources. A multipronged approach involving multiple sectors ensures that interventions are relevant and result in optimal outcomes.

FIGURE 28.1 Framework of Community Resilience

Community Risk Factors		
Social	**Environmental**	**Behavioural**
Economic disadvantage	Isolation	Communal apathy
Unemployment	- geographical	Community anger
Educational disadvantage	- social	Low participation in
Cultural barriers	Disasters	community development

+

Community Protective Factors			
Social Support	**Empowerment**	**Community Connectedness**	**Communal Coping**
Communal support	Communal responsibility	Shared history and culture	Problem focused
Family and friends	and action	Residents "know everyone"	Emotion focused
Volunteers	Retraining	Schools and churches	
Lay support	Educational services		
Community organizations			

↓

Community (Positive) Resilient Outcomes			
Growth	**Residents' Health**	**Community Tone/Outlook**	**Community Development**
New economic and	Physical health	Hope	Community participation
cultural initiatives	Mental health	Optimism	and connectedness
	Healthy behaviours	Embrace opportunities	Organizations survive
			Acquire resources

Source: Statistical Report on the Health of Canadians, Health Canada. (1999). Cat. no. 82-570X1E. http://www.statcan.gc.ca/pub/82-570-x/4227734-eng.pdf. Reproduced with the permission of the Minister of Public Works and Government Services Canada, 2007.

CHNs should have the knowledge and skills to leverage resources that will optimize and support healthy individuals, families, and communities. Doing so requires a good understanding of the interconnectedness between the use, misuse, and abuse of substances and social determinants of health.

Paying attention to issues that impact a community and the factors that may influence individuals who need information and/or professional assistance for a substance abuse-related problem is paramount to finding the right solution, for the right people, and at the right place and time.

CASE STUDY

A local Junior A hockey team plays in your community's municipally owned arena. Team officials have been selling beer during home games as a means of generating revenue for the team. There have been recent and well-publicized complaints about people becoming intoxicated and creating disturbances during and after games. Community officials and private entrepreneurs are looking for the support of the local police department and your public health unit in order to effectively address this issue and prevent further disturbances. The well-attended hockey games represent the main source of entertainment for many families during the long winter season. Your public health board has requested a substance abuse program to explore this issue and develop an appropriate strategy to reduce these emerging alcohol-related problems.

Discussion Questions

1. Discuss the health, social, and legal risks that are commonly associated with the practice of serving alcohol during sports events in municipally owned facilities.

2. Explore various prevention and enforcement strategies that can be adopted to minimize the risks that are associated with the service of alcohol.

3. Identify the various groups of stakeholders that should be targeted as part of these strategies.

SUMMARY

In this chapter, we have explored the impact that substance abuse can have on the health of individuals and communities. Three types of drug consumption, including the use and abuse of drugs, and the concept of dependency, were briefly presented. The reasons people use and abuse drugs were discussed, as well as how a maladaptive pattern of substance abuse progresses toward physical and psychological dependence.

The scope of alcohol, tobacco, and illicit and licit drug use and abuse was discussed. Sociodemographic characteristics commonly associated with certain prevalence patterns were examined because it is essential to understand that substance abuse can cause poor health, just as poor health and other social, health, and economic disadvantages can contribute to substance abuse. The data presented confirm that substance abuse affects many Canadians, with some groups of people being particularly vulnerable, including women, infants, children, adolescents, people who come into contact with the criminal justice system, and the Aboriginal population. Harms commonly associated with substance abuse were identified, including fetal alcohol spectrum disorder, impaired driving, chronic cycles of dependency and relapse, suicides, fatal accidents, and interpersonal violence. The important linkage between mental illness and substance abuse disorders, referred to as concurrent disorders, was also discussed.

Responding to substance abuse problems in the community requires sound data, a plan grounded in theoretical models, and strong intersectoral collaboration. The "four pillars" of Canada's Federal Drug Strategy and other theoretical models presented in this chapter reflect the importance of responding to substance abuse with behavioural and socioenvironmental approaches. Identifying and exploring risk factors that contribute to substance abuse problems in a community was emphasized as these help to ensure that strategies correspond to conditions of the community, the type of drug, and the nature and extent of its consumption. Planning strategies to address substance abuse in a community was described, and activities such as education, policy, environmental support and controls, screening, and treatment and rehabilitation were defined. It was reinforced that no single activity can be effective on its own—that they are mutually complementary and optimize the potential for positive outcomes. The theory of harm reduction was presented with a focus on special programs such as drug treatment courts and methadone maintenance treatment programs. The application of the conceptual frameworks and models presented in this chapter can serve to guide the CHN in the development of relevant interventions that are based on evidence; make important linkages between the individual, the drug, and the environment; and reflect the practice standards of community health nursing.

KEY TERMS

drug, p. 435
psychoactive substance, p. 435
alcohol, p. 435
tobacco, p. 435
illicit drugs, p. 435
inhalants, p. 435
licit drugs, p. 435
substance use, p. 435
substance abuse, p. 435
dependence, p. 435
physical dependence, p. 435
psychological dependence, p. 435
injectable drugs, p. 437
prescription drugs, p. 437
concurrent disorders, p. 437
fetal alcohol spectrum disorder, p. 438
Canada's Federal Drug Strategy, p. 439
prevention and health promotion, p. 439
policies, p. 439
environmental support and controls, p. 439
screening, p. 440
early identification, p. 440
treatment, p. 440
rehabilitation, p. 440
stigma, p. 440
drug treatment courts, p. 440
treatment service continuum, p. 440
enforcement, p. 440
harm reduction, p. 441
methadone maintenance treatment, p. 441
complementary interventions, p. 442
resiliency, p. 442
risk factors, p. 442
protective factors, p. 442
guiding principles, p. 442
person centered, p. 442
inclusiveness, p. 442
non-stigmatizing, p. 442
knowledge and best practices, p. 442
total community, p. 442
collaboration, p. 442

REVIEW QUESTIONS

1. The most prevalent psychoactive substances in Canada are
   a) alcohol and injectable drugs.
   b) tobacco and cannabis.
   c) opioid prescriptions and alcohol.
   d) tobacco, alcohol and cannabis.

2. People use drugs for different reasons. Which of the following reasons would have the most relevance for discussion during an education session with a young group of pre-adolescents?
   a) relieve stress and tension
   b) resolve physical discomforts
   c) boost self-confidence, imitate adults, wanting peer acceptance
   d) reduce insomnia

3. Which of the following is a harm reduction intervention?

   a) drug testing at work

   b) the availability of low or "light" alcohol beverages

   c) a zero tolerance drug use school policy

   d) refusal skills and abstinence training for teens

4. Which of the following are characteristics of an effective continuum of addiction treatment and rehabilitation services?

   a) The diverse needs of people with concurrent disorders are identified and addressed.

   b) Services are run by private clinics.

   c) Screening and early detection are done by addiction specialists only.

   d) Services are solely based on abstinence models.

5. Which of the following determinants are linked to the use and abuse of substances in a community?

   a) urban communities

   b) achievement of higher education

   c) large families

   d) poverty, social isolation, and unemployment

STUDY QUESTIONS

1. Describe the "four pillars" of Canada's Federal Drug Strategy.

2. Why do people use drugs?

3. What is drug dependence? Discriminate between physical and psychological dependence.

4. What are the harmful consequences of substance abuse?

5. Describe important aspects of developing interventions to address substance abuse issues in communities.

6. What are the six principles that should guide a CHN's work in community-based substance abuse interventions?

7. What are the limitations of exclusively focusing on law enforcement?

8. Explain two harm reduction programs available in Canada.

After working through these questions, go to the MyNursingLab at www.pearsoned.ca/mynursinglab to check your answers.

INDIVIDUAL CRITICAL THINKING EXERCISES

1. Privately explore the first thing that comes to mind when you read each of the following expressions. Then, explore your reactions to each expression. Do they differ from each other? If so, consider the reasons why. Did any of your reactions surprise you? If yes, reflect on how your personal values may influence your professional practice.

   - a homeless alcoholic
   - needle exchange program
   - abstinence-based treatment
   - problem drinker
   - methadone treatment
   - parent with hangover
   - IV drug user
   - crack dealer
   - professor smoking marijuana
   - pregnant methadone client
   - crystal meth addict
   - chain (tobacco) smoker
   - demale cocaine user
   - drunk driver
   - twenty-year-old buying booze for underage sibling
   - person with HIV
   - gas sniffer
   - underage drunk
   - coffee drinker

2. Read your local newspaper or a magazine, or watch the news, a television program, or a movie. Pay attention to the images and messages about the consumption of alcohol, tobacco, and illicit or licit drugs. Who are these messages aimed at? What are they portraying? Consider the degree of influence that these images and messages have on drug consumption patterns in society.

3. Think of a community you have lived in and consider the factors that were attributed to that community's health status. What was the prevalence of psychoactive substances in that community? You may want to focus on one or more substances. Explore the factors that placed that community at risk and/or those that protected it, or acted as buffers.

4. In the community you are living in now, think about where screening for the use of psychoactive substances might take place. As a CHN, how might you introduce the concept of screening in a primary health clinic?

5. Thinking of your university or college, think about the activities that should be provided to reduce the abuse of alcohol on campus.

GROUP CRITICAL THINKING EXERCISES

1. Select a particular issue or harm that is associated with substance abuse in your community (e.g., the misuse and abuse of opioid prescription drugs, impaired driving, FASD). What sources of information (local, regional, provincial, and national) can be used to help your group accurately define the problem?

2. For the issue identified in question 1, have your group map your community's current capacity in terms of substance abuse prevention and treatment (health promotion and health recovery/rehabilitation) services and programs. You may use the telephone directory or contact local health and social service agencies. For example, you should highlight any screening and prevention programs, how people access general information about the issue, and, if appropriate,

where people access treatment services. Make note of any service or program gaps your group observes.

3. Using the results of the mapping exercise in question 2 and referring to the Framework for Community Resilience, discuss and analyze as a group the risk factors that you believe have contributed to the development of the issue or harm identified in question 1. Additionally, your group should explore the protective factors that have acted as buffers or that will have the capacity to create positive outcomes for your target population or for the community.

REFERENCES

Adlaf, E. M., Begin, P. & Sawka, E. (Eds.). (2005). *Canadian addiction survey: A national survey of Canadians' use of alcohol and other drugs: Prevalence of use and related harms: Detailed report.* Ottawa, ON: Canadian Centre on Substance Abuse.

American Psychiatric Association. (1994). *Diagnostic and statistical manual of mental disorders* (4th ed.). Washington, DC: Author.

Beirness, D. J., Jesseman, R. Notarandrea, R., & Perron, M. (2008). *Harm reduction: What's in a name?* Ottawa, ON: Canadian Centre on Substance Abuse.

Butterfield, P. (1997). Thinking upstream: Conceptualizing health from a health population perspective. In J. Swanson & M. Nies (Eds.), *Community health nursing: Promoting the health of the aggregate* (pp. 69–92). Philadelphia, PA: W. B. Saunders.

Canadian Centre on Substance Abuse. (2009). *Clearing the smoke on cannabis: Cannabis use and driving.* Ottawa, ON: Author.

Canadian Paediatric Society. (2005). Indian and Inuit Health Committee: Inhalant abuse. *Paediatrics and Child Health, 3*(2), 1998, reaffirmed January 2005.

Collin, C. (2006). *Substance abuse issues and public policy in Canada: Canada's federal drug strategy.* Parliamentary Information and Research Service: Political and Social Affairs Division. Retrieved from http://www.parl.gc.ca/information/library/PRBpubs/prb0615-e.pdf

Dhalla, I. A., Mamdani, M. M., Sivilotti, M. L. A., Kopp, A., Qureshi, O., & Juurlink, D. N. (2009). Prescribing of opioid analgesics and related mortality before and after the introduction of long-acting oxycodone. *Canadian Medical Association Journal, 181,* 891–896.

Harrell, A. *Drug courts and the role of graduated sanctions.* Retrieved from http://www.ncjrs.gov/pdffiles/fs000219.pdf

Haydon, E., Rehm, J., Fischer, B., Monga, N., & Adlaf, E. (2005). Prescription drug abuse in Canada and the diversion of prescription drugs into the illicit drug market. *Canadian Journal of Public Health,* November/December, 459–461.

Health Canada. (2002a). *Best practices: Concurrent mental health and substance use disorders.* Ottawa, ON: Author.

Health Canada. (2002b). *Best practices: Methadone maintenance treatment.* Ottawa, ON: Author.

Health Canada. (2008a). *Canadian alcohol and drug use monitoring survey* [CADUMS]. Ottawa, ON: Author.

Health Canada. (2008b). *Canadian tobacco use monitoring survey [CTUMS].* Ottawa, ON: Author.

Mangham, C., McGrath, P., Reid, G., & Stewart, M. (1995). *Resiliency: Relevance to health promotion: Discussion paper.* Ottawa, ON: Health Canada.

Mulgrew, I., (2003). Drug court measures small success. *Vancouver Sun,* April 19.

Ontario Ministry of Health, Health Promotion Branch. (1991). *A guide for community health promotion planning.* Toronto, ON: Author.

Registered Nurses' Association of Ontario [RNAO]. (2007). *Integrating smoking cessation into daily nursing practice.* Revised. Toronto, ON: Author. Retrieved from http://www.tobaccofreernao.ca/sites/tobaccofreernao.ca/files/1104_Final_revised_smoking.pdf

Registered Nurses' Association of Ontario [RNAO]. (2009). *Supporting clients on methadone maintenance treatment.* Toronto, ON: Author. Retrieved from http://www.rnao.org/Storage/58/5254_BPG_Managing_Methadone_Treatment.pdf

Rehm, J., Ballunas, D., Brochu, S., Fischer, B., Gnam, W., Patra, J., . . . Taylor, B. (2006). The costs of substance abuse in Canada, 2002 highlights. Retrieved from http://www.risqtoxico.ca/documents/2006_Brochu_ReportCost.pdf

Single, E. (1999). *Substance abuse and population health: Workshop on addiction and population health. Edmonton, Alberta, June, 1999.* Ottawa, ON: Canadian Centre on Substance Abuse. Retrieved from http://www.ccsa.ca/NR/rdonlyres/5CC1D7F6-4C32-49A3-8C7E-2F5E53690105/0/ccsa0003891999.pdf

Skinner, W., O'Grady, C., Bartha, C., et al. (2004) *Concurrent substance use and mental health disorders: An information guide.* Toronto, ON: Centre for Addiction and Mental Health.

Traffic Injury Research Foundation [TIRF]. (2009). *The alcohol crash problem in Canada: 2006.* Ottawa, ON: Traffic Injury Research Foundation.

ADDITIONAL RESOURCES

Classic Study

Fischer, B., Rehm, J., Brissette, S., Brochu, S., Bruneau, J., El-Guebaly, N., . . . Baliunas, D. (2005, June). Illicit opioid use in Canada: Comparing social, health, and drug use characteristics of untreated users in five cities. *Journal of Urban Health, 82*(2), 250–266.

National Websites

Canada's Drug Strategy
http://www.parl.gc.ca/information/library/PRBpubs/prb0615-e.pdf

Canadian Centre for Ethics in Sport
http://www.cces.ca

Canadian Centre on Substance Abuse (CCSA)
http://www.ccsa.ca

Canadian Foundation for Drug Policy
http://www.cfdp.ca

Canadian Network of Substance Abuse and Allied Professionals
http://www.cnsaap.ca/ENG/Pages/index.aspx

Drug Rehabilitation Centres in Canada
http://www.drugrehab.ca

FASD Databases
http://www.ccsa.ca/Eng/KnowledgeCentre/OurDatabases/FASD/Pages/default.aspx

Health Canada, First Nations and Inuit Health, Treatment Centre Directory
http://www.hc-sc.gc.ca/fniah-spnia/substan/ads/nnadap-pnlaada_dir-rep-eng.php

MADD Canada Mothers Against Drunk Driving
http://www.madd.ca

National Database of FASD and Substance Use During Pregnancy Resources
http://www.ccsa.ca/fas/

National Native Alcohol and Drug Abuse Program (NNADAP)
http://www.hc-sc.gc.ca/fniah-spnia/pubs/substan/_ads/nnadap_rev-pnlaada_exam/index-eng.php

National Strategy: Moving Forward. The 2006 Progress Report on Tobacco Control in Canada.
http://www.hc-sc.gc.ca/hc-ps/pubs/tobac-tabac/prtc-relct-2006/index-eng.php

Provincial Websites

Addictions Foundation of Manitoba
http://www.afm.mb.ca/

Alberta Alcohol and Drug Abuse Commission (AADAC)
http://www.aadac.com/79.asp

British Columbia Ministry of Health, Mental Health and Addictions
http://www.health.gov.bc.ca/mhd/

Centre for Addictions Research British Columbia
http://www.carbc.ca/

Government of the Northwest Territories, Department of Health and Social Services
http://www.hlthss.gov.nt.ca/english/default.htm

New Brunswick Department of Health and Wellness, Addiction and Mental Health Services
http://www.gnb.ca/0378/poster-e.asp

Newfoundland and Labrador Department of Health and Community Services, Addictions Services
http://www.health.gov.nl.ca/health/commhlth_old/factlist/drugdepts.htm

Nova Scotia Department of Health, Addictions Services
http://www.addictionservices.ns.ca/

Nunavut Department of Health and Social Services
http://www.gov.nu.ca/health/

Ontario Centre for Addiction and Mental Health
http://www.camh.net

Prince Edward Island Addiction Services
http://www.gov.pe.ca/health/index.php3?number=1020507&lang=E

Québec Ministère de la Santé et des Services Sociaux
http://www.dependances.gouv.qc.ca/index.php?toxicomanie-en

Saskatchewan Health, Alcohol and Drug Services
http://www.health.gov.sk.ca/alcohol-and-drug-services

Yukon Department of Health and Social Services, Alcohol and Drug Services Division
http://www.hss.gov.yk.ca/programs/alcohol_drugs

About the Author

Hélène Philbin Wilkinson, BScN, Reg. N., MN. After spending the early part of her nursing career in hospital and public health nursing, Hélène turned to the community, working at the Centre for Addiction and Mental Health as a senior program consultant in policy and service development, and applied research and program evaluations projects. In 1999, she joined the Northern Shores District Health Council as a senior health systems planner overseeing the planning portfolios of addiction, mental health, and French-language health services. Following the closure of the Ontario District Health Councils in 2005, Hélène returned to the hospital sector where she is currently working as the Forensic Program Director at the Northeast Mental Health Centre. She dedicates her chapter to her godmother Ella, who was a pioneer public health nurse in Northeastern Ontario.

Sexually Transmitted Infections and Blood Borne Pathogens

Wendi Lokanc-Diluzio, Alison Nelson, Janet L. Wayne, and Janet B. Hettler

OBJECTIVES

After studying this chapter, you should be able to:

1. Understand the different types of sexually transmitted infections and blood borne pathogens, and the issues surrounding their transmission, testing, treatment, and prevention.

2. Recognize the potential physical, psychological, and financial implications of sexually transmitted infections and blood borne pathogens through analysis of Canadian statistical trends and issues raised in the literature.

3. Identify population-specific issues related to sexually transmitted infections and blood borne pathogens.

4. Identify various applications of the population health promotion model when developing health promotion and prevention strategies for sexually transmitted infections and blood borne pathogens.

5. Describe innovative interventions involving community health nurses that address sexually transmitted infections and blood borne pathogens in different regions of Canada.

INTRODUCTION

Sexually transmitted infections (STIs) and **blood borne pathogens (BBPs)** are significant public health issues in Canada. STIs are infections that are spread through various types of sexual contact (vaginal, anal, or oral) with an infected person. BBPs, on the other hand, are infections that are carried and transmitted by blood (Manitoba Health, 2009). **Human immunodeficiency virus (HIV)** is one of the most common and devastating BBPs.

Historically and currently, those affected by STIs and HIV have encountered stigmatization and discrimination as STIs and HIV often elicit emotional reactions such as anxiety, fear, and shame. The continued stigma of STIs and HIV may impede people from protecting themselves, as well as from seeking testing and treatment. Societal reactions of intolerance toward people at risk for contracting STIs and HIV, as well as those living with HIV and acquired immune deficiency syndrome (AIDS) may further marginalize specific populations who already experience inequities in health status.

In this chapter, community health nurses (CHNs) are challenged to promote health, build capacity, and facilitate access and equity through innovative community strategies to address STIs and BBPs. Historical and current challenges regarding the prevention of STIs and BBPs and the development of healthy public policies are discussed. Additionally, an overview of the main categories of STIs and their incidence and/or prevalence in Canada is presented along with a review of selected BBPs, their transmission, and prevalence. Implications for CHNs working with marginalized populations related to STI and BBP prevention and risk reduction are discussed. Examples of innovative prevention strategies to address STIs and BBPs are presented.

HISTORY OF STIS AND BBPS AND THEIR EFFECTS ON HEALTHY PUBLIC POLICY

Over the years, STIs have been labelled in different ways including *venereal disease* (VD), which referred to Venus, the Roman goddess of love. In the 1970s, the term VD was viewed as inaccurate and replaced by sexually transmitted disease (STD), because "love often plays little or no role in the transmission of such diseases" (Shriver et al., 2002, p. 136). Recently in Canada, STI has become the preferred term, as STI is viewed as an encompassing term that includes infections which may be asymptomatic (Public Health Agency of Canada [PHAC], 2009a).

Healthy public policies and guidelines need to be constantly revisited and updated based on research to assist in protecting the public from the consequences of STI and BBP. Currently, researchers are investigating the complex relationship between STI and HIV. To date, what is known about STI and HIV co-infection is that STI and HIV infections often coexist. In other words, having an STI likely increases the susceptibility to HIV infection (PHAC, 2008). Community health nursing interventions that support people to take precautions to prevent STI may also reduce the risk of HIV infection.

Prior to the discovery of antibiotics, STIs were not treatable, and serious illness was common. Healthy public policies were implemented to test men and women for syphilis prior to marriage and to test women during pregnancy to prevent neonatal infection. With the advent of antibiotic treatment, new policies were developed. For example, for more than 100 years, silver nitrate eye drops, or more recently other antibiotics such as erythromycin, have been recommended by the Canadian Pediatric Society (CPS) for all newborns to prevent blindness from gonorrhea (CPS, 2008). As well, the CPS advises that all pregnant women be screened for gonorrhea and chlamydia and treated as needed (CPS, 2008).

Currently, all Canadian provinces and territories have developed recommendations and/or guidelines for prenatal HIV testing to promote informed decision making related to neonatal HIV prevention (PHAC, 2007). Antiretroviral medications are an effective way to reduce the risk of HIV transmission to newborns and young children when given to HIV-positive women during pregnancy and/or before birth (PHAC, 2007).

Healthy public policies have also been developed in response to community action. For example, the infection of people with HIV through blood transfusions prompted a national response to implement strict blood bank surveillance guidelines. Since 1985, all blood donors are screened for HIV. The risk of HIV transmission via blood transfusion has decreased considerably from 1985 to 2003 from roughly 1 in 16 000 to 1 in greater than a million (PHAC, 2009b).

SEXUALLY TRANSMITTED INFECTIONS AND BLOOD BORNE PATHOGENS

STIs can be categorized as bacterial, viral, or ectoparasitic infections. Some viral diseases such as HIV and hepatitis B are found in the blood and are spread through unprotected (condomless) sexual contact as well as contact with infected blood. The following is a brief summary of the most common STIs and BBPs in Canada.

Bacterial STIs

The most common bacterial STIs are chlamydia, gonorrhea, and syphilis. *Chlamydia* and *gonorrhea* are primarily transmitted through unprotected vaginal and anal intercourse, and less often through unprotected oral intercourse. The infections can also pass from mother to newborn baby during delivery (PHAC, 2008). Symptoms in females may include abnormal vaginal discharge or bleeding, lower abdominal pain, or burning during urination (PHAC, 2008). Symptoms in males may include unusual penile discharge, burning while urinating, or pain or swelling of the testes. Additionally, rectal pain and discharge may indicate infection through anal intercourse. Most often, however, individuals do not experience any symptoms, resulting in the ongoing spread of infection and/or serious complications (PHAC, 2008). In women, untreated chlamydia and/or gonorrhea infections may lead to pelvic inflammatory disease (PID), which is an inflammation of the upper female genital tract (PHAC, 2008). Complications of PID may include chronic pelvic pain, infertility, and ectopic pregnancy (PHAC, 2008).

Many people avoid having STI testing because of their fear of pain and embarrassment. Within a supportive and non-judgmental environment, however, those fears can be alleviated. Chlamydial and gonorrheal infections are detected via urine testing and/or cervical/penile/anal/throat swabbing (PHAC, 2008). Both infections are relatively easy to treat with antibiotics if detected early (PHAC, 2008).

In Canada, chlamydia is the most prevalent reportable STI. From 1997 to 2008, the chlamydia rate increased by 118% from 113.9 to 248.9 per 100 000 population (PHAC, 2010a). A disproportionate number of women and youth are infected with chlamydia (PHAC, 2010a). Gonorrhea is the second most prevalent reportable STI in Canada. From 1997 to 2008, the reported rate more than doubled, from 14.9 to 38.2 per 100 000 population (PHAC, 2010b). Males have higher rates of gonorrhea than females (PHAC, 2010b).

Syphilis is primarily transmitted via unprotected vaginal, oral, or anal sexual contact (PHAC, 2008). The signs and symptoms of syphilis are often overlooked because in the early stages it manifests as painless sores (chancres) with flu-like symptoms. Diagnosis is often delayed until later stages, when there is already extensive damage to the central nervous or cardiovascular system, resulting in complications such as paralysis or mental illness (PHAC, 2008). Syphilis is diagnosed through blood tests, swabs with dark-field microscopy, and clinical symptoms (e.g., chancres and rash) (PHAC, 2008). Syphilis infections are treated with antibiotics, and negative long-term outcomes are reduced with early diagnosis (PHAC, 2008).

Syphilis can also be passed from mother to baby during pregnancy or childbirth, resulting in congenital syphilis or fetal death (PHAC, 2008; PHAC, 2009c). *The Canadian Guidelines on Sexually Transmitted Infections* (PHAC, 2008) recommends that all pregnant women be screened for infectious syphilis during the first trimester of pregnancy. Women who are considered "high risk" for contracting syphilis should also be screened at 28–32 weeks' gestation and at delivery (PHAC, 2008). Pregnant women testing positive for syphilis are treated with antibiotics (PHAC, 2008).

In Canada, syphilis is the least common of the reportable STIs. That said, from 1996 to 2008 the rate of infectious syphilis increased by 950% from 0.4 to 4.2 per 100 000 population (PHAC, 2010c). Over the past decade, there have been several syphilis outbreaks across Canada. Some outbreaks have

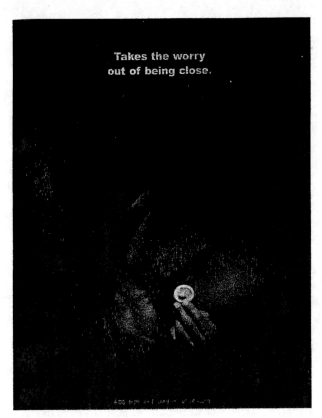

Takes the worry out of being close.

Photo 29.1

An AIDS awareness campaign

Credit: Bill Aron / PhotoEdit

been linked to the sex-trade worker and men who have sex with men populations (PHAC, 2008) (see Photo 29.1).

In 2007, Alberta Health and Wellness declared a syphilis outbreak in Alberta. From 1997 to 2006, the syphilis rate in Alberta increased by over 3000%. Furthermore, 14 Albertan babies were diagnosed with congenital syphilis from 2005 to 2007. This has changed prenatal re-screening practices in Alberta. It is recommended that *all* pregnant Albertan women are rescreened for syphilis at 24–28 weeks' gestation and at delivery (Alberta Health and Wellness & Alberta Health Services, 2009).

Viral STIs

Genital herpes and *human papillomavirus (HPV)* are highly prevalent **viral STIs** among sexually active people. These viruses are easy to spread, difficult to prevent and detect, and non-reportable. Herpes and HPV are transmitted through vaginal, oral, and/or anal sexual intercourse but mostly through skin-to-skin sexual contact (PHAC, 2008). Herpes can also be spread from mother to baby through childbirth and can cause serious complications (PHAC, 2008).

Genital herpes often appears as one or a group of painful, itchy, fluid-filled blisters in or around the genitals, buttocks, and/or thighs. People may experience burning during urination, fever, flu-like symptoms, and swollen glands. After becoming infected with genital herpes, some people experience only one herpes outbreak while others can have an outbreak

every month or so. It is important to note that 60% of infections are asymptomatic (PHAC, 2008).

Herpes is diagnosed through clinical examination or a culture of the fluid drawn from a sore (PHAC, 2008). There are two types of herpes: type 1 (most commonly found on the mouth) and type 2 (most commonly found on the genitals) (PHAC, 2008). Both types 1 and 2 are found on the genitals and/or mouth due to the increased occurrence of oral sex. There is no cure for herpes; however, outbreaks can be managed through intensive and/or preventive doses of antiviral medication (PHAC, 2008).

The incidence and prevalence of genital herpes is unknown in Canada. However, according to the Public Health Agency of Canada (2008), its incidence and prevalence is increasing worldwide.

Many people infected with HPV have no symptoms. There are more than 140 strains of HPV (PHAC, 2008). Some HPV strains cause genital warts; others cause abnormal cell changes on the cervix, which may lead to cervical cancer if left untreated. Abnormal cervical changes as a result of HPV infection are detected through having Pap tests on a regular basis (PHAC, 2008). Abnormal cervical changes may be monitored by repeat Pap tests, or through referral for colposcopy for more intensive diagnostic testing and treatment. Genital warts appear as groups of cauliflower-like growths in the genital area. Clinical examinations and special testing are used to visualize genital warts. Freezing, burning, or laser therapies are used to treat genital warts.

Because HPV is non-reportable, its incidence is unknown. It is estimated that approximately 70% of adults will experience at least one type of HPV infection in their lifetime. This viral infection usually clears up on its own within two years (PHAC, 2008).

Ectoparasites

Ectoparasites include pubic lice (crabs) and scabies, both of which can be transmitted through sexual or non-sexual (e.g., contact with infected towels or bed linens) contact. *Pubic lice* are most commonly found in genital and surrounding hair; however, they can also be found in chest, armpit, or facial hair (PHAC, 2008). The adult louse lays nits (eggs) in the hair, and within 5 to 10 days the nits hatch. Symptoms of lice include itching and skin irritation.

Scabies are parasites that burrow under the skin, leaving red bumps that cause symptoms of irritation and itchiness (PHAC, 2008). Scabies can be found on any part of the body; however, they prefer warm moist places such as the genital area. Both conditions can be diagnosed through careful examination of infected areas and are treated with over-the-counter products containing insecticides such as permethrin (PHAC, 2008).

Vaginal Infections

Vaginal infections include bacterial vaginosis, candidiasis (yeast), and trichomoniasis. Not all these infections are transmitted sexually, but they are often included in the category of STIs. For more information on these conditions, please refer to *Canadian Guidelines on Sexually Transmitted Infections* (PHAC, 2008).

Blood Borne Pathogens

BBPs such as HIV and hepatitis B need special consideration as they are not solely transmitted by sexual activity. Transmission can also occur by reusing drug, tattooing, or piercing equipment that has residual traces of infected blood and from mother to neonate during pregnancy or birth (PHAC, 2008). Additionally, HIV can be transmitted through breast milk, and hepatitis B can be transmitted by sharing razors or toothbrushes with an infected person (Canadian AIDS Society, 2004; PHAC, 2008).

Many people live with HIV for several years without feeling seriously ill. Even with treatment, however, HIV will eventually progress into AIDS. It is estimated that up to 90% of those infected experience primary or acute HIV symptoms, which occur two to four weeks after infection (PHAC, 2008). Symptoms are generally mild and include flu-like symptoms such as sore throat, fatigue, fever, and nausea (PHAC, 2008). The chronic symptomatic phase occurs when the HIV weakens the immune system and the body exhibits long-term symptoms such as swollen lymph nodes, skin lesions, fever, and diarrhea. AIDS is diagnosed when multiple opportunistic infections occur, such as pneumonia, lymphomas, and fungal infections (PHAC, 2008).

HIV is diagnosed through a special blood test that became available in Canada in 1985. There is a window period of three to six months during which HIV antibodies may remain undetectable, requiring an individual to return for follow-up testing (PHAC, 2008). Pre- and post-test counselling by CHNs is important because they can engage clients, prepare them for the potential impact of test results, and raise awareness of risk-reduction practices such as condom use. Some provinces regrettably forgo pre- and post-test counselling as it is assumed to be time-consuming and costly. Unfortunately, there is no cure for HIV infection, but there is treatment. A variety of antiretroviral drugs are now available that delay the progression of HIV infection to AIDS (PHAC, 2008).

From 1985 to 2008, approximately 67 442 positive HIV tests were reported in Canada (PHAC, 2009d). In 2008, 45.1% of all positive adult HIV tests were among the men who have sex with men (MSM) population, 30.8% were among the heterosexual population, and 19.1% were among injection drug users (PHAC, 2009d). Though Aboriginal people comprise only 3.3% of Canada's population (PHAC, 2007), in 2008, 29.4% of all new HIV infections were among Aboriginal people (PHAC, 2009d). It is estimated that over a quarter of the individuals living with HIV do not know their HIV status (PHAC, 2009d). This is a matter for concern as they cannot take advantage of counselling and therapy services and may unknowingly spread the virus (PHAC, 2008).

Many people are infected with hepatitis B without knowing it because they often do not experience any symptoms. Approximately 30% to 50% of adults infected with hepatitis B will show non-specific symptoms including fatigue, nausea, vomiting, jaundice (yellowing of the skin or whites of the eyes), decreased appetite, and joint swelling or pain (PHAC, 2006a, 2008). Most people infected with hepatitis B recover; however, some people become chronic carriers. Most carriers have no symptoms but can infect others. Carriers may eventually develop liver cancer or cirrhosis (PHAC, 2006a, 2008). Hepatitis B is diagnosed through blood testing. Combination antiviral drugs are available for those with chronic active hepatitis B (PHAC, 2008).

It is estimated that fewer than 5% of Canadians have markers of past hepatitis B infection, and fewer than 1% are carriers of hepatitis B (PHAC, 2006a). Certain sub-populations tend to be at greater risk for the virus, including those who were born in endemic areas, men who have sex with men, sex-trade workers, and injection drug users (PHAC, 2006a). The widespread availability of hepatitis B vaccine has assisted in prevention of the infection. Publicly funded vaccination programs are offered in all Canadian provinces and territories. Hepatitis B vaccine is routinely offered to all Canadian children/adolescents. If parents are hepatitis B carriers and/or they were born in endemic areas, the vaccination is offered to children during the first year of life (PHAC, 2006a).

IMPLICATIONS OF STI AND BBP

All STIs and BBPs are underreported, as many Canadians do not go for testing or do not know they are infected (PHAC, 2008). There are large numbers of people living with incurable, non-reportable STIs such as herpes and HPV. Rates of reportable STIs (e.g., chlamydia) and BBPs (e.g., HIV) provide CHNs with some understanding regarding the scope of the problem. If STIs and BBPs remain inadequately addressed and treated, they can lead to ongoing spread of the infection, infertility, neonatal complications, pelvic inflammatory disease, or even death (PHAC, 2008; PHAC, 2009c). STIs can negatively impact a person's relationships, self-esteem, mental health, coping abilities, and work productivity. Additionally, there are societal economic implications due to the medical costs associated with diagnosis and treatment (McKay, 2006), especially if there are complications such as infertility and neonatal infection.

CHNs must attempt to address not only medical issues such as testing and treatment, but also the social and economic issues. For example, CHNs can advocate for the development of support groups that can assist people to cope with their diagnosis of herpes or HIV while supporting them to pursue loving, sexual relationships with an understanding partner. Additionally, CHNs can raise awareness in the workplace and community to increase the funding for HIV medication, research, and alternative employment during times of intense treatment.

STI and BBP Prevention and Risk Reduction

Accurate and consistent use of **male condoms** or **female condoms** (see Photo 29.2) is important to decrease the transmission

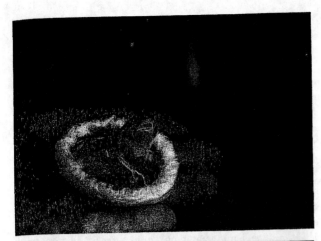

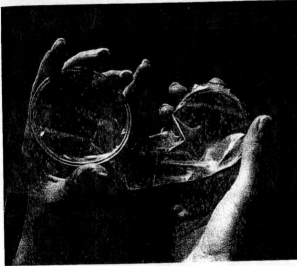

Photo 29.2

Male and female condoms

Credit: CORDELIA MOLLOY / SCIENCE PHOTO LIBRARY; Scott Camazine / Photo Researchers, Inc.

of STIs (PHAC, 2007, 2008). A male condom is a disposable latex or polyurethane sheath worn on the penis (Society of Obstetricians and Gynecologists of Canada [SOGC], 2009a). A female condom is a disposable polyurethane sheath placed inside the vagina (SOGC, 2009a). Both male and female condoms prevent direct contact between the vagina and penis, inhibiting the exchange of bodily fluids such as semen, pre-ejaculate fluid, and vaginal secretions (SOGC, 2009a). Condoms help to protect against pregnancy, STIs, and BBPs (SOGC, 2009a).

It is important to note that condoms are not 100% effective in protecting against herpes or HPV (e.g., genital warts on the testicles or labia). Abstinence from all types of sexual activity (e.g., genital to genital contact) is the only 100% effective method of preventing these STIs. Between 2006 and 2010, Health Canada approved two HPV vaccines that will prevent between two and four types of HPV infections. More information on HPV vaccine is discussed further in this chapter.

Infection by BBPs, such as HIV and hepatitis B, is prevented by condom use and by using clean needles and equipment for tattooing, piercing, and injecting drugs. Condoms and/or dental dams should always be used for oral sex (PHAC, 2007, 2008). As mentioned previously, hepatitis B is also prevented through vaccination.

CHNs are challenged with the issue of "**safer sex fatigue**," which is a term used to describe an individual's apathy regarding complying with and hearing about safer sex messages, resulting in an increase in risky behaviour (Canadian AIDS Society, 2004). Interventions such as sexual health education are important, but to have an impact they must be timely and relevant to the target population. It is vital to find innovative ways to promote the use of male and female condoms and dental dams. CHNs must "think upstream" and use health promotion approaches that address the issues of their target population. CHNs can reach individuals through street outreach, counselling, and peer mentoring programs. Furthermore, CHNs can explore innovative ways to make these risk reduction measures appealing to groups or communities through poster and social marketing campaigns. CHNs can work with other sectors and multidisciplinary groups to develop healthy public policy to address STI and BBP issues. Offering chlamydia urine testing in outreach vans and putting condom machines in schools are examples of health promotion activities resulting from healthy public policies.

CANADIAN RESEARCH BOX

What is the condom use behaviour at last sexual intercourse among 20- to 34-year-old Canadian young adults?

Rotermann, M., & McKay, A. (2009). Condom use at last sexual intercourse among unmarried, not living common-law 20- to 34-year-old Canadian young adults. *The Canadian Journal of Human Sexuality, 18*(3),75–87.

The objectives of the research were (a) to provide Canadian data on the "sexual and condom use behavior of UMNCL [unmarried and not living common-law] Canadian males and females aged 20–34" (p. 76); and (b) to establish if "the inverse association between age and condom use at last intercourse seen in Canadian teens also persists among Canadian young adults aged 20–24, 25–29, and 30–34." (p. 76).

The researchers analyzed data from the Canadian Community Health Survey (CCHS), which consists of cross-sectional surveys conducted in 2003 and 2005. The CCHS collects information from individuals aged 12 and over, living in private residences. Data were collected either in person or over the phone. For the purpose of this study, the researchers included respondents between the ages of 20 and 34, those who were UMNCL, and those who had stated they had sexual intercourse a minimum of once in the past year. A total of 19 455 participants were included in the research.

The findings revealed the following:

(a) Approximately 85% of UMNCL individuals indicated they had had sexual intercourse at least once.

(b) Approximately 41% of males and 29% of females had multiple (more than one) sexual partners in the past year.

(c) Females (49.9%) were significantly less likely than males (59.9%) to state they used a condom during their last sexual intercourse.

(d) The percentage of females using a condom during their last sexual intercourse was significantly higher among 20- to 24-year-olds (53.8%) compared to 25- to 29-year-olds (47.1%). The percentage was also significantly higher among 25- to 29-year-olds compared to those aged 30–34 (42.2%).

(e) The percentage of males using a condom during their last sexual intercourse was significantly higher among 20- to 24-year-olds (63.7%) compared to 25- to 29-year-olds (56.0%). However, there was no significant difference among males aged 25–29 and those aged 30–34 (54.7%).

(f) Males and females were more likely to use condoms if they had multiple partners (males: 69.8%; females 57.0%) in the past year versus one partner (males: 52.8%; females: 47.0%).

The researchers concluded that the findings suggest that many sexually active UMNCL Canadians are at risk for STI and HIV.

Discussion Questions

1. What should a CHN consider when counselling a young adult with regard to condom use?

2. How can a CHN use the Internet to promote the use of condoms with young adults?

Special Populations

The following is not an exhaustive discussion of all the hard-to-reach or marginalized populations in Canada. However, it is meant to raise awareness of some special groups and their risk for acquiring or transmitting STIs and BBPs.

Men Who Have Sex with Men In Canada, the MSM population has the highest proportion of HIV/AIDS when compared to other subpopulations (PHAC, 2008). A survey of Ontario self-identified gay and bisexual MSM determined 35% to 40% of respondents had participated in unprotected anal intercourse within the last year; approximately 17% had unprotected anal intercourse with a partner whose HIV status was unknown; and 4% had unprotected anal intercourse with a partner who tested positive for HIV (Myers et al., 2004).

Although health education messages addressing condom use are constantly being reinforced, it is clear from this study that certain cohorts of MSM are still not being reached with current prevention strategies. It is important for CHNs to *work with* the MSM population to develop messaging that is innovative and relevant. Additionally, it is important for CHNs to deliver messaging at venues frequented by the MSM

population. For example, Myers et al. (2004) noted that MSM search for sexual relations in a number of different sites including gay bars (60.3%), the Internet (35.3%), and bath houses (31.4%). These sites can therefore serve as venues for prevention messaging.

Sex-Trade Workers Sex-trade workers are at increased risk for contracting and spreading STIs and BBPs for several reasons, including their high numbers of sexual partners; limited ability to access social, health, and legal services; lifestyle risks such as substance use; and limited economic resources (PHAC, 2008). Condom use varies among sex-trade workers and the choice to use condoms is frequently controlled by the customer (HIV Prevention Research Team University of Ottawa, Provincial Women and HIV Group, & Ontario Women's Study Research Design Committee, 2007; Rekart, 2005). Customers often refuse to use condoms or offer additional money for "condomless" sex (HIV Prevention Research Team University of Ottawa et al., 2007; Rekart, 2005).

CHNs working with this group can promote a variety of risk-reduction strategies (e.g., correct use of male or female condoms) to prevent this population from acquiring and/or spreading STIs and BBPs. Since access to and the cost of condoms may deter sex-trade workers from using them, it is paramount that condoms are available for free. Peer education strategies have proven promising in terms of increasing knowledge related to STIs and HIV and safer sex practices (Rekart, 2005). CHNs can work with sex-trade workers to educate their peers regarding risk-reduction strategies such as condom negotiation. Overall, it is important that the services developed for sex-trade workers (e.g., peer education, hepatitis B vaccinations, STI testing and/or treatment) are delivered innovatively (e.g., from a mobile van, hotel room, community centre) with the workers' input (Rekart, 2005).

Street-Involved Youth It is estimated that approximately 150 000 youth in Canada live on the streets on any given day (PHAC, 2006b). This population is extremely vulnerable because, for many, addressing the basic necessities of life is of greater priority than preventing or addressing potential health risks (PHAC, 2006c). As a result, youth involved in street culture often do not take effective action in preventing STIs and BBPs (PHAC, 2006c).

In a 2003 Canadian-based study of street youth, it was determined that street youth had a chlamydia rate that was approximately 10 times more, and a gonorrhea rate that was 20 to 30 times more, than that of mainstream youth, and that approximately 25% of street youth were involved in the sex trade at some point (PHAC, 2006c). Resources must be allocated for both sufficient outreach with this population and comprehensive programming that entails prevention, screening, and treatment services (PHAC, 2006c).

Injection Drug Users Injection drug users represent a growing concern for CHNs, as the craving for "another hit" overrides the importance of using a clean needle to prevent the transmission of HIV or hepatitis B. Offering better access to condoms and clean needles/drug equipment via needle exchange

CANADIAN RESEARCH BOX

What are the experiences of youth accessing STI services?

Shoveller, J., Johnson, J., Rosenberg, M., Greaves, L., Patrick, D. M., Oliffe, J. L., & Knight, R. (2009). Youth's experiences with STI testing in four communities in British Columbia, Canada. *Sexually Transmitted Infections, 85,* 397–401.

The purpose of the research was to investigate youths' experiences with accessing STI services; and service providers' experiences regarding the provision of STI testing services.

Data were collected in four British Columbia communities: Vancouver, Richmond, Prince George, and Quesnel. The researchers collected data via interviews and naturalistic observations. Seventy youth (ages 15–24) and 22 service providers participated in in-depth interviews. Additionally, the researchers made observational visits to 11 youth and sexual health clinics. The researchers made note of the clinic design and the level of privacy for clients in the waiting area. Additionally, they observed youth entering the clinic.

Participants identified three factors impacting experiences in relation to STI testing:

(a) *Physical and social aspects of the community.* Participants indicated that lack of privacy, confidentiality, and anonymity were barriers to accessing STI services. Some youth traveled to clinics outside of their community to minimize their risk of seeing someone they knew. Participants also identified that social norms related to heterosexism and homophobia were concerns. Some service providers felt that LGBT (lesbian, gay, bisexual, transgendered) youth do not access STI testing in the communities of Prince George and Quesnel. Youth reported that they felt that it was assumed they were heterosexual.

(b) *Clinic characteristics.* An obstacle to accessing STI services was clinic hours. Additionally, some participants expressed that the clinics were 'feminised' areas because of the décor and because the waiting area was occupied with women.

(c) *Gaps in knowledge.* The majority of the male participants did not know that that urine-based gonorrhea tests were available in many clinic settings, therefore decreasing the need for urethral swabs, which was identified as a barrier for male STI testing. Additionally, female participants did not know the difference between STI and Papanicolaou (Pap) testing.

The researchers provided the following recommendations to improve youth access to STI testing services: (a) clinics need to be located in places accessible to youth (e.g., schools) and clinic hours should cater to their schedules; (b) services that are LGBT-friendly are needed particularly in the cultural and geographical contexts that are homophobic; (c) the clinic décor needs to be both youth friendly and gender neutral; (d) offer male-only clinic hours; and (e) enhance awareness regarding urine-based testing and the difference between STI and Pap testing.

Discussion Questions

1. How can CHNs help improve access to STI services for youth?
2. Consider the last time you accessed a primary care setting. Did the setting provide "LGBT-friendly" services? Explain.

programs and safer injection facilities may help these populations lower their risk of contracting HIV while they search for effective treatment (PHAC, 2008). Needle exchange programs and safer injection facilities are discussed further below.

New Immigrants In 2009, more than 250 000 immigrants became permanent Canadian residents (Citizenship and Immigration Canada, 2010). Citizenship and Immigration Canada (CIC) requires syphilis and HIV testing for immigrants and refugees, over the age of 15, seeking Canadian citizenship. HIV testing is also required for children born to a mother infected with HIV, those with blood/blood product exposure, or those who may be an international adoptee (Health Management Branch, 2009; PHAC, 2008). Presently, syphilis and HIV testing are the only compulsory STI tests for immigrants and refugees applying to become citizens (PHAC, 2008).

Language, cultural, socioeconomic, and educational barriers may deter certain immigrant sub-populations from seeking health services (PHAC, 2008). New immigrants are overwhelmed with adapting to new cultural and healthcare practices. Many come from countries where HIV, hepatitis, and other STIs are more prevalent and treatment is inaccessible (PHAC, 2008). Cultural beliefs may also influence a person's motivation to access health services. Some may try a variety of herbs or culturally accepted medications before seeking medical treatment for an STI or HIV. Many Canadian provinces lack services and resources that are translated, culturally sensitive, and accessible to newcomers (PHAC, 2008). It is important that CHNs be attentive to the stressful and complex issues faced by immigrants as they integrate into Canadian culture (PHAC, 2008).

Unwilling or Unable Population Researchers have identified that some HIV-positive individuals are recalcitrant or "unwilling or unable" (e.g., refuse to disclose HIV-positive status to sexual partners) to prevent the spread of HIV. The research has determined these individuals often present with one or more of the following issues: psychiatric issues (e.g., depression, fetal alcohol spectrum disorder); addictions; social deficits (e.g., lack of support and housing, involvement in the sex trade); and health deficits (e.g., lack of HIV knowledge) (Calgary Coalition on HIV/AIDS, 2004). Researchers believe these variables contribute to higher-risk activities (e.g., having sex without a condom) and can impede a person's efficacy at implementing risk-reduction practices. Health regions across Canada are addressing this issue in different ways, ranging from implementing comprehensive referral systems to providing housing and treatment.

With any of these special populations, it is important for CHNs to forge new partnerships with the agencies these populations access (HIV Prevention Research Team University of Ottawa et al., 2007). For example, to promote the health of new immigrants, CHNs can partner with cultural organizations, public health centres, community groups, or religious centres. For street-involved youth, CHNs can collaborate with sexual and reproductive health centres, mental health services, social services, detox/drug treatment programs, and community groups. Moreover, it is important to actively involve clients in the development, dissemination, and evaluation of promotion/prevention programs.

Innovative STI and BBP Prevention Interventions in Canada

The PHP model (Hamilton & Bhatti, 1996) provides a comprehensive tool for CHNs to utilize when planning STI and BBP prevention interventions with individuals, groups, and populations. (Refer to Chapter 6 for more information on the PHP model.) Novel and innovative strategies are being implemented across Canada in an attempt to lower the prevalence of STIs and BBPs.

Needle Exchange Programs and Safer Injection Facilities Injection drug use is a mounting public health concern in Canada. Individuals who participate in high-risk drug injection behaviours (e.g., sharing needles) pose a number of potential health risks to themselves and others, such as transmission of HIV/AIDS and hepatitis B and C (Elliott, Malkin, & Gold, 2002). Some Canadian communities have addressed the issue of needle sharing with harm-reduction strategies such as needle exchange programs and safer injection facilities. The harm-reduction model acknowledges that abstinence from all drugs is not realistic for all people and therefore, although drug use is not condoned, it is seen as essential to implement risk-reduction strategies to reduce harmful outcomes related to drug use (Elliott et al., 2002).

Needle exchange programs (NEPs) provide injection drug users with free, sterile injecting equipment to reduce their risk of contracting and/or spreading infection (Elliott et al., 2002). Evaluation research conducted on a Vancouver-based NEP demonstrated a reduction in needle sharing (Wood et al., 2002). Although NEPs are controversial, they are widely accepted as a method for minimizing the spread of blood borne diseases (Elliott et al., 2002; Wood et al., 2002).

Safer injection facilities (SIFs) provide a safe location for drug users to inject their own drugs with clean equipment under the supervision of medically trained professionals (Health Canada, 2008). The main objectives of SIFs are to decrease the spread of infectious disease, improve contact between the healthcare system and injection drug users, decrease the use of drugs in public places, decrease fatal and

CASE STUDY

A fictitious community called Homeville has a large population of transient male workers living in remote camps. Several CHNs work in the area of the health authority with this population. The men's income levels are high and their education levels are varied. They are often far away from home, involved in the sex and drug trades, and are heavy users of the Internet, especially for social networking. The CHNs understand, through a review of the literature, and by talking with the company and camp leaders, that appropriate accessible sexual health services are lacking for this population who are at high risk of STIs and BBPs.

Using the PHP model, the CHNs focus on addressing access to health services that considers the men's Internet and social networking practices. They collaborate with a group of representatives from health, social services, and business sectors to discuss the lack of services for this group. The group conducts an assessment to determine any gaps in health services for the transient workers. They work together to apply for and secure sustained funding to develop appropriate Internet-based STI/BBP education and outreach services.

Discussion Questions

1. What determinants of health will the CHNs need to be aware of when working with the transient male workers living in camps?

2. What health promotion strategies can the CHNs and community agencies implement to address the issues of these clients?

3. How can the CHNs involve the men, companies, and community agencies that work with the camp workers in the development of these strategies?

non-fatal drug overdoses, and increase enrolment of injection drug users into addiction treatment and rehabilitation programs (Wood et al., 2004a). Although SIFs are an innovative public health intervention, they are extremely controversial in various countries, including Canada.

In 2003, healthcare providers in Vancouver piloted the first medically supervised SIF in North America (Kerr, Tyndall, Montaner, & Wood, 2005). Evaluation research of this program indicated several positive outcomes including decreased syringe sharing (Kerr et al., 2005), decreased injection-related litter, decreased numbers of individuals injecting in public, and decreased numbers of syringes discarded in public (Wood et al., 2004b).

Social Marketing Campaigns *Social marketing* can be defined as "a program-planning process that applies commercial marketing concepts and techniques to promote voluntary behavior change" (Grier & Bryant, 2005, p. 319). In Canada, these types of campaigns are becoming more innovative as they provide blatant and, at times, provocative messages to different segments of the population (see Photo 29.3). Unfortunately, many of these campaigns are not properly evaluated for their short- or long-term impact on the target population.

One campaign that had evaluation results was launched by AIDS Vancouver and partners across six Canadian cities. The *Assumptions Campaign* was initially launched by the San Francisco AIDS Foundation in 2001. The campaign was then adapted and launched in Canada in 2004 (Trussler & Marchand, 2005). The goal of the campaign was to "reduce the incidence of unprotected anal intercourse with unknown status partners by challenging gay men to reconsider their assumptions about the sero-status of their partners, with the ultimate aim of reducing the number of new HIV infections in the Canadian gay male population" (Trussler & Marchand, 2005, p. 1). The campaign was based upon research with the MSM population, which suggests that gay men have unprotected intercourse with the assumption that they "know" their partner's HIV status (Trussler & Marchand, 2005).

A variety of campaign materials (brochures, postcards, posters, stickers, and washroom, transit, newspaper and magazine advertisements, etc.) were produced, many of which were available in both French and English. The images in the materials were grainy and "designed to be read in the cultural code of contemporary gay men. The texts represent[ed] the interior monologues of men depicted in the images and [made] liberal use of irony to destabilize the certainty of their assertions" (Trussler & Marchand, 2005, p. 1). The campaign's slogan was "How do you know what you know?" and campaign materials directed the audience to a website (www.think-again.ca). The campaign received television and radio, newspaper, and gay press coverage across Canada.

A total of 417 men participated in the evaluation of the campaign. Intercept surveys were completed at the end of the campaign to determine the results. The surveys revealed: (a) 79% of the respondents had been exposed to the campaign; (b) 52% had seen the campaign over 10 times; (c) 56% of those who saw the campaign conversed about it with other gay men; (d) 73% of the respondents rated the message as appealing; (e) 76% stated that the message provoked them to think about safer sex; and (f) 48% of the respondents indicated that the message provoked them to modify something related to their sexual practices (Trussler & Marchand, 2005). From June until November 2004, there were nearly 37 000 individual visits to the www.think-again.ca website (Trussler & Marchand, 2005).

Telehealth and Internet Resources *Telehealth* and *Internet resources* have become important in terms of health education and prevention of STIs and BBPs, as well as support for those living with HIV or AIDS (Kalichman et al., 2003; White & Dorman, 2001). Telehealth is the utilization of advanced telecommunications technology in order to exchange health-related information and administer health services that transcend cultural, time, social, and geographical barriers (Care et al., 2003). Email and the Internet are means of providing telehealth services to those seeking information (Care et al., 2003) about STIs and BBPs. Individuals may experience increased comfort utilizing email as a form of communicating, especially if their questions or concerns are personal or sensitive in nature (Care et al., 2003).

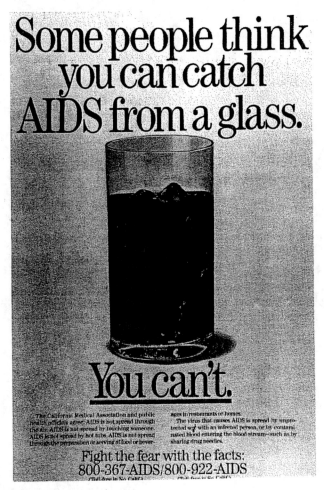

Photo 29.3

The "Fight the Fear with the Facts" campaign

Credit: Mary Kate Denny / PhotoEdit

Although telehealth is promising for sexual health promotion, it is important for CHNs to acknowledge its downfalls. First, "liability for care practices and potential misdiagnosis . . . provided through the medium of distance or electronic technologies are issues warranting careful exploration" (Care et al., 2003, p. 249). Second, this technology may be inaccessible to those who cannot afford computers. Finally, when communication is conducted electronically, the contextualization of the client's situation may be lost.

Internet sites can also be used to disseminate information on STI and BBP signs and symptoms, prevention, treatment and referral. For example, www.teachingsexualhealth.ca (see Photo 29.4) was developed to provide accurate, relevant, and timely resources for Alberta-based sexual health educators, parents, and students. As a provincial Alberta Education (Ministry of Education) approved learning resource, coordinated by Alberta Health Services, the Internet resource provides educators with teaching strategies while considering diversity issues such as ethnicity, differing abilities, and gender in the learning setting.

HPV Vaccination In July 2006, Health Canada approved a vaccine (**Gardasil**) that protects against four strains of HPV.

Photo 29.4

Website that promotes sexual health

Credit: Copyright 2010 Alberta Health Services, www.teachingsexualhealth.ca

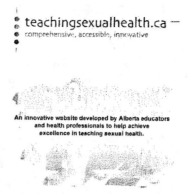

An innovative website developed by Alberta educators and health professionals to help achieve excellence in teaching sexual health.

Now an Alberta Education Authorized Resource

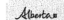 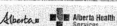

parents   teachers   students

Financial contribution from Alberta Health and Wellness, Alberta Health Services and Alberta Society for the Promotion of Sexual Health.

Two of the strains are responsible for approximately 70% of cervical cancer cases (HPV 16 and 18), whereas the other two strains are responsible for around 90% of genital warts cases (HPV 6 and 11) (Picard, 2010; Shier & Bryson, 2007). In February 2010, a second HPV vaccine, **Cervarix**, was approved by Health Canada (GlaxoSmithKline, 2010; Picard, 2010). Cervarix was designed to protect against two strains of HPV (HPV 16 and 18) causing cervical cancer. It also provides some protection from two additional strains (HPV 45 and 31). Together, the four strains account for 80% of cervical cancer cases. Although Cervarix does not protect against genital warts, it may offer longer-term protection against HPV causing cervical cancer (GlaxoSmithKline, 2010; Picard, 2010).

HPV vaccination is considered a medical milestone in terms of cancer prevention. It is anticipated that the long-term implications of the vaccine will result in a reduction of cervical cancer cases, although the need for women to have regular Pap tests will continue (Shier & Bryson, 2007).

The National Advisory Council on Immunization (NACI) released a *Statement on Human Papillomavirus Immunization* in 2007 to inform Canadian healthcare providers regarding appropriate use of HPV vaccine (NACI, 2007). The Society of Obstetricians and Gynecologists of Canada (SOGC, 2009b) has developed a website, (http://www.hpvinfo.ca) to provide HPV information to teens, adults, parents, teachers, and health professionals.

Gardasil HPV vaccine is available for males and females ages 9–26 (Shier & Bryson, 2007). Cervarix HPV vaccine is available for females ages 10–25 (GlaxoSmithKline, 2010). Currently, all Canadian provinces have publicly funded vaccination strategies in place for school aged girls in grades five to nine, depending on where they reside (SOGC, 2009b). For females and males who do not qualify for the publicly funded programs, but are within the recommended age group, the vaccination is available for a cost of $400–$500 for the three doses (SOGC, 2009b). Women and men older than 26 who are interested in HPV vaccination should be encouraged to speak to their healthcare provider.

SUMMARY

This chapter discusses the complex issues surrounding STIs and BBPs in Canada. The history of STIs and how healthy public policy addresses STI and BBP prevention are briefly outlined. A review of STI and BBP statistical trends and epidemiology are presented. The special needs of marginalized populations who may present unique challenges to CHNs related to STI and BBP are illustrated. Suggestions on how CHNs can use the PHP model to plan innovative prevention strategies are made. In conclusion, the PHP model provides a strong guide for CHNs when planning future STI and BBP promotion and prevention programs within communities.

KEY TERMS

sexually transmitted infections (STIs), p. 449
blood borne pathogens (BBPs), p. 449
human immunodeficiency virus (HIV), p. 449
bacterial STIs, p. 450
viral STIs, p. 451
male condoms, p. 452
female condoms, p. 452
safer sex fatigue, p. 452
needle exchange programs (NEPs), p. 456
safer injection facilities (SIFs), p. 456
Gardasil, p. 457
Cervarix, p. 458

REVIEW QUESTIONS

1. Syphilis can be passed from mother to baby during pregnancy or childbirth, resulting in congenital syphilis or death. In order to demonstrate the Canadian CHN Standard of professional responsibility and accountability, which is the correct current public policy that a CHN

would want to fully implement within the community to protect the health of newborn babies against syphilis?

a) Currently, there are no such policies in place.

b) High-risk women (e.g., sex-trade workers) are screened for syphilis during the second trimester of pregnancy.

c) All pregnant women are screened for syphilis during their first trimester.

d) All babies are given one dose of penicillin at birth.

2. Chlamydia, gonorrhea, and syphilis are the most common reportable sexually transmitted infections (STIs) in Canada. What is the key message that a CHN would want to include when planning an education session on how these STIs are spread?

a) The most common reportable STIs are spread through unprotected vaginal, anal, and oral sex.

b) The most common reportable STIs are spread through unprotected vaginal, anal, and oral sex and skin-to-skin sexual contact.

c) The most common reportable STIs are spread through sharing of needles and other drug paraphernalia.

d) The most common reportable STIs are spread through unprotected vaginal sex.

3. When counselling a young client, what is the most important information about chlamydia that the CHN would want to make sure the client understood?

a) Abnormal vaginal discharge/bleeding is symptom.

b) Burning during urination is often a symptom.

c) Lower abdominal pain is a symptom.

d) Not having symptoms is very common.

4. A CHN is planning a review of the community health centre's education resources for the public. Up-to-date HPV resources would include which of the following as a serious outcome of an HPV (human papillomavirus) infection?

a) genital warts

b) pelvic inflammatory disease (PID)

c) cervical cancer

d) infertility

5. How would a CHN explain Gardasil to a community health council member when planning an upcoming community campaign?

a) Gardasil is a vaccine that protects against all strains of HPV (human papillomavirus).

b) Gardasil is a vaccine that protects against four strains of HPV (human papillomavirus).

c) Gardasil is a viral sexually transmitted infection.

d) Gardasil is a bacterial sexually transmitted infection.

6. A CHN is fulfilling the Canadian CHN Standard of Promoting Health by writing an editorial for the local health magazine on STIs. What information would she/he want to include as the best way to prevent the spread of viral sexually transmitted infections (STIs) such as herpes and HPV (human papillomavirus)?

a) The use of a male or female condom.

b) The use of a male condom and a female condom together.

c) Abstinence from vaginal, oral, and anal sex.

d) Abstinence from vaginal, oral, and anal sex, and skin-to-skin sexual contact.

STUDY QUESTIONS

1. When developing an information sheet on STIs, what are the three most common bacterial STIs and their symptoms that a CHN would need to include?

2. What three key messages about HIV transmission would a CHN want to include in a community presentation on "Protecting your Children from HIV"?

3. When working in a community sexual health clinic, what are three main points plus supporting evidence that a CHN could integrate into client counselling guidelines to potentially reduce the transmission of STIs and BBPs?

4. What measures can a CHN ensure are in place within primary health services to prevent the consequences of congenital syphilis?

5. How would a CHN describe safer injection facilities when planning a community harm reduction strategy?

6. When writing an Internet article on HPV vaccine, how would a CHN answer the question "What is Cervarix?"

> *After working through these questions, go to the MyNursingLab at www.pearsoned.ca/mynursinglab to check your answers.*

INDIVIDUAL CRITICAL THINKING EXERCISES

1. Go to www.teachingsexualhealth.ca and complete the "your values quiz" (http://www.teachingsexualhealth.ca/teacher/howtoteach/quickquiz.html). What did you learn from completing the quiz? How do personal values impact sexual health education provided by CHNs?

2. STI rates are increasing in males 15–24 years old. The Public Health Agency of Canada (2008) states that testing and education are important to prevent STIs. Unfortunately, many youth at risk for STIs leave school early and become street involved, thus missing the benefit of sexual health education opportunities. What determinants of health could be addressed by CHNs related to the issues of street youth and STI?

3. Search the Internet and find one STI prevention resource that can be used with teens. How can CHNs use this resource in a teen clinic?

4. The recommendation to vaccinate elementary school girls against HPV has caused controversy in Canada. What can CHNs say to parents who are uncertain of whether or not to have their daughters vaccinated?

5. Women involved in the sex trade participate in high-risk sexual behaviors (e.g., sex without a condom, sex with multiple partners), placing them at risk for STIs and HIV. How can CHNs protect and promote the sexual health of this population?

GROUP CRITICAL THINKING EXERCISES

1. Gay youth often face rejection from significant support systems such as family and friends when they "come out." Some youth quit school and leave home to live on the street. Some rely on panhandling and prostitution to support themselves or to pay for drugs that help them cope. High-risk activities and a lack of resources increase gay youths' risk for STIs and HIV. How can a CHN use the *Canadian Community Health Nursing Standards of Practice (CCHNSP)* to plan care for gay youth within a sexual health clinic?

2. To address the complications associated with STIs and HIV, healthy public policy has been initiated and developed by policymakers and health professionals, but often with little input from the public. How can CHNs use primary health care's principle of public participation to inform the development of healthy public policy related to STI and HIV?

3. Social marketing campaigns can be effective in raising awareness about public health issues, such as STIs and HIV.

   a) Create an idea for a social marketing campaign addressing STIs and/or HIV.
   b) What is the objective(s) of the campaign?
   c) What is the message of the campaign?
   d) How will the message be delivered?

REFERENCES

Alberta Health and Wellness & Alberta Health Services. (2009). *Frequently asked questions for health professionals: Universal prenatal syphilis rescreening.* Edmonton, AB: Author.

Calgary Coalition on HIV/AIDS. (2004). *Phase two: Guidelines for working with U2 clients.* Calgary, AB: Author.

Canadian AIDS Society. (2004). *HIV transmission: Guidelines for assessing risk* (5th ed.). Retrieved from http://www.cdnaids.ca/web/repguide.nsf/pages/cas-rep-0307

Canadian Pediatric Society (CPS). (2008). *Position statement: Recommendations for the prevention of neonatal ophthalmia.* Retrieved from http://www.cps.ca/english/statements/ID/ID02-03.htm

Care, W. D., Gregory, D., Whittaker, C., & Chernomas, W. (2003). Nursing, technology, and informatics: An easy or uneasy alliance? In M. McIntyre & E. Thomlinson (Eds.), *Realities of Canadian nursing: Professional, practice and power issues* (pp. 243–261). Philadelphia, PA: Lippincott Williams & Wilkins.

Citizenship and Immigration Canada. (2010). *Facts and figures 2009: Preliminary tables—Permanent and temporary residents.* Retrieved from http://www.cic.gc.ca/english/resources/statistics/menu-fact.asp

Elliott, R., Malkin, I., & Gold, J. (2002). *Establishing safe injection facilities in Canada: Legal and ethical issues.* Ottawa, ON: Canadian HIV/AIDS Legal Network.

GlaxoSmithKline. (2010). *Product monograph: Cervarix.* Retrieved from http://www.cervarix.ca/pdf/Cervarix%20Prescribing%20Information.pdf

Grier, S., & Bryant, C. A. (2005). Social marketing in public health. *Annual Review of Public Health, 26,* 319–339.

Hamilton, N., & Bhatti, T. (1996). *Population health promotion: An integrated model of population health and health promotion.* Ottawa, ON: Public Health Agency of Canada, Health Promotion Development Division. Retrieved from http://www.phac-aspc.gc.ca/ph-sp/php-psp/index-eng.php

Health Canada. (2008). *Vancouver's INSITE service and other supervised injection sites: What has been learned from research?* Retrieved from http://www.hc-sc.gc.ca/ahc-asc/pubs/_sites-lieux/insite/index-eng.php#ack

Health Management Branch. (2009). *Handbook for designated medical practitioners.* Retrieved from http://www.cic.gc.ca/english//pdf/pub/dmp-handbook2009.pdf

HIV Prevention Research Team University of Ottawa, Provincial Women and HIV Group, & Ontario Women's Study Research Design Committee. (2007). *Women and HIV prevention: A scoping review.* Retrieved from http://www.health.gov.on.ca/english/providers/pub/aids/reports/women_hivprevention.pdf

Kalichman, S. C., Benotsch, E. G., Weinhardt, L., Austin, J., Luke, W., & Cherry, C. (2003). Health-related internet use, coping, social support, and health indicators in people living with HIV/AIDS: Preliminary results from a community survey. *Health Psychology, 22*(1), 111–116.

Kerr, T., Tyndall, M., Montaner, J., & Wood, E. (2005). Safer injection facility use and syringe sharing in injection drug users. *Lancet, 366,* 316–318.

Manitoba Health. (2009). *Sexually transmitted infections and bloodborne pathogens.* Retrieved from http://www.manitoba.ca/health/publichealth/cdc/sti.html

McKay, A. (2006). Chlamydia screening programs: A review of the literature. Part 1: Issues in the promotion of chlamydia testing of youth by primary care physicians. *The Canadian Journal of Human Sexuality, 15,* 111.

Myers, T., Allman, D., Calzavara, L., Maxwell, J., Remia, R., Swantee, C., et al. (2004). *Ontario's men survey final report.* Retrieved from http://cbr.cbrc.net/modules.php?name=News&file=article&sid=275

National Advisory Council on Immunization (NACI). (2007). Statement on human papillomavirus vaccine. *Canadian Communicable Disease Report, 33* (ACS-2), 1–32. Retrieved from http://www.phac-aspc.gc.ca/publicat/ccdr-rmtc/07pdf/acs33-02.pdf

Picard, A. (2010). *Health Canada approves a second vaccine against HPV.* Retrieved from http://www.theglobeandmail.com/life/health/health-canada-approves-a-second-vaccine-against-hpv/article1462104/

Public Health Agency of Canada (PHAC). (2006a). *Canadian immunization guide* (7th ed.). Retrieved from http://www.phac-aspc.gc.ca/publicat/cig-gci/index-eng.php

Public Health Agency of Canada (PHAC). (2006b). *Street youth in Canada: Findings from enhanced surveillance of Canadian street youth, 1999–2003.* Retrieved from http://www.phac-aspc.gc.ca/std-mts/reports_06/pdf/street_youth_e.pdf

Public Health Agency of Canada (PHAC). (2006c). *Sexually transmitted infection in Canadian street youth: Findings from enhanced surveillance of Canadian street youth, 1999–2003.* Retrieved from http://www.phac-aspc.gc.ca/std-mts/reports_06/sti-youth_e.html

Public Health Agency of Canada (PHAC). (2007a). *HIV/AIDS epi updates November 2007.* Retrieved from http://www.phac-aspc.gc.ca/aids-sida/publication/epi/epi2007-eng.php

Public Health Agency of Canada (PHAC). (2007a). *2004 Canadian sexually transmitted infections surveillance report, 2004: Pre-release.* Retrieved from http://www.phac-aspc.gc.ca/publicat/ccdr-rmtc/07vol33/33s1/index-eng.php

Public Health Agency of Canada (PHAC). (2008). *Canadian guidelines on sexually transmitted infections.* Retrieved from http://www.phac-aspc.gc.ca/std-mts/sti-its/guide-lignesdir-eng.php

Public Health Agency of Canada (PHAC). (2009a). *Sexual health and sexually transmitted infections.* Retrieved from http://www.phac-aspc.gc.ca/std-mts/

Public Health Agency of Canada (PHAC). (2009b). *Transfusion transmitted injuries section: Transfusion transmitted diseases/infections.* Retrieved from http://www.phac-aspc.gc.ca/hcai-iamss/tti-it/ttdi_e.html.

Public Health Agency of Canada (PHAC). (2009c). *Brief report on sexually transmitted infections in Canada: 2006.* Retrieved from http://www.phac-aspc.gc.ca/publicat/2008/sti-its/index-eng.php

Public Health Agency of Canada (PHAC). (2009d). *HIV and AIDS in Canada: Surveillance report to December 31, 2008.* Ottawa: Surveillance and Risk Assessment Division, Centre for Communicable Diseases and Infection Control, Public Health Agency of Canada.

Public Health Agency of Canada (PHAC). (2010a). *Reported cases and rates of chlamydia by age and sex, 1991 to 2008.* Retrieved from http://www.phac-aspc.gc.ca/std-mts/sti-its_tab/chlamydia1991-08-eng.php

Public Health Agency of Canada (PHAC). (2010b). *Reported cases and rates of gonorrhea by age group and sex, 1980 to 2008.* Retrieved from http://www.phac-aspc.gc.ca/std-mts/sti-its_tab/gonorrhea1980-08-eng.php

Public Health Agency of Canada (PHAC). (2010c). *Reported cases and rates if infectious syphilis by age group and sex, 1993 to 2008.* Retrieved from http://www.phac-aspc.gc.ca/std-mts/sti-its_tab/syphilis1993-08-eng.php

Rekart, M. L. (2005). Sex work harm reduction. *Lancet, 366,* 2123–2134.

Shier, M., & Bryson, P. (2007). Vaccines. *Journal of Obstetrics and Gynaecology Canada, 29*(8), S51–S54.

Shriver, S. P., Byer, C. O., Shainberg, L. W., & Galliano, G. (2002). *Dimensions of human sexuality* (6th ed.). Boston, MA: McGraw-Hill.

Society of Obstetricians and Gynaecologists of Canada (SOGC). (2009a). *Contraception: Contraception methods.* Retrieved from http://sexualityandu.ca/adults/contraception-2.aspx

Society of Obstetricians and Gynaecologists of Canada (SOGC). (2009b). *HPV immunization strategies by province.* Retrieved from http://www.hpvinfo.ca/hpvinfo/parents/vaccination-4.aspx

Trussler, T., & Marchand, R. (2005). *Prevention revived: Evaluating the Assumptions Campaign.* Retrieved from http://cbr.cbrc.net/files/1113357097/AssumptionsRpt_Eng.pdf

White, M., & Dorman, S. M. (2001). Receiving social support online: Implications for health education. *Health Education Research: Theory and Practice, 16*(6), 693–707.

Wood, E., Kerr, T., Montaner, J. S., Strathdee, S. A., Wodak, A., Hankins, C. A., et al. (2004a). Rationale for evaluating North America's first medically supervised safer-injecting facility. *The Lancet Infectious Diseases, 4*(5), 301–306.

Wood, E., Kerr, T., Small, W., Li, K., Marsh, D. C., Montaner, J. S. G., et al. (2004b). Changes in public order after the opening of a medically supervised safer injecting facility for illicit injection drug users. *Canadian Medical Association Journal, 171*(7), 731–734.

Wood, E., Tyndall, M. W., Spittal, P. M., Li, K., Hogg, R. S., Montaner, J. S., et al. (2002). Factors associated with persistent high-risk syringe sharing in the presence of an established needle exchange programme. *AIDS, 16*(6), 941–943.

ADDITIONAL RESOURCES

Websites

Alberta Health Services
http://www.teachingsexualhealth.ca
Canadian AIDS Society
http://www.cdnaids.ca
Canadian Federation for Sexual Health
http://www.cfsh.ca
Canadian HIV/AIDS Legal Network
http://www.aidslaw.ca
Public Health Agency of Canada: Canadian Guidelines on Sexually Transmitted Infections
http://www.phac-aspc.gc.ca/std-mts/sti-its/guide-lignesdir-eng.php
Public Health Agency of Canada, Sexual Health and Sexually Transmitted Infections
http://www.phac-aspc.gc.ca/std-mts
Sex Information and Education Council of Canada
http://www.sieccan.org
The Society of Obstetricians and Gynecologists of Canada
http://www.sexualityandu.ca

About the Authors

Wendi Lokanc-Diluzio, BN (University of Calgary), MN (University of Calgary), is a doctoral candidate from the University of Calgary, Faculty of Nursing. Wendi has worked in public health since 1997. Since 2002, she has worked as a Sexual and Reproductive Health Specialist for Alberta Health Services where she provides leadership in the area of child and youth sexual health promotion and service provider education and training. In 2005, Wendi commenced her doctoral studies. The focus of her research is the sexual health promotion capacity development of service providers working with street youth.

Alison Nelson, BScN (University of Alberta), MN (University of Calgary) worked as a public/community health nurse in rural and urban Alberta and B.C. from 1991 to 2001. From 2001 to 2006, she was an Instructor with the Faculty of Nursing, University of Calgary teaching community health nursing and sexual health promotion. Alison was the Board Chair of the Alberta Society for the Promotion of Sexual Health (www.aspsh.ca) from 2006 to 2008 and co-chaired two Biennial Western Canadian Sexual Health Conferences. She has been the President of the Community Health Nurses of Alberta (www.chnalberta.ca) since 2006. Alison has also worked as the Manager of Sexual and Reproductive Health in the Calgary Health Region and is currently the Manager of Health Promotion, Cancer Screening Programs with Alberta Health Services.

Janet L. Wayne, BScN (University of Alberta), MN (University of Calgary), is currently the Director of Accreditation for Southern Alberta (Alberta Health Services). Janet previously worked in the area of sexual and reproductive health and communicable disease for more than a decade. She has spearheaded and managed a number of large, innovative health promotion and telehealth projects involving community and cross-ministry partners such as teachingsexualhealth.ca. Janet has presented these sexual health projects at various conferences across Canada and to university classes in Calgary.

Janet B. Hettler, DipN (Kelsey Institute of Applied Arts and Sciences, Saskatoon), BScN (University of Saskatchewan), MN (University of Calgary), is currently the Manager of the Crisis Nursery at Calgary Children's Cottage Society. Janet has worked in public health since 1981, initially as a public health nurse in rural Alberta. In 1988, she began working in the area of sexual and reproductive health, first in a rural health unit outside Calgary then with the Calgary Health Region as a Sexual and Reproductive Health Clinical Nurse Specialist. During her time in sexual and reproductive health she oversaw a number of sexual health promotion projects.

Emergency Preparedness and Disaster Nursing

Betty Schepens and Lucia Yiu

OBJECTIVES

After studying this chapter, you should be able to:

1. Define the various types of disasters and their consequences.
2. Describe some of the key activities involved in public safety and emergency preparedness in Canada.
3. Understand the roles and responsibilities of the Public Health Agency of Canada in emergency preparedness.
4. Identify the key functions of community health nurses before, during, and following a disaster.
5. Discuss the skill set required for community health nurses to respond effectively to emergencies.

INTRODUCTION

Each year, one in five countries worldwide has a disaster or an emergency that results in massive health, social, and economic consequences and enormous efforts required to save lives and reduce illness and suffering (World Health Organization, 2007). The consequences of different types of disasters also vary in severity, each with its own degree of death, mass injury, illness, and loss. The way in which a disaster will impact a community depends upon the individual community's social, cultural, economic, and health makeup. In order to respond effectively in a disaster situation across different communities, special expertise in emergency management is required.

Emergency preparedness and disaster nursing is an emerging specialty. Since Florence Nightingale demonstrated to the world that nurses have a critical front line role in responding to disasters, emergency preparedness and disaster nursing has continued to expand its scope and define its significance (Jakeway, LaRosa, Cary, & Schoenfisch, 2008). As part of a public health workforce, community health nurses (CHNs) must be well prepared to respond and provide essential services to people affected by disasters. This chapter provides an overview of the role of CHNs in community emergency preparedness planning and in a disaster situation. It highlights different types of disasters, and how the Incident Management System (IMS) functions as a comprehensive model to manage major incidents. The Jennings Disaster

Nursing Management Model will be introduced to guide nurses in understanding disaster nursing.

DISASTERS IN CANADA

According to the Canadian Disaster Database (Public Safety Canada, 2009), chemical and fuel spills, floods, snowstorms, and forest fires were the most common disasters recorded in Canada in the last decade (see Table 30.1). Emergencies and disasters never fail to impact and alter the lives of people and their environment.

WHAT IS A DISASTER?

Disastrous events typically occur suddenly and can be caused by nature, human error, biological hazards, or infectious diseases. They include earthquakes, floods, fires, hurricanes, cyclones, major storms, volcanic eruptions, spills, air crashes, droughts, epidemics, food shortages, and civil strife (Landesman, 2005). Disasters often are perceived as random killers. When disasters strike, they affect everyone in the community in which they occur. Individuals at greatest risk include vulnerable groups such as women, children, the elderly, the poor, and people with mental and physical disabilities (Cohen, 2000). Life-threatening conditions brought on by disasters and the adverse health effects borne of these conditions often result in increased mortality and morbidity.

TABLE 30.1 Selected Canadian Disasters

Date and Location	Disaster	Human Consequences
1900—Ottawa & Hull	Fire	15 000 evacuated 7 died
1910—British Columbia (Rogers Pass)	Snow avalanche	62 railway workers died
1918 to 1925—Canada	Spanish flu	2 million people ill over 50 000 died
1927—Newfoundland	Hurricane	56 died
1936—Canada	Heat Wave (2-Week)	1180 died
1991—Alberta	Fuel spill/collision	4 died
1886—Quebec	Flood	10 died 15 825 people evacuated
1998—Nova Scotia (Peggy's Cove)	Aircraft accident	229 died
2000—Ontario (Walkerton)	Drinking water contamination	7 died 2300 people injured
2003—Canada (Toronto)	SARS epidemic	44 died (of 438 cases)
2003—Southeastern B.C. and Southwestern Alberta	Forest fires (started by lightning, careless fire use)	~50 000 residents evacuated
2005—Saskatchewan (Cumberland House, Cree First Nation)	Flood	~2000 residents evacuated
2005—Alberta (16 communities)	Floods	2 dead 7028 residents evacuated ~40 000 homes damaged

Source: *Public Safety Canada. (2009).* Canadian Disaster Database. *Retrieved from http://www.publicsafety.gc.ca/prg/em/cdd/srch-eng.aspx*

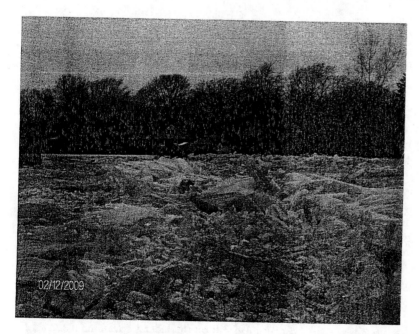

Photo 30.1

Ice jam in the Sydenham River, Wallaceburg, Ontario (February 2009). The ice jam led to the declaration of a municipal emergency after ice quickly mounted to a height of over 30 feet within an hour. Homes, businesses, and local streets were flooded within minutes. Evacuation of the local hospital situated on the banks of the river was imminent until the ice jam broke away on its own before the arrival of an ice breaker.

Credit: Staff of the Municipality of Chatham-Kent. Reproduced with the permission of Dennis Floin.

Types of Disasters

Natural Disasters Natural disasters are unpredictable; they can happen very quickly or slowly. However, with advance warning such as weather reports, the impacts can sometimes be mitigated. Some examples of natural disasters include droughts, heat waves, blizzards, cold waves, heavy snowfalls, earthquakes, cyclones, tsunamis, tornadoes, flood or thunderstorms, volcanoes, and wildfires. On December 24, 2004, the world was shocked when a strong earthquake triggered a massive tsunami that hit Southeast Asia in Indonesia, Sri Lanka, southern India, Thailand, Malaysia, the Maldives, Bangladesh, Burma, Mauritius, Somalia, Kenya, Seychelles, and Tanzania, leaving 280 931 dead. On January 12, 2010, the under-developed and poverty-stricken region of Port-au-Prince, in the country of Haiti, suffered a massive 7.0 earthquake, leaving approximately 150 000 dead. (See MyNursingLab.)

Man-Made Disasters Man-made disasters may result—and have resulted—in mass numbers of civilian injuries and deaths, leaving the affected communities with long-term adverse socioeconomical, health, and environmental effects. Bioterrorism, bombings, and technical disasters, such as nuclear disasters and oil spills, are all examples of man-made disasters. **Bioterrorism** is "the use of a microorganism with the deliberate intent of causing infection in order to achieve certain goals" (Public Health Agency of Canada [PHAC], 2001). The release of a biological agent, such as smallpox or anthrax, with the intent to infect humans is an example of a bioterrorist attack. Ideologically or politically inspired bombings, civil and political disorder as seen in countries at war, riots, and economic emergencies resulting in social instability are also examples of man-made disasters.

The terrorist attacks on the World Trade Center in New York and the Pentagon in Washington in the United States on September 11, 2001, represent one of the most recent and well-watched examples of a man-made disaster of this type (Rodriguez & Long, 2006). Twenty-four Canadians were among the 2823 killed when terrorists flew commercial airliners into the World Trade Center towers in New York City. This attack, combined with the anthrax exposures that followed, prompted an increased awareness of the need for bioterrorism preparedness. The threat of bioterrorism remains even more concerning today when more than 30 diseases previously unknown have emerged as viruses or bacteria, including for example Ebola virus, Legionnaire's disease, E-coli O157:H7 associated with hemolytic uremic syndrome, HIV/AIDS, hepatitis C, and H5N1 Influenza A or avian influenza (Naylor, 2003).

Technological malfunctions resulting from man-made disaster most often occur in communities with industrial sites and can be triggered by a natural disaster. Contamination of the water or food supply; the unintentional release of deadly airborne substances such as anthrax; fires; explosions; oil spills; and exposure to hazardous materials are all conduits for technological disasters. Building or bridge collapses, transportation crashes, dam or levee failures, nuclear reactor accidents, and breaks in water, gas, or deep sea oil drilling and sewer lines may also result in a disaster of this type (CBC, 2010; Landesman, 2005). Both man-made and natural disasters leave people injured, put emergency responders at risk, and have a lasting impact on the health of the communities they affect.

Epidemics Epidemic is another type of disaster that is brought about by the spread of infectious disease. An **epidemic** can occur when an infectious disease spreads rapidly, affecting a large number of individuals within a population, community, or region. Transmission of an infectious disease that is easily transmitted or highly contagious can quickly result in an emergency situation if the right conditions exist. Conditions such as a densely populated area, lack/loss of proper sanitation and hygiene practices, and lack of or disrupted public health services may provide a breeding ground for an epidemic. Even if these conditions are not present, the nature of the disease itself may still result in a disaster situation if the disease is sufficiently serious that there will be high levels of morbidity and mortality. This is particularly so if social and economic disruption occurs once the disease is present, if there is a lack of trained professional personnel with experience available to manage the epidemic, and if there is a lack of equipment and supplies. Epidemics are further complicated if the disease is or may become susceptible to international transmission.

Epidemics become **pandemics** when the infection becomes widespread in different parts of the globe, and affects a significantly higher proportion of the population than normal. The emergence of a novel swine-origin influenza A (H1N1) virus in humans in Mexico in early 2009 that quickly spread around the world is the most recent example of how quickly an infectious disease response can escalate to the declaration of a global influenza pandemic within a period of months. The WHO (2010) explains that an **influenza pandemic:**

> may occur when a new influenza virus appears against which the human population has no immunity. With the increase in global transport, as well as urbanization and overcrowded conditions in some areas, epidemics due to a new influenza virus are likely to take hold around the world, and become a pandemic faster than before. . . . . Pandemics can be either mild or severe in the illness and death they cause, and the severity of a pandemic can change over the course of that pandemic. (para 1)

PUBLIC SAFETY AND EMERGENCY PREPAREDNESS IN CANADA

Disaster preparedness and response at a national and provincial/territorial level ensures support for public health authorities and other officials who are responsible for managing the health of their community before, during, and after a disaster occurs. Public health officials attend to prevention of infectious disease and injury. They routinely conduct surveillance for infectious disease and they work in collaboration with other agencies within the health sector. They have governmental jurisdiction to oversee the public's health, and they use triage skills in disaster situations (Landesman, 2005).

Emergency management and preparedness responses in Canada begin at the local level. Local municipalities have the first responsibility in managing an emergency and if their capacity is exceeded they call on their respective province, which in turn can call on the federal government for assistance. Therefore, local emergency preparedness plans are key to the success in managing emergencies. Some countries have an opposite response chain of command in place. All responses to large-scale emergencies and disasters are initiated at the federal level, as was the case in the United States with the Federal Emergency Management Agency (FEMA) initiating the response to Hurricane Katrina in 2005.

Government Authority and Legislative Framework

Federal legislation with respect to emergencies and emergency preparedness is found in three complementary acts, the *Emergencies Act*, the *Emergency Preparedness Act*, and the *Emergency Management Act*. The first two pieces of legislation were enacted in 1988, at which time the *Emergencies Act* replaced the *War Measures Act* as the source of the federal government's authority to act in the event of a national emergency. The Emergency Management Act replaces parts of the Emergency Preparedness Act.

The Emergencies Act The **Emergencies Act** (Department of Justice Canada, 2007a) allows the federal government to grant the use of special powers to ensure the safety and security of Canadians during a national emergency. The Emergencies Act defines a **national emergency** as

> an urgent and critical situation of a temporary nature that seriously endangers the lives, health or safety of Canadians and is of such proportions or nature as to exceed the capacity or authority of a province to deal with it, or seriously threatens the ability of the Government of Canada to preserve the sovereignty, security and territorial integrity of Canada, and cannot be effectively dealt with under any other law of Canada. (p. 1)

The federal government intervention is restricted to only the most serious of emergency situations, while respecting the authority of the provinces and territories to govern accordingly within their own geographical jurisdictions.

There are four categories of *national emergency*:

1. *public welfare emergencies*, such as a major natural disaster or accident, which are beyond the authority of the province or territory in which the disaster occurs to address;

2. *public order emergencies*, wherein there is a serious security threat to the nation;

3. *international emergencies* arising from acts of coercion or intimidation or the serious use of force or violence, which threaten the sovereignty, security, or territorial integrity of Canada or its allies; and

4. *a state of war*, either active or imminent, involving Canada or its allies.

It is important to note that the extraordinary powers extended by the federal government must be tailored to the specific disaster event, and may not exceed what is necessary to deal with the particulars of the situation at hand. The Emergencies Act is not designed to justify the arbitrary or excessive use of power on the part of the federal government.

The Emergency Preparedness Act The **Emergency Preparedness Act** (Department of Justice Canada, 2007b) functions as companion legislation to the Emergencies Act. Where the Emergencies Act provides the authority for government action, the Emergency Preparedness Act provides a basis for the planning and programming necessary to address disasters of all kinds. Specifically, the Emergency Preparedness Act addresses the need for co-operation between the provinces and territories at the federal level to establish responsibilities and the need for public awareness, as well as providing a structure for training and education.

The Emergency Management Act The **Emergency Management Act** (Department of Justice Canada, 2007c) replaces parts of the Emergency Preparedness Act. This new Act strengthens the Government of Canada's readiness to respond to major emergencies by establishing clear roles and responsibilities for all federal Ministers and enhances information sharing with other levels of government and with the private sector. It provides direction for critical infrastructure protection as this is one of the emerging challenges of modern emergency management (Public Safety Canada, 2009). Critical infrastructure consists of physical and information technology facilities, networks, services, and assets that are vital to the health, safety, security, or economic well-being of Canadians and for the effective functioning of governments in Canada. Public Safety Canada developed the Federal Emergency Response Plan, which is the Government of Canada's "all-hazards" response plan. This plan applies to domestic emergencies and to international emergencies with a domestic impact.

Emergency Management

Emergency management is an essential discipline involving a diverse group of skilled professionals, with the ultimate responsibility resting with the government to assess and deal with risk in an effort to protect the health and safety of the public (Haddow & Bullock, 2006). A crisis or emergency is a threatening condition that requires urgent action. Effective emergency management action can avoid the escalation of an event into a disaster. Emergency management involves plans and institutional arrangements to engage and guide the efforts of government, non-government, voluntary, and private agencies in comprehensive and coordinated ways to respond to the entire spectrum of emergency needs (United Nations/International Strategy for Disaster Reduction, 2009).

The four areas of emergency management in the lifecycle process of a disaster include (Veenema, 2007)

1. mitigating or preventing the effects of an emergency;

2. preparing for emergencies or disasters;

3. responding to an emergency or disaster to reduce the impact on public loss; and

4. recovering from an emergency or disaster by assisting communities to return to normal.

Hazard Identification Risk Assessment (HIRA)

Emergency response plans are generally created using an all-hazards approach. This means that the emergency response plan activities are applicable to any type of emergency. Communication and media plans, business continuity plans, employee health and safety plans, and procurement of supplies and purchasing plans are examples of strategies generic to all response plans.

In addition to an all-hazards approach, planning and preparedness strategies for specific types of emergencies are also required. By completing a Hazard Identification Risk Assessment (HIRA), organizations can prioritize specific threats based on risk of probability and consequence or impact. Probability is the likelihood of an event occurring within a given time period. Impact assesses the level or degree to which the hazard will affect three critical dimensions: human, physical infrastructure, and business impacts. (See MyNursingLab for an example of an assessment tool.)

All levels of government as well as public health agencies and hospitals use this process. Community-level response organizations, such as public health units and hospitals, need to incorporate the individual response plans into a local coordinated community response plan. For example, a fire services agency is the lead for responding to a hazardous materials spill in the community, whereas the public health unit and the hospital would have supporting roles. In comparison, public health would be the lead in responding to a community infectious disease outbreak, or a pandemic, and the local first responder agencies would have supporting roles.

Effective hazard identification risk assessment strategies combined with interagency coordination can and will prepare an agency for response, mitigate the effects of the emergency, and assist in recovery and evaluation activities.

Organizational Structure and Chain of Command: National Incident Management System

An international system known as the **National Incident Management System** (NIMS) was developed by the Department of Homeland Security in the United States and released in March 2004. The NIMS was quickly adopted by the Government of Canada as the Incident Management System (IMS) and now provides the framework for all levels of government in Canada to develop emergency response plans. The NIMS supports an effective management system for disaster preparedness regardless of the nature of the incident or its level of complexity (Qureshi, Gebbie, & Gebbie, 2006).

Incident Management System

The **Incident Management System** (IMS) is a standardized function driven model utilized by agencies throughout North America to manage and respond to emergencies. A similar version, the Incident Command System (ICS), is utilized at on-site emergency scenes by first responders using a formal command approach.

The Incident Management System (IMS) (2008) doctrine for use in Ontario was developed by Emergency Management Ontario (EMO). Public health authorities use the IMS as an operational framework for emergency preparedness

and response planning. The benefits of the IMS are to enhance capacity, streamline resources, improve communication, and facilitate the co-operation of activities and interoperability among organizations.

The Ontario Health Pandemic Influenza Plan (Ontario Ministry of Health and Long-Term Care [OMOHLTC] 2008a) recommends that all health organizations use the IMS model. The basic command structure consists of five components: command, operations, planning, logistics, and finance and administration (Bochenek, Kristjanson, & Schwartz, 2009). (See Table 30.2 and MyNursingLab.) The pertinent functional components are established only when necessary, depending on the magnitude of the emergency.

By using the IMS framework in a health emergency, staff are able to communicate directly with their peers in other healthcare settings and jurisdictions, and with other emergency response organizations. For example, during an influenza pandemic, health organizations can use the IMS to coordinate the distribution of medical supplies from federal and provincial stockpiles to the front line, by utilizing the logistics section personnel at federal, provincial, and local health unit levels.

CRISES IN PUBLIC HEALTH: THE WALKERTON E-COLI EXPERIENCE AND SARS

The face of emergency preparedness in Canada has also been shaped by two recent events that highlighted the gaps and weaknesses in the Canadian public health system and infection control capacity. In 2000, improper execution of safe water practices in Walkerton, Ontario, led to the contamination of the town's water supply by E-coli O157:H7 and *Campylobacter jejuni* bacteria. One year later, the same strain of E-coli contaminated the drinking water in North Battleford, Saskatchewan. The *Walkerton Commission of Inquiry Reports* (O'Connor, 2002) called for 93 recommendations that would ensure the quality of drinking water and reduce the risk of infection and death. A similar inquiry was called on account of the breakdown in the town water filtration plant in North Battleford. In 2003, Canadians again faced the need for emergency response following the outbreak of sudden acute respiratory syndrome (SARS). SARS emerged from China in 2002 and spread quickly across the globe to Toronto (Naylor, 2003).

Since these events, four comprehensive reports have been released, each of which calls for a renewal in the national public health system. Both *The Health of Canadians—The Federal Role* (Kirby & LeBreton, 2002) and *Reforming Health Protection and Promotion in Canada: Time to Act* (Kirby, 2003) called for the federal government to provide funding support and to take a stronger leadership role to strengthen the public health infrastructure and health promotion efforts in Canada.

Learning from SARS: Renewal of Public Health in Canada: A report of the National Advisory Committee on SARS and Public Health, known as the Naylor Report (2003), addressed a lack of capacity in the clinical and public health systems and

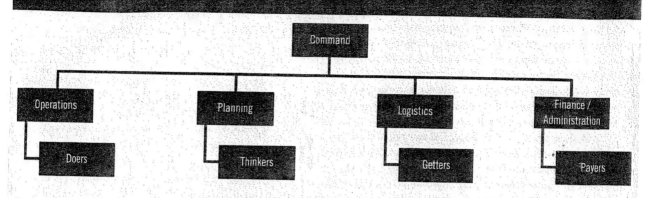

TABLE 30.2   The IMS Structure

The **Command** section includes key positions such as an Incident Commander, Safety Officer, Public Information Officer, and an external community partner Liaison Officer.

The Incident Commander will consult with, and report directly to, administrative authorities such as a Board, Commissioner, or to members of a regional control group.

The **Planning** section assesses the situation, identifies objectives, and creates action plans.

The **Operations** section implements all activities identified by the Command section. For example, public health operations may include mass immunization clinics and the operation of telephone hotlines.

The **Logistics** section is responsible for the procurement and maintenance of required supplies, physical space, and technological support for all sections.

The **Finance and Administration** section co-ordinates and manages human resources and volunteers, all purchases and expenditures, and maintains a record of all activities during the emergency.

Source: Bochenek, R., Kristjanson, E., & Schwartz, B. (2009). Incident Management System (IMS) in the public health response: From SARS to pandemic H1N1. Ontario Agency for Health Protection & Promotion. http://www.oahpp.ca/

epidemiological investigation of the outbreak; dysfunctional relationships between various orders of governments; absence of protocols for data or information-sharing among different government levels; and inadequate business processes between and across jurisdictions for outbreak management and emergency response. The report recommends the need for a Canadian Agency for Public Health, with a chief Public Health Officer of Canada heading the agency and reporting to the Minister of Health; development of a National Health Strategy with specific health targets and benchmarks; public health partnership programs to build capacity in public health at the local/municipal level; and a national strategy to renew and sustain public health human resources (including public health nurses, public health physicians, infection control practitioners, and microbiologists). The report draws specific attention to the role of CHNs in emergency preparedness. He notes that the essential contributions by public health nurses during the SARS outbreak have received little public attention.

In the *Second Interim Report; SARS and Public Health Legislation* (Campbell, 2005), the SARS Commission noted that even though many emergency response organizations were using some form of the incident management system, there should be one common emergency response system "to bring an orderly, consistent, and flexible chain of command and control within an emergency response" (p. 322).

The Walker Report or *For the Public's Health: A Plan of Action* (Walker, 2004) targeted all sectors of Ontario's healthcare system involved in planning for, funding, and delivering public health programs and services in Ontario. The recommendations directly impacted local public health and emergency medical services to build a public health model, establish infection control networks and standards, improve emergency preparedness, develop a communications infrastructure in the event of an emergency, enhance surveillance, and increase enrolment in key public health professions.

THE PUBLIC HEALTH AGENCY OF CANADA

Following the terrorist attacks of September 11, 2001, and the outbreak of Severe Acute Respiratory Syndrome (SARS), the Government of Canada recognized that the country needed to be ready for future public health emergencies. As a result, Public Safety and Emergency Preparedness Canada was created, and renamed Public Safety Canada (PS) in 2003, to ensure that federal departments and agencies responsible for national security and the safety of Canadians could work more closely together.

On September 24, 2004, the Government of Canada established the Public Health Agency of Canada (PHAC) and appointed the first Chief Public Health Officer (CPHO) of Canada. The Agency provides leadership in promoting health, investigating and controlling disease outbreaks, supporting public health infrastructure, and fostering collaboration across and between governments. PHAC and PS are working with the provincial and territorial governments to co-ordinate a unified response to any national public health emergency (Public Health Agency of Canada [PHAC], 2006a).

On December 16, 2006, the *Public Health Agency of Canada Act* (PHAC, 2006b) was given Royal Assent, recognizing the Agency with enabling legislation and establishing the dual role of the CPHO as head of the PHAC and lead public health professional in Canada. Several branches, centres, and directorates report to the Chief Public Health Officer, including the Centre for Emergency Preparedness and Response (CEPR), the National Microbiology Laboratory, the Laboratory for Foodborne Zoonoses, the Pandemic Preparedness Secretariat, the Infectious Disease and Emergency Preparedness (IDEP) Centre, and the Office of Public Health Safety. The agency shares Canadian expertise and works with global partners including the World Health Organization, the United States Centers for Disease Control and Prevention, and the new European Centre for Disease Prevention and Control.

PUBLIC HEALTH RESPONSE IN A DISASTER

Public health preparedness for all types of disasters, especially infectious disease emergencies, has become essential in today's world. According to Rebmann, Carrico, and English (2008), lessons learned and gaps from past disasters that public health can address include infection prevention/control in mass casualty incidents, public education, internal and external communication, and building partnerships with outside agencies. Public health nurses and emergency and disaster preparedness planners must continue to address these gaps. Nurses make up the largest group of healthcare professionals in any given jurisdiction and have often in the past been underutilized particularly in the planning and preparedness stages. With emergency preparedness programming and disaster response planning at the forefront of many healthcare agency and professional agendas, nurses must play pivotal advocacy and leadership roles to facilitate agency-specific and community-wide preparations for health-related emergencies and disasters.

Phases of Disaster Response

Federal, provincial/territorial, and local public health professionals are responsible for the health of their communities in both preparing for a disaster and responding once a disaster has occurred. The seven phases of a disaster response for public health activities in preparing and responding to a disaster are as follows (Landesman, 2005):

1. *Planning*—apply basic concepts of local public health to disaster management;

2. *Prevention*—control/prevent outbreaks, organize services and treatment, manage injuries, and provide long-term counselling and mental health interventions;
3. *Assessment*—determine the incidence of disease and causal factors;
4. *Response*—communicate plans and needs;
5. *Surveillance*—establish syndromic surveillance information systems;
6. *Recovery*—mobilize resources; and
7. *Evaluation*—determine whether emergency plans and disaster response are effective and efficient.

Each phase is linked to specific responsibilities and skill sets possessed by a network of public health professionals for disaster planning and relief.

Stages of Emergency Management

In some provinces in Canada, such as in Ontario, emergency management programming is organized into five stages: prevention, mitigation, preparedness, response, and recovery (OMOHLTC, 2008a).

1. *Prevention* involves activities taken to prevent or avoid an emergency or disaster. The eradication of smallpox is an example of a prevention strategy.
2. *Mitigation* involves actions that can reduce the impact of an emergency or disaster. Influenza vaccination and infection prevention and control measures are health-specific examples of mitigation.
3. *Preparedness* involves measures that are in place before an emergency occurs and that will enhance the effectiveness of response and recovery activities, such as developing plans, tools, and protocols; establishing communication systems; conducting training; and testing response plans.
4. Response involves the co-ordinated actions that would be undertaken to respond to an emergency or disaster. This could include the mobilization of providers, the coordination of healthcare services, and the acquisition of necessary equipment and supplies.
5. *Recovery* involves activities that help communities recover from an emergency or disaster and return to a state of normalcy. This includes activities to restore services, rebuild infrastructure, and carry out the ongoing treatment and care for the sick or injured. It may also include prevention or mitigation measures designed to avert a future emergency (e.g., vaccination to prevent a future outbreak).

Integrated Community Emergency Preparedness

While provincial and federal emergency preparedness and response planning parameters can provide local community emergency planners with a variety of tools, templates, and structure, local community emergency response mechanisms are often led by first responder agencies, such as police, fire, and emergency medical services to manage incidents related to health or non-health types of emergencies. As infectious disease-related emergencies begin to appear more often, local planners must engage all healthcare professionals and agencies in planning for a health-related emergency. In this instance, the healthcare sector becomes the lead or command agency with emergency response agencies having a supporting role. There needs to be consensus and collaboration as to agency and professional roles in advance of any emergency. Public health agencies may facilitate these discussions and challenge key community stakeholders to develop, implement, and maintain a comprehensive preparation, response, and recovery plan for health emergencies. CHNs need to become familiar with local agency emergency plans and key agency personnel, and utilize their community mobilization skills to assist in identifying and developing the required health infrastructure to ensure emergency response readiness, surge capacity, and sustainability. (See MyNursingLab for a schematic diagram outlining active ver-

sus supporting roles for healthcare providers, OMOHLTC, Emergency Response Plan.)

Public Health Emergency Preparedness Program Standard

Public health units or departments in provinces across Canada have mandated requirements for fundamental public health programs and services. In Ontario, a review of the 1997 Mandatory Program and Services Guidelines identified a need to add new standards and protocols. In 2008, the Emergency Preparedness Program Standard was added to the revised and newly named Ontario Public Health Standards (OPHS) (OMOHLTC, 2008b).

The goal of the Public Health Emergency Preparedness Program is to enable and ensure a consistent and effective response to public health emergencies and emergencies with public health impacts. The Emergency Preparedness Standards and Protocol (OMOHLTC, 2009) identifies the minimum expectations for programs and services by providing direction on how health units must operationalize specific requirements. Key components of the Emergency Preparedness Standard and Protocol include

- identifying and assessing the relevant hazards and risks to public health;
- developing a continuity of operations plan;
- developing an emergency response plan utilizing the Incident Management System (IMS);
- developing and implementing 24/7 notification protocols for communications with staff, community partners, and government bodies;
- increasing public awareness regarding emergency preparedness activities;
- delivering emergency preparedness and response education and training for board of health staff and officials; and
- exercising or testing the continuity of the operations plan, the emergency response plan, and the 24/7 notification protocols.

ROLE OF COMMUNITY HEALTH NURSING ORGANIZATIONS IN DISASTERS

International Council of Nurses

The International Council of Nurses (ICN) represents more than 124 national nurses' associations worldwide. It works to establish sound policies that condemn violations of human rights commonly seen during and after a disaster (ICN, 2006). The ICN provides assistance to countries in disaster planning by promoting social justice and equity of access strategies, such as influencing banks and international financial institutions to ensure that countries at increased risk for disasters have quick access to other care services. It urges countries to include disaster planning in their assistance programs, and promotes and facilitates disaster information,

---

CANADIAN RESEARCH BOX

How to plan for a coordinated local healthcare response to a pandemic?

Stalker, S. A., Weir, E., Vessel, S. L., & Mikail, J. (2009). Planning a coordinated Delphi technique: Phase 1. *Canadian Journal of Public Health, 100*(1), 65–69.

The study illustrates how the York Region Health Services Department in Ontario used a Delphi exercise as a first step in planning for a coordinated local healthcare system response to a pandemic. Twenty-seven stakeholders/decision makers from nine categories of healthcare organizations in Ontario acted as expert panel and participated in three rounds of this exercise. The objectives were to identify their local roles and responsibilities and options to enhance capacity during a pandemic. In round 1, stakeholders listed a series of questions pertaining to the subject. In round 2, participants formulated issue-related statements outlining possible strategies or solutions and indicated the level of agreement regarding the statements. In round 3, the participants met face-to-face and discussed their views on the allowed statements. Their questions were generated into statements, collated into categories, and developed into a total of 72 unique statements. Agreement was obtained for 56 of the statements.

This planning approach proved that the Delphi technique was useful in identifying major issues, enhancing familiarity with the issues, strengthening community relationships, and creating consensus on "big picture" issues.

Discussion Questions

1. Would you use the Delphi technique for emergency preparedness planning? Why? Discuss the pros and cons of using this approach.
2. What do you think the next step would be after this exercise?

TABLE 30.3 Responsibilities for Canadian Health Professionals and for National, Provincial, and Territorial Organizations in Emergency Preparedness and Response	
Responsibilities of Health Professionals Including Nurses	**Responsibilities of National, Provincial, and Territorial Nursing Organizations (including professional, regulatory, educational, government, and union organizations)**

■ Participate in developing and evaluating emergency plans and link organization and community plans to provincial and national plans
■ Deliver emergency healthcare services at all points of the continuum: mitigation, preparedness, response, and recovery
■ Articulate their role and the value of being involved in emergency planning
■ Advocate for involving vulnerable groups and other stakeholders in emergency planning
■ Address factors that contribute to emergencies, such as climate change, violence, and poverty, through their roles in clinical practice, education, research, administration, and policy
■ Develop personal emergency plans that reflect the ethical values of their profession and recognize the needs of family members and pets
■ Before an emergency, think through and discuss ethical issues and questions with colleagues, employers, union representatives, and others
■ Maintain the competencies required to participate in emergency management
■ Before an emergency, join registries of volunteer healthcare providers
	■ Identify their roles in emergency preparedness and the value of being involved
	■ Develop and maintain relationships with others in emergency management
	■ Support nurses' practice in emergency management through, for example:
	  ■ practice standards
	  ■ mobility agreements
	  ■ procedures for rapid registration and verification of credentials, and
	  ■ registries of volunteer healthcare providers and procedures to verify their competencies
	■ Provide opportunities for nurses to obtain the knowledge and skills necessary to respond to emergencies through basic and continuing education programs, and support and provide appropriate education to student and retired nurses involved in responding to emergencies

Source: Canadian Nurses Association. (2007). Emergency Preparedness and Response {Position Statement}. *Ottawa, ON: Author.*

training, and technology while encouraging international networks. The ICN states that

> nurses with their technical skills and knowledge of epidemiology, physiology, pharmacology, cultural-familial structures, and psychosocial issues can assist in disaster preparedness programs, as well as during disasters. [They] can play a strategic role cooperating with health and social disciplines, government bodies, community groups, and non-governmental agencies, including humanitarian organizations. (p. 2)

Canadian Nurses Association

The Canadian Nurses Association (CNA) provides information related to global nursing issues including disasters. CNA has partnered with PHAC's Centre for Emergency Preparedness and Response to provide expertise and consultation in developing the role of nurses in a national emergency plan. The CNA's (2007) position statement on the role of nurses in emergency preparedness and response articulates the importance of communication skills, patient teaching, community building, and engagement interventions. In order for an

effective, coordinated community emergency response to take place, effective inter-professional collaboration and shared responsibilities among professionals in non-governmental organizations, such as the health, social services, safety, transportation, meteorology, and voluntary sectors, must be developed and nurtured before emergencies occur. See Table 30.3 for these responsibilities for Canadian health professionals and for national, provincial, and territorial organizations. The next section describes the Jennings Disaster Nursing Management Model, the nursing process used and core competencies required in various phases of a disaster.

THE JENNINGS DISASTER NURSING MANAGEMENT MODEL

The literature has a limited number of disaster planning models to guide nurses in responding to a disaster. The Jennings Disaster Nursing Management Model, originally introduced to teach disaster nursing to nursing students, is an effective framework to assist CHNs in planning for and managing disasters (Jennings-Sanders, 2004). Nursing process is used in the four phases of the Jennings Disaster Nursing Management model to assess, plan, implement, and evaluate provision of care in a community's response to disasters.

Phases of a Disaster

Phase I (Pre-Disaster) This phase involves assessing resources and risks, and planning to achieve primary prevention, such as providing information to help the public at large prepare for a disaster. During this phase, the nurse must be able to respond effectively by identifying and allocating human resources and material resources such as shelters, planning co-operative agreements with other community agencies, defining the roles of everyone involved, assisting special needs groups to develop plans, and developing or activating the disaster plan.

Phase II (Disaster Occurs) In this phase the nurse assumes multiple roles: providing care, education, and case management to disaster victims using a holistic approach that considers emotional, physical, psychosocial, and cultural aspects of care to improve the overall health of disaster victims. The impact of a disaster varies in time and severity. Children, older adults, and people with mental illness are among the highest-risk groups for serious mental health morbidity and mortality. CHNs must recognize symptoms of serious mental illness and depression, and must make every effort to reduce devastating outcomes (Landesman, 2005). Their own family safety, pet care, and personal safety at work, as well as food, water, sleep, shelter, and rest periods while at work, are also of concern to nurses responding in the event of an emergency (Jennings-Sanders, 2004).

CHNs may find themselves working in different roles, such as operating a walk-in clinic, working in a shelter or evacuation centre, and triaging people at mass clinics while providing prophylactic medication or administering vaccine. They act as a case manager to liaise between the victim and a community agency or clinic. Nurses must recognize problems through diagnosis and, through secondary prevention, provide immediate treatment, including making referrals to an emergency room or community site where a clinic has been organized.

Phase III (Post-Disaster) During this phase, the nurse performs tertiary prevention through assessment, planning, and implementation. Nurses ensure that victims in the disaster are receiving treatment, and they decrease disabilities through tertiary preventive interventions such as rehabilitation. Nurses will also assess the emergency disaster plan and evaluate the severity of the disaster on the community. They will coordinate recovery operations to help local residents of the community reduce their exposure to risk and disease. They will apply epidemiological principles to ensure that the community does not become infected with disease, and they will implement infection control measures.

Phase IV (Positive Client/Population Outcomes) In this phase, nurses must measure the overall impact of the disaster to organize the coordination of community services to help residents in their recovery, reduce mortality rates, and reduce healthcare costs while improving the health status of the client/population.

CANADIAN RESEARCH BOX

How willing are nursing students to volunteer during a pandemic?

Yonge, O., Rosychuk, R., Bailey, T., Lake, R., & Marrie, T. (2010). Willingness of university nursing students to volunteer during a pandemic. *Public Health Nursing, 27*(2), 174–180. doi:10.1111/j.1525-1446.2010.00839.x

In response to the growing global threat of influenza pandemic, various communities including universities have begun emergency preparedness planning. Researchers from the University of Alberta conducted a cross-sectional survey to examine the stakeholder's knowledge, risk-perception, and willingness to volunteer. In this study, the subgroup, 484 of 1512 or 32% of the nursing students, responded to a web-based questionnaire regarding pandemic influenza.

Most respondents were year 3 and year 4 undergraduate students (63.4%) with 20.4% of the respondents in their first year and 15.2% in their second year.

The survey results showed that 67.9% of the nursing students said they were likely to volunteer in the event of a pandemic, and 77.4% said they would volunteer if provided protective garments. Overall, these nursing students stated that they had a wealth of volunteer experience; of these, 70.7% expressed their professional obligation to volunteer during a pandemic situation. These students, however, may be ill-prepared to fill front-line nursing roles. The authors concluded that emergency preparedness competencies should be integrated into existing nursing curricula and other health science programs and plans need to be developed to create protocol for recruitment, practice, and protection of volunteers.

Discussion Questions

1. Discuss if you feel that you are well prepared to participate in the event of a pandemic through the preparation you received in your nursing program. Give suggestions if any.
2. How can one maximize the potential for a volunteer workforce in the event of a pandemic?

Positive outcomes include increased community relations, improved knowledge of disasters, improved disaster nursing plans, and decreased costs related to the disaster.

The Nursing Process

The work of public health nurses in the response and recovery phases is often times more visible to the general public and therefore better understood by the public than the equally important contributions of nurses in the mitigation and preparedness phases. Community mobilization skills and collaboration competencies are crucial to these first two phases. Table 30.4 illustrates how the phases of a disaster are linked to the nursing process.

TABLE 30.4 Phases of Disaster Linked to the Nursing Process

Disaster Phase	Definition	Assessment	Planning	Implementation	Evaluation
Mitigation	Prevent a disaster or emergency; minimize vulnerability to effects of an event.	Assess a group of elderly citizens for their awareness about preventing heat stroke.	Develop community education plan to increase awareness about preventing heat stroke.	Conduct community education activities to increase awareness about preventing heat stroke.	Evaluate community education activities on preventing heat stroke.
Preparedness	Assure capacity to respond effectively to disasters and emergencies.	Assess the populations at risk for special needs during a disaster.	Develop plans to care for special-needs populations during a disaster.	Conduct training, drills and exercises related to care of special-needs persons.	Evaluate plans for serving populations with special needs.
Response	Provide support to persons and communities affected by disasters and emergencies.	Serve on a response team to determine the impact and specific health needs of hurricane survivors. Triage victims.	Develop plans to rotate staff on response teams to prevent stress and burnout among responders.	Deploy staff to shelters after a hurricane, in accordance with local and/or state emergency response plans.	Participate in after-action reviews and/or debriefings to evaluate quality of health services provided and lessons learned.
Recovery	Restore systems to functional level.	Serve on team to assess community assets and potential for recovery from a recent flood.	Collaborate with partners and community leaders to plan long-term recovery priorities after a flood.	Participate in restoring community services after a flood.	Serve on team to evaluate long-term impact on persons displaced by a flood.

Sources: The Association of State and Territorial Directors of Nursing (ASTDN). (2007, October 29). The Role of Public Health Nurses in Emergency Preparedness and Response. *Centers for Disease Control and Prevention: Author. (p. 6). Retrieved from http://www.astdn.org/downloadablefiles/ASTDN%20EP%20Paper%20final%2010%2029%2007.pdf*

Core Competencies

Nurses play a critical role during all phases of a disaster emergency response system. They need to be knowledgeable of current emergency preparedness frameworks, structures, and responses within their own professional practice and place of employment. To effectively contribute during a disaster, CHNs must be competent to respond in an emergency. CHNs are accountable to have a basic understanding and knowledge of core competencies related to emergency preparedness, management, and response activities.

Jennings-Sanders (2004) described **disaster nursing** as the systematic and flexible utilization of knowledge and skills specific to disaster-related nursing, and the promotion of a wide range of activities to minimize the health hazards and life threatening damage caused by disasters in collaboration with other specialized fields. (p. 69)

A set of core competencies to educate nursing students related to mass casualty incidents, with examples, should be incorporated into the nursing curriculum (Jennings-Sanders,

Core Competencies Related to Mass Casualty Incidents

1. Critical thinking: Uses an approved ethical framework to support decision making and prioritizing needed in disaster situations.
2. Assessment: Assesses the safety issues for self, the response team, and victims in any given response situation in collaboration with the incident response.
3. Technical skills: Demonstrates safe administration of immunizations, including smallpox vaccination.
4. Communication: Describes the local chain of command and management system for emergency response during a mass casualty incident.

Frisch, & Wing, 2005). (See "Core Competencies Related to Mass Casualty Incidents,") (Also see MyNursingLab for the emergency preparedness core competencies that specifically apply to public health nurses, nurses, and nurse practitioners.)

TABLE 30.5 Core Competencies and Skills and Essential Public Health Services (Jennings-Sanders, 2004)

Eight Domains of Core Competencies and Skills	Ten Essential Public Health Services
■ Analytic assessment skill	■ Monitor health status to identify community health problems
■ Policy development/program planning	■ Diagnose and investigate health problems and health hazards in the community
■ Communication	■ Educate and empower people about health issues
■ Cultural competency	■ Mobilize community partnerships to identify and solve health problems
■ Community dimensions of practice	■ Develop policies and plans that support individual and community health efforts
■ Basic public health sciences	■ Enforce laws and regulations that protect health and ensure safety
■ Financial planning and management	■ Link people to needed personal health service and ensure the provision of health care when otherwise unavailable
■ Leadership and systems thinking	■ Ensure a competent public health and personal health care work force
	■ Evaluate effectiveness, accessibility, and quality of personal and population-based health services
	■ Research for new insights and innovative solutions to health problems

Public Health Nurses in Public Health Surge Events Public health nursing skills and competencies are critical to bioterrorism preparedness and a public health nurse response (Berkowitz, 2002; Patillo, 2003). Eight domains of core competencies and skills were developed by a council of major public health and healthcare organizations to provide essential public health services to respond during an emergency. These skills were cross-referenced with 10 essential services. (See Table 30.5)

These competencies could be applied to generalist registered nurses, and not just public health nurses for public health surge events related to a disaster (Polivka, Stanley, Gordon, Taulbee, Kieffer, & McCorkle, 2008). (See MyNursingLab.) **Surge capacity** has been defined as the "healthcare system's ability to expand quickly beyond normal services to meet an increased demand for medical care in the event of bioterrorism or other large-scale public health emergencies" (Agency for Healthcare Research and Quality, 2004). Surge capacity typically addresses acute care facility issues such as

equipment, supplies, and personnel. It does not, however, address public health's role in population-based care.

Public health surge interventions are those that "improve access and availability of limited health resources for the entire population" (Burkle, 2006). Mass immunization clinics during a pandemic is an example of a public health surge event. The operations of mass immunization clinics during a pandemic would overwhelm public health agencies but would have a minimal effect on hospital systems. Medical triage differs from public health triage in that **medical triage** sorts individuals to maximize the number of lives saved, and **public health triage** is the sorting or identifying of populations for priority interventions (Polivka et al., 2008). The population-based model of care used in public health practice during non-surge events needs to continue during surge events associated with public health triage.

SAFETY OF VULNERABLE POPULATIONS

Nursing organizations and home health nurses (HHNs) must know the types of disasters and biological agents that could occur or be released in their community to provide medical management for their clients while ensuring their own personal protection when responding to an emergency. Management must provide education and training of HHNs to understand the agency emergency preparedness plan, document skill sets of each staff member, know how to answer questions, and establish a clear communication plan in an emergency response (Sawyer, 2003).

Clients receiving home care may be ventilator dependent, so their life is threatened if an electrical failure should occur. Many clients may be hearing impaired, be unable to access a telephone due to physical limitations, and have no close support from their family members who may live out of town. The "Hazard Vulnerability Analysis" assessment tool can be used by HHNs to determine the level of risk to their caseload of clients by focusing on *preparation* and *prevention* (Rodriguez & Long, 2006). In the event of an emergency, HHNs are in an excellent position to provide increased surveillance of those patients who make up their caseload. After assessing the client's home environment, family, social support networks, and community partners, the HHN can develop a plan to ensure communication, protect the client from death, and reduce the impact of a disaster on those most susceptible. As participants in a community emergency, HHNs can also report any suspected evidence of a biological agent, monitor and support those individuals who are quarantined in their homes, and offer skills in health screening and administer vaccines at community sites.

In order to ensure that vulnerable populations are protected in the event of an emergency or disaster, long-term care facilities and community-based support services must be integrated into local and regional disaster planning to provide for clear communication and appropriate response plans. These organizations often deal with low staffing ratios and are not well coordinated with hospitals, yet share common resources during a disaster and can make unique contributions

(Saliba et al., 2004). Knowledge of the current and evolving health status of vulnerable populations within a community will assist in the response and recovery outcomes for those affected by an emergency or disaster.

To date, there has been limited guidance on preparedness activities addressing at-risk populations. However, efforts are being made to provide emergency preparedness information to at-risk populations and many innovative practices to better serve at-risk communities are being developed. For example, in 2008, the Association of State and Territorial Health Officials (ASTHO) (2008) provided a summary of best practice evidence-based models and tools specific to the protection of at-risk populations during an influenza pandemic in its report, "At-Risk Populations in Emergencies: A Review of State and Local Stories, Tools and Practices." The Emergency Preparedness Guide for People with Disabilities and/or Special Needs (OMOHLTC, 2007) details prescriptive preparedness actions for consideration and implementation in preparation to be self-reliant for at least three days immediately after or during an emergency. (See MyNursingLab for a complete list of tools and practices and a list of high-risk population groups in Canada.)

The need for information exchange is valuable in all phases of emergency management, and is particularly important in the case of vulnerable populations. Nurses play a critical role in facilitating this exchange of knowledge and information and are often the advocacy voice for at-risk and vulnerable populations. Health and social service agencies are starting to incorporate emergency preparedness activities into their high-risk client's care plans. Information and education on the contents of a 72-hour personal or family emergency preparedness kit is provided by nurses as part of home visiting care plans.

SUMMARY

This chapter has outlined the types of disasters and challenges to which the nursing profession must learn to competently respond during a community disaster. An explanation for the renewed infrastructure of public health in Canada provides knowledge about the PHAC, leadership from the chief public health officer, and established emergency procedures, legislation, regulations, and processes that continue to build the current framework and legislation essential to healthcare delivery during any emergency.

Canadian nurses must develop an agenda that strengthens education in disaster nursing. An understanding of disaster training combined with community health, public health nursing experience, and technological knowledge strengthens the role of public health nurses in emergency preparedness and response. This can happen only when nursing research is applied to emergency response practice, education, and health policy. CHNs play a vital role in emergency preparedness. Nurses have an important role in community planning and collaboration initiatives and are often key facilitators in the community mobilization process. Nurses comprise the largest group of health professionals in any given jurisdiction.

A strong, effective public health workforce of CHNs must be established to meet the challenges of unpredictable threats on the community. By becoming knowledgeable and competent in emergency preparedness and disaster nursing concepts, principles, and skills, nurses can participate in healthcare policy development processes at the local community, provincial, and federal levels and within the nursing profession.

CASE STUDY

In February 2007, the Public Health Agency of Canada was notified by the World Health Organization (WHO) that a pandemic influenza emergency had been declared in the world. The WHO confirmed that the avian influenza (H5N1) virus had killed 1 million people in Asia as a result of human-to-human transmission. The virus was spreading across Europe. It was estimated that in three months the strain would arrive in North America from Asia and Europe. The Public Health Agency of Canada had informed provincial and territorial governments that they needed to implement their pandemic plans at the provincial/territorial and community levels. Local public health units were taking the lead in each community to implement pandemic plans.

Discussion Questions

1. Determine the type of disaster in an avian influenza pandemic.

2. Describe the steps you would take to prepare for this pandemic situation.

KEY TERMS

REVIEW QUESTIONS

Choose the one alternative that best completes the statement or answers the question.

1. To manage emergencies effectively, emergency management and preparedness responses should begin at the
   a) local level.
   b) regional level.
   c) provincial level.
   d) federal level.

2. After thousands of lives were lost in an earthquake and in the aftermath of rescue efforts and medical aid to the people in need, what should the emergency workers focus on next?
   a) plans to prevent the effects of an emergency
   b) preparations for another possible emergency
   c) continuing to work on how to reduce the impact on the community loss
   d) assisting the community to return to normal

3. A truckload of biological waste was spilled near a densely populated community. A number of people began experiencing nausea and breathing difficulties. Who should be taking a lead role in managing this disaster?
   a) fire department
   b) hospital
   c) public health unit
   d) physicians and nurses

4. During a flu pandemic in an urban community, hundreds of people had fallen ill. Some had to be quarantined and some were gravely ill. Which of the following best describes the nursing role when responding to this pandemic?
   a) working with the federal government officials for logistics instructions
   b) working with the Canadian Nurses Association for practice guidelines and standards
   c) working with the person in charge of the local operations for instructions
   d) working with the ill and carrying out the needed nursing care

5. Which of the following lists the priority groups for care in disasters?
   a) the poor
   b) the children, older adults, women, and people with mental illness
   c) the government leaders
   d) the healthcare professionals

STUDY QUESTIONS

1. Describe the types of disasters and their consequences.
2. What are the essential elements to respond effectively in a disaster situation?

3. Distinguish the Emergencies Act, the Emergency Preparedness Act, and the Emergency Management Act.
4. Explain the four areas of emergency management in the life-cycle process of a disaster.
5. What expertise should nurses possess in order to respond effectively in a disaster situation?
6. List the core competencies and skills and public health services required for pandemic planning.
7. Distinguish medical triage from public health triage.

> After working through these questions, go to the MyNursingLab at **www.pearsoned.ca/mynursinglab** to check your answers.

INDIVIDUAL CRITICAL THINKING EXERCISES

1. What competencies do beginning nurses require to be able to respond to mass casualty incidents?
2. What technical skills do nurses require to respond during an emergency?
3. What must CHNs do in the event of a disaster?
4. Discuss what CHNs must consider following a disaster.
5. How does the Public Health Agency of Canada play a key role in emergency preparedness?

GROUP CRITICAL THINKING EXERCISES

1. A tornado has left many families without homes. Local politicians and emergency response planners have declared a disaster in the area and ordered citizens to evacuate to a shelter.
   a) Discuss what essential public health services are needed in this situation.
   b) How would nursing students assist in this emergency response?
2. What special considerations need to be given when a disaster takes place in developing countries or communities?
3. Discuss what lessons were learned from disasters such as the SARS crisis for emergency preparedness planning.

REFERENCES

Agency for Healthcare Research and Quality. (2004). *Bioterrorism and health system preparedness*. Retrieved from http://www.archive.ahrq.gov/news/ulp/btbriefs/btbrief6.pdf

Association of State and Territorial Health Officials. (2008). *At-risk populations in emergencies: A review of state and local* stories, tools, and practices. Retrieved from http://www.astho .org/Programs/Infectious-Disease/At-Risk-Populations/ ARPP-State—

Berkowitz, B. (2002). One year later: The impact and aftermath of September 11: Public health nursing practice: Aftermath of September 11, 2001. Online Journal of Issues in Nursing, 7(3), Manuscript 4. Retrieved from http://www .nursingworld.org/ojin/topic19/tpc19_4.htm

Bochenek, R., Kristjanson, E., & Schwartz, B. (2009, Sept. 23–24). Incident Management System (IMS) in the public health response: From SARS to pandemic H1N1. Retrieved from http://www.oahpp.ca/resources/documents/ presentations/2009oct5/OAHPP%20re%20IMS%20in% 20Public%20Health%20-%20OAEM%20Oct% 2009.pdf

Burkle, F. M. (2006). Population-based triage management in response to surge-capacity requirements during a large-scale bioevent disaster. Academic Emergency Medicine: Official Journal of the Society for Academic Emergency Medicine, 13(11), 1118–1129.

Campbell, A. (2005). The SARS Commission second interim report: SARS and public health legislation. Retrieved from http://www.health.gov.on.ca/english/public/pub/ ministry_reports/campbell05/campbell05.pdf

Canadian Nurses Association. (2007). Emergency preparedness and response. [Position Statement]. Ottawa, ON: Author.

CBC News. (2010). Oil spills: How they're cleaned up. Retrieved from http://www.cbc.ca/technology/story/2010/ 04/28/f-oil-spill-cleanup-how-its-done.html

Cohen, R. E. (2000). Mental health services in disasters: Instructor's guide. Washington, DC: Pan American Health Organization.

Department of Justice Canada. (2007a). Emergencies Act, R.S., 1985, c. 22 (4th Supp.). Retrieved from http://laws.justice .gc.ca/en/showtdm/cs/E-4.5

Department of Justice Canada. (2007b). Emergency Preparedness Act, R.S., 1985, c. 6 (4th Supp.). Retrieved from http://laws.justice.gc.ca/en/showtdm/cs/E-4.6

Department of Justice Canada. (2007c). Emergency Management Act, S.C., 2007, c.15. Retrieved from http://laws.justice.gc.ca/en/ShowTdm/cs/E-4.56/

Government of Canada. (December 2009). Federal emergency response plan. Ottawa, ON: Her Majesty the Queen in Right of Canada, 2010. Retrieved from http://www .publicsafety.gc.ca/prg/em/_fl/ferp-eng.pdf

Haddow, G. D., & Bullock, J. A. (2006). Introduction to emergency management (2nd ed.). Burlington, MA: Elsevier Butterworth-Heinemann.

Incident Management System (IMS). (2008). Doctrine for use in Ontario. Emergency Management Ontario. Retrieved from http://www.emergencymanagementontario.ca/stellent/ groups/public/@mcscs/@www/@emo/documents/webasset/ ec077494.pdf

International Council of Nurses. (2006, revised). ICN position statement: Nurses and disaster preparedness. Retrieved from http://www.icn.ch/psdisasterprep01.htm

Jakeway, C., LaRosa, G., Cary, A., & Schoenfisch, S. (2008). The role of public health nurses in emergency preparedness and response: A position paper of the Association of State and Territorial Directors of Nursing. Public Health Nursing, 25(4), 353–361.

Jennings-Sanders, A. (2004). Teaching disaster nursing by utilizing the Jennings Disaster Nursing management model. Nurse Education in Practice, 4, 69–76.

Jennings-Sanders, A., Frisch, N., & Wing, S. (2005). Nursing students' perception about disaster nursing. Disaster Management and Response, 3, 80–85.

Kirby, M., & LeBreton, M. (2002, October). The health of Canadians—The Federal Role Final Report. Vol. 6: Recommendations for Reform. The Standing Senate Committee on Social Affairs, Science and Technology. Retrieved from http://www.parl.gc.ca/37/2/parlbus/ commbus/senate/com-e/soci-e/rep-e/repoct02vol6-e.htm

Kirby, M. (2003, November). Reforming health protection and promotion in Canada: Time to act. The Standing Senate Committee on Social Affairs, Science and Technology. Retrieved from http://www.parl.gc.ca/37/2/paribus/ commbus/senate/com-e/soci-e/rep-e/repfinnov-3-e.htm

Landesman, L. Y. (2005). Public health management of disasters: The practice guide (2nd ed.). Washington, DC: American Public Health Association.

Ministry of Environment, British Columbia. (2007). Introduction to the Incident Command System. Retrieved from http://www.env.gov.bc.ca/eemp/resources/icsintro.htm

Naylor, D. (2003). Learning from SARS: Renewal of public health in Canada: A report of the National Advisory Committee on SARS and Public Health. Ottawa, ON: Health Canada.

O'Connor, D. R. (2002). Walkerton Commission of Inquiry reports: A strategy for safe drinking water. Toronto, ON: Ontario Ministry of the Attorney General. Retrieved from http://www.attorneygeneral.jus.gov.on.ca/english/about/ pubs/walkerton/

Ontario Ministry of Health and Long-Term Care. (2007). The emergency preparedness guide for people with disabilities and/or special needs. Retrieved from http://www .emergencymanagementontario.ca/stellent/groups/public/ @mcscs/@www/@emo/documents/abstract/ec078180 .pdf

Ontario Ministry of Health and Long-Term Care. (2008a). Health plan for an influenza pandemic. Retrieved from http://www.health.gov.on.ca/english/providers/program/ emu/pan_flu/ohpip2/ch_02.pdf

Ontario Ministry of Health and Long-Term Care. (2008b). Ontario public health standards. Toronto, ON: Queen's Printer for Ontario. Retrieved from http://www.health.gov .on.ca/english/providers/program/puhealth/oph_standards/ ophs/progstds/pdfs/ophs_2008.pdf

Ontario Ministry of Health and Long-Term Care. (2009). Emergency preparedness protocol. Toronto, ON: Queen's Printer for Ontario. Retrieved from http://www.health.gov .on.ca/english/providers/program/pubhealth/oph_standards/ ophs/progstds/protocols/ep_protocol_09.pdf

Patillo, M. M. (2003). Mass casualty disaster nursing course. Nurse Educator, 28(6), 271–275.

Polivka, B. J., Stanley, S. A. R., Gordon, D., Taulbee K., Kieffer, G., & McCorkle, S. M. (2008). Public health nursing competencies for public health surge events. Public Health Nursing, 25(2), 159–165.

Public Health Agency of Canada. (2001). Bioterrorism and public health. *Canada Communicable Disease Report, 27*(4). Retrieved from http://www.phac-aspc.gc.ca/publicat/ccdr-rmtc/01vol27/dr2704ea.html

Public Health Agency of Canada. (2006a). *Highlights from the Canadian pandemic influenza plan for the health sector 2006.* Retrieved from http://www.phac-aspc.gc.ca/cpip-cplcpi/hl-ps/index-eng.php

Public Health Agency of Canada. (2006b). *Act to establish public health agency comes into force.* Retrieved from http://www.phac-aspc.gc.ca/media/nr-rp/2006/2006_11_e.html

Public Safety Canada (2009). *New Emergency Management Act.* Retrieved from http://www.publicsafety.gc.ca/media/nr/2007/bk20070807-eng.aspx

Public Safety Canada. (2009). *Canadian disaster database.* Retrieved from http://www.publicsafety.gc.ca/prg/em/cdd/srch-eng.aspx

Qureshi, K., Gebbie, K. M., & Gebbie, E. N. (2006, Oct. 27). *Public health Incident Command System: A guide for the management of emergencies or other unusual incidents within public health agencies.* New York, NY: University of Albany.

Rebmann, T., Carrico, R., & English, J. F. (2008). Lessons public health professionals learned from past disasters. *Public Health Nursing, 25*(4), 344–352.

Rodriguez, D., & Long, C. O. (2006). Preparedness for the home healthcare nurse. *Home Healthcare Nurse, 24*(1), 21–27.

Saliba, D., Buchanan, J., & Kington, R. S. (2004). Function and response of nursing facilities during community disaster. *American Journal of Public Health, 94*(8), 1436–1441.

Sawyer, P. P. (2003). Bioterrorism: Are we prepared? *Home Healthcare Nurse, 21*(4), 220–223.

Stanley, J. M. (2005). Disaster competency development and integration in nursing education. *The Nursing Clinics of North America, 40*(3), 453–467.

United Nations/International strategy for disaster reduction. (2009). *UNISDR terminology on disaster risk reduction.* Retrieved from http://www.unisdr.org/eng/terminology/terminology-2009-eng.html

Veenema, T. G. (Ed.). (2007). *Disaster nursing and emergency preparedness for chemical, biological, and radiological terrorism and other hazards* (2nd ed.). New York, NY: Springer.

Walker, D. (2004, April). *For the public's health: A plan of action. Final report of the Ontario expert panel on SARS and infectious disease control.* Toronto, ON: Ontario, Ministry of Health and Long-Term Care.

World Health Organization. (2007). *The contribution of nursing and midwifery in emergencies: Report of a WHO consultation.* Geneva, Switzerland: Author. Retrieved from http://www.who.int/entity/hac/events/2006/nursing_consultation_report-sept07.pdf

World Health Organization Regional Office for Europe. (2010). *Pandemic preparedness.* Retrieved from http://www.who.int/csr/disease/influenza/pandemic

ADDITIONAL RESOURCES

Readings

Canadian Nurses Association. (2008). *Ethical nursing practice in a pandemic: A national nursing perspective.* Retrieved from http://www.cna-aiic.ca/cna/documents/pdf/Ethical_Nursing_Practice-Poster_e.pdf

Danna, D., & Cordray, S. E. (2010). *Nursing in the storm: Voices from Hurricane Katrina.* New York, NY: Springer.

Goodwin Veenema, T. (2007). *Disaster nursing and emergency preparedness for chemical, biological, and radiological terrorism and other hazards* (2nd ed.). New York, NY: Springer.

Health Canada. (2009). *Emergency management: Taking a health perspective.* Retrieved from http://www.hc-sc.gc.ca/sr-sr/pubs/hpr-rpms/bull/2009-emergency-urgence/index-eng.php#a9

Sullivan T. L., Dow, D., Turner, M. C., Lemyre, L., Corneil, W., Krewski, D., Phillips, K. P., & Amaratunga, A. (2008). Disaster and emergency medicine: Canadian nurses' perceptions of preparedness on hospital front lines. *Prehospital and Disaster Medicine, 23*, 8–11.

Wynd, C. (2006). A proposed model for military disaster nursing. *OJIN: The Online Journal of Issues in Nursing, 11*(3). Available from http://www.nursingworld.org/ojin/topic31/tpc31_4.htm

Videos

Rose Charities/AMDA Canada emergency relief experts interview

(Interviews with Rose Charities foremost emergency disaster relief directors. They discuss the Myanmar Cylone and Sichuan China earthquake.)
http://www.youtube.com/watch?v=z4ws4-rT1LU

Pandemic in the Ontario public health services: Part I (2008)
http://www.youtube.com/watch?v=ToXKYsDENTc

Pandemic in the Ontario public health services: Part II (2008)
http://www.youtube.com/watch?v=B2uyL6P3EI4&feature=related

Websites

CDC Bioterrorism Preparedness & Response
http://www.bt.cdc.gov/

http://www.bt.cdc.gov/Documents/Planning/PlanningGuidance.PDF

Center for Research on the Epidemiology of Disasters (CRED)
http://www.cred.be/

International Federation of the Red Cross (IFRC)
http://www.ifrc.org

Public Health Agency of Canada-Emergency Preparedness and Response
http://www.phac-aspc.gc.ca/ep-mu/index-eng.php

About the Authors

Betty Schepens, RN (St. Clair College), BScN (University of Windsor), DPA (University of Western Ontario), is a Public Health Nurse and the Emergency Preparedness Coordinator at the Chatham-Kent Public Health Unit (Chatham, Ontario) where she worked as a Supervisor in Adult Health, in Chronic Disease and Injury Prevention Programs, and as a Program Manager for the Communicable Disease Control programs. During her 15-year tenure in public health, she was seconded to work with the Human Resources Department of the Municipality of Chatham-Kent as the Corporate Wellness Coordinator to develop a municipal corporate wellness program.

She began her nursing career as a registered nurse at Sydenham District Hospital (Chatham-Kent Health Alliance) where she worked for 15 years. She was a classroom and clinical nursing instructor for the nursing program with St. Clair College, Thames Campus. She served as the municipal representative on the Essex Kent and Lambton District Health Council.

Betty is a member of the Registered Nurses' Association of Ontario (RNAO), the Ontario Association of Emergency Managers (OAEM), the Ontario Nurses' Association (ONA), and the Community and Hospital Infection Control Association (CHICA). She has been involved in local emergency response situations including the coordination of the public health response to the February 2009 flood in Wallaceburg, Ontario, and to the Pandemic H1N1 2009. She is often called to provide consultation on public health emergency preparedness programming best practice strategies by colleagues and organizations from across the province. She was recognized by the Ministry of Health and Long-Term Care when asked to present best practices on community partnerships in emergency preparedness programming to all Ontario Public Health Units during the launch of the revised public health standards and protocols in 2008.

Lucia Yiu, BScN, BA (University of Windsor), BSc (University of Toronto), MScN (University of Western Ontario), is an Associate Professor in the Faculty of Nursing, University of Windsor, and an Educational and Training Consultant in community nursing. Her practice and research include multicultural health, international health, experiential learning, community development, breast health, and program planning and evaluation.

chapter 31

Global Health

Freida S. Chavez, Amy Bender, and Denise Gastaldo

OBJECTIVES

After studying this chapter, you should be able to:

1. Explain the relationship of the Health for All movement and globalization.
2. Explain global health, international health, public health, majority world, and minority world in the context of globalization of health.
3. Describe the impact of globalization on the development of the Millennium Development Goals.
4. Become familiar with the concepts associated with the globalizing of nursing, global citizenship, and post-colonial feminist perspective as relevant to global health.
5. Address the consequences of globalization for nursing, nurse migration, and global spread of infections.
6. Discuss international nursing research and global health ethics.

INTRODUCTION

Globalization presents community health nurses (CHNs) with the challenge and ethical responsibility of being competent caregivers for a "global village." Providing competent care is a professional obligation for nurses; however, providing care in an increasingly dynamic, diverse, and borderless society requires CHNs to address enormous complexity when serving concomitantly individuals, families, groups, and populations. This chapter provides an introduction to global health and presents selected global health issues that impact communities as well as the nursing profession. Using the notion of global citizenship to conceptualize nursing practice, community health nursing roles and practices locally and globally will be critically examined.

HEALTH FOR ALL MOVEMENT

In 1978, the United Nations stated that by 2000, health would be a possibility for all human beings (World Health Organization [WHO], 1978). According to WHO, Health for All means that resources for health are evenly distributed and that essential healthcare is accessible to everyone. However, today, this noble aim is only a reality for a small number of people, mostly in the minority world. While the original goal is yet to be achieved, the Health for All strategy sets an important direction for health equity policy and health programming.

In recognition of the link between health, society, and globalization, Messias (2001) proposes a broad **framework for global health** to achieve health for all. The framework includes (1) elimination of poverty and social and economic disparities; (2) sustainable and environmentally responsible economic development; (3) the creation and introduction of public policies for health; (4) the protection of human and reproductive rights; (5) the empowerment and the rights recognition of women, youth, and communities; and (6) the provision of accessible, affordable, and culturally sensitive healthcare services. In other words, global health can be seen as a new framework to achieve health for all (WHO, 1978).

GLOBALIZATION

Globalization has been defined as "a constellation of processes by which nations, businesses, and people are becoming more connected and interdependent via increased economic integration, communication exchange, and cultural diffusion" (Labonte & Togerson, 2005, p.158). These interdependent processes have far-reaching effects, and taken together, the globalization process generates unbalanced outcomes for populations both between and within countries. While there is nothing inherently good or bad about the flow of capital, labour, and knowledge around the world, questions of this nature arise in regard to who governs this flow and who benefits from it (Navarro, 1999). Thus far, the evidence indicates that while globalization has promoted advances in technology, science, communication, and cross-national interdependencies, it has also increased wide disparities in access to the societal resources and the opportunities they afford (Leuning, 2001; Taylor, 2009). Disparities in access have given rise to much discussion and debate regarding the implications of globalization for health and health for all.

Furthermore, according to Woodward, Drager, Beaglehole, and Lipson (2001), globalization exerts direct and indirect effects on health. Globalization and international markets can directly impact health systems and health policies in addition to the health impacts at the population level resulting from issues like infectious diseases. Indirect effects of globalization affect the availability of publicly funded health expenditures via changes in the health sector economy as well as population risks due to declining household spending on nutrition and living conditions.

Neoliberalism refers to promoting free trade between nations so that goods, resources, and enterprises would be cheaper and profits and efficiency maximized. The goal of neoliberalism is to achieve successful market-based economies through a natural balance of market demands (Shah, 2009). Neoliberalism has been a crucial force toward the intensification of globalization (Breda, 2009). Through neoliberal principles, many markets have been made wider and more dynamic, but such growth has been driven by individualism, privatization of public services, and market self-regulation, which means privileging private business over public social welfare systems. The inequities caused by globalization have important inferences, and are revealed through the language used to describe the world in terms of who benefits and who is burdened by globalization. For this reason, we need to rethink the way we use the terminologies: "majority" world and "minority" world (see Table 31.1).

GLOBALIZATION OF HEALTH

As we witness such rising global concerns as emerging infectious diseases, pandemics, bioterrorism, advancing technologies, and migration of health professionals, the traditionally nationalistic focus of the health sector urgently needs to make greater shifts in order to provide health services across borders and to remote regions within the countries in equitable ways. Areas of healthcare that are often identified as explicitly associated with understanding and addressing the effects of globalization on health are public health, international health, and global health (see Table 31.2). While differentiations are made among these terms, which have implications for understanding the unique primary objectives of each, overall public, international, and global health share a common concern for preventing disease, and promoting health for communities and whole populations. The distinctions exist in terms of geographical considerations and how people and organizations work together.

The concept of global health is evolving with a growing recognition that international social, political, economic, environmental, and cultural issues affect health and healthcare around the world (Carlton, Ryan, Ali, & Kelsy, 2007). While many definitions of global health exist, Koplan et al. (2009) define **global health** as an area for study, research, and practice that places a priority on improving health and achieving equity in health for all people worldwide. Global health implies constant attention to the social determinants of health. Allen and Ogilvie (2004) argue that any examination of the social determinants of health ought to include a critical appraisal of issues related to social justice, human rights, and sustainability on both local and international levels. In the spirit of such appraisal, the Bangkok Charter of Health Promotion explicated the link between health, society, and globalization, and the need for action to improve health based on these interrelationships (WHO, 2005a).

TABLE 31.1 Comparison between Majority World and Minority World

	Alternate Terms	Population	Average Annual Income	Access to Health Care
Majority World (Most of Africa, Asia, and Latin America)	"Third World" or "Rest of the World"	5.4 billion people	U.S. $3500/person 3 billion people under U.S. $2/day	800 million people with no access to healthcare 4.6 billion with very limited to full access, depending on their socio-economic status
Minority World (e.g., Europe, U.S.A., Canada, Australia)	"First World" or "Advanced Liberal Nations"	900 million people	U.S. $26 000/person	Access varies, from emergency care only to full access through private insurance and/or public healthcare systems

Source: Adapted from Rajan, R. S., & Park, Y. (2000). Postcolonial feminism/postcolonial and feminism. In H. Schwarz & S. Ray (Eds.), A companion for postcolonial studies. Oxford, UK: Blackwell, pp. 53–71; and Thibeault, R. (2006). Globalisation, universities and the future of occupational therapy: Dispatches for the Majority World. Australian Occupational Therapy Journal, 53, 159–165.

TABLE 31.2 Comparison of Global Health, International Health, and Public Health

	Global Health	International Health	Public Health
Geographical reach	Focuses on issues that directly affect health but that can transcend national boundaries	Focuses on health issues of countries other than one's own, especially those of low income and middle income	Focuses on issues that affect the health of the population of a particular community or country
Level of co-operation	Development and implementation of solutions often requires global co-operation	Development and implementation of solutions usually requires bi-national co-operation	Development and implementation of solutions does not usually require global co-operation
Individuals or populations	Embraces both prevention in populations and clinical care of individuals	Embraces both prevention in populations and clinical care of individuals	Mainly focused on prevention programs for populations
Access to health	Health equity among nations and for all people is a major objective	Seeks to help people of other nations	Health equity within a nation or community is a major objective
Range of discipline	Highly interdisciplinary and multidisciplinary within and beyond health sciences	Embraces a few disciplines but has not emphasized multidisciplinary	Encourages multidisciplinary approaches, particularly within health sciences and with social sciences

Source: Reprinted from *The Lancet*, Vol. 373, Issue 9679 Koplan, J. P., Bond, T. C., Merson, M. H., Reddy, K. S., Rodriguez, M. H., Sewankambo, N. K., Wasserheit, J. N. Towards a common definition of global health. Pages 1993–1995, Copyright 2009, with permission from Elsevier.

There is strong evidence indicating that most of the world's global burden of disease and, more specifically, health inequalities are caused by social determinants of health (Labonte & Torgerson, 2005). The Bangkok Charter (WHO, 2005a) identifies global factors affecting health as increasing inequalities within and between countries; new patterns of consumption and communication; commercialization; global environmental change; and urbanization. These factors compound the negative effects of the already existing social determinants of health, or those social factors influencing health such as income, shelter, peace, education, and food access. As the new millennium approached, the UN held a summit with the purpose of discussing how best to address poverty as arguably the most pressing social determinant of health globally, and specifically in majority world countries. Out of this meeting came the Millennium Development Goals (MDGs). Together they form an action plan of sorts that includes considerations for evaluating the work done to achieve each one of the goals. There are some MDGs in particular that have explicit health outcomes identified (see Table 31.3). All this highlights that a new "globalized" perspective has been added to the Health for All vision, thereby also raising questions for nursing practice in a globalized world.

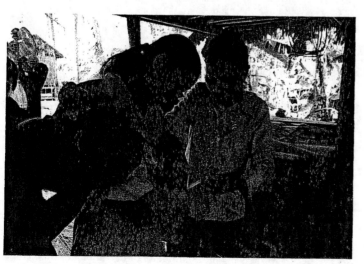

Photo 31.1

Vaccination administration to children in a minority county.

Credit: © Borderlands / Alamy

TABLE 31.3   Millennium Development Goals and Their Health-Related Targets and Health Outcome Indicators

Goal	Health-Related Targets	Health Outcome Indicators
1. Eradicate extreme poverty and hunger	• Between 1990 and 2015, halve the proportion of people who suffer from hunger.	• Prevalence of underweight children under five years of age • Proportion of population below minimum level of dietary energy consumption
2. Achieve universal primary education	• By 2015, ensure all children will be able to complete a full course of primary schooling.	• Proportion of people with full course of primary education
3. Promote gender equality and empower women	• Eliminate gender disparity in primary and secondary schooling by 2005, and in all levels of education by 2015.	• Number of educated women
4. Reduce child mortality	• Reduce by two-thirds, between 1990 and 2015, the under-five mortality rate.	• Under-five mortality rate • Infant mortality rate • Proportion of one-year-old children immunized against measles
5. Improve maternal health	• Reduce by three-quarters, between 1990 and 2015, the maternal mortality ratio.	• Maternal mortality ratio • Proportion of births attended by skilled health personnel
6. Combat HIV/AIDS, malaria and other diseases	• Have halted by 2015 and begun to reverse the spread of HIV/AIDS. • Have halted by 2015 and begun to reverse the incidence of malaria and other major diseases.	• HIV prevalence among pregnant women aged 15–24 years • Condom use rate of the contraceptive prevalence rate • Ratio of school attendance of orphans to school attendance of non-orphans aged 10–14 years • Prevalence and death rates associated with malaria • Proportion of population in malaria-risk areas using effective malaria prevention and treatment measures • Prevalence and death rates associated with tuberculosis • Proportion of tuberculosis cases detected and cured under Direct Observation Treatments (DOTs)
7. Ensure environmental sustainability	• Halve by 2015 the proportion of people without sustainable access to safe drinking water and sanitation. • By 2020 to have achieved a significant improvement in the lives of at least 100 million slum dwellers.	• Proportion of population using solid fuels • Proportion of population with sustainable access to an improved water source, urban and rural • Proportion of population with access to improved sanitation, urban, and rural
8. Develop a global partnership for development	• In co-operation with pharmaceutical companies, provide access to affordable, essential drugs in developing countries.	• Proportion of population with access to affordable essential drugs on a sustainable basis

Source: Adapted from United Nations. (2008). Millennium Development Goals Indicator. *Retrieved from http://unstats.un.org/unsd/mdg/ Host.aspx?Content=Indicators/OfficialList.htm*

CONSEQUENCES OF GLOBALIZATION FOR NURSING

Nurse Migration

Globalization has had far-reaching effects in terms of the nursing workforce as evidenced by the migration of nurses from majority world countries to minority world countries (Dwyer, 2007; Kingma, 2006; McElmurry et al., 2006). This movement of nurses from already resource constrained countries is contrary to primary health care equity and inconsistent with the "Health for All" principles. Health worker migration and international recruitment have a very particular significance to primary health care (PHC). The World Health report in 2006 estimated that the world lacks about 4 million health workers if a minimum level of health outcomes is to be achieved, significantly hindering the attainment of the health-related MDGs (Painter, 2000).

For the past several decades, international recruiting has been a strategy to relieve nurse shortages in recipient countries. This takes nurses away from where they are needed the most (from their source countries) and may mask problems in recipient countries (Bach, 2003; Tejada de Rivero, 2003). McElmurry et al. (2006) argue that in order to satisfy the philosophical approaches to primary health care (see Chapter 7), nurse migration needs to (1) leave majority world countries enhanced rather than depleted, (2) contribute to country health outcomes consistent with essential care for all people, (3) be based on community participation, (4) address common nursing labour issues, and (5) involve equitable and clear financial arrangements. Managing nurse migration will facilitate the achievement of health equity in primary health care.

The nursing labour force is a commodity operating within a capitalist world economy (Herdman, 2004), with the potential to become exploited and oppressed in an environment whose focus has been on economic factors rather than the social and cultural outcomes of globalization. Hence, any examination of the social determinants of health requires critical appraisal of issues related to social justice, human rights, and sustainability on a local and international level (Allen & Ogilvie, 2004).

Since the debates about international health worker recruitment and its impact on the health system has been increasingly pronounced, the WHO has been working on a Code of Practice on the International Recruitment of Health Personnel. Workforce migration is a complex and multidimensional global health challenge and a number of issues, including international recruitment practices, mutuality of employment benefits, and national health workforce sustainability are being discussed (WHO, 2009). The International Council of Nurses (ICN) issued a position statement on Ethical Nurse Recruitment that condemns recruitment of nurses from countries that do not have sound human resource planning and denounces unethical recruitment practices that exploit nurses (ICN, 2007, 2008). The ICN's position statement on retention and migration respects nurses rights and the potential benefits of migration but identifies migration as a symptom of the problem of dysfunctional health systems (see Chapter 8).

Global Spread of Infections

The lessons from Severe Acute Respiratory Syndrome (SARS) and the recent HINI outbreak illustrate the threat from diseases that may rapidly spread from one country to another. These outbreaks have major implications on human life, economies, and societies (Drager & Sutherland, 2007). The revised International Health Regulations issued in 2005 by the WHO were updated to prevent, protect from, and control the international spread of the disease (WHO, 2005b). While it also provides a public health response when disease does spread internationally, the effectiveness of the regulation depends on the country's pandemic preparedness and their ability to have a system to identify and manage outbreaks (Bennett, 2009). This highlights the critical importance for nurses to be aware not only of their own country's landscape since bacteria, viruses, and trends impacting on health do not respect borders. In collaboration with other health professions, nurses not only need to know infectious disease prevention and management, but also need to understand how best to forestall negative impacts locally and globally (Hirschfeld, 2008). (See Chapter 12.)

Globalization of Nursing and Global Citizenship

In the current of increased globalization, nurses need to be educated as global citizens who have a moral responsibility and professional competency to care and promote health beyond their local communities and national institutions (Chavez, Peter, & Gastaldo, 2008). The new global interdependence calls for all persons across the globe to extend their thinking about moral responsibility and health beyond their local communities and national citizenship and to become citizens of the world (Crigger, Branningan, & Barid, 2006). Nussbaum (1997) describes three necessary capacities for the cultivation of global citizenship. The first is the capacity to examine ourselves and our traditions critically, which is known as **reflexivity**, and it involves scrutinizing our beliefs, traditions, and habits to ensure that they are consistent and justifiable. Specific to nursing, Crigger et al. (2006) suggest that global citizenship begins in nursing training when nursing students become sensitized to their own culturally established perspectives on healthcare. These nursing students become capable of identifying and challenging underlying values and assumptions of their nursing education and practice, as well as the healthcare system.

Nussbaum's (1997) second capacity for global citizenship entails the notion of **moral cosmopolitanism**, meaning adopting the fundamental view of all persons as fellow citizens who have equal moral worth and deserve equal moral consideration (Friedman, 2000). **Global citizenship**, however, does not mean that we need to give up our unique local preferences and familial, ethnic, or religious responsibilities. Instead, as fellow citizens of the world, all persons are part of our community of respect and concern, which at times means that such concern may constrain our local interests.

The third capacity is **narrative imagination**, which requires the ability to imagine what it might be like to be a person different from oneself, and to allow such imagination to inform understanding of others' experiences, emotions, desires, and their life stories (Nussbaum, 1997). Being exposed to other cultures and people is one aspect of developing this kind of narrative imagination as part of cultivating global citizenship. It also requires a politicized understanding of how we are all situated in relation to one another across the globe. Global citizenship, then, comes partly through critical thinking skills expressly focused on challenging oppressive power relations along with a commitment to social change, social justice, and reflexivity (Painter, 2000). Global citizenship may be

A Canadian nurse working for a European NGO medical clinic in rural Kenya makes home visits to several elderly community members. During one of these visits, the client tells the nurse that his traditional healer, who charges for his services beyond what the nurse knows this man can afford, has told him that he should stop taking the medication prescribed by the clinic physician because it has been causing drowsiness, leading to sleeping during the day. The client understands that this may open him to the influence of evil spirits. He tells the nurse that his daughter is angry with him for listening to the healer, and he is afraid to mention this to the physician at the next clinic visit because, like his daughter, she will not understand.

Discussion Questions

1. List the health and relational concerns that the nurse must consider. How are they perhaps different in this international context than they might be if she were at home in her own country?

2. Taking into consideration global health ethics, how does the nurse best go about addressing this client's situation?

3. Identify some potential cultural challenges for this nurse. What might the nurse do and/or say that would demonstrate an awareness of being an international visitor and her cultural sensitivity in this regard?

cultivated through various critical theoretical lenses, one of which is postcolonial feminism.

POSTCOLONIAL FEMINISM

Postcolonialism may be described as a theory and political movement that challenges Western authority and its ethnocentric ideas that naturalize the current global economic and political order rather than problematize them as the consequence of centuries of colonialism (Loomba, 2005). Postcolonialism seeks to explain people's lives in places and times other than "the West," celebrate pluralism, and strongly critique any assumptions about universal knowledge. Given that nations and communities are social constructs supported by particular notions of gender, race, and class, postcolonial feminism (PCF) offers a theoretical lens through which to address the intersections of such social locations and to explore their corresponding forms of oppression that are inherently part of everyday experiences (Anderson et al., 2003; Loomba, 2005).

The usefulness of this perspective for cultivating global citizenship is that it sheds light on inequities in any global context and facilitates examination of the complex nature of health issues. It explicitly calls on nurses to critique current global (including Canadian) disparities in health and healthcare arising from such phenomena as sexism, racism, or the imposition of Eurocentric colonialist views over Aboriginal Canadian knowledge and other indigenous ways of understanding health and healing (Chavez et al., 2008).

PCF represents an opportunity for nurses to acknowledge their multiple social and cultural locations as individuals and healthcare professionals. It challenges deeply held certainties about the "right way" to provide care and considers all knowledge as being situated with a given place and within the power relations therein. Using this perspective enables us to consider multiple perspectives on meanings of health and illness (Anderson & McCann, 2002), as well as the complex issues associated with the global locations of nursing practice and care-giving. For instance, as an international profession, nursing faces invisibility in the healthcare decision-making processes and nurses' working conditions are difficult (Lunardi, Peter, & Gastaldo, 2002); however, nurses are subjected to much lower wages and appalling working conditions in certain nations and there is considerable variation in such conditions among institutions within the same country.

Through its focus on gender, PCF is also a useful framework to examine the common unpaid and low-prestige nature of care-giving, despite being an essential activity for the well-being and health of nations (Bover & Gastaldo, 2005). For example, the inclusion of women in the paid labour market in high-income countries has not been accompanied by increased care-giving roles for men but was rather followed by the migration of women from middle- and low-income countries, such as Filipina nannies coming to Canada and Latin American caregivers for the elderly going to Spain.

INTERNATIONALIZATION OF NURSING RESEARCH

Nursing research worldwide is highly influenced by, among others, the availability of professionals, access to research training and graduate programs, and working conditions for academics and practitioners. Some nursing research is situated within the domain of biomedical research, which has been criticized for its lack of commitment toward the disease treatment and prevention for the pathologies that affect the majority of the world's population. This phenomenon is known as the 90/10 divide, which refers to the fact that only 10% of all international funding for biomedical research is dedicated to studying problems associated with 90% of the world's global burden of disease (Resnik, 2004).

Another element to be considered is that high-income countries' researchers are the majority of the world's nursing scientists, who are educated and funded to study local and national issues. In addition, studies are frequently published in English, which is called now the 21st-century language of science (Gennaro, 2009), constituting a barrier for nurses from low- and medium-income countries. In this context, English-speaking scientists become producers of knowledge, while researchers and practitioners in other countries are reduced to being the consumers or are altogether disconnected from new findings or knowledge exchange (Mancia & Gastaldo, 2004).

In order to address these issues, nurse researchers need to work on building networks that employ PCF lenses, or other equitable frameworks, to guide their collaborations and set research agendas that tackle health promotion and healthcare needs of diverse populations, including the issues faced by communities and professionals in resource-constrained settings.

CANADIAN RESEARCH BOX

How to promote student and new researcher participation in global health in Quebec?

Ridde, V., Mohindra, K. S., & LaBossiere, F. (2008). Driving the global public health research agenda forward by promoting the participation of students and new researchers. *Canadian Journal of Public Health, 99*(6), 460–465.

These authors set out to explore how to promote the participation of students and new researchers in global health in Quebec by carrying out a study that focused on documenting the state of teaching and research in global health and gathering the perspectives of key actors in this research arena in Quebec. The "10/90 gap" (only 10% of all U.S. research funds are used to investigate health problems affecting 90% of the world's population) has been a central concern of global health researchers, and while this ratio has improved since it first appeared in a 1990 report, the metaphor continues to capture well the gross inequities in health research worldwide.

In Canada, the establishment of several federal and provincial initiatives has helped to address this. Two noted federal bodies are the Global Health Research Initiative (GHRI) of CIHR and other federal partners, and the not-for-profit group, Canadian Coalition for Global Health Research (CCGHR). The focus for this study was the Global Health Research Axis (GHRA) of the Quebec Population Health Research Network. "Key to promoting and maintaining this enthusiasm for global health research at the provincial and national levels is the role that students and new researchers will play . . . . and a variety of strategies should be pursued to ensure that new researchers are genuine partners in this endeavour" (p. 461).

The authors reviewed the global health work in the public health programs of five Quebec universities, and surveyed and interviewed professors and students/new researchers. They found 36 global health researchers and noted that "researchers generally do not work exclusively on global health projects" (p. 462). There were 76 projects over the past five years—most undertaken in sub-Saharan Africa and Asia. Dominant themes were health services and health policy, and infectious/parasitic diseases. Study participants reported a number of strengths and weaknesses in global health teaching and research in Quebec, as well as opportunities and threats to conducting research in global health. The presence of research units and support from faculties along with competent professors and highly motivated students were listed as strengths. Weaknesses included such issues as lack of courses specific to global health; insufficient numbers of professors; lack of opportunity for global health intervention training; insufficient funding; lack of scientific activities; and little/no involvement of professors from low- and middle-income countries (LMICs) or members of the community/public. The opportunities identified were the relevance of health issues to globalization; Quebec universities have the will to internationalize; seem to be ahead in this area compared to other provinces; the importance of intercultural experiences; conducting research that is 'close to populations.' Finally, threats to global health teaching and research are the difficulty in getting innovative projects funded; the development of long-term partnerships is stifled by lack of young professors/researchers; the potential of distracting students from other aspects of their basic training; the risk of inequitable partnerships reinforcing the Majority World-Minority World divide.

The authors concluded that "there is a strong and growing presence of global health in Quebec universities—although the situation varies according to the institution" (p. 463). Two key trends have supported this: increases in federal funding to global health initiatives and Quebec's growing reputation for academic excellence in global health. The authors recommended (1) that provincial donors follow the federal bodies funding arrangements; (2) putting emphasis on capacity building—bring together researchers from LMICs and Canada for research and to build global health curriculum; and (3) developing global health at the graduate level by seeking out long-term initiatives with universities across provinces, and across disciplines.

Discussion Questions

1. What are the global health initiatives/opportunities at your university? In your nursing school (both in terms of coursework and intervention training, and research)? Share examples in light of the strengths, weaknesses, opportunities, and threats identified in this study.

2. What are the benefits and limitations of nursing-specific global health courses and/or research projects compared to multidisciplinary initiatives?

GLOBAL HEALTH ETHICS

Community health nursing necessarily involves making ethical decisions in daily practice (see Chapter 4). Ethical theory helps to guide such decisions and has been expressed in codes of ethics and standards of practice. **Global health ethics** is a particular avenue of ethical theory that closely aligns with public health ethics, moves beyond traditional bioethical principles, draws from the philosophy of health as a human right, and acknowledges work in this area as largely involving vulnerable populations (Pinto & Upshur, 2009). Benatar, Daar, and Singer (2003) argue that it is imperative to move beyond individually focused biomedical ethical principles to a more comprehensive approach that focuses on improving health globally: a shift in mindset that requires "a realization that health, human rights, economic opportunities, good governance, peace and development are all intimately linked within a complex interdependent world" (p. 108).

Global health ethics can guide moral decision-making in settings other than one's home community, from the perspective of the nurse as global citizen. Situations involving moral dilemmas for researchers and practitioners alike in international settings are innumerable. Some examples include using the already scant resources of host agencies to become culturally familiar with primary health care practices, working through translators, which places a burden on locals who are already overworked and may impede natural flow of care, and balancing learning local standards of care with drawing from one's own ethno-centric knowledge so that interventions are culturally appropriate without being problematic. Pinto and Upshur (2009) suggest four principles for global health research ethics that also apply to primary health care nursing work: humility, introspection, solidarity, and social justice. **Humility** refers to "recognizing one's limitations and being open to learning from all sources" (p. 7). **Introspection**, or reflection, is a "rigorous examination of one's motives and being aware of one's own privilege" (p. 8). **Solidarity** refers to "working to ensure that goals and values are aligned with those of the community and seeing indigenous views of health and healthcare as an opportunity to understand a problem from the perspective of those receiving care" (p. 8). Finally, **social justice** addresses the "need to diminish the gross inequities observed, to understand power relationships and networks at interpersonal, organizational, and international levels, to explicitly consider equity in examining health systems, and to always familiarize oneself with the political and human rights conditions of the places visited" (p. 9).

study brought with it a number of questions regarding its implementation in Uganda, a very different cultural context than the researcher's own as a Canadian.

One question is how best to gain participant acceptance of and input into the project prior to conducting the research, particularly by distance. Nurse researchers are challenged by engaging in research related to globalization. Specifically, they must confront three key ethical issues arising when researchers are from high-income countries planning to conduct projects in LMICs. These issues are vulnerability and exploitation; community considerations; and doing good. Vulnerability and exploitation refer to "the degree of cultural difference between the involved countries and the potential for exploitation." Providing informed consent is one example of where the participants' vulnerability and potential for exploitation are high (p. 73). For example, "language barriers, high illiteracy rates and a lack of formal education may result in difficulty obtaining a meaningful informed consent," which leads to the need for ample time and thorough explanation of the study signing the consent form. Exploitation is avoided only when the researcher articulates clearly the direct benefit of participation and when any actions in the study that prove successful are affordable and sustainable for that particular community. The researcher must also know or be willing to learn about the region in which the research will be conducted (p. 73).

The second issue is community considerations. Traditional research ethics, focused on individual rights, do not necessarily address the role of the community in research, but such ought to be considered in the context of LMIC. This includes paying attention to traditions, history, interpersonal relations, and power relations (p. 75). Doing good is the third ethical issue, which refers to considerations of what good might be done beyond the obligations outlined in the study itself, which touches on the personal values of the researcher and how s/he responds to the participants as collaborators.

The authors suggest that the principles of respect for persons and communities, justice, contextual caring, and beneficence be adhered to. Most importantly, they stress the value of a "communitarian relational philosophy" for research in LMICs that first acknowledges the irreducibility of community.

CANADIAN RESEARCH BOX

What are the ethical considerations for nurses in global nursing research?

Harrowing, J. N., Mill, J., Spiers, J., Kuling, J., & Kipp, W. (2010). Culture, context and community: Ethical considerations for global nursing research. *International Nursing Review, 57,* 70–77.

This article argues that in the current age of globalization it is vital that nurse researchers develop and implement ethical guidelines for research in LMICs, particularly when that research is carried out by non-resident investigators. This study aimed to examine the impact of an education program for Ugandan registered nurses and nurse-midwives caring for persons living with HIV and AIDS. Planning this

Discussion Questions

1. Name the three key issues to consider in conducting global health research according to these authors. Discuss examples of each that you have either experienced directly or read in the media.

2. What aspects of regional knowledge should a researcher have and understand before beginning the study? How much time do you think needs to be spent in the field in order for the research to be considered ethical? Why? How does being familiar with the region lessen vulnerability and exploitation?

SUMMARY

CHNs as global citizens look past the dominant emphasis on individual care (commonly disconnected from social, economic, and cultural contexts); engage critically and reflexively with social, historical, and political issues; and develop their capacity in identifying tensions between personal professional interests and global interests. A nurse who can exercise her or his global citizenship professionally works from the premise that people's experiences of health and illness are culturally and geographically located; that the majority of the world live under severe social and economic inequities and suffer from preventable or curable diseases and experience an enormous amount of unnecessary human suffering; that global health nurses should have the ability to address the health concerns of the majority of the world population; that nursing labour has become a market commodity; and that projects related to "Health for All" are those that engage in the construction of sustainable, publicly run sanitation and safe water programs; affordable, healthy food and housing initiatives; and that build national healthcare systems (Chavez et al., 2008). Nurses, the biggest group of health professionals in the world, are strategically located and needed to leverage this position to advocate for global health in this globalized world.

KEY TERMS

globalization, p. 480
framework for global health, p. 480
neoliberalism, p. 481
global health, p. 481
reflexivity, p. 484
global citizenship, p. 484
moral cosmopolitanism, p. 484
narrative imagination, p. 484
postcolonialism, p. 485
postcolonial feminism (PCF), p. 485
90/10 divide, p. 485
global health ethics, p. 486
humility, p. 486
introspection, p. 486
solidarity, p. 486
social justice, p. 486

REVIEW QUESTIONS

Choose the one alternative that best completes the statement or answers the question.

1. Global health
   a) is synonymous to international health.
   b) focuses on health issues other than one's own.
   c) focuses on issues that affect the health of the population.
   d) transcends national boundaries.

2. Nurses as global citizens
   a) look past the dominant emphasis on individual care.
   b) work solely internationally.
   c) give up unique local preferences.
   d) speak many languages.

3. Global health ethics, closely tied to public health ethics, predominantly involves the principles of
   a) autonomy, benevolence, non-malificence, and justice.
   b) solidarity, social justice, introspection, and humility.
   c) social justice, justice, duty to care, and compassion.
   d) community autonomy, empowerment, reciprocity, and human rights.

4. Which of the following most clearly represents a moral dilemma for a Canadian nurse working in an international setting?
   a) drawing information about the culture and healthcare practices from someone of that culture in preparing for the work term prior to departure
   b) working through a Canadian translator who comes as part of the team for the work term
   c) providing good care with the culturally appropriate resources that are available
   d) needing to adopt questionable local standards of care while working within one's scope of practice and Western medical knowledge-base

5. What is not necessary to cultivate global citizenship?
   a) reflexivity
   b) moral cosmopolitanism
   c) narrative imagination
   d) autonomy

STUDY QUESTIONS

1. Differentiate global health and international health.
2. Describe a global health issue arising out of the globalization of nursing.
3. In your nursing practice, how can you think globally and act locally?
4. Identify the three capacities needed to develop global citizenship.
5. How can the notion of global citizenship guide your nursing practice?
6. Describe social determinants of health that impact on individual and community health.

INDIVIDUAL CRITICAL THINKING EXERCISES

1. Define global citizenship in your own words and describe it using examples from your own life story or that of those close to you.

2. Imagine you are working in a First Nations community in Canada.

   a) In what ways might you see the effects of globalization on the community?

   b) How might the Millennium Development Goals apply to First Nations Canadian communities?

3. As you have come to understand the role of CHNs throughout the whole textbook, how do you now understand this role specific to a global health perspective?

4. Write a brief rebuttal to the following statement: "Public health, international health, and global health are really all the same anyway, so making distinctions in language is not meaningful or useful."

After working through these questions, go to the MyNursingLab at **www.pearsoned.ca/mynursinglab** *to check your answers.*

GROUP CRITICAL THINKING EXERCISES

1. When spider-webs unite, they can tie up an elephant

   —Ethiopian proverb

Imagine forming a web of connections among global health topics raised in this chapter that brings together the health issues, the sociopolitical global context, and corresponding concerns for nursing. Take a few minutes to individually draw a "global health and nursing" web representing what you have imagined, labelling/identifying its various strands. Share your drawings with the group, explaining the following:

- Your identification of the central strands that give strength to the whole web (i.e., foundational ideas) and those strands that may be further out in the web; those that are important but not central.

- Your understanding of the points where the strands connect as points where nurses may take action (i.e., how issues, context, and nursing concerns come together to direct care in global health).

2. Mrs. Chen is waiting to be seen in the outpatient clinic with her granddaughter, who looks to be about 10 years old. It is about 6:30 p.m. when a primary health care nurse invites them into her office for assessment and discovers that Mrs. Chen has only recently arrived in Canada and speaks no English. The nurse does not like to use family members as interpreters but the hospital interpreters and the Cantonese-speaking receptionist have left for the day. Not knowing what else to do, the nurse begins the interview with the help of the granddaughter acting as interpreter. In carrying out some open-ended questions, the nurse realizes that Mrs. Chen may be seriously depressed. She wants to ask more focused questions to assess the risk of suicide, but feels uncomfortable about posing these questions through Mrs. Chen's granddaughter. As a group, discuss the following:

   a) What global health issues arise in this situation?

   b) What are the implications for nursing practice that would reflect global citizenship?

3. Imagine that you are in a remote, resource-constrained area of a majority world country, working in a health clinic staffed only by one nurse and two lay health workers. Write a letter home describing your imagined experience. Tell the person to whom you are writing about situations in which your taken-for-granted assumptions have been challenged; you felt discomfort in taking action or felt great confidence; and/or you felt marginalized in some way. Read your letters to one another in the group and discuss how these experiences can be understood through postcolonial feminism.

REFERENCES

Allen, M., & Ogilvie, L. (2004). Internationalization of higher education: Potential and pitfalls for nursing education. *International Nursing Review*, 73–80.

Anderson, J., Perry, J., Blue, C., Brown, A., Henderson, A., Khan, K. B., et al. (2003). Rewriting cultural safety within the postcolonial and postnational feminist project: Toward new epistemologies of healing. *Advances in Nursing Science*, *26*(3), 196–214.

Anderson, J. M., & McCann, E. K. (2002). Toward a postcolonial feminist methodology in nursing research: Exploring the convergence of post-colonial and black feminist scholarship. *Nurse Researcher*, *9*(3), 7–27.

Bach, S. (2003). *International migration of health workers: Labour and social issues*. Geneva, Switzerland: International Labour Office.

Benatar, S. R., Daar, A. S., & Singer, P. A. (2003). Global health ethics. The rational for mutual caring. *International Affairs*, *79*(1), 107–138.

Bennett, C. (2009). Lessons from SARS: Past practice, future innovation. In J. J. Kirton & M. Schreurs (Eds.), *Innovation in global health governance* (pp. 49–62). Aldershot, UK: Ashgate.

Bover, A., & Gastaldo, D. (2005). La centralidad de la familia como recurso en el cuidado domiciliario: Perspectivas de género y generación [The centrality of the family as a resource in home care: Gender and generational perspectives]. *Revista Brasileira de Enfermagem*, *58*(1), 9–16.

Breda, K. L. (Ed.). (2009). *Nursing and globalization in the Americas: A critical perspective*. New York, NY: Baywood.

Carlton, K. H., Ryan, M., Ali, N. S., & Kelsy, B. (2007). Integration of global health concepts in nursing curricula: A national study. *Nursing Education Perspectives*, *28*(3), 124–129.

Chavez, F. S., Peter E., & Gastaldo, D. (2008). Nurses as global citizens: A global health curriculum at the University of Toronto, Canada. In V. Tschudin & A. J. Davis (Eds.), *The globalisation of nursing* (pp. 175–186). Oxford, UK: Radcliffe.

Crigger, N., Brannigan, M., & Baird, M. (2006). Compassionate nursing professionals as good citizens of the world. *Advances in Nursing Science, 29*(4), 15–26.

Drager, N., & Sunderland, L. (2007). Public health in a globalizing world: The perspective from the World Health Organization. In A. F. Cooper, J. J. Kirton, & T. Schrecker (Eds.), *Governing global health: Challenge, response, innovation* (pp. 67–78). Aldershot, UK: Ashgate.

Dwyer, J. (2007). What's wrong with the global migration of health care professionals? Individual rights and international justice. *Hastings Center Report, 37*(5), 36–43.

Friedman, M. (2000). Educating for world citizenship. *Ethics, 110*(3), 586–601.

Gennaro, S. (2009). Searching for knowledge. *Journal of Nursing Scholarship, 41*(1), 1–2.

Herdman, E. (2004). Globalization, internationalism and nursing. *Nursing and Health Sciences, 6*, 237–238.

Hirschfeld, M. J. (2008). Globalization: Good or bad, for whom? In V. Tschudin & A. J. Davis (Eds.), *The globalisation of nursing* (pp. 12–26). Oxford, U.K.: Radcliffe.

ICN. (2007). *Ethical nurse recruitment: Position statement.* Geneva, Switzerland: Author. Retrieved from http://www.icn.ch/PS_C03_Ethical%20Nurse%20Recruitment.pdf

ICN. (2008). *Nurse retention and migration: Position statement.* Geneva, Switzerland: Author. Retrieved from http://www.icn.ch/PS_C06_NurseRetenMigration.pdf

Kingma, M. (2006). *Nurses on the move: Migration and the global health care economy.* Ithaca, NY: Cornell University Press.

Koplan, J. P., Bond, T. C., Merson, M. H., Reddy, K. S., Rodriguez, M. H., Sewankambo, N. K., & Wasserheit, J. N. (2009). Towards a common definition of global health. *The Lancet, 373*, 1993–1995.

Labonte, R., & Torgerson, R. (2005). Interrogating globalization, health and development: Towards a comprehensive framework for research, policy, and political action. *Critical Public Health, 15*(2), 157–179.

Leuning, C. J. (2001). Advancing a global perspective: The world as classroom. *Nursing Science Quarterly, 14*, 298–303.

Loomba, A. (2005). *Colonialism/Postcolonialism* (2nd ed.). New York, NY: Routledge.

Lunardi, V., Peter, E., & Gastaldo, D. (2002). Are submissive nurses ethical? Reflecting on power anorexia. *Revista Brasileira de Enfermagem, 55*(2), 183–188.

Mancia, J. R., & Gastaldo, D. (2004). Production and consumption of science in a global context. *Nursing Inquiry, 11*(2), 65–66.

McElmurry, B. J., Solheim, K., Kishi, R., Coffia, M. A., Woith, W., & Janepanish, P. (2006). Ethical concerns in nurse migration. *Journal of Professional Nursing, 22*(4), 226–235.

Messias, D. K. H. (2001). Globalization, nursing and health for all. *Journal of Nursing Scholarship, 33*(1), 9–11.

Navarro, V. (1999). Health and equity in the world in the era of "globalization." *International Journal of Health Services, 29*(2), 215–226.

Nussbaum, M. C. (1997). *Cultivating humanity: A classical defense of reform in liberal education.* Cambridge, MA: Harvard University Press.

Painter, J. (2000). Critical human geography. In R. J. Johnston, D. Gregory, G. Pratt, & M. Watts (Eds.), *The dictionary of human geography* (4th ed., pp. 126–128). Oxford, UK: Blackwell.

Pinto, A. D., & Upshur, R. E. (2009). Global health ethics for students. *Developing World Bioethics, 9*(1), 1–10.

Rajan, R. S., & Park, Y. (2000). Postcolonial feminism/postcolonial and feminism. In H. Schwarz & S. Ray (Eds.), *A companion for postcolonial studies* (pp. 53–71). Oxford, UK: Blackwell.

Resnik, D. B. (2004). The distribution of biomedical research resources and international justice. *Developing World Bioethics, 4*(1), 42–57.

Shah, A. (2009). *A primer on neoliberalism.* Retrieved from http://bing.search.sympatico.ca/?q=Neoliberalism%20&mkt=en-ca&setLang=en-CA

Taylor, S. (2009). Wealth, health and equity: Convergence to divergence in late 20th century globalization. *British Medical Bulletin, 91*(1), 29–48.

Tejada de Rivero, D. A. (2003). Alma-Alta revisited. *Perspectives in Health, 8*, 3–7.

United Nations. (2008). Millennium Development Goals Indicator. Retrieved from http://unstats.un.org/unsd/mdg/Host.aspx?Content=Indicators/OfficialList.htm

Woodward, D., Drager, N., Beaglehold, R., & Lipson, D. (2001). Globalization and health: A framework for analysis and action. *Bulletin of the World Health Organization, 79*, 875–881.

World Health Organization. (1978). Declaration of Alma Alta: International conference on primary health care, Alma-Ata, USSR, 6-12. Europe: Author. Retrieved from http://www.who.int/topics/primary_health_care/en/

World Health Organization (WHO). (2005a). Bangkok Charter of Health Promotion. From the 6th Global Conference on Health Promotion, Bangkok, Thailand, August 11, 2005. Retrieved from http://www.who.int/healthpromotion/conferences/6gchp/hpr_050829_%20BCHP.pdf

World Health Organization (WHO). (2005b). *International health regulations 2005* (2nd ed.). Retrieved from http://www.who.int/ihr/9789241596664/en/index.html

World Health Organization (WHO). (2009). *A World Health Organization code of practice on the international recruitment of health personnel: Background paper.* Geneva, Switzerland: Author.

ADDITIONAL RESOURCES

Readings

Hanefeld, J. (2008). How have global health initiatives impacted on health equity? *Promotion and Education, 15*(1), pp. 19–23.

Kirkham, S. R., & Browne, A. J. (2006). Toward a critical theoretical interpretation of social justice discourses in nursing. *Advances in Nursing Science, 29*(4), 324–339.

Levine, R. (2007). *Case studies in global health: Millions saved.* Sudbury, MA: Jones and Bartlett.

Pam Baker, P., Gilden, D., Kher, U., Mastandrea, A., Otrompke, J., & Perilstein, J. D. (2009). *Case studies for global health: Building relationship, sharing knowledge.* Deerfield, IL: Alliance for Case Studies for Global Health. (Can download full book from http://www.casestudiesforglobalhealth.org)/

Skolnik, R. (2008). *Essentials of global health.* Sudbury, MA: Jones and Bartlett.

Walraven, G. (2010). *Health and poverty: Global health problems and solutions.* Stirling, VA: Stylus.

Websites

The Canadian Nurses Association's Global Health and Equity Position Statement
http://www.can-aiic.ca/CNA/documents/pdf/publications/PS106_Global_Health_Equity_Aug_2009_e.pdf

Canadian Nurses Association
http://www.cna-nurses.ca/cna/default_e.aspx

Center for Global Development
http://www.cgdev.org

Consortium of Universities for Global Health
http://www.cugh.org

Doctors Without Borders
http://www.msf.org

Global Health Action
http://www.globalhealthaction.org

Global Health Alliance of Nursing and Midwifery
http://knowledge-gateway.org/ganm

Global Health Education Consortium
http://www.globalhealthedu.org

Health Canada
http://www.hc-sc.gc.ca/english/

International Council of Nurses
http://www.icn-apnetwork.org

The Nightingale Inititative for Global Health (NIGH)
http://www.dosseydossey.com/barbara/nigh.html

Pan American Health Organization
http://www.paho.org

United Nations Millennium Development Goals
http://www.unmillenniumproject.org

World Health Organization
http://www.who.int/en

About the Authors

Freida Chavez, RN, MHSc, CHE is a Senior Lecturer and Director of the International Office at the Lawrence S. Bloomberg Faculty of Nursing (LSBFON), University of Toronto. Freida champions the integration of global health and the notion of global citizenship in the nursing curriculum, created the Global Health section in the undergraduate course "Primary Health Care, Nursing Perspectives," and "Critical Perspectives in Global Health Nursing: An Elective Practicum," where students are prepared practically and theoretically for an enhanced experience in resource-constrained areas nationally and internationally. She also leads the first nursing partnership between LSBFON and the Brazil Ministry of Health in Primary Health Care Nursing.

Amy Bender, RN, PhD, is an Assistant Professor at the Lawrence S. Bloomberg Faculty of Nursing, University of Toronto. She teaches in the areas of psychiatry/mental health, community health, nursing theory, and global health. Her research interests centre on the mental health dimensions of infectious diseases, specifically tuberculosis, and nurses' relationship skills as part of public health core competencies.

Denise Gastaldo, PhD, is an Associate Professor at the Lawrence S. Bloomberg Faculty of Nursing and Associate Director of the Centre for Critical Qualitative Health Research, University of Toronto. She studies migration and gender as social determinants of health, using predominantly participatory and community-based methodologies. She is the co-creator and former general coordinator of the International Nursing PhD Collaboration, a partnership among doctoral programs from Australia, Brazil, Canada, Finland, Mexico, and Spain.

chapter
32

Challenges and Future Directions

Lynnette Leeseberg Stamler and Lucia Yiu

"The future is here—it's just not everywhere."

Marilyn Chow, RN, DNSc, FAAN
Executive Leadership Conference, June 2010

In Villeneuve and MacDonald's discussion paper *Towards 2020: Visions for Nursing* (2006), we find scenarios of nursing in a future that looks quite different from what the majority of your teachers were taught, as well as what you will see as you graduate in the near future from basic nursing programs. In describing the healthcare system, Rosemary Goodyear (as cited in Villeneuve & MacDonald, 2006) suggests that "communities are moving away from doctors as primary care providers and are more open to alternative providers like NPs and RNs" (p. 94).

Primary health care is the way to achieve health for all. (See Chapter 7.) The *Towards 2020* discussion paper identifies self-care as the "largest contributor to the creation and maintenance of health" (Villeneuve & MacDonald, 2006, p. 95). Self-care is described as taking place "in the socioenvironmental–political–cultural context of the individual and is influenced by resources available" (p. 95). The second largest contributor is identified as "all the community health and social resources in place to support health and keep people well" (p. 95). In other words, nurses play a key role in providing a supportive environment for people to attain good health in their own communities—where they live, work, learn, and play.

According to the Canadian Institute for Health Information (2010), almost 63% of nurses currently work in hospital settings, and just over 14% work in community settings. Villeneuve and MacDonald (2006) suggest that by 2020 the percentages will have reversed, with two-thirds working in community-based care. Further, they identify that nurses will "develop and implement broad programs of health promotion and illness prevention in schools, workplaces, and communities, and [be] a strong, visible presence" (p. 99). Finally, they identify that nursing research will "place less emphasis on nurses and nursing processes than was the case 20 years ago, focusing instead on health, the needs of patients and communities, and providing sound evidence to guide policy and practice" (p. 99).

While some of the issues identified, e.g., place of employment of nurses, seem to have changed little in the years since publication, there are other areas where changes are more easily detected. For example, the Canadian Institutes of Health Research recently published a "Strategy on Patient Oriented Research" (CIHR, 2010). While still in the development stage, this strategy "aims to create a more cost-effective delivery of healthcare in fields such as primary care and chronic disease management as well as an overall improved health system" (CIHR). It is clear that if the futuristic picture is an accurate one, the changes in the next few years will be profound. There are implications for nursing education as well as nursing practice.

How are we preparing for such changes? First, let's look at changes in nursing practice, specifically community nursing practice. We know that the demographics of the Canadian population are changing, as seen in the age stratifications, the cultural mix, and the increase in Aboriginal populations. The "one-size" approach will no longer fit all. Strategies to improve population health will need to be targeted to specific groups. As the Canadian population becomes increasingly diverse, nurses must be mindful to move beyond cultural sensitization and awareness and direct their care to promoting cultural harmony and acceptance of individual cultural differences. As the largest group of healthcare workers in community settings, nurses will be required to be politically savvy and provide leadership in promoting equality and social justice in their local community and around the globe.

With longer life expectancy, we encounter various illnesses such as cancer, diabetes, heart conditions, or Alzheimer's disease during our life course. New advances in genetics and other treatments will radically change how we adapt and age. The need for emergency preparedness will not diminish, but will be always present, albeit with a variety of concerns, from HIV/AIDS to H1N1, or from natural to man-made disasters. In the pursuit of social justice and equity to achieve health for all, nurses face new health challenges in helping individuals and populations through chronic disease management, reducing dependence on hospital services, and supporting people at home. We need to work interprofessionally and intraprofessionally to create a seamless health system. This system is expected to provide timely access to appropriate services and care to the clients. While several provinces have initiated strategies to examine and improve timely access to acute care services, considerably less attention has been paid to access to community services, Yet, health promotion and illness prevention will be key to reducing healthcare costs and to ensuring our communities are in the healthiest state possible. CHNs must envision what role they can play as leaders and change agents as they plan and implement appropriate care for their community clients.

We must stress the importance of using frameworks such as the determinants of health to assist CHNs in proactively planning for the future and positioning ourselves as co-creators of change in practice. We must envision what community health is and go beyond local and national needs. CHNs must be well informed of how socioeconomic and political trends and environmental changes such as global warming may impact the health of various communities.

Some steps have already been taken at the national level. In response to many factors, including public inquiries into specific disease outbreaks and other reports, investments were accomplished in public health at the national level. Thus there was the creation of the Public Health Agency of Canada (PHAC), the creation of the position of Chief Public Health Officer, and also the identification of a federal cabinet minister for public health. The PHAC has been working with practitioners to develop a set of core competencies for all workers in public health, as well as specific competencies for individual professions, in collaboration with the Community Health Nurses Association of Canada (CHNAC) Standards of Practice (2008) (see Appendix A). The standards and competencies are complementary documents, describing the desired practice of a nurse with two years of experience in community health. Since the second edition of this book, the renamed Community Health Nurses of Canada (CHNC) has published *Public Health Nursing Discipline Specific Competencies* (2009) and *Home Health Nursing Competencies* (2010) (see Appendices B and C). Finally, CHNC has partnered with the Canadian Nurses Association (CNA) to create a nursing certification in community health nursing, incorporating both public health and home health nursing. Nursing graduates have the opportunity to achieve initial and continuing certification through examination and continuing education.

Concerns about nursing shortages are not limited to acute-care facilities. Community health nurses are particularly disadvantaged in that nurses in this practice area have a higher average age than nurses in other practice arenas (Underwood, et al., 2009). At this time there are difficulties providing sufficient numbers of practitioners to fulfill current needs, much less a new future. One way to accomplish this task is to increase the number of nursing students in basic programs. However, this capacity building is not limited to increasing the numbers of nursing students, but also to increasing the number of faculty members (and, in some cases, enhancing their skills) to produce the numbers of community nurses required to influence the health of Canadians. Further, increased globalization has forced our profession to consider such things as ethical hiring practices for international nurses, and global standards for basic nursing education.

As well, there are changes in community nursing education. Community nursing has always been part of a baccalaureate nursing curriculum, with a broad-based approach and the individual, family, group, aggregate, and population identified as clients. Public health nursing is identified as having a stronger focus on population health. However, there are both challenges and new opportunities peeking over the horizon. The Canadian Association of Schools of Nursing created a task force that has since become a permanent sub-committee specifically related to public health education. Members of the sub-committee are working with nurse educators, employers, and other stakeholders to examine the competencies and standards as they apply to new graduates, and how that might change basic nursing curricula. They have also created guidelines for the selection of appropriate clinical sites for students engaged in community nursing courses (CASN, 2010). The Canadian Nurse Practitioner Initiative (CNPI) from the CNA has worked with provincial organizations and schools of nursing to create curricula for primary health care nurse practitioner programs. A progress report with recommendations was published in 2009, and CNA appointed a task force to continue this work. Once again, leadership by nurses is contributing to the competence of the profession and healthcare for all.

Graduate opportunities are also increasing in number, scope, and variety. Specific to community nursing, graduate nursing students have opportunities to tailor Master's in Nursing degrees to a community specialty or to consider one of the new interdisciplinary Master's in Public Health programs that are springing up across the country. In addition, schools of public health are recently begun in several universities—representing additional opportunities for advanced interdisciplinary work and research in community health with a strong nursing contribution. Research in community nursing is also increasing. Throughout this book you have seen examples of Canadian nursing research addressing various aspects of community nursing care. You will notice that there are some areas where very recent Canadian nursing research is simply not available, a testament to the need for additional researchers and research funding to support studies. It is research into excellence in both practice and education that assists nursing to be proactive in building capacity and in translating knowledge to practice, in line with the patient-oriented research strategy mentioned earlier. This translation is one of community nursing's strengths. We add to the national picture and research efforts through the knowledge and data of our local communities, and then, when national priorities and strategies have been formulated, we tailor them to our local communities to enhance success. We are the health profession that clearly contributes to both arenas. At the end, the concerted efforts played by all community nursing educators, researchers, and practitioners will benefit the communities we care for.

So, what of the future? As each of us gazes into our cloudy crystal ball, a few things are discernable. One is that nurses, including CHNs, have the skills and knowledge to be a political force for the health of Canadians, if we so choose. By supporting our professional organizations at home and globally, by being proactive in the political process, and by using our knowledge to affect and effect healthy public policy, we can contribute significantly to influencing the movement and direction of healthcare in Canada.

In addition, CHNs now nurse a global community. Though it will be up to us to make a concerted effort to ensure that our voices are heard and that we stand together to protect the health of Canadians, we must, at the same time, position ourselves and partner with nurses in other countries to influence and support healthcare on a global scale. The challenges of preparing practitioners in community health nursing and producing the evidence on which our practice is based will continue to arise. And at the heart of it all will be our nurse–client relationships, with a focus to promote and protect the health of the community. What an exciting future to behold!

REFERENCES

Canadian Association of Schools of Nursing. (2010). *Guidelines for quality community health nursing clinical placements.* Retrieved from http://casn.ca/en/Public_Health_123/items/5.html

Canadian Institute for Health Information. (CIHI). (2010). Regulated nurses in Canada: Trends of registered nurses. In *CIHIR regulated nurses: Canadian trends.* Retrieved from http://secure.cihi.ca/cihiweb/products/chapter_1_rn_2004_to_2008_e.pdf

Canadian Institutes of Health Research (CIHR). (2010). *Strategy on patient-oriented research.* Retrieved from http://www.cihr-irsc.gc.ca/e/41204.html

Canadian Nurses Association (CNA). (2009). *Recommendations of the Canadian nurse practitioner initiative: Progress report.* Retrieved from http://www.cna-aiic.ca/can/documents/pdf/publications/CNPI_report_2009_e.pdf

Community Health Nurses of Canada. (2009). *Public health nurses discipline specific competencies.* Retrieved from http://www.chnc.ca/documents/competencies_june_2009_english.pdf

Community Health Nurses of Canada. (2010). *Home health nursing competencies.* Retrieved from http://www.chnc.ca/documents/HomeHealthNursingCompetenciesVersion 1March2010.pdf

Underwood, J. M., Mowat, D. L., Meagher-Stewart, D. M., Deber, R. B., Baumann, A. O., MacDonald, M. B., . . . Munroe, V. J. (2009, September/October). Building community and public health nursing capacity: A synthesis report of the national community health nursing study. *Canadian Journal of Public Health, 100*(5), 11.

Villeneuve, M., & MacDonald, J. (2006). *Towards 2020: Visions for nursing.* Ottawa, ON: Canadian Nurses Association.

About the Authors

Lynnette Leeseberg Stamler, RN, PhD, is a Full Professor and Assistant Dean, College of Nursing, University of Saskatchewan. She has degrees from Olaf College, Minnesota (BSN), the University of Manitoba (MEd – Health Education), and the University of Cincinnati (PhD – Nursing). Her research interests include patient/health education, breast health, diabetes education, nursing education, and most recently, quality care. She was a VON nurse for four years prior to her career in nursing education. She has been active in research and professional nursing organizations including Sigma Theta Tau International, the Nursing Honor Society. She was President of the Canadian Association of Schools of Nursing from 2008–2010.

Lucia Yiu, BScN, BA (University of Windsor), BSc (University of Toronto), MScN (University of Western Ontario), is an Associate Professor in the Faculty of Nursing, University of Windsor, and an Educational and Training Consultant in community nursing. Her practice and research include multicultural health, international health, experiential learning, community development, breast health, and program planning and evaluation.

Appendix A: Canadian Community Health Nursing Standards of Practice

COMMUNITY HEALTH NURSING

Evolving from centuries of community care by laywomen and members of religious orders, community health nursing started to gain recognition as a nursing specialty in the mid-1800s. Community health nursing has been indelibly shaped by such remarkable nurses as Florence Nightingale and Lillian Wald and organizations such as the Victorian Order of Nurses, the Henry Street Settlement and the Canadian Red Cross Society. During the 20th century public health and home health nursing emerged from common roots to represent the ideals of community health nursing. Community health nursing respects its roots and traditions while embracing advances and continually evolving as a dynamic nursing specialty.

Community health nurses are registered nurses whose practice specialty promotes the health of individuals, families, communities and populations, and an environment that supports health. They practice in diverse settings such as homes, schools, shelters, churches, community health centres and on the street. Their position titles may vary as much as their practice settings.

The practice of community health nursing combines nursing theory and knowledge, social sciences and public health science with primary health care. Community health nurses view disease prevention, health protection and health promotion as goals of professional nursing practice (Smith, 1990). They collaborate with individuals, families, groups, communities and populations to design and carry out community development, health promotion and disease prevention strategies. They identify and promote care decisions that build on the capacity of the individual or community. A critical part of their practice is to mobilize resources to support health by coordinating care and planning services, programs and policies with individuals, caregivers, families, other disciplines, organizations, communities and government(s).

Community health nursing is rooted in caring (Canadian Nurses Association, 1998). The social conscience expressed in community health nursing has been reflected in public policies such as the Canada Health Act (Government of Canada, 1984), the Ottawa Charter for Health Promotion (World Health Organization, Canadian Public Health Association, Health and Welfare Canada, 1986) and the Jakarta Declaration (World Health Organization, 1997).

Community health nursing concepts and competencies are essential to community-focused nursing practice and the practices of all nurses concerned with promoting and preserving the health of populations.

Mission

Community health nurses view health as a resource for everyday living. Their practice promotes, protects and preserves the health of individuals, families, groups, communities and populations wherever they live, work, learn, worship and play, in an ongoing rather than an episodic process (Cradduck, 2000). Their practice is based on a unique understanding of how the environmental context influences health. Community health nurses work at a high level of autonomy and build partnerships based on the principles of primary health care, caring and empowerment.

Values and Beliefs

The following values and beliefs are based on Canadian Nurses Association's Code of Ethics for Registered Nurses (2002a) and interpreted from the community health nursing perspective. The community health nurse values and believes in

Caring Community health nurses recognize that caring is an essential and universal human need and that its expression in practice varies across cultures and practice domains. In community health nursing practice in Canada, caring is based on the principle of social justice. Community health nurses support equity and the fundamental right of all humans to accessible, competent health care and essential determinants of health. Caring community health nursing practice acknowledges the physical, spiritual, emotional and cognitive nature of individuals, families, groups and communities. Caring is expressed through competent practice and development of relationships that value the individual and community as unique and worthy of a nurse's "presence" and attention. Community health nurses preserve, protect and enhance human dignity in all of their interactions.

The Principles of Primary Health Care Primary health care represents a fundamentally different way of thinking about health and health care for community health nurses and their practice. Primary health care differs significantly from primary care (first point of access to care) and is an integral part of the Canadian health care system. Community health nurses value the following key principles of primary health care as described by the World Health Organization (1978):

- universal access to health care services
- focus on the determinants of health
- active participation by individuals and communities in decisions that affect their health and life

- partnership with other disciplines, communities and sectors for health
- appropriate use of knowledge, skills, strategies, technology and resources
- focus on health promotion and illness prevention throughout the life experience

Community health nurses recognize the impact of the social, political and economic environment on the health of individuals and the community, and on their own practice.

Multiple Ways of Knowing Community health nurses integrate multiple types of knowledge into their practice. Five fundamental ways of knowing in nursing have been identified: aesthetics, empirics, personal knowledge, ethics and socio-political knowledge (Carper, 1978; White, 1995). Each type is an essential part of the integrated knowledge base of community health nursing practice:

- *Aesthetics*, the art of nursing, means adapting knowledge and practice to particular rather than universal circumstances. It encourages nurses to explore possibilities, promotes individual creativity and style, and contributes to the transformative power of community health nursing.
- *Empirics*, the science of community health nursing, includes research, epidemiology and theories and models (incorporating publicly verifiable, factual descriptions, explanations and predictions based on subjective and objective data). Empirical knowledge is generated and tested by scientific research (Fawcett, Watson, Neuman & Hinton, 2001).
- *Personal knowledge*, the most fundamental way of knowing, comes from discovery of self, values and morals and lived experience. It involves continuous learning through reflective practice. Reflective practice in community health nursing combines critical examination of practice, interpersonal relationships and intuition to evaluate, adapt and enhance practice.
- *Ethics*, or moral knowledge, describes the moral obligations, values and goals of community health nursing. It is guided by moral principles and ethical standards set by the Canadian Nurses Association (2002). Ethical inquiry clarifies values and beliefs and uses dialogue to examine the social and political impact of community health nursing on the health environment (Fawcett et al., 2001).
- *Socio-political knowledge*, or emancipatory knowing, goes beyond personal knowing and nurse–client introspection. It places nursing within the broader social, political and economic context where nursing and health care happen. It equips the nurse to question the status quo and structures of domination in society that affect the health of individuals and communities.

Each way of knowing is necessary to understand the complexity and diversity of nursing in the community. By integrating multiple ways of knowing into the practice of community health nursing, the individual nurse becomes a co-creator of nursing knowledge. Critical examination of this nursing knowledge contributes to evidence-based community health nursing practice. By recognizing diverse evidence for practice, community health nursing is able to question and move beyond the status quo, evolve and create relevant and effective action for community health.

Individual and Community Partnership Community health nurses believe that the individual or community must be an active partner in decisions that affect their health and well-being. Their participation is essential throughout the nursing process: to define their own health needs during assessment, set their own priorities among health goals, control the choice and use of various actions to improve their health and lives, and evaluate the efforts made. Community health nurses identify the health values of the individual or community throughout the nursing process, including what health means to that particular individual or community.

Community health nurses work with individuals and communities to build capacity so they can participate in and make decisions about their health. For community health nurses this participation is the basis of therapeutic, professional, caring relationships that promote empowerment. Community health nurses also make their expertise available as a resource to people they work with. Along with capacity building work, community health nurses have an advocacy role and responsibility. Their knowledge and experience equip them to advocate in partnership with clients who are vulnerable or intimidated in a particular situation and help them to access services (case advocacy). Community health nurses also advocate for changes in policies, systems and resource allocation (class advocacy) to increase opportunities for health within society (Pope, Snyder & Mood, 1995).

Empowerment Community health nurses recognize that empowerment is an active, involved process where people, groups and communities move towards increased individual and community control, political efficacy, improved quality of community life and social justice. Empowerment is a community concept because individual empowerment builds from working with others to produce change and wanting increased freedom of choice for others and society. Empowerment is not something that can be done to or for people—it involves people discovering and using their own strengths.

Empowering strategies or environments (e.g., healthy workplaces that support flex time or exercise) build capacity by helping individuals, groups and communities discover their strengths and ability to take action to improve their quality of life.

Community Health Nursing

While community health nursing concepts and competencies are part of the practices of nurses with varied functions and position titles across Canada, these practice standards apply directly to home health and public health nursing. Home health and public health nursing are linked historically through common beliefs, values, traditions, skills and above all their unique focus on promoting and protecting community health. Home health and public health nursing differ in their client and program emphasis.

A home health nurse is a community health nurse who

- combines knowledge from primary health care (including the determinants of health), nursing science and social sciences
- focuses on prevention, health restoration, maintenance or palliation
- focuses on clients, their designated caregivers and their families
- integrates health promotion, teaching and counseling in clinical care and treatment
- initiates, manages and evaluates the resources needed for the client to reach optimal well-being and function
- provides care in the client's home, school or workplace
- has a nursing diploma or a degree (a baccalaureate degree in nursing is preferred)

A public health nurse is a community health nurse who

- combines knowledge from public health science, primary health care (including the determinants of health), nursing science and social sciences
- focuses on promoting, protecting and preserving the health of populations
- focuses on populations and links health and illness experiences of individuals, families and communities to population health promotion practice
- recognizes that a community's health is closely linked with the health of its members and is often reflected first in individual and family health experiences
- recognizes that healthy communities and systems that support health contribute to opportunities for health for individuals, families, groups and populations

- practices in increasingly diverse settings, such as community health centres, schools, street clinics, youth centres and nursing outposts—and with diverse partners—to meet the health needs of specific populations
- has a baccalaureate degree in nursing

The relationship between home health nursing and public health nursing practice is like the shifting lens of a camera. Home health nurses begin with a close-up lens, zooming in and focusing on the individual client and family, and then shift to a wide-angle lens to include groups and supports in the community. Public health nurses shift from a wide-angle lens looking at systems, population health and intersectoral partnerships to a close-up lens focusing on the health of individual clients and families.

THE CANADIAN COMMUNITY HEALTH NURSING PRACTICE MODEL

Understanding the community health nursing process and its evidence and knowledge base is essential for practicing community health nursing. The Canadian Community Health Nursing Practice Model (Figure 1) has been developed specifically for this standards document to reflect the knowledge and experience of community health nurses in practice, education, research and administration across Canada. The model illustrates the dynamic nature of community health nursing practice, embracing the present and projecting into the future.

The model shows the five standards of practice embracing the values and beliefs of community health nurses [dark orange], the community health nursing process [light orange] and the environmental context of community health nursing practice. The focus of community health nursing is always on

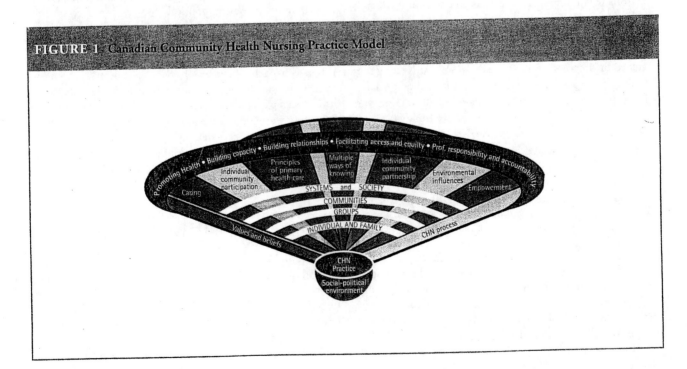

FIGURE 1 Canadian Community Health Nursing Practice Model

improving the health of people in the community and encouraging change in systems or society to support health.

The Canadian Community Health Nursing Standards of Practice form the core expectations for community health nursing practice. The five interrelated standards for community health nursing are

1. Promoting health
2. Building individual and community capacity
3. Building relationships
4. Facilitating access and equity
5. Demonstrating professional responsibility and accountability

These standards are based on the values and beliefs of community health nursing, nursing knowledge and partnerships with people in the community. They apply to practice in all settings where people live, work, learn, worship and play.

The values and beliefs ground community health nursing practice in the present and guide its development over time. The practice standards and community health nursing process reflect community health nursing's philosophical base and foundational values and beliefs: caring, the principles of primary health care, multiple ways of knowing, individual and community partnerships and empowerment.

The community health nursing process (CHN process) represents how community health nurses work with people and put the standards into practice. The community health nursing process includes the traditional nursing process components of assessment, planning, intervention and evaluation. Community health nurses enhance this process through

- individual or community participation in each component multiple ways of knowing
- awareness of the influence of the broader environment on the individual or community that is the focus of their care (e.g., the community will be affected by provincial or territorial policies, its own economic status and the actions of its individual citizens)

Community health nursing practice does not happen in isolation but within an environmental context (socio-political environment). It is influenced by social, economic and political forces that shape legislation and public policies. Community health nursing practice is delivered through several agencies such as provincial or municipal departments of health, regional health authorities and non-governmental organizations. Community health nurses are accountable to a variety of authorities and stakeholders (e.g., regulatory bodies, employers and the public). Their practice is influenced by multiple legislative and policy mandates (mostly provincial or territorial in nature and both internal and external to their work situation). The organizations community health nurses work for also influence their practice through their organizational structures, processes, values and principles, policies, goals, objectives, standards and outcomes. These diverse influences can be enabling factors, or they may constrain how community health nursing is practiced.

COMMUNITY HEALTH NURSING PRACTICE

All community health nurses are expected to know and use the following standards of practice:

1. Promoting health
   a) Health promotion
   b) Prevention and health protection
   c) Health maintenance, restoration and palliation
2. Building individual and community capacity
3. Building relationships
4. Facilitating access and equity
5. Demonstrating professional responsibility and accountability

These standards apply to community health nurses working in practice, education, administration or research. The standards set a benchmark for new community health nurses and become basic practice expectations after two years of experience. The practice of expert community health nurses will extend beyond these standards. Each standard applies to the practice of home health nurses and public health nurses—nurses may emphasize different elements of specific standards according to their practice focus.

Each practice standard contains

- the standard statement
- a description of the standard in the context of community health nursing
- indicators (activities) that show how community health nurses apply and meet this standard

The list of indicators or activities for each standard begins with the heading "The community health nurse." They are based on the four components of the nursing process—assessment, planning, intervention and evaluation—and provide criteria for measuring the actual performance of an individual nurse. The standards and indicators combine to describe and distinguish the specific practice of community health nursing.

Standard 1: Promoting Health

Community health nurses view health as a dynamic process of physical, mental, spiritual and social well-being. Health includes self-determination and a sense of connection to the community. Community health nurses believe that individuals and communities realize hopes and satisfy needs within their cultural, social, economic and physical environments. They consider health as a resource for everyday life that is influenced by circumstances, beliefs and the determinants of health. Social, economic and environmental health determinants include: (Health Canada, 2000)

- income and social status
- social support networks
- education
- employment and working conditions
- social environments
- physical environments
- biology and genetic endowment
- personal health practices and coping skills
- healthy child development
- health services
- gender
- culture

Community health nurses promote health using the following strategies: (a) health promotion, (b) prevention and health protection and (c) health maintenance, restoration and palliation. They recognize they may need to use these strategies together when providing care and services. This standard incorporates these strategies from the frameworks of primary health care (World Health Organization, 1978), the Ottawa Charter for Health Promotion (World Health Organization, 1986) and the Population Health Promotion Model (Health Canada, 2000).

a) Health Promotion Community health nurses focus on health promotion and the health of populations. Health promotion is a mediating strategy between people and their environments. It is a positive, dynamic, empowering and unifying concept based in the socio-environmental approach to health. It recognizes that basic resources and conditions for health are critical for achieving health. The population's health is closely linked with the health of its members and is often reflected first in individual and family experiences from birth to death. Community health nurses also consider socio-political issues that may be underlying individual and community problems. Healthy communities and systems support increased options for well-being in society.

The Community Health Nurse
1. Collaborates with individual, community and other stakeholders to do a holistic assessment of assets and needs of the individual or community.
2. Uses a variety of information sources to access data and research findings related to health at the national, provincial, territorial, regional and local levels.
3. Identifies and seeks to address root causes of illness and disease.
4. Facilitates planned change with the individual, community or population by applying the Population Health Promotion Model.
   - Identifies the level of intervention necessary to promote health.
   - Identifies which determinants of health require action or change to promote health.
   - Uses a comprehensive range of strategies to address health-related issues.

5. Demonstrates knowledge of and effectively implements health promotion strategies based on the Ottawa Charter for Health Promotion.
   - Incorporates multiple strategies: promoting healthy public policy, strengthening community action, creating supportive environments, developing personal skills and reorienting the health system.
   - Identifies strategies for change that will make it easier for people to make healthier choices.
6. Collaborates with the individual and community to help them take responsibility for maintaining or improving their health by increasing their knowledge, influence and control over the determinants of health.
7. Understands and uses social marketing, media and advocacy strategies to raise awareness of health issues, place issues on the public agenda, shift social norms and change behaviours if other enabling factors are present.
8. Helps the individual and community to identify their strengths and available resources and take action to address their needs.
9. Recognizes the broad impact of specific issues on health promotion such as political climate and will, values and culture, individual and community readiness, and social and systemic structures.
10. Evaluates and modifies population health promotion programs in partnership with the individual, community and other stakeholders.

b) Prevention and Health Protection The community health nurse applies a range of activities to minimize the occurrence of diseases or injuries and their consequences for individuals and communities. Governments often make health protection strategies mandated programs and laws for their overall jurisdictions.

The Community Health Nurse
1. Recognizes the differences between the levels of prevention (primary, secondary, tertiary).
2. Selects the appropriate level of preventive intervention.
3. Helps individuals and communities make informed choices about protective and preventive health measures such as immunization, birth control, breastfeeding and palliative care.
4. Helps individuals, groups, families and communities to identify potential risks to health.
5. Uses harm reduction principles to identify, reduce or remove risk factors in a variety of contexts including the home, neighbourhood, workplace, school and street.
6. Applies epidemiological principles when using strategies such as screening, surveillance, immunization, communicable disease response and outbreak management, and education.
7. Engages collaborative, interdisciplinary and intersectoral partnerships to address risks to individual, family, community or population health and to address prevention and protection issues such as communicable disease, injury and chronic disease.

8. Collaborates on developing and using follow-up systems in the practice setting to ensure that the individual or community receives appropriate and effective service.
9. Practices in accordance with legislation relevant to community health practice (e.g., public health legislation and child protection legislation).
10. Evaluates collaborative practice (personal, team and intersectoral) for achieving individual and community outcomes such as reduced communicable disease, injury, chronic disease or impacts of a disease process.

c) Health Maintenance, Restoration and Palliation

Community health nurses provide clinical nursing care, health education and counselling to individuals, families, groups and populations whether they are seeking to maintain their health or dealing with acute, chronic or terminal illness. Community health nurses practice in health centres, homes, schools and other community-based settings. They link people to community resources and coordinate or facilitate other care needs and supports. The activities of the community health nurse may range from health screening and care planning at an individual level to intersectoral collaboration and resource development at the community and population level.

The Community Health Nurse

1. Assesses the health status and functional competence of the individual, family or population within the context of their environmental and social supports.
2. Develops a mutually agreed upon plan and priorities for care with the individual and family.
3. Identifies a range of interventions including health promotion, disease prevention and direct clinical care strategies (including palliation), along with short- and long-term goals and outcomes.
4. Maximizes the ability of an individual, family or community to take responsibility for and manage their health needs according to resources and personal skills available.
5. Supports informed choice and respects the individual, family or community's specific requests while acknowledging diversity, unique characteristics and abilities.
6. Adapts community health nursing techniques, approaches and procedures as appropriate to the challenges in a particular community situation or setting.
7. Uses knowledge of the community to link with, refer to or develop appropriate community resources.
8. Recognizes patterns and trends in epidemiological data and service delivery and initiates strategies for improvement.
9. Facilitates maintenance of health and the healing process for individuals, families and communities in response to significant health emergencies or other community situations that negatively impact health.
10. Evaluates individual, family and community outcomes systematically and continuously in collaboration with individuals, families, significant others, community partners and other health practitioners.

Standard 2: Building Individual and Community Capacity

Building capacity is the process of actively involving individuals, groups, organizations and communities in all phases of planned change to increase their skills, knowledge and willingness to take action on their own in the future. The community health nurse works collaboratively with the individual or community affected by health-compromising situations and with the people and organizations that control resources. Starting where the individual or community is, community health nurses identify relevant issues, assess resources and strengths, and determine readiness for change and priorities for action. They take collaborative action by building on identified strengths and involving key stakeholders such as individuals, organizations, community leaders. They work with people to improve the determinants of health and "make it easier to make the healthier choice." Community health nurses use supportive and empowering strategies to move individuals and communities toward maximum autonomy.

The Community Health Nurse

1. Works collaboratively with the individual, community, other professionals, agencies and sectors to identify needs, strengths and available resources.
2. Facilitates action in support of the five priorities of the Jakarta Declaration to
   - promote social responsibility for health
   - increase investments for health development
   - expand partnerships for health promotion
   - increase individual and community capacity
   - secure an infrastructure for health promotion
3. Uses community development principles.
   - Engages the individual and community in a consultative process.
   - Recognizes and builds on the readiness of the group or community to participate.
   - Uses empowering strategies such as mutual goal setting, visioning and facilitation.
   - Understands group dynamics and effectively uses facilitation skills to support group development.
   - Helps the individual and community to participate in the resolution of their issues.
   - Helps the group and community to gather available resources to support taking action on their health issues.
4. Uses a comprehensive mix of community and population-based strategies such as coalition building, intersectoral partnerships and networking to address concerns of groups or populations.
5. Supports the individual, family, community or population to develop skills for self-advocacy.
6. Applies principles of social justice and engages in advocacy to support those who are not yet able to take action for themselves.
7. Uses a comprehensive mix of interventions and strategies to customize actions to address unique needs and build individual and community capacity.

8. Supports community action to influence policy change in support of health.
9. Actively works with health professionals and community partners to build capacity for health promotion.
10. Evaluates the impact of change on individual or community control and health outcomes.

Standard 3: Building Relationships

Community health nurses build relationships based on the principles of connecting and caring. Connecting involves establishing and nurturing relationships and a supportive environment that promotes the maximum participation and self-determination of the individual, family and community. Caring involves developing empowering relationships that preserve, protect and enhance human dignity. Community health nurses build caring relationships based on mutual respect and understanding of the power inherent in their position and its potential impact on relationships and practice. One of the unique challenges of community health nursing is building a network of relationships and partnerships with a wide variety of relevant groups, communities and organizations. These relationships happen within a complex, changing and often ambiguous environment with sometimes conflicting and unpredictable circumstances.

The Community Health Nurse

1. Recognizes her or his personal beliefs, attitudes, assumptions, feelings and values about health and their potential effect on interventions with individuals and communities.
2. Identifies the individual and community beliefs, attitudes, feelings and values about health and their potential effect on the relationship and intervention.
3. Is aware of and uses culturally relevant communication when building relationships. Communication may be verbal or non-verbal, written or graphic. It may involve face-to-face, telephone, group facilitation, print or electronic methods.
4. Respects and trusts the ability of the individual or community to know the issue they are addressing and solve their own problems.
5. Involves the individual, family and community as an active partner to identify relevant needs, perspectives and expectations.
6. Establishes connections and collaborative relationships with health professionals, community organizations, businesses, faith communities, volunteer service organizations and other sectors to address health-related issues.
7. Maintains awareness of community resources, values and characteristics.
8. Promotes and supports linkages with appropriate community resources when the individual or community is ready to receive them (e.g., hospice or palliative care, parenting groups).

9. Maintains professional boundaries in often long-term relationships in the home or other community settings where professional and social relationships may become blurred.
10. Negotiates an end to the relationship when appropriate (e.g., when the client assumes self-care or when the goals for the relationship have been achieved).

Standard 4: Facilitating Access and Equity

Community health nurses embrace the philosophy of primary health care. They collaboratively identify and facilitate universal and equitable access to available services. They collaborate with colleagues and with other members of the health care team to promote effective working relationships that contribute to comprehensive client care and optimal client care outcomes. They are keenly aware of the impact of the determinants of health on individuals, families, groups, communities and populations. The practice of community health nursing considers the financial resources, geography and culture of the individual and community.

Community health nurses engage in advocacy by analyzing the determinants of health and influencing other sectors to ensure their policies and programs have a positive impact on health. Community health nurses use advocacy as a key strategy to meet identified needs and enhance individual and community capacity for self-advocacy.

The Community Health Nurse

1. Assesses and understands individual and community capacities including norms, values, beliefs, knowledge, resources and power structures.
2. Provides culturally sensitive care in diverse communities and settings.
3. Supports individuals and communities in their choice to access alternate health care options.
4. Advocates for appropriate resource allocation for individuals, groups and populations to support access to conditions for health and health services.
5. Refers, coordinates or facilitates access to services in the health sector and other sectors.
6. Adapts practice in response to the changing health needs of the individual and community.
7. Collaborates with individuals and communities to identify and provide programs and delivery methods that are acceptable to them and responsive to their needs across the life span and in different circumstances.
8. Uses strategies such as home visits, outreach and case finding to ensure access to services and health-supporting conditions for potentially vulnerable populations (e.g., persons who are ill, elderly, young, poor, immigrants, isolated or have communication barriers).
9. Assesses the impact of the determinants of health on the opportunity for health for individuals, families, communities and populations.

10. Advocates for healthy public policy by participating in legislative and policy-making activities that influence health determinants and access to services.
11. Takes action with and for individuals and communities at the organizational, municipal, provincial, territorial and federal levels to address service gaps and accessibility issues.
12. Monitors and evaluates changes and progress in access to the determinants of health and appropriate community services.

Standard 5: Demonstrating Professional Responsibility and Accountability

Community health nurses work with a high degree of autonomy when providing programs and services. Their professional accountability includes striving for excellence, ensuring that their knowledge is evidence-based and current, and maintaining competence and the overall quality of their practice. Community health nurses are responsible for initiating strategies that will help address the determinants of health and generate a positive impact on people and systems.

Community health nurses are accountable to a variety of authorities and stakeholders as well as to the individual and community they serve. This range of accountabilities places them in a variety of situations with unique ethical dilemmas. One dilemma might be whether responsibility for an issue lies with the individual, family, community or population, or with the nurse or the nurse's employer. Other dilemmas include the priority of one individual's rights over the rights of another, individual or societal good, allocation of scarce resources and quality versus quantity of life.

The Community Health Nurse
1. Takes preventive or corrective action individually or in partnership to protect individuals and communities from unsafe or unethical circumstances.
2. Advocates for societal change in support of health for all.
3. Uses nursing informatics (including information and communication technology) to generate, manage and process relevant data to support nursing practice.
4. Identifies and takes action on factors which affect autonomy of practice and quality of care.
5. Participates in the advancement of community health nursing by mentoring students and new practitioners.
6. Participates in research and professional activities.
7. Makes decisions using ethical standards and principles, taking into consideration the tension between individual versus societal good and the responsibility to uphold the greater good of all people or the population as a whole.
8. Seeks help with problem solving as needed to determine the best course of action in response to ethical dilemmas, risks to human rights and freedoms, new situations and new knowledge.
9. Identifies and works proactively—through personal advocacy and participation in relevant professional associations—to address nursing issues that will affect the population.
10. Contributes proactively to the quality of the work environment by identifying needs, issues and solutions, mobilizing colleagues and actively participating in team and organizational structures and mechanisms.
11. Provides constructive feedback to peers as appropriate to enhance community health nursing practice.
12. Documents community health nursing activities in a timely and thorough manner, including telephone advice and work with communities and groups.
13. Advocates for effective and efficient use of community health nursing resources.
14. Uses reflective practice to continually assess and improve personal community health nursing practice.
15. Seeks professional development experiences that are consistent with current community health nursing practice, new and emerging issues, the changing needs of the population, the evolving impact of the determinants of health and emerging research.
16. Acts upon legal obligations to report to appropriate authorities any situations of unsafe or unethical care provided by family, friends or other individuals to children or vulnerable adults.
17. Uses available resources to systematically evaluate the availability, acceptability, quality, efficiency and effectiveness of community health nursing practice.

Appendix B: Public Health Nursing Discipline Specific Competencies

Public Health Nursing Competencies are the integrated knowledge, skills, judgement and attributes required of a public health nurse to practice safely and ethically. Attributes include, but are not limited to attitudes, values and beliefs. (Canadian Nurses Association Code of Ethics, 2008)

1. PUBLIC HEALTH AND NURSING SCIENCES

This category includes key knowledge and critical thinking skills related to: the public health sciences (behavioural and social sciences, biostatistics, epidemiology, environmental public health, demography, workplace health, prevention of chronic diseases, infectious diseases, psychosocial problems and injuries) as well as nursing theory, change theory, economics, politics, public health administration, community assessment, management theory, program planning and evaluation, population health principles, community development theory, and the history of public health. Competency in this category requires the ability to apply knowledge in practice.

A public health nurse is able to . . .

1.1 Apply knowledge about the following concepts: the health status of populations; inequities in health; the determinants of health and illness; social justice; principles of primary health care; strategies for health promotion; disease and injury prevention; health protection, as well as the factors that influence the delivery and use of health services.

1.2 Apply knowledge about the history, structure and interaction of public health and health care services at local, provincial/territorial, national, and international levels.

1.3 Apply public health and nursing sciences to practice and synthesize knowledge from a broad range of theories, models and frameworks.

1.4 Critically appraise knowledge gathered from a variety of sources.

1.5 Use evidence and research to inform health policies, programs and practice:

  ▪ contribute to the development and generation of evidence-based nursing
  ▪ use available resources to systematically plan and evaluate public health nursing practice

1.6 Pursue lifelong learning opportunities in the field of public health that are consistent with: current public health nursing practice; new and emerging issues; the changing needs of individuals, families, groups and communities; emerging research and evolving information about the impact of the determinants of health.

1.7 Integrate multiple ways of knowing into practice.

2. ASSESSMENT AND ANALYSIS

This category describes the core competencies needed to collect, assess, analyze and apply information (including data, facts, concepts and theories). These competencies are required to make evidence-based decisions, prepare budgets and reports, conduct investigations and make recommendations for policy and program development. Community members are involved in identifying and reinforcing those aspects of everyday life, culture and political activity that are conducive to health.

A public health nurse is able to . . .

2.1 Recognize that a health concern or issue exists:

  ▪ apply principles of epidemiology
  ▪ conduct comprehensive community assessments with individuals, families, groups and communities using quantitative and qualitative strategies
  ▪ recognize patterns and trends in epidemiological data and service delivery
  ▪ assess the impact of the broad social, cultural, political and economic determinants of health.

2.2 Identify relevant and appropriate sources of information, including community assets, resources and values in collaboration with individuals, families, groups, communities and stakeholders.

2.3 Collect, store, retrieve and use accurate and appropriate information on public health issues.

2.4 Analyze information to determine appropriate implications, uses, gaps and limitations.

2.5 Assess impact of specific issues on health such as political climate and will; values and culture; social and systemic structures; settings; as well as the individual, family, group, and community's readiness and capacity.

2.6 Assess the health status and functional competence of individuals, families, groups, communities or populations within the context of their environmental and social supports.

2.7 Determine the meaning of information, considering the ethical, political, scientific, socio-cultural and economic contexts:

  ▪ identify attitudes, beliefs, feelings and values about health and their effect on relationships and interventions

- support individuals, families, groups and communities to identify risks to health and make informed choices about protective and preventive health measures
- describe the role of power in relationships by giving voice to the vulnerable
- demonstrate skill in dealing with diversity and high levels of ambiguity.

2.8 Recommend specific actions based on the analysis of information:

- identify a range of appropriate interventions including health promotion; health protection; disease and injury prevention and clinical care using a multi strategy and multi target approach
- identify short and long term goals
- identify outcome indicators
- identify research questions.

2.9 Recognize opportunities to promote social justice.

3. POLICY AND PROGRAM PLANNING, IMPLEMENTATION AND EVALUATION

This category describes the core competencies needed to effectively choose options, and to plan, implement and evaluate policies and/or programs in public health. This includes the management of incidents such as outbreaks and emergencies.

3(A). Policy Development

A public health nurse is able to . . .

3A.1 Describe selected policy options to address a specific public health issue.

3A.2 Describe the implications of each policy option, especially as they apply to the determinants of health and recommend or decide on a course of action.

3A.3 Develop a plan to implement a course of action taking into account relevant evidence, legislation, emergency planning procedures, regulations and policies.

3A.4 Implement a policy.

3A.5 Support community action to influence policy change.

3A.6 Build community capacity to improve health and address health inequities.

3A.7 Advocate for healthy public policy and services that promote and protect the health and well-being of individuals, families, groups and communities.

3A.8 Advocate for the reduction of inequities in health through legislative and policy making activities.

3(B). Program Planning

A public health nurse is able to . . .

3B.1 Describe selected program options to address a specific public health issue.

3B.2 Describe the implications of each option, especially as they apply to the determinants of health and recommend or decide on a course of action.

3B.3 Develop a plan in collaboration with individuals, families, groups and communities to implement a course of action that is responsive to needs taking into account relevant evidence, legislation, emergency planning procedures, regulations and policies.

3(C). Implementation and Intervention

A public health nurse is able to . . .

3C.1 Take action, across multiple levels, to address specific public health issues by using a comprehensive mix of public health strategies to address unique needs and to build individual, family, group and community capacity.

3C.2 Facilitate planned change with individuals, families, groups, communities, systems or population(s) by applying the Population Health Promotion Model, primary health care principles and appropriate change theory.

3C.3 Demonstrate the ability to integrate relevant research and implement evidence informed practice.

3C.4 Participate in collaborative, interdisciplinary and intersectoral partnerships to enhance the health of individuals, families, groups, communities and populations.

3C.5 Maximize the capacity of the individual, family, group or community to take responsibility for and to manage their health needs according to resources available and personal skills.

3C.6 Set and follow priorities and maximize outcomes based on available resources.

3C.7 Fulfill functional roles in response to a public health emergency.

3C.8 Facilitate access to services in the health sector and other sectors.

3C.9 Adapt practice in response to the changing health needs of the individual, family, group and community and in response to the unique characteristics of the setting.

3C.10 Take action to protect individuals, families, groups and communities from unsafe or unethical circumstances.

3C.11 Advocate in collaboration with, and on behalf of, and with individuals, families, groups and communities on social justice related issues.

3(D). Evaluation

A public health nurse is able to . . .

3D.1 Evaluate an action, policy or program in a systematic and continuous manner by measuring its effect on individuals, families, groups or communities.

3D.2 Evaluate programs in relation to determinants of health and health outcomes.

3D.3 Evaluate programs in partnership with individuals, families, groups, communities and other stakeholders.

4. PARTNERSHIPS, COLLABORATION AND ADVOCACY

This category captures the competencies required to influence and work with others to improve the health and well-being of the public through the pursuit of a common goal. This includes the concepts of: social justice, which is the fair distribution of society's benefits and responsibilities and their consequences (Canadian Nurses Association, Code of Ethics, 2008); partnership and collaboration, which is to optimize performance through shared resources and responsibilities; advocacy, which is to speak, write or act in favour of a particular cause, policy or group of people and aims to reduce inequities in health status or access to health services.

A public health nurse is able to . . .
4.1 Advocate for societal change in support of health for all:
- collaborate with partners to address public health issues and service gaps in order to achieve improved health outcomes
- build coalitions, intersectoral partnerships and networks
- facilitate the change process to impact the determinants of health and improve health outcomes.
4.2 Use skills such as team building, negotiation, conflict management and group facilitation to build partnerships and to support group development.
4.3 Mediate between differing interests in the pursuit of health and well-being, and advocate for appropriate resource allocation and equitable access to resources.
4.4 Advocate for healthy public policies and services that promote and protect the health and well-being of individuals and communities.
4.5 Involve individuals, families, groups and communities as active partners to identify assets, strengths and available resources and to take action to address health inequities, needs, deficits and gaps.

5. DIVERSITY AND INCLUSIVENESS

This category identifies the competencies required to interact effectively with diverse individuals, families, groups and communities in relation to others in society as well to recognize the root causes of disparities and what can be done to eliminate them (Canadian Nurses Association, Code of Ethics, 2008). It is the embodiment of attitudes and actions that result in inclusive behaviours, practices, programs and policies.

A public health nurse is able to . . .
5.1 Recognize how the determinants of health (biological, social, cultural, economic and physical) influence the health and well-being of specific population groups.

5.2 Address population diversity when planning, implementing, adapting and evaluating public health programs and policies.
5.3 Apply culturally-relevant and appropriate approaches with people from diverse cultural, socioeconomic and educational backgrounds, and persons of all ages, genders, health status, sexual orientations and abilities.

6. COMMUNICATION

Communication involves an interchange of ideas, opinions and information. This category addresses numerous dimensions of communication including internal and external exchanges; written, verbal, non-verbal and listening skills; computer literacy; providing appropriate information to different audiences; working with the media and social marketing techniques.

A public health nurse is able to . . .
6.1 Communicate effectively with individuals, families, groups, communities and colleagues:
- use verbal, non-verbal and written or graphic communication skills
- speak and write in plain language
- use multi-sensory forms of communication to address unique communication styles
- use culturally relevant communication when building relationships.
6.2 Interpret information for professional, nonprofessional and community audiences.
6.3 Mobilize individuals, families, groups and communities by using appropriate media, community resources and social marketing techniques.
6.4 Use current technology to communicate effectively.

7. LEADERSHIP

This category focuses on leadership competencies that build capacity, improve performance and enhance the quality of the working environment. They also enable organizations and communities to create, communicate and apply shared visions, missions and values.

A public health nurse is able to . . .
7.1 Describe the mission and priorities of the public health organization where one works, and apply them in practice.
7.2 Contribute to developing key values and a shared vision to assess, plan and implement public health programs and policies in the community by actively working with health professionals and in partnership with community partners to build capacity.
7.3 Use public health and nursing ethics to manage self, others, information and resources and practice in accordance with all relevant legislation, regulating body standards and codes (e.g., provincial health legislation, child welfare

legislation, privacy legislation, Canadian Nurses Association Code of Ethics for registered nurses).

7.4 Contribute to team and organizational learning in order to advance public health goals.

7.5 Contribute to the maintenance of organizational performance standards.

7.6 Demonstrate an ability to build capacity by sharing knowledge, tools, expertise and experience:

- participate in professional development and practice development activities
- mentor students and orient new staff
- participate in research and quality assurance initiatives.

8. PROFESSIONAL RESPONSIBILITY AND ACCOUNTABILITY

This category addresses a number of dimensions including the recognition that nurses are accountable for their actions and are responsible for making sure they have the required knowledge and skills needed to ensure the delivery of safe, compassionate, competent and ethical care. It includes the competencies required to maintain quality work environments and relationships needed in a professional practice. Public Health nurses are responsible for initiating strategies that will address the determinants of health and generate a positive impact on people and systems. They are accountable to a variety of authorities and stakeholders as well as to the individual and community they serve. This range of accountabilities places them in a variety of situations with unique ethical dilemmas.

A public health nurse is able to . . .

8.1 Demonstrate professionalism in independent practice in multiple settings with multiple stakeholders.

8.2 Apply ethical standards and principles taking into consideration appropriate public health and nursing ethics.

8.3 Consult as needed to determine the best course of action in response to: ethical dilemmas, safety issues, risks to human rights and freedoms, new situations and new knowledge.

8.4 Use reflective practice to continually assess and improve practice:

- examine practice in relation to personal and individual, family, group or community attributes, existing knowledge and context
- adapt public health nursing techniques, approaches and procedures to the challenges in a particular community situation or setting.

8.5 Advocate for effective, efficient and responsible use of resources.

8.6 Act upon legal and professional obligations, and practices in accordance with relevant legislation.

8.7 Contribute to the quality of public health nursing work environments by identifying needs, issues, solutions and mobilizing colleagues by actively participating in team and organizational structures and mechanisms.

Appendix C: Home Health Nursing Competencies

1. ELEMENTS OF HOME HEALTH NURSING

These elements and associated competencies focus on the nursing activities, functions, goals and outcomes that are central to home health nursing practice.

a. Assessment, Monitoring and Clinical Decision Making

The home health nurse is able to . . .

i. conduct comprehensive autonomous and/or collaborative health assessments to determine the health status, functional and psychosocial needs and competence of clients and their families within the context of their environment and social supports

ii. apply critical thinking skills and creative problem-solving analysis when making clinical decisions

iii. analyze information to determine appropriate nursing actions, implications, applications, gaps and limitations

iv. collaborate with health care team members and others who are involved with the client, to determine appropriateness and availability of required services

v. incorporate a combination of basic and advanced knowledge of health and nursing across the lifespan and the health-illness continuum

vi. keep knowledge current and use evidence to inform practice to ensure optimal case management

vii. assess the safety of the home environment with the goal of optimizing client safety and taking actions to support a safe work environment for all members of the home health care team

b. Care Planning and Care Coordination

The home health nurse is able to . . .

i. plan and prioritize visits to meet the health and scheduling needs of clients

ii. use the nursing process to collaboratively develop, coordinate and implement mutually agreed upon care plans, negotiating priorities in care with clear treatment and outcome goals and supporting client navigation and transition through the continuum of care

iii. support clients and families to build on their strengths to attain or maintain a desired health status within available resources

iv. anticipate the need for alternative ways of providing services and use creative problem solving skills to overcome obstacles in delivery of client care, i.e., weather, lack of resources, etc.

v. ensure discharge planning is integrated within the care plan and occurs in collaboration with the client, family, health care team and community

vi. promote an integrated assessment and develop a unified care and treatment plan that is collaboratively carried out by team members to maximize continuity of care within a client-centered approach

vii. appreciate and understand the roles and responsibilities and the contributions of other regulated and unregulated health workers involved in the client care plan

viii. facilitate and coordinate access to other members of the multidisciplinary team such as primary care providers, specialist physician, community pharmacist, nurses, and other allied health professionals to address a specific health issue

ix. collaboratively evaluate care plan interventions through reassessment and ongoing evaluation of results and adapt them to the changing conditions of the client and the client's family

c. Health Maintenance, Restoration and Palliation

The home health nurse is able to . . .

i. assist clients and families to maintain and/or restore health by using a comprehensive mix of strategies to address their health needs across the life span and illness continuum

ii. understand and/or educate clients, their families/caregivers and colleagues in the safe and appropriate use and maintenance of various types of equipment, technology and treatments to maintain health and assist clients and families to integrate them into their everyday life/routine

iii. communicate effectively with clients and families while supporting them through the decision making process about end of life issues

iv. use basic and advanced nursing skills to perform and adapt complex procedures in the home health setting

v. recognize when specialized counselling beyond the scope of nursing is required and facilitate an appropriate referral

vi. respond to the ever-changing and evolving health care needs of the client and family by strategically revising interventions and therapies

vii. self-identify the need for assistance when not familiar with care requirements and seek support to assure continued excellence in care

d. Teaching and Education

The home health nurse is able to . . .

i. assess the knowledge, attitudes, level of motivation, values, beliefs, behaviours, practices, stage of change, and skills of the client/family

ii. consider and integrate into educational planning the factors that may impact the client/family's ability to learn. For example: environment, readiness, willingness, literacy level, educational background, socioeconomic situation, health status, etc.

iii. interpret and explain complex information for clients and families

iv. apply appropriate learning principles, teaching methods and educational theories to educational activities

v. include family, volunteers and caregivers in teaching and education

vi. evaluate the effectiveness of health education interventions

e. Communication

The home health nurse is able to . . .

i. use effective listening, verbal and non-verbal communication skills to understand the client's perspective and be understood by the client, family and other caregivers involved in the care

ii. use effective interviewing skills and strategies to engage in constructive dialogue with clients and their families

iii. use effective communication skills to engage, connect, appreciate, respond, empathize and support the empowerment of others

iv. identify and use strategies to overcome language and communication barriers

v. maintain a focused approach amidst multiple distractions within the home environment

vi. employ negotiation and conflict management skills

vii. use techniques that are client-centered, client-driven, and strength-based when counselling clients

viii. use documentation as an effective communication tool

ix. use technology to effectively communicate and manage client care in a confidential manner

f. Relationships

The home health nurse is able to . . .

i. optimize the health of the client and caregiver(s) by establishing and maintaining a therapeutic nurse–client relationship based on mutual trust, respect, caring, and listening within the context of being "a guest in the house"

ii. acknowledge the contribution that the family/caregiver provides to client health in a way that makes them feel valued and respected and support them to maintain relationships that support effective care

iii. work effectively and non-judgementally in a wide range of environments with varying conditions of cleanliness

iv. use skills such as team building, negotiation, conflict management and group facilitation to build and sustain partnerships

v. involve clients and families as active partners to identify assets, strengths and available resources

g. Access and Equity

The home health nurse is able to . . .

i. advocate for healthy public policies and accessible, inclusive and integrated services that promote and protect the health and well-being of all individuals and communities

ii. apply culturally-relevant and appropriate approaches with people of diverse cultural, socioeconomic and educational backgrounds, and persons of all ages, genders, health status, sexual orientations and abilities

iii. recognize opportunities to promote social justice and advocate in collaboration with, and on behalf of clients and families on related issues to give voice to the vulnerable

iv. optimize allocation of human, financial, and infrastructure resources in order to provide a safe and accessible health delivery system

v. advocate for the reduction of inequities in health by participating in legislative and policy making activities

h. Building Capacity

The home health nurse is able to . . .

i. mobilize clients, families and others to take action to address health needs, deficits and gaps accessing and using available resources

ii. assist the client and their family to recognize their capacity for managing their own health needs according to available resources

iii. assist colleagues, partners and/or clients to support and build on the capacities that are inherent in the individual, families and the communities to influence policy change

iv. demonstrate cultural competency when addressing client care issues and when working in an environment where there may be levels of ambiguity

v. adapt and be flexible and responsive to the changing health needs of the client and family

2. FOUNDATIONS OF HOME HEALTH NURSING

These competencies focus on the core knowledge and primary health care philosophy that is central to home health nursing practice.

a. Health Promotion

The home health nurse is able to . . .

i. facilitate planned change with clients and families by applying and incorporating health promotion theory, primary health care principles and change theory into practice

ii. recognize how the determinants of health influence the health and well-being of clients and families

iii. assess the impact specific issues may have on the client's health such as political climate; priorities, values and culture; social and systemic structures and settings

iv. assess the readiness and capacity of the client and family to make changes to promote their health

b. Illness Prevention and Health Protection

The home health nurse is able to . . .

i. apply nursing sciences to practice and evaluate, synthesize and apply knowledge from a broad range of theories, models, frameworks and practice

ii. use critical thinking to consider the ethical, political, scientific, socio-cultural and economic contexts to determine the meaning of information related to client health care needs

iii. support clients and families to identify risks to health and make informed choices about protective and preventive health measures

iv. take action to protect clients, families and groups from unsafe or unethical circumstances

v. participate in collaborative, interdisciplinary and intersectoral partnerships to enhance the health of clients and families

3. QUALITY AND PROFESSIONAL RESPONSIBILITY

These competencies focus on practice activities and/or strategies by which the home health nurse promotes quality of care and demonstrates professional responsibility.

a. Quality Care

The home health nurse is able to . . .

i. initiate, lead and participate in risk management and quality improvement activities to measure effectiveness of services, cost implications and processes

ii. initiate and participate in critical incident reviews

iii. evaluate nursing interventions in a systematic and continuous manner by measuring their effect on clients and families

iv. evaluate programs in relation to determinants of health and health outcomes

v. contribute to the quality of work environments by identifying needs, issues, solutions and actively participating in team and organizational quality improvement processes

vi. understand the financial aspects of care and be accountable for effective, efficient and responsible use of time and resources when delivering care to clients and families

b. Professional Responsibility

The home health nurse is able to . . .

i. demonstrate professionalism, leadership, judgement and accountability in independent practice in multiple settings with multiple stakeholders

ii. practice independently and autonomously providing client centered services in a wide variety of settings where nursing care and services are needed

iii. use reflective practice to continually assess and improve practice

iv. integrate multiple ways of knowing into practice

v. contribute to the development and generation of evidence-informed nursing practice

vi. pursue lifelong learning opportunities to support professional practice

vii. use nursing ethics, ethical standards and principles and self-awareness to manage self and practice in accordance with all relevant legislation, regulatory body standards, codes and organizational policies

viii. describe the mission, values and priorities of the health organization where one works

ix. participate in the advancement of home health nursing by mentoring students and new practitioners

x. recognize and understand that one's attitudes, beliefs, feelings and values about health can have an effect on relationships and interventions

Answers to Review and Study Questions

CHAPTER 1

Review Questions

1. Correct: (c) Charitable organizations were employing nurses to work with them as early as 1885 (McKay, 2009). Incorrect: (a) Visiting nurses were employed by charitable organizations; health departments did not use the term "visiting nurse" to describe their employees. (b) The rationale is the same as for (a). (d) Self-employed nurses were called private duty nurses. They were one of the three types of nurses described by McPherson (1996). The other two types were public health nurses (PHNs), which included visiting nurses and hospital nurses.

2. Correct: (b) In 1900, the mortality rate for tuberculosis was 180 per 100 000 population. Incorrect: (a) Cardiovascular disease is a chronic illness associated with a high life expectancy, and in 1900, a Canadian's life expectancy at birth was 47 years. (c) Typhoid fever outbreaks could kill high numbers of people, but outbreaks were sporadic, unlike the steady rate of tuberculosis infections experienced in 1900. (d) Diagnosed cancer was not as high as tuberculosis.

3. Correct: (a) Urban PHNs were employed in specialist practices in the early 20th century. In 1914, the Toronto Health Department became the first health department to reorganize PHNs into districts and have them work as generalist practitioners to meet the needs of the families living in that district. Incorrect: (b) Early PHNs worked only in specialist programs. (c) Bedside nursing services were delivered by visiting nurses employed by agencies such as the Victorian Order of Nurses (VON) or the Margaret Scott Nursing Mission. (d) Public health departments were publicly funded and their employees were paid from these funds.

4. Correct: (c) For example, in Winnipeg, the VON contracted with the provincial government to provide child hygiene, prenatal, and mothercraft services in suburban Winnipeg when the government was unable to employ PHNs to provide these services. Incorrect: (a) The VON was established to provide nursing care to the sick living in both town and country districts. (b) Most VON branches depended on charitable donations, patient fees, and government grants to remain in business. (d) Until 1921, the VON operated training centres in several large Canadian cities to provide post-diploma public health programs for hospital-trained nurses.

5. Correct: (d) In the United States, community-based nurses focus on the provision of acute and long-term care to individuals and families living in the community. Incorrect: (a) In both the American and Canadian definitions, a PHN is responsible for promoting, protecting, and preserving the health of populations. (b) In the Canadian definition, PHNs and home health nurses are included under this broader category. In the American definition, a community health nurse (CHN) preserves, protects, promotes, or maintains the health of individuals, families, and groups in the community. (c) This American term defines a community-oriented nurse as a nurse who focuses on the care of either the whole community or a population of individuals, families, and groups living in the community. Both PHNs and CHNs fall under this definition.

Study Questions

1. The two forms of community health nursing that evolved in Canada in the early 20th century were public health nursing and visiting/district nursing. PHNs were employed by civic, provincial, or federal health departments to carry out preventive programs in the community. In the later part of the 20th century, PHNs took on new roles in health promotion and community development. Visiting/district nurses offered bedside nursing services in the home. They were most frequently employed by charitable organizations. Visiting nursing is now more commonly referred to as home care nursing.

2. The social gospel movement was one important impetus for the development of community-based social services. It was an ecumenical and evangelical stream within the Protestant churches that had as its goal the establishment of God's kingdom on earth. Another important social movement was maternal feminism. Maternal feminists had a particular interest in the health and welfare of women and children. The social gospel movement and maternal feminism created an important strategic alliance after World War I, and their efforts are theorized to have had an important influence on the rise of the Canadian welfare state. The last important social movement was the public health movement. Sanitarianism, bacteriology, and health education were all important paradigms within the early public health movement. All contributed to the overarching belief that the application of scientific knowledge would create a healthy nation.

3. Early community health nursing programs focused on women, children, the poor, the working class, and immigrants. There were several interrelated reasons for this emphasis. All these groups were vulnerable within a society where political and economic power was held by elite and middle-class males. Their vulnerability was clearly demonstrated by the higher mortality rates these groups experienced. Another reason for the focus on these groups was the need to create a strong and healthy pool of future citizens to establish Canada's pre-eminence in the 20th century. Immigrants were an important target group because elite and middle-class reformers believed that they needed to adopt Canadian beliefs and practices rather than retain those of their countries of origin.

4. The earliest public health programs that employed nurses were tuberculosis (TB) control, school health, and infant

welfare. TB was a leading cause of death in early 20th-century Canada and a particular problem among the urban poor. Early efforts to control TB were based on the belief that a reduction in the incidence of this disease would, as well as alleviating suffering, reduce the costs of public welfare and healthcare programs.

School-health programs were established to identify health problems among school-age children. As working-class children entered the public school system, it became apparent that they suffered from many preventable health problems that detracted from their capacity to learn.

Infant welfare programs were established to reduce infant mortality rates. In the early 20th century, immigration, industrialization, and urbanization created unprecedented urban squalor.

5. The British North America Act reflected 19th-century beliefs about the role of the state. In keeping with the philosophy of laissez faire, the state had no role to play in the provision of healthcare and social welfare for its citizens. These were private matters, which were the responsibility of individuals and families. Those who could not provide for their families were compelled to obtain charitable assistance from local governments or, more likely, voluntary philanthropic agencies. The BNA Act left responsibility for healthcare in the hands of the provinces, which also took only a limited interest in this area. Enabling legislation for the establishment of health departments was passed by several provinces prior to the end of the 19th century, but permanent health departments were not established in most Canadian cities and provinces until the 20th century. Prior to the end of World War II, local and provincial health departments received no assistance from the federal government. Their capacity to respond to the health needs of the communities for which they were responsible was constrained by their ability to fund programs from local tax revenues.

6. The Canadian welfare state had its origins in the early 20th century as provincial and municipal departments of health began to provide publicly funded public health programs at the local level. Some provinces, cities, and municipalities, particularly in Western Canada, were virtually bankrupted by their attempts to respond to widespread unemployment and poverty. They put pressure on the federal government to assist them. However, other provinces, more concerned about maintaining strict divisions between provincial and federal powers, opposed any initiatives that would enable the federal government to intervene into what had previously been provincial responsibilities. Several attempts by the federal government to take a greater role in health and welfare programs were stopped by the Supreme Court, which used the BNA Act as the basis of its decisions. In 1940, the Royal Commission on Dominion–Provincial Relations recommended that the federal government undertake responsibility for old-age pensions and unemployment insurance, but leave responsibility for health with the provinces.

In the 1940s, 1950s, and 1960s, a series of cost-sharing arrangements enabled the federal government to establish a national healthcare system by creating incentives for the provinces to spend more money in this area and to extend those services to all citizens regardless of their ability to pay. The National Health Grants Program (1948), the National Hospital Insurance and Diagnostic Services Act (1957), and the Medical Care Insurance Act (1968) were key elements in the increased federal role in the provision of healthcare.

7. First, they often pioneered community health nursing programs, thus demonstrating both the need for and the effectiveness of these programs. Second, they provided community health programs in communities where local governments were either unable or unwilling to do so. Third, they created educational programs to prepare nurses to practise in this area. Fourth, they provided funding to support local initiatives to create community health nursing programs.

CHAPTER 2
Review Questions

1. Correct: (c) Transformational leadership practices focus on building relationships and trust both individually and collectively, in turn fostering work environments that empower individuals and groups to anticipate the need for change and begin to look for new ways of approaching situations. An environment where new ideas are encouraged and rewarded results in nurses actively participating in problem solving and change. Incorrect: (a) Although there are many positive attributes of non-governmental organizations, their limitations generally include a focused/narrow mandate and unstable funding. (b) Although strong mandates are often useful in driving an organizational direction (such as health promotion), when such mandates are narrowly focused on only a component of the larger issue, overall effectiveness is limited. Similarly, as nurses value "holistic practice," a narrow focus holds back their ability to provide optimal nursing care. (d) Organizations that have multiple visions of the direction of their organization establish an environment of uncertainty and conflict. Groups within the organization tend to work against each other as they compete for scarce resources and attention.

2. Correct: (c) Primary care reform has resulted in the establishment of Family Health Teams. A Family Health Team is a group of interprofessional healthcare professionals who provide care to a community. In Ontario, over 170 teams have been established as one of many strategies to improve primary care. They have many similarities to Community Health Centres established in the 1970s and the CLSCs in Quebec. Incorrect: (a) Community Health Centres have actually increased throughout the last decade from 69 to 74. They are distinct in that they focus their work on a determinants of health model. Many are established to serve specific priority populations such as multicultural communities or homeless individuals. (b) and (d) Although in some parts of the country community nursing care has been privatized and some physicians' offices have closed, this is a result of other government and policy issues (e.g., home care) or because physicians have decided to join FHTs, CHCs, and so on.

3. Correct: (b) Protective, promotive, and preventive services as well as home health are not required to meet the five criteria of Medicare and are not subject to the conditions of the CHA. Each province, territory, and region considers them as additional or extended services and as such makes its own choices as to which ones (or how much) will be funded. As a result, there is significant diversity across the

country in prevention and promotion services available. Incorrect: (a) Formal education opportunities abound for CHNs, with online courses now widely available. (c) CHNs consistently express their difficulty in explaining to clients and communities their role in the healthcare system. The provision of greater role clarity will form the basis for nurses and others being able to describe the valuable services they provide. (d) Recent studies identify the decreased number of CHN leaders. As we have moved toward interdisciplinary practice and program teams, steps often have not been taken to ensure nurses continue to have opportunities to meet to ensure nursing practice issues are addressed and guided by nursing leaders.

4. Correct: (b) Contextual factors that produce an environment that supports lifelong learning include organizational supports and personal resources. Organizational supports include components such as designated resources and nurse leaders who model and promote ongoing learning, stated and lived values that express the value of nursing to the effectiveness of the organization, and formalized systems in place that ensure nurses have a meaningful role in decision making. Personal resources are those which speak to the attributes individual nurses, or groups of nurses, bring to the organization. They include professional identity, social support, and previous professional and personal experience that have shaped values and attitudes. These predisposing factors strongly influence the quality of nursing practice within organizations. Incorrect: (a) Although bureaucratic and government bodies have been known to be responsive to public demands for nurses, there is no correlation between the increase in jobs for nurses and establishing a working environment for nurses that predisposes or promotes lifelong learning. (c) The key to lifelong learning is establishing a relationship with professional nursing organizations. However, if one waits for "time to permit" such involvements, the connections may not be forged or at best will be weak. (d) Agencies that promote and support meaningful connections to professional organizations demonstrate leadership by encouraging nurses to develop on multiple professional levels.

5. Correct: (c) One of the key limitations of the Canada Health Act is the focus on essential hospital and medical services. Incorrect: (a), (b), and (d) The CHA is federally funded to cover essential medical services (in hospital, medical and surgical services). It is available after three months' residency in all provinces and no user fees are allowed. The Act identifies only essential services listed above as qualifying for federal cost-sharing. These conditions have not changed throughout the more than 25 years of its history.

Study Questions

1. North America's first universal health insurance program was initially implemented in 1947 at a provincial level in Saskatchewan. It was not until 1957 that similar legislation, the Hospital Insurance and Diagnostic Services Act (HIDS), was passed by the federal government. The HIDS provided financial incentives for the provinces to establish hospital insurance plans.

In 1962, Saskatchewan led the country again with legislation providing universal, publicly funded medical insurance. In 1966, the federal government followed suit with the passage of the National Medical Care Insurance Act (Medicare). This Act was implemented in 1968, and by 1971 all provinces were fully participating.

As a result of the strain on the federal budgets caused by the blanket 50/50 cost-sharing between the federal and provincial/territorial governments, in 1977 the federal government passed the Established Programs Financing Act (EPF), which changed the federal share of health costs to per capita block grants assigned to provinces and tied to economic performance.

As our understanding of what factors determine healthy individuals and communities grew, it became clear a number of other services were critical to ensuring the health of Canadians. Phase 2 of the implementation of Medicare was intended to address protective, preventive, and promotion services. In addition, home care and a universal drug plan were identified as important components to be addressed. These healthcare components, which would add balance to the treatment-focused delivery system, were left unprotected by federal legislation. This remains the case today.

2. When Monique Begin was appointed Federal Minister of Health and Welfare, she became aware that extra-billing and user fees by institutions and physicians were rising dramatically in Canada. This growing practice undermined key criteria by which provinces were to receive federal funding for health services. The cornerstones or pillars upon which funding was issued included accessibility and universality of coverage related to physician and institutional care. These criteria could not be met as long as extra-billing practices were allowed. She therefore developed Bill C-3, also known as the Canada Health Act, which reasserted the five criteria required to receive federal funding. It was passed in 1984.

3. The Canadian Nurses Association intensely lobbied for the Bill's passage into law. In addition, they were successful in amending it. As it was introduced into Parliament in 1983, Bill C-3 identified only physicians as providers of insurable services. The CNA amendment changed the language to include other healthcare workers as potential providers of insurable services, opening the door for the public to have direct access to nursing care through insured services.

4. Although the 1867 Constitution Act did not explicitly assign responsibility for health policy to either the federal or provincial governments, historically both levels of government have been involved in ensuring the availability of health services for Canadians, and in funding those services. Responsibility for hospitals is assigned by the Act exclusively to provinces and, as a result, healthcare in Canada has sometimes been erroneously interpreted to fall under provincial jurisdiction. The federal government assumes responsibility for delivery of a few direct health services, e.g., to Aboriginal populations, veterans, and military personnel. Provincial governments are responsible for the delivery of the remainder of healthcare services, including public health.

Funding for healthcare is another matter, however. The federal government's involvement in funding healthcare relates both to its mandate to equalize services among provinces and to its responsibilities to ensure provinces are in compliance with the Canada Health Act. The federal government has carried this out in two main ways. First, it has transferred money from wealthier provinces to poorer provinces and territories. Second, it has stipulated specific conditions that must be met in order for funds to be transferred.

5. Public health in Canada is funded by a combination of provincial and/or municipal tax dollars, although federal grants may be available for specific initiatives. Without a national public health program, however, provinces are free to make changes in funding mechanisms that can further destabilize the system and deepen disparities among and within provinces.

   In all 13 provinces/territories, the ministries or departments of health and/or social/community services maintain control over home care budgets and funding levels. However, contrary to other forms of healthcare provided in Canada, home care has retained a significant private-sector component. So while all provincial governments finance home care services to some extent, often user fees or co-payments are required. As funding mechanisms and intensity vary from province to province, this has resulted in a patchwork of programs and services not consistent with the underpinning five principles of a national health program.

6. With respect to stopping the practices of extra-billing and charging user fees, the CHA fulfilled its purpose. However, the issue of provincial/territorial non-compliance with the five criteria of the Act remains to be adequately addressed.

   ▪ The intent of the Act was to relate federal cash contributions not only to insured health services but also to extended healthcare services. In that respect the CHA has not been effective. Furthermore, the Act endorsed health promotion but limited its focus to medically necessary hospital and physicians' services. Health promotion services, largely provided by provincial public health, were left unprotected by federal legislation. The resulting variability of health promotion and disease prevention services within and among jurisdictions violates the Act's principle of portability.

   ▪ Canadians enjoy relatively good health when compared with other countries. Canada also spends less per capita and less of its gross domestic product on health than some other countries, including the United States. However, there is room for improvement, particularly with respect to outcomes such as infant mortality rates, which are still higher than in a number of other developed countries.

CHAPTER 3

Review Questions

1. Correct: (a) CHNs' professional practice competencies are defined in the text and contrasted with other competencies listed. Incorrect: (b), (c), and (d) While these are plausible uses for the CHNs, they are not as correct as (a), which is more definitional.

2. Correct: (c) Community health nursing practice is guided by health promotion and the principles of primary health care. Incorrect: (a), (b), and (d) These are all part of community health nursing but are not the major underpinning foundational concepts outlined in the text.

3. Correct: (b) Under Nurse–Person Relationship competencies, "care in the home is adapted according to the client's environment and direction." Incorrect: (a) This is not as relevant to the "individual as client" situation. (c) This is not a realistic premise. (d) This is not really relevant to the nurse–person therapeutic relationship.

4. Correct: (b) Primary Health Care Nurse Practitioners are registered nurses who practise at an advanced level, functioning within the full scope of nursing practice, and as such are not second-level physicians, nor are they doctors' assistants. Incorrect: (a), (c), and (d) These are all aspects of practice that fall within the legislated scope of the PHCNP scope of practice.

5. Correct: (a) PHNs work within the community often invisibly. Incorrect: (b) and (c) While this may be true, these are not major features of public health nursing and are not exclusive to some other community nursing roles, such as faith community nursing or nurse entrepreneurs. (d) This is not an absolute fact.

6. Correct: (a) Within Nursing Practice: Health and Wellness, "practice reflects changes in cultural composition, demographics, health trends, and economic factors (aging population, globalization)" is a global answer that transverses all aspects of CHNng. Incorrect: (b), (c), and (d) These are micro aspects of societal trends.

Study Questions

1. Ten types of practice settings for nurses working in CHNng are public health units/departments; workplaces; schools; homes; street health; community health centres; emergency departments such as SANE or community outreach program such as diabetes clinics, maternal and newborn follow-up clinics; NP-led clinics; military base; parishes/churches; outpost; and medical office.

2. Some broad roles nurses working in CHNng may perform in the various practice areas discussed in this chapter are
   ▪ Teacher/educator: Having the ability to impart knowledge and skills with clients, families, groups, and communities is foundational to educating the public. Nurses teach clients and their families how to manage their illnesses or injuries; explain post-treatment home care needs; advise on diet, nutrition, and exercise programs; explain medication self-administration; and provide physical therapy. They promote general health by educating the public on warning signs and symptoms of disease and ways to stay healthy. Nurses are also teachers/educators/mentors of new staff and nursing students.
   ▪ Facilitator: Often in group settings (e.g., families, community groups, etc.), nurses act as facilitators to maintain order and to keep conversations flowing.
   ▪ Primary health care provider: Nurses provide healthcare to clients to prevent illness and promote health.
   ▪ Planner: Whether planning care for a client/family or a program in public health, planning is critical to achieving desired goals and outcomes.
   ▪ Policy developer: Policy development is an important strategy to ensure equal opportunities for health.
   ▪ Advocate: Often nurses have knowledge of community resources or awareness of how various systems work and are well positioned to advocate on behalf of clients.
   ▪ Presenter: Nurses often share knowledge and information in group settings.

- Community mobilizer: CHNs and PHNs working in a community can bring people together to mobilize on particular health issues.
- Evaluator: To ensure that programs are effective or health improvements are being achieved, it is important to undertake evaluations.

3. Determining the various learning styles in class can be challenging, but the PHN can take some measures to facilitate and encourage all types of learners. Consideration of adult learning principles and the variety of learning styles highlights the need for order, structure, creativity, group work, and practical exercises. The PHN must incorporate as much variety as possible into educational sessions. The exercises/discussions should have a purpose, enhance understanding, and develop new knowledge. The following is a list of strategies to assist the PHN.

- Class preparation: As adult learners come from varied backgrounds, life experiences, and educational attainment, it is necessary to state clearly if there are any prerequisites for a particular class. Are there assumptions of the learners having any particular skills or abilities? It is important to determine whether certain characteristics (e.g., age, culture, language, social circumstance) will impact how the PHN approaches the session(s).
- Clear goals and outcomes: Clear learning outcomes, some of which are negotiated and agreed upon by both PHNs and learners, ensure that everyone works toward the same goal(s). When learning outcomes are mutually agreed upon, learners feel more involved in the learning process, which helps focus attention and promotes a unified sense of purpose. This also helps the PHN to organize the session(s).
- Organization of content: Learning is facilitated when content and skills to be learned are organized in a meaningful way. Learners will understand and remember material longer if it is organized logically, following a sequenced progress to the new knowledge or skill. Also, the rate at which information is to be presented by the PHN should be determined in terms of its complexity and by gauging the learner's readiness. It is important to provide the signposts that will help learners to perceive the structure.
- Consideration of emotions: It is important to note that learning involves emotions and personal feelings, as well as the intellect. If learners have not been involved in formal learning for some time, they may feel vulnerable. It is important to make learning fun.
- Active participation: Optimal learning involves active participation. Participation means engaging in mental and/or physical activity that will help the learner to understand and retain the information. Sharing personal stories, small group discussions, or group work are examples.
- Ongoing feedback: Providing ongoing feedback and encouragement assists with learning. Learning motivated by success is rewarding; it builds confidence and positively affects behaviour.
- Linkages and associations: In order to learn and remember information, it is better if associations are made with it. For example, the PHN can ask participants to associate information with the learner's prior knowledge or life experiences.

- Practice and repetition: Opportunity for practice and repetition ensures that the knowledge/skill is learned.
- Attention: The 90:20:8 rule. Adults can listen with understanding for 90 minutes and with retention for 20 minutes, so try to involve them every 8 minutes.

From Wlodkowski, R. J. (2008). *Enhancing adult motivation to learn: A comprehensive guide for teaching all adults* (3rd ed.). San Francisco, CA: Jossey-Bass.

4. Responses should be linked to the standards of practice and core competencies (e.g., reflective practice, lifelong learning, etc.).

5. Trends in community health nursing that may have an impact on education include
- Technology: documentation, searches, course options (e.g., WebCT)
- Determinants of health impacted: curriculum content
- Infectious diseases: practice guidelines and curriculum
- Diverse placement options in a community

6. This is an individual response. Ensure that the examples reflect the five community health nursing standards (see Appendix A).

CHAPTER 4

Review Questions

1. Correct: (a) Advocating for broad social change, such as housing policy, enables groups within society to achieve well-being. Incorrect: (b) This intervention is beneficial in the short term for clients but does not address broad social inequities. (c) Allocating time equally does not address inequalities among social groups. (d) This intervention does not address broad social inequities.

2. Correct: (d) This intervention gets at the source of inequities and barriers that might exist so that they can be addressed. Incorrect: (a), (b), and (c) Without knowing the barriers, the actions may not address the problems that exist for these women in obtaining PAP smears.

3. Correct: (d) This explanation clarifies the nature of the relationship while maintaining a positive, caring relationship. Incorrect: (a) The action is too severe and would unnecessarily destroy a caring relationship. (b) Accepting a large sum of money from a client is a violation of professional boundaries. (c) While clarifying professional boundaries is important, long-term relationships in home care generally are not entirely clinically focused.

4. Correct: (b) Mrs. Black's autonomy is preserved with this response and a relationship between Mrs. Black and her neighbour could be fostered. Incorrect: (a) Providing this kind of medical information is a violation of privacy and confidentiality. (c) The nurse cannot assume Mrs. Black will want the neighbour's company. (d) While this is true, it does not foster a potentially caring relationship between Mrs. Black and her neighbour.

5. Correct: (d) This response has the potential to support Mrs. Black and does judge her behaviour. Incorrect: (a) This option does not provide direction to the student regarding how to help Mrs. Black. (b) Learning more about addictions will not help the immediate need to support Mrs. Black. (c) This approach would be harmful to the nurse–client relationship.

Study Questions

1. See Table 4.1.
2. See Table 4.2.
3. CHNAC's five standards of practice are
   i. Promoting health
   ii. Building individual/community capacity
   iii. Building relationships
   iv. Facilitating access and equity
   v. Demonstrating professional responsibility and accountability

   See Appendix A.

4. The first, the harm principle, requires that power be exercised over individuals against their will only to prevent harm to others. Restricting the liberty of mentally competent people to protect their own well-being is not a sufficient justification.

   The second principle, least restrictive or coercive means, stipulates that the full force of governmental authority and power should not be used, unless less coercive methods are unavailable or have failed. Education, negotiation, and discussion should come before regulation and incarceration (Upshur, 2002).

   The third, the reciprocity principle, indicates that if a public action is warranted, social entities, such as a public health department, are obligated to assist individuals in meeting their ethical responsibilities. In addition, because complying with the requests of the public health department may impose burdens on individuals, such as time and money, the reciprocity principle demands that compensation be given (Upshur, 2002).

   The fourth, the transparency principle, refers to the way in which decisions are made. All relevant stakeholders should participate in decision making in an accountable and equitable fashion that is free of political interference or coercion (Upshur, 2002).

5. In order for CHNs to assist clients in making informed choices, at least two elements must be considered: the exchange of information between the client and CHN, and respect for the client's autonomy. The process of consent includes CHNs disclosing, unasked, whatever a reasonable person would want to know if they were in the position of the client. The nurse must provide the information that the average prudent person in the client's particular position would want to know. CHNs must provide information about the nature of the treatment/procedures, including benefits and risks, alternative treatments, and consequences if the treatment is not given. The presentation of this information must consider the client's education, language, age, values, culture, disease state, and mental capacity. When clients provide consent it must be done voluntarily (i.e., without being coerced) and they must have the capacity (i.e., mental competence) to do so. The only exceptions to consent for treatment are in emergency situations and as required by law.

6. There are four key elements that must be proven to make a finding of negligence: (a) that there was a relationship between the person bringing the claim (i.e., plaintiff, e.g., client, family) and the person being sued (i.e., defendant, e.g., nurse); (b) that the defendant breached the standard of care; (c) that the plaintiff suffered a harm; and (d) that the harm suffered was caused by the defendant's breach of the standard of care.

CHAPTER 5

Review Questions

1. Correct: (b) In the chapter, it is noted that discourses shape relations of power, citing Foucault and Habermas. Rather than encouraging innovative thinking, discourses operate in such a way as to discourage thinking that does not align with the patterns of thinking foundational to a particular discourse. Incorrect: (a) This answer demonstrates a lack of understanding of the concept. (c) and (d) These could be potential outcomes of qualitative data analysis. (e) Identifying thinking is not a social function.

2. Correct: (c) In the chapter, it is noted that the systems view is a competing discourse to the medical view. Incorrect: (a) The health system is simply a picture of the elements of the system, not a way of looking at change. (b) The medical community is only beginning to look at system patterns and changes. (d) The systems view of health could be used to examine and improve the experience of people with heart disease. (e) Many lay people do not view healthcare from a systems perspective, but focus on their own perceptions.

3. Correct: (d) All of these items are within the social determinants of health. Incorrect: (a), (b), and (c) Biology, genetics, and pharmacology were not identified in the literature cited in the chapter as key social determinants. (e) Place of residence is missing.

4. Correct: (a) It is only in (a) that all the strategies suggested in the chapter appear. Incorrect: (b) The social determinants of health are missing. (c) Educating patients/clients is missing. (d) It is necessary to re-orient the health system, not just the medical system. (e) Social determinants of health are missing.

5. Correct: (d) The chapter suggests that nurses need to be cognizant of the effects of the social determinants of health on lifestyle behaviours. The only way that nurses can begin to understand this is to ask the women about their conditions of living and listen carefully to what they say. Incorrect: (a) Here the nurse focuses on the behaviour without considering the life context. (b) This action does not advance the nurse–client relationship without accompanying conversation. (c) Again, this would follow discussion and assessment of needs from the client perspective. (e) This has nothing to do with the topic of the question.

Study Questions

1. A discourse is a patterned system of texts, messages, talk, dialogue, or conversations that can be identified in communications and located in social structures. Key ideas are patterned expressions that can be located within social structures.

2. Primary health care is a balanced combination of medical care, health promotion and prevention, consumer protection, effective healthcare systems, appropriate technology, and inter-sectoral co-operation organized to ensure effective action on the determinants of health and to shape environments in support of healthful living and healthy lifestyles.

The Primary Health Care Model suggests a balanced combination of medical care, health promotion and prevention, consumer protection, effective healthcare systems, appropriate technology, and inter-sectoral co-operation.

3. The difference between these two views originates in how each perspective conceptualizes health. Traditionally, the medical model defines health as the absence of disease, whereas the systems view envisions health as shaped by myriad physical, social, environmental, and organizational factors.

4. The challenge to nurses is to be aware of the view of health that dominates in their practice environment and to begin practice from the client's perspectives on health, working collaboratively within this view in the interest of the client.

5. The Lalonde Report shifted perspectives on health from illness care to healthcare by suggesting that health is embedded in a web of factors, including physical, social, and environmental factors.

6. In the ecological perspective, health is viewed as a consequence of the interdependence between the individual and the family, community, culture, and physical and social environments.

7. In a relational nursing practice, the nurse builds trusting relationships, collaborates with clients to identify and address their health-related issues, fosters clients' strengths, promotes and protects clients' rights, practises in an inter-sectoral manner to address the determinants of health, and strives for a respectful, integrated, and accessible system of healthcare delivery.

8. Through the development of a series of charters and frameworks that flesh out the elements of systems views of health, Canada has played a leading role in shaping discourses of health toward a systems view. These works, in combination with the scholarly and advocacy efforts of an army of academics and health advocates, have been fundamental in arguing to maintain a single-payer system for healthcare in Canada—a system consistent in its philosophy with a systems view of health rather than a biomedical model view of health. Canada's charters and framework of health promotion, population health, and primary health care, along with the related healthcare system, are models in the international arena for a healthcare system that advances a systems view of health.

9. The authors invite students to offer their views on the metaphors of nursing practice provided in this chapter by e-mail communication to the first author, Lynne Young, at leyoung@uvic.ca. The author will model a relational process while facilitating the discussion by ensuring that all voices are heard and all opinions are respected. The facilitator will share her observations and reactions and summarize the discussion.

CHAPTER 6

Review Questions

1. Correct: (a) It was the first time that a national government had made an official statement regarding the importance of health promotion as a key strategy for improving population health. Incorrect: (b) The Lalonde Report expanded the concept of health to include physical–functional ability and physical–emotional well-being. Social well-being at the individual and community levels was a concept of health that emerged in the 1980s with the Ottawa Charter. (c) It challenged the dominant thinking of the time that access to medical/healthcare was the key to population health. (d) The Lalonde Report argued that the focus of health promotion efforts should be on strategies that encourage the adoption of behaviours or lifestyles that promote functional ability and well-being.

2. Correct: (c) The Ottawa Charter focused on equity as a focus of health promotion. Incorrect: (a) The Ottawa Charter was signed by delegates from 38 countries, including Canada, in 1986. (b) It outlined five central strategies for promoting population health: strengthening community action, creating supportive environments, developing personal skills, building healthy public policy, and reorienting health systems. (d) The essential prerequisites for health in the Charter are peace, education, shelter, food, income, a stable ecosystem, sustainable resources, social justice, and equity.

3. Correct: (b) The prerequisites for health identified in the Ottawa Charter are focused on social and environmental influences on health. Incorrect: (a) The behavioural approach to health promotion continues to be very popular. Public health departments frequently rely on communication campaigns to deliver "healthy lifestyle" messages; social marketing techniques have been used in HIV/AIDS prevention; health education programs are commonly used within the school system; and health teaching remains a major part of healthcare professionals' practice. (c) The use of the mass media, direct mail, product labels, pamphlets, or posters to communicate a health message to the public is an example of health communication—a strategy that is focused on changing individual behaviours. (d) Laws requiring the use of seatbelts or banning smoking in public places are an example of the Ottawa Charter strategy of healthy public policy.

4. Correct: (d) CHNs can contribute to the promotion of health equity by monitoring the impact of public policies related to housing, transportation, social assistance, etc., on families, and reporting them to their employers, the public, and/or the media. Incorrect: (a) "Healthy Living" programs that encourage increased physical activity among the population as a whole may increase inequities in health because there is greater uptake by more socially advantaged groups. (b) It is part of the CHN's role to make decision makers aware of the research on the links between socio-economic factors and inequities in health. (c) The term "health inequities" is often used synonymously with "health disparities" or "health inequalities." However, a health inequity is a disparity or inequality in health that is linked to social disadvantage.

5. Correct: (d) The use of a critical social approach to health promotion by CHNs involves empowering strategies at the personal/individual, interpersonal (small group), community, and policy levels. Incorrect: (a) Changing perceptions and attitudes that are viewed as non-health-enhancing and assisting the client to develop, carry out, and evaluate a behaviour-change plan are the main focus of the nurse's role in Pender's Health Promotion Model. Falk-Rafael's Critical Caring theory aims to reincorporate the social justice agenda into public health nursing. A core carative process of PHNs' practice is contributing to the creation of supportive and sustainable physical, social, political, and

economic environments. (b) This is an example of a macroscopic ("upstream") approach in community health nursing. A microscopic ("downstream") approach focuses on assessing individual/family responses to health and illness. (c) The Canadian Community Health Nursing Standards of Practice are based on a socio-environmental perspective of health and health promotion.

Study Questions

1. See Table 6.1.

2. Approaches that focus solely on individual behaviour change and individual responsibility for health can lead to "victim-blaming," whereby individuals end up being implicitly blamed for being sick because they have "chosen" unhealthy lifestyles or they have unhealthy coping styles when, in fact, their social and economic circumstances have often left them with limited options.

3. Empowerment is the central concept. It refers to the process or outcome of individuals, communities, and populations gaining power, knowledge, skills, and/or other resources that allow them to achieve positive change, including increased self-efficacy. Empowerment relates directly to the concept of health promotion as a process of enabling individuals, communities, and populations to increase control over the determinants of health.

4. Health promotion
   - involves the population as a whole and the context of their everyday lives, rather than focusing on people at risk for specific diseases;
   - is directed toward action on the determinants or causes of health;
   - combines diverse, but complementary, methods or approaches;
   - aims particularly at effective and concrete public participation; and
   - recognizes that health professionals, particularly those in primary health care, have an important role in nurturing and enabling health promotion.

5. Nurses can play an important role in addressing social determinants of health
   - by working on their individual practices (e.g., including SDOH in client assessments and treatment and follow-up plans);
   - by helping to reorient the healthcare system (e.g., ensuring that health promotion programs go beyond lifestyle and behaviour to include SDOH);
   - by advocating for healthy public policies (e.g., using stories from patients to help advocate for policies that address SDOH); and
   - by making decision makers aware of the research on the links between socioeconomic factors and health.

6. The five guidelines are focus on health and building capacity for health; promote health equity; think "upstream"; look for partnership opportunities; and be patient.

CHAPTER 7

Review Questions

1. Correct: (d) Collaboration with other agencies is supported by intersectoral co-operation, which is one of the Canadian Nurses Association's five Principles of Primary Health Care. Incorrect: (a) and (b) These are too limited in the range of services offered, as both prevention and health promotion services need to be included. (c) This goes against public participation.

2. Correct: (a) All other options are inconsistent with population health approach. Incorrect: (b) This goes against intersectoral collaboration. (c) This does not include other system levels that impact social determinants of health. (d) This does not support a population health approach, as it is more of a primary care model.

3. Correct: (d) Collaboration with key stakeholders that are invested in planning and evaluation of health services toward a common goal demonstrate intersectoral cooperation, one of the PHC principles. This option includes various stakeholders within the community, and actions of working with a collaborative group might lead to change as compared to one level of stakeholders. Incorrect: (a), (b), and (c) These are less than optimal choices because they involve one stakeholder group.

4. Correct: (d) This demonstrates public participation, one of the PHC principles. The other options do not demonstrate public participation. Incorrect: (a) This includes only nurses. (b) This includes experts, but does not involve community members' participation in decision making. (c) This is inconsistent with the primary health care notion that clients and communities are experts in their own health.

5. Correct: (c) All other options demonstrate a CHN using social determinants of health to examine the structural causes of homelessness. Incorrect: (a) This affects accessibility of services and lack of social support networks. (b) This speaks to lack of income and social status. (d) This addresses living conditions that can impact physical and social environments.

6. Answer: (d) This demonstrates public participation, one of the PHC principles, and supports clients' engagement within their own care. (a) This does not support clients being involved within their environment. (b) This goes against public participation. (c) This does not support the client to be involved in care.

Study Questions

1. Primary care is narrower in scope than primary health care and denotes the first entry point to healthcare and therefore is generally biomedical in focus. Access to primary care is an essential component of primary health care.

2. There is a close relationship between health promotion and primary health care in both philosophy and methods. However, primary health care also involves curative, rehabilitative, and palliative care methods as a part of provision of first-line contact with the community. Population health focuses on maintaining and improving the health of entire populations and reducing inequities in health status among population groups. It is often associated with a "top down" approach to reducing inequities in health, such as developing healthy public policy. This approach to population health is congruent with the original thinking of primary health care outlined in the *Declaration of Alma Ata*; it has a strong orientation to evidence-based interventions.

3. See definitions in the box on page 110.

4. CHNs often encounter significant social issues in their work, including, but not limited to, inadequate housing, poverty, accessibility to healthcare, violence, etc.

5. Facilitate discussions using examples of strategies for each level of involvement and action from local, provincial, national, or international efforts to reduce inequities in health.

CHAPTER 8

Review Questions

1. Correct: (b) This nurse is assuming that she/he can determine the "correct" plan and that the nurse's conclusions are best. Nursing care needs to be developed in partnership and collaboration with clients. Incorrect: (a) Stereotyping occurs when background information is never checked with the client and is assumed to be true for all. (c) Generalizations can be useful in providing background information about meanings of care and health practices, but they must be used with caution and sensitivity. (d) Cultural competence is seen as the mechanism to address culturally specific health needs.

2. Correct: (d) Values and beliefs regarding positive expressions of multiculturalism are diverse. Incorrect: (a) When groups come together there will be diversity of values, meanings, and opinions, particularly regarding the complexities and conflicts inherent in the representations of difference. (b) Committees or groups will not reach unanimous agreement in all areas; they need to reach enough of a consensus in order to set some of their goals and proceed with their proposed actions. (c) The goal of Canada's multiculturalism policy is not assimilation, nor is this likely possible.

3. Answer: (a) The concept of race has been used to create and sustain subordinate groups. Nurses should be aware that historically, the concept of race has been used to maintain the dominant social order and this continues to occur today. Race is a powerful social construct, not objective biological categories. There is more biological variation within "races" than between them. Incorrect: (b), (c), and (d) These do not question the assumptions underlying racial categorizations.

4. Correct: (a) The family's traditions and values are strengths in a situation currently shared by many Canadians. Helpful personal and family health strategies are strengths that need to be identified and supported within a context of detrimental conditions that may be affecting many people. The nurse needs to approach the family in partnership, with empathy and sensitivity to the uniqueness of the client. Incorrect: (b) Given the significant potential for reduced health or illness due to language barriers, poverty, lack of work, and poor housing, the nurse should not expect that personal health strategies will be sufficient. The larger structural context of people's lives also needs to be addressed. (c) All people acculturate to greater or lesser degrees in a new situation—some of the family's values and beliefs will change over time. (d) Language barriers are a major difficulty for new immigrants; however, successful adjustment is linked to many of the determinants of health.

5. Correct: (d) A culturally safe approach explicitly addresses issues of power; a culturally competent approach does not. It is an expectation that nursing professional practice includes the ability to provide culturally safe care. Incorrect: (a) and (b) Neither cultural competence nor cultural safety makes explicit that all the characteristics of culture are systematically addressed. (c) Cultural safety has some elements in common with cultural competence; however, cultural safety makes explicit issues of power and the context of power relations.

6. Correct: (d) Awareness of the intersections of the community's cultural values and the social determinants of health should be demonstrated throughout the assessment. In order to recognize the health and wellness values of the community, the nurse needs to be aware of the interactions and interventions that arise from attention to the effects of determinants of health. Incorrect: (a) The nurse needs to engage in a self-reflective process with community members, not focus on the differences between the nurse and the community. (b) A characteristic of culture is that it is fluid and dynamic. A nurse who exclusively focuses on the culture(s) of origin will not be attuned to the culture of the community that has been created. (c) It is not possible (or necessary) to have complete knowledge of cultures before or after an assessment.

Study Questions

1. See "Assumptions and Characteristics of Culture" in Chapter 8.

2. These terms are defined in the chapter. Students should focus on the similarities and differences within and between these concepts. Culture is often conflated with ethnicity and race. There can be many cultures within a larger group history and tradition, and vice versa. Though race may seem to be a neutral category or designation, it is a socially constructed concept that is often used for the purposes of domination and oppression.

3. Cultural values, beliefs, and practices are linked to our assumptions and expectations of what it means to be healthy or ill and what constitutes acceptable health/illness behaviour and responsibilities, as well as to our assumptions and expectations of personal and professional care and appropriate caring behaviours and responsibilities. It is important to remember that socioeconomic status may influence health more than culture.

4. Current conceptualizations of cultural competence and cultural safety share an awareness and valuing of the process of approaching relationships with openness and humility. The nurse is the learner in culturally competent and safe relationships. A culturally safe approach is one where the recognition of the context of power relations and structural inequities is made explicit. Proponents of cultural safety consider that cultural awareness, sensitivity, and competence provide a starting place for comprehending cultural complexities, and that cultural safety is particularly congruent with social justice and advocacy.

5. Clients and nurses are both shaped by multiple cultures, with the potential for both enhanced relationship-building and misunderstandings. Clients are shaped by their cultures of origin, education, life experiences, and the social determinants of health. CHNs' cultures of origin, professional and organizational cultures, and life experiences influence how they define health and illness and the interventions they are comfortable promoting.

6. See "Touchstones for Working with Diverse Communities" in MyNursingLab.

CHAPTER 9
Review Questions

1. Correct: (c) Mortality statistics are death statistics, and represent the ultimate threat of any health challenge. One could argue that PYLL statistics represent the loss to society. Incorrect: (a) Morbidity statistics are illness statistics. (b) Survival rates are the percentage of individuals with the health challenge who tend to live a set number of years, usually set at five years. (d) Stratified prevalence tells you only the category of population most affected.

2. Correct: (b) A cross-sectional design gives the researcher a snapshot of the present. This design is commonly used as a base line for future interventions or to measure change at a later date. Incorrect: (a) A cohort study looks at those who have a common factor, such as all women with breast cancer in a given geographical area, or those who have enrolled in a support group for persons with diabetes. (c) The researcher pairs individuals who exhibit a specific factor or illness with those who do not, to compare the effect on several variables. (d) A trial is applying an intervention of some sort to a population and comparing that result to one shown by another population not receiving the intervention.

3. Correct: (c) Reportable diseases are generally infectious diseases that have the capacity to severely affect a population. This means that healthcare practitioners have the legal responsibility to report on the number of new cases they see in given amounts of time, such as monthly or quarterly. This information informs national and international healthcare leaders as to the potential threat of that specific disease. Incorrect: (a) These are both examples of infectious diseases. (b) Case studies are usually reports on a single case that represents either the common course of the disease or a unique example. (d) The census is the count of the population as well as the answers to questions that help us to describe the population, such as language, ethnicity, work, housing, and health status.

4. Correct: (a) Not everyone who is exposed to a stressor such as a disease will respond in exactly the same manner. Genetic, lifestyle, and environmental factors strongly influence the response. Incorrect: (b) Health professionals also will be at risk, but risk is not limited to them. (c) It is impossible to remove all risk from a population. (d) Risk and survival rates are not really related.

5. Correct: (d) There are always ethical questions to consider when conducting intervention research in healthcare. The reason for the research is that the researcher has cause to believe that the new treatment or way of doing things is better, so withholding it from an individual or population must be examined for ethical reasons. Sometimes this is solved by the population itself functioning as the control group by measuring the factor of interest before applying the intervention. Incorrect: (a) While it is often difficult to get high participation or response rates, this is not a valid reason for not conducting the research. (b) While this is true, it is not a reason to avoid the research. (c) This is also true; however, researchers learn to apply for funding for portions of the total project, so they are able to demonstrate progress and results in subsequent funding applications, thus achieving their goal.

Study Questions

1. See Table 9.1.

2. Mortality statistics look at the deaths due to specific diseases/conditions; morbidity looks at people who become ill with specific diseases/conditions. Morbidity tells epidemiologists how frequently the illness occurs, while mortality tells them how likely it is that the person will die from the illness. Both types of data assist in planning future foci for health professionals and health promotion, as well as in evaluating the usefulness of interventions.

3. ■ Cohort: a study in which the researcher examines the individual characteristics of a group of people who manifest a particular disease or health challenge, to find out what common factors they share and what differences can be discerned. Example research questions: (1) What factors are common or different in a group of teens who are involved in front-end automobile collisions? (2) What are the dietary habits and hygiene practices of 10-year-olds with no dental caries?
   ■ Case-control: the individuals in the cohort with a disease or health choice are matched to individuals who are similar in some characteristics (for example, age, gender, time, geographic residence) but who have not manifested the disease or health choice in question. The health histories or characteristics of the individuals in both groups are then obtained. These data are compared and any common and different factors are identified between the two populations. Example research questions: (1) What are the similarities and differences in maternal age, presence of family support system, education, and level of anxiety between teen mothers who choose to breastfeed and those who do not? (2) What are the differences and similarities between women in province X who have multiple sclerosis and those who do not?
   ■ Cross-sectional: snapshots of the present that are used to suggest relationships that can be tested in future research. Example research questions: (1) What coping behaviours do nursing students use to manage community clinical practice and what are their anxiety levels? (2) Are stress scores for people who exercise regularly three or more times a week high or low?

4. ■ Environment: the context in which the event occurs. Examples of environments are physical, economic, and psychological
   ■ Agent: the contagious or non-contagious force that begins or continues a health challenge
   ■ Host: the human being in which the event occurs

5. *Incidence* is a measure of the new cases of a particular disease/health condition in a given space of time (usually one year); *prevalence* is the number of persons in a given population who have a given condition/disease at the current time. If prevalence and incidence are different, the disease may be chronic, with death or recovery frequently experienced a long time after diagnosis, e.g., rheumatoid arthritis. If prevalence and incidence are similar, the disease is probably short lived, with recovery or death a short time after diagnosis, e.g., the flu or Ebola virus.

6. *Prospective* is a study in which individuals are followed for a period of time to see if they acquire the disease in question or to find out what happens to them. Example research questions: (1) What illnesses/injuries are experienced by women working in an automobile manufacturing plant compared with women working in a food-processing plant over a 10-year period? (2) Is the use of health professionals different over time between women who are in professional university programs and those who are not?

Retrospective is a study in which individuals are grouped in the present relative to a particular issue or disease and then examined for past events or situations that may or may not have influenced their susceptibility to the present issue or disease. Example research questions: (1) What are the common factors in the histories of a group of women who required hysterectomies for non-malignant causes in their third decade? (2) What are common wellness strategies that a group of octogenarians have used over their lifetimes?

CHAPTER 10

Review Questions

1. Correct: (d) The Canadian Nurse is a source of primary studies, not pre-processed. Incorrect: (a), (b), (c), and (e) These are all examples of sources of pre-appraised evidence.

2. Correct: (b) The methods chosen should match the research question. Incorrect: (a) The population will influence the data collection strategy more than the method. (c) Study outcomes come after the methodology is chosen. (d) Sample size is dependent on the methodology, rather than the other way around. (e) Type of data is dependent on the methodology.

3. Correct: (a) Randomized trials allow the least possibility of bias of all designs and are therefore best for answering effectiveness questions. Incorrect: (b) Grounded theory is used to develop descriptions and explanations for a given phenomenon. (c) This type of study compares one group with another on variables of interest. (d) In this type of study subjects with the health issue are matched with others who have the same demographics (e.g., age, gender, geographic residence) but do not have the health issue present. (e) This type of study is a snapshot of the present.

4. Correct: (d) Intention to treat includes all dropouts to allow for the most conservative analysis. Incorrect: (a) Here the preciseness of the measurement is the question to be answered. (b) This is the ability of a screening test to correctly identify those who do not have a disease. (c) This describes the number of people who must be treated with the intervention in order to prevent one additional negative outcome or promote one additional positive outcome. (e) Reliability is the consistency of measures with a specific instrument.

Study Questions

1. For evidence-based decision making, consider research evidence, patient preferences, nurse skills, and resources available.

2. The most critical attitude for a nurse practising in an evidence-based way is a critical questioning approach to care planning and evaluation.

3. You might
   - collect data for outcomes of care or for process indicators such as number of visits, hours of care, attendance at a session, or number of sessions delivered;
   - deliver experimental intervention, e.g., smoking cessation, sexual health intervention, comprehensive stroke care; or
   - work collaboratively to develop an important clinical question and to write a proposal to conduct the research.

4. Individual studies can produce different results, including no significant effect of treatment if the sample size was not large enough. By reading a systematic review, you get a more complete picture of the literature, both published and unpublished, compiled in a way that minimizes bias. This pre-appraised literature will save you time, money, and resources from doing the complete literature review yourself.

5. Factors to consider when planning to implement a clinical practice or policy change:
   - characteristics of the change (or innovation) itself, e.g., how different it is from current practice, whether it will save time or add to the time needed to give care
   - characteristics of the people involved in adopting the change, e.g., how open they are to change and their attitudes toward research and research utilization, their age, the time since graduation, and their level of education
   - characteristics of the organization where the change will take place, e.g., how research-intensive the organization is, its culture of using research and "keeping up to date," and its culture of evaluating care given
   - characteristics of the organization's environment, e.g., rural or urban, in an academic setting

6. There are thousands of patient questions that are relevant to qualitative research. Here are a few examples:

   Phenomenology
   - What is the experience of stroke for elderly women?
   - What is the experience of fetal loss for couples?
   - What is the lived experience of watching a loved one being resuscitated?

   Grounded theory
   - What is the process by which diabetics achieve acceptance of their diagnosis?
   - What is the central process for deciding about disclosure of intimate partner violence to a public health nurse during a home visit?

   Ethnography
   - What is the understanding of gender roles in urban core youth?
   - "Playing the slots"—how do people who regularly gamble describe the risks/benefits of gambling?

CHAPTER 11

Review Questions

1. Correct: (a) Viral marketing relies on person-to-person electronic communications about a topic, which are self-generating—an electronic version of "word of mouth" communication. The aim is to target whole populations or segments of a population to spread a message or messages rapidly and effectively. Incorrect: (b) This sentence is

correct as it stands, but has nothing to do with viral marketing. (c) This situation exists but has nothing to do with viral marketing. (d) This has nothing to do with viral marketing.

2. Correct: (c) Providing clients with clear criteria of credible online information is the best means of enabling them to assess its quality. The Health Information Technology Institute (HITI) provides a set of criteria that evaluate health information websites for consumers, such as credibility, content, disclosures, links, design, and interactivity. Incorrect: (a) Running the URL of a health information website through an accessibility checker does not assess its quality of information, but it does assess the usability of the website for people with disabilities. (b) Encourage clients to look for a HON code logo on websites. This logo indicates that the site has been certified to have met an ethical standard for quality health information and the author intends to publish useful, objective, and accurate information. (d) SMOG criteria deal with readability of the site.

3. Correct: (a) Although sick or disabled adults are less likely to use the Internet, they do search for online health information. Incorrect: (b) Although seniors are not heavy Internet users, Internet health resources exist that are tailored for them. (c) Since Web accessibility guidelines have been instituted, many websites are accessible to the visually impaired. Nurses should, therefore, teach all clients to assess the quality of health information regardless of their state of health or age. (d) Since there are very good sources of health information beyond government websites, nurses should not restrict clients to only one source.

4. Correct: (a) Websites with features that enhance interactivity have long been known to enhance learning. Interactivity refers to a process where a user is an active participant in using technology and information exchange occurs (i.e., chat rooms, calorie calculators, and links). Incorrect: (b) Tailored messages are typically enhanced when they are presented with self-comparison and recommendations that are based on authoritative research. (c) The reading level required to ensure accessibility for laypersons should be focused at about a Grade 9 level. (d) Testimonials are helpful, but accurate information is more important.

5. Correct: (c) Three types of electronic documentation systems that have been developed include the electronic medical record (EMR), the electronic patient record (EPR), and the electronic health record (EHR). The EHR is a more comprehensive record that includes contents from the EPR and EMR. It typically includes most information gathered from encounters with the healthcare system, such as primary care and diagnostic imaging units. The EHR is being tested in numerous provinces by Canada Health Infoway, although the goal to have a pan-Canadian EHR by 2010 is still at a stage of infancy. Incorrect: (a) This could be seen as correct, but it is rarely found in Canada at this time. (b) If used, the EPR would be found in institutions. (d) This option is a possibility for the future.

6. Correct: (b) The Canadian Nursing Informatics Association (CNIA) has made recommendations concerning basic Internet and computer competencies of nursing graduates (CNIA, 2003). Incorrect: (a) The Canadian Community Health Nursing Standards of Practice are based on the principles of primary health care, which include the appropriate use of technology and resources. (c) A set of public health informatics competencies have been developed in the United States that are aimed at front-line staff, supervisory and management staff, and senior-level technical staff. (d) The CHNAC Nursing Practice Standards do not include specific competencies for informatics.

Study Questions

1. The digital divide was first identified in the late 1990s as the "haves" and "have nots," referring to populations with no access to digital information. Since its initial use, the term has been refined to describe people with no access at all, compared with those with modest access (slow dial-up connections) and the broadband elite (fast connections). Others have also revised the categories to provide more contextual information, including the following: "net-evaders" live in connected homes but do not connect to the Web themselves; "net-dropouts" used the Internet in the past but have stopped due to technical problems or dislike of the Web; "intermittent users" dropped out for a while and are back using the Internet; "truly disconnected" have never used the Internet and do not know any or many Internet users.

2. Screen readers turn text into speech and are therefore very useful to support individuals with visual impairments. OCR (optical character recognition) software is useful for visually impaired individuals who want to read text not available in digital form. They can scan the document, and with the OCR software convert the scan to digital text; they can then use a screen reader to have it read aloud. Windows users can adjust the operating system in the Control Panel's accessibility tools to adjust various settings such as text magnification, screen resolution, and image contrast. There are many other tools to enhance accessibility. A reputable Canadian source of information to stay updated on software and products is the Canadian Adaptec Network Project website.

3. The HON code is a set of criteria developed by a group of Internet experts to assess the credibility of health information websites. The code comprises eight criteria: authority, complementarity, confidentiality, attribution, justifiability, transparency of authorship, transparency of sponsorship, and honesty in advertising and editorial policy. These criteria can be used to judge the usefulness of the information provided to health information consumers and healthcare professionals. The criteria reflect an emphasis on evidence-informed practice and the use of health information that is provided in an objective, unbiased format to support client decision making. This code has been widely accepted as a means of evaluating health information websites. It is made more useful to public consumers through the "WRAPIN" website (http://www.wrapin.org), which applies these criteria to website URLs that users submit to the website for assessment.

4. There are many e-health promotion interventions that are gaining popularity and show promising results. They generally enable individuals, groups, and/or communities to take control over their own health. A few such interventions that will be interesting to continue to watch and study are online social support groups; online screening tools, especially those that use tailored messaging; e-counselling; and interactive websites that involve local citizens in driving policy change. It is important to note that many

of these interventions have not been rigorously evaluated, and further research is needed to draw firm conclusions about their effectiveness.

5. This is bit of a moving target as repositories of research findings, communities of practice, and portals continue to develop and evolve over time. There are some key Web services and sites to visit, including the Canadian Best Practices Portal for Health Promotion and Chronic Disease Prevention, the Canadian Nurses Association's NurseONE portal, the Effective Public Health Practice Program Health-Evidence.ca: Promoting Evidence-Based Decision-Making, and the CHNET Works! Community of Practice.

6. Review Table 11.1. Some of the key actions include developing your own skills in online health information retrieval and evaluation, fostering discussions with clients regarding health information they found online, and teaching clients how to evaluate the quality and appropriateness of health information on the Internet.

CHAPTER 12

Review Questions

1. Correct: (c) The first recorded worldwide threat from a communicable disease was bubonic plague, which killed about one-third of the population in Europe in the 13th century. Incorrect: (a) Although typhoid was recorded earlier than bubonic plague, it was not recorded as causing worldwide outbreaks until the 19th century. (b) Although evidence of TB disease was found in skeletal remains from a Neolithic settlement in the Eastern Mediterranean dating back to 7000 BC, and tubercular decay has been found in the spines of mummies from 3000–2400 BC, worldwide threat was not evident. (d) The use of the word "leprosy" before the mid-19th century, when microscopic examination of skin for medical diagnosis was first developed, can seldom be correlated reliably with Hansen's disease as we understand it today.

2. Correct: (c) In order to identify an emerging infection, a surveillance program is vital for ongoing detection of changes in prevalence and incidence of disease. Incorrect: (a) Healthcare professional awareness is not a key component of creating disease data; the healthcare professional is required to report disease. (b) The public is not generally aware of the reporting requirements and does not have the required information or authority to report. Public awareness is necessary for creating disease data. (d) Immunization uptake rates are not a contributing factor since an emerging infection occurs prior to vaccine availability.

3. Correct: (d) The host must be infected for the infectious organism to be passed directly or indirectly. Excretions are considered an indirect route of transmission. Incorrect: (a) Infectious toxins is not an accurate term; the infectious agent may have associated toxic products. (b) The transmission of a communicable disease is to a susceptible person, not from a vulnerable person. (c) This is only partially incorrect. The exposure is to either the infectious agent or its toxic products and either directly or indirectly through an intermediate plant or animal host, vector, or the inanimate environment.

4. Correct: (c) Influenza is spread by droplets through coughing, sneezing, or singing. Incorrect: (a) Between 2000 and 8000 Canadians die of influenza and its complications annually. (b) Human influenza is a respiratory infection caused by influenza virus. (d) Vaccination is routinely given annually at the onset of the influenza season, typically in October or November.

5. Correct: (d) As of yet there is no West Nile virus vaccine. Incorrect: (a) HPV vaccine was licensed for use in Canada in July 2006. (b) Pandemic influenza H1N1 vaccine was licensed for use in Canada in October 2009. (c) Rotavirus vaccine was licensed for use in Canada in August 2006.

6. Correct: (a) E. coli were found in the Ontario town of Walkerton's water supply, raising awareness of the importance of safe municipal water systems across Canada. Incorrect: (b) There have been small outbreaks of listeria associated with soft cheese or milk products. (c) Outbreaks of cryptosporidium occurred in North Battleford, Saskatchewan. (d) Legionella outbreaks have occurred but have been associated with air conditioning systems or cooling towers.

7. Correct: (c) Vector-borne diseases most commonly seen in Canada include Eastern equine encephalitis, Lyme disease, and West Nile virus. Incorrect: (a) Rabies is a zoonotic infection. (b) Pertussis is a respiratory infection passed by airborne route. (d) Hantavirus is a zoonotic infection.

Study Questions

1. Communicable diseases are illnesses caused by a specific agent that arise from direct or indirect transmission from an infected host through an intermediate environment. The control and management of communicable diseases is based on a sound understanding of epidemiological investigation and the interplay of the host–agent–environmental factors.

2. There are two modes of transmission: direct and indirect contact with infected hosts or with their excretions. Most diseases are transmitted, or spread, through contact or close proximity because the causative bacteria or virus is airborne.

3. Contact tracing begins with interviewing this student (initial case definition) to gather data to confirm the exhibiting signs and symptoms and place and time of exposure to TB. Usually, the investigation is done by CHNs at the local health unit. A list of contacts will be gathered to identify the index case or first case. The follow-up will include investigation and surveillance of each of these contacts for the needed screening, diagnosis, and treatment as deemed necessary.

4. First, validate that meningitis is a confirmed medical diagnosis. If the diagnosis is confirmed, work with the daycare staff to ensure that you have all the information necessary for your investigation with follow-up to be carried out in a timely manner. Provide information on meningitis re: mode of transmission, incubation period, signs and symptoms, period of communicability, and control measures (see Table 12.1). Educate the staff and parents in the control and management of the disease.

5. ▪ Review the principles of communicable disease and epidemiology and evidence from the latest research studies to ensure that you will have a sound theoretical base to guide your practice.
   ▪ Understand your role by reviewing the agency guidelines and protocol in communicable disease control and

management, including the latest directives from the Public Health Agency of Canada for communicable disease control measures.

- Conduct your own community assessment to better understand the health and risks of residents in your community. Assess the agent, host, and environmental factors by conducting a community scan and by examining local health data. Assess the relationship of your community to the larger communities for mortality and morbidity data to see how healthy your community is and why your community is at risk for hepatitis. Validate and conclude your assessment of the hepatitis situation in your community by discussing your findings and questions with your team to formulate a community plan of action with a focus on hepatitis A prevention.

6. You would need full disclosure of all the contacts and the nature of the contacts in a timely manner. This will enable you to identify whether these contacts are at risk through confidential contact tracing. Health education on the disease and its mode of transmission can be carried out at the same time to avoid further spread of the infection and to encourage early treatment.

CHAPTER 13

Review Questions

1. Correct: (a) This is a population indicator that describes the population characteristics of the community. Incorrect: (b) Patient satisfaction is an acceptability indicator for the health system performance. (c) Exposure to air pollution is an environmental indicator for non-medical determinants of health. (d) Number of low-birthweight babies is a health status indicator that describes the health condition of the community population. (See Table 13.2.)

2. Correct: (a) While all other determinants can impact on the health of individuals in one way or other, people who cannot access health services are usually those who are too frail or poor and who live in rural communities. Thus, whether transportation is available is the most important social determinant of health for people requiring home services. Accessibility is also one of the key primary health care principles. Incorrect: (b) Government and policies help to form the structure of the service delivery system and related healthcare funding allocations. (c) Education gives the people the needed and appropriate level of health information so they are well informed. (d) Culture and religion provide people with culturally sensitive care.

3. Correct: (d) This option is based on the Public Health Agency of Canada's statement that the main goals of a population health approach are to maintain and improve the health status of the entire population and to reduce inequities in health status among population groups. CHNs must focus on how to empower the community so they have the needed skills to advance to a higher level of functioning. Various population health actions are described in Appendix 13A. Incorrect: (a) Where income is the most important determinant of health, eliminating the unemployment rate is an unrealistic goal. (b) This addresses only a segment of the population. (c) While mobilizing the community to make participatory healthcare decisions is sound, making the decision alone is only a

process for community engagement; it is not the goal of the population health approach.

4. Correct: (b) CHNs can select a valid risk assessment tool to assess prenatal and postnatal women who may be at risk for postpartum depression and then plan for the interventions as per evidence-based practice and agency policies. Incorrect: (a) Assessing and interviewing all prenatal and postnatal women would not be cost effective and efficient. In providing population healthcare, CHNs do not necessarily work with every member (of the population group) in the community. Rather, they assess the conditions of risks and benefits that apply to the entire population or to its significant aggregates and deliver health services to those who are at risk. (c) and (d) These are tertiary prevention activities. They are not early identification and screening protocols to assess risk and thereby to reduce the likelihood for the disease occurrence. Also, a focus group is not an appropriate intervention for women who were just diagnosed with postpartum depression. One-to-one counselling would be more appropriate.

5a. Correct: (c) Figure 13.2 shows that Canada has a rapidly aging population. If one reviews the Canadian cancer statistics as well as mortality, morbidity, and hospital admission rates, there is a high incidence/prevalence for prostate cancer, breast cancer, colon cancer, lung cancer, heart disease, hip fractures, and falls among older adults.

5b. Correct: (b) The community forum approach allows community members to discuss issues, opinions, or concerns with the decision makers through two-way dialogue. It is an inexpensive way to collect community data concerning the people who are either directly involved in or affected by the topic being discussed. Incorrect: (a) Although a community survey can produce a wide range of questions, it can be expensive to administer and the response rate tends to be low. (c) A focus group is smaller in scale and is a more feasible approach once specific groups (e.g., healthcare providers or caregivers) are identified for further dialogue. (d) Census data collect information about every member of some population; they do not give the needed information to specific service utilization.

6. Correct: (a) The Senate of Canada (2009) endorses a new style of governance in which the federal, provincial, territorial, and local governments must take a leadership role to implement population health policies with clear program goals and targets. Incorrect: (b) Local government must work with federal and provincial governments. Local government has the responsibility to engage its community members by encouraging participation of the community and reinforcing citizens' capacities and expertise. By doing so, a healthy and inclusive community will be created and the community members will be empowered. (c) and (d) These represent only a segment of the population. Co-ordination and implementation of population policies for various programs must be a concerted effort by all community members involved, and the co-ordination process is a mix of top-down and bottom-up approaches.

7. Correct: (a) The fundraising event engages the community in a marathon run to raise money for cancer research. All participants share this common goal to raise awareness about cancer care. Such activities can strengthen community resources; raise social consciousness about their goal for change; and empower, reinforce,

and further expand social networks and support within a community and beyond. Incorrect: (b) A food bank program is a service available for use by the population in need. (c) A community health survey is a community data collection method. (d) Construction of a sport centre is a sign of economic growth in the community and provides a place for socialization, not for community development.

Study Questions

1. CHNs work in many settings: homes, schools, health clinics, community centres, physicians' offices, family health teams, and health units.
   - Most CHNs work as home health nurses (HHNs) and public health nurses (PHNs). HHNs care for individuals and families, and PHNs care for the community or population at large. Both groups of nurses apply nursing process with a focus to promote the health of community residents. See Chapter 3 for the roles and functions of other CHNs such as nurse practitioners, occupational health nurses, and nurses working in the faith community or correctional setting.
   - HHNs may be employed by VONs, St. Elizabeth, ParaMed, or ComCare. They provide mainly direct care, from managing acute or post-surgical problems to rehabilitative or palliative care.
   - Some other CHNs work in public health for official health agencies such as health units. They carry out services as set by the Health Protection and Promotion Act and provide population-focused care.
   - Depending on the settings and the nature of the work, CHNs carry out various functions in consultation, counselling, health teaching, case management, referral and follow-up, screening, outreach, disease surveillance, policy development and enforcement, social marketing, advocacy, community organizing, coalition building, and collaboration.

2. Healthy communities are those with competent community dynamics that foster public participation, mutual support, and community action to promote optimal community growth. Characteristics of healthy communities are provided in the box on page 214.

3. To promote the health of the community, CHNs must understand the characteristics and needs of their populations and the community. They need to possess strong community assessment skills to get a realistic profile of community dynamics and to critically analyze and explore the roots of the community strengths or problems, and assess the effects of various social determinants of health on the health of the population.

   CHNs need to develop a community plan to mobilize resources to help the community attain optimal health. These population-focused health promotion strategies include, but are not limited to, advocacy for healthy public policy, strengthening of community action, and the creation of supportive environments. The ability to work in partnership with the stakeholders and engage them at the grassroots level is critical throughout the nursing process.

   Overall, CHNs must possess a sound knowledge base of community health promotion strategies to guide their practice. Strong research and critical thinking skills are essential for CHNs to analyze the problems and strengths and help translate knowledge to practice from their evidence-based practice.

4. CHNs systematically assess all components that will affect the health of the population and the community dynamics and functions. These components are outlined in Figure 13.1 as follows: population, physical environments, socioeconomic environments, education and healthy child development, culture and religion, health and social services, and transportation.

5. Population health aims to maintain and improve the health status of the entire population (i.e., community-focused); a specific target population (i.e., systems-focused); or the individuals (i.e., individual-focused) within the community. It strives to reduce inequities in health status between population groups by addressing what determines their health.

   Community engagement is a process involving citizens at various levels of participation based on interpersonal communication and trust and a common understanding and purpose.

   Community governance is a method of community engagement that ensures effective involvement and empowerment of local community representatives in the planning, direction setting, and monitoring of health organizations to meet the health needs and priorities of the populations within local neighbourhood communities.

   Community development is the process of involving a community in the identification and reinforcement of those aspects of everyday life, culture, and political activity that are conducive to health. This might include support for political action to modify the total environment and strengthen resources for healthy living, as well as reinforcing social networks and social support within a community and developing the material resources and economic base available to the community.

   Capacity building is a process that strengthens the ability of an individual, organization, community, or health system to develop and implement health promotion initiatives and sustain positive health outcomes over time. It involves organizational development, human resource development, leadership, partnership, resource allocation, and policy formulation.

6. Community dialogue encourages two-way communication among community members to share and discuss their experiences, lessons learned, problems, needs, visions, and goals. Members engage in the discussions, exchange information, and become an open learning community and support for one another. When working with a population that the CHNs are not familiar with or when there is a need to introduce new information or resolve old community issues, community dialogue is an effective way for both parties to learn about each other's cultures, needs, values, expectations, and reasons why differences exist. Once a common understanding is reached, mutual goals can be developed and community partnership for actions can be built.

CHAPTER 14

Review Questions

1. Correct: (c) The steps in this cycle may need to be repeated as one develops a better understanding of an issue and

obtains additional input from partners. It may be necessary to cycle back to other steps in the process to try to develop a more complete picture of the factors that are affecting the problem, and the potential solutions that need to be considered. Incorrect: (a) The cycle is not linear, steps may be repeated or cycled back to. (b) Partners should be involved throughout the process. The authentic engagement of the community in planning, monitoring, and evaluating community health programs is essential. (d) More than one alternative may be selected.

2. Correct: (b) The logic model is unique among tools for its simplicity in demonstrating program interrelationships and linkages. Incorrect: (a) A logic model is a diagram or visual representation of what a program is supposed to do, with who, and why. (c) Logic models should be developed in collaboration with community and academic partners. In this way, both experiential learning and research findings can inform model development. Joint preparation of a logic model will help build consensus about program priorities among the planning team. (d) In using a logic model, one should avoid positioning it as a rigid guideline, which prevents iterative evolution or lateral exploration of the program under review.

3. Correct: (c) Short-term outcomes are the immediate and direct results of the program. Incorrect: (a) Training youth workers in crisis management is an "activity." Activities are the specific intervention strategies to be used for each component. Therefore, with the suicide prevention example, the crisis intervention component includes the activity of training youth workers in crisis management. (b) Reducing suicide rates is a long-term outcome. (d) Target groups are the intended recipients of the program and should be identified in the first planning stage (CAT) when developing a logic model.

4. Correct: (b) This principle is transparency, whereby the process for selecting priorities is made apparent to those who were not directly involved in the process. In other words, key stakeholders are able to understand how you got from point A (understanding problem and considering possible intervention strategies) to point B (priority definition of the problem and strategies). Incorrect: (a) Setting priorities means that one can neither address all of the identified needs nor operationalize all of the proposed interventions. (c) Both objective and subjective criteria are important to identify priority interventions. (d) It is not realistic to involve a large community in a priority-setting exercise; however, one can invite input from selected community members.

5. Correct: (b) Refer to Table 14. 2. Incorrect: (a), (c), and (d) Refer to Table 14.2 for examples of determinants at each level of the socioecological model.

6. Correct: (b) The authentic engagement of the community (parents, teachers, and children) in planning, monitoring, and evaluating the program will be essential to address underlying social determinants of health, to ensure "buy-in" and transparency. Incorrect: (a), (c), and (d) Community input on the feasibility of implementing interventions in their setting and the need to adapt interventions to ensure cultural and geographic relevance are required prior to the selection and implementation of interventions.

Study Questions

1. The steps in a planning-evaluation cycle do not always occur in a linear fashion. Previous steps may need to be repeated or undertaken in more depth as one develops a better understanding of an issue and obtains additional input from collaborators and partners.

2. Four factors influencing selection of program planning and evaluation framework are
   - A standard planning framework may be used within departments of a healthcare agency to promote a more coherent and consistent approach to planning.
   - Use of a particular framework may be a requirement of those who fund programs as this allows them to compare results across funded programs.
   - A framework may be chosen because it helps detail a particular aspect of the planning process that is vexing or challenging.
   - The selection of a framework may be influenced by a set of underlying values or principles such as an intention to use participatory approaches.

3. Tools commonly used in planning programs include
   - Environmental scans using an assessment of strengths, weaknesses, opportunities, and threats; key informant interviews, focus groups, and round tables are examples of ways to engage partners efficiently and fully in a planning process.
   - Examples of tools used to organize information include matrices, content analysis of qualitative data, graphs and tables to display quantitative data, priority-setting, and Gantt charts.

4. Three uses of quantitative data in program planning and evaluation are
   - Document the magnitude of the problem and contributing factors.
   - Help estimate program costs and the potential return on investments.
   - Evaluate short-term and long-term results of the program.

5. Three principles of priority setting are buy-in, transparency, and communication.

6. Five main elements of the multiple intervention program framework are identify community health issue; describe socioecological determinants; consider and select intervention options; optimize intervention strategies; and monitor and evaluate impacts, spin-offs, and sustainability.

CHAPTER 15

Review Questions

1. Correct: (d) The complex interplay of genetic, biology, and behaviour and the environment shapes women's health. Incorrect: (a) Although genetic endowment influences women's health, it cannot be assumed to be the single most important factor. (b) Although biology shapes women's health, it does not act alone to do that. (c) Behavioural influences never act alone to impact women's health.

2. Correct: (a) Poverty is a material deprivation that threatens adequate childhood nutrition. Incorrect: (b) Poverty is a political issue. Because gender social welfare politics create the context for gender differences in access to employment, pay equity, and primary care-giving roles, women are vulnerable to living in poverty. (c) Poverty is a social

and economic determinant of health and is therefore a critical aspect of public health policy. (d) Poverty impacts children's nutrition, health, and growth and development well into adolescence.

3. Correct: (d) A lack of access to the social determinants of health in pregnancy can worsen existing poor health status. Incorrect: (a) Material deprivation is known to create adverse birth outcomes. (b) Poverty and homelessness act as barriers to accessing adequate prenatal care. (c) Access to the social determinants of health is a fundamental basis for primary health care provision and public health interventions.

4. Correct: (a) Screening for antenatal depression provides information about the risk for postpartum depression (PPD); CHNs can mobilize support and resources for women during the antenatal period. Incorrect: (b) Antenatal screening cannot prevent PPD, but it can help anticipate women's potential risk for PPD. (c) Depression can be treated in pregnancy; for example, nonpharmacological therapies are available. (d) Antenatal depression is responsive to nonpharmacological treatment (i.e., exercise, cognitive behavioural therapy).

5. Correct: (c) We know that, regardless of stressors in a child's life or genetic qualities, sustained and healthy relationships with caring adults are essential for infants' and children's physical and emotional development. Incorrect: (a) Although access to material resources has been linked to children's opportunities for development and is a vital determinant of child well-being, access to all the resources in the world without sustained, healthy relationships with caring adults will not ensure a child's optimal development. (b) While genetic predisposition is an important determinant of child development, it is only one piece of the complex influences on that development. (d) All infants and children experience stress; in fact, stress is a stimulus for development.

6. Correct: (a) Research has shown that toxic stress influences the physiology of the infant's or child's developing brain. Toxic stress takes many forms, including the lack of sustained, healthy relationships with caring adults. Incorrect: (b) Although toxic stress may disrupt relationships with adults, this answer does not acknowledge the wide range of sources of stress or the range of capacities of caring adults. (c) This is based on an assumption that toxic stress is related to child maltreatment or other sources of physical injury. (d) Although toxic stress may influence an infant's or child's capacity to engage with other children, there are many other factors that may influence these relationships. Exposure to toxic stress may influence but will not determine the infant's or child's capacity to engage in relationships with others.

7. Correct: (b) In all provinces, nurses have the responsibility to report suspected cases of child abuse or neglect to the appropriate provincial authority. Incorrect: (a) Although CHNs may be involved in family assessment and intervention when child abuse or neglect is suspected, this will depend on the organization of resources and the particular CHN's role. (c) Although (in some instances) it may be appropriate for the CHN to discuss the issue with the child, this will depend on the role of the particular CHN and the organization of services for the child. (d) Although the CHN will often have the responsibility to inquire about the history of past incidents of abuse or neglect within the specific family, and in fact will require this information in order to provide support to particular infants, children, and their families, this is not the first and primary responsibility.

Study Questions

1. The health of mothers in Canada is shaped by contemporary discourses, ideals, and social values related to what constitutes "good mothering." Such discourses rely upon the often invisible but powerful ideal of "exclusive" mothering, the idea being that good mothers devote themselves to mothering that necessitates a withdrawal from the labour force, thereby creating situations of economic dependence. Given that in 2000, 83% of lone-parent families were headed by females, there is a greater chance that single mothers will live with some form of material and/or economic disadvantage, both of which are known social determinants of maternal health.

2. Social isolation following childbirth has been described by new mothers over several decades, and it is known that social support has a positive impact on reducing at-risk women's potential for postpartum depression. CHNs can consider tailoring postpartum support and care to include ways to connect new mothers to one another so they can benefit from the "buffering" effects of social inclusion, connection, and community. Knowledge about infant safety, nutrition, and play and development, among other topics, can also be shared among new mothers to enhance the health promotion work of CHNs.

3. "Critical periods" refer to a specific limited time wherein crucial developmental advancement takes place. One critical period for healthy child development is the prenatal period, where intense physical growth takes place and the foundations of the child's physical and intellectual capacities are developed. Stressors during the prenatal period (including excessive maternal stress, exposure to toxic substances, or poor nutrition) may have lifelong consequences from birth onward. Other critical periods in relation to specific aspects of child development (including social development, language acquisition, and physical growth) have been identified by various researchers. For example, infancy is a critical period for language acquisition, a time when the child begins to absorb sound stimuli and copy some of the sounds they hear.

4. The term "inequality" is generally used to describe differences of any sort in health and access to healthcare within a population. An example of this might be that children with diabetes have access to a greater portion of our healthcare resources than children without chronic illness. "Inequity" is a term used to refer to differences in health and access to healthcare that are unjust or unfair. This might be the difference in the availability of maternal healthcare in rural and remote settings compared to urban settings. CHNs may have no responsibilities in relation to inequalities, except where an inequality might be considered unfair. In the development of programs and in advocating for services, CNHs have opportunities to draw attention to inequities in health and access to healthcare and to advocate for a more just, fair system.

5. A social determinants of health perspective can help CHNs identify and act upon the conditions that impact

women's/children's power, choice, and ability to achieve health. A relational approach focuses attention on the inseparability of experience, health, and context; that is, CHNs can simultaneously examine individual health behaviours, lifestyles, genetic endowment, etc., and the broader socio-environmental conditions that create risk in pregnancy, result in adverse birth outcomes, and become barriers to healthy childhood development.

CHAPTER 16

Review Questions

1. Correct: (d) Family form includes any combination of two or more persons who are bound together over time by ties of mutual consent, birth and/or adoption or placement: nuclear families, extended families, single-parent families, blended families, and homosexual families. Incorrect: (a) Family forms are not limited to nuclear families. (b) Family forms are not limited to homosexual families. (c) Family forms are not limited to single-parent families.

2. Correct: (d) In fact, the number of childless couples is now surpassing those with children. Incorrect: (a) Married couples are now in the minority. (b) The population is aging. (c) We are in a period when life expectancy is increasing.

3. Correct: (d) When used appropriately, "commending a family's competence, resilience, and strengths and offering them a new opinion or view of themselves creates a context for change that allows families to discover their own solutions to problems and enhance healing" (Wright & Leahey, 2009, p. 151). Family commendations can be interventions that demonstrate the standard of Promoting Health. Incorrect: (a) The quotation best describes the standard of Professional Responsibility and Accountability. (b) This best describes the standard of Facilitating Access and Equity. (c) This best describes the standard of Building Relationships.

4. Correct: (d) Nurses must have the conviction to assist the family to identify their strengths, to secure extra-familial resources, and to identify their potential for growth through use of family protective and recovery factors. Incorrect: (a) This best describes the standard of Professional Responsibility and Accountability. (b) This best describes the standard of Facilitating Access and Equity. (c) This best describes the standard of Building Relationships.

5. Correct: (c) A collaborative relationship facilitates an assessment of family strengths; promotes an understanding of the family fears, issues, and concerns; and identifies opportunities to collaboratively plan, intervene, and evaluate the desired goals. Incorrect: (a) This best describes the standard of Professional Responsibility and Accountability. (b) This best describes the standard of Facilitating Access and Equity. (d) This best describes the standard of Building Family Capacity.

6. Correct: (b) Access to resources and services should be based on the needs of the family, with an understanding of those needs in a cultural context. Incorrect: (a) This best describes the standard of Professional Responsibility and Accountability. (c) This best describes the standard of Building Relationships. (d) Bomar (2004) defines family health promotion as "the process of achieving family well-being in the biological, emotional, physical, and spiritual realms for individual members and the family

unit" (p. 11). Assessment, in and of itself, is not sufficient to demonstrate the standard of Facilitating Access and Equity.

7. Correct: (d) The goal of case management is to arrive at quality, cost-effective client/family outcomes. Incorrect: (a) The goal is to achieve the provision of quality, cost-effective services. (b) The goal is focused on client/family outcomes, not cost-containment. (c) A structured care plan may or may not suit the needs of clients and families and may or may not result in quality, cost-effective services.

Study Questions

1. A family is "a social group whose members share common values and interact with each other over time" (Hunt, 2009, p. 81). Family functions include
   - physical maintenance and care of group members;
   - addition of new members through procreation or adoption;
   - socialization of children;
   - social control of members;
   - production, consumption, distribution of goods and services; and
   - affective nurturance–love (Vanier Institute of the Family, 2006).

2. The demographic shifts that are changing the composition of Canadian families include
   - The declining proportion of "traditional" families.
   - Increasing numbers of families with no children living at home. This may be due to lower fertility rates, decisions to delay having children or choosing as a couple not to have children, and marrying later in life.
   - More couples and families living in common-law relationships, meaning that people are not waiting for marriage to have children.
   - Canadian legislation recognizing same-sex marriages.
   - Children moving back home between school, jobs, and marriages.
   - Two parents working in paid employment outside of the home, resulting in very busy lives of families and lack of free time.
   - Single-parent families headed by women experiencing financial stress.
   - Round-the-clock consumer services.
   - Increased life expectancy.
   - Divorce and re-marriage, resulting in increased numbers of blended families.

   For more information, visit Statistics Canada and The Vanier Institute of the Family online (listed in the chapter references).

3.
   - First: family as context to the client. The CHN focuses nursing care on the individual, with the family as a secondary focus.
   - Second: family is viewed as a sum of its individual family members or parts. Healthcare is provided to each individual family member and this is viewed as providing family healthcare. This is not the same as viewing the whole family as the focus of care.
   - Third: family subsystems. Family dyads, triads, and other family subsystems are the focus of care.
   - Fourth: family as client. The unit of care is the entire family. The nurse does not focus on either the individual or the family, but concentrates on both the individual

and the family simultaneously. The interaction that occurs among members of the family is emphasized.

- ■ Fifth: family as a component of society. The family is seen as one of society's basic institutions. (Friedman et al., 2003)

4. A genogram (see Figure 16.3) is used to build a picture of family structure, relationships, and boundaries. Another tool that is especially useful for CHNs is the ecomap (see Figure 16.4), which visually represents a family's connections and the nature of relationships with the larger community and can be used to assess resources and strengths (Tarko & Reed, 2004; Wright & Leahy, 2009).

5. The components of a family home visit are building relationships; maintain confidentiality; reflective questioning; setting mutual goals; family assessment tools; and negotiate plan of care and identify parameters for relationship.

6. Case management is a collaborative approach used by CHNs to co-ordinate and facilitate the delivery of health-care services. Consider the benefits of adopting a family-centred case-management approach versus a client-centred approach.

CHAPTER 17

Review Questions

1. Correct: (b) Children and youth living in poverty are disadvantaged in almost every way. Aboriginal children are the poorest in the country. An example of high-risk behaviour contributing to leading causes of mortality is driving a car after drinking alcohol. Car crashes are the main cause of injury and death in children and youth. Incorrect: (a) Today, infectious diseases cause fewer than 5% of all deaths. Sporting injuries usually limit activity but are not a leading cause of morbidity and mortality. (c) ADHD is a health concern but does not put teens at greatest risk for early death. (d) Smoking and unprotected sex are considered risky behaviours but do not affect health status as much as drinking and car crashes, poverty, and Aboriginal status.

2. Correct: (b) Youth-led initiatives foster youth engagement. Focus groups can be very effective in gathering community views. They encourage community participation in the identification of assets and needs. Incorrect: (a) This does not involve youth in the planning process. (c) This engages youth but does not allow for youth to assist in the initial planning of the program. (d) This is an important part of the planning process but does not engage the youth.

3. Correct: (d) A healthy social environment is not emphasized in this scenario; however, teaching and learning, health and other support services, and healthy physical environment are the three components illustrated in this scenario. Incorrect: (a) A supportive social environment is not emphasized. (b) Health promotion is not one of the four components of CSH. (c) While health promotion is a key element of a CHN's work, it is not one of the four components of CSH.

4. Correct: (b) To collect data about the strengths and areas of need of the school community, a variety of tools and approaches can be used. Interviews, focus groups, community forums, and surveys such as the Healthy School Profile with students, staff, principals, and community members gives key people in the school community the opportunity to provide input. Incorrect: (a) A health status report would not provide information that is specific to this school's area of focus. (c) At this point in the process the nurse is working with her school partners to assess the nutrition issue fully. They are not getting into planning activities. (d) The nurse is in the process of assessment and would consult the dietitian in planning possible solutions.

5. Correct: (a) It is important and more effective to involve as many stakeholders as possible to begin a comprehensive assessment of the situation. Incorrect: (b) This is more of a downstream approach and does not fully address a prevention strategy. (c) This strategy could be part of an overall strategy but is not a first step in establishing an effective prevention initiative. (d) Posters can increase awareness among students and teachers and are part of an overall prevention strategy; however, they would be considered following a comprehensive assessment of the situation.

Study Questions

1. The principles of health promotion, including empowerment, fostering meaningful participation, and building on the strengths of individuals and communities, are relevant whether working with individuals, families, or whole school communities. CHNs generally view the individual or community within an ecological framework (i.e., in the context of their environment). Health promotion strategies, such as community action, building health public policy, and creating supportive environments, are appropriate for health promotion at the school level. Developing personal skills to increase self-care and healthy habits are often supported in one-to-one or group education/training sessions. These skills can in turn contribute to creating a healthy school environment.

2. While CHNs across Canada have provided leadership in promoting the benefits of socio-environmental approaches for school-based health promotion, they have encountered a number of challenges. In the last 15 years, significant reductions in the financing of health and social services eroded public health services across the country. Health service restructuring and changing public health mandates at the provincial/territorial level reduced or eliminated CHNs in schools or placed constraints on their practice. A lack of stable funding for health promotion and prevention programs reduced PHN staffing. The fragmentation of these programs into a restructured health service often contributed to the invisibility of CHNs and other staff.

While individual attention and the counselling role of the CHN can make important contributions to adolescent health—i.e., personal skill building, optimizing the problem-solving and coping abilities of young people—such services are rarely included within mandated public health services. Even in jurisdictions supportive of this CHN role, most CHNs are on-site only a few hours per week, so it is important that additional counselling services be provided by other professionals such as social workers, guidance counsellors, and psychologists.

The Comprehensive School Health framework facilitates interventions on many levels: individual- or group-focused interventions, including one-to-one counselling in an office or school-based clinic; classroom education; small group facilitation; school-wide health promotion; and community-wide action. CHNs are quite capable and skilled to practise across this continuum of service provision, but this needs to be recognized in the mandatory programs for school-based health promotion.

3. The term Comprehensive School Health (CSH) was coined in the 1980s to describe the socioecological approach to school-based health promotion in Canada and the United States. In Canada, CSH is now defined as "a multifaceted approach that includes teaching health knowledge and skills in the classroom, creating health-enabling social and physical environments, and developing linkages with parents and the wider community to support optimal health and learning" (CASH, 2007). The four main components are teaching and learning; health and other support services; supportive social environment; and healthy physical environment. This approach emphasizes the creation of dynamic, collaborative partnerships among children and youth, parents, teachers, principals, school councils, and members of community agencies concerned about the health and learning of children. Partnerships and policies are viewed as integral within all four elements of CSH.

The concept of the Health Promoting School (HPS) began in Scotland in 1986 and provided the World Health Organization (WHO) with an opportunity to test the principles and strategies set out in the Ottawa Charter. Since that time, the HPS movement has further broadened and refined these initial ideas through the lens of "a settings approach" endorsed in the Jakarta Declaration on Health Promotion into the 21st century. The HPS movement has emphasized national policy formation, community mobilization, and intersectoral partnerships that are reflected in the 10 key principles guiding the development of HPS: democracy, equity, empowerment and action competence, school environment, curriculum, teacher training, measuring success, collaboration, communities, and sustainability.

The Coordinated School Health Program (CSHP) includes eight components to effectively address major health risks identified among the school-aged population: health education; physical education; health services; nutrition services; health promotion for staff; counselling, psychological and social services; healthy school environment (physical and psychosocial); and parent and community involvement.

4. More than a decade of work in the healthy school field points to the need for a team or committee that is composed of teachers/school staff, a critical mass of students, parents and community members that lead and coordinate efforts in addressing health and social issues in the school. To ensure the sustainability of school-based health promotion activities, a working committee or "action team" of dedicated representatives or school champions is necessary. This composition facilitates the entire school community living out the values of democracy, equitable access, and respect for all school stakeholders within the school community. It is also consistent with the principles of community development, mobilization, and empowerment, where work with a core community group enables the building of capacity that enhances the health of the community-at-large.

5. Poverty; unintentional injuries related to falls, burns, suffocation, traffic mishaps, sports injuries; communicable diseases; inactivity and unhealthy eating; mental health problems such as depressive and anxiety mood disorders, disordered eating, sleep deprivation; risky behaviours related to sexual activity, drug and substance use and abuse, excessive speed in driving motor vehicles, all-terrain vehicles and water crafts; coping with chronic diseases such as diabetes; allergic reactions to foods, insects, environmental pollen, dust, mould, and chemicals.

6. The Health Council of Canada (2006) identifies the following ten key ingredients for effective child and youth health programs:
   i. Act early, act often [e.g., build strengths from preconception and through pregnancy, through early child development programs, and by promoting life skills through adolescence; act quickly to address problems that arise in children and youth].
   ii. Involve parents and families [e.g., promote good parenting and supportive positive relationships with parents].
   iii. Involve youth [e.g., engage young people to identify needs as well as plan and deliver services; promote youth leadership opportunities and peer-based approaches].
   iv. Harness the energy of the community [e.g., work closely with all relevant sectors and promote collaboration amongst community partners].
   v. Use a variety of approaches [e.g., policy, legislation, regulation, education, and services].
   vi. Integrate policy and practice [e.g., reduce fragmented programs and promote integrated initiatives at the local, provincial, and federal levels].
   vii. Make programs accessible and equitable [e.g., remove barriers to accessing programs, such as income, distance, language, or lack of awareness].
   viii. Adapt programs to meet community needs [e.g., involve community members in tailoring and customizing child and youth programs to meet the needs and priorities of specific communities].
   ix. Modify programs based on what works [e.g., build mechanisms to share the growing body of knowledge about what works and plan interventions accordingly].
   x. Maintain political commitment and sustain good programs [e.g., ensure sustainable funding from multiple ministries to widely support and adopt effective child and youth health initiatives]. (pp. 38–43)

CHAPTER 18

Review Questions

1. Correct: (b) Many clinics are feminized spaces where boys and men are not comfortable. Efforts need to be made to make them feel welcome and address barriers to attendance. Incorrect: (a), (c), and (d) These actions do not address the boys' reluctance to attend the clinic.

2. Correct: (b) False: Sex is biological and gender is social. Incorrect: (a) True: One's biological sex affects one's gender identity. (c) True: Gender refers to a social construct. (d) True: Sex is made up of chromosomal, hormonal, and physical factors. Gender includes identities and relations.

3. Correct: (b) It is important to develop a gender-sensitive approach that considers the unique ways that obesity

affects men and the role of food in their lives. Incorrect: (a) While some people may think of body image as a "women's issue," it is incorrect to assume men are not concerned with their weight and shape. (c) It is a gender bias to assume that men like exercise. (d) One does not need to be a man to develop or run a gender-sensitive program for men.

4. Correct: (d) Social norms for men suggest that help-seeking is a form of weakness. Incorrect: (a) Men and women both experience illness that requires medical attention. Both men and women can benefit from preventive services. (b) There is no evidence that men are more resilient and require less healthcare. (c) Men are less likely to engage in preventive health practices.

5. Correct: (d) The healthcare needs of men and women can differ and so we must tailor our programs accordingly. Incorrect: (a) and (b) Men and women are similar in many regards. While one should be gender sensitive, it is incorrect to assume men and women require different care in all regards. (c) One should be gender sensitive and consider the ways that men and women may differ and require different approaches.

Study Questions

1. Sex refers to the biological makeup of and differences between females and males. It is a concept that encompasses anatomy, physiology, genes, and hormones that all influence how we function and see ourselves. Gender refers to the array of socially constructed roles and relationships, personality traits, attitudes, behaviours, values, and relative power and influence that society ascribes men and women on a differential basis.

2. The use of a gender lens is one way to ensure that nursing programs and interventions are appropriate for women and men, and girls and boys. You can liken the use of a gender lens to putting on a pair of eyeglasses. Through one lens of the glasses, you see the participation, needs, and realities of women. Through the other lens, you see the participation, needs, and realities of men. Your sight or vision is the combination of what each eye sees. It is applied by considering a series of questions in relation to a program or an intervention.

3. Mortality figures show that as of 2005, Canadian women had an average life expectancy at birth of 82.7 years while Canadian men live to an average of 78 years. Women continue to outlive men, although men have recently made greater gains in life expectancy. While the top 10 causes of death are the same for men and women, the ranking of these causes differs. Men are more likely to die from accidents and self-harm. Women are more likely to die of Alzheimer's disease and chronic respiratory disease.

4. Biologically, men and women differ in terms of the diseases they develop, the symptoms they experience, and the ways they respond to medicines and other treatments. Likewise, women's and men's varying alignments to gender ideals mediate their experiences and expressions about health and illness.

5. Gender considerations are relevant to all community health nursing programming and practice. By applying a gender lens, we can start to consider the ways programs and practices can better meet the needs of men and women.

CHAPTER 19
Review Questions

1. Correct: (c) This is based on CHN practice of referral to support groups that strengthen social networks, enhance client resilience, and promote self-mastery and autonomy. Incorrect: (a) This is inappropriate in that it assumes that memory function is a major determinant of how a family member will understand the experience of AD. (b) This presumes that written information about brain changes associated with AD in isolation of explanation and dialogue with the client will enhance overall understanding of the dementia process. (d) This depersonalizes the relationship between the CHN and the client. While referral may ultimately be helpful and necessary, the first choice in this context is providing information and encouraging the client's spouse to become an active member of a support group.

2. Correct: (c) This option best acknowledges the role of the CHN in establishing collaborative, trust-based relationships. It also acknowledges the principles of person-centred care outlined as a major philosophical principle supporting older adult healthcare in Chapter 19. Incorrect: (a) and (b) These are paternalistic responses that reinforce a unidirectional communication pathway that puts the nurse in control. (d) This does not acknowledge the need to uncover the meaning or lived experience behind the older person's behaviour, nor does it establish the collaborative nature of what it is to engage in person-centred care relationships.

3. Correct: (d) This supports the role of the CHN as building capacity and mobilizing the strengths of the client/family for action. Incorrect: (a), (b), and (c) Each undermines the centrality of the family as an integrated whole, and places the family in a position of dependence with an inappropriate paternalism on the part of the CHN.

4. Correct: (c) This is most correct based on the information provided in the chapter section "Assessments and Resources Needed for Aged-Care Support" (see MyNursingLab). It is an easily modifiable risk factor that can be quickly identified and acted upon. Incorrect: (a), (b), and (d) These contain some inaccuracies and absolute statements that suggest a value judgment on the part of the nurse. For example, (a) suggests low body mass is a main reason for falls in the elderly, and this is incorrect. Option (b) presumes that alcohol must be entirely eliminated from Mr. Ho's daily intake, without any supportive evidence that he is abusing alcohol or that his intake of alcohol requires modification. Option (d) is incorrect because it is not the financial status itself that results in falls; rather is it the outcomes associated with low-income status such as malnutrition and unsafe environmental circumstances that contribute to a higher fall rate among low-income groups.

5. Correct: (d) This is based on the notion that there are frequently physiological reasons behind changes in behaviour associated with dementia. Incorrect: (a) It is not appropriate for the CHN to assume that any changes in behaviour are based on a progression of the disease itself. Depression is under-diagnosed in older adults and is easily treated. The CHN will play a significant role in screening for depression in those older adults living in the community. (b) Although somewhat helpful in determining the scope of a sleep–wake disturbance, this is a limited option, given

that sleep disturbance is only one symptom associated with depression in the elderly. (c) This course of action is premature and based on the values of the healthcare professional. It also does not take into account the unique cultural practices and preferences of this family. There are many interventions that could be put in place to help manage this behaviour prior to giving serious consideration to transition into long-term care. Families are often reluctant to consider this option and require much counselling, support, and discussion before transfer to long-term care takes place.

Study Questions

1. In order to answer this question fully, students should go to the Statistics Canada website and access information on population growth for older adults. Students should also access additional resources available through MyNursingLab. The key components in response to this question should include the following:
   - the number of older adults over the age of 65 living in Canada has increased dramatically between 1981–2005. This increase is estimated to have been by 2.2 million.
   - By 2036, this demographic is expected to increase by an additional 5 million people, bringing the anticipated numbers up to 9.8 million older adults over the age of 65.
   - This has significance for healthcare planning, given that many of these individuals will be living with illnesses that will require services to manage their healthcare needs (see "Population Trends" in the chapter).

2. Four societal myths about older adults are that they are of inferior intelligence, poor, unhealthy, and a burden to the healthcare system and the general community. These myths contribute to the stigmatization of older adults so that they are marginalized and must advocate for continued access to healthcare services. Thus, CHNs must be in a position to contribute to public education and assist with developing and implementing strategic advocacy that influences policy about healthcare for older adults.

3. The main philosophical tenets that underpin exemplary aged care are person-centred care, unconditional positive regard, maximization of remaining strengths, and partnerships. Person-centred care is the grounding principle. CHNs validate the personhood of older adults through behaviours and interactions that provide recognition, respect, support, and acceptance of the older person. The beliefs that CHNs would hold that facilitate person-centred care include valuing older adults, treating them as individuals, looking at the world through their unique perspective, and providing an interpersonal environment in which the older adult can experience well-being. These values form the basis of unconditional positive regard, whereby the CHN works in partnership with the older person so that health needs can be identified and implemented collaboratively, according to their own healthcare goals.

4. The principle behind building an age-friendly community is based on the notion of "active aging," whereby older persons are engaged in all aspects of the life of a community according to their personal preferences and interests. In this context, community is broadly defined, and could refer to neighbourhoods, social groups, or political organizations or could reach further to interests at a macro level such as federal policy groups on aging. The age-friendly community recognizes the role that older adults play in sustaining the ultimate health of the community. There are several complex, inter-related determinants of active aging. These include economic, service, behavioural, personal, physical, and social determinants within the context of gender and culture. In order to ensure active aging, the age-friendly community purposefully plans for those mechanisms that will ensure participation of older adults. A checklist of the features of an age-friendly community includes the following:
   - outdoor spaces and buildings,
   - transportation,
   - housing,
   - respect and social inclusion,
   - social participation,
   - communication and information,
   - civic participation and employment, and
   - community support and health services.

5. Depending on the unique healthcare status and needs of a specific older adult, there will be many interrelated assessment/resource areas that must be implemented. These areas cannot be prioritized. Rather, each must be addressed to determine the probability and level of risk associated. Therefore, CHNs must assess older adults for each of the following potential healthcare issues:
   - Physical activity and fall prevention: relates strongly to maintaining independence. If the older person is physically inactive, the higher the likelihood that he or she will fall and sustain an injury that will contribute to mortality, morbidity.
   - Mental health: relates to assessment for depression, delirium, dementia, anxiety disorders, medication and substance abuse, as well as elder abuse.
   - Polypharmacy: related to assessment for inaccurate self-administration of medications that can lead to drug interactions and ineffective treatment.
   - Social isolation: related to assessment for the adequacy of social supports and social networks.
   - Sexual expression and sexual health: related to the assessment for health risk associated with sexual behaviour and the quality of intimate relationships.
   - Food security: related to the assessment of the accessibility of food that is preferred, safe, nutritious, and affordable.
   - Elder abuse: related to the assessment for relationships that are at risk for being dangerous and exploitive because they are based on physical, psychosocial, financial, sexual, or mental abuse.
   - End-of-life care: related to the assessment of older adults whose healthcare needs are in the domain of palliation and related to pain, comfort, and symptom management.

6. The CHN role focuses on identifying healthcare needs that have emerged from an evidence-informed approach to health assessment. The CHN works collaboratively with older people and their support networks to provide educational support, counselling, and health system navigation. The CHN actively participates with older adults in the context of their communities to engage in informed and

strategic political advocacy. Advocacy frequently involves public education about the healthcare issues that are of concern to older adults. The CHN thus serves as a conduit between evidence-based literature and research and the general public as well as older adults themselves.

7. There are two main components of long-term care services available for older adults. These services are available to older adults through the community-based healthcare sector and the facility-based healthcare sector. In both sectors there is a broad range with respect to the cost, funding sources, and standards of healthcare provision. In both sectors there are professional services available. However, in the community-based sector, access to professional services for care delivery may be restricted by availability and cost. In both community- and facility-based care sectors, family may be required to provide financial supplementation if funding levels are insufficient. In most regions of Canada, access to free healthcare for older adults is controlled by a regulatory body such as a Regional Health Authority or Community Care Access Centre. In the community-based care sector, services can involve respite care, meal provision, professional care for bathing and grooming, subsidized transportation, adult day programs, and recreational services. All are intended to provide infrastructure support so that the older person can remain at home. In the facility-based care sector, services can include accommodation, meals, and professional care services up to and including extensive advanced practice technical and medical care supports in the face of chronic illnesses that impact on respiratory, cardiac, and palliative care needs. The main difference between these two sectors is the frequency with which care can be offered. Those older adults who require 24-hour services are most likely to be living in facility-based care. However, there is striking similarity with respect to the complexity of care that both community-based and facility-based services can provide to older adults.

CHAPTER 20

Review Questions

1. Correct: (b) Lesbians are often assumed to be less likely to contract STIs and so are less likely to be offered STI screening. Incorrect: (a) There is no evidence that lesbians have fewer mammograms. (c) Lesbians may in fact be screened for depression more often. (d) STI screening is needed unless they have unprotected sex with men.

2. Correct: (a) The evidence suggests that these youth are expelled from their home rather than leaving of their own volition. Incorrect: (b) Not all home situations are abusive. (c) There is no research evidence to support this. (d) Not all gay youth are victims of emotional abuse.

3. Correct: (a) Delayed coming out puts gays at increased risk of suicide and depression, both of which are regarded as poor health outcomes. Incorrect: (b) and (d) There is no evidence to support this. (c) This is only partly true.

4. Correct: (b) Lesbians are at greater risk of these cancers because they usually do not experience pregnancy or use oral contraceptives that are protective for both these cancers. Incorrect: (a) and (d) There is no evidence to support this. (c) There are risks for STIs unless they have unprotected sex with men.

5. Correct: (b) The evidence suggests that the use of inclusive forms and language increases satisfaction with care. Incorrect: (a) There is no evidence to support this. (c) This is a practice in the U.S. military. (d) Not all gay, lesbian, bisexual, and transgender individuals are at risk for STIs; it depends on their sexual orientation and lifestyle practices.

Study Questions

1. Homophobia is often manifested in derogatory language, jokes, and discriminatory treatment of those individuals perceived or known to be gay or lesbian. At its very worst, it may involve extreme violence (gay bashing) toward those perceived to be homosexual. More often it is manifested as bullying in schools and social situations when young persons are seen to be "different" from their peers or identify themselves as lesbian, gay, or bisexual.

2. Being neutral about homosexuality may result in healthcare providers not asking about sexual orientation when meeting a new client or ignoring disclosure in an attempt to appear accepting. It is more appropriate to acknowledge this disclosure and reflect acceptance and caring, which will further encourage the client to share sensitive information that may influence care. Acting in a neutral manner may in fact be seen as a negative response.

3. Internalized homophobia is negative because if individuals find it difficult to accept who they are because of negative societal messages that have been absorbed, this causes a significant amount of self-doubt and self-loathing, resulting in destructive behaviours and high-risk activities. The stresses that many in this population are exposed to have been termed "minority stress," referring to the negative effects on mental health of stigma, prejudice, and discrimination. Encompassed in this concept is the expectation of rejection, the need to hide and conceal internalized homophobia, and coping mechanisms used to adapt to the hostile environment that is created.

4. Gay youth are more likely to be self-destructive in their behaviours; this is theorized to occur because of psychological distress and shame.

5. Risk of suicide has been noted to be highest for gay youth around the time when disclosure to parents is being planned or has occurred.

6. Healthcare settings can become more accepting of gay, lesbian, and transgender clients through the creation of a welcoming environment (brochures and posters showing same-sex couples); use of inclusive forms, languages, and discussions; the development of a written confidentiality policy that outlines what information is collected and how it is shared; and training and evaluation of staff to maintain standards of respect and confidentiality.

7. CHNs can advocate for social inclusion and equity in health in our diverse nation by influencing the attitudes and knowledge of community members. This may start at the level of the family, where nurses can help a young gay person come out to his or her family and support the family in accepting this. This work can then extend to the school, the community centre, and perhaps even to the level of civic and provincial politics.

8. Nurses who work in schools have a particularly important role to play in affecting the health and physical and mental

safety of gay, lesbian, bisexual, or transgender youth. It is vitally important that the needs of this vulnerable and invisible population are identified and addressed both on an individual and school-based level. There is much work to be done in sensitizing teachers, coaches, aides, and other youth to the challenges facing these youth every day in our schools and playgrounds.

9. Risk of suicide among gay, lesbian, bisexual, and transgender youth has been noted to be highest around the time when disclosure to parents is being planned or has occurred.

10. Gay men, lesbians, and bisexuals of colour and/or with visible or invisible disabilities face additional challenges both within larger society and within the gay/lesbian community. They have to confront the norms of both the majority and minority communities and cultures in which they live. Aboriginal or First Nations people who are gay or lesbian face additional challenges based on historical and familial patterns of abuse and trauma with high levels of psychological distress and increased use of mental health services.

CHAPTER 21

Review Questions

1. Correct: (b) In the recovery model a multifaceted approach to life problems works best. While Jake's wandering is not causing any harm, he is not receiving services that could help him to regain more of his life. A team that focuses on his strengths and potential could assist him. Incorrect: (a) AA will not be an appropriate resource related to Jake's thought disorder. He will require more specialized and sensitive treatment for his mental illness issues. (c) Leaving Jake to wander may not be in his best interests and may not allow him to reach his potential in a recovery model. (d) Consulting with psychiatry may be an important part of the multidisciplinary team approach, but medications will not be the sole answer to Jake's situation.

2. Correct: (c) The best resource for a person with a mental illness and a substance abuse problem is CODI. These services recognize both disorders and are sensitive to treatment issues that may arise due to the interrelatedness of the two disorders. Incorrect: (a), (b), and (d) These are not appropriate for a person with schizophrenia. Providing a rationale for abstaining is unlikely to motivate Jake. His thinking is concrete and he will likely not be motivated by this rationale. Meditation will be difficult to practise and likely beyond his capabilities at this point. AA will not be sensitive to issues related to mental illness.

3. Correct: (d) It is important to assess what has happened and ensure that Jake's rights are not being violated. Stigma and discrimination are ongoing factors in Canadian society that may be present in this situation. People with schizophrenia are vulnerable and require someone to ensure that they are being treated fairly. Incorrect: (a) This may be interpreted as threatening and punitive. (b) and (c) These may be reasonable at some point but it is first important to assess what has happened and if there are any violations of human rights.

4. Correct: (c) The behaviours that are described are indicative of a psychotic break and indicate a change in behav-

iour. It is important to intervene early in order to prevent further decompensation and regression. Incorrect: (a), (b), and (d) While these may be a concern at some point, the priority is assessing the meaning of the behaviour in order to intervene appropriately. The nurse would be cognizant of symptoms of an exacerbation of mental illness.

5. Correct: (d) Jake will benefit from some structure in his day. Due to the nature of his illness and recent discharge from hospital, he could benefit from a para-professional helper. This helper can assist him in a daily routine and ensure he is available for long-acting medication appointments. Having a daily destination such as a community meal program may provide nutrition and structure to his afternoons. This would be chosen carefully so as to not overwhelm him. Incorrect: (a) This could be interpreted as threatening and punitive. (b) This could make Jake paranoid and more uncomfortable in his home. (c) This is impractical as people with schizophrenia generally have problems with motivation and Jake will likely need more concrete assistance at this time.

Study Questions

1. There has been much debate about the effects of deinstitutionalization on the current mental health system. The most debated topic is homelessness. Some would argue that closing the larger psychiatric hospitals contributed to the current societal problems related to stigma, discrimination, marginalization, and homelessness. People who had lived there for many years became vulnerable when placed in the community without adequate supports that they needed to be part of society. In addition, there is discussion positing that the warehousing of the mentally ill in jails and prisons has also occurred, largely due to insufficient resources to support people with mental illness in the community.

2. Strategies to decrease suicide:
   - Aboriginal youth: Develop culturally sensitive information about suicide, engage culturally appropriate counsellors, mentor youth peer buddies to befriend vulnerable youth, advocate for recreation programs.
   - Elderly Caucasian males living alone: Educate community members of this high-risk population; reach out to include and engage this population in supportive community programs; discuss and reform gun control laws to prevent suicides.
   - Gay, bisexual, and transgender youth: Target homophobic attitudes and organize discussion sessions; develop safe drop-in places for youth where they can feel respected and receive sensitive counselling.
   - Drug and alcohol dependent individuals: Use screening tools that will recognize early development of drug/alcohol dependencies; help individuals get treatment, target advertisements that glamorize use of drugs and alcohol.

3. Mental health promotion is the process of enabling individuals and communities to increase control over the determinants of health and thereby improve their health. Supportive strategies: foster supportive environments, individual resilience; show respect for equity and social justice; foster connections and personal dignity.
   i. Frail elderly living in the community: Think about the needs of the frail elderly and systemic issues that might

affect them. Use their ideas to consider program development:

- ▪ Isolation: transportation issues—develop community interconnections (church, volunteer drivers, community development organizations) to assist the frail elderly with transportation issues that may preclude their involvement.
- ▪ Nutrition: develop a nutrition program and "meet your neighbour" lunch program with interested community organizations.
- ▪ Liaison with police services to teach seniors about safety precautions in their neighbourhoods.

ii. Immigrant mothers

- ▪ Develop relationships with key community members in the immigrant population to gain an understanding of the immigrants' mothers' concerns.
- ▪ Develop a community program where mothers can meet, relax, and get information about life in Canada. Provide information about child health services, nutrition, car seats, stress management, postpartum depression, and English language circles. Organize activities to help the mothers and their children learn about Canadian society. Listen to the mothers and work with them to develop the program.

iii. Suburban high school students

- ▪ Identify needs of the students by conversing with teachers and with the students.
- ▪ Ensure that programs have an element of fun and pique students' interest.
- ▪ Mental health promotion ideas: safe sex seminar, sports challenge day, drug awareness campaigns, safe and responsible driving, accident prevention, depression and suicide workshop.

4. MCMHN must first be aware of evidence-based risk factors related to mental illness. Some risk factors will require political action to draw attention to the issues, i.e., poverty and inadequate housing. Others may need community action efforts such as Neighbourhood Watch to keep children and youth safe from exploitation. Service reorientation, i.e., early screening and intervention to detect learning and emotional problems, may be needed to manage other risk factors.

5. Four recommendations from the national report on the state of mental health services in Canada include

i. Develop a comprehensive basket of services that will provide a co-ordinated holistic approach to care. The current system is often fragmented and it is difficult to obtain co-ordinated services that will address the holistic needs of the person, not just the biomedical needs.

ii. Implement the recovery principles in mental health treatment. There is a need to change the focus of care to a recovery philosophy that provides hope for individuals living with mental illness and allows them to experience life in a fuller fashion.

iii. Stigma and discrimination occur within Canadian society. A national campaign to decrease stigma toward people with mental illness is needed to address this problem.

iv. Children's mental health services should be incorporated within a national health strategy. They require additional public funds and mental health professionals.

CHAPTER 22

Review Questions

1. Correct: (c) The Canadian constitution uses the term "Aboriginal" to refer to First Nations, Métis, and Inuit as the original inhabitants of Canada. Incorrect: (a) First Nations leaves out the Métis and Inuit. (b) Registered Indian refers only to the First Nations population, once again leaving out the Métis and Inuit. (d) Status Indian, another term for First Nations, leaves out Métis and Inuit.

2. Correct: (d) The Indian Act was originally established to protect the land base, also referred to as reserves, of Status Indians brought about through the signing of the treaties. Reserve land could not be bought or sold by anyone except the federal government. Incorrect: (a) The Indian Act quickly became a grab bag of social policies that were intended to assimilate First Nations people into the mainstream society, such as mandatory attendance at residential schools and involuntary enfranchisement if one received a university education, married a non-status man, served in the armed forces, lived off reserve for a certain period of time, etc., but this was not the original intent of the Indian Act. (b) The Supreme Court of Canada has ruled that provision of healthcare services to treaty Indians is not a treaty right. The only signed treaty that mentions healthcare was Treaty #6, known as the Medicine Chest Clause, which only specified that a medicine chest would be kept at the Indian agent's house, and that the Queen would provide assistance in times of pestilence and famine. (c) The Indian Act was used as a method of controlling the First Nations attempts to integrate into society. For example, when those in the prairies became adept at farming, the Indian Act was changed to prevent them from selling any produce or animals without the permission of the Indian agent; they were also required to get permission from the Indian agent to leave the reserve for any length of time. The land that was set aside for reserves was usually economically unviable and any minerals were still owned by the federal government. But once again, this was not the original intent.

3. Correct: (a) Residential schools were originally established by missionaries in the eastern provinces, usually of Jesuit or Roman Catholic background. Incorrect: (b) The federal government assisted the running of the schools financially once the First Nations communities started demanding education for their children as part of their treaty negotiations. (c) There were residential schools operated by the United Church, mostly in the western provinces and later during the time period, but they were not the initial ones. (d) Same answer as (c).

4. Correct: (b) Establishing partnerships with Elders would facilitate uptake of new information as Elders are the traditional knowledge keepers in Aboriginal communities. This process would also indicate respect for Elders by working with them from the outset. Incorrect: (a) A literature review could be part of the process to find out what works and what doesn't, but any program needs to incorporate that particular community's ways of knowing and being. (c) This would likely be the second step, after consultation and working with the Elders and other community members to create the program. Testing it out would need to be carried out to assess for effectiveness. (d) This could

also be a step later on in the process, depending on what the team comes up with in their planning.

5. Correct: (c) The human concepts of spiritual, physical, emotional, and mental are in the four quadrants of the medicine wheel. Incorrect: (a) Environment is not part of the human being. (b) Only three aspects and the medicine wheel has four. (d) Although all components are included in the medicine wheel teachings, they do not specifically refer to the humanness of the individual.

Study Questions

1. A Status Indian is an individual whose ancestors signed the treaties in the early 20th century or a woman who married a status Indian male before 1985 and is registered under the Indian Registration List in Ottawa and receives treaty rights such as housing on a reserve, education, health services including uninsured health benefits such as eye glasses, dental care, medication, travel expenses, and interpreter/helper assistance.

   A non-status Indian is someone whose ancestors did not sign the treaties or whose ancestors lost their treaty rights during enfranchisement prior to 1985, or who cannot access treaty rights due to the limitations of Bill C-31 but still maintains all the cultural and possibly physical traits of being an Indian.

2. Aboriginal women are more likely to be overweight or obese than men, which is a risk factor for diabetes. The rates of gestational diabetes are higher among Aboriginal women, which is another predictor for Type II diabetes. Women seek healthcare more often than men, which can mean that diabetes can be diagnosed sooner.

3. Healthcare is considered a treaty right among First Nations due to the Medicine Chest clause in Treaty #6; however, the Supreme Court of Canada has ruled that healthcare is not a treaty right. The federal government provides healthcare services as part of its responsibility to First Nations peoples.

4. The 1969 White Paper proposed the dissolution of the Indian Act, the Department of Indian and Northern Affairs, and the treaties. The outcome was an unprecedented show of force and solidarity among First Nations peoples in Canada and a resurgence in cultural pride.

5. Effects of the residential school legacy are seen in not only the generations that attended but also the generations that came after, also known as Intergenerational Impacts. The most common effects are alcohol and drug abuse; fetal alcohol syndrome (FAS) and fetal alcohol effect (FAE); sexual abuse (past and ongoing); physical abuse (past and ongoing); psychological/emotional abuse; low self-esteem; dysfunctional families and interpersonal relationships; parenting issues; suicide (and the threat of suicide); and teen pregnancy.

   The more insidious characteristics are numerous and long-lasting. See http://www.wherearethechildren.ca/en/exhibit/impacts.html for a list of impacts on intergenerational survivors.

6. Bill C-31 was enacted in response to the involuntary enfranchisement of First Nations women and their children when women married a non-status man according to the Indian Act. Women who had lost their status due to marriage could reclaim their status from this bill, along with their children and grandchildren.

CHAPTER 23

Review Questions

1. Correct: (b) This would be blurring the roles of nurse and friend. Incorrect: (a) It would not be unethical to offer a phone number to a client. (c) Unions generally do not have rules about contact with clients outside of the practice setting. (d) There may or may not be rules—more likely the rules would state not to cross professional boundaries.

2. Correct: (b) Rates are higher in rural areas. Incorrect: (a) Mortality rates in circulatory diseases can often be altered by lifestyle changes. (c) They are not the same between rural and urban areas. (d) High mortality rates for circulatory diseases are high in rural areas.

3. Correct: (a) Nursing practice standards can guide nurses in identifying unsafe working conditions. Incorrect: (b) Professional boundaries look at the relationship of the nurses to the clients. (c) Principles of teaching and learning would assist the nurse to provide patient teaching. (d) Community capacity looks at the strengths of the community for participating in care.

4. Correct: (d) In this answer Anita is reminding Mrs. Hewett that she does not disclose confidential information about Mrs. Nyl; she will also keep Mrs. Hewett's information confidential. Incorrect: (a) This may be helpful information, but may just serve to irritate Mrs. Hewett. (b) This will again be poor communication and not contribute to a trust relationship. (c) This is sure to negatively impact on any relationship with Mrs. Hewett.

5. Correct: (c) The rationale is found in the chapter. Incorrect: (a), (b), and (d) These choices are simply alternative choices.

Study Questions

1. Establish trust and rapport with Maria as well as with her immediate family members; ensure the presence of a High German–speaking interpreter, being careful about sensitive topics; assist Maria to attend at least some of her follow-up appointments.

2. Work with the band council to update and revise the disaster plan as necessary; identify all individuals who are at risk for lingering chronic health issues such as respiratory conditions; develop and present public information sessions about disaster management and mitigation; advocate for families who lost their homes to ensure that they have appropriate lodging.

3. Read local history books; conduct a community assessment; spend time getting to know local community members by attending local events; talk to key stakeholders in the community.

4. Factors to take into consideration include the time of year for the project (e.g., avoiding seedtime and harvest; the length of the project); no overlap with the times mentioned above; and ensuring it meets a farming community need, not just a rural need.

5. Accessibility of health services; similarities among rural communities; the impact of place on health status; communicating and diagnosing at a distance with mechanisms such as telehealth.

6. Working alone; lack of access to other health professionals; lack of access to continuing education; lack of access to technology.

CHAPTER 24

Review Questions

1. Correct: (b) See "The DPSEEA Framework" in the chapter. Incorrect: (a), (c), and (d) These choices simply contain other words that fit the acronym.

2. Correct: (c) See Figure 24.1. Diarrhoea, lower respiratory tract infections, unintentional injuries (i.e., workplace injuries, industrial accidents, pedestrian and cycling accidents, and radiation), and malaria have the largest burden of attributable environmental factors. Incorrect: (a), (b), and (d) These choices simply contain diseases that are not part of the figure in the chapter at all.

3. Correct: (b) See "Defining Environmental Health" in the chapter. Incorrect: (a) and (c) The WHO definition is based on human health outcomes related to environmental factors, not ecosystem health or animal health. (d) Although low levels of harmful agents in the environment are an important aspect of environmental health, it does not define environmental health.

4. Correct: (d) See "Defining Environmental Health." Driving forces are factors that create pressures, which can influence the state of the environment. Other examples include poverty, population density, age structure, urbanization, and technology. Incorrect: (a), (b) and (c) Indoor air pollution, water quality, and occupational exposures are all exposures.

5. Correct: (b) See "Categorization of Environmental Factors." Other physical factors include ionizing and non-ionizing radiation, vibration, and extremes in temperature and pressure. Incorrect: (a) Chemical factors are vapours, gases, dusts, etc. (c) Biological factors include any living organism that can cause adverse health effects. (d) Psychological factors individual stress or distress events. (e) Ergonomic factors are those elements that affect the "fit" of the person to the environment.

6. Correct: (c) See "Routes of Entry." The four common routes of entry for individual environmental factors (chemical, physical, or biological) are inhalation, absorption, injection, and ingestion. Incorrect: (a), (b), and (d) These are all possible routes for diffusion, but not common routes of entry as described.

7. Correct: (c) See "Risk Assessment, Risk Management, and Risk Communication." Risk communication is defined as the process of making risk assessment and risk management information comprehensible and taking the necessary steps to distribute and present that information accordingly. Incorrect: (a) A press conference delivers any information to the public—it might be used as a strategy within risk communication. (b) Editorials are opinion pieces in news media—again, they may be used as a strategy within risk communication. (d) This is an umbrella term related to making information more available.

8. Correct: (b) See "Hazard Control." The three strategies that are typically employed to control for exposure include engineering controls, administrative controls, and use of personal protective equipment. Incorrect: (a) This was part of the initial assessment for CPR. (c) These are parts of the DPSEEA Framework.

9. Correct: (c) See "Occupational Health Nursing." Incorrect: (a) Environmental Health Nurses may work in institutions, but their work is broader and would also contain elements, for example, of making the workplace "green." (b) CHNs apply the practice of nursing in a wide variety of community settings. (d) Clinical nursing refers to any setting with patients or clients.

Study Questions

1. The driving force is that the population in a small rural town is 65% over age 65 and 5% under the age of 5. The pressure generated by this driving force is that there are very few working individuals to support the community and community activities and to drive the economic and social vitality of the community. In addition, there will be increased pressure on healthcare services for the aged, including housing, support services (i.e., home care or meals on wheels), and travel accommodations for services unavailable in the community. One possible hazard is that older individuals may engage in activities beyond the scope of their abilities and these actions may put them or others in harm (i.e., driving a vehicle or operating farm equipment without the sight or reaction time) for these activities to be undertaken safely. The possible routes of exposure for this hazard are on the roadways. An action to improve the issue would be to have alternative sources of transportation available for seniors (i.e., weekly bus service) or having a pool of labourers to call for agricultural assistance.

2. The five categories of environmental factors are physical, chemical, biological, psychological, and ergonomic.
   - Chemical factors: household cleaners, hazardous chemicals
   - Physical factors: noise, radiation, natural hazards, road safety, housing quality
   - Biological factors: water safety, waste management, food safety, insect-borne diseases, agricultural dusts, air quality
   - Psychological factors: stress
   - Ergonomic factors: workstation design, repetitive motion

3. The four routes of entry for environmental factors are inhalation, absorption, injection, and ingestion.

4. Three hazard control strategies for environmental factors in order of preferred use are engineering, administrative, and personal protective equipment.

5. The three categories of information gathered during an individual interview are occupational, residential, and recreational.

6. Five challenges to environmental health assessments are as follows. First, environmental exposures may be associated with latent health conditions. Second, the combined effect of one or more exposures from home, work, and social activities can make it difficult to attribute one particular exposure to a particular effect. Third, many environmentally related conditions and illnesses are characterized by signs and symptoms that are very similar to those of more typical "non-environmental" illnesses. Fourth, in the case of low-level environmental exposures and mild or uncertain health effects, attempts to attribute cause to a particular exposure may be extremely difficult. Fifth, considerable "background noise" in the form of co-existing health conditions, other exposures (i.e., workplaces, smoking) and inherited factors may be present.

7. The three environmental indicators measured by the federal government are air quality, water quality, and greenhouse gases.

8. Examples of primary, secondary, and tertiary prevention in terms of environmental health are as follows:
   - Primary prevention: immunization, counselling about reducing exposures, supporting development of policy and standards related to environmental health, education, supporting and practising positive activities (i.e., washing fruit and vegetables under running water before eating).
   - Secondary prevention: assessing for blood lead levels in at-risk young children, assessing urine for arsenic in individuals with arsenic content in their water supply, and recommending x-rays for individuals occupationally exposed to asbestos.
   - Tertiary prevention: assisting in distribution of information as well as taking action (treatment, medical management) in the event of an acute environmental health–related incident.

CHAPTER 25

Review Questions

1. Correct: (b) The Corrections and Conditional Release Act is a legal framework for the correctional system. It covers among other things correctional health service provision. Incorrect: (a) The Canada Health Act deals with how provincial and territorial health insurance programs are financed. (c) The Provincial or Territorial Mental Health Acts covers legislation for people with mental health problems in the general population. (d) There is no Canadian Public Health Act; the provincial Acts cover legislation and services for people in the general population.

2. Correct: (b) Presently, testing for infectious diseases is not mandatory in correctional services. Incorrect: (a) Even if resources were in place, mandatory screening is not legislated. (c) While this may be somewhat true, screening is voluntary. (d) Harm-reduction strategies are not in place in all facilities and they remain a controversial issue.

3. Correct: (a) Policies, staffing patterns, and methods of operation are an example of dynamic security. Incorrect: (b), (c), and (d) The examples are static.

4. Correct: (d) Participating in a community-based committee is focused on avoiding the development of interpersonal violence, and thus would be the best example. Incorrect: (a) Relapse prevention is a tertiary prevention strategy. (b) and (c) Medication management and crisis intervention are examples of secondary prevention.

5. Correct: (d) Parole by exception allows for offenders to be granted parole under exceptional circumstances, when they are terminally ill, or if remaining confined would seriously affect their health. Incorrect: (a) Probation is a community-based sentence in lieu of incarceration. (b) Medical leave refers to sick leave that an employee would take. (c) Clemency is the forgiveness of a crime and the penalty associated with it.

Study Questions

1. MMT is a controversial harm-reduction strategy that has been adopted in most Canadian correctional facilities since 2002. Stigma associated with MMT is common, and correctional nurses need to work diligently to overcome the stigma that surrounds MMT in correctional facilities. Nursing awareness, understanding, and promotion of MMT in corrections is important to dispel misunderstandings, foster acceptance and cooperation among correctional staff, and provide unbiased treatment and education.

According to the Registered Nurses Association of Ontario (2009) best practice guideline, Supporting clients on methadone maintenance treatment, common issues and implications related to MMT include
   i. perceptions of methadone: education re: MMT as a harm reduction program for all correctional staff; education for offenders re: the fact that they will not be punished for admitting they have an opioid problem; urine samples that are collected as part of the program are confidential and will not be used for punitive reasons
   ii. administration of methadone: diversion of methadone is a major issue in correctional institutions. Nurses need to be aware that a common strategy for diversion of methadone is regurgitation (to give to others).
   iii. discharge/release planning: clients need to be monitored for a minimum of 20 minutes following administration to reduce risk of diversion
   iv. related issues: awareness of signs and symptoms of methadone withdrawal

2. The primary focus for correctional services is the custody of those they house. Providing healthcare in an environment in which healthcare delivery is not the primary goal is fraught with many trials and tribulations, and correctional nurses are continually challenged to negotiate the goals of healthcare vis-à-vis the goals of confinement and security. These obligations are often framed as a debate, i.e., custody versus caring. Custody and caring represents a paradox for correctional nurses. As such, it is not uncommon for them to struggle to meet the expectations of their profession, their employer, their clients, and the community at large.

Correctional systems focus on confinement and security, and matters of security often take precedence over healthcare. However, regardless of the setting, correctional nurses must meet the competing demands of custody (confinement and security) and caring (nursing care). In essence, correctional nurses are charged with providing social goods (healthcare) within institutions dedicated to social necessities (confinement). As such, nurses are often faced with clinical issues and moral dilemmas not encountered in other, more traditional healthcare settings. The Code of Ethics for Registered Nurses (CNA, 2008) and various provincial standards and practice documents are a good source of guidance for matters related to the provision of nursing care. The need for nurses to provide both custody and caring distinguishes nursing care in corrections from other specialized areas of practice.

3. When working with women who are incarcerated, it is important to adopt gender-sensitive strategies that take into account their vulnerabilities as incarcerated women. This means developing programs targeted specifically for women and not simply adopting those that have been developed for men. Healthcare challenges for incarcerated women include
   - Physical and sexual abuse (50 to 70%)
   - Substance abuse

- Infectious diseases (HIV/AIDS, HBV, HCV)
- Reproductive issues including pregnancy-related concerns
- Chronic health concerns and disorders (asthma, hypertension, diabetes, heart disease)
- Mental health concerns (anxiety disorders/PTSD, depression, self-injurious behaviour, schizophrenia, borderline personality disorder)

4. Correctional environments can be tough places to work and are not suited for all nurses. Nurses choosing to work in corrections should have good communication skills, as well as physical and psychological assessment skills. They also need to be able to work independently as well as part of a team. Nurses require a broad knowledge base—including mental health nursing, public health nursing, geriatric nursing, general medical surgical nursing, and trauma nursing—but more importantly, they need to be able to be consult appropriately with other nurses, physicians, and correctional staff.

    Nurses have to be able to apply the nursing process in their interactions with offenders, and be knowledgeable regarding primary, secondary, and tertiary interventions. They must also be able to self-reflect and demonstrate self-awareness, particularly around therapeutic engagement with offenders. This includes being able to manage their therapeutic boundaries while providing appropriate care. Furthermore, they must be able to demonstrate non-judgmental attitudes, and see the person as a person, who requires care, and not solely as an inmate who has broken the law. Finally, they must be able to transcend the phenomenon of "custody and caring."

5. The prevalence of communicable diseases within correctional populations such as HIV, TB, Hepatitis B and C, and sexually transmitted infections provides opportunities for correctional health to participate and contribute to public health.

    Offenders typically have had limited access to healthcare prior to incarceration, coupled with poor treatment adherence. As such they may be difficult to identify and treat within the community. Incarceration does provide an opportunity of sorts for nurses to identify and treat offenders prior to their return to the community. This is particularly important in areas where there is a high turnover of offenders, especially among provincial and territorial facilities (particularly offenders on remand).

    Correctional nurses can participate in this public health opportunity by providing offenders with education, counselling, early detection, and treatment. In short, good correctional healthcare contributes to good public health.

6. Harm-reduction strategies such as accessible bleach, distribution of condoms, methadone maintenance programs, and safe tattooing projects are controversial, and their discussion will raise a variety of opinions for and against their adoption. Opinions may be based in science (e.g., harm reduction prevents the spread of disease); may be seen as promoting illegal activities while incarcerated (e.g., illicit or recreational drug use); and may be socially and politically motivated (e.g., methadone maintenance may not be seen as a medical treatment, and tattooing projects seen as "pampering" those who are incarcerated). To be most effective, harm-reduction strategies should be used in conjunction with other correctional rehabilitation programs;

together, they may prevent future disease associated with drug use, sexual activity, and tattooing, and may assist the individual with ceasing or decreasing criminal activity. To date, no Canadian jurisdiction has adopted a PNSPs. The pros and cons of such approaches should be discussed and debated. Students should also consider whether there are limits to harm-reduction approaches within correctional facilities.

CHAPTER 26

Review Questions

1. Correct: (a) While community health nurses are frequently the first members of healthcare teams to encounter individuals experiencing violence and abuse and there are expectations for an active response by healthcare practitioners, Wathen et al. (2009, p. 1) found that these expectations "may not match the realities of professional preparation." Given the prevalence of violence in societies, there is an urgent need for professional nursing education about violence, especially for socially excluded, marginalized, and/or at-risk populations. Incorrect: (b) While cultural and language barriers often exist, the question is about what CHNs need to learn about violence in societies and working to decrease barriers to effective healthcare. (c) While there may be lack of institutional support, healthcare practitioners need to learn about violence, regardless of whether there is institutional support. Nurses may function in many different healthcare settings over time, and, if they are already informed about the issues regarding violence, they can advocate for healthy social change at the institutional level. (d) Certainly it is important for nurses to be aware of the pervasiveness of violence, but awareness is not enough if the expectation is that healthcare practitioners are already prepared to work to prevent violence and to decrease barriers to effective healthcare for those at risk.

2. Correct: (a) Violence also cuts across genders, social classes, races, abilities, education levels, sexualities, age brackets, ethnicities, cultures, religions and spiritualities, and nationalities. Yet to date the statistics seldom focus on these intersecting factors and their implication for the health of socially excluded, marginalized, and at-risk individuals, groups, communities, and populations. CHNs need to be critically aware of these limitations so they can attend to the specific health needs in terms of violence of those with whom we work. Moreover, without attention to these marginalized groups, the larger health and social costs in relation to the occurrence of violence will not be addressed, nor will the potential for health promotion in marginalized populations.

    Incorrect: (b) While cultural safety is needed in CHNing practice related to violence, the question addresses the lack of specific data. (c) There can be difficulties in defining violence, but the question deals with cultural diversity in Canada and the lack of data addressing differing experiences of violence and its implications. (d) Without specific data addressing differing experiences of violence, health needs can be overlooked and the reporting of these health needs may also be overlooked, complicating the overall data collection.

3. Correct: (d) Connecting individual harm with social, cultural, environmental, and political contexts makes violence

public and political. CHNs can initiate political actions, supported by critical theoretical frameworks, including intersectionality and cultural safety and, as argued by Stevens and Hall (1992), take a stand with diverse communities vulnerable to the oppressive, health-damaging effects of violence. When CHNs make the connections between individual harm and social context, the focus is shifted, e.g., from personal blaming for the violence experienced to the larger context in which it takes place. CHNs then can see the interconnections between the pervasiveness of violence against women and how it can vary by gender, race, class, and sexualities, among other intersecting factors, and work together for healthy social change. Incorrect: (a) When we aim strategies at the individual level, individuals are often left with the problem, and may feel responsible for the violence perpetrated against them. When we consider the collective social level, we can see the interconnections between individual experience and context. The choice of approach must consider social and cultural circumstances; CHNs also must work collaboratively to develop broad-based, comprehensive health promoting strategies that address prevention as well as health promotion. (b) While it is important to build connections with local members of parliament, they too need to know more about violence against women and its social and health implications. Taking a stand with diverse populations in relation to violence helps to build the needed community support to begin health social change. CHNs together with community members have more power when they engage with members of parliament. (c) Working primarily with healthcare professionals, many of whom have not had education about violence in their preparation and may not have had professional in-service education or workshops related to violence, will not add the strength needed to lobby for change. Working with diverse, socially isolated, marginalized, and at-risk populations, and bringing their issues to the front and centre would give more weight and legitimacy to the political efforts needed to bring about healthy social change.

4. Correct: (c) The safety of the individual is key in the assessment of the individual related to violence. Poorly designed and implemented assessment strategies put women, children, and elders in violent, abusive, or neglectful relationships at substantial risk. Within the context of cultural safety and cultural humility, the environment must be safe and individuals must feel safe before they can discuss their experiences. A short-form ABCD-ER Mnemonic Tool can help to guide this process (see the box on p. 410). Incorrect: (a) Certainly the attitude of the CHN is important in assessing for violence. But more important is being sure that the assessment is carried out from the start with the safety of the individual uppermost in the CHN's mind. It is the responsibility of the CHN to ensure, before any assessment is begun, that all related safety factors are considered to protect the individual from harm. Incorrect: (b) The attitude of the CHN is important, as is respecting the individual, but each is superseded by consideration of the safety of the individual. When CHNs attend to cultural safety while including cultural humility, they remain critically aware of the need for ongoing self-reflection and self-critique, including identifying and examining their own patterns of unintentional or intentional racism and classism, and addressing power relations that can occur between client and the healthcare provider. (d) Confidentiality is also very important when CHNs assess for violence. As noted in the two preceding responses, all of these are required within the context of the primacy of the safety of the individual.

5. Correct: (b) Critical social theories include liberation work against poverty and illiteracy; feminist scholarship on oppression of women; lesbian and gay studies; and critical perspectives on race and ethnic relations, gender inequalities, and health promotion. These include theories of violence and encompass intersectional theory, theories of empowerment, and cultural safety. In defining violent societies, critical theorists (i) analyze the social, economic, political, cultural, and environmental ways individuals and groups are harmed by social institutions and states and (ii) act on these health-damaging effects at the community level for structural change. Incorrect: (a) Empowerment is an important health promotion strategy and approach. But critical social theory and its perspectives can help guide the processes involved in creating the conditions in which one can feel empowered, i.e., the understandings emerging from critical theories set the context for beginning to work on empowering strategies. (c) As noted above, cultural safety and its processes emerge from the analysis informed and guided by critical theory, especially for those who are socially isolated, marginalized, and/or rendered at risk due to violence. (d) Intersectional theory, as a perspective, has also emerged within the context of critical social theories that preceded it. Understanding the intersections of gender, race, class, abilities, sexualities, and age, among others, helps to bring front and centre those who have been devalued, marginalized, and socially excluded, e.g., by violence. In defining violent societies, critical theorists analyze the social, economic, political, cultural, and environmental ways individuals and groups are harmed by social institutions and states and act on these damaging effects at the community level for health structural change. Informed by critical social theory, intersectional analysis helps in this process.

Study Questions

1. Three of the four concepts are key terms bolded in the chapter with their defining characteristics. Violence and violence against women are defined on the first page of this chapter; root causes in the section, "Strategies to Eliminate Violence in Societies"; and violence in societies is addressed in the introduction to this chapter.

2. These three concepts are also key terms, defined in the section "Intersectionality." The critical analysis related to these concepts is in the same location.

3. Answers to this question will depend on the choices made by the students. Marginalized and/or at-risk populations (six options) addressed in this chapter can be found in the section "Critical Analysis of Violence in Societies and Health Implications."

4. Framing the analysis of violence in societies with critical theories, while attending to socially excluded, marginalized, and at-risk populations, brings their experiences to the front and centre so that the needed work to address the health and social cost of violence to each individual, family, group, community, and society can be highlighted.

Critical theories, together with the theory of intersectionality, help to maintain a focus on the intersections of gender, race, class, sexualities, and age, among other factors, and the underlying power relations in which they are embedded. When the blame, responsibility, and explanations of violence are shifted from the individual to the social context, including the culture of violence that, as Hankivsky and Varcoe (2007, p. 482) argue, "encompasses the violence of racism, poverty, heterosexism, and other forms of inequity," CHNs can see possibilities for political action for healthy social change. CHNs must hear and understand the experiences and concerns of marginalized, socially excluded, and at-risk populations and provide culturally safe and sensitive health and social services to those who have experienced violence in their communities.

These theoretical perspectives provide CHNs with frameworks to guide assessment, prevention, and health promotion strategies, beginning with analysis of their own biases and beliefs. Cultural safety shifts the focus from the competencies of nurses to enabling an environment for community members to, among other possibilities, indicate whether they feel safe, which can lead to a shift in behaviours of the healthcare practitioners where needed (Israel et al., 2005). These theories also draw attention to the communities' own capacities and agency to work for healthy social change in relation to violence, and to how CHNs can be more fully engaged in working with communities to bring culturally safe awareness of violence, assess for it, and work to prevent violence while promoting health.

5. Universal screening and case finding are key terms in this chapter and are addressed in the introduction. These concepts are compared and analyzed more fully in the section "Assessment, Prevention, and Health Promoting Strategies."

6. For CHNs, becoming aware of violence in societies is essential. A critical reading of the current statistics on violence in societies, for who is visible and who is less visible, is a beginning to enable the possibility of bringing to the forefront groups or people who have been marginalized, socially excluded, or rendered at risk. See "Theoretical Frameworks and Approaches" to guide CHN practice. The strategies CHNs can use are outlined in detail in "Assessment, Prevention, and Health Promoting Strategies." The "Summary" outlines the importance of working collaboratively with allies to facilitate healthy social change at the individual, family, group, community, and societal levels in the collective work to eradicate violence in societies.

CHAPTER 27

Review Questions

1. Correct: (b) The LICO measure works best here because it considers geographical setting. Housing costs vary considerably across geographic settings and, in fact, according to neighbourhoods. Incorrect: (a) The market basket measure does include housing, but not the relative cost of items within the basket. (c) The LIM differentiates between adults and children, but not geographical residence. (d) For all the reasons stated in the chapter, conducting a survey among homeless people is difficult in itself, and it would be even more difficult to find the data to compare across Canada.

2. Correct: (d) The assessment of this family centres around nutrition and food safety. Therefore, helping the mother to access food is a top priority. Incorrect: (a) There are no data to suggest physical safety or issues with housing. (b) This would be a secondary concern, and Mrs. Bennet may earn just enough to be not eligible. (c) This is a good idea if the school in question is close to them and school transfers are possible within the municipal bylaws.

3. Correct: (c) Part of your goal with Charlie is to establish a therapeutic relationship that includes trust. He has accepted a nursing assessment at this visit; encouraging him to establish an ongoing relationship with the clinic will allow for early assessment of ongoing problems. Incorrect: (a) We don't have data about Charlie's family and the relationship with them; this may be highly non-therapeutic. (b) The first part about immediate health concerns is good; however, giving a homeless person additional belongings to manage may be problematic. There are no data to suggest he has prescription drugs to manage. (d) Again, the first part is good, although the referral to the physician could be overwhelming unless Charlie has identified a problem for which he is willing to undergo medical intervention.

4. Correct: (d) Absolute homelessness is when the individual lives on the street or in shelters most of the time. Incorrect: (a) The individual moves often, and is homeless part of the time. (b) The homelessness occurs in relationship to an event, such as a fire or domestic violence. (c) The individual finds housing (not temporary shelters) over the winter months or when required.

5. Correct: (b) At this point, you still know very little about Charlie, but given the retail cost of condoms, his knowledge of where and when he can access free condoms is the most important choice. Incorrect: (a) This is important but may not change his behaviour, and the use of condoms will be a safer alternative. (c) If he hasn't asked about testing at this point, it may not be his worry, or he may be afraid of the cost, especially since laboratories may ask for an address or how to contact him for the results. (d) Keeping him as safe as possible within his activities is a higher priority.

Study Questions

1. Murphy (2000) chose to define homelessness in its narrowest and most limiting terms, which is "those using emergency shelters and those sleeping in the street" (p. 12). The Niagara District Health Council (1997, pp. i–ii) identified four categories of homelessness: episodic (moves often, has periods of no housing); situational (absence of housing due to significant life event such as violence, illness, fire); seasonal (able to find housing during winter or other inclement weather); and absolute (lives on the street or in shelters for the majority of any given time). Stearman (1999, p. 5) chose four other categories to describe this population: inadequate or inferior housing (lack of basic facilities); insecure housing (squatters in buildings or refugee camps); houselessness (people who use shelters, institutions, or other short-term accommodation like hotels); and rooflessness (living and sleeping outdoors).

2. The low-income cut-off measure (LICO) and low-income measure (LIM) are both based on family income rather

than family costs. Both measures are based on the assumption that poverty is relative rather than absolute. The LIM is based directly on income and is calculated based on what a single person requires, with the assumption that food, clothing, and shelter should account for 50% of the median income for one person. The LIM stratifies the amounts by number of adults and children in the household. The better known of these two measures, the LICO, is based on the premise that the average Canadian family spends half its after-tax income on food, clothing, and shelter. The LICO stratifies by number of persons in the household and geography, but not by children and adults.

3. People can have working income and still be considered poor. A working poor person has been defined as "someone who works the equivalent of full-time for at least half of the year but whose family income is below a low-income threshold" (Human Resources and Skills Development Canada, 2007, p. 6). Several factors contribute to a perception of middle class moving into working poor: Recent tax policies have shifted the burden of federal and provincial income taxes onto lower-income workers. A second tax is the consumption tax, such as the sales tax. The required outlay for basic necessities takes a larger percentage of the poor family's income; thus, they bear a higher burden from consumption taxes. Wages, including low-income wages, have only been increasing at or below the rate of inflation.

4. Food banks, before-school breakfast programs, and other social activities to encourage healthy eating, where available, are making some inroads to better food security in Canada.

5. This assumption is generally based on perceptions of lower housing costs, lower property taxes, and more opportunities to grow one's own food or barter with others for services and goods. However, transportation, some foods, and fewer services for individuals with special needs may offset those advantages. The LICO (see Table 27.1) is based on this assumption.

6. ■ Income and social status: Our income often dictates where we can afford to live, what we can afford to eat, and the activities we enjoy. Single parents, especially women, have historically made less money than their male counterparts, but still have dependents to care for.
   ■ Social support networks: Historically, Canadians have looked out for each other. This is evident in the way our healthcare and social support systems have evolved. However, some may not be able to meet these needs, i.e., a poor family's circle of friends and relatives may have exhausted the assistance they are able to give, putting strain on the relationships. Obtaining money for travel or long-distance communication to continue the relationships may be problematic.
   ■ Education and literacy: People who are poorly educated are less likely to qualify for high-paying jobs.
   ■ Employment/working conditions: Persons with no fixed address and little or no income have difficulty getting ID, applying for jobs, or maintaining employment. The jobs they do get are often transitory, hourly wage jobs with few benefits, forcing them to choose, for instance, between going to a health professional for a personal or family health problem, and going to work.
   ■ Social environments: Poverty can be viewed as a social exclusionary factor. Many persons who are poor and/or

homeless are victims of violence or have been deinstitutionalized. Thus, social supports previously available may not be in place. Further, the social definition of poverty can be internalized, contributing to a sense of stigma, feelings of shame, inferiority, and low self-esteem.

CHAPTER 28

Review Questions

1. Correct: (d) Tobacco and alcohol are the most commonly used legal substances and cannabis is the most widely used illicit drug in Canada. Incorrect: (a), (b), and (c) Canada is also one of the top 10 countries that have the highest rates for opioid prescriptions and benzodiazepines. And experts are warning that as the abuse of prescription opiates grows, prescription drug abuse may exceed the abuse of illicit street drugs as more and more of them are making their way into the illicit drug market. However, opioids are part of the licit drug category, which is not as a group one of the top three psychoactive substances used in Canada.

2. Correct: (c) These are the most common reasons that are likely to influence young people to experiment with and/or use drugs. It is important to initiate an open and ongoing dialogue about these reasons. Adolescence is an important milestone involving the formation of social values and psychological traits that can be strongly influenced by wanting to imitate adults, increasing one's self-confidence, and having a strong sense of belonging to and acceptance by peer groups. These are important sources of influence to begin discussing with children as they enter adolescence. Incorrect: (a), (b), and (d) While these are also reasons for using, they have less relevance for young pre-adolescents. Relieving tension and insomnia, resolving physical discomfort such as pain, and forgetting about a traumatic event are reasons people use drugs but are more often reasons reported by adults.

3. Correct: (b) Providing low or light alcohol beverages is an intervention aimed at minimizing or reducing the harms associated with the consumption of alcohol vs. taking a total abstinence or zero tolerance approach. Incorrect: (a), (c), and (d) Drug testing in the workplace and a zero tolerance drug use policy in a school are both enforcement and control strategies, teaching refusal skills to teens is a prevention and health promotion activity, and teaching abstinence from psychoactive substances is an abstinence-based health promotion model. Harm reduction focuses on lowering the risk and severity of adverse consequences without necessarily reducing use or consumption.

4. Correct: (a) An effective service continuum should meet the diverse needs of individuals with concurrent disorders given its high prevalence. An effective continuum should also have services to address the unique needs of women, youth, and Aboriginal people, and any other population group that tends to be marginalized. Incorrect: (b) Access to treatment and rehabilitation services is made more effective and efficient when services are integrated within various sectors including health, mental health, social services, education, and the criminal justice system vs. being offered by a single point of access such as private clinics, which are also cost-prohibitive for many people. (c) Addiction specialists are health and social service professionals with additional expertise in the field of substance abuse treatment.

They can lend their expertise to allied professionals working in various services sectors so that screening and early detection are done at various points of entry across multiple systems, including schools, correctional facilities, and primary health care clinics. (d) A service continuum should have a variety of treatment models to meet the various needs of individuals; while some may need an abstinent-based treatment; others may benefit from a harm reduction program.

5. Correct: (d) Poverty, social isolation, disasters, a sense of hopelessness, high unemployment rates, and the lack of healthy alternatives such as positive recreational activities are determinants of health and socioeconomic conditions that may adversely affect a community's capacity to cope successfully with adversities and predispose its citizens to problematic patterns of substance use and abuse, which in turn can stress the community so that it is left with risk factors that overwhelm and overshadow its buffers or protective factors. Substance use and abuse is multifactorial and requires a socio-environmental approach that recognizes the interrelationships between the person, the substance, and the environment. Incorrect: (a) Both small rural and large urban communities face substance abuse problems; smaller rural and isolated communities may have higher rates of binge drinking and inhalant use, while larger urban communities may have higher rates of illicit drug use and crimes associated with trafficking. (b) Although education may be associated with various rates of some substances, overall people with lower levels of education are more likely to experience determinants making them more susceptible to substance use/abuse problems. (c) There is no evidence to support that being a member of a large family is a social determinant of health linked to substance use and abuse in a community.

Study Questions

1. The "four pillars" of Canada's Federal Drug Strategy are prevention and health promotion, treatment, enforcement, and harm reduction. Prevention and health promotion consists of interventions that seek to prevent or delay the onset of substance use as well as avoid problems before they occur, but it is more than education. It includes strengthening the health, social, and economic factors that can reduce the risk of substance use, such as creating alternative activities for youth groups. The main focus of prevention and health promotion is to help people avoid the use of harmful substances, and in the case of those who are using, the goal is to enhance their ability to control their use and prevent the development of substance abuse problems. Awareness campaigns and other education initiatives help people make healthy decisions and participate in health activities. These activities typically consist of programs and services that impart information about substances and help develop refusal skills. They can be developed to target the whole community and/or specific at-risk or high-risk populations.

Prevention and health promotion activities may also include policies, health warning labels, and even elements of harm reduction. Policies such as tobacco by-laws or alcohol and drug legislation can create healthy social and physical environments. Environmental support and controls help to ensure healthy conditions, practices, and policies that make it easier for people to achieve and maintain their health. For example, the presence of recreational activities and self-help groups can provide important environmental supports for a community. Policy changes are intended to create an environment that is conducive to healthy practices by making it easier to adopt healthy behaviours and more difficult to adopt unhealthy practices.

Treatment or health recovery is for people who have started to experience problems related to their substance use. Screening and early identification help detect signs and symptoms in order to intervene and reduce consumption levels and effectively manage the problems that have developed. Treatment and rehabilitation are intended to assist people with substance abuse problems as their consumption is considered to be "high risk." These individuals should be provided with a range of options in order to match their recovery needs and personal circumstances with appropriate treatment services. Overall, the purpose in health recovery is to prevent further deterioration and reduce the harms that have resulted from a problematic consumption pattern. Community treatment services typically include detoxification services, screening, assessment, inpatient and outpatient treatment, and aftercare and follow-up.

The goal of enforcement is to strengthen community health and safety by responding to the crimes and community disorder issues associated with the supply, distribution, possession, and use of legal and illegal substances. Effective enforcement also means being visible in communities, understanding local issues, being aware of community resources, and participating in improving social conditions and attitudes while upholding public safety.

Harm reduction is a public health philosophy that has gained popularity in the last two decades; however, some claim that it is a new name for an old concept. It is described as a program or policy designed to reduce drug-related harm without requiring the cessation of drug use. Examples include the availability of "light" alcoholic beverages, alcohol server training programs, and impaired driving countermeasures. In the treatment field, the most pre-eminent harm-reduction strategies are supervised injection sites, street outreach, needle exchange, and methadone maintenance treatment (MMT) programs, all of which allow the individual to live with a certain level of dependency while minimizing risks and other disruptive effects to the person and the community. It is often said that harm reduction is not "what's nice, it's what works." The focus is not on the use or the extent of use, but on the harms associated with the use. While becoming drug free may be the ultimate goal, it is not required from the outset. The goal is to reduce more immediate and tangible harms.

2. People use different drugs for different reasons, and the reasons vary from drug to drug, from person to person, and from circumstance to circumstance. While certain psychoactive drugs may be prescribed to relieve anxiety, tension, stress, or insomnia, some people may self-medicate to improve performance or to resolve physical or emotional discomfort. The mere availability of a drug may cause individuals to be curious enough to experiment. The danger, however, is that experimental use may lead to other reasons for using, which may in turn result in abuse and/or dependence.

Other people may take drugs to boost their self-confidence or to forget about or cope with traumatic life events or situations. Immediate gratification from drugs may make people feel good and/or can quickly reduce or eliminate uncomfortable emotions, albeit temporarily. Social pressures to use drugs can be very strong for both young people and adults. However, children are especially vulnerable as they may imitate and interpret their parents' use as a necessary part of having fun or relaxing. Young people may use drugs to rebel against unhappy situations or because they feel alienated, have an identity crisis, or need to be accepted by their peers. The media are also considered a powerful source of influence. Ads often promote drinking or smoking as a social activity or as a factor in the achievement of success.

3. Drug dependence is progressive in nature and affects the physiological, cognitive, behavioural, and psychological dimensions of a person's health. It is manifested by continuous use despite the presence of problems that are caused by the pattern of repeated self-administration that results in tolerance, withdrawal, and compulsive substance-taking behaviour. Dependence can be physical and/or psychological. Physical dependence occurs when an individual's body reacts to the absence of a drug, and psychological dependence occurs when drug use becomes central to a person's thoughts and emotions.

4. Children living with parents who use substances, children and youth who have friends who use substances, and children who themselves use substances suffer negative physical, cognitive, emotional, and social consequences. The harmful consequences extend far beyond individuals using substances, their families, and friends. Substance abuse affects community health, safety, and quality of life, and because it impacts the whole community, it requires the total community effort to ensure collective health and well-being.

The long-term use of tobacco can cause lung damage; exposure to second-hand smoke among neonates, infants, children, and adults is associated with an increased risk of a number of acute and chronic conditions. Tobacco surpasses alcohol and illicit drugs as the leading cause of death, hospitalization, and lost years of life. Nicotine dependence of tobacco addiction is the most lethal of all addictions; it is a chronic and relapsing disorder with at least half of smokers dying of tobacco-related illnesses.

Alcohol abuse can cause liver damage and heavy drinking raises blood pressure and can also increase the risk of stroke and heart failure. The consumption of alcohol during pregnancy can result in fetal alcohol spectrum disorder (FASD), which is manifested by developmental, neurological, and behavioural delays in infants and young children.

Alcohol remains the primary cause of motor vehicle fatalities in Canada. Alcohol is also frequently involved in snowmobiling and boating accidents. Other associated harms can include an increase in crime and violent acts; strained relationships; workplace and school absenteeism; and health problems such as ulcers, liver and kidney damage, pancreatic diseases, heart disease, cancer, sexual and reproductive issues, and pre- and post-natal complications.

Sniffing cocaine can damage nasal passages, and people who inject drugs intravenously can become infected with blood borne pathogens such as HIV and hepatitis B and C.

Many injection drug users share needles and drug injection equipment, and engage in unprotected commercial sex. Ecstasy and crystal meth, both of which belong to the amphetamine family, can be easily manufactured in unregulated illegal labs. As a result, the chemicals and processes vary, affecting the strength, purity, and effect of the final product. The consequences can be devastating, including severe dependency and drug reactions, and fatal overdoses. Mortality rates due to opioids are also sharply increasing in our country.

Having a mental health problem increases the risk of having a substance use problem, just as having a substance use problem increases the risk of having a mental health problem. And the use of substances can cause behaviours that mimic symptoms of mental health problems. Research on concurrent disorders suggests that these substance-induced problems may improve as substance use is decreased or stopped; however, almost three of every ten people who have a mental illness will be dependent on alcohol or drugs, and about four of every 10 people who use alcohol in a harmful way, and over half of people who use other substances in a harmful way will have a mental illness at some time in their lives.

5. Communities should have a combination of complementary interventions such as education, policy, enforcement, screening, early intervention, and various types of treatment and rehabilitation options, all of which are consistent with the various practice expectations of community health nursing. Developing interventions should be informed by research, best practices, existing community knowledge, and the insight and experience of those affected by the issue. Taking stock of community conditions that can play a major role in substance abuse and addiction is an important first step to understand the unique challenges and opportunities facing the community. Social and economic conditions such as limited income; living in unsafe neighbourhoods; and lack of leisure, recreation, job, and training opportunities are known to increase the risk of substance abuse and addiction. Assessing the community's conditions is an essential step the CHN should take before defining, supporting, or moving ahead with any intervention. CHNs working to introduce community interventions should do so according to type of substance, and the nature and extent of the substance use and/or abuse. It is important to have a solid understanding of the community before pursuing the development of any strategy. Substance abuse is not one dimensional; it requires a multipronged approach involving multiple sectors. The CHN should explore collaborative partnerships with various other health professionals, volunteers, parents, schools, workplaces, municipal governments, recreational organizations, and enforcement and justice officials to ensure that the proposed community strategies are relevant and can result in optimal outcomes.

6. Six principles that should guide CHNs' work in community-based substance abuse interventions are person-centred, inclusiveness, non-stigmatizing, knowledge and best practices, total community, and collaboration (see p. 443).

7. The risk of focusing exclusively on enforcement is that the social, economic, and emotional complexities of drug use are ignored and we tend to respond with punishment and legal sanctions without considering and offering rehabilitation options. Although different from other components of a comprehensive community strategy, enforcement

should be seen as complementary, with each type of activity having an important role in correcting substance abuse problems and improving the health status of our communities.

8. Drug treatment courts offer alternatives to incarceration for repeat drug-involved offenders. Currently, there are six drug treatment courts operating in Canada including Edmonton, Ottawa, Regina, Toronto, Vancouver, and Winnipeg. These courts facilitate access to treatment and help reduce the harms and risk of ongoing dependence and criminal recidivism by helping offenders reduce the number of crimes committed to support their drug dependence, and providing them with judicial supervision, comprehensive substance abuse treatment, random and frequent drug testing, incentives and sanctions, clinical case management, and social support services.

Methadone maintenance treatment programs were introduced in Canada in response to the increasing use of opioids and the extensive cycle of this devastating drug dependency. Methadone alleviates the symptoms of opioid withdrawal by creating stable and sufficient blood levels of methadone. These programs have been demonstrated to improve physical and mental health status; reduce illicit drug use, infectious disease risks, and crime involvement among those involved in treatment; and offer a significant cost benefit to the community given the costs associated with untreated opioid dependency. They are available in most provinces and in some correctional facilities.

CHAPTER 29

Review Questions

1. Correct: (c) All pregnant women are screened for syphilis during the first trimester of pregnancy. Incorrect: (a) There are policies in place to protect the health of newborn babies at risk for contracting syphilis. (b) High-risk women would be screened during the first trimester of pregnancy, at 28–32 weeks' gestation, and at delivery. (d) All babies are not given penicillin at birth to protect against syphilis.

2. Correct: (a) Chlamydia, gonorrhea, and syphilis are bacterial STIs spread through unprotected vaginal, anal, and oral sex. Incorrect: (b) Chlamydia, gonorrhea, and syphilis are not spread through skin-to-skin (genital-to-genital) sexual contact. HPV and herpes are spread through skin-to-skin sexual contact. (c) Chlamydia, gonorrhea, and syphilis are not spread through sharing of needles and other blood paraphernalia. Blood borne pathogens such as HIV and hepatitis B are spread through sharing needles and other drug paraphernalia. (d) Although this is correct, (a) is the better answer.

3. Correct: (d) Most often there are no symptoms. Incorrect: (a), (b), and (c) Although abnormal vaginal discharge and bleeding, burning during urination, and lower abdominal pain are all symptoms of chlamydia in females, most commonly there are no symptoms.

4. Correct: (c) HPV causes cervical cancer. An HPV infection can lead to abnormal cell changes of the cervix, which may turn into cervical cancer if not detected early. Incorrect: (a) Although HPV can lead to genital warts, warts are not considered serious. (b) and (d) HPV cannot lead to pelvic inflammatory disease or infertility. PID and

infertility are possible consequences of untreated chlamydia and gonorrhea.

5. Correct: (b) Gardasil is a vaccine that protects against four strains of HPV (human papillomavirus) that cause the majority of cervical cancers and genital warts. Incorrect: (a) Gardasil does not protect against all strains of HPV. (c) Gardasil is not a viral sexually transmitted infection. (d) Gardasil is not a bacterial sexually transmitted infection.

6. Answer: (d) Viral STIs such as HPV and genital herpes are spread through unprotected vaginal, oral, and anal sex and skin-to-skin (genital-to-genital) sexual contact. The best way to prevent the spread of these infections is through abstaining from all these activities. Incorrect: (a) The use of male and female condoms can help to prevent the spread of these STIs; however, condoms are not 100% effective. Sometimes genital herpes or warts are on an area of the body not covered by the condom (e.g., testicles). (b) Male and female condoms should not be used together. Using two condoms together may cause them to break. (c) HPV and genital herpes are also spread through skin-to-skin sexual contact.

Study Questions

1. The three most common bacterial STIs and their symptoms are:
   - Chlamydia: Commonly there are no symptoms. Females may experience abnormal vaginal discharge or bleeding, lower abdominal pain, or burning during urination. Males may experience unusual penile discharge, burning while urinating, or pain and swelling of the testes. Anal pain and discharge may indicate infection through anal intercourse.
   - Gonorrhea: Commonly there are no symptoms. Females may experience abnormal vaginal discharge or bleeding, lower abdominal pain, or burning during urination. Males may experience unusual penile discharge, burning while urinating, or pain and swelling of the testes. Anal pain and discharge may indicate infection through anal intercourse.
   - Syphilis: During the early stages of syphilis, individuals experience painless sores (chancres) and flu-like symptoms. During the later stages of syphilis, individuals may experience central nervous system and cardiovascular system damage.

2. HIV can be transmitted through unprotected sexual activity such as vaginal and anal sex. HIV can be transmitted by reusing drug, tattooing, or piercing equipment that has residual traces of infected blood. HIV can be passed from mother to neonate during pregnancy, birth, or breastfeeding.

3. STIs and BBPs may be reduced by
   - practising abstinence from all types of sexual activity
   - accurately and consistently using latex or polyurethane male condoms or polyurethane female condoms
   - using clean needles and equipment for tattooing, piercing, and injecting drugs
   - always using condoms and/or dental dams for oral sex

4. All pregnant women should be screened for infectious syphilis during the first trimester of pregnancy. Women, who are considered "high risk" for contracting syphilis should also be screened at 28–32 weeks' gestation and at delivery.

5. Safer injection facilities (SIFs) provide a safe location for drug users to inject their own drugs with clean equipment under the supervision of medically trained professionals. The main objectives of SIFs are to decrease the spread of infectious disease, improve contact between the healthcare system and injection drug users, decrease the use of drugs in public places, decrease fatal and non-fatal drug over-doses, and increase recruitment of injection drug users into addiction treatment and rehabilitation programs.

6. Cervarix is a vaccine against certain types of cancer-causing human papillomavirus (HPV). Cervarix is designed to pre-vent infection from HPV types 16 and 18, which currently cause about 70% of cervical cancer cases. Some cross-protection against virus strains 45 and 31 were shown in clinical trials. Cervarix also contains an adjuvant that has been found to boost protection against HPV for a longer period of time. Cervarix is manufactured by Glaxo-SmithKline. An alternative HPV vaccine from Merck & Co. is known as Gardasil.

CHAPTER 30
Review Questions

1. Correct: (a) Local municipalities have the first responsibil-ity in managing an emergency, and if their capacity is exceeded they call on their respective province, which in turn can call on the federal government for assistance. Therefore, local emergency preparedness plans are key to the success in managing emergencies. Incorrect: (b), (c), and (d).

2. Correct: (d) It is important to assist the community to recover from the disaster and enable people to return to their normal lives as quickly as possible. Incorrect: (a) and (b) These are important activities for emergency preparedness. (c) This is an activity used to respond during the disaster.

3. Correct: (a) Fire departments have the responsibility to take the lead role in managing all Hazardous Material emergencies within their jurisdiction. Incorrect: (b), (c), and (d) These all play a supportive role in this situation. Public health units are mandated to protect the health of the communities, from surveillance of infectious control to monitoring air quality. Effective hazard identification risk assessment strategies combined with interagency co-ordination can and will prepare an agency for response, mitigate the effects of the emergency, and assist in recovery and evaluation activities.

4. Correct: (c) In referring to Table 30.2, the Incident Man-agement System (IMS) outlines a chain of commands with specific responsibilities in each section, from operations, planning, and logistics to finances/administration. All lev-els of government as well as public health agencies and hospitals utilize this process. Community-level response organizations including public health units and hospitals collaborate on incorporating the individual response plans into a local co-ordinated community response plan. Incor-rect: (a) Nurses must first follow the emergency prepared-ness procedures of their own employers. (b) The Canadian Nurses Association provides expertise and consultation with the government in developing the role of nurses in a national emergency plan. (d) This response provides only a limited scope in an overall emergency management plan.

During any disasters or emergencies, CHNs may find themselves working in different roles, such as operating a walk-in clinic, working in a shelter or evacuation centre, and triaging people at mass clinics while providing prophylactic medication or administering vaccine. They act as case manager to liaise between the victim and a com-munity agency or clinic. Nurses must recognize problems through diagnosis and, through secondary prevention, provide immediate treatment, and make referrals to an emergency room or community site where a clinic has been organized.

5. Correct: (b) These are the vulnerable populations with little or no resources to care for themselves. Incorrect: (a) Disasters affect all people regardless of their social status or income levels. (c) and (d) These are key people in lead-ing, planning, resourcing, and participating in disaster situations. While they need to attend to their own needs as well as their own families', their professional obligations are to care for the people they chose to serve and care for.

Study Questions

1. Natural disasters are unpredictable and can happen slowly or quickly. Some examples of natural disasters include droughts, heat waves, blizzards, cold waves, heavy snow-falls, earthquakes, cyclones, tsunamis, tornadoes, floods or thunderstorms, volcanoes, and wildfires. Man-made disas-ters can be bioterrorism, bombings, nuclear disasters, and technical malfunctions that result in civilian injuries and deaths. Both man-made and natural disasters leave people injured, put emergency responders at risk, and have a last-ing impact on the health of the communities they affect. Epidemics and pandemics refer to the transmission of a highly infectious disease from a defined community or region to different parts around the globe, affecting a large number of people. They can result in emergency situations with high levels of morbidity and mortality as well as social and economic disruptions.

2. Special expertise in emergency management is required. Preventing, preparing for, responding to, and recovering from an emergency or disaster requires individual and pro-fessional expertise combined with collaboration among agencies and across communities.

3. The Emergencies Act allows the federal government to grant the use of special powers to ensure the safety and security of Canadians during a national emergency to pre-serve the sovereignty, security, and territorial integrity of Canada. The federal government intervention is restricted to only the most serious of emergency situations, while respecting the authority of the provinces and territories to govern accordingly within their own geographical jurisdictions.

   The Emergency Preparedness Act is a companion legis-lation to the Emergencies Act. It provides a basis for the planning and programming necessary to address disasters of all kinds. Specifically, this Act addresses the need for cooperation between the provinces and territories at the federal level to establish responsibilities and the need for public awareness, as well as providing a structure for train-ing and education.

   The Emergency Management Act replaces parts of the Emergency Preparedness Act. This Act strengthens the

Government of Canada's readiness to respond to major emergencies by establishing clear roles and responsibilities for all federal ministers and enhances information sharing with other levels of government and with the private sector. It provides direction for critical infrastructure protection, as this is one of the emerging challenges of modern emergency management. Critical infrastructure consists of physical and information technology facilities, networks, services, and assets that are vital to the health, safety, security, or economic well-being of Canadians and for the effective functioning of governments in Canada.

4. The life-cycle process refers to the following areas: mitigating or preventing the effects of an emergency; preparing for emergencies or disasters; responding to an emergency or disaster to reduce the impact on public loss; and recovering from an emergency or disaster by assisting communities to return to normal.

5. Nurses should have special individual and professional expertise in emergency management. This includes preventing, preparing for, responding to, and recovering from an emergency or disaster. They should display a leadership role and be able to work collaboratively with agencies and across communities.

6. Refer to Table 30.5 for the eight domains of core competencies and skills and ten essential public health services for pandemic planning.

CHAPTER 31

Review Questions

1. Correct: (d) This question seeks the understanding of students' ability to distinguish the geographical reach between global health, international health, and public health. International health focuses on health issues other than one's own, whereas the specific focus on health issues affecting a population lies in the realm of public health. Global health, on the other hand, has a particular focus on health issues that can transcend national boundaries. Incorrect: (a) Global health and international health are not synonymous. Rather, they differ in their geographical reach, level of cooperation, focus on individuals or populations, access to health, and range of discipline. (b) Focusing on health issues other than one's own is an international health idea related to focusing on the health of countries above and beyond that of your own. (c) The focus of health issues affecting populations is a matter under public health and can include the population health of a particular community or country.

2. Correct: (a) The idea of promoting nurses as global citizens is to encourage nurses to assume the moral responsibility and professional competency to address health issues beyond the focus on individualized care. Nurses as global citizens extend their thinking and world beyond local communities and national citizenship both through work internationally and nationally. As suggested by Nussbaum's (1997) idea of moral cosmopolitanism, nurses can still be global citizens without having to give up their unique local preferences. The importance is being able to view all persons, with different preferences, as fellow citizens who deserve equal consideration. Incorrect: (b) Being a global citizen is not related to whether you work abroad or not. It is a matter of how you approach your work to demonstrate your role as a global citizen. (c) You are not expected to give up your own unique preference; instead, you can continue to have unique preferences, while accepting the views of others. (d) While speaking numerous languages may be beneficial, it is not a requirement.

3. Correct: (b) Pinto and Upshur (2009) perceived global health ethics to include humility (recognizing own limitations and openness to learn), introspection (reflective of own motives and privilege), solidarity (ensuring alignment of goals and values to understand health in the perspective of those receiving care), and social justice (understanding power relationships and gross inequalities). Incorrect: (a), (c) and (d) These responses do not contain all the elements of global health ethics as suggested by Pinto and Upshur.

4. Correct: (d) A moral dilemma is most prominent when nurses must evaluate local standards of care against their own beliefs in their scope of practice and Western medical knowledge base. The ability to balance the potentially different standards of care may present a dilemma to nurses, particularly if local standards are questionable according to the nurse. However, acknowledging local standards of care is important because of the need to incorporate culturally appropriate interventions in care. Incorrect: (a) The gathering of information on the culture and health practices from another culture does not present any dilemma; rather, it is encouraged to help prepare nurses in their work prior to departure. (b) A translator is a facilitator for communication and can be beneficial for working, particularly in situations where language barriers are prevalent. (c) Providing good care is a basic expectation of nurses.

5. Correct: (d) According to Nussbaum (1997), the three capacities to cultivate global citizenship are reflexivity (scrutinizing one's own beliefs and traditions to ensure they are justifiable), moral cosmopolitanism (adopting the view that all persons are fellow citizens with equal moral worth), and narrative imagination (ability to perceive what it might be like to be a person different than oneself. Incorrect: (a), (b), and (c) These are actually components necessary to cultivate global citizenship.

Study Questions

1. For a differentiation between global health and international health, refer to the comparison in Table 31.2.

2. Issues arising out of the globalization of nursing include nurse migration and the global spread of infections. Nurse migration generally occurs in the direction of nurses from the majority work migrating to the minority world, thus resulting in a shortage of nurses from already resource-constrained countries. The resulting inadequacy in healthcare workers contradicts the Health for All principles of ensuring that health resources be evenly distributed and that essential healthcare be accessible to everyone. The global spread of infectious diseases requires nurses working in international and global health to be vigilant of the impact of health, which transcends borders. The spread and outbreak of such infectious diseases have tremendous impact on the health of populations and the capacity of nurses to provide healthcare to infected populations.

3. This is a self-reflection question on thinking globally and acting locally; responses will be individual.

4. The three capacities useful for developing global citizenship are reflexivity, moral cosmopolitanism, and narrative imagination. Reflexivity requires individuals to be able to critically examine their own beliefs, traditions, and habits to ensure that they are consistent and justifiable. Moral cosmopolitanism means to adopt the view that all persons are fellow citizens who have equal moral worth and deserve equal moral consideration, without giving up each individual's unique local preferences and responsibilities. Narrative imagination requires imagining what it might be like to be a person different than oneself, and to allow such imagination to inform understanding of others' experiences, emotions and desires, and life stories.

5. The notion of global citizenship can guide nurses to acknowledge their role as a global citizen and to exert moral responsibility and professional competency to care and promote health beyond their local communities and national institutions. In an increasingly globalized world, where health transcends national borders, nurses who engage the notion of global citizenship into their practice can recognize the increasing disparities in access to healthcare and the resulting unbalanced health outcomes for populations both between and within countries. Furthermore, nurses can be depended on to acknowledge that experiences of health and illness differ culturally and geographically so that they can develop the capacity to identify possible tensions between personal professional interests and global interests.

6. Social determinants of health that impact on individual and community health may include poverty, housing, living standards, peace, employment, food access, and education.

Index

public health nursing, 43, 124
vs. standards, 43
complementary interventions, 442
comprehensive, 22
Comprehensive School Health (CSH), 286–288, 287*t*, 289*t*, 291, 292
compulsory treatment orders, 343
concurrent disorders, 437–438
confidence intervals, 161
Constitution Act of 1867. *See* British North America Act (BNA Act)
Constitution of Canada, 126, 353
consumer, 335
consumption tax, 422
contact tracing, 204–205
contacts, 204
control, 240*f*
Controlled Drugs and Substances Act, 435
Cooperative Commonwealth Federation (CCF), 22
Coordinated School Health Program (CSHP), 286
coping skills, 426
correctional health
    aging offender, 393
    common health challenges, 395–397
    communicable diseases, 395–397, 399–400
    community connection, 397–398
    culturally diverse offenders, 394
    healthcare of correctional population, 391–395
    mental illness, 340, 392–393
    policy development, 398
    practice setting, 397
    prevention levels, 390–391
    special populations, 391–394
    substance abuse, 395
    women's issues, 393–394
    youth, 394
correctional nursing
    see also correctional health
    defined, 390
    professional development and research, 398
Corrections and Conditional Release Act (CCRA), 390
Corrections nursing: Scope and standards of practice (ANA), 398
Courage, M.L., 225
Cournoyer, D., 436
The Crazy Race, 173
creating supportive environments, 93
Creutzfeldt-Jakob disease, 190, 205
criminalization of the mentally ill, 391
crisis stabilization units, 343
critical appraisal
    critical appraisal skills, 158
    data analysis, 164
    of qualitative research, 163–164
    results, meaning of, 160–161, 163–164
    of studies of interventions, 158–161
    of systematic reviews, 161–163
    use of results, 161, 163, 164
    validity of results, 158–160, 162, 164

critical appraisal skills, 158
critical caring theory, 99
critical incident technique (CIT), 132
critical social nursing, 98–99
critical social theories, 409
Crockett, M., 201
Crooks, C., 411
cross-sectional studies, 149
Crowe, Cathy, 116, 213, 429
Crowe, T., 379
Crowsnest Pass, Alberta, 369
crude mortality rates, 145
Csiernik, R., 150
cultural assessments, 133, 134
cultural competence, 131–133, 410
cultural diversity. *See* diversity
cultural humility, 410
cultural pluralism, 126
cultural safety, 124, 132, 277, 410
cultural sensitivities, 46
culture
    assumptions and characteristics, 125–126
    and community assessment, 220–221
    concept of, 125–127
    defined, 125
    as determinant of health, 130–131
    ethnocentrism, 125
    extended families, 277
    and gender equity, 302
    intersections, 126–127
    poverty and homelessness, effect of, 426
Culture Care Diversity and University (Leininger), 125
cumulative incidence, 148
Cumulative Index of Nursing and Allied Health Literature (CINAHL), 158

D

Danish-Newfoundland PHC Project, 114
D'Arcy, C., 368
data analysis, 163, 164, 239–240
data collection, 222
dating violence prevention, 411–412
Davies, B., 117
death rates, 145–147, 146*f*
death statistics, 148
Declaration of Alma Ata (WHO), 24, 26, 44, 93–109, 112, 113
    see also Alma Ata Conference
DeCorby, K., 159
degree of exposure, 204
degree of hazard, 380
deinstitutionalization movement, 391
delivery
    community health services, 26–28
    home care, 27–28
    mental health service delivery models, 344–345
    mental health services, 342–343
    primary health care and primary care, 26–27
    public health, 27
    treatment focus, 23

Delphi technique, 470
dengue fever, 200
density of population, 218
Department of Indian Affairs and Northern Development, 351
dependence, 336*t*, 435
depression, 257–258, 304
determinants of health
    and causation, 143–144
    culture, 130–131
    and healthcare reform, 80
    maternal, fetal, and infant health, 256
    shift of focus to, 22
    social determinants of health. *See* social determinants of health
Determinants of Health: Empowering Strategies for Nursing Practice, 78
developing personal skills, 94
developmental assets, 293
Developmental Model of Health and Nursing, 269
diabetes (type 2), 84
diagnostic analysis, 165
Diagnostic and Statistical Manual (DSM-IV TR), 336
Dietitians of Canada, 294
digital divide, 173
dignity, 64
diphtheria, 189, 190
direct observed therapy (DOT), 207
direct transmission, 142
Directory of Plain Language Health Information, 178
disabled populations, and Internet access, 174
disaster nursing
    community health nursing organizations, role of, 470–474
    core competencies, 473–474
    described, 473
    disasters in Canada, 463, 464*t*
    Jennings Disaster Nursing Management Model, 471, 472
    nursing process, 472, 473*t*
    phases of disaster response, 469
    public health surge events, 474
    safety of vulnerable populations, 474–475
    types of disasters, 464–465
disclosure of information, 70–71
discourses
    defined, 77
    discourses of health, 77
    medical discourse, 79
    mothering, 255
    "risk" discourses and childbearing, 255
    and role of community health nurse, 83–84
    social determinants of health. *See* social determinants of health
    systems discourse, 79
disease prevention, 24
district nursing, 2
diversion programs, 392, 440